Bill Gibbons, DO, FAWM

610-608-5482 cell

DIAGNOSTIC IMAGING FOR THE EMERGENCY PHYSICIAN

DIAGNOSTIC IMAGING FOR THE EMERGENCY PHYSICIAN

Joshua Broder, MD, FACEP
Associate Professor
Associate Residency Program Director
Division of Emergency Medicine
Duke University Medical Center
Durham, North Carolina

1600 John F. Kennedy Blvd.
Ste 1800
Philadelphia, PA 19103-2899

DIAGNOSTIC IMAGING FOR THE EMERGENCY PHYSICIAN

ISBN: 978-1-4160-6113-7

Notices

Library of Congress Cataloging-in-Publication Data
Diagnostic imaging for the emergency physician / edited by Joshua Broder.
    p. ; cm.
  ISBN 978-1-4160-6113-7 (pbk. : alk. paper) 1. Medical emergencies—Imaging. 2. Emergency medicine—Diagnosis. 3. Emergency physicians. I. Broder, Joshua.
  RC86.7.D49 2011
  616.02'5—dc23   2011014644

Acquisitions Editor: Stefanie Jewell-Thomas
Developmental Editor: Rachel Miller
Publishing Services Manager: Anne Altepeter
Project Manager: Cindy Thoms
Design Direction: Louis Forgione

Printed in the United States of America

Last digit is the print number: 9 8 7 6 5 4 3 2

To my family

Acknowledgments

This book would not have been possible without the aid of my mentors, colleagues, and loving family.

Many thanks to Amal Mattu, David Jerrard, Michael Witting, and the entire teaching faculty at the University of Maryland Department of Emergency Medicine for the outstanding training they provided to me in residency and for the mentorship and encouragement they continue to provide.

I also owe much to the faculty and residents of the Duke University Division of Emergency Medicine. They inspire me every day with their dedication to quality patient care and their enthusiasm for evidence-based medicine.

Thanks to Ryan Martiniuk for his work in cataloging and preparing images for the extremity chapter. Ryan, you have a great future in medicine.

My thanks also to Robert Preston, with whom I have had the pleasure of working for many years. Rob's passion for emergency medicine is evident to all who know him.

My parents, Michael and Susan Broder, are responsible for so many wonderful things in my life. My father is a board-certified radiologist who introduced me to diagnostic imaging and also to emergency medicine. He dedicated his career to the patients of my hometown of Thomasville, North Carolina, and inspired me to share with others the lessons I have learned. My mother is a human geneticist whose greatest experiments were my sister, my brother, and me. The three of us benefited enormously from her intelligence and unfailing belief that we would achieve any goal we undertook. Thank you for all of your support through the development of this book and for everything you have done for me.

My sister, Elena, and brother, Daniel, were also essential to this book. Both set a remarkable standard through their work in law and software engineering, making difficult tasks appear easy. Their humor and love helped me to continue when the job seemed to have no end in sight.

My wife, Pek, and sons, Spencer and Isaac, have borne the greatest burden during the development of this book. My deadline was Spencer's birth; 18 months later, Pek sternly reminded me that I had better be done before Isaac was born. Thank you for your love and devotion and for the joy the three of you bring me.

Finally, thank you to patients—people—whose suffering from disease and injury is visible throughout this book. I hope that readers will provide better care through the lessons you have taught.

Joshua Broder

Foreword

It is often said that a picture is worth a thousand words. Although this quote originated in the advertising industry, it certainly applies to the field of medicine as well. Visual findings are the cornerstone of diagnosis for many medical conditions. One might argue, in fact, that the field of radiology was borne out of the need to look beyond a patient's *external* findings—essentially, *internal* visual diagnosis—without the need for surgical exploration.

The first x-ray of the human body was performed in 1895 and allowed the first noninvasive look inside the body. Since that first x-ray was performed, advances in technology have produced incredible developments in radiologic imaging. Modern radiologic techniques allow cancers that were once diagnosable only after metastasis to now be detected at stages when most are still localized and treatable. Appendicitis, a condition that had always been ruled out only by exploratory laparotomy, is now routinely excluded by computed tomography (CT). Coronary artery disease, the major cause of death in Western societies, had always been diagnosed by cardiac catheterization, but now noninvasive methods such as CT-angiography are routinely used to stratify a patient's risk of disease. Even the stethoscope, the primary diagnostic tool of physicians for more than 100 years, is slowly being pushed aside by portable ultrasound (US) machines.

Radiographic imaging has certainly become an intrinsic part of the field of emergency medicine. Almost all of the major journals in emergency medicine routinely include research publications focused on emergency imaging, and recently an entire journal dedicated to emergency imaging was initiated. All of the major educational and research conferences in emergency medicine include sessions focused on emergency radiology, and residency training programs in emergency medicine universally include *some* training in use and interpretation of imaging studies. However, there remains a significant shortcoming in the current level of radiology knowledge that most emergency physicians possess. All too often we find ourselves dependent on radiologists for diagnoses of life-threatening diseases. Often the radiologists are not immediately available, and the result is that patient care is compromised. Given the frequency with which emergency physicians depend on radiologic tests for diagnoses, it stands to reason that we should be more knowledgeable about interpreting these tests on our own.

Thankfully, there are certain members of our specialty who have committed their academic careers to becoming experts at emergency radiology and *teaching* this skill to the rest of us. Dr. Joshua Broder is one of those physicians. Dr. Broder is one of the brightest and most talented educators in emergency medicine, having won numerous local and national teaching awards. The majority of his academic work has been focused on the study and teaching of emergency radiology. He routinely teaches at national conferences on this topic, and he always finds a way of making the most complicated concepts simple and understandable. He has now turned his enormous talent toward writing, and the result lies before you: arguably *the* best textbook on the topic of emergency radiology ever written for our specialty.

Dr. Broder's textbook covers every aspect of imaging, from head to toe; and from x-ray to CT to magnetic resonance imaging to US. His writing style, much like his teaching style, is simple, practical, and understandable. Although there are several other textbooks on the market focused on emergency radiology, there are notable characteristics of this text that set it apart from the rest. First and foremost, the images in this text are truly *outstanding* in quality. These images tell the complete story. The reader will note that the images themselves contain text, arrows, highlights—all the usual features that other textbooks relegate to hard-to-read legends. These images can truly stand alone.

Dr. Broder's textbook also is written in a prose that demonstrates the consistency of a single writer. Many other texts suffer from inconsistencies in writing style and image format from chapter to chapter because multiple authors are used. The result is that some chapters always "read" or look better than others. That is not the case here. Dr. Broder's writing style is smooth, simple, and unambiguous; and the image quality is consistent throughout the text.

Another strength of this text lies in the fact that it has been written by a master educator. The clear purpose of the text is to teach the reader how to use and interpret images in the diagnosis of emergency conditions, not to simply dump loads of information onto the printed page for the reader to sort through on his or her own. Dr. Broder, for example, provides clear direction for how and when to order specific tests, and he systematically describes how to read CTs.

Although I could certainly continue doling out praise for Dr. Broder's book, I would instead prefer to simply invite you to turn the page and experience this text for yourself. I have no doubt that this text is destined to become one of our specialty's landmark textbooks, a classic that will be considered a must-have resource for all emergency physicians and emergency departments. My kudos go to Dr. Broder for his tremendous work. This textbook represents a valuable addition to the emergency medicine literature. Now, turn the page and enjoy!

Amal Mattu, MD, FAAEM, FACEP
Director, Emergency Medicine Residency
Director, Faculty Development Fellowship
Professor of Emergency Medicine
Department of Emergency Medicine
University of Maryland School of Medicine
Baltimore, Maryland

Preface

This is a book for emergency physicians, by an emergency physician. I set out to create a book that would differ from other available texts and be targeted to the specific needs of board-certified emergency physicians, emergency medicine residents, and students interested in emergency medicine. This book may also serve any provider attending to patients in urgent and emergent settings. I've attempted to provide clinical information valuable to practitioners at multiple levels of training, with or without prior training in diagnostic imaging. I've intentionally avoided discussions of physics behind diagnostic imaging, focusing instead on the clinical application of imaging technology. The book is designed to be used in several different ways, recognizing that emergency physicians are unlikely to read the book cover to cover. Here's what you can look for in this text:

1. Chapters organized by body region rather than by imaging modalities. My goal is to convey information tailored to the approach of an emergency physician in evaluating a patient.
2. Meticulously annotated images, designed to allow you to interpret imaging studies yourself and to understand the findings described by the radiologist. Each figure in the book tells a clinical story and can be used to understand a disease process without reference to the text. Whenever possible, I have included multiple imaging modalities from the same patient to demonstrate the strengths and weaknesses of different imaging techniques and to emphasize the similarities and differences in findings using different modalities. Throughout the book, I insisted on illustrating only those findings that I myself—an emergency physician—could identify. We've all experienced the frustration of scrutinizing an illustration and being unable to decipher the finding, or wondering what that open arrowhead is really pointing at. I've spent 2 years selecting and labeling images for maximum clarity.
3. Detailed strategies for the systematic interpretation of imaging studies, including computed tomography (CT). These discussions are meant to augment the information provided in the figure legends. Today's emergency physicians need to be able to recognize time-dependent conditions themselves, before the interpretation of a radiologist is available. My approach focuses on imaging findings requiring immediate interventions. Recognizing the time limits of emergency medicine practice, I've tried to encapsulate the discussions of important medical conditions so that each section stands alone. For readers with time to read whole sections, the discussion is meant to build upon earlier sections, leading to a more advanced interpretation ability.
4. Critical analysis of the evidence behind imaging techniques. Although this is not a book on research methodology, statistics, or evidence-based medicine, modern emergency physicians are sophisticated medical practitioners who need to know the reliability of the diagnostic strategies they employ. Without dwelling on technical detail, I attempt to uncover weaknesses of evidence, particularly when these might mislead the physician, leading to misdiagnosis or unnecessary additional workup. I briefly review some evidence-based medicine concepts when necessary to the discussion.
5. Clinically oriented discussions of frequently asked questions I've encountered in my practice, such as the indications for oral and IV contrast in abdominal CT and the differences between CT pulmonary angiography and aortography. I've attempted to equip the emergency physician with evidence to facilitate discussions with the radiologist. Throughout the book, I've highlighted areas where strong evidence and expert consensus guidelines from major emergency medicine and radiology professional organizations support the elimination of contrast agents, potentially benefiting patients by reducing risks of allergy, contrast nephropathy, and diagnostic delay.
6. Detailed discussions of the indications for diagnostic imaging and application of clinical decision rules to limit unnecessary diagnostic imaging and radiation exposure. I've emphasized areas in which clinical decision rules can achieve the goals of patient safety, faster throughput, decreased patient exposure to radiation, and reduced cost.
7. Discussion of risks of ionizing radiation from diagnostic imaging. I had originally considered a separate chapter on radiation risks but instead chose to incorporate this discussion into each chapter on

body regions. Emergency physicians need to understand the risks and benefits of diagnostic imaging, which has become a major source of radiation exposure in the U.S. population.

8. Discussions of the economics of various imaging strategies. Because much of the diagnostic workup occurs in emergency departments today, a few hours in an emergency department can result in significant expenditures on diagnostic imaging. Knowledgeable emergency physicians can provide high-quality care while managing expense.

I've written and edited the entire text myself, with help along the way from colleagues in emergency medicine and radiology. I hope that this decision results in a more integrated text than books with chapters authored by a multitude of practitioners.

If these features would benefit your practice and your patients, read on.

Joshua Broder, MD, FACEP

Contents

---

*For the complete chapter text, go to expertconsult.com. To access your account, look for your activation instructions on the inside front cover of this book.

---

*For the complete chapter text, go to expertconsult.com. To access your account, look for your activation instructions on the inside front cover of this book.

CHAPTER 1 Imaging the Head and Brain

Joshua Broder, MD, FACEP, and Robert Preston, MD

Emergency physicians frequently evaluate patients with complaints requiring brain imaging for diagnosis and treatment. The diversity of imaging modalities and variations of these modalities may be daunting, creating uncertainty about the most appropriate, sensitive, and specific modality to evaluate the presenting complaint. An evidence-based approach is essential, with modality and technique chosen based on patient characteristics and differential diagnosis. In this chapter, we begin with a brief summary of computed tomography (CT) and magnetic resonance (MR) technology. Next, we present a systematic approach to interpretation of head CT, along with evidence for interpretation by emergency physicians. Then, we discuss the cost and radiation exposure from neuroimaging, as these are important reasons to limit imaging. We review the evidence supporting the use of CT and magnetic resonance imaging (MRI) for diagnosis and treatment of emergency brain disorders, concentrating on clinical decision rules to target imaging to high-risk patients. We also consider adjunctive imaging techniques, including conventional angiography, plain films, and ultrasound. By chapter's end, we consider the role of neuroimaging in the evaluation of headache, transient ischemic attacks (TIAs) and stroke, seizure, syncope, subarachnoid hemorrhage (SAH), meningitis, hydrocephalus and shunt malfunction, and head trauma.

NEUROIMAGING MODALITIES

Indications for neuroimaging are diverse, including traumatic and nontraumatic conditions (Table 1-1). The major brain neuroimaging modalities today are CT and MRI, with adjunctive roles for conventional angiography and ultrasound. Plain films of the calvarium have an extremely limited role, as they can detect bony injury but cannot detect underlying brain injury, which may be present even in the absence of fracture.

Computed Tomography

CT has been in general clinical use in emergency departments (EDs) in the United States since the early 1980s. The modality was simultaneously and independently developed by the British physicist Godfrey N. Hounsfield and the American Allan M. Cormack in 1973, and the two were corecipients of the Nobel Prize for Medicine in 1979.[1,2] Advances in computers and the introduction of multislice helical technology (described in

detail in Chapter 8 in the context of cardiac imaging) have dramatically enhanced the resolution and diagnostic utility of CT since its introduction. CT relies on the differential attenuation of x-ray by body tissues of differing density. The image acquisition occurs by rapid movement of the patient through a circular gantry opening equipped with an x-ray source and multiple detectors. A three-dimensional volume of image data is acquired; this volume can be displayed as axial, sagittal, or coronal planar slices or as a three-dimensional image. CT does raise some safety concerns with regard to long-term biologic effects of ionizing radiation and carcinogenesis, which we describe later. The radiation exposure to the fetus in a pregnant patient undergoing head CT is minimal.[3] Most commercially available CT scanners have a weight capacity of approximately 450 pounds (200 kg), although some manufacturers now offer units with capacities up to 660 pounds (300 kg).[4] Portable dedicated head CT scanners with acceptable diagnostic quality and no weight limits are now available.[4a]

Noncontrast Head CT

Noncontrast CT is the most commonly ordered head imaging test in the ED, used in up to 12% of all adult ED visits.[5,6] It provides information about hemorrhage, ischemic infarction, masses and mass effect, ventricular abnormalities such as hydrocephalus, cerebral edema, sinus abnormalities, and bone abnormalities such as fractures. Although dedicated facial CT provides more detail by acquiring thinner slices through the region of interest or by changing the patient's position in the scanner during image acquisition, general information about the face and sinuses can be gleaned from a generic noncontrast head CT, as described in detail in Chapter 4 on facial imaging. The American College of Radiology recommends acquisition of contiguous or overlapping slices with slice thickness no greater than 5mm. For imaging of the cranial base, the ACR recommends the thinnest slices possible. If multiplanar or three-dimensional reconstruction is planned, slice thickness should be as thin as possible and no greater than 2-3 mm.[6a]

Contrast-Enhanced Head Computed Tomography

Contrast-enhanced head CT is usually performed following a noncontrast CT, and the two are then compared. In a contrast-enhanced head CT, IV contrast is injected, usually through an upper extremity intravenous catheter.

TABLE 1-1. Clinical Indications, Differential Diagnoses, and Initial Imaging Modality

Clinical Indication	Differential Diagnosis	Initial Imaging Modality
Headache	Mass, traumatic or spontaneous hemorrhage, meningitis, brain abscess, sinusitis, hydrocephalus	Noncontrast CT
Altered mental status or coma	Mass, traumatic or spontaneous hemorrhage, meningitis, brain abscess, hydrocephalus	Noncontrast CT
Fever	Meningitis (assessment of ICP), brain abscess	Noncontrast CT
Focal neurologic deficit—motor, sensory, or language deficit	Mass, ischemic infarct, traumatic or spontaneous hemorrhage, meningitis, brain abscess, sinusitis, hydrocephalus	Noncontrast CT, possibly followed by MRI, MRA, or CTA, depending on context
Focal neurologic complaint—ataxia or cranial nerve abnormalities	Posterior fossa or brainstem abnormalities, vascular dissections	MRI or MRA of brain and neck; CT or CTA of brain and neck if MR is not rapidly available
Seizure	Mass, traumatic or spontaneous hemorrhage, meningitis, brain abscess, sinusitis, hydrocephalus	Noncontrast CT, possibly followed by CT with IV contrast or MR
Syncope	Trauma	Little indication for imaging for cause of syncope, only for resulting trauma
Trauma	Hemorrhage, mass effect, cerebral edema	Noncontrast CT—if clinical decision rules suggest need for any imaging
Traumatic loss of consciousness	Hemorrhage, DAI, mass effect, cerebral edema	Little indication when transient loss of consciousness is isolated complaint
Planned LP	Increased ICP	Noncontrast head CT—limited indications

A time delay is introduced to allow the venous contrast to pass to the brain. Depending on the delay between contrast injection and image acquisition, the resulting CT may be a CT cerebral angiogram (CTA) or a CT cerebral venogram (CTV). The CT data may be reconstructed in any of several planes (typically axial, sagittal, or coronal) or even three-dimensionally. Cerebral perfusion can be mapped with IV contrast, using a technique described in more detail later. Contrast CT is useful for depicting abnormal vascular structures, such as aneurysms or arteriovenous malformations; for demonstrating abnormal failure of filling of vascular structures, such as sagittal sinus thrombosis (akin to demonstrating a filling defect in chest CT for pulmonary embolism); and for demonstrating neoplastic, inflammatory, and infectious processes. These latter abnormalities typically have increased regional blood flow, consequently receive abnormally high levels of vascular contrast agents, and may demonstrate ring enhancement, a circumferential increase in density around a lesion on CT occurring after IV contrast administration.

Magnetic Resonance

MR has been in wide clinical use in the United States since the late 1980s. The modality was coinvented by the American Paul C. Lauterbur and the British physicist Sir Peter Mansfield, who shared the 2003 Nobel Prize in Medicine for their work.[7] MR allows imaging of the brain by creating variations in the gradient of a magnetic field and analyzing the radio waves emitted in response by hydrogen ions (protons) within the field. MR provides outstanding soft-tissue contrast that is superior to that obtained from CT. MR can be performed with or without intravenous contrast agents. Advantages of MRI include the noninvasive nature of the test and its apparent safety in pregnancy.[8] It does not employ ionizing radiation and has no known permanent harmful biologic effects.[9] Traditionally, contraindications have been thought to include the presence of ferromagnetic material within the body, including electronic devices such as pacemakers or metallic debris such as shrapnel, especially in sensitive structures such as the eye or brain. However, there are now more than 230 published prospective cases of patients with pacemakers safely having undergone low-field MRI, so MRI may be an imaging option in these patients.[10] Magnetic effects on tattoos, including first-degree burns and burning sensation, have been reported, although these appear rare and more likely to interfere with completion of MR than to cause significant harm.[11–13]

Can Emergency Physicians Accurately Interpret Head CT Images? What Are the Potential Benefits to Patients?

Head CT is rapid to obtain, but delays in interpretation could result in adverse patient outcomes if clinical treatment decisions cannot be made in a timely fashion. Surveys of emergency medicine residency programs suggest that, in many cases, radiology interpretation is not rapidly available for clinical decisions and that emergency physicians often perform the initial interpretation of radiographic studies. A study simulating a teleradiology support system estimated the time to interpretation of a noncontrast head CT at 39 minutes, potentially wasting precious time in patients with intracranial hemorrhage or ischemic stroke.[14] The ability of the on-scene emergency physician to interpret the CT could be extremely valuable.

Multiple studies have examined the ability of emergency medicine residents and attending physicians to interpret head CT. A 1995 study showed that in an emergency medicine residency program, although up to 24% of potentially significant CT abnormalities were not identified by the emergency medicine residents, only 0.6% of patients appear to have been mismanaged as a result.[15] Studies have shown that substantial and sustained improvements in interpretation ability can occur with brief training. Perron et al.[16] showed an immediate improvement from 60% to 78% accuracy after a 2-hour training session based on a mnemonic, sustained at 3 months. In the setting of stroke, emergency medicine attending physicians perform relatively poorly in the recognition of both hemorrhage and early ischemic changes, which may contraindicate tissue plasminogen activator (t-PA) administration, with accuracy of approximately 60%. However, neurologists and general radiologists achieve only about 80% accuracy compared with the gold-standard interpretation

by neuroradiologists.[17,18] Undoubtedly, improvements in training are needed, but the pragmatic limitations on the availability of subspecialist radiologists, even with teleradiology, mean that emergency physicians must become proficient first-line readers of emergency CT.

INTERPRETATION OF NONCONTRAST HEAD CT

Several systematic methods for interpretation of noncontrast head CT have been described. The mnemonic "Blood Can Be Very Bad" has been shown to assist in the sustained improvement of interpretation by emergency medicine residents.[16] The mnemonic reminds the interpreter to look for blood (blood), abnormalities of cisterns and ventricles (can and very, respectively), abnormalities of the brain parenchyma (be), and fractures of bone (bad).

Broder used the familiar ABC paradigm to drive the assessment of the head CT (see "A Mnemonic for Head CT Interpretation: ABBBC").[5]

Hounsfield Units and Windows

The density of a tissue is represented using the Hounsfield scale, with water having a value of zero Hounsfield units (HU), tissues denser than water having positive values, and tissues less dense than water having negative values (Figure 1-1). By convention, low-density

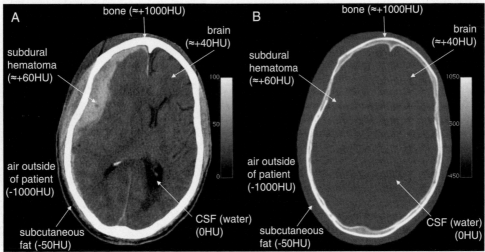

Figure 1-1. **The CT Hounsfield scale and window settings.** The CT Hounsfield scale places water density at a value of zero with air and bone at opposite extreme values of -1000HU and +1000HU. Fat is less dense than water and has a density around -50HU. Other soft tissues are slightly more dense than water and have densities ranging from around +20 to +100HU. The colors associated with these density values can be reassigned to highlight particular tissues, a process called "windowing." **A,** Axial CT slice, viewed with brain window settings. Notice in the grayscale bar at the right side of the figure that the full range of shades from black to white has been distributed over a narrow HU range, from zero (pure black) to +100HU (pure white). This allows fine discrimination of tissues within this density range, but at the expense of evaluation of tissues outside of this range. A large subdural hematoma is easily discriminated from normal brain, even though the two tissues differ in density by less than 100HU. Any tissues greater than +100HU in density will appear pure white, even if their densities are dramatically different. Consequently, the internal structure of bone cannot be seen with this window setting. Fat (-50HU) and air (-1000HU) cannot be distinguished with this setting, as both have densities less than zero HU and are pure black. **B,** The same axial CT slice viewed with a bone window setting. Now the scale bar at the right side of the figure shows the grayscale to be distributed over a very wide HU range, from -450HU (pure black) to +1050HU (pure white). Air can easily be discriminated from soft tissues on this setting because it is assigned pure black, while soft tissues are dark gray. Details of bone can be seen, because a large portion of the total range of gray shades is devoted to densities in the range of bone. Soft tissue detail is lost in this window setting, because the range of soft tissue densities (-50HU to around +100HU) represents a narrow portion of the gray scale.

tissues are assigned darker (blacker) colors and high-density structures are assigned brighter (whiter) colors. Because the human eye can perceive only a limited number of gray shades, the full range of density values is typically not displayed for a given image. Instead, the tissues of interest are highlighted by devoting the visible gray shades to a narrow portion of the full density range, a process called "windowing" (Figures 1-1 and 1-2). The same image data can be displayed in different window settings to allow evaluation of injury to different tissues. In general, head CT images are viewed on *brain* or *bone windows* to allow most emergency pathology to be assessed (see Figure 1-2).

Bone windows are useful for evaluation in the setting of trauma. By shifting the gray scale to center on the range of densities typical of bone bone windows allow detection of abnormalities such as subtle fracture lines. At the same time, they sacrifice detailed evaluation of structures less dense than bone (brain, cerebrospinal fluid, and blood vessels). Air remains black on bone windows and can be readily identified—for example, intracranial air can easily be seen on bone window settings. Sinus spaces are also nicely delineated on bone windows because of the contrast between air (black) and all other tissues (gray shades).

Brain windows are useful for evaluation of brain hemorrhage, fluid-filled structures including blood vessels and ventricles, and air-filled spaces. The majority of our evaluations will be done using this window setting. On brain windows, bone and other dense or calcified structures (e.g., surgical clips and calcified pineal glands) all appear bright white, and internal detail of these high-density structures is lost.

Right–Left Orientation of Computed Tomography Images

By convention, axial CT images are displayed with the patient's right side on the left side of the video screen or printed image. The point of view is as follows. Imagine yourself standing at the foot of the CT gantry, gazing toward the patient's head, with the patient positioned supine. Your left hand is placed on the patient's right foot. The patient is virtually "sectioned" into slices like a loaf of bread (Figure 1-3).

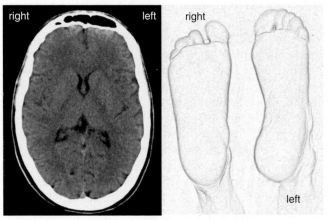

Figure 1-3. Right–left orientation in computed tomography (CT). Axial CT images are displayed with the patient's right side on the left side of the video screen or printed image **(A)**. The point of view is that of an observer standing at the feet of a supine patient, gazing toward the patient's head. The volume of the patient's head is divided into a stack of axial slices for review. **(B)**. *(From Broder J. Midnight radiology: Emergency CT of the head. (Accessed at http://emedhome.com/.)*

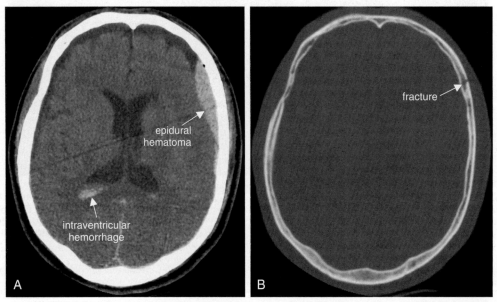

Figure 1-2. Hounsfield units and windows. A single noncontrast computed tomography slice, shown in brain windows **(A)** and bone windows **(B)**. Brain windows allow evaluation of the brain parenchyma, hemorrhage, cerebrospinal fluid (CSF) spaces, and other soft tissue at the expense of bony detail. Gross fractures may be seen. Bone windows allow detailed examination for fractures but obscure most soft-tissue detail. *(From Broder J, Preston R: An evidence-based approach to imaging of acute neurological conditions.* Emerg Med Pract 9(12):4, 2007.)

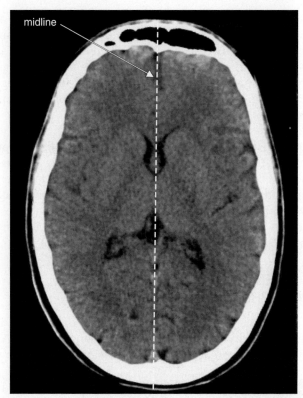

Figure 1-4. Normal brain symmetry brain windows. Abnormal masses or hemorrhage may deviate brain structures across an imaginary line dividing the brain, creating midline shift. The degree of midline shift is more important acutely than the exact etiology of the shift, since shift is an indication of threatened subfalcine herniation and may require surgical intervention. *(From Broder J, Preston R: An evidence-based approach to imaging of acute neurological conditions.* Emerg Med Pract *9(12):6, 2007.)*

Brain Symmetry

The brain, air and cerebrospinal fluid (CSF) spaces and the surrounding bone are normally symmetrical structures (Figure 1-4; see also Figures 1-7 and 1-19). A head CT should be inspected for normal symmetry, as deviation from this norm often indicates pathology (Figure 1-5; see also Figure 1-4). If the patient's head is not centered symmetrically in the CT gantry, the resulting images can create a false sense of asymmetry. It is critical to note that some life-threatening pathological conditions such as diffuse subarachnoid hemorrhage, cerebral edema, and hydrocephalus can have a symmetrical CT appearance, so symmetry does not guarantee normalcy.

Abnormal Asymmetry: Mass Effect and Midline Shift

The compression or displacement of normal brain structures (including ventricles and sulci) by adjacent masses is called *mass effect*. This displacement may occur due to tumor, hemorrhage, edema, or obstruction of CSF flow, to name but a few common causes. When this effect becomes extreme, shift of brain structures across the midline of the skull can occur, a finding called *midline shift*. Midline shift can indicate significant pathology, including threatened subfalcine herniation (Figure 1-5), and it should be carefully sought, as it may be more important than the underlying etiology of the shift in determining initial management. The degree of displacement of structures across the normal midline of the brain can be easily measured using digital tools on the

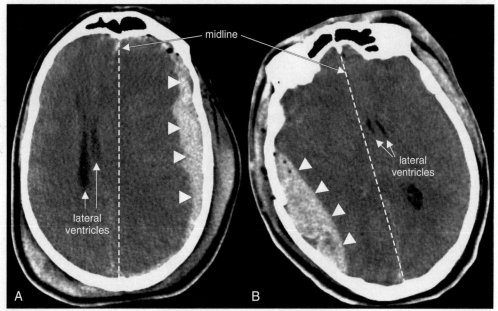

Figure 1-5. Mass effect and midline shift, brain windows. Abnormal masses such as hemorrhage create mass effect, displacing other structures from their normal positions. When mass effect drives structures across the brain midline, midline shift is present. The degree of mass effect or midline shift is more important than the underlying etiology. Guidelines call significant midline shift (5 mm or greater) a neurosurgical emergency, although the clinical status of the patient is the more important parameter. **A,** A large subdural hematoma *(arrowheads)* creates a mass effect and is displacing brain structures, including the lateral ventricles *(arrowheads),* across the midline *(dotted line)* to the patient's right. **B,** A large epidural hematoma *(arrowheads)* creates mass effect. The lateral ventricles *(arrowheads)* are shifted across the midline *(dotted line)* to the patient's left.

picture archiving and communication system (PACS), a computer viewing system. Midline shift may have some prognostic value in determining the likelihood of regaining consciousness after surgical decompression; patients with significant shift, greater than 10 mm, are more likely to benefit from decompression than are those with lesser degrees of shift.[19] Patients with shift of 5 mm or greater are more likely to have neurologic deficits requiring long-term supervision than are those with lesser midline shift.[20] Midline shift is also linked to probability of death after traumatic brain injury.[21] Published guidelines on surgical indications for brain lesions include midline shift as one of several parameters (as shown later), so recognizing and measuring midline shift is important.

Artifacts: Motion and Metal

A brain CT should be examined for artifacts that may limit interpretation, including motion and *streak artifact* or *beam-hardening artifact* from high-density structures such as metal (Figure 1-6). Although artifact may degrade the overall quality of the study, useful diagnostic information can often still be gleaned from an imperfect scan. Modern CT scanners acquire images at a very fast rate—a 64-slice CT can scan the entire brain in approximately 5 seconds.[22] As a consequence, CT is less subject to motion artifact than in the past, although significant patient motion may still render images uninterpretable. Just as in standard photographs, motion results in a blurry CT image.

Very dense objects create distortion on CT, called streak artifact. Examples include implanted metallic devices, such as cochlear implants and dental fillings; metallic foreign bodies, such as bullets; and even dense bone, such as occipital bone surrounding the posterior fossa. These artifacts may make it difficult or impossible to identify pathologic changes in the region (see Figure 1-6).

A MNEMONIC FOR HEAD CT INTERPRETATION: ABBBC

A systematic approach to interpretation of head CT is necessary to avoid missing important abnormalities. We review one approach, with a discussion of the normal

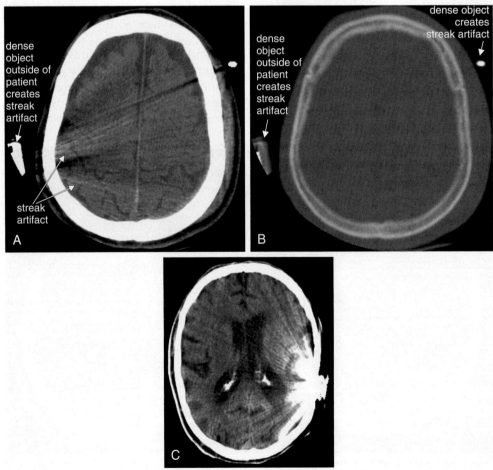

Figure 1-6. Streak artifacts. Streak artifacts may result from extremely high-density structures, such as dental fillings, implanted devices, or metal objects outside of the patient. **A,** Streak artifacts are most evident on brain windows. **B,** It is evident that the source of the artifact is very high-density material on bone windows. Notice how the external objects are denser (whiter) than the patient's calvarium. C, A cochlear implant (in another patient) also creates significant streak artifact. Although streak artifact may obscure some important details, relevant clinical information may be obtained from an imperfect scan. For example, in these scans, no midline shift is visible. *(From Broder J, Preston R: An evidence-based approach to imaging of acute neurological conditions.* Emerg Med Pract 9(12):6, 2007.)

appearance of the brain. Although a detailed understanding of neuroanatomy will improve your head CT interpretation, our mnemonic avoids significant anatomic detail, as many clinical decisions don't require this level of sophistication. Table 1-2 gives an overview of the mnemonic, with images illustrating each finding in the figures that follow.

A Is for Air Spaces

Our mnemonic starts with *A*, for air-filled spaces in the head. The normal head contains air-filled spaces: the frontal, maxillary, ethmoid, and sphenoid sinuses and the mastoid air cells (Figure 1-7). Opacification of an air space may occur because of fluids such as pus, mucus, or blood; mucosal edema; or because of tumor invasion of the space. In the setting of trauma, opacification of an

air space may indicate bleeding into that space, raising suspicion of a fracture of the surrounding bone (Figure 1-8). In the absence of trauma, opacification may indicate sinus infection or inflammation, although this is a nonspecific finding that may require no treatment in the absence of symptoms.

Normal air spaces appear black on either brain or bone windows, because air has the lowest Hounsfield density, negative 1000 HU. The frontal, maxillary, ethmoid, and sphenoid sinuses are normally air-filled, with no thickening of mucosa or air–fluid levels. The mastoid processes are normally spongy bone filled with tiny pockets of air, the mastoid air cells. If these air spaces become partially or totally opacified with fluid, this is easily recognized as a gray shade. Dense bone surrounding the small mastoid air cells creates a "bloom artifact" that can obscure the actual air spaces when viewed on brain windows, making assessment for abnormal fluid more difficult. This is minimized by viewing this region using bone windows. Abnormal fluid appears gray on this setting as well. The relatively small ethmoid air cells are also best-assessed for fluid using bone windows. For larger air-spaces, bloom artifact is minimal and brain or bone windows will usually reveal fluid. Recognizing abnormalities of normally air-filled structures requires some basic knowledge of their normal location and configuration (see Figure 1-7). Box 1-1 summarizes abnormalities of sinus air spaces, which are discussed in more detail later.

Sinus Trauma

Facial fractures are discussed in more detail in the dedicated chapter on facial imaging (Chapter 2). In trauma, fractures through the bony walls of sinuses result in bleeding into the sinus cavity. While the trauma patient remains in a supine position, this blood accumulates in the dependent portion of the sinus, forming an air–fluid level visible on CT. Previously existing sinus disease may be visible as circumferential sinus mucosal

TABLE 1-2. A Mnemonic for Systematic Interpretation of Non-Contrast Head CT: ABBBC

Assess These Structures…	For Signs of This Pathology

Air-filled spaces
  Mastoid air-cells
  Sinuses
	Fractures
	Infections

Bones	Fractures
Blood	Epidural hemorrhage Intraparenchymal hemorrhage Subarachnoid hemorrhage Subdural hemorrhage
Brain	Midline shift or mass effect Edema Infarction Masses

CSF spaces
  Cisterns
  Sulci
  Ventricles
	Atrophy
	Edema
	Hydrocephalus
	Subarachnoid hemorrhage in these
	  structures

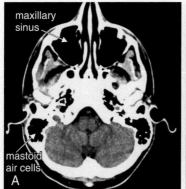 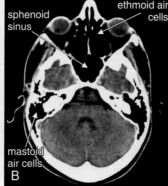 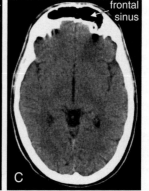

Figure 1-7. Air-filled spaces. The normal location and appearance of air-filled spaces when viewed on brain windows. Air-filled spaces are normally black on both brain and bone windows. Even more detail of fine bony partitions can be seen by selecting bone windows. **A** through **C** move progressively from caudad to cephalad. The structures are labeled on one side. Try to identify the same structure on the opposite side. *(From Broder J, Preston R: An evidence-based approach to imaging of acute neurological conditions.* Emerg Med Pract *9(12):5, 2007.)*

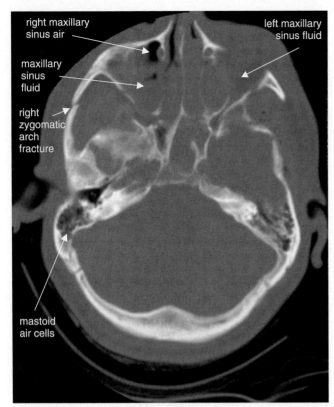

right maxillary sinus air

left maxillary sinus fluid

maxillary sinus fluid

right zygomatic arch fracture

mastoid air cells

Figure 1-8. Fluid in normally air-filled spaces. Fractures of the bony walls of normally air-filled structures, including the sinuses and mastoid air cells, can result in hemorrhage. Blood pooling in the dependent portion of these air-filled chambers results in an air–fluid level or sometimes in complete opacification. This may be the only evidence of fracture. If no history of trauma is present, fluid in an air space may indicate infection, such as sinusitis or mastoiditis. Viewed here on bone windows, the patient's right maxillary sinus has an air *(black)*–fluid *(gray)* level. The left maxillary sinus is completely opacified. The fractures of the sinuses themselves are hard to identify, though a right zygomatic arch fracture is visible. The mastoid air cells are normal and have no fluid. Following trauma, opacification of the mastoid air cells is a sign of temporal bone fracture. *(From Broder J, Preston R: An evidence-based approach to imaging of acute neurological conditions.* Emerg Med Pract *9(12):6, 2007.)*

thickening, rather than as an air–fluid level. Inspect the sinuses carefully for air–fluid levels, as these may indicate occult fractures. In trauma, opacification of sinuses should be considered evidence of fracture until proven otherwise, as the fracture itself may be hard to identify (Figures 1-8 and 1-9). The ethmoid sinuses are small and may be completely opacified by blood in the event of fracture. Opacified ethmoid sinuses should increase suspicion of a medial orbital blowout fracture. Air–fluid levels in the maxillary sinus may be associated with inferior orbital blowout fractures, because the inferior wall of the orbit is the superior wall of the maxillary sinus. The frontal sinus is less easily fractured, as its anterior and posterior plates are thick and resistant to trauma. Fracture of the anterior wall of the frontal sinus is relatively less concerning, requiring plastic surgery or otolaryngology consultation. Fracture of the posterior wall of the frontal sinus is a potential neurosurgical emergency due to communication of the sinus space with the CSF. Look for intracranial air whenever frontal

Box 1-1: CT Findings of: Sinus and Mastoid Pathology

● **Window setting: Bone windows helpful for smaller air-space evaluation.**
● **CT Appearance: Normally air filled (black), no air–fluid levels**
● **Significance**
  ○ Air–fluid levels or opacification in the setting of trauma may indicate fracture.
  ○ In the absence of trauma, air–fluid levels or mucosal thickening may be too sensitive and should not necessarily be equated to bacterial sinusitis in the absence of strong clinical evidence.
  ○ Mastoid opacification without trauma may indicate mastoiditis when clinical signs and symptoms are present.

sinus air–fluid levels are present and disruption of the posterior plate is suspected. When the mastoid air cells are obliterated or opacified, suspect temporal bone fracture. The normal side is a useful comparison.

Sinus Infections

In the absence of trauma, sinus mucosal thickening and air–fluid levels *may* be normal findings. They should not be used to make a diagnosis of bacterial sinusitis in the absence of strong clinical evidence, as they are nonspecific and may occur in allergic sinusitis or even asymptomatic patients. The mastoid air cells are not normally fluid filled, and in the presence of mastoid tenderness and erythema, their opacification on CT is evidence of mastoiditis (Figure 1-10). Sinus infections are discussed in more detail in Chapter 2, Imaging the Face.

B Is for Bone

The first *B* in our mnemonic is for bone. Following trauma, bony fractures should be suspected, although they are often of less clinical significance than any underlying brain injury. Abnormalities of bone including acute fractures are best identified on bone windows. Defects in the cortex of bone may indicate fracture, but these must be distinguished from normal suture lines (Figure 1-11). Comparing the contralateral side to the side in question may help to distinguish fractures from normal sutures. Air–fluid levels within sinuses following trauma are likely blood resulting from fracture (see Figures 1-8 and 1-9). Pneumocephalus (air within the calvarium) may also be present and may provide an additional clue to fractures communicating with sinus spaces or the outside world (Figures 1-12 and 1-13). Air may take the form of large amorphous collections abutting the calvarium or small black spheres within hemorrhage associated with the fracture.

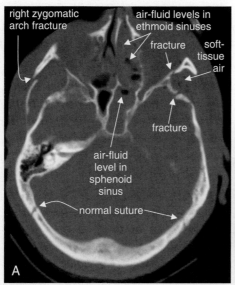

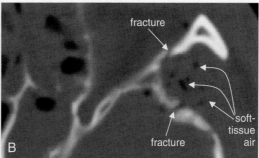

Figure 1-9. Fractures. A, Fractures, viewed on bone windows. **B,** Close-up from **A.** Fractures are sometimes evident as discontinuities in the bony cortex. It is important to compare the contralateral side to ensure that a normal suture is not misidentified as a fracture. Air in soft tissues and air–fluid levels or opacification of sinus air spaces are additional clues to minimally or nondisplaced fractures. *(From Broder J, Preston R: An evidence-based approach to imaging of acute neurological conditions.* Emerg Med Pract *9(12):9, 2007.)*

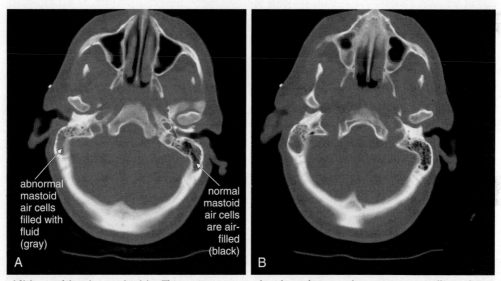

Figure 1-10. Mastoiditis resulting in meningitis. This patient presented with confusion and nystagmus, as well as a history of right ear pain. Noncontrast Computed tomography (CT) showed opacification of the right mastoid air cells, consistent with mastoiditis. Given the patient's confusion, meningitis as a complication of mastoiditis was suspected. Cerebrospinal fluid ultimately grew *Streptococcus pneumoniae.* The mastoid air cells are best viewed on bone windows **(A and B),** as soft-tissue windows are subject to bloom artifact from dense bone, which often obscures the small air spaces. A normal mastoid process is a spongy, air-filled bony lattice. Fluid in the mastoids air cells is abnormal. In the setting of trauma, fluid may indicate blood filling air cells from a temporal bone fracture. With no history of trauma, infectious mastoiditis should be suspected. Mastoiditis can be recognized on a noncontrast head CT and does not require special temporal bone views or facial CT series.

When a fracture is identified, look carefully for associated brain abnormalities using brain windows. Inspect for any of the types of hemorrhage described later. Look for soft-tissue swelling outside the calvarium overlying the fracture.

B Is for Blood

The second *B* in our mnemonic is for blood. A brain CT should be carefully inspected for the presence of subarachnoid, epidural, subdural, and intraparenchymal blood using brain windows. Multiple hemorrhage types may coexist. On noncontrast head CT, acute hemorrhage appears hyperdense (brighter or whiter) compared with brain tissue. As time elapses, blood darkens, indicating lower density. This is likely due to a number of factors, including the absorption of water by hematoma, changes in oxidation state, and the dispersion of blood within the subarachnoid space. As discussed later, the sensitivity of CT to detect subarachnoid hemorrhage is thought to decline as time elapses from the moment of hemorrhage. Debate exists about the accuracy of CT in dating blood.[23]

Hemorrhage can occur in any of several spaces within or around the brain. The shape of blood collections on CT depends on the anatomic location, as described in the sections that follow.

Subarachnoid Hemorrhage

SAH is blood within the subarachnoid space, which includes the sulci, Sylvian fissure, ventricles, and basilar cisterns surrounding the brainstem (Figure 1-14).

Fresh SAH appears white, although the appearance varies depending on the ratio of blood to CSF.[24] CT is

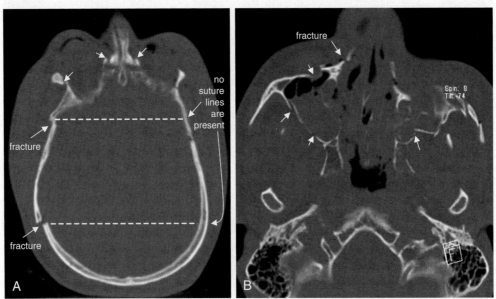

Figure 1-11. **Distinguishing fractures from normal sutures.** Fractures, viewed on bone windows. **A,** Multiple fractures are visible *(arrows)*. The *dotted line* connecting to the contralateral side confirms that no sutures are present in these locations. **B,** Multiple displaced fractures are present *(arrows)*. The patient's left maxillary sinus is badly comminuted. The associated air–fluid levels and opacification are additional clues to the presence of fractures.

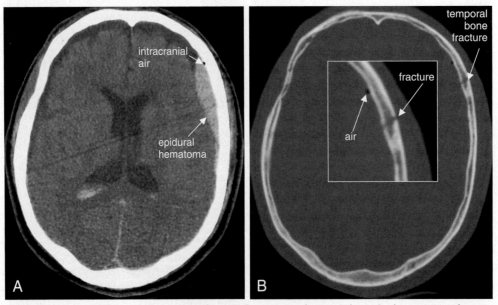

Figure 1-12. **Pneumocephalus, noncontrast CT. A,** Brain windows. **B,** Same image, bone windows. In this patient with a temporal bone fracture and associated epidural hematoma, air has entered the calvarium and is visible as a small black area on brain windows. On this setting, cerebrospinal fluid, fat, and and air all appear nearly black, so fine adjustment of the window setting may sometimes be necessary to confirm that this finding is air. Air may be more visible on bone or lung windows. In this case, the location, adjacent to the fracture, and the rounded shape, typical of air bubbles, are confirmatory. Finally, the actual density of the tissue can be measured using tools on a digital picture archiving and communication system (PACS). Air has a density of -1000HU, far lower than any other tissue. *(From Broder J, Preston R: An evidence-based approach to imaging of acute neurological conditions. Emerg Med Pract 9(12):6, 2007.)*

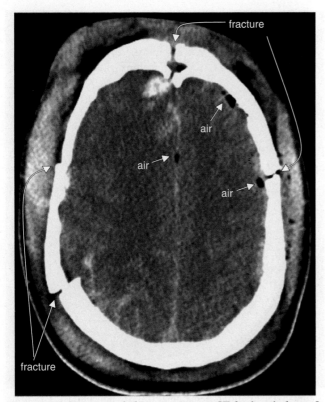

Figure 1-13. Pneumocephalus, noncontrast CT, brain windows. In this patient with multiple skull fractures, air *(arrows)* has entered the calvarium and is visible as *black areas* on brain windows. On this setting, cerebrospinal fluid (CSF) and air both appear nearly black, so fine adjustment of the window setting may sometimes be necessary to confirm that this finding is air. Air (-1000 HU) will remain black on all window settings, while CSF is much denser (0 HU) and will become lighter in color with adjustment of the window level. The density of the tissues can be measured directly using PACS tools when uncertainty exists. In this case, the location, immediately adjacent to fractures, and the rounded shape, typical of air bubbles, are confirmatory.

believed to be greater than 95% sensitive for SAH within the first 12 hours but to decline to 80% or less after 12 hours.[25-27] SAH may result from trauma or may occur spontaneously after rupture of an abnormal vascular structure such as an aneurysm. When looking for SAH, inspect the entire subarachnoid space, including the sulci, ventricles, Sylvian fissure, and cisterns for blood. Because subarachnoid blood may diffuse into adjacent regions, it may defy the guideline that hemorrhage and other abnormalities disturb normal brain symmetry. In other words, large amounts of SAH, including hemorrhage into cisterns, may actually result in a symmetrical-appearing head CT. Beware of this possibility when inspecting the brain for abnormalities. Familiarity with the black appearance of normal CSF spaces (see Figure 1-32) can help to avoid confusion. CSF spaces are reviewed in detail later with the "C" in our mnemonic. However, two CSF spaces deserve special mention here with respect to SAH. The suprasellar cistern lies just above the sella turcica (home of the pituitary gland) at the level of the brainstem. This cistern usually is CSF-filled and has the appearance of a symmetrical black "star." When filled with blood, it appears as a symmetrical white star (see Figure 1-14). The quadrigeminal plate cistern is usually visible on the same axial CT slice and has the appearance of a black "smile" when filled normally with CSF. When filled with subarachnoid blood, it becomes a white "smile."

As time elapses from the moment of hemorrhage, blood will diffuse through the subarachnoid spaces, like a drop of food coloring dropped into a glass of water. Thus a bright white punctate finding on head CT is not

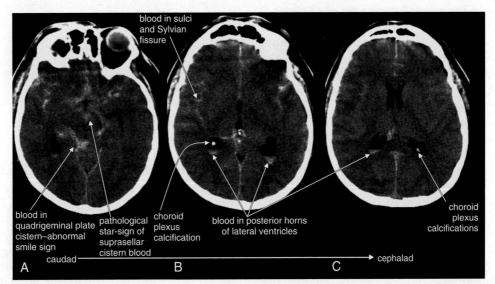

Figure 1-14. Subarachnoid hemorrhage (SAH), noncontrast CT, brain windows. Acute SAH appears white on noncontrast computed tomography (CT) brain windows. **A** through **C,** nonconsecutive axial slices, progressing from caudad to cephalad. In this case of diffuse SAH, note the presence of subarachnoid blood filling the sulci, as well as extending into the cisterns, Sylvian fissures, and even lateral ventricles. In **A,** blood (white) fills the suprasellar cistern. This star-shaped structure is normally filled with CSF (black). The quadrigeminal plate cistern is normally a smile-shaped black crescent, filled with CSF--but in this case is filled with blood. Extremely bright calcifications in the choroid plexus of the posterior horns of the lateral ventricles are common, normal findings—do not mistake these for hemorrhage. Note their similarity in density to bone of the calvarium.

Box 1-2: CT Findings of Subarachnoid Hemorrhage

- **Appearance: White on brain windows**
- **Location: Localized or diffuse**
  - ○ Sulci
  - ○ Fissures
  - ○ Ventricles
  - ○ Cisterns
- **Shape: Assumes shape of surroundings**
- **Pearl: Suspect increased ICP, look for signs of diffuse edema**
- **Pearl: Look for abnormal white "star" sign and "smile" sign from SAH in suprasellar and quadrigeminal plate cisterns**

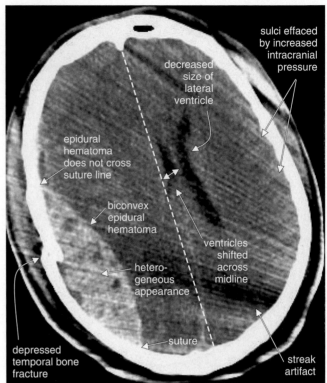

Figure 1-15. **Epidural hematoma (EDH), noncontrast CT, brain windows.** EDHs are frequently the result of traumatic injury to the middle meningeal artery at the site of a temporal bone fracture. They characteristically have a biconvex (lens) shape. Because they lie between the calvarium and the dura, they are restricted from extending beyond suture lines, where the dura is tightly adherent to the skull. Sutures are not actually visible on this brain window setting but could be readily identified by use of bone windows. Suture locations are pointed out in this figure for reference. In this CT, image quality is somewhat degraded by streak artifact emanating from an object outside of the patient to the left side (cropped out of the field of image). Despite this, several classic features of EDH are visible:
- Lenslike or biconvex disc shape
- Temporal location, with associated depressed temporal bone fracture
- No crossing of suture lines
- Mass effect with midline shift
- Swirl sign (heterogeneous appearance suggesting active bleeding)
- Elevated intracranial pressure, with small ventricles and no visible sulci
(From Broder J, Preston R: An evidence-based approach to imaging of acute neurological conditions. Emerg Med Pract 9(12):7, 2007.)

likely to be SAH, especially hours after the onset of clinical symptoms. Figure 1-14 shows several examples of SAH, involving different brain regions. SAH may be accompanied by other important changes, including hydrocephalus and cerebral edema, discussed later. Box 1-2 summarizes findings of SAH.

Epidural Hematoma
Epidural hematoma (EDH) is a collection of blood lying outside the dura mater, between the dura and the calvarium. It is almost always a traumatic injury, commonly resulting from injury to the middle meningeal artery. Because blood is extravasating from an artery under high pressure, rapid enlargement of the hematoma may occur, leading to significant mass effect, midline shift, and herniation. The common CT appearance is a biconvex disc or lens, collecting in the potential space between the calvarium and the dura mater.[28] This shape occurs because the more superficial aspect of the EDH conforms to the curve of the calvarium, while the inner aspect expands and presses into the dura. The dura is usually tethered to the calvarium at sutures, so EDHs usually do not cross suture lines on CT. EDHs may cross the midline, because there are no midline sutures in the frontal and occipital regions. The usual location of an EDH is temporal, although EDHs occasional occur in other locations. Transfalcine herniation may occur with EDHs, so the midline of the brain should be carefully inspected on CT for midline shift or compression of the lateral ventricle. The *swirl sign*, described as a bright white vortex or "swirl" within the EDH, has long been considered a finding of active bleeding and should be interpreted as a sign of continued expansion, although recent studies have questioned the prognostic significance of this finding.[29-32] Figures 1-15 and 1-16 show several examples of EDHs, with the classic findings described earlier. Interestingly, the volume of hematoma has not been shown to correlate with preoperative neurologic status or 6-month postoperative status.[33] Box 1-3 summarizes findings of EDH.

Indications for Surgery in Epidural Hematoma. Published criteria for surgical evacuation of an acute EDH include volume greater than 30 cm[3] (regardless of Glasgow Coma Score, or GCS). Many PACS toolkits allow automated computation of volumes from two-dimensional datasets by measuring the thickness of a structure or outlining it. For patients with a GCS greater than 8 and no focal deficit, an EDH smaller than 30 cm[3], less than 15 mm thick, and with less than 5 mm of midline shift can be managed nonoperatively. Anisocoria with a GCS below 9 is an indication for surgery, regardless of EDH size.[34]

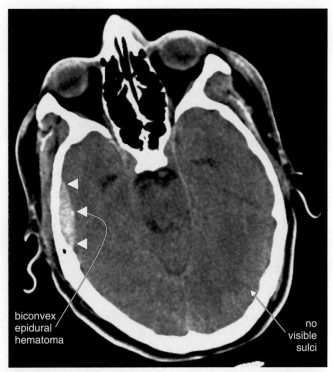

biconvex
epidural
hematoma

no
visible
sulci

Figure 1-16. Epidural hematoma (EDH), noncontrast CT, brain windows. This EDH *(arrowheads)* demonstrates several classic features, including a lenslike or biconvex disc shape and a temporal location. Although it appears small on this slice, the entire CT may reveal a different story. On this slice, sulci are absent, raising concern for elevated intracranial pressure.

Box 1-3: CT Findings of Epidural Hematoma

- **CT Appearance: Variable white to gray on brain windows**
- **Location: peripheral to brain, variable but usually temporal region**
- **Shape: Biconvex disc or lens**
- **Pearl: Does not cross suture lines**
- **White swirl sign means active bleeding**
- **Significance: May cause mass effect and herniation**
  - ○   Look for midline shift
  - ○   Look for effacement of ventricles and sulci
- **Surgical indications[34]: 15-mm thickness or 5-mm midline shift**

Subdural Hematoma

Subdural hematoma (SDH) (Figures 1-17 and 1-18) is a collection of blood between the dura mater and the brain surface. SDHs usually occur from traumatic injury to bridging dural veins, although a history of trauma is not always found. SDHs may be self-limited in size due to the lower pressure of venous bleeding, but they can become enormous, causing significant mass effect, midline shift, and herniation. They may also rebleed after an initial delay, resulting in expansion. Moreover, they are frequently markers of significant head trauma, and patient outcomes may be compromised by associated diffuse axonal injury (DAI) (described later) or edema. The typical CT appearance of an SDH is a crescent, with the convex side facing the calvarium and the concave surface abutting the brain surface. The shape of SDHs results from their accumulation between the dura and the brain surface. Because they lie between the dura and the brain, they are not restricted by attachment sites between the dura and the calvarium at sutures. Consequently, SDHs may cross suture lines. Moreover, each cerebral hemisphere is wrapped in its own dura, so SDHs typically do not cross the midline but instead may continue to follow the brain surface into the interhemispheric fissure.

The color may vary depending on the age of the SDH (see Figure 1-18). Fresh subdurals are typically brighter white (or lighter gray) than the adjacent brain. Older

SDHs, or acute hematomas in anemic patients, may become similar in density (isodense) to the adjacent brain and thus may be difficult to detect.[35,36] Clues to their presence include the obliteration of sulci on the brain surface and mass effect resulting from the SDH. Still older SDHs may become similar in density or color to the CSF surrounding the brain and thus may be difficult to recognize. Sometimes SDHs are multicolored or layered, indicating blood of varying ages. Box 1-4 summarizes findings of SDH.

Indications for Surgery in Subdural Hematoma. Published criteria for surgical evacuation of an acute SDH include thickness greater than 10 mm or midline shift greater than 5 mm, regardless of GCS. Surgery may be indicated with smaller SDHs and lesser degrees of shift in patients with a GCS score less than 9, based on intracranial pressure (ICP), pupillary findings, and worsening GCS.[37]

Intraparenchymal Hemorrhage

Intraparenchymal hemorrhage (Figures 1-19 and 1-20), or hemorrhage within the substance of the brain matter, may occur in trauma or spontaneously, perhaps as a complication of hypertension. The appearance is generally bright white acutely. The size may vary from punctate to catastrophically large, with associated mass effect and midline shift. For intraparenchmyal hemorrhage, mass effect such as midline shift or ventricular effacement should be assessed. Signs of increased ICP should be identified. Particularly for smaller punctate hemorrhages, care must be taken not to mistake hemorrhage for normal benign calcifications of the pineal gland, choroid plexus, and meninges, or vice versa. Calcifications can usually be distinguished from hemorrhage as the former remain bright white on bone windows. In addition, if the density is measured with PACS tools, calcifications have very high density, near +1000HU, while hemorrhage has a density around +40 to +70HU. Pineal

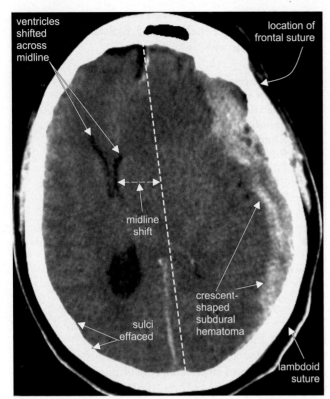

Figure 1-17. Subdural hematoma (SDH), noncontrast CT, brain windows. SDHs are most often the result of shearing of dural veins from blunt trauma. They usually have a crescent shape and may cross suture lines, as they lie within the dura and are thus free to extend along the brain surface, rather than being restricted by the tethering of the dura to the calvarium at sutures. In this figure, the sutures themselves are not visible due to the window setting, but their locations are labeled to illustrate this point. This SDH demonstrates several classic features:
- Crescent shape
- Crossing of suture lines
- Mass effect with midline shift
- Elevated intracranial pressure (ICP), with small ventricles
- No visible sulci (due to effacement from elevated ICP)

(From Broder J, Preston R: An evidence-based approach to imaging of acute neurological conditions. Emerg Med Pract *9(12):5, 2007.)*

gland and choroid plexus calcifications also have stereo-typical locations (Figure 1-21) that aid in their recognition. Calcifications are shown in Figure 1-21.

Indications for Surgery in Parenchymal Hemorrhage. Published criteria for surgical treatment of traumatic intraparenchymal hematoma are complex. They include size greater than 20 cm³ with midline shift greater than 5 mm, cisternal compression, or both if the GCS score is 6 to 8. Lesions greater than 50 cm³ in size should be managed operatively, regardless of the GCS score.[37a]

B Is for Brain

The third *B* in our mnemonic is for brain. Brain abnormalities include neoplastic masses, localized vasogenic edema, abscesses, ischemic infarction, global brain edema, and DAI.

Masses

Masses are best delineated on CT with IV contrast or on MRI. However, noncontrast CT can demonstrate a variety of masses if they are of sufficient size. In some cases, the mass itself may not be seen, but secondary findings such as mass effect, calcification (see Figure 1-21), or vasogenic edema (Figure 1-22) (see the discussion in the next section) may occur. IV contrast is useful in detecting masses because they are generally extremely vascular and thus enhance in the presence of contrast material. On noncontrast CT, masses may be denser than surrounding brain if they are calcified. Examples are meningiomas, which are often seen as midline structures emanating from the falx cerebri.

Vasogenic Edema

Malignant primary brain neoplasms or metastatic lesions often appear *hypodense* (darker or blacker) compared with normal brain. This appearance is typical of localized

Figure 1-18. Three variations of subdural hematoma (SDH) from different patients, noncontrast CT, brain windows. A, A small SDH. **B,** Bilateral SDHs, likely subacute or chronic, as they are hypodense relative to brain. **C,** Bilateral SDHs with varying density, likely indicating hemorrhage at different times. Bright white hemorrhage is acute, while dark hemorrhage is subacute or chronic. Also notice that the window settings for panels **A** through **C** are not identical. CSF within the lateral ventricles appears darker in panel **A** than in panel **C** due to differences in the window setting. Windows can be varied to accentuate various tissues.

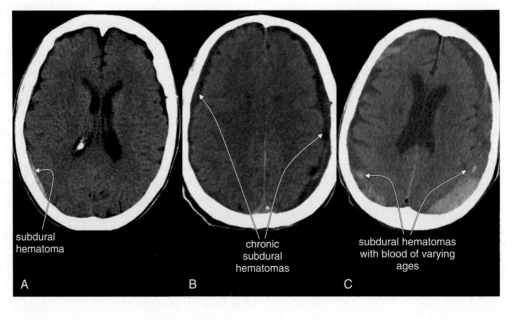

Box 1-4: CT Findings of Subdural Hematoma

- **Appearance: Variable white to gray on brain windows**
- **Location: peripheral to brain or interhemispheric; variable location around brain perimeter**
- **Shape: Crescent**
- **Pearl: May cross suture lines**
- **Significance: May cause mass effect and herniation**
  - ○ Look for midline shift
  - ○ Associated with other brain injuries, look for effacement of ventricles and sulci
- **Surgical indications[37]: 10-mm thickness or 5-mm midline shift**

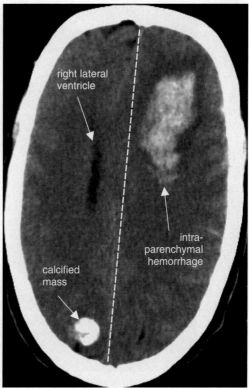

Figure 1-19. Intraparenchymal hemorrhage, noncontrast CT, brain windows. Acute intraparenchymal hemorrhage appears white on CT brain windows. Hemorrhage in the patient's left frontal region is creating mass effect with midline shift. The left lateral ventricle has been completely effaced. The single visible ventricle is the right lateral ventricle. A calcified mass in the right occipital region must be differentiated from acute hemorrhage. Calcifications are extremely bright white on brain windows—as white and dense as bone. On bone windows, they remain white, while hemorrhage does not. The density can also be measured using PACS tools. Bone has a density near +1000HU, while blood has a density closer to +50HU, easily differentiating the two in most cases. *(From Broder J, Preston R: An evidence-based approach to imaging of acute neurological conditions.* Emerg Med Pract *9(12):6, 2007.)*

vasogenic edema surrounding a lesion. Neoplasms often secrete vascular endothelial growth factor, resulting in the development of immature blood vessels that perfuse the tumor. These immature vessels have leaky endothelial junctions, allowing fluid to extravasate into the interstitium, which causes vasogenic edema. This increased fluid content reduces the density of brain tissues toward that of water (zero on the Hounsfield scale), resulting in a hypodense appearance on CT. In addition, the mass itself and associated local edema increase the volume of brain tissue, resulting in local mass effect, including the effacement of ventricles (see Figure 1-22, effacement of the posterior horn of the lateral ventricle) and effacement of sulci as adjacent gyri expand in size (see Figure 1-22).

Vasogenic edema must be differentiated from infarction, which may also cause a hypodense appearance. Vasogenic edema does not need to conform to a normal vascular territory within the brain, whereas hypodensity associated with ischemic stroke does. Vasogenic edema responds to treatment with dexamethasone, whereas steroids are not indicated for other forms of cerebral edema such as traumatic edema do not. In fact, a multicenter randomized controlled trial of corticosteroid therapy in patients with traumatic brain injury showed an increased risk of death and severe disability from steroid use.[38]

As described earlier, midline shift associated with a mass should be carefully assessed during inspection of the brain on brain windows.

Abscesses

Abscesses may be visible on noncontrast CT as hypodense regions (Figure 1-23), occasionally with air within them. This appearance may be nonspecific, and a differential diagnosis including toxoplasmosis, mass with vasogenic edema, or central nervous system lymphoma should be considered, depending on the patient's

clinical scenario. Abscesses, toxoplasmosis, neurocysticercosis (Figure 1-24), and masses all may undergo *ring enhancement,* an increase in density around a lesion after administration of IV contrast (Box 1-5). This reflects increased blood flow in the vicinity of the lesion, as well as leaky vascular structures that allow extravasation of contrast in the region.

Ischemic Stroke and Infarction

Ischemic stroke accounts for 85% of strokes.[39] It is potentially one of the most important indications for head CT and is an area in which the interpretation of CT by emergency physicians might play the greatest role by shortening the time to diagnosis. One obvious reason is the 3-hour or 4.5-hour window for administration of IV t-PA—an intervention that is still fiercely debated in the emergency medicine community and that has been reviewed elsewhere.[40]

Understanding CT findings of acute ischemic stroke is important—for those who do not believe in

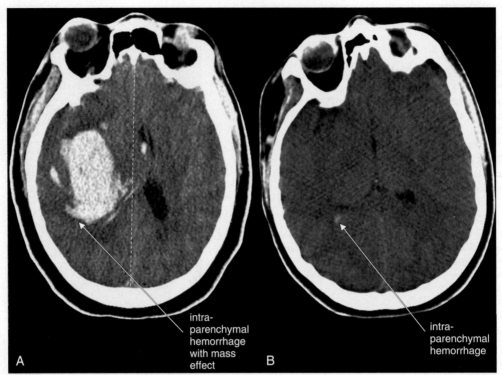

Figure 1-20. Spectrum of intraparenchymal hemorrhage, noncontrast CT, brain windows. Intraparenchymal hemorrhage may be grossly obvious or subtle. **A,** A large hemorrhage with midline shift and mass effect. **B,** A small amount of hemorrhage *(arrow)*.

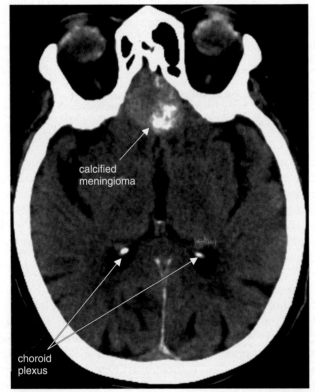

Figure 1-21. Calcifications, noncontrast CT, brain windows. Calcification of the choroid plexi is a frequent incidental finding that may resemble punctate intraparenchymal hemorrhage. Clues are bright white density (equal to that of bone), location in the posterior horns of the lateral ventricles, and frequent bilaterality. This patient also has a calcified meningioma. Meningiomas are common benign neoplasms that may become quite large. A well-circumscribed, rounded appearance and calcification are common. *(From Broder J, Preston R: An evidence-based approach to imaging of acute neurological conditions. Emerg Med Pract 9(12):8, 2007.)*

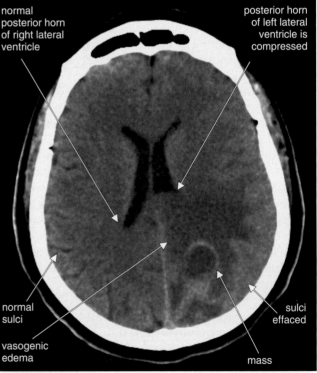

Figure 1-22. Masses, noncontrast CT, brain windows. A mass with surrounding vasogenic edema, which has a hypodense *(dark gray)* appearance. Neoplasms frequently are associated with vasogenic edema, named for the putative cause, which is abnormal blood vessels that allow extravasation of fluid. This form of edema appears hypodense, like an ischemic infarct, but is not restricted to a vascular territory. An abscess might appear similar. Masses often exert mass effect. Here, the edema surrounding the mass is compressing the posterior horn of the left lateral ventricle. Notice also the effacement of the sulci in the region of the mass. *(From Broder J, Preston R: An evidence-based approach to imaging of acute neurological conditions. Emerg Med Pract 9(12):8, 2007.)*

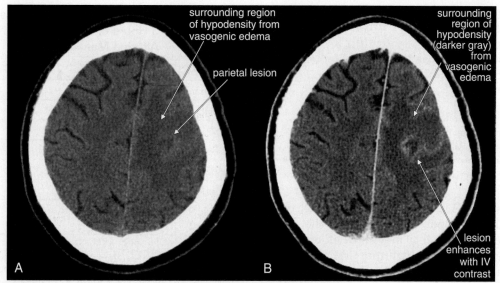

Figure 1-23. Brain abscess. This 48-year-old male presented with status epilepticus. CT showed a parietal mass, which at brain biopsy was found to be an abscess. Cultures grew mixed gram-positive and gram-negative organisms and anaerobes. The patient was subsequently found to be human immunodeficiency virus positive. **A,** Noncontrast head CT, brain windows. **B,** CT with intravenous (IV) contrast moments later, brain windows. Abscesses and other infectious, inflammatory, or neoplastic lesions typically have surrounding hypodense regions representing vasogenic edema. When IV contrast is administered **(B),** the lesion may enhance peripherally, often referred to as ring enhancement.

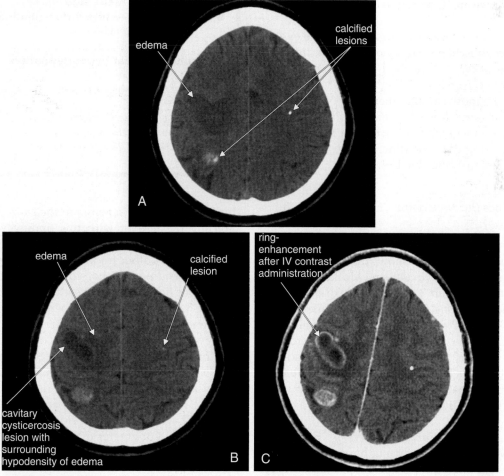

Figure 1-24. Neurocysticercosis. This 40-year-old Bolivian male presented with left-hand weakness. **A, B,** Noncontrast head CT, brain windows. **C,** CT with contrast moments later—compare this with image **B,** a slice through the same level of the brain before contrast administration. Hypodense lesions are present, with surrounding hypodensity *(dark gray)* representing edema. Scattered calcifications are also seen, which are a common feature of old neurocysticercosis lesions. Administration of IV contrast leads to ring enhancement, a feature of many infectious and inflammatory conditions, including neurocysticercosis, brain abscess, and toxoplasmosis.

Box 1-5: CT Findings of Enhancement

- **Increased brightness (Hounsfield units) after IV contrast administration**
- **Seen in**
    - ○   Infection
    - ○   Inflammation
    - ○   Neoplasm
    - ○   Vascular lesions

TABLE 1-3. Early Ischemic CT Changes Within 3 Hours of symptom onset, Possibly Altering Management

Type of Change	Percentage
Any change	31%
GWMD loss	27%
Hypodensity	9%
CSF space compression	14%
GWMD loss > ⅓ MCA territory	13%
Hypodensity > ⅓ MCA territory	2%
CSF space compression > ⅓ MCA territory	9%

GWMD, Gray–white matter differentiation.
From NINDS; Patel SC, Levine SR, Tilley BC, et al: Lack of clinical significance of early ischemic changes on computed tomography in acute stroke. *JAMA* 286:2830–2838, 2001.

administration of t-PA, they provide yet another argument against the treatment, while for those who would use t-PA in select patients, they may allow more rational and safer patient selection. Apart from t-PA administration, rapid diagnosis of ischemic stroke may allow the emergency physician to make better-informed decisions about patient management and disposition. If new stroke therapies such as intra arterial thrombolysis and clot retrieval become widely accepted and available, rapid CT interpretation for ischemic stroke may become even more valuable. Interventional radiologic therapies for ischemic stroke are reviewed in Chapter 16.

A complex cascade of events occurs to cause the evolving appearance of ischemic stroke on head CT. Initially, at the moment of onset of cerebral ischemia, no abnormalities may be seen on head CT—thus, this is one of the most difficult diagnoses for the emergency physician, as a normal CT may correlate with significant pathology. Studies have shown emergency physicians to be relatively poor at recognizing early ischemic changes, which we review here (Table 1-3 and Box 1-6).

Box 1-6: Early CT Findings of Acute Ischemia

- **Hyperdense MCA sign**
- **Loss of gray–white differentiation**
    - ○   Insular ribbon sign
    - ○   Cortical sulcal effacement
- **Ischemic focal hypoattenuation**
    - ○   MCA territory
    - ○   Basal ganglia

From Patel SC, Levine SR, Tilley BC, et al: Lack of clinical significance of early ischemic changes on computed tomography in acute stroke. *JAMA* 286:2830-2838, 2001.

How Early Does the Noncontrast Head CT Indicate Ischemic Stroke?

Analysis of the National Institute of Neurological Disorders and Stroke (NINDS) data shows that early ischemic changes are quite common in ischemic stroke, occurring in 31% of patients within 3 hours of stroke onset,[41] in contrast to the widely held belief that ischemic strokes become visible on CT only after 6 hours.[42] Some findings may occur immediately, such as the hyperdense middle cerebral artery (MCA) sign, while other findings may require time to elapse, with the gradual failure of adenosine triphosphate (ATP)–dependent ion pumps and resulting fluid shifts.

Hyperdense Middle Cerebral Artery Sign. The hyperdense MCA sign is a finding of hyperacute stroke, indicating thrombotic occlusion of the proximal MCA. This may be present on the initial noncontrast head CT *immediately following symptom onset*, since the finding does not require the failure of ion pumps and fluid shifts that lead to other ischemic changes on head CT. Because

this lesion leads to ischemia in the *entire MCA territory*, typically the patient with this finding will have profound hemiparesis or hemiplegia on the contralateral side, as well as other findings such as language impairment, depending on the side of the lesion. In other words, this finding is not associated with mild or subtle strokes. The presence of a hyperdense MCA sign is an independent predictor of neurologic deterioration.[43] However, the dense MCA sign is only visible in 30% to 40% of patients with stroke affecting the MCA territory.[71,72] It may seem surprising that this vascular abnormality is visible on noncontrast head CT. As the name implies, the MCA appears hyperdense (bright white) compared with the normal side. A specific Hounsfield unit threshold of greater than 43 units has been recommended to avoid false positives.[44]

Use your knowledge of the location of the patient's neurologic deficits to direct you to the likely side of the lesion, which will be on the contralateral side. Then use the normal symmetry of the brain to help you identify this

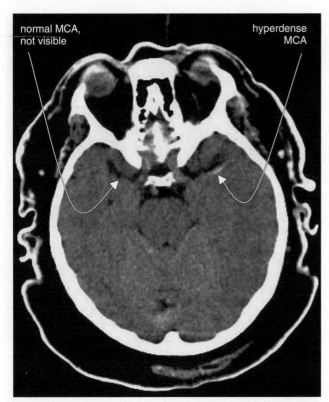

normal MCA, not visible

hyperdense MCA

Figure 1-25. Hyperdense middle cerebral artery (MCA) sign, noncontrast CT, brain windows. The hyperdense MCA sign is a CT finding of thrombosis of the MCA. Importantly, this is a sign seen on noncontrast CT—the typical initial imaging study obtained in patients with suspected acute stroke. It can be seen in the immediate hyperacute stages of thrombotic–ischemic stroke and may guide therapy, such as intra arterial tissue plasminogen activator administration. On CT, the hyperdense MCA appears as a white line or point representing the thrombosed vessel. Care must be taken not to confuse this with the white appearance of fresh extravascular blood in hemorrhagic stroke. In this patient, who presented within 30 minutes of onset of right hemiplegia, the normal MCA is not visible while the left MCA is thrombosed and demonstrates the hyperdense MCA sign. *(From Broder J, Preston R: An evidence-based approach to imaging of acute neurological conditions. Emerg Med Pract 9(12):12, 2007.)*

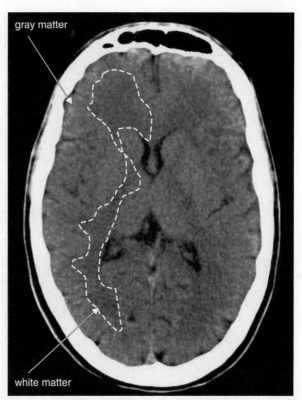

gray matter

white matter

Figure 1-26. Normal gray–white matter differentiation, noncontrast CT, brain windows. Myelinated regions (white matter) have a greater fat content than unmyelinated regions (gray matter). As a consequence, and perhaps counterintuitively, white matter has lower density and appears darker than gray matter on computed tomography. The *dotted line* on the patient's right outlines the border between gray and white matter. Trace this interface yourself on the patient's left.

abnormality. A related finding, the MCA "dot" sign, has been validated by angiography and found to be a specific marker of branch occlusion of the MCA. This sign appears as a bright white dot in the sylvian fissure on the affected side.[45] Figure 1-25 shows the hyperdense MCA sign.

Gray–White Differentiation. Understanding this finding of stroke requires a brief and simple review of neuroanatomy. Gray matter is brain tissue without myelin—examples include the cerebral cortex, lentiform nucleus, caudate, and thalamus. White matter is composed of myelinated axons in brain tissue—rendered white on gross pathologic section by the high lipid content of the myelin sheath. Recall from our earlier discussion of Hounsfield units that lower density on CT means a darker color—low-density fat appears a darker gray than does higher-density water. Thus, the higher fat content of white matter makes it appear darker on CT. In other words, on a normal head CT, gray matter is whiter

and white matter is grayer. Figure 1-26 shows the normal gray–white matter boundary.

Loss of Gray–White Matter Differentiation. In an ischemic stroke, as brain tissue consumes ATP and is unable to replenish it, ATP-dependent ion pumps stop working. Ions equilibrate across membranes, and fluid shifts occur. Gray matter gains fluid, lowering its density, and as it does, its density becomes more similar to that of white matter. White matter also gains fluid, increasing its density slightly. Since differences in density are the reason that these tissues look different on CT, as their densities converge, their appearances become more similar, and it becomes more difficult to discern where gray matter ends and white matter begins. This change is called *loss of gray–white matter differentiation*, and it is an early finding of ischemic stroke, occurring within 3 hours after onset of ischemia.[41] Figures 1-27 and 1-28 show an abnormal gray–white matter boundary.

Insular Ribbon Sign (Loss of Insular Ribbon). The insula (or insular cortex) is a thin ribbon of gray matter tissue that lies just deep to the lateral brain surface, separating the temporal lobe from the inferior parietal cortex. On CT, it is visible as the tissue layer lining the

Figure 1-27. Early ischemic hypodensity, noncontrast CT, brain windows. Three examples of subtle hypoattenuation in early stroke (*dotted circles*). Compare the abnormal side to the normal side in each image. Large areas of hypoattenuation predict an increased risk of hemorrhage and are relative contraindications for tissue plasminogen activator.

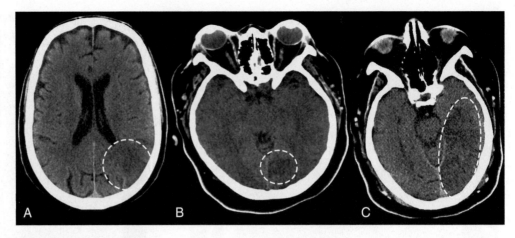

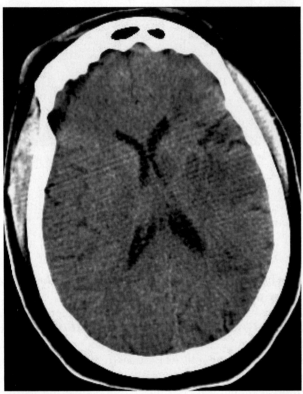

Figure 1-28. Gray and white matter differentiation, noncontrast CT, brain windows. When ischemia renders the gray–white interface less discrete, the computed tomography appearance is called loss of gray–white differentiation. In this example, the differentiation is normal on the patient's right but is being lost on the patient's left. The patient has progressed beyond early hypoattenuation (Figure 1-27) and is developing the frank hypodensity of ischemic stroke.

Sylvian fissure. This region is subject to early ischemic changes in the form of loss of gray–white matter differentiation, often called the insular ribbon sign or loss of the insular ribbon, as this area becomes less distinct.

Hypodensity in Ischemic Stroke. Ischemic brain looks hypodense, or darker than normal brain in the same anatomic region. This change occurs for the same general reasons as does loss of gray–white differentiation. As neurons deplete stores of ATP, cytotoxic and

vasogenic edema both occur. Ion gradients run back toward equilibrium, and water shifts into gray matter, making it less dense relative to normal tissue. The appearance of an infarct becomes progressively more hypodense over the first several days to weeks of an ischemic stroke. Again, this finding can occur as an early change within 3 hours of symptom onset.[41] Figures 1-27 through 1-30 show examples of hypodensity. Figure 1-31 shows the progressive hypodensity of an ischemic stroke over several days.

Hypodensity of Ischemic Stroke Versus Vasogenic Edema of Masses. Hypodensity in an ischemic stroke follows a vascular distribution, whereas hypodensity caused by vasogenic edema around a mass need not respect vascular territories.

Are Ischemic Changes a Contraindication to t-PA?

Early ischemic stroke findings were *not* used as exclusion criteria in the NINDS trial, which required only the absence of hemorrhage on initial head CT.[46] However, multiple studies following NINDS have shown an increased risk of intracranial hemorrhage, bad neurologic outcomes, and death in patients with early ischemic changes on head CT.[47,48] Ischemic changes are relative contraindications to t-PA administration, and their presence may suggest that greater than 3 hours have elapsed from symptom onset, in which case systemic t-PA may be contraindicated. In addition, *the Food and Drug Administration, American Heart Association, and American Academy of Neurology specifically recommend against administering t-PA if early signs of major infarction are present, because of increased risk of intracranial hemorrhage.*[49–51] MCA infarction greater than one third of the MCA territory predicts increased bleeding risk if t-PA is given, and it was poorly detected by radiologists, neurologists, and emergency physicians in past studies.[18,52,53] In addition, the greater the extent of ischemic changes on CT, the higher the risk of bleeding, as demonstrated in the second multinational European Cooperative Acute Stroke Study (ECASS-II).[48]

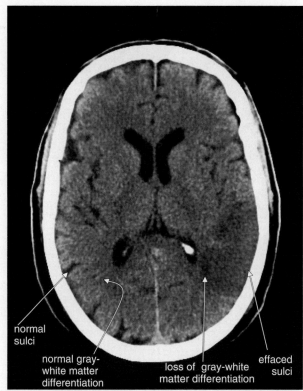

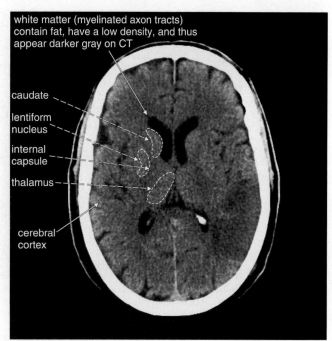

Figure 1-30. Early ischemic changes, noncontrast CT, brain windows. (Same image as Figure 1-29.) Image contrast has been increased to accentuate gray–white matter differentiation. On a PACS image, you can adjust the window level and contrast. In a normal brain, you should be able to discern several white and gray matter structures. Normal gray–white matter differentiation is subtle. Gray matter has lower lipid content than myelinated white matter and therefore appears brighter on computed tomography (CT). On CT, this leads counterintuitively to gray matter appearing whiter and white matter appearing grayer. Normal gray matter areas include the cerebral cortex, lentiform nucleus, caudate, and thalamus. White matter tracks, including the internal capsule, separate these structures. *(From Broder J, Preston R: An evidence-based approach to imaging of acute neurological conditions.* Emerg Med Pract 9(12):12, 2007.)

Figure 1-29. Early ischemic changes, noncontrast CT, brain windows. Early ischemic changes may be visible within 3 hours of onset of ischemic stroke. They include sulcal effacement, loss of gray–white matter differentiation, and the insular ribbon sign. Sulcal effacement occurs as local edema develops, swelling brain matter and displacing the cerebrospinal fluid that normally fills sulci as the adjacent gyri become edematous. Loss of gray–white matter differentiation occurs as ion pumps fail, leading to equilibration of diffusion gradients and shift of fluid. The normal ability of computed tomography (CT) to differentiate gray from white matter relies on differences in their density due to differences in their fluid and lipid content. White matter contains more fat, is less dense, and therefore appears darker on CT. Gray matter contains less lipid, is denser, and therefore appears whiter on CT. Local edema in the region of a developing infarct renders the region darker on CT because of the presence of increasing amounts of fluid. This masks the normal differentiation between white and gray matter. The insular ribbon sign is another manifestation of this loss of gray–white matter differentiation. The insula is a region of gray matter lining the lateral sulcus, in which ischemic strokes of the middle cerebral artery distribution may demonstrate early abnormalities. In this patient, both sulcal effacement and loss of gray–white matter differentiation have occurred. The frank hypodensity of ischemic stroke is also becoming visible. Compare these to similar regions on the patient's right side, where normal sulci and normal gray–white matter differentiation are seen. *(From Broder J, Preston R: An evidence-based approach to imaging of acute neurological conditions.* Emerg Med Pract 9(12):12, 2007.)

The many noncontrast CT findings of ischemic stroke may seem too much to hope to remember, and their clinical relevance may appear unclear. A few simple rules can make sense of this. First, a normal head CT is perhaps the most likely finding if the patient presents within 3 hours of symptom onset. In this setting, the most important job of the emergency physician in interpreting the head CT is to rule out hemorrhage. Second, in the presence of significant unilateral neurologic abnormalities, the hyperdense MCA sign should be sought. Third, early changes such as loss of gray–white

differentiation and hypodensity should be identified, again using the patient's clinical symptoms to direct you to the likely abnormal side of the brain. These early changes may imply either an earlier time of onset than suggested by the history or a massive stroke in progress.

Cerebral Edema

Diffuse cerebral edema is an abnormality of the brain, but it is manifest through compression of CSF spaces. It can logically be evaluated under *B* or *C* in our mnemonic. Cerebral edema can result from many pathologic processes, including trauma, anoxic brain injury, carbon monoxide poisoning, and systemic fluid and electrolyte abnormalities. The appearance is therefore not diagnostic of the underlying etiology. As the brain swells, several visible changes occur on noncontrast CT. CSF spaces become collapsed as they give way to the increasing volume of solid brain tissue. As a result, the lateral ventricles become slitlike and ultimately become obliterated. In addition, the sulci become effaced as the gyri swell. The normal rim of CSF surrounding the brain disappears. The cisterns surrounding the brainstem become compressed, and risk of herniation rises. Moreover, as the ICP rises, the cerebral perfusion pressure falls

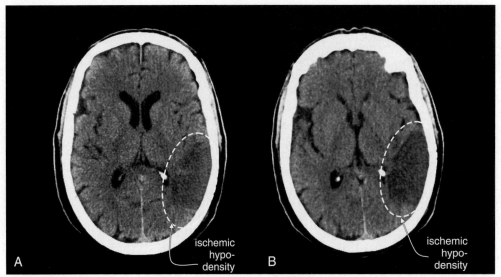

Figure 1-31. Progression of ischemic hypodensity over days, noncontrast CT, brain windows. A left middle cerebral artery distribution stroke, day 2 **(A)** and day 4 **(B)** after symptom onset. Early ischemic changes may be visible within 3 hours of symptom onset. The rate of progression of computed tomography findings may depend on the degree of ischemia or infarction and thus may vary between patients. Unlike vasogenic edema, this hypodense region follows a vascular territory and has a wedge-shaped appearance. Also note the local effacement of sulci in the region of the infarct due to local edema. *(From Broder J, Preston R: An evidence-based approach to imaging of acute neurological conditions.* Emerg Med Pract *9(12):8, 2007.)*

Box 1-7: Relationship Among Intracranial Pressure, Arterial Blood Pressure, and Cerebral Perfusion Pressure

As ICP rises, blood flow to the brain decreases unless a compensatory rise in blood pressure occurs:

(cerebral perfusion pressure) =
(mean arterial pressure) − ICP

Box 1-8: CT Findings of Cerebral Edema

- **Loss of CSF-containing spaces**
  - Sulci effacement
  - Ventricular effacement
  - Cistern effacement
- **Loss of gray–white differentiation**
- **Significance**
  - Increased ICP
  - Global brain ischemia from decreased cerebral perfusion pressure

---

(in the absence of a compensatory rise in mean arterial pressure) and global brain ischemia occurs (Box 1-7). Just as with focal ischemia (stroke), ion pumps fail and loss of gray–white matter differentiation occurs. Figure 1-35 later in this chapter shows changes of diffuse cerebral edema. Box 1-8 summarizes findings of cerebral edema.

Diffuse Axonal Injury
DAI is the widespread shearing of long axons that occurs as the result of deceleration injury. Common clinical scenarios include high-speed motor vehicle collisions and falls from great height. This injury is not typical of blows to the head or penetrating brain injury. The CT appearance is nonspecific: normal in the hyperacute phase, often followed by cerebral edema over hours to days. Punctate intraparenchymal hemorrhage may occur as well. Often, other traumatic brain injury will be evident, such as SDH or EDH.

The prognosis is poor, and resolution of CT findings may not equate with clinical improvement. MRI is thought to be more diagnostic.[54]

Normal Findings That May Simulate Disease
Several common incidental findings may simulate disease. These include calcifications in the choroid plexus of the posterior horns of the lateral ventricles (recall that the choroid plexus secretes CSF) (see Figure 1-21) and calcifications in the pineal gland.[55] These should not be confused with hemorrhage, because they have a greater density (brighter white appearance) and a stereo typical location. The significance of these findings is unknown, although choroid calcifications have been associated with hallucinations in schizophrenia.[56]

Why Can Two Patients With the Same CT Findings Have Markedly Different Neurologic Examinations?

Remember that CT offers a macroscopic snapshot in time of complex pathologic changes. It may be that a patient with severe neurologic impairment but a relative

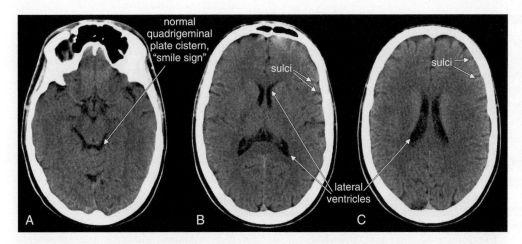

Figure 1-32. **Normal cerebro-spinal fluid spaces, noncontrast CT, brain windows.** Images are from the same patient, progressing from caudad to cephalad. **A,** In a normal brain, the basilar cistern is patent and filled with black CSF (sometimes referred to as the "smile sign"). **B, C,** The lateral ventricles are open but not enlarged. In all panels, sulci are visible but not excessive. *(From Broder J, Preston R: An evidence-based approach to imaging of acute neurological conditions. Emerg Med Pract 9(12):5, 2007.)*

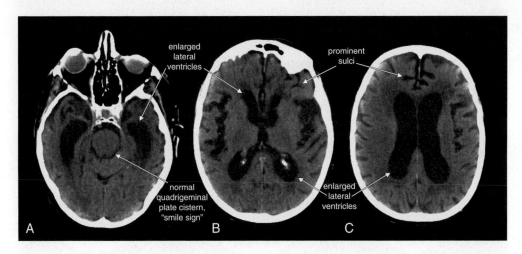

Figure 1-33. **Cerebral atrophy, noncontrast CT, brain windows.** Images are from the same patient, progressing from caudad to cephalad. In cerebral atrophy, all cerebrospinal fluid spaces become prominent. **A,** The quadrigeminal plate cistern is open. **A–C,** The lateral ventricles are enlarged and sulci are prominent, helping to distinguish this condition from hydrocephalus, where ventricles are large but sulci are effaced. *(From Broder J, Preston R: An evidence-based approach to imaging of acute neurological conditions. Emerg Med Pract 9(12):9, 2007.)*

benign–looking head CT will soon develop changes such as cerebral edema due to neuronal injury that has already occurred or is ongoing. In other cases, a patient with a large SDH may appear surprisingly neurologically intact, whereas another patient with similar head CT findings is severely impaired. One explanation is the degree of DAI that may accompany abnormalities such as SDH. The patient with minimal deficits may have no DAI, whereas the patient with severe deficits may have severe DAI, which is not as evident on CT. Another of many factors that may determine clinical status is the amount of cerebral atrophy present before the injury. Atrophy is loss of brain volume and compensatory increase in the size of CSF-containing spaces, such as ventricles, cisterns, and sulci. When an injury occurs and cerebral edema or a space-occupying lesion such as an SDH develops, the presence of atrophy (see Figure 1-33) may be protective by allowing room for expansion of the pathologic lesion without leading to herniation or precipitous rises in ICP.

C Is for CSF Spaces

The final letter in our mnemonic, *C,* reminds us to inspect CSF spaces. *This is critical, even in cases in which other pathology, such as intracranial hemorrhage, has already*

been found. The CSF spaces offer clues to ICP and may reveal a neurosurgical emergency. In addition, as discussed earlier, SAH may accumulate in CSF spaces, including sulci, cisterns, and ventricles. Normal CSF spaces (Figure 1-32) show symmetrical lateral ventricles that are neither enlarged nor effaced, patent sulci, and patent basilar cisterns. Deviations from this norm are best appreciated by understanding the normal pattern. In cerebral atrophy (Figure 1-33), all CSF spaces are enlarged. In obstructive hydrocephalus (Figure 1-34), the enlarging ventricles compress other CSF spaces, causing effacement of the sulci and basilar cisterns. In diffuse cerebral edema (discussed earlier under "*B* is for Brain") (Figure 1-35), the swelling brain parenchyma compresses and effaces all CSF spaces, including sulci, ventricles, and cisterns. Figure 1-36 compares various combinations of CSF spaces and their diagnostic correlates. Table 1-4 summarizes changes in CSF spaces and the accompanying change in ICP.

Because the volume of the calvarium is fixed in patients whose fontanelles and sutures have closed, as the size of one component of skull contents (brain, CSF, and blood) increases, the volume of other components must diminish. Once the compressible skull contents (CSF spaces

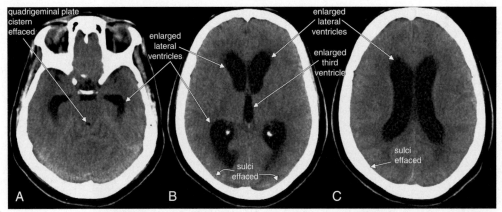

Figure 1-34. Hydrocephalus, noncontrast CT, brain windows. Images are from the same patient, progressing from caudad to cephalad. In hydrocephalus, the quadrigeminal plate cistern is effaced, resulting in loss of the normal smile sign. **A–C,** Because the total volume of intracranial contents is fixed in patients whose fontanelles and sutures have closed, as the ventricles enlarge, the sulci become effaced. **B,** The lateral ventricles and third ventricle are enlarged. *(From Broder J, Preston R: An evidence-based approach to imaging of acute neurological conditions. Emerg Med Pract 9(12):9, 2007.)*

Figure 1-35. Cerebral edema, noncontrast CT, brain windows. Images are from the same patient, progressing from caudad to cephalad. **A,** The quadrigeminal plate cistern becomes effaced, resulting in loss of the normal smile sign. **B, C,** The lateral ventricles become compressed and slitlike, or even completely effaced. Sulci become effaced. *(From Broder J, Preston R: An evidence-based approach to imaging of acute neurological conditions. Emerg Med Pract 9(12):9, 2007.)*

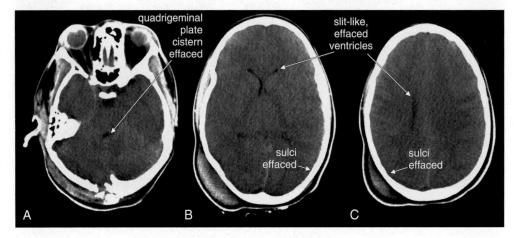

and circulating blood volume) have been reduced to their minimum volumes, ICP rises rapidly if other cranial contents continue to enlarge.

Sulci

Sulci, the CSF spaces between the undulating gyri of the brain surface, should appear black on brain windows. Normal sulci are visible but not prominent, and a thin ribbon of CSF should outline the entire brain. In cases of cerebral edema, the sulci may be completely effaced as the brain swells. In hydrocephalus, the volume of brain remains fixed but ventricles increase in size, leading to compression of the sulci. In cases of cerebral atrophy, loss of brain tissue volume leads to a compensatory increase in the size of sulci (Figures 1-32 through 1-36).

Ventricles and Hydrocephalus

Hydrocephalus is an important finding for emergency physicians because of its potential as a neurosurgical emergency. Untreated, hydrocephalus can result in tonsillar herniation, brainstem compression, and respiratory arrest.[57] In general, as hydrocephalus becomes severe, the lateral ventricles become significantly

enlarged. Because the volume of the calvarium is fixed, and solid brain tissue is essentially incompressible, as the ventricles expand, other CSF spaces become compressed—consequently, the sulci become effaced. In contrast, in the patient with atrophy, the ventricles may appear dilated but sulci appear similarly enlarged. In communicating hydrocephalus, the axial CT at the level of the lateral ventricles and third ventricle can resemble the face of a Halloween pumpkin. The enlarged anterior horns of the lateral ventricles are the rounded eyes, and the normally slitlike midline third ventricle dilates to a rounded nose. The posterior horns of the two lateral ventricles resemble corners of a grin, though they do not connect in the midline. Depending on the location of obstruction to CSF flow, the fourth ventricle just posterior to the quadrigeminal plate cistern may become dilated, producing an O-shaped mouth. The quadrigeminal plate cistern itself may be effaced if significant downward herniation is occurring. This appearance has also been described as a cartwheel, with 5 spokes (the 2 anterior and 2 posterior horns of the lateral ventricles, plus the fourth ventricle) radiating from an axle (the third ventricle). In noncommunicating hydrocephalus,

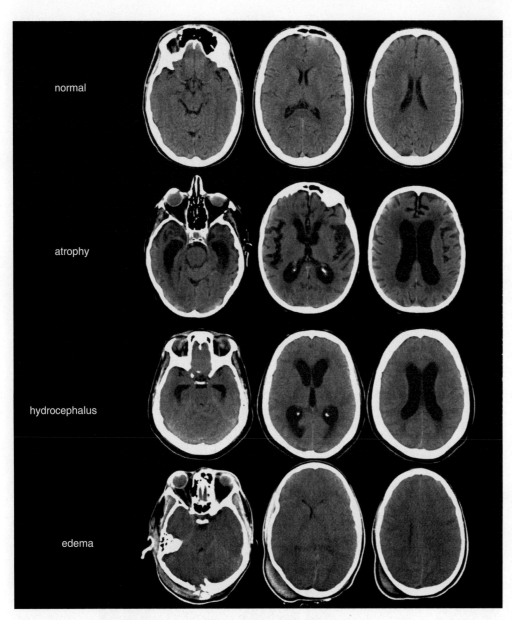

Figure 1-36. Comparison of cerebrospinal fluid (CSF) spaces.
- Overview of CSF spaces
  - Normal brain
    - All CSF spaces are present, neither effaced nor enlarged
  - Atrophy
    - All CSF spaces are enlarged
  - Hydrocephalus
    - Ventricles expand
    - Sulci and cisterns are compressed
  - Edema
    - All CSF spaces are compressed

(From Broder J, Preston R: An evidence-based approach to imaging of acute neurological conditions. Emerg Med Pract 9(12):9, 2007.)

the obstruction may lie proximal to the fourth ventricle, which will then not appear dilated. Comparison with a prior head CT is always valuable in assessing for hydrocephalus, because ventricular size alone is a relatively poor predictor of ICP.[58] Normal ventricular size does not completely exclude the possibility of increased intracranial pressure.

A variety of CT criteria for acute and chronic hydrocephalus have been described (Box 1-9). Figure 1-34 shows CT findings of hydrocephalus. Figure 1-37 shows a disconnected ventriculoperitoneal shunt, which can result in hydrocephalus.

Atrophy

In cerebral atrophy, loss of brain volume results in relatively symmetrical increase in size of sulci and ventricles. The basilar cisterns should also remain patent (see Figure 1-33).

Computed Tomography Findings of Elevated Intracranial Pressure

A variety of CT findings may indicate elevated ICP, though none are completely predictive. Findings that suggest increased ICP are decreased ventricle size, decreased basilar cistern size, effacement of sulci, degree of transfalcine herniation (midline shift), and loss of gray–white matter differentiation (Box 1-10).[59]

What CT Findings Are Contraindications to Lumbar Puncture?

Before performing lumbar puncture, confirm that findings of midline shift or elevated ICP are not present. The midline should be midline, the sulci should be evident, and the cisterns should be open. Ventricle size should not be excessive, particularly when compared to sulci. The evidence basis for assessment of ICP using CT is reviewed later in this chapter.

DETERMINATION OF NEED FOR IMAGING

We have discussed interpretation of head CT in detail, which prepares us for the harder task we face as emergency physicians: determining which patients actually require imaging. We begin this assessment with a review of the costs and radiation risks of imaging, because these are important factors in deferring imaging when possible.

Costs of Imaging

Costs of CT and MR tests are listed in Table 1-5. These Medicare reimbursement figures may dramatically underestimate the cost billed to the patient. An industry survey of imaging costs in New Jersey found a wide variation in consumer costs, ranging from $1000 to $4750 for brain MRI or magnetic resonance angiography (MRA).[60] The American Hospital Directory reports

TABLE 1-4. Assessment of Cerebrospinal Fluid Spaces and Intracranial Pressure

Condition	Sulci	Ventricles	Cisterns
Atrophy	Enlarged	Enlarged	Enlarged
Hydrocephalus	Effaced	Enlarged	Effaced
Cerebral edema	Effaced	Effaced	Effaced

the national average charge for head CT as $996 and for MRI as $2283.[61] Additional radiologist physician fees may apply. Some authors have concluded that, in the setting of traumatic brain injury, the extreme cost of a missed injury justifies the use of CT in all patients, rather than a more selective imaging policy based on clinical criteria.[62] However, with an annual cost of emergency head CT in the United States estimated to exceed $130 million, others have estimated the savings from selective use of CT to be high and the risk of missed injury to be low using validated clinical decision rules such as the Canadian CT Head Rule (CCHR), discussed later in this chapter.[63]

Radiation

Radiation dose from head CT is approximately 60 mGy.[64,65] Attributable mortality risk varies, depending on age of exposure. A single head CT in a neonate would be expected to contribute less than a 1 in 2000 lifetime risk of fatal cancer, whereas in adults the risk declines even further, to less than 1 in 10,000.[65] However, head CT may have other risks—one study of patients undergoing external beam radiation therapy for scalp hemangiomas, with a radiation exposure similar to that from CT, found an association with lower high school graduation rates.[66] This study, although large (more than 2000 subjects followed over time), was retrospective and therefore can demonstrate only association, not

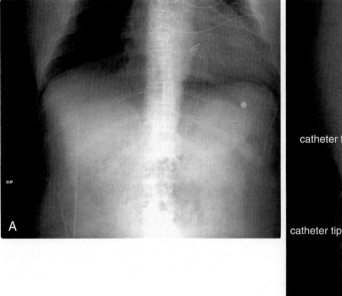
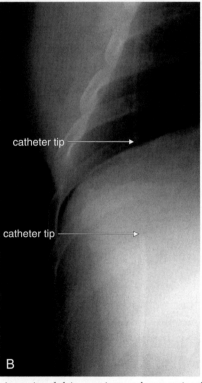

Figure 1-37. Ventriculoperitoneal shunt failure. A ventriculoperitoneal shunt series is a series of plain x-ray images documenting the course of a shunt from brain to peritoneum. Rarely, a shunt series may reveal an abnormality despite a normal brain CT. Much more frequently, the shunt series will be abnormal only if the head CT shows hydrocephalus. **A,** Chest x-ray from a shunt series. **B,** Close-up from the same image. In this patient, a discontinuity is faintly visible between the shunt catheter in the chest and that in the abdomen. The patient's head CT demonstrated hydrocephalus. *(From Broder J, Preston R: An evidence-based approach to imaging of acute neurological conditions.* Emerg Med Pract *9(12):17, 2007.)*

TABLE 1-5. Costs of Computed Tomography and Magnetic Resonance Tests*

Diagnostic Procedure	Cost ($)
CT head or brain without contrast	230.54
CTA head without contrast, followed by contrast, further sections, and postprocessing	382.19
MRA, head with contrast	386.64
MRA, neck with contrast	386.64
MRI, brain with contrast	386.64
MRA, neck without contrast material(s), followed by contrast material(s) and further sequences	522.54

*Based on 2007 Medicare reimbursement national averages.
From Reginald D, Williams AR II, Glaudemans J: Pricing Variations in the Consumer Market for Diagnostic Imaging Services. Avalere Health LLC, CareCore National, December 2005; American Hospital Directory. (Accessed at http://www.ahd.com/sample_outpatient.html.)

causation. In general, the radiation exposure from head CT likely poses a very low level of risk for deleterious biologic effects, but care should be taken to perform testing only when indicated, as radiation effects are cumulative and not fully understood.

Emergency Department Evaluation

Before imaging can be considered, basic principles of emergency medicine must be applied, including management of the patient's airway and hemodynamic stabilization as indicated. An unstable patient is not appropriate for imaging tests that will take the patient out of the ED for extended periods, such as MRI. The history and physical examination can guide imaging decisions. A thorough neurologic examination, including assessment of orientation, strength, sensation, deep tendon reflexes, cerebellar function, and language, may help localize the neurologic lesion to assist in choice of imaging modality. Motor and sensory deficits that are unilateral may be more suggestive of an anterior fossa brain abnormality, imaged by CT or MRI, whereas a bilateral motor and sensory level may suggest a spinal lesion. Symptoms of vertigo, ataxia, and dysmetria may suggest posterior fossa cerebellar abnormalities, best imaged by MRI. Acute onset of these symptoms could suggest posterior circulation stroke, for which imaging options would include MRI with MRA and CT angiography (CTA) of the head and neck, described in more detail later. Symptoms of cranial nerve dysfunction, including dysarthria, dysphagia, and abnormalities of extraocular muscles, suggest brainstem pathology better imaged with MRI than with CT. A motor deficit with ptosis and miosis may suggest carotid artery aneurysm or dissection, imaged by CTA, MRA, or carotid ultrasound. Table 1-1 correlates chief complaints, the differential diagnosis, and the suggested initial imaging test. A complete review of neuroanatomic localization is beyond the scope of this chapter.

Critical Appraisal of the Literature

A large number of studies have examined indications for imaging, as well as the test characteristics (including sensitivity, specificity, and positive and negative likelihood ratios) of the available imaging modalities. When possible, this chapter focuses on large, multicenter, prospective trials; unfortunately, for many of the clinical questions addressed, strong evidence is lacking. In the sections that follow, we discuss many studies, addressing methodologic strengths and weaknesses. Before we begin, we briefly review some common principles of evidence-based medicine.

Principles of Evidence-Based Medicine for Imaging Studies

Imaging studies for neurologic emergencies share a common problem in that the gold standard for diagnosis is often another imaging study, with no clear independent means of settling discrepancies. It is unclear what strategy should be used when two imaging studies yield divergent results. For example, if CT is compared to MR for evaluation of acute intracranial hemorrhage, which test should serve as the gold standard? Given a negative CT in the context of a positive MR, is the CT a false negative or the MR a false positive? Alternative gold standards may include clinical follow-up for mortality, readmission, neurosurgical intervention, or neurologic outcome. The most stringent reference standard might be autopsy findings, compared with imaging findings. When evaluating a study's relevance to clinical practice, the strength of the gold standard must be considered.

Another important concept when interpreting the results of a study is *point estimate* versus *95% confidence interval (CI)*. Take the example of a study with a point estimate sensitivity of 99% and a CI of 66% to 100%. The 95% CI indicates that the true sensitivity of the test in an infinitely large sample has a 95% chance of lying between the extreme values of 66% and 100%. Although the likelihood of the test having either of these extreme values is low, it cannot be ruled out on the basis of the data. Small studies often have broad 95% CIs for their results, whereas large studies usually have narrower CIs. For a test to be reliable for ruling out a disease process, it must have both a high sensitivity and a narrow CI. To rule in pathology, the specificity must be high and the CI narrow. The lower boundary of the CI can be considered a "worst-case scenario" for the test characteristic.

Another means of reporting a test's ability to "rule in" or "rule out" pathology is the likelihood ratio (Box 1-11). The likelihood ratio positive (LR$^+$) is the factor by which the odds of disease increases when the test result is positive. The likelihood ratio negative (LR$^-$) is the factor by which the odds of disease decreases when the test result is negative. The pretest odds multiplied by the likelihood ratio (positive or negative) yields the posttest odds.

Positive and negative predictive values are not emphasized in this chapter in that they are heavily influenced by disease prevalence and thus must be used cautiously in clinical practice.

Which ED Patients With Acute Headache Require Emergency Imaging?

The American College of Emergency Physicians (ACEP) published an update to its clinical policy on evaluation of acute headache in 2008.[67] Based on the available evidence, no level A recommendations could be made for indications for imaging. Level B and C recommendations are listed in Box 1-12. Overall, the sensitivity and specificity of history and physical are limited in identifying patients who require emergency imaging.

Imaging for Suspected Stroke

Stroke is the leading cause of disability in the United States[68] and may be ischemic (85%) or hemorrhagic (15%) in nature. When presented with signs and symptoms suggestive of stroke, the emergency physician must take steps to differentiate ischemic stroke from intraparenchymal hemorrhage while entertaining the possibility of *stroke mimics* (e.g., hypoglycemia or Todd's paralysis). A number of neuroimaging modalities may aid in this task. Some techniques may yield additional information, including the vascular territory affected, the extent of injury, clues to the underlying precipitant cause or causes, and identification of tissue that, though ischemic, might still be viable. This information is critical when contemplating the use of thrombolytic or neuroprotective therapies. Unfortunately, many imaging modalities are not currently available at all institutions during all

---

Box 1-12: Guidelines for Imaging in Adult Patients Presenting With Acute Headache

- ● **Level A recommendations: None**
- ● **Level B recommendations**
  1. Patients presenting to the ED with headache and new abnormal findings in a neurologic examination (e.g., focal deficit, altered mental status, and altered cognitive function) should undergo emergent* noncontrast head CT.
  2. Patients presenting with new sudden-onset severe headache should undergo emergent* head CT.
  3. Human immunodeficiency virus–positive patients with a new type of headache should be considered for an emergent* imaging study.
- ● **Level C recommendations**
  - ○ Patients who are older than 50 years and presenting with a new type of headache but with a normal neurologic examination should be considered for an urgent† imaging study.

From ACEP; Edlow JA, Panagos PD, Godwin SA et al. Clinical policy: Critical issues in the evaluation and management of adult patients presenting to the emergency department with acute headache. *Ann Emerg Med* 52:407-436, 2008.
*Emergent is defined as CT before ED disposition.
†Urgent is defined as scheduled as part of ED disposition or performed in ED if follow-up cannot be assured.

Box 1-11: Likelihood Ratio

$$LR^+ = sensitivity / (1 - specificity)$$
$$LR^- = (1 - sensitivity) / specificity$$
$$odds_{post} = odds_{pre} \times LR$$

hours of the day. Furthermore, many theoretically useful options remain untested or inconclusive with regard to their utility in guiding intervention and disposition.

Computed Tomography for Stroke

CT is the most widely available, immediate imaging technique for patients presenting to the ED with signs and symptoms of stroke. Noncontrast head CT is rapid, taking less than 5 seconds for image acquisition using some 64-slice scanners.[22] It is sensitive for detecting intracranial hemorrhage,[26] and immediate imaging is more cost effective than either delayed or selective imaging strategies.[69] Limitations do exist, however. Surrounding bone can obscure evidence of ischemic stroke, an artifact effect known as beam hardening. This problem can be minimized by requesting fine thickness cuts (~1 mm), but the risk of false negatives for stroke detection still exists—particularly when a vertebral–basilar distribution is present, because beam hardening is worsened by thick bone surrounding the posterior fossa.[70]

Noncontrast CT findings of ischemic stroke were reviewed earlier in the section on head CT interpretation. The prognostic importance of these findings and implications for t-PA therapy are also discussed there. Although the sensitivity of noncontrast head CT for ischemic stroke increases beyond 24 hours, the sensitivity for ischemia-induced changes in the first six hours is relatively low at 66%. Thus, a normal CT is consistent with the diagnosis of acute ischemic stroke in a patient presenting with suggestive signs and symptoms.[47]

For the emergency physician, several points about early ischemic changes should be emphasized. First, in contrast to the assertion in some emergency medicine texts that ischemic stroke becomes visible on noncontrast head CT only after 6 hours,[42] the NINDS trial upon which t-PA therapy is largely based demonstrated that 31% of patients had early findings of ischemia within 3 hours of symptom onset (see Table 1-3).[41] Although early ischemic changes were not an exclusion criterion for t-PA in the original NINDS trial,[46] subsequent research has shown a heightened risk of hemorrhagic conversion of ischemic stroke, poor neurologic outcomes, and death in patients with these changes.[47,48] As a consequence, and as mentioned earlier, the Food and Drug Administration, American Heart Association, and American Academy of Neurology recommend against use of t-PA in the patients with major early ischemic changes.[73] Specifically, early ischemic changes occupying an area one third the size of the MCA territory or one third of a cerebral hemisphere, cerebral edema, and midline shift are considered relative contraindications to t-PA because of the increased risk for hemorrhage.[74] When discussing the head CT findings with a radiologist before administration of t-PA, it is important to ask specifically about the presence and extent of these changes, in addition to asking about hemorrhage.

Standard contrast-enhanced head CT is rarely used for evaluation of stroke since it provides little additional information compared with noncontrast head CT. With the advent of multidetector CT scanners and spiral CT technology, however, CT angiography (CTA) can be performed to obtain images of the extracranial and intracranial vasculature from the aortic arch to the cranial vertex (Figs. 1-38 through 1-42). Images are acquired by administering a rapid bolus of IV contrast

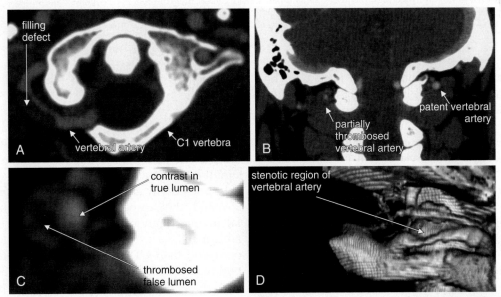

Figure 1-38. Computed tomography angiography (CTA). CTA can identify dissections of cervical arteries. **A,** Axial image. **B,** Coronal image. **C,** Enlarged region from **B. D,** Three-dimensional reconstruction. In this case, the false lumen has thrombosed, so a filling defect is seen where thrombus prevents contrast from entering the false lumen. If the false lumen had not thrombosed, an intimal flap would be seen separating the true and false lumens. Although the three-dimensional reconstruction **(D)** provides useful anatomic context here, it does not reveal the etiology of the stenosis. Instead, the thrombosed dissection itself is evident from the cross-sectional images **(A–C).**

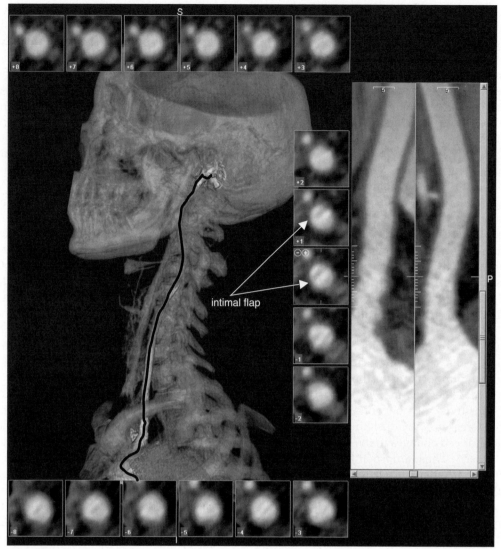

Figure 1-39.   Computed tomography angiography (CTA).   In this patient with carotid artery dissection, CTA allows three-dimensional reconstruction of the vessel, with cross sections displayed at intervals around the periphery. An intimal flap is faintly visible on several of these cross sections *(arrows). (From Broder J, Preston R: An evidence-based approach to imaging of acute neurological conditions.* Emerg Med Pract *9(12):13, 2007.)*

immediately after standard noncontrast head CT. The raw images can be acquired in as little as 60 seconds, and three-dimensional computer reconstructions can be performed in less than 15 minutes. The results might profoundly alter the course of management, because large artery occlusions correlate with National Institutes of Health Stroke Scale scores[75] and may indicate a need for endovascular intervention (Discussed in Chapter 16). Generally, agreement between CTA and catheter angiography—still the gold standard for diagnosis of vessel stenosis—approaches 95%. For severe carotid artery stenosis, sensitivity for CTA approaches 100%, whereas the sensitivity for diminished flow in the circle of Willis is 89%.[76] Although traditional angiography may have subtle, additional benefits related to characterization of the plaque lesion, the noninvasive and rapid nature of CTA renders it an attractive option to the emergency physician, assuming that the risks

of exposure to contrast and additional radiation are acceptable to the patient.

CTA uses enhancement of the cerebral vasculature as a surrogate for estimating perfusion of the parenchyma. Targeted CT perfusion studies (CTPSs) can be performed simultaneously using the same bolus of contrast[77] and have a sensitivity and specificity for detecting ischemia of 95% and 100%, respectively.[78] By measuring the rise and fall in concentration of injected contrast over time, CTPSs are capable of even more direct estimates of cerebral perfusion than CTA, including measurements of cerebral blood volume and cerebral blood flow (see Figure 1-41). Quantifying these variables may allow clinicians to identify areas of the brain that, although ischemic, are potentially still viable—the so-called ischemic penumbra. This has implications for the clinician attempting to weigh the benefits of administering IV or intraarterial

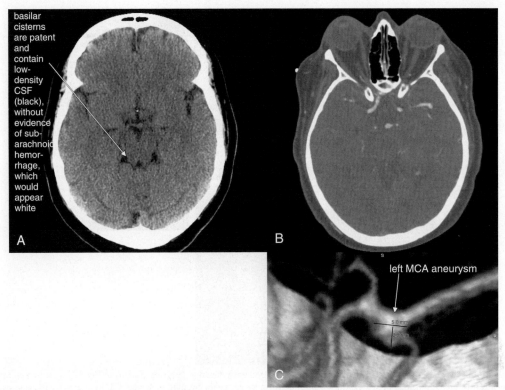

basilar cisterns are patent and contain low-density CSF (black), without evidence of sub-arachnoid hemor-rhage, which would appear white

A

B

left MCA aneurysm

C

Figure 1-40. **Computed tomography angiography (CTA) of intracranial vessels. A,** Noncontrast head CT. **B,** CT angiogram, axial image. **C,** Three-dimensional reconstruction rendered from axial CT dataset. CTA can identify berry aneurysms and arterial–venous malformations. This 53-year-old female awoke at 4 AM with a severe headache. Noncontrast head CT was normal, but lumbar puncture showed xanthochromia and more than 20,000 red blood cells per cubic millimeter. CTA confirmed an aneurysm of the left middle cerebral artery (MCA) trifurcation, with one of the MCA branches arising from the aneurysm. The patient underwent clipping of the aneurysm rather than angiographic coiling because of this configuration.

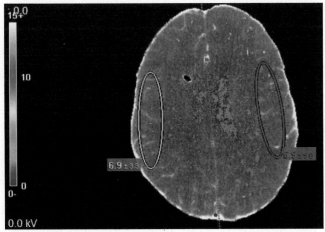

Figure 1-41. **Computed tomography (CT) perfusion scan.** A CT perfusion scan provides a map of blood flow in ischemic stroke, potentially identifying ischemic areas that could be salvaged by reperfusion. Here, blood flow in similar regions of the two cerebral hemispheres is compared. This is an imaging technique that continues to be developed in the research setting but is not a routine part of most clinical practice. Erroneously programmed CT perfusion scans have been the cause of iatrogenic radiation injury to patients undergoing stroke evaluations. *(From Broder J, Preston R: An evidence-based approach to imaging of acute neurological conditions. Emerg Med Pract 9(12):13, 2007.)*

thrombolytic drugs against the risk of intracranial hemorrhage. Routine use of CTPSs could potentially allow a more precise prediction of outcome[79] and could even herald a paradigm shift in one of the indications for thrombolytic administration: rather than excluding the use of thrombolytics in patients presenting after an arbitrary time interval (e.g., 3 hours), thrombolytic therapy could be initiated or excluded based on actual visualization or absence of a penumbral area likely to benefit from such intervention.

However, routine use of CTPSs in the hospital setting (much less in the ED) is not without challenges. First, the usual difficulties of imaging the posterior fossa with CT techniques persist.[70,80] Second, only limited volumes of brain can be imaged at one time with each bolus of contrast, so ischemia located outside the scanning level of interest can be missed,[81] although this is partially alleviated by the use of multislice scanners or repeated contrast boluses. Third, despite the theoretical appeal, only small studies in limited populations exist that confirm the ability of CTPSs to detect infarct,[82] to predict infarct location[83] and size,[84] and to predict final outcomes.[82,84] We await large study confirmation of these findings before routinely recommending their use in the ED setting. Because CT perfusion studies require that the same regions of the brain be repeatedly scanned over a period of a few minutes to acquire data about perfusion over time, focal areas of the brain receive higher levels of radiation exposure. Widely publicized accounts exist of patients receiving dangerous radiation exposures when CT scanners were misprogrammed, prompting lawsuits and an investigation by the US Food and Drug Administration.[84a]

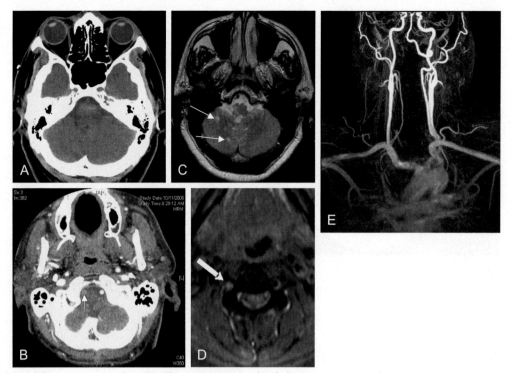

Figure 1-42. Multimodality assessment of stroke. This patient presented with dizziness, nausea, and vomiting. Noncontrast computed tomography of the brain **(A)** was interpreted as normal, but symptoms were concerning for posterior circulation stroke. CT angiography **(B)** suggested right vertebral artery dissection *(arrow)*. Magnetic resonance imaging **(C)** revealed posterior inferior cerebellar artery–territory ischemic stroke *(arrows)* and magnetic resonance angiography (MRA) **(D)** confirmed vertebral dissection *(arrow)*. **E,** A three-dimensional view from the MRA. *(From Broder J, Preston R: An evidence-based approach to imaging of acute neurological conditions.* Emerg Med Pract *9(12):15, 2007.)*

Magnetic Resonance Imaging for Acute Stroke
Standard MRI for stroke includes scout images, T1- and T2-weighted images and MRA. Increasingly available new-generation scanners incorporate additional high-sensitivity methods such as diffusion-weighted imaging (DWI), gradient echo pulse sequencing (GEPS), and perfusion-weighted imaging (PWI).

Obtaining DWI has been possible since 1985.[85] In brief, the technique involves detecting and processing a signal in response to the movement of water molecules caused by two pulses of radiofrequency. Ischemic changes can be detected in as little as 3 to 30 minutes after insult, and in a small study of 22 patients who presented within 6 hours of symptom onset, DWI was found to be 100% sensitive and specific.[86] In a subsequent study, DWI was found to have a far superior sensitivity compared to CT (91% vs. 61%).[87] When MRA is done simultaneous with DWI as part of a fast protocol to detect vascular stenosis, their combined use within 24 hours of hospitalization substantially improved the early diagnostic accuracy of ischemic stroke subtypes.[88] DWI may also be useful when the clinician encounters a patient with remote-onset neurologic defects. In patients presenting with a median delay of 17 days after symptom onset, clinicians gained additional clinical information one third of the time (including clarification of the vascular territory affected) by performing DWI in addition to conventional T2-weighted images. Of this third, the information was designated as "highly likely" to affect management strategy in 38%.[89]

MRI is superior to CT at both detecting acute ischemic change[85,87] and visualizing the posterior fossa.[70,80] However, MRI has failed to supplant CT as the imaging modality of choice for stroke in the ED due to cost, availability of the requisite personnel, time, and a long-standing belief that MRI is not reliable for detecting intracerebral hemorrhage. At least the last two factors are being surmounted. New scanners are faster, with acquisition times in the range of 3 to 5 minutes, compared to 15 to 20 minutes previously.[90] With respect to hemorrhage, DWI has proved sufficient to exclude intracerebral hemorrhage,[91] and in studies comparing GEPS with CT, GEPS was at least as useful for detecting acute intracranial hemorrhage and actually better at elucidating chronic hemorrhagic changes,[92-94] with sensitivity approaching 100% when interpreted by trained personnel.[92] The issues of cost and personnel are more complex, however. MRI hardware costs and costs associated with imaging are roughly double those of CT.[95] Whether these costs will fall in the future or can be justified in the form of better outcomes, shorter hospital stays, or other measurable end points is unknown. Personnel issues are related not only to sheer manpower but also to qualitative training demands. MRI requires specially trained technicians spending more time per study compared to CT, and expert-level radiologists with extensive training in MRI interpretation must be employed, because interpretation is still not reproducible (though advocates of DWI point out that there is virtually *no* intra-observer or interobserver variability with this modality).[87]

Similar to the ability of CTPSs to identify the ischemic penumbra, the combination of DWI and PWI makes it possible to make inferences about ischemia before permanent injury (infarction) has occurred. DWI provides a map of brain tissue that is ischemic and at high risk for infarction. PWI provides a map of brain tissue that is threatened by decreased blood flow but not yet demonstrating cellular injury marked by changes in diffusion. Typically, the hypoperfused region (PWI defect) is larger than the area of diffusion abnormality (DWI defect) early in stroke. The DWI–PWI mismatch is thought to represent the ischemic penumbra, a region that is potentially salvageable with aggressive reperfusion (either by thrombolytic therapy or by catheter-based mechanical interventions).[96]

PWI is performed with standard MRI and MRA using gadolinium and requires a total imaging time of less than 15 minutes. PWI can be performed in cases of contraindication to gadolinium (a rare event, as gadolinium has been found safe in most instances, though recent fatal nephrogenic systemic fibrosis has been noted in patients with advanced renal disease; see Chapter 15[97]), by magnetically labeling the blood as the blood enters the brain, a technique known as continuous arterial spin labeling.[98] Patients with large perfusion defects[96,99] detected by PWI or occluded arteries detected by MRA[100] are at heightened risk for enlarging regions of frank infarction, leading some to suggest that these findings should prompt early revascularization, either with thrombolytic agents pharmacologically or with mechanical devices. The volume of abnormalities on DWI and PWI during acute stroke correlates with acute National Institutes of Health Stroke Scales and with chronic neurologic scores, and lesion size may predict early neurologic deterioration.[101–102] Still another benefit of advanced techniques like DWI and PWI is, as is the case for CTPSs, the potential to identify areas of ischemia that have not yet progressed to infarction, potentially permitting extension of the traditional 3-hour window for thrombolytic administration.[103,104] However, PWI and DWI have yet to prove practical and reliable in defining the ischemic penumbra and infarct core,[105] and head-to-head trials comparing MRI diffusion–perfusion studies to CTPSs are limited.

Figure 1-42 shows images from a single patient in various modalities, including CT, CTA, MRI, and MRA.

Ultrasonography for Ischemic Stroke

Ultrasound techniques include Doppler (used to assess flow rate and presence of stenosis), brightness mode (permitting anatomic and structural details of the tissue to be illuminated), and duplex (a combination of the two). Carotid duplex ultrasound has traditionally been deployed electively (i.e., nonemergently) to investigate whether the origin of an acute ischemic event in a given patient could be due to carotid artery stenosis. Studies show conflicting results, with some showing poorer performance of ultrasound (65% sensitivity, 95% specificity) compared with MRA (82%-100% sensitivity, 95%-100% specificity) and the gold standard (by definition 100% sensitive and specific) of digital subtraction angiography.[106,107] Transcranial ultrasound can be used to visualize the vessels in and near the circle of Willis. Here, it is possible to identify stenosis with reasonable success, though less well for the vertebral–basilar system. In the internal carotid artery distribution, the sensitivity and specificity for stenosis are 85% and 95%, respectively. Sensitivity and specificity are only 75% and 85%, respectively, in the vertebral–basilar system. Additional benefits of transcranial ultrasound reportedly include the ability to identify collateral pathways, visualize in real time harmful emboli and in the postthrombolysis state, judge the success of therapy.[108–110] In addition, ultrasound is being used therapeutically in trials to augment the thrombolytic effect of medications.[111]

Studies have focused on the use of ultrasound to select patients for thrombolytic drug therapy or endovascular treatment. Ultrasound is inexpensive relative to other imaging modalities, noninvasive, and does not expose the patient to ionizing radiation, but the validity of the results is highly operator-dependent. In addition, it is impossible to differentiate reliably between complete and high-grade stenosis, and contralateral stenosis can result in falsely reassuring flow velocities ipsilaterally, resulting in a false-negative interpretation for stenosis.[112–115]

Conventional Catheter Angiography for Stroke

Still considered the gold standard for diagnosing arterial stenosis, conventional catheter angiography has been substantially improved with the advent of digital subtraction techniques permitting visualization of even small, cortical branches of intracranial arteries. Endovascular techniques permit administration of intraarterial thrombolysis, and some users have the ability to perform clot retrieval and angioplasty with or without stenting.[116] However, despite its utility when noninvasive diagnostic techniques are equivocal or conflicting, angiography is still used only sparingly in the acute stroke setting because of its invasive nature and the approximate 1% risk of iatrogenic stroke associated with the procedure.[117]

Stroke Neuroimaging Summary

The goals of neuroimaging in the ED patient presenting with signs and symptoms consistent with stroke include the exclusion of intraparenchymal hemorrhage, space-occupying lesions, and other stroke "mimics." Ideally, the imaging technique would also highlight areas of ischemia, identify underlying causes of ischemia (i.e., vessel occlusion), and delineate those areas that are ischemic but salvageable. Currently, no single imaging modality can accomplish all of these goals quickly and at low cost, and no combination of studies is widely available in all centers.

When stroke is the suspected diagnosis, the patient must be imaged as quickly as possible with the most readily available neuroimaging modality to rule out hemorrhage and other stroke mimics. Typically, this is with noncontrast CT. In the absence of contraindication to the use of contrast, simultaneous CTA can evaluate for large vessel occlusion. Provided that it does not delay other indicated therapy, CTPS may be useful for prognosis and to guide therapeutic decisions, including the use of thrombolytic drug therapy. In specialized centers with the required expertise and resources, MR stroke protocols including MRI, MRA, DWI, and PWI may be feasible from the ED without the need for prior CT imaging.

Clinical Questions in Stroke Imaging

What Is the Risk of Progression to Stroke in Acute TIA? What Imaging Studies Are Indicated?

Large studies in multiple settings have demonstrated that patients diagnosed with TIA in the ED progress to stroke at a high rate of 10% in 3 months, with half of those strokes occurring within 48 hours.[118,120] In addition, some evidence suggests that patients with TIA may be at higher risk for subsequent adverse clinical outcomes than patients with minor ischemic strokes—possibly because of a higher rate of large vessel atherosclerosis as the cause of TIA. In TIA, large artery atherosclerosis (including carotid artery disease) may account for up to 34% of cases. The 3-month risk for stroke, myocardial infarction, and vascular death is higher for TIA patients than for minor stroke patients (15% vs. 3%; hazard ratio = 4.6; 95% CI = 2.3-9.3 in multivariate analysis).[121] The result has been a significant impetus to admit patients with TIA or to perform urgent diagnostic testing in the outpatient setting. A variety of neuroimaging strategies have been proposed to identify patients at high risk.

Is Noncontrast CT Valuable in Apparent TIA?

In patients presenting with apparent TIA, head CT might be expected to be normal, and the value of CT in the context of resolved neurologic symptoms could be questioned. Yet 4% of patients clinically diagnosed with TIA in the ED have evidence of new infarct on noncontrast head CT. Moreover, those patients have a fourfold increased 90-day risk of subsequent stroke.[118] Thus, head CT may be warranted in TIA as a risk stratification tool. If MRI with or without MRA will be performed in

the ED, CT is not necessary as MR can evaluate for hemorrhage, infarct, and other brain pathology.

Is MRI Useful in Apparent TIA?

MRI may be a useful alternative imaging modality when available for patients with apparent TIA. The age of ischemic lesions can be judged with DWI based on measurement of the apparent diffusion coefficient, which varies with time from onset of ischemia. Ischemic lesions of varying ages on DWI MRI predict a substantially higher risk of new lesions on 30-day follow-up MRI (relative risk = 3.6; 95% CI = 1.9-6.8), so MRI may be useful for risk stratification.[122] Ischemic lesions of varying ages suggest an embolic source of TIA and future stroke. A negative diffusion weighted MRI within 24 hours of apparent TIA predicts a low risk of disabling ischemic stroke within 90 days in patients with moderate or high risk ABCD(2) scores (described later).[122a]

What Percentage of Patients with TIA or Stroke Have a Cardioembolic Source? Is Echocardiogram Indicated?

Studies show that 51% to 61% of patients with TIA or stroke in whom a clear cause had not yet been identified after initial workup had a cardiac abnormality potentially warranting anticoagulation identified on echocardiography. Transesophageal echocardiography was superior to transthoracic echocardiography, identifying an abnormality in 40% of those with a normal transthoracic echocardiography. An absolute indication for anticoagulation was identified by echocardiography in 20% of patients, and 80% of those were identified only on transesophageal echocardiography.[123,124] Another study demonstrated that coexisting cardiac and carotid artery lesions are quite common in TIA and stroke patients, occurring in 11%, so imaging of both the heart and the cervical vessels is likely indicated.[125]

Does a Clinical Prediction Rule Exist to Identify High-Risk TIA Patients Who Require Further Imaging?

The ABCD score has been described to identify patients at low risk of progression to TIA. The rule incorporates age, blood pressure, unilateral weakness, speech disturbance, and duration to generate a score, which has been correlated with 7-day risk for stroke. A dichotomized version of the ABCD score, with patients scoring five or more points being at high risk, has been validated for the ED. Unfortunately, the small numbers in these studies result in wide CIs for the sensitivity of the score, with lower 95% CIs as low as 60%. Some studies have shown the ABCD score to have only limited value, as patients with relatively low risk scores (predicted to correlate with low risk for stroke) had adverse outcomes

Box 1-13: ABCD(2) Score for Predicting Progression from Transient Ischemic Attacks to Stroke[*]

- Age ≥60 years (1 point)
- Systolic blood pressure ≥140 mm Hg and/or diastolic blood pressure ≥90 mm Hg (1 point)
- Unilateral weakness (2 points)
- Speech disturbance without weakness (1 point)
- Duration of symptoms
  - ○ ≥60 minutes (2 points)
  - ○ 10–59 minutes (1 point)
  - ○ <10 minutes (0 points)
- Diabetes (1 point)

From Asimos AW, Johnson AM, Rosamond WD, et al. A multicenter evaluation of the ABCD2 score's accuracy for predicting early ischemic stroke in admitted patients with transient ischemic attack. *Ann Emerg Med* 55:201-210 e5, 2010; Bray JE, Coughlan K, Bladin C. Can the ABCD score be dichotomised to identify high-risk patients with transient ischaemic attack in the emergency department? *Emerg Med J* 24:92-95, 2007; Cucchiara BL, Messe SR, Taylor RA, et al. Is the ABCD score useful for risk stratification of patients with acute transient ischemic attack? *Stroke* 37:1710-1714, 2006; Johnston SC, Rothwell PM, Nguyen-Huynh MN, et al. Validation and refinement of scores to predict very early stroke risk after transient ischaemic attack. *Lancet* 369:283-292, 2007; Rothwell PM, Giles MF, Flossmann E, et al. A simple score (ABCD) to identify individuals at high early risk of stroke after transient ischaemic attack. *Lancet* 366:29-36, 2005; Tsivgoulis G, Spengos K, Manta P, et al. Validation of the ABCD score in identifying individuals at high early risk of stroke after a transient ischemic attack: A hospital-based case series study. *Stroke* 37:2892-2897, 2006.
[*]In validation studies, ABCD(2) poorly predicts short-term stroke risk.

in external validation.[126–129] A recent extended version of the ABCD score including diabetes as a risk factor, known as ABCD(2), attempts to predict 2-day risk for stroke but requires further validation (Box 1-13).[130] A multicenter study demonstrated a low 7-day risk for progression from TIA to disabling stroke in patients with an ABCD(2) score of no more than three. However, risk for more minor stroke was poorly predicted, limiting applicability in the ED.[131] Another prospective study suggested a 5-fold higher 90-day risk of stroke in patients with an ABCD(2) score >2.[131a]

What Is the Yield of CTA, Ultrasound, or MRA in TIA?

As stated earlier in the discussion of stroke, CTA has been shown to be 100% sensitive for high-grade carotid stenosis. MRA and carotid ultrasonography are alternative studies with similar sensitivity.[132]

Suspected Subarachnoid Hemorrhage

Traditional practice in the evaluation for suspected SAH has been lumbar puncture (LP) following negative CT, a practice still advocated by major textbooks of emergency medicine.[133] The reported sensitivity of CT (third generation or higher) for SAH is in the range of 90% in the first 24 hours, declining afterward.[134] A recent study of fifth-generation CT found no SAH in patients undergoing LP after negative CT.[27] However, this retrospective review examined only 177 ED patients undergoing both CT and LP. Records and follow-up were not reviewed for patients who underwent CT but not LP, so it is possible that cases of SAH with negative head CT occurred but were not detected. In addition, the interval between headache onset and CT or LP was not recorded, so this study provides no information on any time dependency of CT sensitivity for SAH. Given an incidence of SAH of only around 3.4% compared with previously reported numbers in the range of 12% of ED acute, severe, nontraumatic headache patients, the true sensitivity of fifth-generation CT may be as low as 61%.[26,27,135] A prospective study of patients presenting with the worst headache of their life reported a sensitivity of 97.5%, but again the small number of patients, 107, yielded a lower CI—as low as 91%.[26] Another retrospective study found the sensitivity of noncontrast head CT for SAH to be 93% (95% CI = 88%-97%).[136] Sensitivity of CT is thought to decline over time due to clearance of blood and is reported to be as low as 50% at 7 days.[137] How good is the combination of CT with LP for ruling out the diagnosis of SAH? A prospective cohort study of 599 patients undergoing both LP and head CT for nontraumatic acute headache found the combination of head CT and LP to be 98% sensitive (95% CI = 91%-100%) for the diagnosis of SAH or aneurysm. The authors calculated a negative likelihood ratio of 0.024, indicating an extremely low posttest probability of SAH when both CT and LP are negative.[138] Emergency medicine physicians are only moderately accurate at predicting SAH based on clinical history,[139] so a conservative approach including LP after negative head CT is probably still warranted based on CT sensitivity. Even the authors of studies of CT sensitivity are reluctant to state that LP is not needed after negative CT.[140] Future advances in CT may eliminate this need, although some have argued on theoretical grounds that CT sensitivity will never reach 100% for SAH.[141]

CT Angiography for Aneurysmal Subarachnoid Hemorrhage

When noncontrast head CT is negative in a patient suspected of SAH, is additional imaging warranted to assess for aneurysmal disease? Is there a role for CTA (see Figure 1-40)? The precise role is as yet undefined. A small study found aneurysms in 5.1% (6/116) of patients with a negative CT and positive LP and in 2.5% (3/116) following a normal CT and LP. Given the incidence of berry aneurysms in the general population, believed to be approximately 1% to 5%,[142,144] it is possible that the aneurysms detected in these patients were incidental, not the acute cause of the patients' symptoms. Wide use of CTA might result in detection of large numbers of asymptomatic aneurysms, resulting in unneeded procedures, including formal angiography and endovascular coiling of aneurysms, with associated morbidity and mortality. Perhaps the best role of CTA would be in patients in whom LP is not feasible—for example, those with coagulopathy. CTA might also be useful in patients with a particularly high pretest probability of disease but negative noncontrast CT and LP.[145] Finally, CTA could be used to evaluate for aneurysm in patients with negative noncontrast CT and equivocal LP results, such as a declining but nonzero number of red blood cells.

How Is Cerebral Dural Sinus Thrombosis best Imaged?

Dural sinus thrombosis is a rare but important cause of headache. An observational study of 1676 consecutive Pakistani patients undergoing a CT or MRI study found dural sinus thrombosis in 3.3%, although the incidence in U.S. ED patients may be quite different.[146] Risk factors include hypercoagulable states. Untreated, the condition leads to rising ICP due to failure of drainage of blood from dural sinuses into the internal jugular venous system. This in turn can lead to intracranial hemorrhage. Both CT venography and MR venography can be used to detect this condition. Only small studies dating from the 1990s have directly compared the two techniques, and without a strong gold standard, it is impossible to state the sensitivity of the techniques accurately.[147,148] The technique for CT venography is the same as for CTA with one exception: in CTV, CT image acquisition is timed to coincide with the arrival of contrast in venous structures.[149,152]

Imaging of Vascular Dissections

Vascular dissections of the carotid and vertebral arteries are a relatively rare cause of acute headache and neurologic symptoms, occurring in an estimated 2.5 to 3 per 100,000 and 1 to 1.5 100,000 annually in the United States.[153,154] They account for only about 2% of all ischemic strokes but as much as 20% of strokes in young adults.[155] Noncontrast head CT is expected to be negative in the setting of these lesions unless ischemic stroke has resulted. In addition, dissection of the vertebral arteries would be expected to result in ischemia in the region of the basilar artery (which forms from the confluence of the vertebral arteries), and the territories supplied by the basilar artery lie within the posterior fossa, an area poorly seen on noncontrast CT. Multiple imaging techniques are available for this diagnosis. CTA, MRA, and conventional angiography all have excellent sensitivity

and specificity, greater than 95%.[156] Imaging of the head and neck should be ordered when these diagnoses are suspected to ensure that the lesion is within the imaged field (see Figures 1-38 and 1-39).

Imaging in Acute Hydrocephalus and Shunt Failure

Noncontrast head CT is the initial study of choice for diagnosis of acute obstructive hydrocephalus. As the ventricles enlarge, due to obstruction of the normal outflow of CSF, other CSF spaces become progressively effaced, because the total volume of all skull contents is fixed (Figures 1-34, 1-36, and 1-37). Large ventricles with small or completely effaced sulci and cisterns are consistent with hydrocephalus. In contrast, in cerebral atrophy all CSF spaces are enlarged, whereas in cerebral edema all spaces are effaced (see Figure 1-36). Occasionally, a mixed picture can occur, with both obstructing hydrocephalus and diffuse cerebral edema. A number of radiographic criteria for hydrocephalus have been described (see Box 1-9).

How Common Is Ventricular Shunt Obstruction Among Children Presenting With Suspected Obstruction Undergoing CT? How Sensitive and Specific Are Computed Tomography and Shunt Series for Shunt Obstruction?

Among children presenting with suspected shunt malfunction, up to 25% may require surgical intervention. The sensitivity of noncontrast head CT is reported to be 83%, with a specificity of 76%. Traditionally, a shunt series (a series of plain x-rays without contrast following the course of the shunt from head to destination, usually peritoneum) is also performed. Shunt series have low sensitivity (20%) but high specificity (98%). Studies do not suggest high utility of this test in patients with normal noncontrast head CT, but occasionally the shunt series may be positive in these patients (see Figure 1-37). In one series, 3 of 233 patients undergoing imaging had normal head CT but abnormal shunt series and documented shunt obstruction.[58,157]

When head CT and standard shunt series are normal but shunt malfunction continues to be suspected, MRI can be used to assess flow within the shunt. The technique is felt to be highly sensitive but not perfectly specific. Some patients may have intermittent flow through a functioning shunt, and if MRI is performed during a period of normal physiologic low flow, the MRI may falsely suggest the shunt to be occluded. However, demonstration of flow by MRI confirms shunt patency.[158,159]

Central Nervous System Infections

When central nervous system infection is suspected, imaging may be indicated for diagnosis. Imaging serves several roles in this setting: it evaluates for other diagnoses, including hemorrhage or masses; it identifies focal infectious processes, such as abscess or toxoplasmosis; and it identifies possible contraindications to LP, such as the presence of elevated ICP.

Assessment of Intracranial Pressure Before Lumbar Puncture: Does CT predict elevated ICP before LP?

Some studies have shown size of ventricles on CT to be only weakly predictive of ICP.[58] Oliver et al. have argued that the evidence that imaging accurately predicts elevated ICP is scant, that some degree of ICP elevation in meningitis is probably ubiquitous, and that examination findings suggesting high ICP, such as stupor, coma, or focal neurologic deficits, are more reliable than CT in identifying patients at risk of herniation.[160] Nonetheless, CT is frequently performed before LP for suspected meningitis, with the goal of ruling out alternative diagnoses and identifying contraindications to LP. A prospective study in 2001 demonstrated an association among age, recent seizure, abnormal neurologic examination findings, and immunocompromise and CT abnormalities before LP, although the majority of the CT abnormalities were felt to be unlikely to contraindicate LP (Table 1-6).[161] Because elevations of ICP may be present that are not detected on head CT, LP should be carefully considered in patients with abnormal mental status or neurologic examinations, even if CT appears normal. Conversely, significant midline shift or findings suggesting herniation on CT may rarely be present in patients with normal neurologic examinations. Following head trauma, 1.9% of patients with CT-diagnosed frank herniation and 4.4% of patients with significant brain shift but no herniation had no neurologic deficit in National Emergency X-radiography Utilization Study (NEXUS) II.[162]

Imaging in Patients With Seizures

Imaging of patients with new-onset seizure who have returned to a normal neurologic baseline is a level B recommendation in the 2004 ACEP clinical policy on seizures (Box 1-14).[163] Level B recommendations generally reflect evidence with moderate certainty based on class II studies (e.g., nonrandomized trials, retrospective or observational studies, and case-control studies) directly addressing a clinical question or reflect broad consensus among experts based on class III studies (e.g., case reports and case series). What is the basis of the ACEP recommendation? Studies on patients with new-onset seizure show a wide range of abnormal head CT results, from 3% to as high as 41%, often unsuspected on the basis of history or examination.[164,166] It is not clear whether there is a causal relationship between some of the CT abnormalities found in these studies and acute seizure or whether any beneficial change in management resulted from CT imaging. A systematic review

TABLE 1-6. Predictors of Head CT Abnormalities Potentially Contraindicating Lumbar Puncture in Patients With Suspected Meningitis

Baseline Patient Characteristic	Risk Ratio (95% CI)
Age ≥60 years	4.3 (2.9-6.4)
Immunocompromised state*	1.8 (1.1-2.8)
History of central nervous system disease†	4.8 (3.3-6.9)
Seizure within 1 week before presentation	3.2 (2.1-5.0)
Neurologic Findings	
Abnormal level of consciousness	3.3 (2.2-4.4)
Inability to answer two questions correctly	3.8 (2.5-5.8)
Inability to follow two commands correctly	3.9 (2.6-5.9)
Gaze palsy	3.2 (1.9-5.4)
Abnormal visual fields	4.0 (2.7-5.9)
Facial palsy	4.9 (3.8-6.3)
Arm drift	4.0 (2.7-5.8)
Leg drift	4.4 (3.0-6.5)
Abnormal language‡	4.3 (2.9-6.5)

From Hasbun R, Abrahams J, Jekel J, Quagliarello VJ: Computed tomography of the head before lumbar puncture in adults with suspected meningitis. *N Engl J Med* 345:1727-1733, 2001.
*Human immunodeficiency virus or AIDS, immunosuppressive therapy, or transplant.
†Mass lesion, stroke, or focal infection.
‡Aphasia, dysarthria, or extinction.

Box 1-14: Indications for Imaging in Adult Patients With New-Onset Seizure

Urgent neuroimaging is *recommended for all* adult patients, even with return to baseline neurologic status. Imaging should be performed in the emergency department for patients with:
- **Age >40 years**
- **AIDS or immune compromise**
- **Anticoagulation**
- **Cancer history**
- **Fever**
- **Focal onset before generalization**
- **New focal deficits**
- **Persistent altered mental status**
- **Persistent headache**
- **Suspected acute intracranial process**
- **Trauma**

From ACEP Clinical Policies Committee, Clinical Policies Subcommittee on Seizures: Clinical policy: Critical issues in the evaluation and management of adult patients presenting to the emergency department with seizures. *Ann Emerg Med* 43:605-625, 2004.

found that among all adult ED patients with new-onset seizure, 17.7% had an abnormal head CT—26.6% of those undergoing head CT. Among patients with acquired immunodeficiency syndrome (AIDS) and new-onset seizure, the risk appears higher still (20%-30%), with frequent CT diagnoses including cerebral toxoplasmosis, progressive multifocal leukoencephalopathy, and central nervous system lymphoma.[167] Whether seizure is new onset or recurrent, emergent CT scanning is recommended for patients with any of the risk factors in Box 1-14.[168] Noncontrast CT is the initial imaging method, as the majority of life-threatening lesions (hemorrhage, edema, mass effect, and hydrocephalus) would be expected to be found with this modality. Enhanced CT or MRI may be indicated if unenhanced CT is normal and suspicion remains of a structural lesion.

Febrile and Typical Recurrent Seizures

Neither emergent nor urgent imaging is recommended for patients with a typical simple febrile seizure (Box 1-15) or recurrent seizures with typical features compared with the patient's prior seizure history.[168] Do complex febrile seizures require emergency imaging? A recent study found that although 16% of children presenting with new-onset complex febrile seizure had abnormal CT or MR findings, none required emergent intervention (0%; 95% CI = 0%–4%).[169]

Do partial seizures suggest a focal structural brain abnormality and thus mandate imaging? A study from South Africa in a region with a high incidence of tuberculosis and neurocysticercosis suggests that the answer is no. This prospective cohort study of 118 children with new-onset partial seizure found abnormal CT scans in only 8 (7%), all of whom were suspected prospectively of having the CT diagnosis. The investigators concluded that routine scanning would require 11 scans and 5 courses of antihelmintic therapy to prevent one case of childhood seizure disorder, versus no scans and 11 courses of drug therapy if all seizure patients were empirically treated.[170] Of course, this study is from a population quite different from the U.S. population, and its results must be viewed in this context.

Head and Brain Imaging in Syncope

Head CT is commonly obtained as part of the evaluation of a patient with syncope, despite little evidence supporting its use. Syncope is a brief, nontraumatic loss of consciousness with loss of postural tone. Syncope is due to global cerebral hypoperfusion, but the brain is generally the "victim" of syncope, not the cause. Syncope is rarely due to stroke, as loss of consciousness requires loss of blood flow to both cerebral hemispheres or to the medullary reticular activating system in the brainstem. Studies of the diagnostic yield of head CT performed for syncope show little pathology clearly related to the syncope episode.[171] In one retrospective study, 34%

Box 1-15: Simple Versus Complex Febrile Seizure

- **Simple febrile seizure (imaging not generally indicated)**
  - age 3 months to 5 years
  - generalized
  - duration <15 minutes
  - do not recur within 24 hours
- **Complex febrile seizure (imaging may be indicated, though recent studies suggest low risk of emergent intervention)**
  - age <3 months or >5 years
  - focal, with or without secondary generalization
  - duration >15 minutes
  - recur within 24 hours

From Greenberg MK, Barsan WG, Starkman S: Neuroimaging in the emergency patient presenting with seizure. *Neurology* 47:26-32, 1996.

---

of patients presenting to a community ED underwent head CT, with only 1 patient (0.7%) having the etiology identified by imaging (posterior circulation infarct).[172] A second retrospective study found that 283 of 649 (44%) patients admitted with syncope at two community teaching hospitals from 1994 to 1998 underwent head CT, with 5 (2%) revealing an apparent causal diagnosis: 10 patients underwent MRI without a diagnosis of a cause of syncope. Utilization of head CT fell from 61% to 33% of syncope patients from 1994 to 1998, but diagnostic yield remained extremely low, under 1% for both groups.[173] A prospective observational study found a 39% rate of head CT in ED syncope patients at Harvard University's Beth Israel Deaconess Medical Center, with only 5% having head CT abnormalities. That research group proposes that a decision rule for head CT in syncope might reduce utilization by 25% to 50%, although such a rule has not been prospectively validated (Box 1-16).[174] Head CT may be warranted when the history and exam do not fully exclude other diagnoses, such as seizure or stroke, or when trauma results from a syncope episode.[175] A 2007 ACEP Clinical Policy found that there is no evidence for routine screening of syncope patients with advanced imaging including CT. That policy gives a Level C recommendation for cranial CT only when indicated by specific findings in the history or physical examination.[175a]

Posterior Reversible Encephalopathy Syndrome (PRES)

Posterior Reversible Encephalopathy Syndrome (PRES) is a state of vasogenic brain edema seen in severe hypertension, eclampsia, lupus, and cyclosporine toxicity, among many other conditions. The mechanism remains

Box 1-16: Proposed Decision Rule for Computed Tomography Head in Syncope*

- **CT head indicated only for patients with one or more of the following**
  - ○ Signs or symptoms of neurologic disease, including headache
  - ○ Trauma above the clavicles
  - ○ Coumadin use
  - ○ Age >60 years

From Grossman SA, Fischer C, Bar JL, et al: The yield of head CT in syncope: A pilot study. *Intern Emerg Med* 2:46-49, 2007.
*Not yet validated.

Box 1-17: National Emergency X-radiography Utilization Study II: Intracranial Injuries Considered Significant

- **Mass effect or sulcal effacement**
- **Signs of herniation**
- **Basal cistern compression or midline shift**
- **Substantial EDHs or SDHs (>1.0 cm in width or causing mass effect)**
- **Substantial cerebral contusion (>1.0 cm in diameter or >one site)**
- **Extensive SAH**
- **Hemorrhage in the posterior fossa**
- **Intraventricular hemorrhage**
- **Bilateral hemorrhage of any type**
- **Depressed or diastatic skull fracture**
- **Pneumocephalus**
- **Diffuse cerebral edema**
- **DAI**

From Mower WR, Hoffman JR, Herbert M, et al: Developing a decision instrument to guide computed tomographic imaging of blunt head injury patients. *J Trauma* 59:954-959, 2005.

in debate, and studies of imaging findings are limited by the lack of a strong diagnostic reference standard. CT and MR can demonstrate focal regions of symmetric hemispheric edema. The most commonly involved regions are the parietal and occipital lobes, followed by the frontal lobes, inferior temporal-occipital junction, and cerebellum. Vascular watershed areas of the brain appear most affected. The basal ganglia, brain stem, and deep white matter (external/internal capsule) can also be involved. Complications such as hydrocephalus and hemorrhage can occur. On MRI, restricted diffusion representing infarction is seen in 11% to 26% of cases. The clinical importance of imaging for the specific diagnosis and management of PRES is not well established, though imaging to rule out hemorrhage, mass or mass effect, hydrocephalus, and ischemic stroke is indicated.[175b]

Imaging of Traumatic Brain Injury

For evaluation of traumatic brain injury, noncontrast CT remains the primary imaging modality. Brain injuries can include traumatic SAH, SDH, EDH, intraparenchymal hemorrhage, DAI, and traumatic cerebral edema. Concurrent injuries may include bony injuries such as skull fracture. More rarely, head and neck trauma may result in vascular dissection of the intracranial or extracranial arteries (carotid or vertebral), with potential catastrophic neurologic outcomes such as ischemic stroke.

Epidemiology of Traumatic Brain Injury

The incidence of an acute intracranial injury seen on CT following a "mild" traumatic brain injury (GCS score = 13–15) is approximately 6% to 9%, but not all detected injuries result in a clinically meaningful change in management.[63,176] Of patients in the derivation phase of the Canadian CT Head Rule (CCHR), 8% had potentially important CT head findings, yet only 1% underwent a neurosurgical intervention.[63] NEXUS II enrolled 13,728 patients at 21 medical centers in the United States, including all ED patients undergoing head CT after blunt head trauma, regardless of GCS score or neurologic examination. Of these, 6.7% to 8.7% had clinically significant traumatic blunt head injury (prospectively defined) (Box 1-17).[177,178] For purposes of NEXUS II, a clinically significant traumatic brain injury was defined based on prior research as an injury that may require neurosurgical intervention (such as craniotomy, invasive ICP monitoring, or mechanical ventilation) or an injury with potential for rapid deterioration or long-term neurologic dysfunction.[179] Based on NEXUS II, an average emergency physician evaluating patients with a range of GCS scores and neurologic examination findings might expect to find a potentially important head CT abnormality in between 1 in 20 and 1 in 10 patients in whom CT head was ordered after blunt trauma.[177–178] Stiell and collaborators in Canada showed a 6% incidence of head injuries in ED patients undergoing CT following blunt head injury, although they also demonstrated great heterogeneity in the ordering practices of ED physicians, from 6.5% to 80% of patients with head trauma undergoing CT, depending on treating physician.[180] As described later, a variety of decision rules have been investigated to reduce unnecessary imaging in patients with a very low risk for intracranial injury.

Skull Films for Blunt Head Trauma

The 2008 ACEP clinical policy on altered mental status and mild blunt head trauma found that "plain films of the skull have essentially no utility" in the emergency evaluation of patients with altered mental status.[181] Surprisingly, they are still widely used in international

TABLE 1-7. Outcomes and Test Characteristics of Three Clinical Decision Rules for Computed Tomography Use Following Minor Blunt Head Injury in Adults*

	GCS or Neurologic Examination	Time to Imaging	Outcome of Interest	Sensitivity and Specificity (95% CI)
NEXUS-II	Any GCS or any examination with or without LOC	Within 24 hours of injury	Clinically important traumatic injuries	98.3% (97.2-99.0) 13.7% (13.1-14.3)
New Orleans Criteria	With LOC, GCS = 15, normal neurologic examination†	Within 24 hours of injury	Any intracranial injury	100% (95-100) 25% (22-28)
CCHR	GCS = 13-15 with LOC, amnesia, or confusion	For patients with GCS <15, 2-hour postinjury observation required to observe for improvement in GCS Clinically important brain injury	Injuries requiring neurosurgical intervention	100% (92-100) 68.7% (67-70) 98.4% (96-99) 49.6% (48-51)

Data from Haydel MJ, Preston CA, Mills TJ, et al: Indications for computed tomography in patients with minor head injury. *N Engl J Med* 343: 100-105, 2000; Mower WR, Hoffman JR, Herbert M, et al: Developing a decision instrument to guide computed tomographic imaging of blunt head injury patients. *J Trauma* 59:954-959, 2005; Stiell IG, Wells GA, Vandemheen K, et al: The Canadian CT Head Rule for patients with minor head injury. *Lancet* 357:1391-1396, 2001.
*Patients with evidence of more severe head injury, defined by GCS lower than 13 or focal neurologic deficits, require head CT.
†Normal neurologic exam is normal strength, sensation, and cranial nerves.
LOC, loss of consciousness.

emergency practice. In the United Kingdom, skull radiographs are obtained in about 20% of blunt head injury patients, a decrease from nearly 50% in the past.[182] Some investigators have argued that this diagnostic test may play a limited role when CT is not available.[183–184]

Clinical Decision Rules for Blunt Head Trauma
Clinical decision rules have been derived by several groups in the United States, Canada, the United Kingdom, and Scandinavia with moderate success. These rules differ in their definitions of clinically significant injuries, the neurologic inclusion criteria (GCS score, loss of consciousness, and neurologic examination), and the time from injury to imaging. Table 1-7 compares three rules, while Boxes 1-19 through 1-23 and Table 1-8 list the specific inclusion and exclusion criteria and specified outcomes of interest. In general, the New Orleans Criteria (NOC) (Box 1-18) seek to identify any acute intracranial injury, while NEXUS II and the CCHR seek to identify injuries most likely to require neurosurgical intervention or to result in serious neurologic deficits. It is a matter of debate as to which definition is most appropriate. For example, is it important to know of the existence of a traumatic brain injury that does not require neurosurgical intervention to follow cognitive function long-term? Moreover, some clinical interventions may not have truly been "needed" but rather may have been driven by the judgment of individual physicians once they became aware of imaging findings.

New Orleans Criteria. The New Orleans Criteria investigators sought a rule with 100% sensitivity, citing prior surveys of emergency physicians indicating that a clinical decision rule with anything less than perfect

---

Box 1-18: New Orleans Criteria: "Positive" Computed Tomography Findings

- **Any acute traumatic intracranial lesion, including:**
  - SDH
  - EDH
  - Parenchymal hematoma
  - SAH
  - Cerebral contusion
  - Depressed skull fracture

From Haydel MJ, Preston CA, Mills TJ, et al: Indications for computed tomography in patients with minor head injury. *N Engl J Med* 343:100-105, 2000.

---

sensitivity would be unacceptable. Their rule achieved this goal of sensitivity (100%; 95% CI = 95%-100%) but has a low specificity (25%; 95% CI = 22%-28%).[176] This rule (see Box 1-20) has been challenged for its lack of specificity, which might lead to increased utilization of head CT for patients with no other indication for imaging beyond headache, vomiting, or minor head and neck trauma such as facial abrasions.

Canadian Computed Tomography Head Rule. The CCHR was 100% sensitive (95% CI 92%-100%) and 68.7% specific (95% CI 67%-70%) for patients with blunt trauma and a GCS score of 13-15 in its original study; subsequent studies have found slightly lower values.[63,185–189] This rule (see Box 1-21) has been criticized for its relative complexity, as well as for end points (see Box 1-19) that

Box 1-19: Canadian Head CT Rule: Outcomes

Primary Outcomes: Neurosurgical Intervention
- **Death within 7 days secondary to head injury**
- **Any of the following procedures within 7 days:**
  - ○ Craniotomy
  - ○ Elevation of skull fracture
  - ○ ICP monitoring
  - ○ Intubation for head injury (demonstrated on CT)

Secondary Outcomes
- **Clinically important brain injury on CT**
  - ○ Any acute brain finding revealed on CT and that would normally require admission to hospital and neurosurgical follow-up
- **Not clinically important**
  - ○ Patient was neurologically intact and had one of the following:
    - ■ Solitary contusion <5 mm in diameter
    - ■ Localized subarachnoid blood <1 mm thick
    - ■ Smear SDH <4 mm thick
    - ■ Closed depressed skull fracture not through the inner table

From Stiell IG, Wells GA, Vandemheen K, et al: The Canadian CT Head Rule for patients with minor head injury. *Lancet* 357:1391-1396, 2001.

Box 1-20: New Orleans Criteria

Head C is required for blunt trauma patients with loss of consciousness, GCS score of 15, a normal neurologic exam,* and any of the following:
- **Headache**
- **Vomiting**
- **Age >60 years**
- **Drug or alcohol intoxication**
- **Deficits in short-term memory**
- **Physical evidence of trauma above the clavicles**
- **Seizure**

From Haydel MJ, Preston CA, Mills TJ, et al: Indications for computed tomography in patients with minor head injury. *N Engl J Med* 343:100-105, 2000.
*Normal cranial nerves and normal strength and sensation in the arms and legs, as determined by a physician on the patient's arrival at the ED.

Box 1-21: Canadian CT Head Rule*

For patients with a GCS score of 13-15 after witnessed traumatic loss of consciousness, definite post-traumatic amnesia, or witnessed post-traumatic disorientation, CT is only required for patients with any one of the following findings:

High Risk for Neurosurgical Intervention
- **GCS score <15 at 2 hours after injury**
- **Suspected open or depressed skull fracture**
- **Any sign of basal skull fracture†**
- **Two or more episodes of vomiting**
- **Age ≥65 years**

Medium Risk for Brain Injury Detection by Computed Tomography
- **Amnesia before impact >30 minutes**
- **Dangerous mechanism‡**

*Exclusion criteria: no history of trauma, GCS <13, age <16 years, warfarin use or coagulopathy, obvious open skull fracture.
†Including hemotympanum, raccoon eyes, cerebrospinal fluid, otorrhea or rhinorrhea, and Battle's sign.
‡A pedestrian struck by a motor vehicle, an occupant ejected from a motor vehicle, or a fall from ≥3-foot elevation or five stairs.
From Stiell IG, Wells GA, Vandemheen K, et al: The Canadian CT Head Rule for patients with minor head injury. *Lancet* 357:1391-1396, 2001.

might be considered unacceptable in some medical practice settings, including the United States, where fears of litigation might make any CT abnormality undesirable to be missed. Nonetheless, in multiple validation studies and subanalyses, the rule appears to perform well in identifying patients who present with normal mental status but require emergent neurosurgical intervention, including in U.S. populations.[190] Remarkably, despite numerous studies in multiple settings, emergency physician awareness of the rule remains low. A recent study found that only 35% of U.S. emergency physicians were aware of the rule (see Table 1-8).[191]

National Emergency X-radiography Utilization Study II. The NEXUS II investigators identified a decision rule with high sensitivity (98.3%; 95% CI = 97.2%–99.0%) but low specificity (13.7%; 95% CI = 13.1%–14.3%) for significant intracranial injury.[177] This rule (see Box 1-22) has limited clinical utility because it would mandate brain CT in the majority of patients following blunt trauma and thus might actually increase CT use when compared with current physician practice. Its clinical outcome benefit is uncertain—no study to date has demonstrated whether application of the NEXUS

II rule instead of current clinical practice would identify important injuries that would otherwise have been missed. Another difficulty with this proposed rule is the potential variability in application of terms such as *scalp hematoma* or *abnormal behavior* by different observers. In addition, coagulopathy, found to be a high-risk factor,

Box 1-22: National Emergency X-radiography Utilization Study II: Variables Associated With Significant Head Injury

- **Evidence of significant skull fracture**
- **Scalp hematoma**
- **Neurologic deficit**
- **Altered level of alertness**
- **Abnormal behavior**
- **Coagulopathy (includes aspirin use)**
- **Persistent vomiting**
- **Age ≥ 65years**

From Mower WR, Hoffman JR, Herbert M, et al: Developing a decision instrum ent to guide computed tomographic imaging of blunt head injury patients. *J Trauma* 59:954-959, 2005.

Box 1-23: Prediction Rule for Head Injury in Children Under 2 Years of Age

CT is not indicated for patients meeting these criteria.
- **No scalp hematoma except frontal**
- **No loss of consciousness or loss of consciousness for less than 5 seconds**
- **Normal mental status**
- **Nonsevere injury mechanism**
- **No palpable skull fracture**
- **Acting normally according to the parents**

From Kuppermann N, Holmes JF, Dayan PS, et al: Identification of children at very low risk of clinically-important brain injuries after head trauma: A prospective cohort study. *Lancet* 374:1160-1170, 2009. Severe mechanism of injury: motor vehicle crash with patient ejection, death of another passenger, or rollover; pedestrian or bicyclist without helmet struck by a motorized vehicle; falls of more than 1.5 m [5 feet]; or head struck by a high-impact object.

TABLE 1-8. Canadian Computed Tomography Head Rule: International Survey Responses

	Australasia	Canada	United Kingdom	United States
Aware of CCHR	83%	87%	63%	35%
Use of CCHR	55%	83%	44%	29%
Consider future use	67%	84%	33%	77%

From Eagles D, Stiell I, Clement C, et al. An international survey of emergency physicians' knowledge, use, and attitudes towards the Canadian CT Head Rule. Acad Emerg Med 2007;14:S86.

would increase CT use and associated costs.[193,194] In German populations, the rules appear to reduce utilization.[195] A prospective Dutch study validated the high sensitivity of both rules but found that the New Orleans Criteria would decrease use by only 3% and the CCHR by 37.3%.[186] These reductions in use are smaller than the estimates from the original New Orleans Criteria publication (20%)[176] and CCHR (50% to 70%).[63] These findings reflect the existing practices in other countries; when baseline CT use for blunt head injury is low, the NEXUS, Canadian, and New Orleans rules may result in smaller decreases in use or could actually increase use.

Is One Rule "Best"?

A retrospective study of 7955 patients with traumatic head injury published in 2009 compared the three rules we've discussed in detail, plus the guidelines of the Neurotraumatology Committee of the World Federation of Neurosurgical Societies, the National Institute of Clinical Excellence (UK), and the Scandinavian Neurotrauma Committee. No statistical difference was found when comparing the sensitivity of the rules for detection of intracranial hematoma requiring surgical treatment. Current ACEP (2008) guidelines continue to endorse the New Orleans Criteria with a level A recommendation and the CCHR with a level B recommendation.[196]

Can We "Mix and Match" the Rules?

It may be tempting to adopt a combination of features of the preceding decision rules to manufacture a superior decision rule. Unfortunately, there is little evidence to support this practice. The NEXUS investigators and the New Orleans investigators tested a variety of other combinations of clinical criteria besides the final suggested rules. [176,177] Eliminating criteria not surprisingly improved specificity but impaired sensitivity, and adding additional criteria improved sensitivity but impaired specificity. A rule with large numbers of criteria fails the original purpose of developing a clinical decision rule;

included aspirin use, potentially increasing the need for head imaging among patients who do not otherwise appear at risk for brain injury. One important finding of NEXUS II is a lack of association among several clinical variables that have traditionally been considered as potential markers of significant clinical injury, including loss of consciousness, seizure, severe headache, and vomiting.

External Validity of Decision Rules for Blunt Head Trauma. The CCHR and the New Orleans Criteria have been prospectively tested in other populations with less success; in Australia, the rules fail to exclude injury while reducing use.[192] In Britain, the CCHR

it detects all injuries by mandating CT for all blunt head trauma patients.

Some Commonalities Among the Rules

An important take-home point for all of the decision rules described earlier is the notable absence of loss of consciousness alone as an indication for head CT. In the CCHR and New Orleans Criteria studies loss of consciousness was a required inclusion criterion, but in none of the studies did isolated loss of consciousness identify patients at risk for significant injury. NEXUS II included patients with or without loss of consciousness in the study population, and did not find that loss of consciousness required head CT in the absence of the other rule critera. Prior studies had shown little association between loss of consciousness and significant traumatic brain injury.[197] Neither NEXUS II nor the CCHR found posttraumatic headache to be an indication for head CT. The New Orleans Criteria did identify headache as a high-risk criterion, though a decision rule omitting headache would have had 97% sensitivity in the derivation phase.[176] Because the New Orleans investigators desired 100% sensitivity, they did not further validate such a rule. Single posttraumatic seizure also does not appear to be a high-risk feature by the CCHR or NEXUS II, though again, it is considered high risk by NOC.

Table 1-9 summarizes the rules for ease of comparison and application.

Decision Rules for Children

Clinical decision rules for children following blunt head injury remain controversial.[198] Predictors of intracranial injury such as scalp hematoma lack specificity, resulting in large numbers of head CT performed to detect an injury. For example, only about 1% of patients under the age of 2 years with scalp hematoma have traumatic brain injury, although large hematomas, nonfrontal location, and accompanying skull fracture increase the risk.[198] In general, acceptably high sensitivity in these studies comes at the price of extremely low specificity, resulting in little reduction in the utilization of CT in pediatric populations. In some settings, application of these rules could actually increase utilization. These rules may also be very sensitive to the care with which they are applied; the NEXUS II rule, for example, falls in sensitivity from approximately 99% to only 90% when the word *headache* is replaced with *severe headache*, so emergency physicians must scrupulously apply the rules if they expect the rules to function as described in the original studies.[199-203]

Palchak et al.[200] prospectively derived a clinical decision rule for pediatric patients using a cohort of 2043 patients at a single center. They excluded patients with trivial trauma such as falls from standing. They identified five predictors, any of which would mandate CT: abnormal mental status, clinical signs of skull fracture (including retroauricular ecchymosis, CSF otorrhea or rhinorrhea, and palpable fracture), history of any vomiting, scalp hematoma (in children ≤2 years of age), or headache. The sensitivity of the rule was 99% (95% CI = 94%-100%) for traumatic brain injury and 100% (95% CI = 97%-100%) for detection of injury requiring acute intervention. This rule would have eliminated 24% of the CT scans performed at the study institution, but the CIs for the result remain wider than would be accepted by some clinicians and parents.

In the largest study of pediatric blunt head injury to date, Kuppermann et al.[204] conducted a prospective study of 42,412 children ages 18 years and younger to derive and validate a clinical decision rule identifying children with extremely low risk for clinically important traumatic head injuries after blunt trauma.[204] Of these, 14,969 (35.3%) underwent head CT, with clinically important head injuries occurring in 376 (0.9%), and neurosurgery occurring in 60 (0.1%). The investigators identified two rules: one for children younger than 2 years and a second for children 2 years and older. For children under 2 years of age, the rule had a negative predictive value of 100% (95% CI = 99.7%-100%) and sensitivity of 100% (95% CI = 86.3%–100%). In children 2 years and older, the negative predictive value was 99.95% (95% CI = 99.81%-99.99%) and sensitivity was 96.8% (95% CI = 89.0%-99.6%). The rules would have eliminated the need for imaging in 24.1% of children younger than 2 years and 20.1% of older children, without missing any children requiring neurosurgery. Thus children meeting all low-risk criteria do not require a head CT. Conversely, children who do not meet all of the low-risk criteria *do not necessarily require an immediate head CT*; the rules had positive predictive values of less than 2.5% for clinical important traumatic brain injury. This underscores a major limitation of clinical decision rules: high sensitivity inevitably comes at the price of poor specificity and potential for overuse. While the Kuppermann rules identify children with very low risk of important brain injury, they are not intended to identify children at high risk. The authors consequently recommend CT *or* clinical observation in those patients not meeting all low-risk criteria.

In the youngest patients, preverbal children 0 to 3 years of age, clinical assessment is particularly difficult. A very low threshold for CT must be applied after any head trauma, especially considering the possibility of nonaccidental trauma.

Decision Rules for Elderly

The elderly have a high rate of injury with few clinical predictors.[205] NEXUS II found that the rate of clinically significant injury in those 65 years of age or older

TABLE 1-9. Criteria for Three Clinical Decision Rules for Computed Tomography Use Following Blunt Head Injury in Adults[*]

	CCHR[†]	New Orleans Criteria	NEXUS II
	CT is only required for patients with GCS of 13-15 after witnessed traumatic loss of consciousness, amnesia, or confusion and any one of the following findings: **High Risk for Neurosurgical Intervention**	Head CT is required for blunt trauma patients with loss of consciousness, GCS 15, a normal neurologic exam,[‡] and any of the following:	Head CT is required for blunt trauma patients with any of the following:
Age	• < 16 years (exclusion criteria in original study) • ≥ 65 years	• <3 years (excluded from original study) • >60 years	• No lower limit • ≥65 years
Vomiting	• Two or more episodes	• Even one episode	• Recurrent (no specific number of episodes)
Traumatic findings on examination	• Suspected open or depressed skull fracture • Any sign of basal skull fracture[§]	• Physical evidence of trauma above the clavicles • Headache	• Evidence of significant skull fracture • Scalp hematoma
Neurologic examination	• GCS <15 at 2 hours after injury	• Deficits in short-term memory • Drug or alcohol intoxication • Seizure	• Altered level of alertness • Abnormal behavior • Neurologic deficit
Coagulopathy	• Warfarin use or coagulopathy (considered a preexclusion criterion; i.e., not tested in original study)	• *Not* part of the final rule (only one patient in the original study met this criterion, preventing evaluation)	• Suspected coagulopathy (includes aspirin use)
	Medium Risk for Brain Injury Detection by CT *(adding these criteria improves sensitivity but reduces specificity)*		
	• Amnesia before impact of ≥30 minutes		
	• Dangerous mechanism[¶]		

Data from Haydel MJ, Preston CA, Mills TJ, et al: Indications for computed tomography in patients with minor head injury. *N Engl J Med* 343: 100-105, 2000; Mower WR, Hoffman JR, Herbert M, et al: Developing a decision instrument to guide computed tomographic imaging of blunt head injury patients. *J Trauma* 59:954-959, 2005; Stiell IG, Wells GA, Vandemheen K, et al: The Canadian CT Head Rule for patients with minor head injury. *Lancet* 357:1391-1396, 2001.

*For convenience of comparison, similar characteristics for the rules are paired. The order of variables is not important, as any single violation of a rule requires CT imaging. Each bulleted item is a separate item requiring consideration.

†Exclusion criteria: No history of trauma, GCS <13, age <16 years, warfarin use or coagulopathy, obvious open skull fracture, unstable vital signs, seizure before presentation.

‡Normal cranial nerves and normal strength and sensation in the arms and legs, as determined by a physician on the patient's arrival at the emergency department

§Including hemotympanum, raccoon eyes, cerebrospinal fluid, otorrhea or rhinorrhea, and Battle's sign.

¶A pedestrian struck by a motor vehicle, an occupant ejected from a motor vehicle, or a fall from ≥3-foot elevation or five stairs.

was 12.6%, compared with 7.8% in those younger than 65 years.[178] The CCHR classifies patients older than 65 years as high risk and therefore in need of imaging in the case of traumatic loss of consciousness.

Is a Repeated Head CT Required for Patients With Abnormal Head CT After Blunt Trauma?

A range of reported progression in CT findings has been published, with few clear-cut indications for safely omitting repeat scan. A systematic review from 2006 found that the range of reported progression of injury on repeat head CT varied from 8% to 67%, with resulting neurosurgical intervention in 0% to 54% of patients.[206] The review's authors cite a variety of explanations for this dramatic variability in study outcomes, including selection bias, spectrum bias (studies with more severely injured patients being more likely to show unfavorable outcomes), and poor definitions of injury progression. Risk factors including coagulopathy, poor GCS score, and high overall injury severity appear to be associated with worsening CT abnormalities, but methodologic flaws in the studies reviewed make more specific recommendations impossible. Since the

Box 1-24: Prediction Rule for Head Injury in Children 2 Years and Older

CT is not indicated for patients meeting these criteria.
- **Normal mental status**
- **No loss of consciousness**
- **No vomiting**
- **Nonsevere injury mechanism**
- **No signs of basilar skull fracture**
- **No severe headache**

From Kuppermann N, Holmes JF, Dayan PS, et al. Identification of children at very low risk of clinically-important brain injuries after head trauma: A prospective cohort study. *Lancet* 374:1160-1170, 2009. Severe mechanism of injury: motor vehicle crash with patient ejection, death of another passenger, or rollover; pedestrian or bicyclist without helmet struck by a motorized vehicle; falls of more than 1.5 m [5 feet]; or head struck by a high-impact object.

publication of that review, a prospective study of level I trauma center patients with an abnormal head CT has addressed some of the issues raised by that review. The study stratified patients according to GCS (mild: GCS = 13-15; moderate: GCS = 9-12; and severe: GCS <9) and indication for repeat CT (routine vs. indicated by neurologic deterioration). Among patients undergoing CT for neurologic deterioration, a medical or surgical intervention followed CT in 38%. In contrast, among patients undergoing routine repeat CT, 1% underwent an intervention—in both cases, in patients with a GCS score below 9. The authors conclude that repeat CT is warranted in any patient with neurologic deterioration and routine repeat CT may be warranted among patients with a GCS score below 9. No interventions occurred in patient with a GCS score of 9 or higher undergoing routine head CT, but this study is too small to conclude with certainty that routine repeat CT is never necessary in this group.[207] Other recent retrospective studies also suggest that routine repeat head CT is not likely to change clinical management in the absence of a deteriorating neurologic examination, but a larger prospective study will be needed to more stringently define those patients with abnormal CT after blunt trauma in whom repeat CT can be deferred.[208]

What Is the Best Imaging Modality for DAI?

As the name implies, DAI is damage to white matter tracts throughout the brain, thought to occur as the result of shearing from rapid deceleration, often with a rotational component.[209] There is some debate as to the clinical scenarios in which this injury occurs, with some arguing that DAI is a feature only of severe injury while others suggesting it as a mechanism underlying postconcussive syndromes in patients with normal CT.[210] Studies in patients with mild head injury are problematic, as it is unclear whether MR abnormalities are truly evidence of CT-negative DAI or, rather, false-positive MR findings. CT is generally thought to be poor in detecting these changes, though a gold standard for comparison is often lacking or limited to comparison with MRI. A prospective study in 1988 compared CT and MR for identification of blunt traumatic head injuries, but advances in both modalities have rendered its results invalid. A 1994 study found the modalities to be complementary for head trauma, with MR substantially more sensitive for DAI.[211] Subsequent studies have often compared new MR image sequences such as fluid attenuated inversion recovery and DWI to other MR sequences, using as a gold standard a clinical definition of DAI (loss of consciousness persisting more than 6 hours after injury, no hemorrhage on CT) plus imaging criteria (presence of white matter injury on MRI). This type of study, in which the gold standard or reference used to determine the accuracy of the experimental test incorporates that test, suffers from *incorporation bias*.[212] The sensitivity of MRI may be overestimated as a result.

SUMMARY

Emergency imaging of the brain is required for a number of presenting chief complaints. Clinical decision rules can guide imaging in some instances, particularly trauma. Noncontrast CT is the most widely used modality, but some processes, such as ischemic stroke, vascular dissection, and SAH, cannot be ruled out by noncontrast CT alone. Emergency physicians should understand when more diagnostic testing is required after a normal CT. A systematic approach to CT interpretation can improve the accuracy of interpretation by emergency physicians.

Facial imaging plays an important role in the evaluation of trauma, as well as in assessment of soft-tissue infections and masses of the face. Facial imaging often overlaps with imaging of the brain, cervical spine, and soft tissues of the neck. These topics are covered in detail in dedicated chapters, though we discuss common themes in this chapter. We begin with a brief discussion of facial computed tomography (CT) protocols, followed by a guide to interpretation of facial CT. In Chapter 1, we discussed clinical decision rules for CT of the brain, based on large multicenter studies. The evidence for facial imaging is less clear. We examine the two major indications for facial imaging, trauma and nontraumatic facial complaints such as pain, swelling, and erythema, framing our discussion with clinically based questions. We answer common questions about facial CT, such as its value relative to other modalities, such as panoramic x-ray.

Arrangement of Figures in This Chapter

Figures in this chapter are generally arranged into traumatic facial conditions and nontraumatic facial conditions. Because many figures illustrate numerous findings, you will often encounter cross-references to figures presented earlier or later in the chapter. For your quick reference, see Table 2-1, which presents the general order of the figures.

Imaging Options

Traditionally, facial x-rays played an important screening role in the evaluation of facial trauma and infection. However, the complex three-dimensional relationship of facial bones and sinus air spaces makes interpretation of plain x-ray difficult. Facial x-ray imaging has limited sensitivity and specificity and has been largely replaced by CT scan. Other modalities such as ultrasound play specialty roles in evaluating injuries such as ocular trauma. We focus our discussion on CT, highlighting the role of other modalities when appropriate.

What Is the Facial CT Protocol? How Does it Differ from Head CT? Is Facial CT for Trauma the Same as Facial CT for Nontrauma? When Is IV Used?

Facial CT differs from noncontrast head CT in several ways. Thinner CT sections are routinely performed to increase sensitivity for fracture. The CT dataset is processed using special bone algorithms, a different process than simply selecting bone windows to view a head CT. In addition, the CT gantry may be repositioned to allow true coronal plane source images to be acquired, in addition to the axial images acquired during noncontrast head CT (Figure 2-1). In facial CT, both axial and coronal views are routinely provided for interpretation; in noncontrast head CT, axial images are the routine series. Facial CT for trauma is performed without intravenous (IV) contrast, as findings of trauma such as bony fracture, blood in sinus spaces (forming air–fluid levels), and soft-tissue swelling do not require IV contrast for identification. When CT is used for evaluation of nontraumatic facial complaints, IV contrast should be administered if possible. Neoplasms, vascular malformations, and infectious and inflammatory conditions all may show enhancement with IV contrast, aiding diagnosis. Facial CT has a narrower field of view than brain CT. For example, Figure 2-2 demonstrates that while the face is seen in detail, the posterior cranial vault and much of the brain are not within the field of view. As a consequence, if brain injury or nonfacial skull fracture is suspected, noncontrast head CT should be obtained.

In the past, true coronal sections acquired with the patient in a prone position offered higher resolution than coronal reconstructions created from axial source images (see Figure 2-1). These high-resolution images have excellent sensitivity for even minimally displaced fractures. Modern multislice helical CT has the ability to create multiplanar sagittal and coronal, as well as three-dimensional, reconstructions from source data acquired

TABLE 2-1. Arrangement of Figures

Content	Figure Number
Comparison of head and face computed tomography	2-1
Facial trauma	
Frontal bone fracture	2-2
Orbital fractures and ocular injuries	2-3 through 2-13
Midface injuries and Le Fort classification	2-14 through 2-23
Mandible injuries	2-24 through 2-26
Nontraumatic facial conditions	
Orbital soft-tissue infections and neoplasms	2-27 through 2-31
Sinusitis and mastoiditis	2-32 through 2-34
Parotid gland disease	2-35

with the patient in a supine position, eliminating the need to acquire true coronal images by patient and gantry repositioning. One cadaver study suggested that coronal plane facial reconstructions generated from axial fine-cut (1.25 mm) head CT images had a sensitivity of 97% for displaced fracture compared with coronally acquired images when interpreted by an experienced radiologist.[1] The true sensitivity of facial CT is difficult to determine, as no independent gold standard for comparison is available to confirm negative CT results. Is a normal CT a true negative, or is it a false negative, having missed a fracture? This study assigns coronally acquired facial CT the role of diagnostic reference standard for comparison with coronal reconstructions from axially acquired images. In this study, facial fractures were generated in the cadavers by striking the cadaver heads in a standardized fashion. However, the exact number of fractures generated by this method is unknown, so it is impossible to determine whether either CT technique actually detected all fractures.

Why should we care about these issues as emergency physicians? Advantages of using coronal reconstructions rather than true coronally acquired images include reduced scan time, reduced radiation exposure (particularly to the radiosensitive lens of the eye), and utility in patients who cannot be repositioned for other clinical reasons, including cervical spine injuries (which prevent prone positioning) and life-threatening injuries that limit additional CT.

INTERPRETATION OF FACIAL COMPUTED TOMOGRAPHY IN THE SETTING OF TRAUMA

The approach to interpretation of facial CT requires a knowledge base similar to that for head CT. Refer to Chapter 1, in which basic features of CT, including right–left orientation, Hounsfield units, and window settings, are explained in detail. For facial CT, we rely on two primary window settings: bone windows for bony injury from facial trauma, and soft-tissue windows for soft-tissue injury from trauma and for other indications, such as assessment of soft-tissue infections and masses. When interpreting facial CT for trauma, review the entire CT using bone windows, and then repeat the process using soft-tissue windows. Throughout this chapter, you will find carefully annotated images depicting a range of pathology. The figure captions lead you through the interpretation of the specific findings, including the optimal choice of window setting. Unlike head CT, in which axial images are often the only image set reviewed, facial CT images are generally acquired and displayed in both axial and coronal planes. Sagittal planes and three-dimensional reconstructions are selectively used to depict injuries and pathology that are incompletely characterized by axial and coronal images.

A few sources of error in interpretation deserve mention here. Use of the wrong window setting prevents detection of important pathology. For example, soft-tissue windows do not allow detailed inspection of bone, so nondisplaced fractures may not be seen. Emergency physicians may not be familiar with detailed anatomy of facial bones, so normal structures such as sutures and foramen may be mistaken for fractures. If a patient has a unilateral complaint or injury, use the normal side for comparison when inspecting the CT images. Recognize that CT reconstructions often have reconstruction artifacts, such as the "seams" where two image sets are pieced together by the computer (see Figure 2-15 on page 62). These artifacts can be distinguished from fractures, as the "step-off" created by reconstruction artifact extends across the entire CT image, not just through bone. Understanding that these artifacts may exist can prevent artifact from being misconstrued as fracture. Asymmetrical positioning of the patient within the CT gantry also results in asymmetry of CT images, which may be misinterpreted by the novice as injury or pathology (see Figure 2-16, B, on page 62 where asymmetry is caused by patient positioning). Note the patient's position on the CT images as you begin your interpretation so that you may take position into account and avoid this pitfall.

CT for facial trauma is performed without IV contrast. Bone windows are used to evaluate most injuries, as they demonstrate both fractures and air–fluid levels well. Soft-tissue windows can depict subcutaneous hematomas and swelling, but these injuries rarely require specific therapy. Two important exceptions must be recognized. First, soft-tissue windows may reveal intracranial injury, although the field of view of facial CT does not include the entire brain, and brain (head) CT should be ordered if intracranial injury is suspected

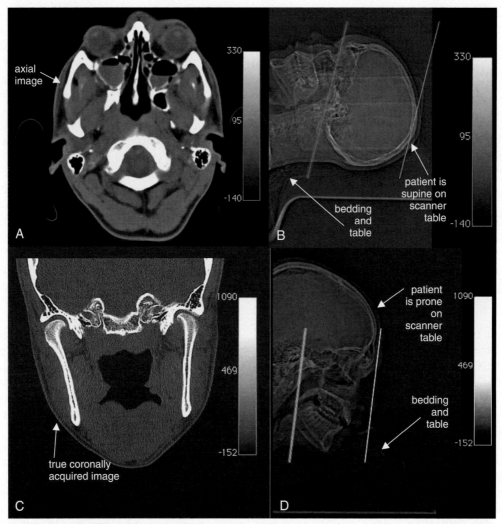

Figure 2-1. Differences between head and face computed tomography (CT). Images are from the same patient. **A,** Head CT is typically acquired with the patient supine, with the scanner gantry tilted slightly to comply with the natural angulation of the cranial vault. This allows brain structures to be imaged in a true axial plane. Slice thickness is commonly around 5 mm. The axial image corresponds to the plane through the left line in the scout image, **B**. Axial facial images are acquired in the same position. **C,** Facial CT requires axial and coronal images to be generated. In the past, patients were often positioned prone for facial CT to allow acquisition of true coronal images. The coronal image in **C** corresponds to the coronal plane through the left line in the scout image, **D**. Today, multislice scanners using fine slice thickness (1.25 to 3 mm) allow high-resolution, reformatted images in multiple planes without repositioning the patient. Patients can be positioned in the usual supine position for a single volumetric data acquisition. The three-dimensional dataset can be "sliced" to produce images in any plane.

(see Chapter 1). Second, injuries to the globe and other orbital contents may require emergency ophthalmologic intervention and are seen on soft-tissue windows. Most remaining traumatic facial injuries are fractures and injuries to sinus spaces, best seen using bone windows. Our approach uses a cephalad to caudad orientation. Consequently, we first discuss frontal bone fractures, followed by orbital and ethmoid sinus injuries; maxillary, zygomatic, tripod, nasal, and Le Fort midface fractures; and finally, dental and mandibular injuries.

Frontal Bone Fractures

Frontal bone fractures (see Figure 2-2) can be isolated facial injuries or can extend intracranially. The frontal sinus has an anterior and posterior wall. Fractures to the anterior plate alone are facial injuries, requiring cosmetic surgical treatment if depressed. Fractures to the

posterior plate are calvarial injuries and carry several risks, including intracranial infection (from contamination of the cerebrospinal fluid with nonsterile air and fluid from the frontal sinus), intracranial hemorrhage, and direct traumatic brain injury if fracture fragments are projected posteriorly. Inspect for frontal sinus injury first using bone windows and then using brain windows. On bone windows, examine the anterior and posterior plates for discontinuities. Anterior plate fractures may require otolaryngology or plastic surgery consultation. Posterior plate fractures require neurosurgical consultation. Some patients have a hypoplastic frontal sinus, with no airspace—the anterior and posterior plates are fused as one bone, so any fracture requires neurosurgical consultation. The normal frontal sinus is air-filled (black). Look for opacification of the frontal sinus (gray on bone windows), indicating traumatic blood. In the absence of

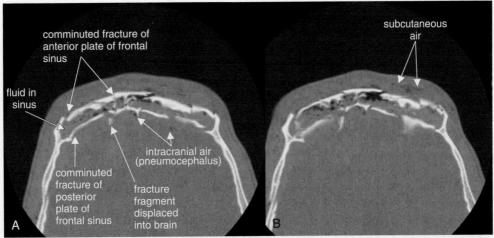

Figure 2-2. Frontal sinus fractures. Facial fractures involving the sinuses are common and are usually not life-threatening injuries. These injuries may dissipate force, preventing intracranial injury. The sinuses could be called "airbags for the brain." However, sometimes enough force is exerted to fracture not only the anterior wall of the sinus but also the posterior wall, which is a shared wall with the calvarium. These injuries are extremely serious, resulting in potential cerebrospinal fluid leak, intracranial hemorrhage, and intracranial infection. **A** and **B,** In this patient, severely comminuted fractures of the anterior and posterior plates of the frontal sinus are present. The frontal sinus is nearly filled with fluid, presumably blood from the acute fractures. Air is present in the subcutaneous tissue, likely having escaped from the frontal sinus but also possibly entering through a facial laceration. Fracture fragments from the posterior wall of the frontal sinus have been displaced posteriorly into the calvarium. Air is also present within the calvarium. Inspection of the brain for hemorrhage should be performed using brain window settings, and dedicated brain computed tomography should be performed. Because the posterior wall of the sinus is fractured, this is a true neurosurgical emergency, not a simple facial fracture.

trauma, frontal sinusitis can have a similar appearance. When fractures of the posterior plate are present, look for intracranial air (pneumocephalus, black) using bone windows. Inspect for bone fragments that have been displaced posteriorly. Switch to brain windows and inspect for intracranial hemorrhage, which will appear white (see Chapter 1). Posterior plate fractures should prompt additional imaging with noncontrast head CT if this has not already been obtained.

Orbital Injuries

Fractures to the orbit are detected by reviewing CT images on bone windows. The plane of the fracture and direction of displacement of fracture fragments varies, so axial and coronal images should be reviewed to ensure detection of any fractures. If the patient has a unilateral injury, use the normal side for comparison. As discussed in Chapter 1, bony injury may be seen directly as a discontinuity in the bone making up the walls of the orbit or adjacent sinus space (sometimes called a cortical defect). However, some minimally displaced fractures may be difficult to recognize directly, and indirect signs of injury may draw your attention to a likely fracture. These signs include fluid in normally air-filled spaces—the ethmoid sinuses medial to the orbit and the maxillary sinuses inferior to the orbit. An air–fluid level may be present, or the sinus space may be completely opacified with blood products. On bone windows, bone appears quite white, air appears completely black, and blood and other soft tissues appear various shades of gray. Another indirect sign of orbital fracture is air within the orbit. Again, on bone windows, air in the orbit will appear black. Air is not normally found within the orbit but may be introduced from adjacent

sinus spaces when fractures occur. Figures 2-3 through 2-6 (see also Figure 2-14) demonstrate common orbital injuries, including medial and inferior orbital fractures with secondary signs of injury to adjacent sinus spaces. Entrapment of extraocular muscles may be seen on CT, with bone fragments directly impinging on muscle soft tissue. Sometimes orbital fat is seen projecting through an orbital fracture. Soft-tissue windows may help to determine whether entrapped soft tissue is muscle or fat. Fat appears nearly black on soft-tissue windows, while extraocular muscles have a light gray appearance. The density in Hounsfield units (HU) can also be measured directly using tools on most digital picture archiving and communication systems. Fat has a density of approximately -50 HU, whereas muscle density is approximately +50 HU.

Injuries to the orbital contents (soft tissues) are best seen using soft-tissue windows. Again, axial and coronal images should be inspected. Normally, the globe is quite round in cross section. The lens appears bright (light gray), while the anterior and posterior chambers are lower in density and appear a darker gray. The choroid and sclera surrounding the eye are similar in density to the lens and appear light gray. Orbital fat is normally dark, nearly black on soft-tissue windows due to its low density. The extraocular muscles are denser than both orbital fat and vitreous humor within the globe and appear light gray. They are normally quite discrete and well margined, as they are surrounded by dark orbital fat, which provides contrast. The optic nerve is also seen in the orbit posterior to the globe—it shares the same "soft tissue" density with extraocular muscles and appears light gray. CT reveals soft-tissue injury,

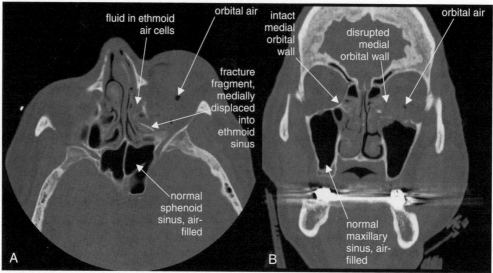

Figure 2-3. Orbital fracture: Medial wall fractures. In this unenhanced computed tomography image, viewed on bone windows, fractures of the medial wall of the orbit are evident. Force directed at the globe often results in fractures of the medial wall, including the paper-thin lamina papyraceae. Several features of this fracture pattern are evident. Here, the fracture itself is visible, although in some cases this may be difficult to see. This sliver of bone has tipped medially into the adjacent ethmoid sinus **(A).** The ethmoid sinus, normally an air-filled space, is fluid-filled—in this case, due to bleeding from the acute fracture. Compare this with the normal sphenoid and maxillary sinuses, which are well aerated. Air has escaped from the ethmoid air cells into the left orbit. An inferior orbital fracture involving the left maxillary sinus is also present, investigated in more detail in Figures 2-4 through 2-6 and Figure 2-14. The bone window setting is ideal for depicting the preceding findings, since air alone appears black on this setting.

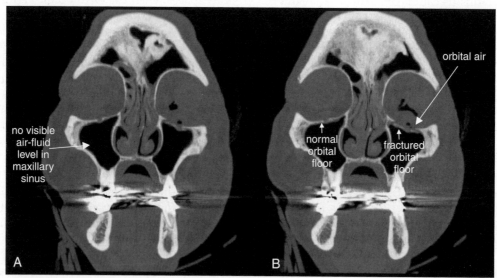

Figure 2-4. Orbital fracture: Subtle inferior wall fractures. A and **B,** Inferior orbital fractures (also called orbital floor fractures) involve the superior wall of the adjacent maxillary sinus. These can be difficult to recognize on axial views, as the fracture fragment may lie in the axial plane. In contrast, these are usually easily recognized on coronal reformations. In this example, minimally displaced fractures of the orbital floor are visible—compare the discontinuity of the left orbital floor with the continuous right orbital floor. Air within the orbit (orbital emphysema) also is evidence of this fracture—air likely leaked from the maxillary sinus into the orbit. A common associated finding would be an air–fluid level in the maxillary sinus due to bleeding into the sinus from the fracture. On these images, no air–fluid level is visible. This may be a function of the patient's position at the time of computed tomography (CT) scan acquisition. Although the coronal reformations may look like the patient is in an upright position, don't be fooled. The patient was supine during the CT scan, and any blood would have pooled posteriorly in the maxillary sinus. These slices were reconstructed at a relatively anterior position through the sinus and could miss pooled blood products.

which can only be suspected with the use of facial x-ray (Figure 2-7). Figures 2-8 through 2-13 show injuries to orbital contents imaged with CT, with the contralateral side providing a good example of normal orbital anatomy.

Important injuries to orbital contents include globe ruptures, particularly related to intraorbital and intraocular foreign bodies; vitreous hemorrhage; lens dislocation; retinal detachment; and retrobulbar emphysema and hematoma.

Global rupture

Globe rupture (see Figures 2-7 through 2-11) may result from either blunt or penetrating trauma. In the setting of penetrating trauma, a radiopaque foreign body may be

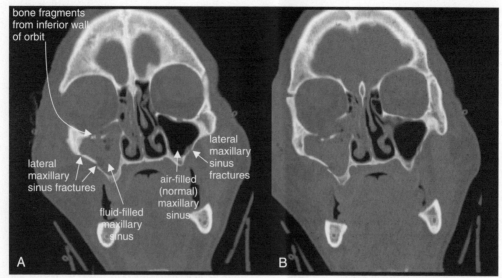

Figure 2-5. Orbital fracture: Blowout. Most orbital fractures are of the "blowout" type: force applied to the globe and orbital rim increases pressure within the orbit, and fractures occur in the weak medial, inferior, or both walls of the orbit, forcing the orbital wall to blow out into the adjacent ethmoid or maxillary sinus. **A** and **B,** In this patient, an inferior blowout has occurred, with bone fragments being displaced inferiorly into the maxillary sinus. Fluid (blood from acute fractures) fills the maxillary sinus, a common finding associated with facial fractures. An air–fluid level is not seen, because this patient was in a supine position during the computed tomography scan and the coronal reformations are parallel to the patient's position in the scanner. In addition, this patient's maxillary sinus is nearly filled with blood. Additional fractures are present, including ethmoid fractures revealed by fluid in the ethmoid air cells and a lateral maxillary sinus fracture.

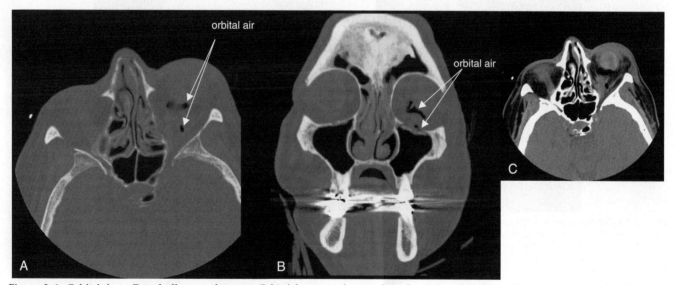

Figure 2-6. Orbit injury: Retrobulbar emphysema. Orbital fractures often result in the escape of air from adjacent sinus spaces into the orbit. Because the orbit does not normally contain air, the presence of air within the orbit should be interpreted as strong evidence of a fracture after trauma, even if the fracture line itself is not visible. **A** (axial view) and **B** (coronal view), In this example, medial (ethmoid) and inferior (maxillary) fractures are present and are likely the sources of the orbital air. A bone window setting is ideal for detecting both the fracture and orbital air. On this setting, bone appears bright white, air appears completely black, and soft tissues are an intermediate gray. A soft-tissue window may make recognition small amounts of air more difficult, because orbital fat is nearly black on this setting (**C,** same image as **A** but viewed on soft-tissue window).

seen within the globe. High-density foreign bodies (e.g., metal, stone, or glass) may be readily seen on CT as bright white intraocular densities. These may also be visible on x-ray (see Figure 2-7), but CT offers more definitive localization within the globe rather than in the orbit (see Figure 2-8). Lower-density materials such as wood may be isodense with normal intraocular contents or with intraocular blood. They may be invisible on x-ray and CT and may require magnetic resonance imaging (MRI)

or ultrasound for detection. Globe rupture may result in disruption of the normal spherical contour of the globe (circular in cross section). The globe may appear irregular and smaller than the normal contralateral side (see Figure 2-9). Intraocular air is also proof of globe rupture following trauma (see Figure 2-11). As with air in other locations, air is black on all window settings and is readily visible within the globe, contrasted against denser (therefore brighter) globe contents.

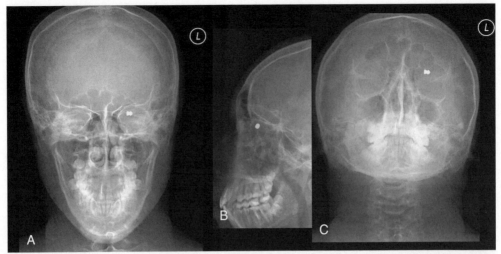

Figure 2-7. Orbit injury: Orbital foreign body. Anterior–posterior **(A)**, lateral **(B)**, and submental **(C)** views of the face using plain x-ray reveal an orbital foreign body. The patient is a 16-year-old man shot with a pellet gun. Although plain film is useful for detecting metallic and other dense orbital foreign bodies, it provides little information about the globe or other structures in the orbit. A computed tomography scan was also performed in this patient (Figure 2-8).

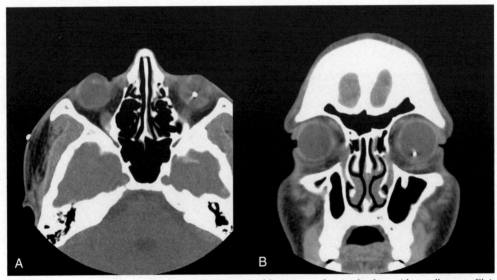

Figure 2-8. Globe rupture with intraocular foreign body. This 16-year-old man was shot in the face with a pellet gun. Plain x-ray (Figure 2-7) demonstrated an orbital radiopaque foreign body. **A** (axial view) and **B** (coronal view), This computed tomography scan confirms that the pellet is within the left globe—an ophthalmologic emergency. The dense object creates some metallic artifact around it. These images use soft-tissue settings to allow inspection of the globe and orbital contents. Amazingly, the remainder of the orbital contents appear normal. Bone windows should also be inspected to allow detection of any associated fractures. The patient was taken to the operating room for removal of the foreign body.

Vitreous hemorrhage

Vitreous hemorrhage (see Figures 2-9 through 2-12) can occur with blunt or penetrating globe trauma and is *not* proof of globe rupture when seen in isolation. Hemorrhage within the globe is higher density than the normal vitreous humor and thus appears brighter against the dark gray background of the vitreous. Blood can be isodense with the lens of the eye, sometimes make it difficult to determine whether the lens is properly located.

Lens dislocation

On soft-tissue windows, the lens is normally found as a biconvex bright disc in the anterior globe (see Figures 2-9 through 2-12). The two pointed edges of the lens should each tangentially contact the globe circumference. A thin crescent of low-density aqueous humor should be visible as a dark gray region anterior to the lens. Lens dislocation is recognized by the absence of the lens from its normal location—the lens may be visible in another region of the eye or may be obscured by intraocular blood (see Figures 2-10 and 2-11). In some patients, the lens is surgically absent, so it is important to take a thorough history when the lens is not found in normal position (see Figure 2-12).

Retinal detachment

Retinal detachment may be seen on CT scan (see Figures 2-12 and 2-27). Normally, the retina is invisible on CT scan, as it is adherent to the periphery of the globe, is extremely thin, and is isodense with other ocular contents. However, when retinal detachment occurs, the

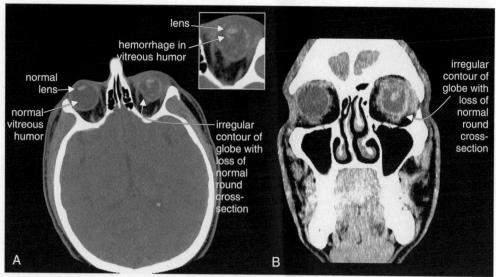

Figure 2-9. Ocular injury with globe laceration and rupture. This patient fell in a bathroom, striking the left globe against an unknown object. **A** (axial view) and **B,** (coronal view) soft-tissue CT images reveal a ruptured globe with associated vitreous hemorrhage. The left globe is obviously not round in cross-section because of rupture and extrusion of some ocular contents. Compare with the normal right globe. The lens appears to be in a relatively normal position. Dense intraocular hemorrhage is visible in the posterior chamber, against the darker background of normal vitreous humor.

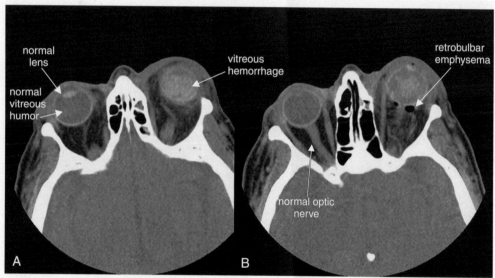

Figure 2-10. Ruptured globe with lens dislocation and intraocular hemorrhage. This patient sustained a ruptured left globe from airbag deployment. **A** and **B,** The axial computed tomography (CT) images viewed on soft-tissue windows reveal several important findings. First, dense material is present in the posterior chamber of the left eye, consistent with intraocular hemorrhage. Compare with the normal right globe. Second, the lens cannot be identified in its normal location in the left eye, suggesting dislocation. Recognize that a patient may not be positioned symmetrically in the CT scanner during scan acquisition, resulting in an asymmetrical appearance of structures in the CT images. This may simulate pathology, so confirmation of this suspected injury requires careful inspection of adjacent slices in the stack of CT images. Fresh blood in the posterior chamber is also isodense with the lens, making detection of the lens difficult. **B,** Air is also visible posterior to the globe. Small amounts of air may be difficult to see against the dark gray background of orbital fat on soft-tissue windows and may be more apparent on bone windows. These should be inspected to detect associated sinus fractures, which are the likely source of orbital air.

retina is lifted up by blood or other soft-tissue material. This can result in a peripheral convexity projecting into the vitreous humor (see Figure 2-27). In some cases, other ocular injury, such as vitreous hemorrhage, may make retinal detachment impossible to recognize. If retinal detachment is the only suspected injury, CT should not be used for evaluation, as radiation to the eye contributes to cataracts (see later discussion), and other modalities including ocular ultrasound can be used for diagnosis without radiation exposure.

Retrobulbar emphysema and hematoma

Retrobulbar emphysema (also called orbital emphysema) (see Figures 2-6 and 2-10) can be seen on both soft-tissue and bone windows, as air appears black on both window settings. It is more easily seen on bone windows, where orbital fat appears gray. On soft-tissue windows, orbital fat appears nearly as black as air. Usually, orbital emphysema requires no specific treatment and is a secondary sign of a fracture to the medial or inferior orbital wall, with air entering the orbit from the ethmoid or maxillary sinus.

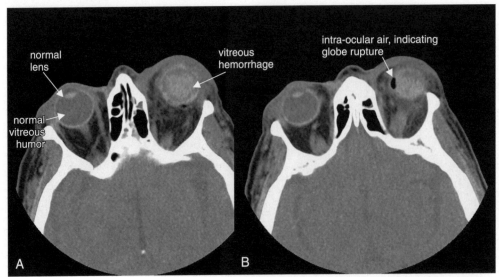

Figure 2-11. Ocular injury: Globe rupture with vitreous hemorrhage and lens dislocation. This patient was struck in the left eye by a deploying airbag, resulting in vitreous hemorrhage and lens dislocation (**A** and **B,** axial CT images, soft-tissue window). These are discussed in detail in Figure 2-10. An additional finding mandates immediate operative therapy: air is present within the globe, indicating globe rupture **(B)**.

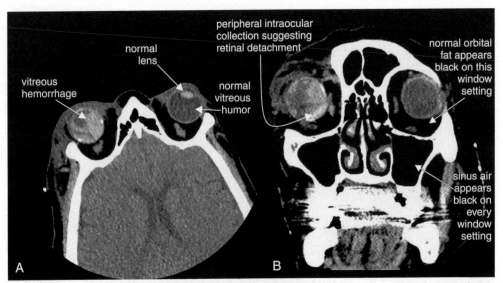

Figure 2-12. Ocular injury with retinal detachment and vitreous hemorrhage. This patient also suffered an ocular injury during airbag deployment. **A** (axial image) and **B** (coronal image), Like the patient described in the preceding figures, this patient has posterior chamber hemorrhage, indicated by dense material posterior to the lens position. This patient had undergone prior ocular surgery and does not have a native lens in the right eye, explaining the absence of a visible lens—though this appearance would also be consistent with lens dislocation. The patient also has retinal detachment with subretinal blood, visible as hyperdense collections on the periphery of the globe. Retinal detachment and vitreous hemorrhage may be indistinguishable by computed tomography, though both would require emergency ophthalmologic consultation. The soft-tissue window setting in this figure would not be appropriate for detection of orbital air, since the window setting has been adjusted in such a manner that orbital fat appears as black as air. Air could be detected by adjusting the window setting, for example, to bone windows.

Retrobulbar hematoma (see Figure 2-13) is a more important injury, as ongoing hemorrhage in this location can result in rising pressure, compressing and injuring the optic nerve. This can progress to orbital compartment syndrome, which can result in blindness unless lateral canthotomy is performed. Retrobulbar blood is visible on soft-tissue windows. Fresh blood is intermediate gray, similar to the appearance of the optic nerve and extraocular muscles. It blurs the contours of these structures, which are normally quite distinct and outlined by dark orbital fat. An additional finding that suggests high orbital pressure in this setting is proptosis of the affected eye.

Ethmoid Sinus Injuries

Ethmoid fractures often accompany other orbital injuries—search for these injuries using bone windows. The ethmoid sinuses lie medial to the orbits, and blows to the orbits can result in medial blowout fractures of the thin lamina papyracea (see Figure 2-3). In addition, direct anterior–posterior blows to the nose often cause ethmoid fractures, as the ethmoid sinuses lie deep to the nose. The

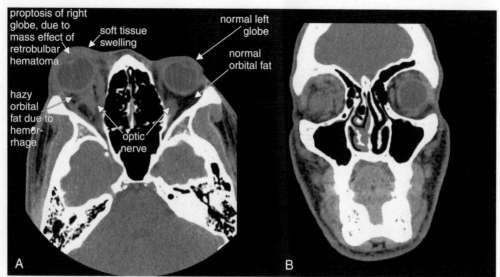

Figure 2-13. Orbit injury: Postbulbar hemorrhage (retrobulbar hematoma). Orbital trauma can result in significant, sight-threatening injury. In this case, hemorrhage posterior to the globe is exerting mass effect, displacing the globe anteriorly and resulting in proptosis. Retrobulbar hematoma can exert pressure on the optic nerve, resulting in permanent blindness. This patient underwent emergency lateral canthotomy to relieve the elevated orbital pressure. **A** (axial) and **B** (coronal) images are shown on soft-tissue windows to highlight the globe and orbital soft tissues. Bone windows should also be reviewed to allow detection of associated fractures. Several computed tomography findings are evident. First, the right globe is proptotic compared with the normal left globe. Second, soft-tissue swelling of the eyelid is evident on the patient's right, compared with the left. Third, the orbital fat appears hazy on the right, compared with the normal black appearance of orbital fat on the patient's left—this is consistent with hemorrhage. The patient's globes are intact bilaterally, with normally positioned lenses and normal vitreous (gray).

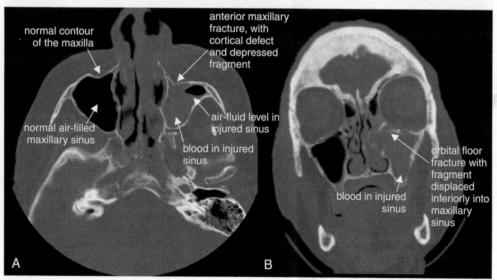

Figure 2-14. Maxillary fracture. This patient has a minimally depressed fracture of the anterior wall of the maxillary sinus, with associated bleeding into the maxillary sinus. **A,** An air–fluid level marks the injured side; compare with the normal right maxillary sinus. **B,** On the coronal reformation, the opacified maxillary sinus is again visible. A fracture of the orbital floor is also visible.

normal ethmoid sinuses are air-filled and appear black (see Figure 2-21). Fractures of the ethmoid sinuses often allow air to escape into the orbits (see Figure 2-3). Infra-orbital air appears black, as described earlier. Bleeding from ethmoid fractures causes opacification of the ethmoid air cells, which then appear gray on both bone and soft-tissue windows (see Figures 2-3 and 2-16).

Midface Fractures

After assessing the orbit, inspect other structures of the midface.

Maxillary fractures

Maxillary fractures (Figure 2-14; see also Figures 2-15, 2-16, 2-18, and 2-19) can be isolated injuries or part of a larger pattern of injury, such as the inferior orbital fractures, tripod fractures, or Le Fort fracture patterns. Figure 2-14 shows unilateral maxillary sinus fractures with a normal contralateral side for comparison. Use bone windows to evaluate the maxillary sinus for fracture. Defects in the thin bony wall can often be seen directly. Fluid in the maxillary sinus appears gray and should be suspected of being blood from a fracture following trauma—even if

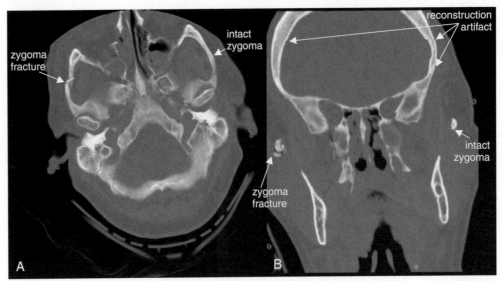

Figure 2-15. Zygoma fracture. Many textbooks emphasize that bony rings rarely break in a single location—when one fracture is detected, a second fracture should be suspected and sought after. In practice, this is often true, but a single fracture location with comminuted fragments may dissipate force sufficiently to prevent a second fracture site. **A,** This patient has a comminuted fracture of the zygomatic arch. Compare the patient's right (fractured) zygoma with the normal left. This patient does have additional fractures, including maxillary sinus and ethmoid sinus fractures, which are described in detail in other figures. **B,** The coronal view is a computer reconstruction, which has visible artifact at several levels. These artifacts can be distinguished from fracture lines because they extend across the entire image in a horizontal line. Try to identify additional reconstruction artifacts in the image.

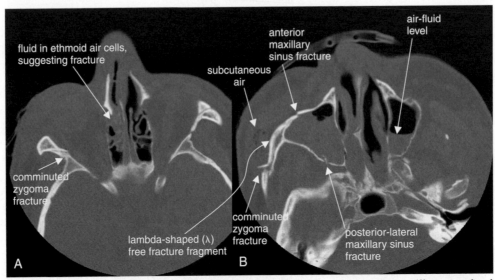

Figure 2-16. Zygomatic complex fracture (also called tripod fracture, malar fracture, or zygomaticomaxillary complex fracture). The bony rings formed by the zygoma and walls of the maxillary sinus and orbit often fracture in a predictable pattern in response to an applied force—although the "real-life" patterns of fracture are often more complex than the textbook descriptions. A tripod fracture involves the zygomatic arch, inferior orbital rim, and anterior and lateral walls of the maxillary sinus. These fractures are depicted in the axial computed tomography images above, viewed on bone windows. **A,** Blood is present in the ethmoid sinuses, suggesting ethmoid fracture. **B,** Notice the lambda-shaped (λ) free fracture fragment, which creates instability of the inferior and lateral orbit. Note the air–fluid levels in the bilateral maxillary sinuses, indicating blood associated with bilateral maxillary sinus fractures.

the fracture itself is not seen. Always consider the differential diagnosis for opacification of the maxillary sinus. This can include both traumatic blood (see Figure 2-14) and preexisting sinus disease (see Figure 2-22). Typically, sinus blood fills the sinus in a dependent position (usually posterior first, as the patient is supine for CT), forming an air–fluid level. Sinusitis from infectious or allergic causes usually creates more circumferential and often lobulated thickening of the soft tissues lining the sinus. Fractures to the anterior and posterior walls of the

maxillary sinus are best recognized on axial images (see Figure 2-14, *A*), whereas fractures of the superior wall of the maxillary sinus (orbital floor) are better seen on coronal images (see Figure 2-14*B*). Both axial and coronal images should be inspected for this reason.

Zygomatic arch fractures

Fractures of the zygomatic arch are common and should be evaluated using bone windows. These are readily apparent on axial images, although coronal images can

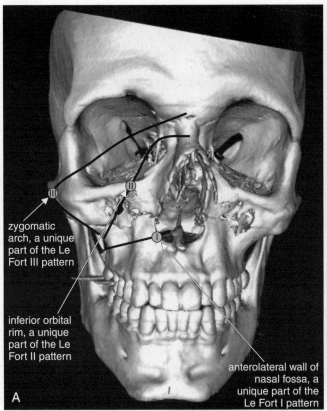

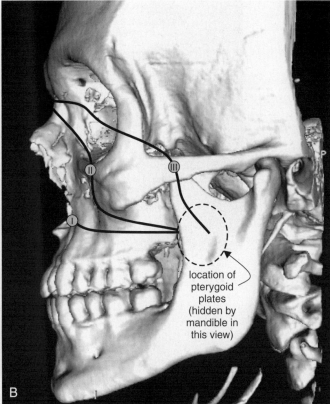

zygomatic arch, a unique part of the Le Fort III pattern

inferior orbital rim, a unique part of the Le Fort II pattern

anterolateral wall of nasal fossa, a unique part of the Le Fort I pattern

location of pterygoid plates (hidden by mandible in this view)

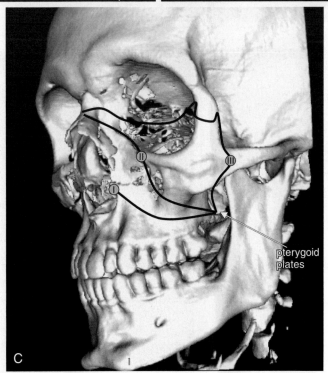

pterygoid plates

Figure 2-17. The Le Fort classification system for facial fractures. All Le Fort fractures involve the pterygoid plates, plus at least one other unique fracture. Le Fort I fractures involve the anterolateral wall of the nasal fossa. Le Fort II fractures involve the inferior orbital rim. Le Fort III fractures involve the zygomatic arch. Inspection of each of these zones and the pterygoid plates can allow you to rule in or rule out each fracture type. Remember that more than one type may be present on each side of the patient's face, and the fractures may or may not be bilaterally symmetrical. Here, anterior–posterior **(A),** lateral **(B),** and oblique **(C)** views of the face are shown, taken from three-dimensional, surface-rendered computed tomography reconstructions. Black lines indicate the general path of the fracture in a Le Fort III–II–I pattern. The lines are intentionally drawn on only half of the figure, as Le Fort fractures need not be bilaterally symmetrical. A *small circle* has been placed along each line to mark a location unique to each fracture pattern, which can be used to help to rule in or rule out that pattern. This patient has visible bilateral Le Fort I fractures. The pterygoid plates are not visible in some views but lie posterior to the maxilla, hidden behind the ramus of the mandible.

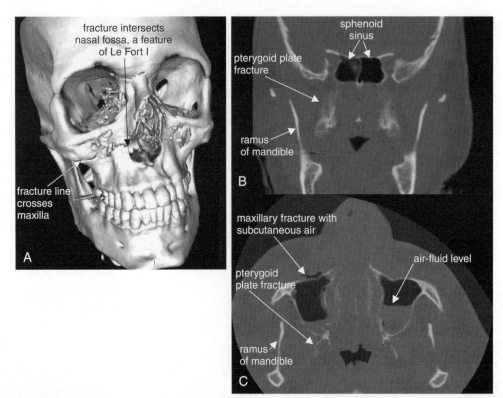

Figure 2-18. Le Fort I fracture. This 30-year-old man was struck in the midface by a baseball at a minor league park. He presented with epistaxis, as well as some instability of the maxillary teeth, which were mobile as a unit. His computed tomography image shows fractures consistent with a bilateral Le Fort I pattern. **A,** A three-dimensional, surface-rendered reconstruction shows the fracture line extending from the anterolateral nasal fossa, across the maxilla, and toward the pterygoid plates (not visible in this image). **B,** Coronal reconstruction, with the pterygoid fracture visible. **C,** Axial view.

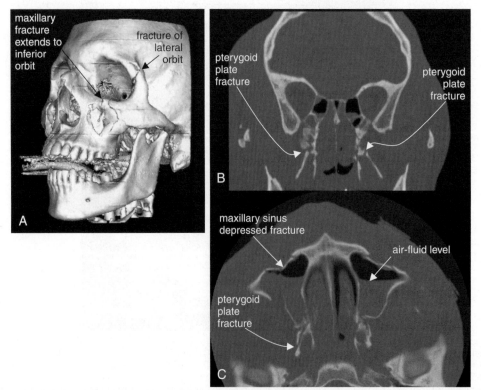

Figure 2-19. Le Fort II fracture. This 24-year-old man was assaulted with the butt of a shotgun and sustained multiple facial fractures, which in general follow the Le Fort II pattern bilaterally. A Le Fort II fracture makes the midface mobile due to fractures through the maxilla, inferior orbital rim, and pterygoid plates. Additional fractures are present in this patient. No single computed tomography image shows the entire scope of the patient's fractures, so selected images have been chosen to depict the most critical injuries. **A,** A three-dimensional, surface-rendered image shows a depressed maxillary fracture involving the inferior orbital rim on the left. This patient also has a fracture of the lateral orbit, a reminder that real-world fractures often do not adhere exactly to a Le Fort pattern. **B,** Coronal view. **C,** Axial view.

also reveal these fractures (Figure 2-15). The normal smooth curve of the zygomatic arch is disrupted by fracture. Like other ring structures, the zygomatic arch rarely fractures in a single location, although a comminuted fracture may dissipate enough force to prevent fracture in a second discrete location. Zygomatic arch fractures are frequently accompanied by other complex fracture patterns, including tripod fractures and Le Fort III fractures (described in detail later).

Tripod fractures

A tripod fracture (Figure 2-16) is also called a zygomatic complex fracture, malar fracture, or zygomaticomaxillary complex fracture. This fracture involves the zygomatic arch, inferior orbital rim, and anterior and lateral walls of the maxillary sinus. Look carefully at Figure 2-16, *B*. The fractures of the zygoma and maxillary sinus have created a lambda-shaped (λ) free fracture fragment—typical of tripod fracture. This fracture requires surgical repair, because it creates instability in the inferior–lateral orbit. Unlike a Le Fort III fracture (described later), the fracture does not extend to the pterygoid processes, so the face is not dissociated completely from the calvarium. When a zygomatic fracture is present, always inspect the inferior orbital rim and maxillary sinus to determine whether a tripod fracture has occurred.

Le Fort injuries

The Le Fort classification of midfacial fractures (Figures 2-17 through 2-20) is based on the work of the French physician Rene Le Fort using cadaver skulls, published in 1901.[2] Le Fort described a series of midface fractures spanning from relatively stable maxillary injuries (Le Fort I) to complete craniofacial dissociation (Le Fort III). Not surprisingly, his description of fractures inflicted on skulls postmortem does not perfectly describe the range of injuries seen in living patients. However, the patterns he observed do form the basis for approaches to surgical repair. In reality, injuries are often combinations of the Le Fort I, II, and III patterns, with additional fractures frequently noted that do not conform to the Le Fort classification. Other midface fracture classifications have been described. From an emergency physician standpoint, critical issues include recognition of isolated facial fractures and those that concurrently involve the calvarium and thus pose risks of cerebrospinal fluid leak and subsequent infection (see the earlier frontal sinus fracture discussion). Patients with these injuries are often severely injured and intubated and thus may not be able to offer useful clinical information about neurologic or sensory complaints. Use of the Le Fort classification system can facilitate communication with physicians in other specialties—although simple description of the involved bones and planes of fracture can suffice and can be more complete and accurate.

Rhea and Novelline[3] have described a simple method for detection of Le Fort fractures on CT scan (Table 2-2). They note that Le Fort I, II, and III fractures have in common fracture of the pterygoid plates, whereas each fracture pattern has a unique additional bony fracture not found in the other patterns. If the unique fracture is not present, the specific Le Fort pattern is ruled out. If the unique fracture is present, the particular Le Fort pattern must be confirmed by inspecting for the additional typical features of that fracture pattern. Le Fort I fractures always involve the anterolateral margin of the nasal fossa. Le Fort II fractures always involve the inferior orbital rim. Le Fort III fractures always involve the zygomatic arch. Remember that more than one type may be present on each side of the patient's face, and the fractures may or may not be bilaterally symmetrical.

To assess systematically for a Le Fort fracture, first inspect for fractures of the pterygoid plates, which must be present. Because these structures may be unfamiliar to emergency physicians, we briefly review their location and appearance. As their name suggests, these plates or processes are thin, winglike (think of the pterodactyl, an ancient winged reptile) projections of the sphenoid bone and thus are located just caudad to the sphenoid sinus on coronal views (see Figure 2-18*B*). They are seen posterior to the maxillary sinuses on axial images (see Figure 2-18*C*). The ramus of the mandible is present lateral to the pterygoid processes, hiding them from view on the three-dimensional reconstructions in Figures 2-17 through 2-20. The proximity of the pterygoids and the mandible is no coincidence—the pterygoid processes are points of attachment for muscles of mastication, which move the mandible.

Once a pterygoid fracture is found, inspect for the unique fracture of each Le Fort pattern described earlier. Figure 2-17 shows the typical path of each Le Fort fracture, always passing through the pterygoid plates. Figures 2-18 through 2-20 explore Le Fort I, II, and III fractures in more detail.

Nasal fractures

Isolated nasal fractures require no imaging (as shown later), but nasal fractures are often found on CT performed for assessment of other facial injuries (Figures 2-21

TABLE 2-2. Features of Le Fort Fractures*

Le Fort Pattern	Fracture Unique to Le Fort Pattern
I	Anterolateral margin of the nasal fossa
II	Inferior orbital rim
III	Zygomatic arch

Rhea JT, Novelline RA: How to simplify the CT diagnosis of Le Fort fractures. *AJR Am J Roentgenol* 184:1700–1705, 2005.
*All Le Fort fractures involve fractures of the pterygoid plates, plus an additional unique fracture.

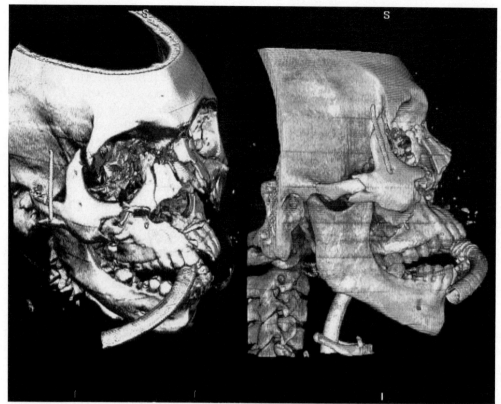

Figure 2-20. Le Fort III fracture and beyond. This 34-year-old man sustained major facial fractures in a motor vehicle collision. Although his fractures could be described using the Le Fort classification, they are not symmetrical and have a complex pattern that defies the Le Fort categories. Three-dimensional, volume-rendered CT images are shown. Such reconstructions are particulary valuable to define spatially complex fractures. **A,** an oblique view from a vantage point superior to the patient's right eye. **B,** a direct lateral view from the patient's right. The patient is intubated and an endotracheal tube is visible entering the mouth and continuing past the hyoid bone.

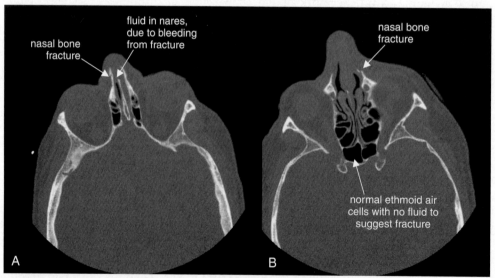

Figure 2-21. Nasal fractures. Isolated nasal fractures require no imaging—neither computed tomography nor plain film. However, sometimes nasal fractures are incidentally noted on imaging performed to evaluate for other suspected head and facial injuries. In this patient, minimally displaced nasal bone fractures are present. Some blood is present in the nares **(A),** but the ethmoid air cells are well aerated, with no fluid to suggest fractures **(B).**

and 2-22). Nasal fractures are evident on bone windows as discontinuities in the thin nasal bones. Often, blood is present in the nares, visible as a dark gray density on bone windows. Always inspect for associated injuries to the ethmoid and maxillary sinuses and orbits. The Le Fort

I fracture pattern (see the earlier detailed description and Figures 2-17 through 2-18) involves the anterolateral nasal fossa and extends across the maxilla to the pterygoid plates, resulting in instability of the maxilla and maxillary teeth relative to the remainder of the face and skull.

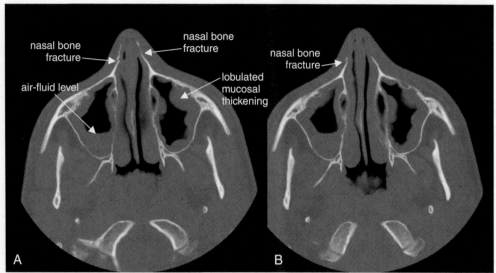

Figure 2-22. Nasal fractures with preexisting maxillary sinus disease. This 14-year-old man struck himself in the nose with his knee while high-jumping, sustaining nasal fractures. As discussed earlier, sinus spaces should be inspected for air–fluid levels, which may indicate bleeding from an underlying fracture. **A** and **B,** axial CT images viewed on bone windows. In this patient's case, the bilateral maxillary sinuses show significant mucosal thickening. In addition, the right maxillary sinus has an air–fluid level. Are these the sequelae of trauma? More likely, they indicate preexisting sinus disease. The bilateral abnormalities and the lobulated appearance are more likely findings of sinus inflammation. Blood from acute fractures would be expected to pool in the dependent portions of the sinuses, while inflamed mucosa (whether from infection or allergy) has a more circumferential appearance. Careful inspection of the bones of the sinuses reveals no fractures. The air–fluid level could represent blood from acute trauma or fluid associated with preexisting sinus disease. Sinus disease is a common incidental finding on computed tomography (CT) of the head performed for other indications. In the absence of clinical symptoms, the CT findings are nonspecific.

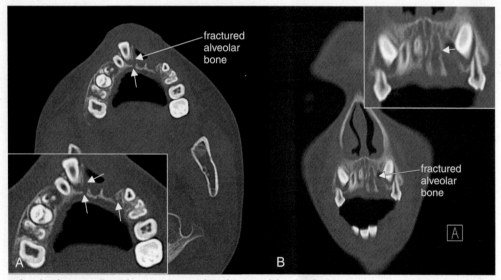

Figure 2-23. Dentoalveolar fracture. Dental trauma can result in fracture of the alveolar bone surrounding the dental root. In this young man, the left central and lateral incisors have been completely avulsed. **A,** On the axial view, the right central incisor is displaced anteriorly and the surrounding alveolar bone is fractured (*arrows*, close-up view). **B,** On the coronal reformation, a fracture of the left maxilla is also seen (*arrow*, close-up view).

Dental and Mandibular Injuries

Facial trauma can result in dental–alveolar injuries—fractures of the alveolar bone surrounding maxillary and mandibular teeth. Traditionally, this has been evaluated with panoramic x-ray (Panorex), although CT performed for evaluation of other facial injuries readily detects dental–alveolar fracture. CT and panorex are compared later. Figure 2-23 demonstrates a maxillary dental–alveolar injury. These injuries are often treated by dentists or oral–maxillofacial surgeons and are not

life threatening. On CT, inspect for cortical bone defects using bone windows. Review both axial and coronal images.

Mandibular fractures (Figures 2-24 through 2-26) can be evaluated by panorex or CT scan (see later comparison). Panorex (see Figure 2-24) uses a moving x-ray tube to generate a flattened planar projection of the curved mandible. As with other x-rays, on panorex, fractures may be visible as cortical defects, step-offs, or linear

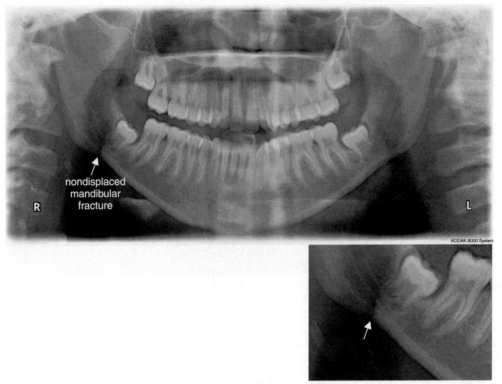

Figure 2-24. Mandibular fracture. Which imaging modality is the gold standard, Panorex or computed tomography (CT)? Traditionally, Panorex plain film has been considered the gold standard for diagnosis of mandibular fractures. The wide availability of CT has encouraged the replacement of Panorex with CT as a common imaging modality for this indication. The two modalities are sometimes complementary. In this case, the Panorex shows a linear lucency adjacent to the right mandibular angle posterior to the posteriormost molar, which represents a fracture (*arrow,* close-up view). The fracture was not recognized on CT, although a left temporomandibular joint dislocation was recognized on CT but not on Panorex.

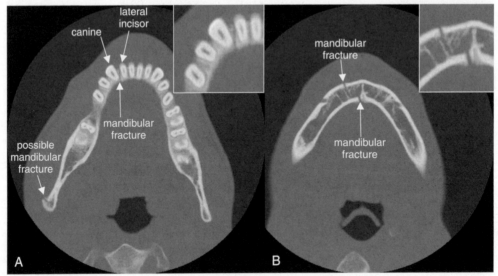

Figure 2-25. Mandible fracture: Nondisplaced. Fractures of the mandible are classically described as rarely solitary, as the mandible forms a rigid ring not easily broken in a single location. Sometimes isolated fractures do occur, but once one fracture has been detected, a careful search should be conducted for additional fractures. Sometimes a single fracture is accompanied by dislocation of one or both mandibular condyles at the temporomandibular joint. **A,** In this patient, an isolated fracture of the anterior mandible is present, dividing between the right canine and the lateral incisor. A possible second fracture is seen at the mandibular ramus. **B,** The original fracture line is again seen, now zigzagging through the mandible. Cortical defects are visible on both mandibular surfaces.

lucencies. On CT scan, inspect for cortical defects using bone windows. Minimally displaced fractures may be subtle. Solitary mandibular fractures are thought to be rare due to the arch or ringlike structure of the mandible. Stress in one location in the arch generates stress at other locations, and multiple fractures are common. Sometimes stress is sufficiently relieved by a single minimally displaced fracture. Displaced fractures (see Figure 2-26) may result in a second fracture location or in dislocation of the mandibular condyles from the

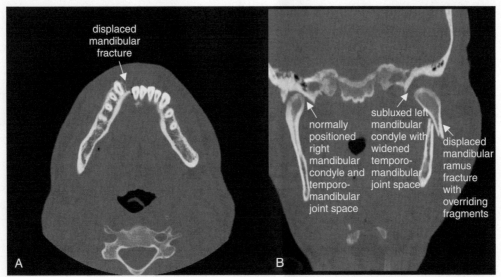

Figure 2-26. Displaced mandibular fracture. When a significantly displaced mandibular fracture occurs, a second fracture or a dislocation of the mandibular condyle is nearly inevitable. This patient has both. **A,** On the axial view, a significantly displaced mandibular symphysis fracture is seen. **B,** On the coronal view, the left mandibular ramus is fractured and overriding, and the left mandibular condyle is subluxed. Compare with the normally positioned right mandibular condyle.

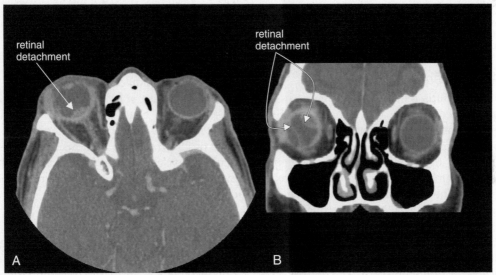

Figure 2-27. Choroidal metastases resulting in retinal detachment. This elderly male presented clinically as though with a periorbital or orbital cellulitis but failed to improve with antibiotics. Computed tomography with intravenous (IV) contrast was performed due to suspicion of orbital infection. IV contrast is not used in the setting of facial trauma, as it is unnecessary for detection of fractures, air, lens dislocation, intraocular hemorrhage, or dense intraorbital or intraocular foreign bodies. When infection or malignancy is suspected, IV contrast should be given to allow enhancement of hypervascular pathology. This patient was found to have choroidal metastases from a known non–small cell lung carcinoma. Several malignancies, including lung and prostate neoplasms and melanoma, can metastasize to the orbit or globe. **A,** In this patient, a lens-shaped region of increased density is seen at the posterior right globe near the optic disc, consistent with retinal detachment in this location. **B,** Additional areas of retinal detachment are seen on the coronal view. Spontaneous or traumatic retinal detachment would have a similar appearance and could be detected without IV contrast.

temporomandibular joints. These joints are seen well on coronal reconstructions (see Figure 2-26), so both axial and coronal images should be reviewed.

INTERPRETATION OF FACIAL COMPUTED TOMOGRAPHY FOR NONTRAUMATIC CONDITIONS

We have discussed interpretation of CT scan for facial trauma in detail. We now turn to interpretation of CT scan performed for evaluation of nontraumatic facial abnormalities. For most of these applications, CT scan is performed with IV contrast. Soft-tissue windows provide the best visualization of important anatomic structures. Bone windows may occasionally provide additional clinically relevant information.

Rarely, metastatic tumors such as melanoma, prostate, and lung tumors can involve the eye, so CT with IV contrast should be considered in evaluation of patients with these conditions who present with eye complaints (Figure 2-27).

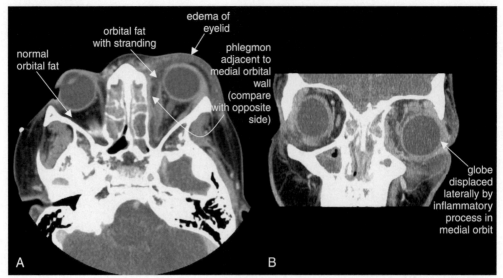

Figure 2-28. Orbital cellulitis. Computed tomography (CT) is often used to distinguish orbital from periorbital cellulitis. Both conditions may have periorbital soft-tissue swelling. However, on CT, orbital cellulitis should also demonstrate stranding of orbital fat. Proptosis may be present if sufficient soft-tissue swelling occurs within the orbit to displace the globe. Intravenous contrast is given when orbital infection is suspected, as it will result in enhancement of hypervascular lesions. Neoplasms invading the orbit can present in a similar fashion to infection and can be detected by contrasted CT. In this patient, soft tissues anterior to the globe are thickened (compare with normal side) **(A)**, though this does not distinguish preseptal from post septal cellulitis. Mild proptosis is present. The orbital fat shows inflammatory stranding, a hazy appearance compared with the normal right orbital fat. A thin enhancing collection is present along the medial wall of the left orbit, possibly representing an early abscess or phlegmon. The ethmoid sinuses are completely opacified, a finding described in detail in the next figure. **B** (coronal view), Lateral displacement of the globe is visible. The patient improved with antibiotics without undergoing surgery.

Orbital Cellulitis and Abscess

Suspected orbital cellulitis or abscess can be assessed with CT scan with IV contrast. A discussion of the clinical indications for imaging is presented later. In the earlier discussion on orbital trauma, we reviewed the normal appearance of the globe and orbital contents. The normal globe is round in cross-section on both axial and coronal images. The vitreous humor is intermediate gray on soft-tissue windows. Normal orbital fat has a dark gray to nearly black appearance on soft-tissue windows. It outlines the extraocular muscles and optic nerve, which usually have discrete margins and a light gray appearance, reflecting their soft-tissue density. The normal orbit contains no air, although occasionally air may become trapped beneath the eyelid following physical examination.

Periorbital (preseptal) cellulitis

In periorbital (preseptal) cellulitis, soft-tissue inflammatory changes are restricted to the region anterior to the septal plate of the eyelids and do not involve other orbital contents. These inflammatory changes may include thickening of the eyelid and periorbital soft tissues, as well as inflammatory stranding of the subcutaneous fat. Stranding is a smoky or light gray appearance found in inflamed fat. Normal subcutaneous fat, such as orbital fat, is nearly black. As inflammation develops, an increase in soft-tissue water content occurs. This increases the density of fat tissue. On CT scan, increasing density results in a brightening of color.

Orbital (postseptal) cellulitis

In orbital (postseptal) cellulitis (Figures 2-28 and 2-29), inflammatory changes involve the orbital contents. Orbital fat develops the brightening or smoky appearance of fat stranding. As a result, the margins of extraocular muscles and the optic nerve become less distinct. Swelling of orbital contents may push the globe anteriorly, resulting in proptosis.

Orbital abscess

If a frank orbital abscess is present (Figures 2-30 and 2-31), IV contrast will result in enhancement of the lesion. Enhancement is an increase in the Hounsfield units of tissue following administration of IV contrast, resulting in a brighter appearance on CT. It reflects increased blood flow and vascular permeability in inflammatory, infectious, or neoplastic conditions. The rim of the abscess typically appears bright due to enhancement. If the abscess contains relatively low-density liquid pus, the center of the abscess will have a dark gray appearance on soft-tissue windows. This will be similar in density to the vitreous humor within the globe. Occasionally, abscesses may contain air, which will appear black on all window settings.

Adjacent sinus infections

Orbital abscesses and cellulitis commonly originate from infections of adjacent sinus spaces (see Figures 2-28 and 2-29). The ethmoid and maxillary sinuses should be carefully inspected for abnormal opacification or mucosal thickening, which may indicate sinusitis. Normally,

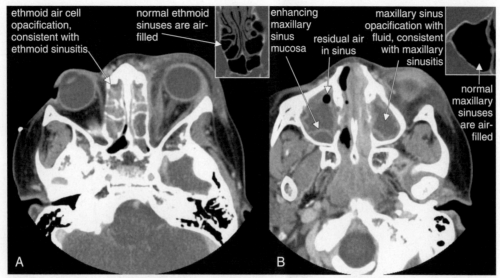

Figure 2-29. Sinus disease leading to orbital cellulitis. This is the same patient depicted in Figure 2-28, with orbital cellulitis confirmed by computed tomography. **A,** The source of this infection is likely ethmoid sinusitis, as the ethmoid and maxillary sinuses are completely opacified with fluid. The ethmoid spaces are separated from the orbit only by the paper-thin lamina papyracea. **B,** Because intravenous contrast was given, the inflamed mucosa of the maxillary sinus is visible as an enhancing serpiginous line on the periphery of the sinus space. This likely separates the inflamed and thickened mucosa from the residual sinus space, which is then secondarily filled with fluid. Normal ethmoid **(A)** and maxillary **(B)** sinuses are shown in small boxes for comparison.

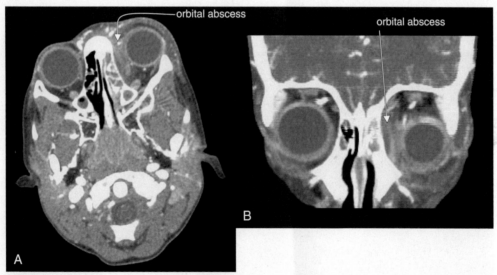

Figure 2-30. Orbital abscess, developing in the setting of ethmoid sinusitis. In these contrast-enhanced facial computed tomography images, a left orbital abscess is visible. Several distinct features are present. **A,** Axial view, soft-tissue windows. The left eye demonstrates proptosis, due to mass effect of the abscess within the left orbit. **B,** Coronal view, soft-tissue windows. The left eye is displaced laterally and inferiorly, again by mass effect of the abscess. The orbital fat normally has a dark, nearly black appearance on soft-tissue windows. Here inflammation leads to fat stranding, giving the orbital fat a smoky gray appearance. Compare the fat of the left orbit to that of the right orbit **(A** and **B)**. The abscess obscures the normal appearance of the extraocular muscles, which appear as gray tissue density. The abscess is visible as a spindle-shaped collection hugging the medial wall of the left orbit, with an enhancing rim. The contents of the abscess are fluid density, similar to the density of fluid in the adjacent ethmoid sinuses—the likely source of the orbital infection. Compare this appearance with the normally air-filled ethmoid sinuses on the patient's right. Figure 2-31 demonstrates these features in detail.

the sinuses are air-filled and black. Findings of sinusitis are discussed next.

Sinusitis

Sinusitis may involve the frontal, maxillary (Figure 2-32; see also Figures 2-22 and 2-29), ethmoid (see Figures 2-28 through 2-31), and sphenoid (see Figure 2-32) sinuses. Controversy remains about the specificity of CT abnormalities for the diagnosis of sinusitis

(see later discussion). The normal sinuses are air-filled and black (see Figure 2-14 for maxillary, Figure 2-21 for ethmoid, and Figure 2-3, *A* for sphenoid). The normal sinus mucosa is extremely thin and essentially invisible on CT scan. In general, sinusitis results in circumferential mucosal thickening in the involved sinuses, appearing gray on both bone and soft-tissue windows. Thickened mucosa may have an undulating or lobulated appearance (Figure 2-33; see also

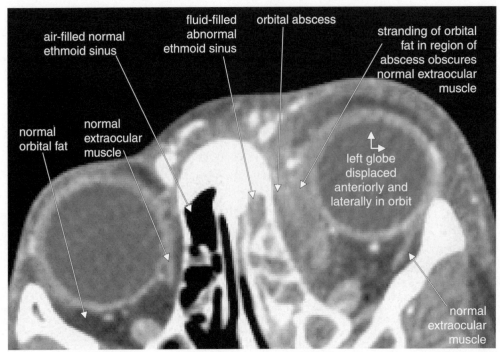

Figure 2-31. Orbital abscess, developing in the setting of ethmoid sinusitis. This contrast-enhanced facial computed tomography image details features of the preceding figure. The left eye is displaced anteriorly and laterally by mass effect of an orbital abscess. Compare the fat of the left and right orbits. The abscess obscures the normal appearance of the extraocular muscles, which appear as a thin slip of gray tissue density.

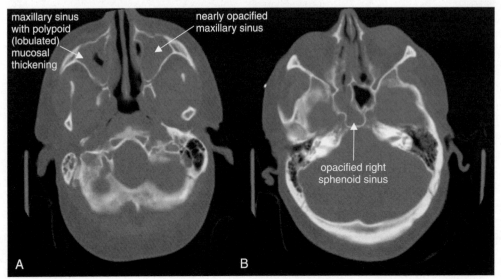

Figure 2-32. Paranasal sinusitis, complicated by development of *Streptococcus pneumoniae* meningitis. This 60-year-old man presented with profoundly altered mental status and vomiting. His head CT demonstrated severe sinus disease, which was correctly recognized as a potential source for meningitis. His cerebrospinal fluid ultimately grew *S. pneumoniae*. When extensive sinus disease is seen, complications such as meningitis or cavernous sinus thrombosis should be considered. The computed tomography (CT) findings here include opacification of the maxillary sinuses **(A)**, ethmoid air cells **(B)**, and right sphenoid sinus **(B)**. The maxillary sinuses have a lobulated or polypoid appearance **(A)**. No intravenous contrast was given, because this was a head CT performed for assessment of altered mental status, not a dedicated sinus CT. Bone windows are useful for inspection of the paranasal sinuses, as fluid and soft tissue appear gray while air appears black.

Figure 2-22). An air–fluid level may also be present, or the sinus may be completely opacified by the combination of mucosal thickening and fluid. With administration of IV contrast, the sinus mucosa may enhance (see Figure 2-29*B*). Figure 2-33 compares normal maxillary sinuses with sinuses showing fluid from fracture and mucosal thickening from sinusitis. CT alone cannot determine the cause of sinus mucosal thickening, as thickening may result from infectious or allergic causes. Patients with CT abnormalities may be asymptomatic—clinical judgment must be used to determine the significance of the CT findings. Sinusitis can result not only in orbital infection, as described earlier, but also in meningitis (see Figure 2-32) or brain abscess.

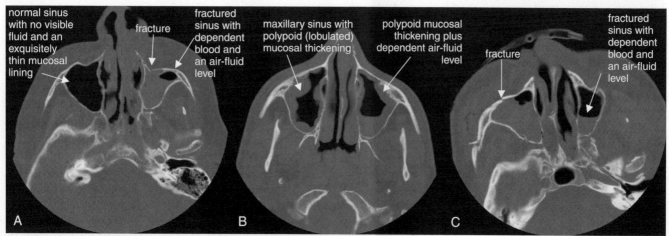

Figure 2-33. Sinus disease: Normal, air–fluid levels, and mucosal thickening. Abnormalities of paranasal sinuses are commonly encountered on head or face computed tomography. A range of findings, from normal (**A,** right maxillary sinus), to mucosal thickening consistent with sinusitis (**B**), to traumatic blood with air–fluid levels (**C,** left maxillary sinus) may be seen. The clinical scenario plays an important role in determining the significance of imaging findings. In the absence of trauma, fluid may represent infection. With a history of trauma, fluid may indicate blood from a sinus fracture. Polypoid thickening is not the result of trauma and indicates preexisting sinus disease, whether infectious or allergic. In the absence of any clinical symptoms, sinus abnormalities may be incidental and may not require specific treatment. Controversy remains over the significance of mucosal thickening and air–fluid levels without fever, facial swelling, or purulent nasal discharge.

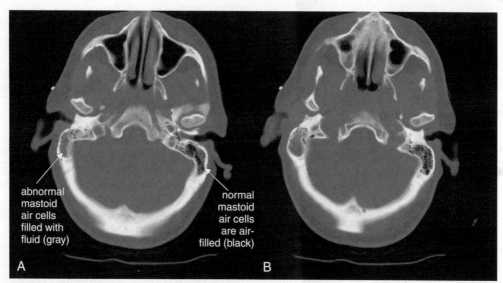

Figure 2-34. Mastoiditis resulting in meningitis. Though technically not part of the face, the mastoid air cells share many common features with facial sinuses. The mastoid air cells are best viewed on bone windows, because soft-tissue windows often obscure the small air spaces. A normal mastoid is a spongy, air-filled lattice, and appears black on CT bone windows. Fluid in the mastoids is abnormal and appears gray on CT bone windows. In the seeting of trauma, fluid may indicate blood filling air cells from a temporal bone fracture. With no history of trauma, fluid should raise suspicion of infectious mastoiditis. Mastoid fluid can be recognized on a noncontrast head CT and does not require special temporal bone view of facial series. This patient presented with confusion and nystagmus, as well as a history of right ear pain. **A** and **B,** Computed tomography (CT) showed opacification of the right mastoid air cells, consistent with mastoiditis. Given the patient's confusion, meningitis as a complication of mastoiditis was suspected. Cerebrospinal fluid ultimately grew *Streptococcus pneumoniae.*

As a result, when a patient is found to have sinus disease on CT scan, the differential diagnosis must continue to be evaluated, as fever and headache may reflect simple sinusitis or more ominous intracranial infection.

Mastoiditis

The mastoid air cells are air-filled spaces like other facial sinuses. The normal mastoid spaces are black, with a multitude of small cells created by fine bony partitions. Mastoiditis can be recognized on facial CT, although the field of view of facial CT often does not fully include the mastoid air cells. Like sinusitis, mastoiditis is characterized by fluid density (gray) replacing the normal air contents (black). Like sinusitis, mastoiditis can be complicated by intracranial extension and meningitis (Figure 2-34). Review the mastoid air cells on bone windows, because soft-tissue windows sometimes obscure the small mastoid air spaces. As with sinusitis, CT findings of fluid in mastoid air cells must be clinically correlated with signs and sympoms to determine their significance.

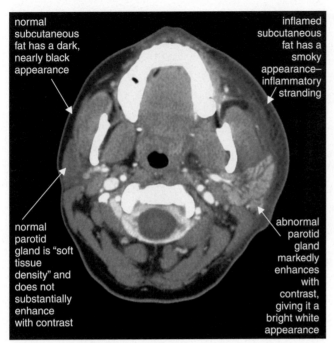

normal subcutaneous fat has a dark, nearly black appearance

inflamed subcutaneous fat has a smoky appearance—inflammatory stranding

normal parotid gland is "soft tissue density" and does not substantially enhance with contrast

abnormal parotid gland markedly enhances with contrast, giving it a bright white appearance

Figure 2-35. Parotitis with overlying cellulitis. This 29-year-old female presented with 2 days of left face and neck swelling, tenderness, and erythema. CT of the face and neck was performed with administration of intravenous (IV) contrast. The image demonstrates enlargement and enhancement of the left parotid gland consistent with sialoadenitis. Compare the abnormal left parotid gland with the normal right parotid gland, which has nearly the same soft-tissue density as adjacent masseter muscle. The abnormal gland enhances due to increased blood flow and inflammatory vascular permeability. Soft-tissue swelling and stranding in the subcutaneous fat are also seen on the left side—again, compare to the normal right side. The CT demonstrated no drainable abscess, and the patient improved with IV antibiotics (clindamycin) alone.

Evaluation of Facial Soft Tissues

Facial soft-tissue infections and masses can be evaluated well with CT with IV contrast. Neck infections are discussed separately in Chapter 4. IV contrast provides enhancement of inflamed tissues, abscesses, and neoplastic masses, as described earlier. Figure 2-35 demonstrates a CT scan of a patient presenting with significant facial swelling. CT confirmed parotitis, as well as surrounding cellulitis. Soft-tissue pathology is best viewed (no surprise) using soft-tissue windows. Axial views may be sufficient, although review of coronal views is prudent.

CLINICAL QUESTIONS IN IMAGING FOLLOWING FACIAL TRAUMA

Who Needs Facial Imaging? Does a Clinical Decision Rule Exist for Facial Trauma?

Facial fractures are common following blunt trauma. Approximately 12% of trauma patients requiring a head CT will have a facial fracture, and 50% of patients with one fracture will have multiple fractures.[4] Well-derived and validated clinical decision rules for facial imaging do not exist. A number of small retrospective

studies have evaluated physical examination findings, that might predict the presence of fractures. Lip laceration, intraoral laceration, periorbital contusion, subconjunctival hemorrhage, and nasal laceration were associated with facial fractures found on CT scan, and the study authors recommended that the presence of these findings be used to determine the need for facial CT.[4-5] However, the weak associations identified in these studies mean that the presence or absence of these findings does not alter the pretest probability of injury to a degree that should drive our medical decision making. For example, extremity fractures were also statistically associated with facial fractures, but clearly the presence of an extremity fracture should not lead to facial CT in a patient without evidence of facial injury. A retrospective study published in the *Journal of Trauma* suggests that physical examination in alert patients detects most facial fractures (91.5%), and that radiographic findings altered management in a minority of patients. Unfortunately, methodologic flaws make this study unreliable. This was a retrospective chart review with no clearly described methods. It is uncertain how the researchers determined whether physical exam had revealed a fracture and, if so, what examination maneuvers or assessments allowed fractures to be recognized. The authors do not describe how they determined the role of diagnostic imaging findings in treatment decisions.[6]

What does this mean in practice? For the moment, the decision to perform facial imaging after trauma depends on your experienced assessment of the likelihood of a fracture, based on the aggregate of many factors, including the mechanism of injury, severity of exam findings, and the planned disposition of the patient. Can the patient receive follow-up if symptoms do not improve? Is a symptom debilitating (e.g., inability to open the mouth sufficiently to chew)? Your clinical gestalt will allow you to categorize the patient as high or low risk.

How Sensitive Is the Routine Noncontrast Head CT for Facial Fractures? If Head CT Is Performed for Evaluation of Intracranial Injury, Is a Dedicated Facial CT Required? Are Facial Reconstructions Required, or Is Review of the Axial Head CT Images Sufficient? Bottom Line: Does a Negative Head CT Rule Out Facial Fracture?

The sensitivity of routine noncontrast head CT to detect facial fractures is excellent when compared with dedicated facial CT, though occasional minimally or nondisplaced fractures may be missed if dedicated facial CT is not obtained (Table 2-3). Review of axial slices alone has a very high sensitivity, compared with additional review of coronal slices. For nonnasal midface fractures, one emergency department retrospective study found that axial noncontrast head CT at 10-mm slice thickness

TABLE 2-3. Diagnostic Tests for Midface Nonnasal Fractures

	Sensitivity	Specificity
Noncontrast head CT axial images	90%–100%	95%
Coronal reconstructions from axial facial CT	97%	Not reported
True facial CT with axial and coronal reconstructions	100%*	100%*

*Gold standard, assumed to be 100% sensitive and specific.

had a sensitivity of 90%, with a 95% confidence interval (CI) of 79% to 96%, and specificity of 95% (95% CI = 84%-95%).[7] When coronal reconstructions are generated from axially acquired images using fine (1.25 mm) slice thickness, the sensitivity of CT is 97% for facial fractures, compared with coronally acquired images.[1] Another retrospective study found that the sensitivity for facial fracture of routine noncontrast axial head CT images at 8-mm slice thickness was 100% when findings of an air–fluid level within the paranasal sinuses or fractures of the maxillary, orbital, or zygomatic bones were assessed. Facial fractures were ruled out by the absence of all of these findings.[8]

Does a Negative Facial CT Rule Out Intracranial Injury In a Patient with Facial Trauma?

We already reviewed studies suggesting that a normal head CT can rule out facial fracture. But the reverse is not true: a normal facial CT alone does not rule out intracranial injury, because the field of view of the scan is limited and does not include the entire brain and calvarium. Indications for head CT are reviewed in Chapter 1. If both brain and facial injuries must be ruled out, and if only one CT can be performed, head CT is the better choice to evaluate both brain and facial injuries.

Does Facial Trauma Predict Brain or Spine Injuries? If Facial CT Is Positive, Should Brain CT be Ordered?

The presence of some types of facial fractures increases the odds of concomitant skull base fracture and may be an indication for head CT. A single study found an increased risk of skull base fractures in patients with orbital rim and wall fractures, although this did not reach statistical significance. Orbital floor and maxillary and zygomatic arch fractures do not appear predictive of skull base fracture. Mandible and nasal fractures are rarely associated with skull base fractures. Increasing numbers of facial fractures increase the risk of coexisting skull base fracture—in one study, 21% of patients with one facial fracture had skull base fracture, whereas more than 30% of patients with two or three facial fractures had skull base fracture.[9] Consider brain imaging if multiple facial fractures are present. As discussed in detail in Chapter 1, the Canadian CT Head Rule does not automatically require head CT for isolated blunt facial trauma unless findings of skull fracture, such as Battle's sign, raccoon eyes, or cerebrospinal fluid otorrhea or rhinorrhea, are present.[10] In contrast, the New Orleans Criteria (echoed in the American College of Emergency Physicians clinical policy for blunt head trauma) call for CT of the head when any "evidence of trauma above the clavicles" is present.[11-12]

How Does the Sensitivity of X-ray Compare to CT for Facial Fracture? Is there Still a Role for Plain Film in the Age of CT?

Facial x-rays have only moderate sensitivity as a screening test for midface fracture, based on limited studies. A systematic review performed in the Best Evidence Topics series found only five relevant studies to address this question.[13] The reported sensitivity of facial x-rays for fractures ranged from 88.6% to 90.9%, although several of the studies had an inadequate or no gold standard, casting doubt on these numbers. One study investigated the sensitivity of a single OM15 view (occipitomental view, taken at 15 degrees), compared with the addition of an OM30 and lateral view. An OM15 x-ray had a sensitivity of 87.5%, with a specificity of 83%. The addition of an OM30 and lateral view increased the specificity to 97% but did not enhance sensitivity. The study authors point out a 50% reduction in use of x-ray and radiation exposures by use of a single OM15 view, omitting the lateral and OM30 views. However, this study was biased by a single reviewer who knew the study hypothesis and may have underestimated the additional yield of the OM30 and lateral views.[14]

Strangely, few studies have directly compared x-ray and CT. A study of 40 consecutive patients undergoing facial x-ray and CT showed the two methods to be equivalent for the diagnosis of zygomatic arch fractures, while CT was superior for orbital and maxillary fractures. This study has no independent gold standard, so the sensitivity of CT cannot be conclusively determined.[15]

A study in 1999 found that 70% of emergency department patients undergoing imaging for blunt facial trauma at Emory University in Atlanta, Georgia, underwent x-ray as the primary imaging study and 30% underwent primary CT. Patients undergoing primary facial CT were more likely to have at least one fracture detected (57% vs. 26%). This may reflect greater sensitivity of CT or selection bias, with patients judged by the emergency physician to be at high risk of fracture being chosen for CT first. Physicians may have opted to perform x-ray first in patients with low pretest probability of fracture. Of patients with a fracture detected on plain film, 29% underwent subsequent CT. Facial imaging charges are discussed later.

Is Diagnostic Imaging Required for Suspected Nasal Bone Fractures?

Treatment decisions for nasal bone fractures are typically based on the presence of external nasal deformity. The presence of nasal bone fractures correlates poorly with physical exam deformity. *Consequently, nasal x-rays are unnecessary and not recommended for the evaluation of patients with nasal trauma.*[16] Despite this, a practice survey in England found that 57.9% of doctors in accident and emergency departments reported using nasal x-rays for a variety of reasons, including medicolegal, detection of unsuspected nasal fracture, compound nasal fracture, and foreign body detection.[17] Surveys in Canada found similar rates of utilization, despite guidelines recommending against use of nasal x-rays.[18] Introduction of a "no x-ray" policy for nasal bone fractures reduces unnecessary x-ray use.[19] Given that CT scan is more costly than and involves a much higher radiation exposure than does x-ray, CT should never be ordered for the sole indication of evaluation of potential nasal bone fracture.

Is Panoramic X-Ray Better than CT for Mandibular Fractures?

Panorex has been the historical gold standard for the diagnosis of mandibular fractures. The technique allows projection of the curved structure of the mandible onto the plane of an x-ray film or digital detector, eliminating overlap of the mandibular rami, which renders standard anterior–posterior and lateral radiographs of the mandible difficult to interpret. CT scan is also useful in the diagnosis of mandibular fractures and has the advantage of being capable of diagnosing other traumatic injuries, including other facial, intracranial, and spinal injuries. Eliminating Panorex from the trauma workup could be valuable in the multitrauma patient, eliminating the need for the patient to be transported for additional diagnostic imaging when CT is already being employed for evaluation of other injuries. A recent study comparing Panorex and helical CT found that the two tests identify similar numbers of fractures. However, CT offered superior interobserver agreement on fracture number and location (96% for CT vs. 91% for Panorex). CT may be considered the new gold standard for radiographic evaluation of mandibular fractures, although Panorex is a reasonable alternative when other injuries to the head and face are not suspected.[20] Panorex delivers about 8 mrem (8.0×10^{-5} Sv) and so carries a very low radiation exposure compared with facial CT, which has a dose of around 1 to 6 mSv depending on the exact CT protocol. Cancer risk depends on radiation dose, tissue sensitivity, and age at exposure. Radiation doses in the range seen with facial CT are predicted to induce cancers at a rate of 1 in 4000 to 1 in 15,000, while doses from Panorex, being about 100-fold lower, would be associated with an extremely low risk of cancer, 1 in 40,000 to 1 in 1,500,000.[20a]

When Should Orbital Imaging Be Performed for a Foreign Body? How Are Orbital Foreign Bodies Best Detected?

Globe injuries from penetrating foreign bodies represent an obvious high-risk injury due to risk of ocular infection, inflammation-mediated injury, and blindness. These injuries have a poor prognosis even when rapidly diagnosed. X-ray can detect small, high-density foreign bodies such as metal fragments with moderate sensitivity. In study of 204 patients with a suspected foreign body, only 70% of intraorbital foreign bodies were detected by x-ray, compared with 100% by CT.[29] High-density orbital foreign bodies may be detected with high sensitivity on CT, but organic foreign bodies such as wood may be difficult to detect on CT or x-ray, because they have similar density to fat and air. MRI is more sensitive and should be used when an organic foreign body is suspected but not visualized on CT.[23] Wood is sometimes visualized on orbital CT.[30] Very-high-density materials such as metal can create streak artifact on CT, which may make determination of their exact size and location more difficult. Ultrasound is useful for evaluation of the globe but should be used with extreme care to evaluate suspected globe rupture, because pressure exerted during the ultrasound examination could result in herniation of globe contents.

If an Intraorbital Foreign Body Is Seen on X-Ray, Does CT Provide Useful Additional Information?

CT may be unnecessary when x-ray localizes a single intraorbital foreign body and if exam findings do not suggest ocular penetration. In addition, if exam findings are highly suggestive of ocular penetration and x-ray confirms a metallic foreign body, operative exploration is required and CT may play a limited role. If questions remain about addition radiolucent foreign bodies not seen on x-ray, CT may be useful.

CLINICAL QUESTIONS IN FACIAL IMAGING WHEN NO HISTORY OF TRAUMA IS PRESENT

Facial imaging is often used to assess patients with nontraumatic pain, swelling, and erythema. The range of potential pathology is broad but generally may include infections, vascular abnormalities, and malignancies. CT is the most useful emergency department imaging modality in most cases, although ultrasound can be used to identify fluid collections. MRI is not usually ordered for this indication in the emergency department due to limited availability and long scan times. We review some of the more common clinical scenarios here, with CT findings demonstrated in the interpretation section earlier in this chapter.

When is CT Needed for Suspected Orbital Cellulitis?

CT is often used to distinguish orbital from periorbital cellulitis. As inflammation or frank abscess develops within the orbit, rising pressure may be exerted on the globe, optic nerve, and extraocular muscles. Increased pressure results in the classic exam findings of orbital cellulitis, which include proptosis, pain with eye movements, restriction of eye movements or frank ophthalmoplegia, diplopia, and change in vision with blurred or diminished visual acuity. The pupil may become unreactive as optic nerve compression increases. Periorbital erythema and edema alone are not suggestive of orbital cellulitis. No large high-quality studies have been conducted to determine the exam findings most predictive of postseptal (orbital) cellulitis. Multiple small retrospective studies have reported findings such as diplopia, ophthalmoplegia, and proptosis to be statistically associated with orbital cellulitis.[21-24] A guideline published in *Clinical Otolaryngology* lists indications for CT, including neurologic abnormalities, inability to assess the eye due to gross periorbital edema, gross proptosis, ophthalmoplegia, abnormal pupillary response, worsening visual acuity or loss of color vision, bilateral eye involvement, failure to improve after 24 hours of therapy for periorbital cellulitis, and recurrent fever not resolved by 36 hours of therapy.[25] The guideline authors recommend against CT unless one or more of these findings is present.

What Kind of CT Should Be Ordered for Orbital Cellulitis?

CT for detection of orbital cellulitis should be performed with IV contrast unless the patient has a contraindication (renal insufficiency or dye allergy). Generally, the CT should include both the orbits and the paranasal sinuses, as these are the source of infection in up to 90% of cases.[21]

What Are the CT Findings of Orbital Cellulitis?

The findings of orbital cellulitis are illustrated in the section on CT interpretation at the beginning of the chapter. What is the evidence for these findings? CT findings of orbital cellulitis include diffuse orbital fat infiltration (increased density or stranding) (seen in 24%), subperiosteal abscess (62%), and orbital abscess (13%).[26] Orbital cellulitis can be a consequence of adjacent sinusitis or odontogenic infections, so the ethmoid and maxillary sinuses should be inspected for signs of sinusitis. The maxillary teeth should be inspected for periapical lucency suggesting dental abscess.[27] Rarely, complications such as thrombosis of the superior ophthalmic vein

may occur. CT with IV contrast can reveal this finding, and orbital MRI with gadolinium enhancement and fat suppression can further delineate this complication.[28]

Is CT Required for the Evaluation of Sinusitis?

CT is not routinely recommended for the diagnosis of sinus infections, unless complications such as orbital infection or intracranial extension are suspected. Guidelines published by the American Academy of Otolaryngology (Head and Neck Surgery) in 2007 support avoiding routine CT.[31] The CT findings of bacterial sinusitis are relatively nonspecific, including air–fluid levels and mucosal thickening, which may be present in allergic or viral sinusitis. While these findings may be quite specific for bacterial infection in the setting of concurrent clinical findings such as facial swelling and erythema, facial pain, fever, and purulent nasal discharge, it is not clear that patient outcomes are changed by diagnostic CT in this scenario. Antibiotic therapy without CT may be appropriate, with guidelines suggesting that symptoms should be present for 10 days beyond the onset of upper respiratory symptoms. Multiple studies suggest that sinus abnormalities noted on CT in an asymptomatic patient (e.g., mucosal thickening and air–fluid levels in a patient undergoing head CT following head trauma) may not indicate acute sinus infection, as they occur incidentally in more than 40% of subjects.[32-33] The Lund-MacKay scoring system evaluates sinus abnormalities on CT in a standardized fashion. Each of five sinuses (anterior ethmoid, posterior ethmoid, maxillary, frontal, and sphenoid) is scored on the following scale: 0 (no opacification), 1 (partial opacification), or 2 (complete opacification). The ostiomeatal complex is scored as 0 (not occluded) or 2 (occluded). The right and left sides are scored independently, for a total score ranging from 0 to 24. Using a Lund-MacKay score of 2 as the cutoff, sensitivity is 94% but specificity is only 41%, meaning that false positive outnumber true positives. At a Lund score of 4, specificity increase to 59%, but sensitivity falls to 85%.

Other authors contend that abnormal sinus CT results should not occur in normal, healthy patients. A retrospective study, they assessed three groups of patients: asymptomatic patients (defined as emergency department patients undergoing CT for indications presumably unrelated to sinus disease, such as syncope, alerted mental status, or stroke), acute headache patients (undergoing CT in the emergency department for assessment of acute headache), and chronically symptomatic patients (being evaluated in an otolaryngology clinic). Of asymptomatic patients, 3% had abnormal CT sinus findings, compared with 5.5% of acutely symptomatic patients and 64% of chronically symptomatic patients.[36] The validity of these findings is questionable. This retrospective review identified patients by ICD9 ninth revision, code, and no additional clinical features were assessed. For example, although patients undergoing CT head for acute headache had a higher rate of sinus abnormalities, it is not clear that sinus disease was the cause of the patients' acute headaches. Clinical guidelines require the presence of 10 days of symptoms for the diagnosis of acute bacterial sinusitis, and it is possible that the CT findings were actually incidental in patients presenting with headaches of other etiologies. The investigators did not review the charts for duration of symptoms or for fever, facial swelling, or nasal discharge. No confirmatory bacterial cultures were obtained in the asymptomatic or acutely symptomatic groups, so the contention that the sinus findings in the second group represent acute sinusitis is unconfirmed.

Are X-Rays Useful in Detection of Nasal Foreign Bodies?

X-rays for detection of nasal foreign bodies are likely to have a low yield. A study of pediatric patients presenting with suspected nasal foreign bodies or unilateral nasal discharge found that plastic beads, foam, paper and tissue fragments, and food matter accounted for 65% of foreign bodies—and none of these is likely to be identified on x-ray. In one small study, 7% of patients had a nasal button battery. The study's authors recommended x-ray when a suspected foreign body is not visible on physical exam due to potential increased morbidity from prolonged presence of button batteries.[37] CT can visualize nasal foreign bodies but may not be required—it may be more practical to examine the nose directly with nasopharyngoscopy or nasal speculum if doubts remain.

What is the Cost of Facial Imaging?

Facial CT scan is more costly than facial x-ray (Table 2-4).[38] Arguments can be made for two strategies: facial bone x-ray first in low-risk patients (assessed clinically as unlikely to have fracture) and CT first in high-risk patients very likely to have fractures based on examination. In one study, patients undergoing facial x-ray as the first imaging test had an average imaging cost of $258, versus $1166 for patients undergoing CT first. If imaging costs are considered on a per-case-of-fracture basis (per patient having at least one facial fracture), an x-ray-first strategy cost $978, versus $2048 for a CT-first strategy. Clearly there is no role for facial x-ray in a patient considered to have very substantial risk of facial fracture, as CT would undoubtedly be performed following abnormal facial x-ray. More recent studies suggest facial CT alone has a cost of between $850 and $1450.[1,5,8] Coronal reconstructions from head CT are somewhat cheaper, around $400 (in addition to the standard cost of head CT).[1] Of course, economic evaluations are complicated by the number of different charges and costs that may

TABLE 2-4. Hospital Charges for Facial Imaging*

Procedure	Cost
Orbital bone x-ray series	$76.23
Facial bone x-ray series	$100.89
Facial computed tomography	$722.70
Coronal and sagittal reconstructions	$776.16

Adapted from Pearl WS. Facial imaging in an urban emergency department. *Am J Emerg Med* 17:235–237, 1999.
*In 1997 U.S. dollars.

occur in different practice settings. Medicare reimburses only about $214 for facial CT, so cost savings would be substantially less when using this figure for comparison.[7] As discussed earlier, if a patient requires CT of the head for other clinical reasons, it may be reasonable to avoid any dedicated facial imaging and to review bone windows from axial head CT for fractures, with no additional cost.

How Much Time Is Required for Facial Imaging?

Facial CT is very rapid with modern CT scanners, taking less than 1 minute. Facial CT is likely more rapid than facial x-ray for most patients.

How Much Radiation Exposure Occurs With Facial CT?

Radiation exposures from facial CT are significant, particularly because the field of view includes the lens of the eye and thyroid. In one study, dedicated axially and coronally acquired CT images of the face delivered 11.7 cGy to the orbit. Axially acquired images alone with reformatted coronal images deliver 6.7 cGy to the orbit.[1] The ocular lens is susceptible to radiation-induced cataracts.[39-44] The thyroid is susceptible to radiation-induced cancers, albeit at a very low rate, estimated to be between 4 and 65 per 1 million patients undergoing CT scan of the head.[45] As a consequence, facial CT should be performed only when moderate suspicion for a clinically important condition exists. If CT is not performed, the patient can be counseled about the possibility of an undiagnosed injury and indications for follow-up.

SUMMARY

CT is the most informative modality for facial imaging, with x-rays playing a limited screening role due to poor sensitivity. Indications for facial imaging have not undergone rigorous study, and clinical judgment will continue to play an important role in identifying patients requiring imaging. Because of the cost and radiation exposure from CT, emergency physicians should carefully consider whether CT findings are likely to change management before obtaining facial imaging.

CHAPTER 3 Imaging the Cervical, Thoracic, and Lumbar Spine

Joshua Broder, MD, FACEP

In this chapter, we discuss imaging of the cervical, thoracic, and lumbar spine. Although differences exist, many common themes are shared in both the selection and the interpretation of diagnostic studies for all regions of the spine. Our discussion of all spinal regions starts with interpretation of images, with a focus on computed tomography (CT) scan. We correlate CT findings with x-ray when possible, and we demonstrate associated soft-tissue abnormalities identified on magnetic resonance imaging (MRI). Don't be daunted by the number of figures in this chapter—we explore injuries and nontraumatic spinal pathology in many imaging planes and in multiple modalities to maximize your three-dimensional understanding. The figure captions are designed to allow the figures to stand alone, so we spend relatively little time discussing specific fracture patterns in the text. The figures in the chapter span a range of important spinal pathology, moving from cephalad to caudad. The list in Table 3-1 can guide you to the relevant figure, where diagnostic features are discussed in detail.

In many ways, the more difficult task for the emergency physician is not the interpretation of the image but the decision to image the spine. We review two well-validated clinical decision rules (CDRs) that can identify patients at low risk of cervical spine injury who do not require any imaging. Similar decision instruments can identify patients who require thoracic and lumbar imaging.

Imaging of the spine has undergone a revolution with the advent of multidetector CT with multiplanar reconstructions. We review the evidence for use of CT and x-ray, comparing their sensitivity for detection of fractures. Remarkably, the latest version of the American College of Radiology (ACR) Appropriate Guidelines for Imaging of Suspected Spine Trauma (2009) advocates thin-section CT as the primary screening study for suspected cervical spine injury in adults, removing plain radiography (x-ray) from this position. The three-view radiograph that has been the long-standing screening test in the emergency department is now recommended by the ACR "only when CT is not readily available."[1] Radiography is described in this document as "not … a substitute for CT."[1] The ACR cites a lack of evidence for recommendations of CT or x-ray as the primary screening tool for suspected cervical spine injury in children. We discuss the radiation burden and cost of cervical CT. The new ACR recommendation for a CT-first strategy guarantees an increase in the radiation exposure resulting from any screening for cervical spine injury. Consequently, an even greater emphasis should be placed on applying reliable CDRs. Let's begin our discussion with the cervical spine, followed by a parallel discussion of the thoracic and lumbar spine.

EPIDEMIOLOGY OF CERVICAL SPINE INJURY

Cervical spine injuries occur in approximately 2% to 4% of blunt trauma cases, and diagnostic imaging plays a pivotal role in the evaluation of patients for these potentially life-threatening or seriously debilitating injuries. In addition, nontraumatic cervical spine pathology occasionally requires imaging in the emergency department. This evaluation differs from the evaluation in trauma, as fractures or other bony pathology may not be present. The incidence of cervical injuries is relatively independent of the setting—level I, II, and III trauma centers (the U.S. designation) all encounter cervical spine injuries with similar frequency, and emergency physicians must be intimately familiar with the imaging required to diagnose these dangerous injuries. In one study of 165 U.S. medical centers involving 111,219 patients, 4.3% of patients had injuries, at similar rates, in both academic and nonacademic centers, regardless of trauma center type (I through III).[2] The National Emergency X-radiography Utilization Study group, which is discussed in more detail later in regard to its CDR, found similar rates of injury: 2.4% of 34,069 patients in 21 U.S. medical centers.[3-5]

IMAGING THE CERVICAL SPINE FOLLOWING TRAUMA: APPLICATION AND INTERPRETATION OF IMAGING MODALITIES

Cervical spine imaging following trauma must perform a number of clinical functions. These include identification of fractures, ligamentous injuries, and injuries to neurologic structures, including the spinal cord and nerve roots. Diagnostic modalities for cervical spine imaging are plain film, CT scan, and MRI. We consider

TABLE 3-1. Imaging Findings and Related Figure Numbers

Content	Figure Number
Three-dimensional CT reconstructions of the normal cervical spine	3-1 through 3-7
X-rays of the normal cervical spine • Lateral • AP • Odontoid • Swimmer's view • Flexion–extension	3-8 through 3-13, 3-19, 3-20 3-8 and 3-14 3-8, 3-15, and 3-16, 3-21 3-17 3-18
Normal sagittal CT views	3-19 and 3-20
Normal coronal CT view	3-21
Normal axial view	3-22
Occipital condyle fractures	3-24 through 3-27
C1 burst (Jefferson) fractures	3-28 through 3-31
Atlantoaxial (C1-C2) rotary fixations	3-32 through 3-38
C1 posterior arch fracture	3-39
C2 dens fractures, type II	3-40 through 3-43
C2 dens fractures, type III	3-44 through 3-48
Hangman's fractures of C2	3-49 through 3-57
Transverse process fractures	3-58 and 3-98
Cervical burst compression fractures	3-59 through 3-62
Teardrop flexion fractures	3-63 through 3-66
Jumped facets, bilateral and unilateral	3-67 through 3-75
Cervical facet fractures with spinal cord injury on MRI	3-76 and 3-77
Cervical lamina fractures	3-78 through 3-80
Acute cervical ligamentous injuries with x-ray, CT, and MRI findings	3-81 through 3-84
Three-column concept of spinal stability	3-85
T2 corner avulsion fractures (extension teardrop)	3-86 and 3-87
Thoracolumbar compression and burst fractures	3-88 through 3-101
Chance fractures	3-99 through 3-101
Thoracic spine metastatic disease with cord compression	3-102 through 3-104
Vertebral osteomyelitis and discitis	3-105 through 3-107
Spinal epidural abscesses	3-108 through 3-110, 3-115, and 3-116
Vertebral tuberculosis (Pott's disease)	3-111 through 3-116
Degenerative joint disease and disc herniation	3-117 through 3-120
Cauda equina, normal and compression	3-119 and 3-120
Osteopetrosis	3-121 and 3-122
Ankylosing spondylitis	3-123 through 3-127
Spinal cord injuries on MRI	3-77 and 3-127
Penetrating spinal trauma	3-128 through 3-131
Motion artifact on MRI	3-132
Syrinx	3-133
Pseudosubluxation	3-134 and 3-135

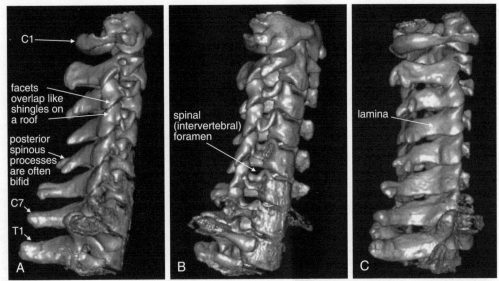

Figure 3-1. Lateral and oblique three-dimensional views of the normal cervical spine. This three-dimensional reconstruction of the cervical spine was generated from standard computed tomography axial images using 1.25-mm slice thickness. Images like this are not routinely reviewed by emergency physicians, but they provide a good starting point for our discussion of cervical spine imaging. **A,** A lateral view, showing the normal relationship of C1 through T1 vertebrae. Compare this with the lateral x-ray in Figures 3-8 and 3-9. Note the overlap of the cervical facet joints, like shingles on a roof. **B,** An anterior oblique view, similar in perspective to an oblique x-ray view sometimes obtained to inspect for narrowing of the spinal foramen through which spinal nerves exit. **C,** A posterior oblique view. This has no routine x-ray equivalent but demonstrates the spinal lamina and posterior processes.

each of these in turn, with examples of the types of pathology detected or ruled out and the limitations of each technique. Although the ACR now recommends CT rather than x-ray as the primary screening tool in adults, plain x-ray is still widely used in children, and CT is not available in all settings. We review the interpretation of x-rays and CT, recognizing that some patients may not undergo both tests. At this time, MRI is more rarely interpreted by emergency physicians, and we thus review MRI interpretation in less detail.

Evaluating for Fracture or Dislocation with Plain X-ray

Plain films in a neutral anatomic position with the patient immobilized in a cervical collar have long been the standard test to evaluate for bony fractures and dislocations. Although plain x-rays are still widely used, CT has increasingly become the primary modality for evaluation of fracture due to its higher sensitivity. Nonetheless, plain x-rays continue to play an important role in screening for fractures. Because of their limited sensitivity, plain x-rays should not be used to "rule out fracture" in cases with a high pretest probability of cervical spine injury.

Plain x-rays of the cervical spine identify fractures by three major methods:

- Direct visualization of fractures (discontinuity of the bony cortex)
- Misalignment of bony structures, suggesting possible fracture or dislocation
- Soft-tissue changes, suggesting underlying fracture

Plain x-rays do not directly identify abnormalities of soft tissues such as spinal ligaments, although gross misalignment of vertebral bodies almost always indicates concurrent ligamentous injury. Plain x-rays also do not directly identify spinal cord injuries, although x-ray abnormalities showing impingement upon the spinal canal imply cord impingement. Direct visualization of ligamentous and cord injuries requires MRI. CT scan is useful in delineating fractures and dislocations in greater detail. As described later, CT with multiplanar reconstructions can visualize some soft-tissue injuries and, when normal, indicates a low likelihood of unstable cervical spine injury.

Standard Plain X-ray, Three Views

Figures 3-1 through 3-7 demonstrate three-dimensional CT models of the cervical spine. Review these, as they will assist you in understanding cervical spine anatomy and the information to be gleaned from the two-dimensional projections obtained in plain x-ray. An adequate cervical spine plain x-ray series consists of three images: a lateral, an anterior–posterior (AP), and an open-mouth odontoid view (Figure 3-8). It is extremely important that adequate x-rays are obtained to maximize the sensitivity of this technique.

Normal Features of the Lateral X-ray. The lateral x-ray (Figures 3-8 through 3-13; see also 3-19 and 3-20) provides information about gross fractures, as well as alignment of vertebral bodies relative to one another. In addition, prevertebral soft tissue widening may suggest soft-tissue hematoma or swelling, a surrogate marker of fractures that may themselves be invisible on plain

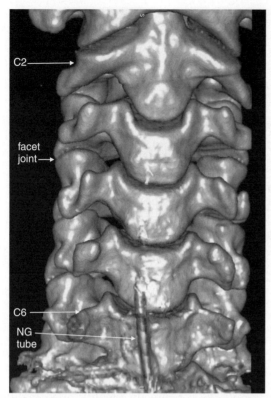

Figure 3-2. Anterior three-dimensional view of the normal cervical spine. This three-dimensional reconstruction from axial cervical spine images shares the same perspective with an anterior–posterior x-ray or coronal computed tomography (CT) views. The C1 vertebrae is cropped from this image—we look at C1 in detail in Figure 3-3. C7 and T1 are also not in this image—as we discuss later, these must be seen in an x-ray series to allow adequate evaluation of the cervical spine. Note how the facet joints are not horizontal but slope caudad from anterior to posterior. As a result, these joints are not fully seen in a single axial CT image, as you will see in future figures. Also note how the spacing of vertebral bodies is symmetrical. The lower portion of this reconstruction shows artifacts from a nasogastric (NG) tube.

film. The x-ray must visualize the cervical spine from the skull base to the C7-T1 (cervical seventh vertebra–thoracic first vertebra) junction. This is not an arbitrary definition of an adequate plain film. An x-ray that fails to visualize the entire cervical spine and its junctions with the adjacent skull and thoracic spine may miss injuries. Widening of the space between the C1 vertebra and the skull base may be a subtle indication of a devastating occipital–cervical dissociation—although this injury is usually clinically evident with a moribund patient with quadriplegia. At the caudad end of the cervical spine, it is essential to visualize the C7-T1 junction to avoid missing subluxation of these vertebral bodies relative to one another. This injury is made more likely by the sudden change in the mobility of the spine, from the highly mobile cervical spine to the relative immobile thoracic spine, which is supported by the buttresses of the ribs.

A normal lateral cervical spine image shows a gentle cervical lordosis—a curve with its convex border oriented anteriorly (see Figure 3-10). This lordosis may be straightened slightly due to the presence of the cervical collar. When all cervical vertebrae are intact and in normal alignment with one another, this cervical lordosis results in four parallel curved lines, for which the lateral x-ray should be inspected (the numbered lines in Figure 3-10):

1. The anterior longitudinal ligament line, which follows the anterior border of the vertebral bodies.
2. The posterior longitudinal ligament line, which follows the posterior border of the vertebral bodies.
3. The spinolaminar line, which follows the anterior border of the posterior spinous processes, where the lamina converge.
4. The spinous processes line, which follows the posterior border of the posterior spinous processes. It does not fully parallel the other lines because of the increasing length of the spinous processes from C1 to C7. The space between the posterior longitudinal ligament line and the spinolaminar line is the spinal canal. If these lines are intact and parallel, the spinal canal should be intact, and the spinal cord should be safely contained within it.

In addition, the lateral film should be examined with attention to the following:

5. The predental space (see Figure 3-11), which separates the dens from the anterior ring of C1. Widening suggests dens or C1 ring fracture, or subluxation of the transverse ligament, which binds the dens to the anterior ring of C1. In adults, this space should be no more than 3 mm, and in children it should be no more than 4 to 5 mm.
6. Prevertebral soft tissues (see Figure 3-12). Widening suggests cervical spine injury with soft-tissue swelling or hematoma. In adults, this distance should be less than 7 mm at C2 and less than 5 mm at C3 and C4. In children, a commonly cited distance is less than half the width of the adjacent vertebral body. False widening may occur in children under the age of 2 years if the image is obtained during expiration. Below C4, the airway moves anteriorly, the esophagus occupies the prevertebral space, and soft-tissue widths vary considerably, usually between 10 and 20 mm in adults. Soft-tissue width exceeding the width of the adjacent vertebral body suggests injury.
7. The spinal facet joints (Figure 3-13), which should overlap like shingles on a roof. Decreased overlap can occur in the case of a jumped or perched facet joint.
8. Widening of the distance between posterior spinous processes, which can indicate fracture or ligamentous injury.

Normal Features of the Anterior-posterior X-ray. The AP x-ray (Figure 3-14) provides information about lateral alignment of vertebral bodies with one another. A small number of additional fractures (particularly

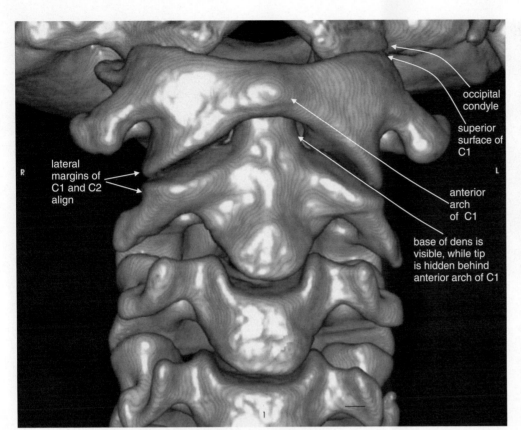

Figure 3-3. C1 and C2 view of the normal cervical spine. This three-dimensional reconstruction from computed tomography (CT) axial images focuses on the occipital–cervical junction and the C1-2 (atlantoaxial) junction. Note how the occipital condyles articulate with the superior surface of C1. The tip of the dens is hidden from view behind the anterior arch of C1. Two-dimensional slices can be more useful in identifying injuries because superficial structures do not obscure the view of deeper structures. The lateral margins of C1 and C2 align. These features will prove important in our discussions of fractures of this region in later figures. The author generated this figure from a standard cervical CT scan using open-source software called OsiriX.

Labels in figure: occipital condyle; superior surface of C1; anterior arch of C1; base of dens is visible, while tip is hidden behind anterior arch of C1; lateral margins of C1 and C2 align; R; L

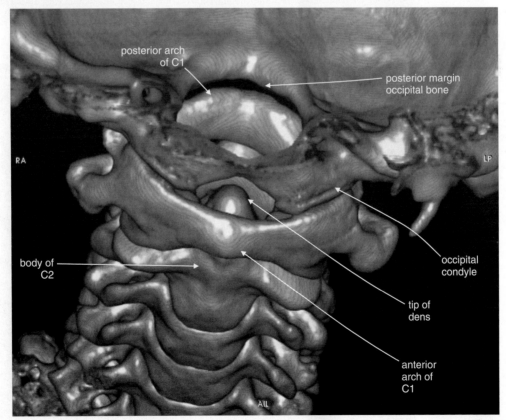

Labels in figure: posterior arch of C1; posterior margin occipital bone; occipital condyle; body of C2; tip of dens; anterior arch of C1; RA; LP; AIL

Figure 3-4. C1 and C2 view of the normal cervical spine. Again, this three-dimensional reconstruction from computed tomography (CT) axial images focuses on the occipital–cervical junction and the C1-2 (atlantoaxial) junction. Compared with Figure 3-3, the view has been shifted to look down slightly upon C1. The tip of the dens is visible behind the anterior arch of C1. The occipital condyles articulate with the superior surface of C1. The skull has been cut away in this model, allowing the posterior ring of C1 to be seen through the foramen magnum. Later in this chapter we examine injuries to this region using multiplanar cross-sectional CT images. Refer to this figure for orientation if the two-dimensional images appear confusing.

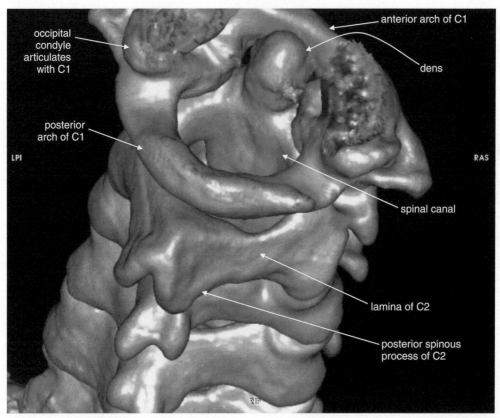

Figure 3-5. C1 and C2 view of the normal cervical spine. The skull base has been cut away nearly completely in this CT model, allowing the ring of C1 and its relationship to the dens of C2 to be seen in detail. Portions of the occipital condyles are still seen articulating with the superior surface of C1. Note that C1 does not have a true vertebral body—instead, the dens occupies the space immediately posterior to the anterior arch of C1. The posterior arch of C1 is in full view, and this perspective gives good views of the spinal canal, lamina of C2, and posterior spinous processes of C2 and more caudad vertebral bodies. C1 does not have a posterior spinous process.

Figure 3-6. C1 and C2 view of the normal cervical spine. As in Figure 3-5, this three dimensional CT model has been rotated and the skull base cut away to allow the ring of C1 and its relationship to the dens of C2 to be seen in detail. The posterior arch of C1 is in full view. The transverse ligament, which holds the dens in position against the anterior arch of C1, is partially calcified in this patient and is therefore visible.

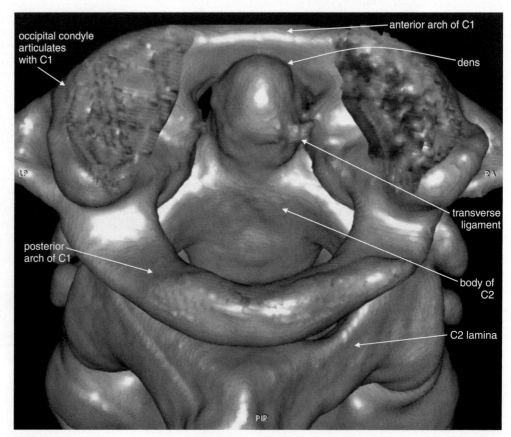

oblique fractures) may be noted on the AP x-ray, and subtle abnormalities from the lateral film may be confirmed. The posterior spinous processes should be centered in the midline and aligned with one another. The cortex of each vertebral body should be intact. The height of and spacing between adjacent vertebral bodies should be uniform.

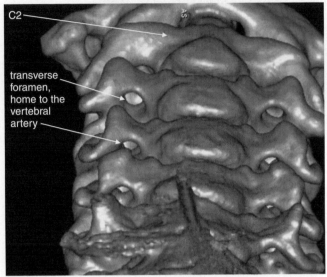

Figure 3-7. Transverse foramen (foramen transversarium). This three-dimensional CT model is oriented with the observer looking cephalad along the anterior surface of the cervical spine. A series of holes perforating the transverse processes of each vertebra can be seen—the transverse foramen. These canals house the vertebral arteries as they ascend to the brain. Fractures through the transverse processes can result in arterial injuries, as can rotational injuries such as unilateral facet dislocation and subluxation injuries such as bilateral jumped facets. These injuries are discussed in detail in later figures, illustrated with the two-dimensional multiplanar computed tomography images routinely available to emergency physicians. Use this figure to understand how fractures and malalignment of vertebral bodies can disrupt the normal canal containing the vertebral arteries.

Open-Mouth Odontoid X-ray. The open-mouth odontoid view (Figures 3-15 and 3-16) is essential for evaluation of two important injury patterns:

- Burst fractures of the C1 ring, also called Jefferson fractures
- Fractures of the odontoid process or dens, which is a structure of C2

The open-mouth odontoid view is so called because it is obtained with the patient's mouth opened as wide as possible, with the x-ray tube aimed into the open mouth. This gives a direct view of C1 and C2. Issues that may prevent adequate visualization include an obtunded or uncooperative patient who is unable to comply with this maneuver; a patient with trismus, temporomandibular joint disease, or other injuries (e.g., mandibular fractures) that prevent full opening of the mouth; and the presence of significant metal dental work. Sometimes, the cervical spine collar may restrict mouth opening too much to allow an adequate open-mouth odontoid view. When an adequate open-mouth odontoid view cannot be obtained, CT should be performed to avoid a missed injury of C1 or C2.

An adequate open-mouth odontoid view visualizes the entire dens and the lateral margins of both C1 and C2. A fully visualized dens is essential for evaluation of dens fractures. The cortex of the dens should be carefully inspected for defects. Shadows of overlying structures such as central incisors can simulate or hide fractures, so a wide-open view with no overlap of teeth with the dens is desirable. When the ring of C1 is intact, the lateral margins of C1 should align with the lateral margins of C2. When fractured, C1 typically "bursts," with the fracture fragments spreading outward. Consequently,

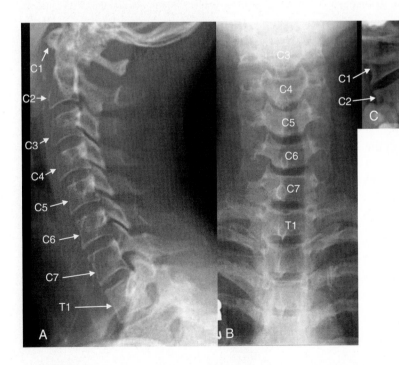

Figure 3-8. Lateral, anterior – posterior (AP) and odontoid view x-rays of the normal cervical spine. A plain x-ray cervical spine series consists of three standard views: lateral **(A)**, AP **(B)**, and odontoid **(C)**. An adequate series requires visualization of the entire cervical spine and its cephalad and caudad borders: the skull base and the first thoracic vertebral body (T1). An adequate odontoid x-ray must include the entire dens and the lateral borders of C1 and C2. We examine each of these views in more detail in the next several figures.

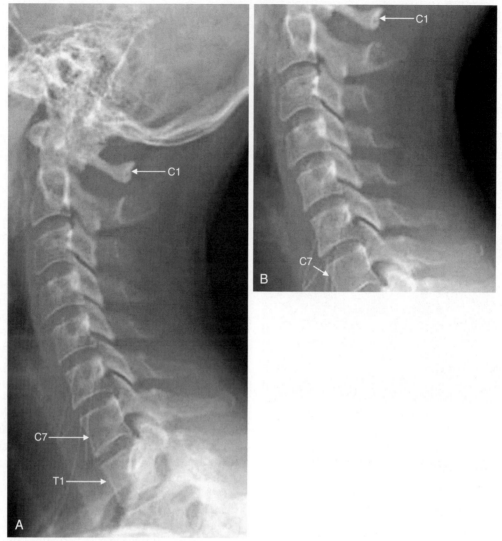

Figure 3-9. Adequate and inadequate lateral cervical spine x-rays. A, An adequate lateral cervical spine x-ray, showing the entire cervical spine and its cephalad border (the skull base) and caudad border (T1). **B,** The image is inadequate because C1 and T1 are not seen fully. Fractures or subluxation at these locations would be missed. The x-ray should be repeated, perhaps using special views such as the swimmer's view to visualize the C7-T1 junction, or computed tomography could be used.

an indirect sign of C1 fracture is misalignment of the lateral margins of C1 with the lateral margins of C2. Frequently, the lateral margins of C1 appear displaced laterally compared with the lateral margins of C2, although medial displacement of C1 is also possible. This finding may be unilateral or bilateral. When C1 is intact and the patient is facing directly forward, the distance between the dens and the medial borders of the C1 ring should be bilaterally symmetrical. When C1 is fractured, displacement of fracture fragments typically renders this distance asymmetrical. The lateral margins of C1 and C2 may be hidden by radiopaque dental fillings, especially if the patient's mouth is not fully opened.

The standard three-view series just described is sometimes augmented with additional plain x-ray views. Adding two oblique views allows visualization of the pedicles, lamina, and neural foramina. Although this

technique may be useful in selected cases, this "five-view" technique has been compared with the standard three views and does not detect additional injuries at a rate high enough to make five views a useful standard. The five-view series was insensitive (44%) compared with CT in a high-risk group of patients with altered mental status and a high rate of cervical spine injury (>10%).[6] CT should be obtained if subtle lamina, pedicle, or neural foramen injuries are suspected.

In cases in which the C7-T1 junction is not visualized on the lateral x-ray, "swimmer's" (Figure 3-17) or "traction" views may allow visualization of this region. In a swimmer's view, the patient is positioned with the arm closer to the x-ray detector raised above the head. This elevates the humeral head above the C7-T1 junction, preventing it from obscuring this area. The opposite arm is held at the patient's side, resulting in that humeral head lying

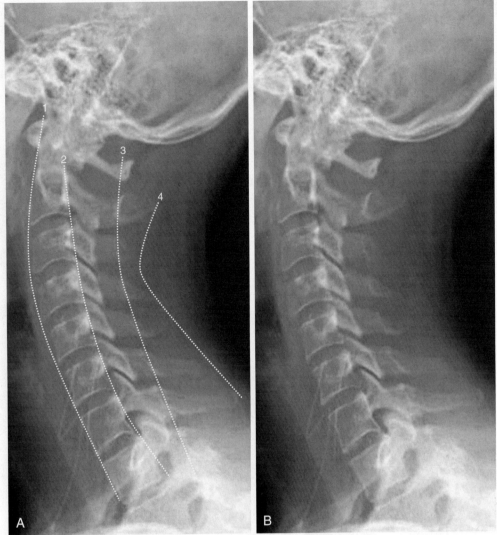

Figure 3-10. Interpretation of the lateral cervical spine x-ray. A normal lateral cervical spine x-ray, with **(A)** and without **(B)** labels. The spine should be inspected for four curved, roughly parallel lines:
1 Anterior longitudinal ligament line (follows the anterior border of the vertebral bodies)
2. Posterior longitudinal ligament line (follows the posterior border of the vertebral bodies)
3. Spinolaminar line (follows the anterior border of the posterior spinous processes, where the lamina converge)
4. Spinous processes line (follows the posterior border of the posterior spinous processes and does not fully parallel the other lines due to the increasing length of the spinous processes from C1 to C7)
The spinal canal, which houses the spinal cord, lies between lines 2 and 3.
If all lines are intact, the vertebral bodies should be properly aligned and the spinal canal should be preserved.

somewhat lower that the C7-T1 junction. Variations on this theme include having the patient raise both arms directly in front of the body or over the head. In a traction view, a health care worker pulls on the patient's arms from a position at the foot of the bed, distracting the humeral heads down to reveal the C7-T1 junction – a method now discouraged because of the possibility of worsening spinal injury. When these maneuvers do not allow adequate visualization of C7-T1, CT is indicated. In many cases, these views are skipped in favor of CT. Flexion and extension views (Figure 3-18) are sometimes obtained to assess for ligamentous instability—the evidence for these views is discussed in detail later.

Computed Tomography of the Cervical Spine

CT scan evaluates for fractures and dislocations with high sensitivity and specificity. Soft-tissue injuries are demonstrated less directly and accurately (Box 3-1). CT scan should be performed in several situations (Box 3-2):

- As a follow-up to plain x-rays to further evaluate any fracture, dislocation, or soft-tissue abnormality on x-ray.
- As a follow-up study when adequate x-rays cannot be obtained. Examples include obese patients, obtunded or intoxicated patients, and patients with pre-existing spine disease.

Figure 3-11. **Evaluation of predental space.** On lateral cervical spine x-ray, the predental space should be evaluated. Several injury patterns can widen this space. Fracture of the ring of C1 can allow the anterior portion of the ring to migrate anteriorly with respect to the dens. Dens fracture can allow posterior migration of the dens relative to the ring of C1. Subluxation of the transverse ligament can allow widening of this space. Patients with rheumatoid arthritis are at particular risk of this latter abnormality.

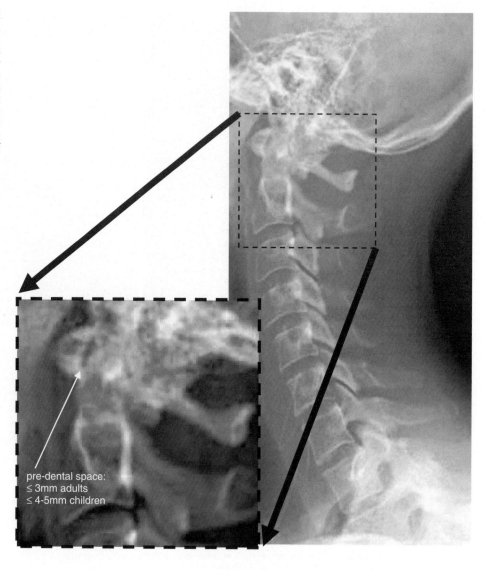

pre-dental space:
≤ 3mm adults
≤ 4-5mm children

- As the primary imaging study (rather than plain x-rays) when high pretest probability of cervical spine injury is present. It makes little sense to perform plain x-rays in this circumstance, because abnormal plain films would mandate CT and because normal plain films should be suspected of having missed cervical spine injury.

Interpreting Cervical Computed Tomography

Interpretation of cervical CT can be based on many of the same criteria used for plain x-ray. We make some direct comparisons of imaging findings on CT and x-ray, so skills you may already have from x-ray can be translated to CT. For those with little experience with either modality, starting with CT may prove easier, with CT findings then clarifying subtle findings on x-ray. We take a step-by-step approach, using the sagittal, coronal, and axial images for different purposes. Each image series should be reviewed, because fractures in the plane of a given image series are difficult to see in that series

but are readily apparent in perpendicular planes. We spend relatively little time up front on normal findings; instead, we concentrate on pointing out abnormalities in the figures that follow, with comparison to normal findings.

CT has high resolution for bony injury and directly detects fractures and dislocations. Modern CT scanners allow multiplanar and three-dimensional reconstructions, facilitating injury characterization. Image data is helically acquired as the patient passes through the CT gantry, typically at 1-mm or submillimeter slice thickness. Reconstructions are performed in sagittal, coronal, and axial planes (Table 3-2). The sagittal plane yields information similar to that from the lateral plain x-ray. The coronal plane yields information similar to that from the AP and odontoid plain x-ray views. Axial views give detailed anatomy of individual vertebral bodies, including clear views of the lamina, pedicles, transverse foramen enclosing the vertebral arteries, and

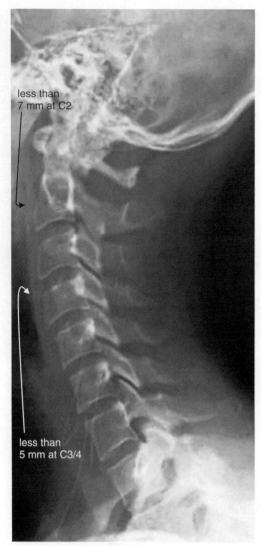

less than
7 mm at C2

less than
5 mm at C3/4

Figure 3-12. Prevertebral soft tissues. The lateral cervical spine x-ray should be examined for the width of prevertebral soft tissues. Widening suggests cervical spine injury with prevertebral soft-tissue swelling or hematoma, even in the absence of visible fracture. Lack of widening is relatively reassuring, as a fracture or ligamentous injury would be expected to be accompanied by some degree of soft-tissue swelling or hemorrhage. In adults, soft tissues should be less than 7 mm in width at C2 and less than 5 mm at C3 and C4. A rule of thumb in children is that the prevertebral soft tissues should be less than half the width of the adjacent vertebral body. False widening may be seen on expiratory films in children younger than 2 years, particularly if images are obtained during crying, which creates forced expiration.

spinal canal. Although the spinal cord is not well visualized on CT, the preceding image sets allow the canal to be carefully inspected for fracture fragments or dislocations that might impinge on the spinal cord. CT is considered to have outstanding sensitivity for fractures and dislocations—a normal CT viewed on bone windows effectively rules out these injuries. Nevertheless, it remains common practice to continue spine immobilization following a normal CT if the patient cannot be clinically evaluated for neurologic complaints or continued pain, though recent studies suggest a low risk of unstable cervical injuries following normal CT (see later discussion).

Step 1: Examine the Sagittal Computed Tomography Reconstructions. The sagittal CT reconstructions provide detailed information about the AP alignment of the cervical spine, as well as fractures or subluxations that may impinge on the spinal canal. Start your evaluation by selecting bone windows, and then move to a slice in the middle of the sagittal series, corresponding to the midsagittal plane (Figure 3-19). If you are experienced in interpreting cervical spine x-rays, this image should look familiar—it strongly resembles the lateral cervical spine x-ray, without the confusing overlay of bones and soft tissues from other planes. Just as with the lateral x-ray view, the midsagittal CT image allows assessment of alignment, using the curves of the anterior and posterior longitudinal ligaments and the spinolaminar line. In this view, the spinal canal can be seen in detail and inspected for any fracture fragments or subluxation of vertebral bodies that could impinge on the spinal cord. Remember that you are only looking at a single plane—you need to scroll laterally to the patient's right and then left to perform these same steps in planes moving away from the patient's midline. In the midsagittal plane, notice how large the dens is—perhaps you did not appreciate this on x-ray, but look now at the lateral x-ray for comparison. Check the contour of the dens for fracture lines, and if fracture is present, inspect for retropulsion of the dens into the spinal canal. Inspect the predental space for widening. Look at prevertebral soft tissues for increased thickness suggesting soft-tissue injury. Inspect each vertebral body for fracture lines. Check the spinal lamina and posterior spinous processes for fracture. Notice that in the midsagittal plane, the facet joints are not visible. These are lateral structures and are seen in the far lateral parasagittal images (Figure 3-20). Inspect these joints for unilateral or bilateral dislocation (jumped facets, shown in a later figure). At the cephalad limit of the cervical spine, inspect the articulation of the occipital condyles with C1 (see Figure 3-20). It may take you some time to become accustomed to imagining the cervical spine in three dimensions as you scroll through it in this plane.

Step 2: Inspect the Coronal Images. Use the coronal CT images (Figure 3-21) to simulate the open-mouth odontoid and AP cervical x-rays. Scroll through the "stack" of coronal images until you see the odontoid process projecting between the lateral masses of C1. Check for the same features you would expect on the open-mouth odontoid view. The lateral masses of C1 and C2 should align along their lateral borders. The spaces between the odontoid process and the lateral masses of C1 should be symmetrical. The odontoid process itself should have a smooth contour, with no fracture lines present. Once you have completed this evaluation, scroll in anterior and posterior directions through the stack of images, inspecting for fractures of the vertebral bodies, facets, and transverse processes. Fractures in the

Figure 3-13. **Assessment of facet joints. A,** Lateral cervical spine x-ray. **B,** Close-up. The facets should overlap like shingles on a roof. In the case of jumped or perched facet joints, the degree of facet overlap at the level of injury will be less than the overlap at uninjured levels. The facets can be recognized by their rhomboid shape in profile. Fracture through the facets and lamina is also common and should be looked for carefully.

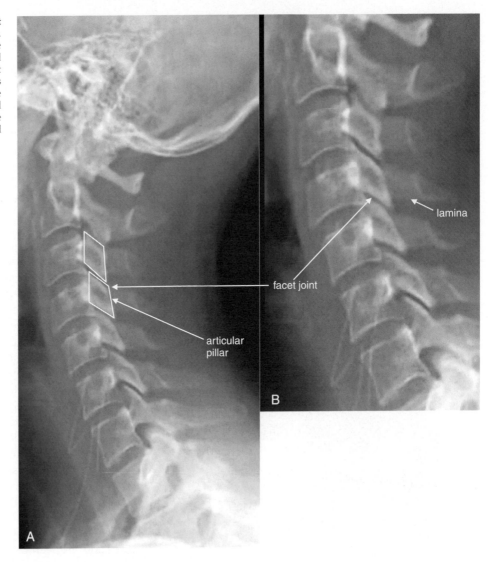

sagittal plane are visible on coronal images, and may be missed on the sagittal images reviewed first. Look for lateral displacement of vertebral bodies with respect to one another. Spend some time reviewing the figures in this chapter to familiarize yourself with the most common fracture patterns.

Step 3: Inspect the Axial Computed Tomography Images. The axial CT images (Figure 3-22) have no immediate analogue in the normal three-view x-ray series. They can provide additional information not readily seen on the sagittal and coronal views. Particularly, they demonstrate fractures of the canals housing the vertebral arteries (foramen transversarium), which are more difficult to assess on other views. They also provide good views of fractures in the sagittal and coronal planes, which may not be seen well on those image series as they lie parallel to the plane of the image. From the sagittal images, you should already have a good idea of the alignment of the cervical spine, although the

axial images can also demonstrate jumped facet joints. The axial images provide an en face view of the spinal canal. As you scroll from the level of C1 to T1, imagine yourself traveling down the spinal canal, and watch for fracture fragments that narrow the canal and may impinge on the spinal cord. Check the body, pedicles, lamina, and transverse and posterior spinous processes for fractures. We review many abnormal findings on the axial images in the figures throughout this chapter (see list, Table 3-1).

CLINICAL DECISION RULES: WHO NEEDS CERVICAL SPINE IMAGING?

Indications for cervical spine imaging have been studied extensively, resulting in two well-validated clinical decision rules (CDRs) to aid the clinician in identifying patients who require cervical spine imaging. We review both rules in detail, discussing their strengths and weaknesses.

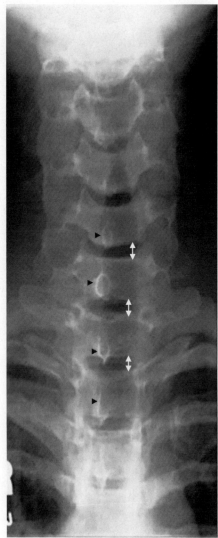

Figure 3-14. Anterior–posterior (AP) normal cervical spine x-ray. The AP cervical spine x-ray should be inspected for gross fractures. The intervertebral spacing *(double arrows)* should be symmetrical if the intervertebral discs (not visible on x-ray) are intact. The posterior spinous processes *(black arrowheads)* should project directly backward out of the plane of the x-ray and should be aligned with one another. In cases of unilateral jumped facet joint, rotation of one vertebral body relative to the adjacent bodies causes the posterior spinous process to project at an angle and thus not be aligned with the processes of other vertebrae.

The National Emergency X-radiography Utilization Study

The National Emergency X-radiography Utilization Study (NEXUS) was a prospective study of 34,069 patients at 21 U.S. medical centers, examining blunt trauma patients undergoing cervical spine imaging (Box 3-3).[4-5] This study was well planned and conducted and identified 818 patients with cervical spine injuries, comprising 2.4% of the study population. The study evaluated a CDR consisting of five clinical criteria, which had been suggested by prior studies (Box 3-4). Cervical spine imaging was considered necessary if any one of the five was present. The investigators prospectively defined a group of clinical unimportant

cervical spine injuries which they did not expect their proposed rule to identify, as they would not be anticipated to lead to patient harm if undetected. This rule proved 99% sensitive, though only 12.9% specific for clinically important acute cervical spine fracture. The negative predictive value of the rule was 99.8%, with a positive predictive value of only 2.7%. Application of the rule would have reduced cervical spine imaging by 12.6%. The rule failed to identify 8 of 818 injuries—2 which would have been clinically significant, 1 of which was treated surgically. Application of this rule is estimated to miss one injury in 125 years of clinical practice by a typical emergency physician.

The Canadian Cervical Spine Rule

The Canadian Cervical Spine Rule (CCR) (Figure 3-23) is a classic example of a methodologically rigorous CDR. CDRs are aids to bedside decision making, intended to reduce the cost, time, and adverse consequences of care, such as radiation exposures from diagnostic imaging. CDRs must be rapid to apply, inexpensive, and sensitive to avoid missing important pathology. They must be specific enough to reduce subsequent test utilization; otherwise, they fail their primary objective. Typically, CDRs use readily available information from the history and physical examination, occasionally supplemented by simple, rapid, and inexpensive bedside tests such as urinalysis.

A CDR goes through three important steps before it is ready for clinical application: derivation, internal validation, and external validation.

In step 1, called the derivation phase, the rule is developed. At this phase, many variables that might predict the presence or absence of a disease state are analyzed, and their contribution to the predictive value of the rule is calculated. Patients with and without the disease or injury in question (such as cervical spine fracture) are studied, and the presence or absence of each variable is recorded. Some variables may be found to have little predictive value and are discarded, while others may be highly predictive and are retained for the final rule. Sophisticated statistical techniques such as multivariate analysis allow the individual predictive characteristics of each variable to be assessed. The final rule must strike a balance among simplicity of application, sensitivity for detection of pathology, and specificity. A rule that is very sensitive and specific but has dozens of variables may be too cumbersome for clinical application. A rule that is simple and specific but insensitive cannot safely be employed, because it would limit testing to just those patients with disease but might miss many patients with pathology. A rule that is simple and sensitive but nonspecific would mandate testing of many patients without disease, at potentially great cost.

Following derivation, the limited number of variables that appear to constitute a simple, sensitive, and specific

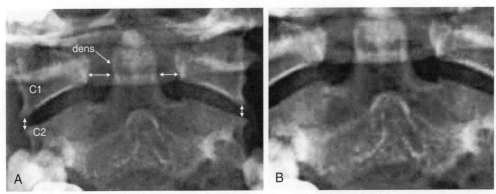

Figure 3-15. **Adequate and inadequate open-mouth odontoid view x-ray.** An adequate open-mouth odontoid view must visualize the entire dens and the lateral borders of C1 and C2. An incompletely visualized dens could result in an undiagnosed dens fracture. The lateral borders of C1 and C2 must be seen to assess for misalignment, which can occur in the setting of C1 burst fracture, in which the lateral masses of C1 are displaced laterally. **A,** An adequate view. The lateral borders of C1 and C2 are visible and align normally. The spaces between the dens and the lateral masses of C1 are symmetrical. The entire dens is visible and appears intact. **B,** An inadequate view with the tip of the dens and the lateral masses of C1 and C2 cropped. Alignment and fracture cannot be assessed.

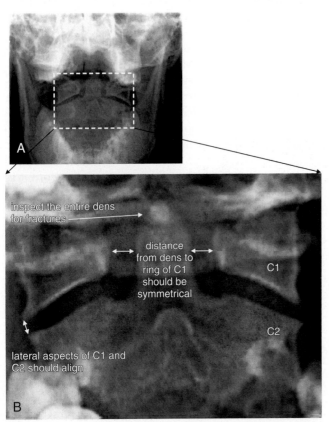

Figure 3-16. **Normal open-mouth odontoid view x-ray.** The open-mouth odontoid view is essential for evaluation of potential dens fractures and fractures of the C1 ring. **A,** Routine open-mouth odontoid image. **B,** Close-up of the region of interest, which includes C2 with the dens, as well as the lateral masses of C1.

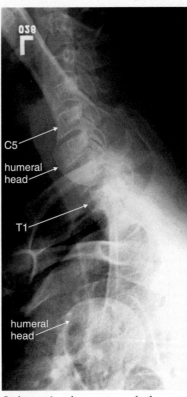

Figure 3-17. **Swimmer's view x-ray of the cervical spine.** A swimmer's view is a lateral cervical spine x-ray in which the patient is positioned with one arm raised above the head. This position tilts the shoulder girdle, elevating one humeral head and depressing the other, thus revealing the C7-T1 junction. Other variations on the swimmer's position are sometimes used, including raising both arms above the head. The swimmer's view is only necessary when the C7-T1 junction is not visualized on a standard lateral x-ray. Today, computed tomography is more commonly used to visualize this region.

rule are retested to ensure that statistical chance did not result in their apparent predictive value. Remember that many variables are assessed in the derivation phase, because the researchers do not yet know which will have predictive value. This methodology is subject to the appearance of false chance associations between variables and endpoints. Conventionally, an association is considered to have statistical significance if the likelihood of the association occurring *by chance* is less than 5%. This corresponds to a p value of less than 0.05. When multiple comparisons or associations are tested, as is the case in the derivation phase, the probability of one or more associations meeting this threshold grows rapidly. When only one association is tested, the chance

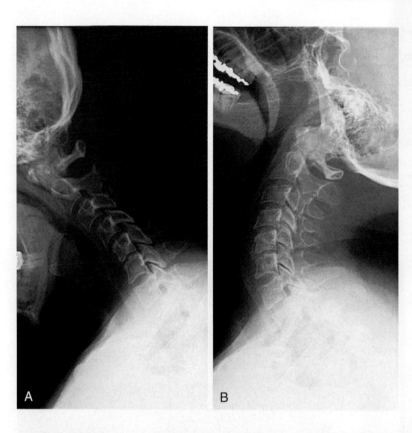

Figure 3-18. **Flexion and extension x-rays of the cervical spine.** Flexion **(A)** and extension **(B)** views may be performed to evaluate for ligamentous injury if plain films in neutral position do not show fractures or subluxation but the patient has persistent pain. The patient is asked to flex and extend the cervical spine actively, stopping if pain or neurologic symptoms develop. Subluxation suggests a ligamentous injury. Passive flexion and extension (in which the patient is manipulated by the examiner) should never be used, because this may cause cervical spinal cord injury. The utility of flexion–extension views is an area of controversy, but generally these are not useful in the evaluation of acute trauma because patients with acute pain are often unable to flex or extend sufficiently to exclude ligamentous injury.

Box 3-1 What Does Cervical Spine Computed Tomography Show?

- Fractures (bones)
- Dislocations (indirectly indicating ligamentous injury)
- Subluxation (indirectly indicating ligamentous injury)
- Widened soft tissues (indirectly indicating ligamentous injury)

Controversy exists about the screening value of CT in assessing spinal cord or ligamentous injury. Some authors advocate that a normal CT scan virtually eliminates these diagnostic possibilities, but MRI remains the diagnostic standard. The evidence for CT is discussed in the text.

Box 3-2 When Should Cervical Spine Computed Tomography Be Performed?*

- High pretest probability of spine injury–skip plain x-ray
- Fracture on plain x-ray
    - Provides more detailed characterization
    - Identifies additional fractures
- Inadequate plain x-ray
    - Degenerative disc disease
    - Osteopenia
    - Failure to visualize the entire spine from C7 to T1
- Negative plain x-ray but high suspicion for fracture* (go directly to CT without plain film if pretest probability is so high that a negative plain film would not be considered sufficient)
- Altered mental status or CT head planned
- Neurologic deficits referrable to the cervical spine following trauma

---

*The ACR now recommends CT as the initial screening modality for all suspected acute cervical spine trauma in patients meeting imaging requirements by NEXUS or the CCR.

---

of a *p* value below 0.05 is, by definition, 0.05 or 5%. This is like rolling a 20-sided die a single time: there is a 5% chance that the number 1 will be rolled, just by chance. But consider the chance of at least one association meeting this threshold as multiple associations are tested. This is equivalent to rolling the 20-sided die many times. It becomes increasingly *unlikely* that the number 1 will *not* be rolled at least once.

All of this is to say that, following the derivation phase, the apparent rule must be carefully tested, as some of

the apparent predictors may have occurred solely by chance. The more exhaustive the derivation phase, with more variables or associations being tested, the more likely that one or more of these associations is false, with no predictive value (or even the opposite

TABLE 3-2. Information Provided by Various Computed Tomography Image Planes

Abnormality	Sagittal Images	Coronal Images	Axial Images
Three-column stability	Yes	No	Yes
AP subluxation	Yes	No	No
Lateral subluxation	No	Yes	No
Loss of vertebral body height	Yes	Yes	No
Loss of disc height	Yes	Yes	No
Burst injury	Yes	Yes	Yes
Nondisplaced fractures	Yes, if not in sagittal plane	Yes, if not in coronal plane	Yes, if not in axial plane
Retropulsion of fragments into spinal canal	Yes	No	Yes

Figure 3-19. **Normal mid-sagittal computed tomography (CT) image, compared with normal lateral cervical spine x-ray.** This 24-year-old female hydroplaned on a wet road at 45 mph and complained of midline cervical spine tenderness. Her CT is reviewed to demonstrate normal findings. **A,** When reviewing CT sagittal images, follow the paradigm of the lateral x-ray. First, select bone windows. Next, select the midsagittal CT image and note the alignment of vertebral bodies, using the same four lines used for evaluating alignment on the lateral x-ray (see Figure 3-10). Then, inspect each vertebra for fractures (shown in subsequent figures). Notice how the facet joints are not visible in the midsagittal plane. Also notice how large the dens is and how small the ring of C1 is. Prevertebral soft tissues can be evaluated using the same criteria as for x-ray. **B,** Lateral x-ray for comparison.

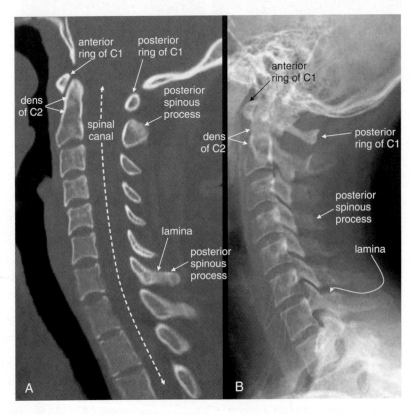

predictive value of that determined in the derivation phase).

In step 2, the internal validation phase, the rule is retested in the same population (or a similar population) to that in which it was derived. If the rule retains its predictive value, it may be safely applied in that population henceforth. If the rule fails to perform as it did in the derivation phase, additional testing and refining of the rule is needed. If the rule withstands internal validation, additional external validation should be performed (step 3) before the rule is widely implemented in populations that differ from the initial population. These external validation phases may vary the patient population, the setting, or the medical practitioner applying the rule. For example, a CDR

that works well when applied by emergency physicians in an emergency department in the United States might work poorly when applied by paramedics in the prehospital setting in another country. Well-validated CDRs are often testing in many settings to ensure that they are robust and impervious to variations of this type.

With this background, let's return to the specific example of the Canadian Cervical Spine Rule (CCR). The CCR was derived and validated in Canada, and it has subsequently undergone additional external validation.[7] The rule is somewhat more complex than the NEXUS criteria but boasts greater specificity, resulting in a greater decrease in cervical spine imaging. The original study was prospectively conducted in 10 Canadian medical

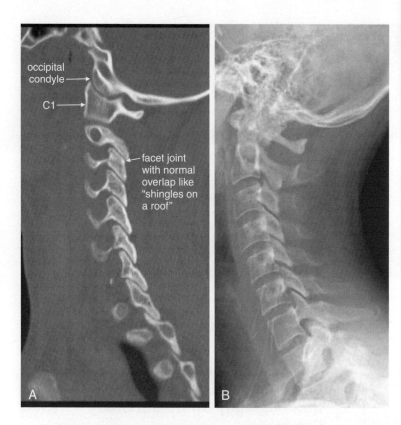

Figure 3-20. **Normal parasagittal computed tomography (CT) image, compared with lateral cervical spine x-ray. A,** In this far lateral parasagittal CT image, the facet joints can be seen articulating normally, like shingles on a roof. The vertebral bodies are not seen in this plane, as we are far from the midline. The occipital condyles are seen articulating with C1. **B,** Lateral x-ray for comparison. Notice how much clearer the occipital–cervical junction is on CT.

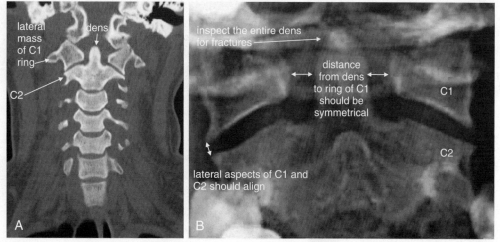

Figure 3-21. **Normal coronal computed tomography image, compared with odontoid view x-ray. A,** Same patient as Figures 3-19 and 3-20. A coronal image centered on the odontoid (dens) and C1, simulating the open-mouth odontoid x-ray. CT findings of a normal dens are the same as those seen on open-mouth odontoid x-ray, and deviation from normal should heighten suspicion for injury, even when a fracture line is not seen. Subluxation without fracture may be present. The lateral borders of the C1 and C2 vertebral bodies should align. Fractures of the ring of C1 (Jefferson fractures) commonly result in radial spread of C1 fragments, disturbing this normal alignment. The spaces between the lateral masses of C1 and the odontoid process should be bilaterally symmetrical. C1 fractures can result in asymmetrical spread of fragments, and subluxation of the transverse ligament can also result in asymmetry. The odontoid process should be smoothly contoured with no visible fracture lines. A slight notched appearance on each side of the base of the dens is normal. **B,** Open-mouth odontoid x-ray for comparison.

centers, enrolling 8924 patients with blunt head and neck injury, stable vital signs, and a normal Glasgow Coma Scale (Box 3-5). It found 151 patients with cervical spine injuries, 1.7% of the enrolled population. The rule was 100% sensitive and 42.5% specific, resulting in an impressive 41.8% reduction in cervical imaging utilization.

The CCR and NEXUS have been prospectively compared in a study conducted by the authors of the CCR (Box 3-6).[8] This study enrolled 8283 patients in nine Canadian medical centers, finding 169 patients with cervical spine injuries, constituting 2% of the population. The CCR outperformed NEXUS, with a sensitivity of 99.4% versus 90.7% for NEXUS. In addition, the CCR was

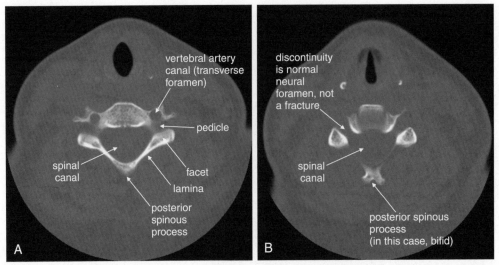

Figure 3-22. Normal axial computed tomography image. Same patient as Figures 3-19 through 3-21. An axial image shows a cervical vertebra in cross section. The vertebral body, spinal canal, pedicles, lamina, and base of the posterior spinous process are visible. It takes some practice to become accustomed to the normal appearance of vertebrae in axial section. They are irregular structures and never lie completely within a single axial plane. Apparent discontinuities in the ring may be visible on some slices but may not represent fractures—instead, they simply reflect the irregular contour of the vertebrae passing in and out of the image plane. **A, B,** Two sequential slices.

Box 3-3 The National Emergency X-radiography Utilization Study

- **Prospective**
- **21 centers**
- **34,069 patients**
- **Blunt trauma patients undergoing cervical spine imaging**
    - 818 injuries (2.4%)
- **Evaluated 5 criteria for cervical spine imaging (Box 3-4)**
    - Sensitivity = 99%
    - Specificity = 12.9%
    - Negative predictive value = 99.8%
    - Positive predictive value = 2.7%
    - Reduces x-ray by 12.6%
    - Missed 8 of 818 injuries
        - 2 clinically significant
        - 1 surgically treated
    - Estimated to miss one injury in 125 years of emergency medicine practice

---

Box 3-4 The National Emergency X-radiography Utilization Study Criteria*

Direct Signs of Spinal Fracture or Spinal Cord Injury
- **No midline cervical tenderness**
- **No focal neurologic deficit**

Factors That Make Examination Unreliable
- **Normal alertness**
- **No intoxication**
- **No painful distracting injury**

---

*Violation of any one criterion mandates cervical imaging.

45.1% specific, versus 36.8% for NEXUS. The Canadian authors have argued that NEXUS is insufficiently sensitive to be applied safely and that their criteria have the additional benefit of superior reductions in imaging use. The American authors of NEXUS have pointed to the outcome of this study as inconsistent with the original NEXUS study, which was conducted in a much larger population of some 30,000 patients. Why, they ask, did NEXUS perform with higher sensitivity in that setting? They argue that it is implausible that NEXUS has a sensitivity of only 90%, as this would have resulted in 80 missed cervical spine injuries in the original NEXUS study.

Which Criteria Should I Use: The National Emergency X-radiography Utilization Study or the Canadian Cervical Spine Rule?

Both NEXUS and the CCR are the result of well-conducted prospective clinical trials—level I evidence under the hierarchy used by the American College of Emergency Physicians (Table 3-3), which does not have a current clinical policy recommending the best CDR for evaluation of the cervical spine. The American College of Radiology (ACR) cites both rules as appropriate for evaluation of the need for cervical spine imaging in its appropriateness criteria.[1] Application of either rule is appropriate.

Can I Mix and Match the Rules?

It may be tempting to mix two well-validated rules in an attempt to capture the best features of both. Unfortunately, it is uncertain what the result of this strategy

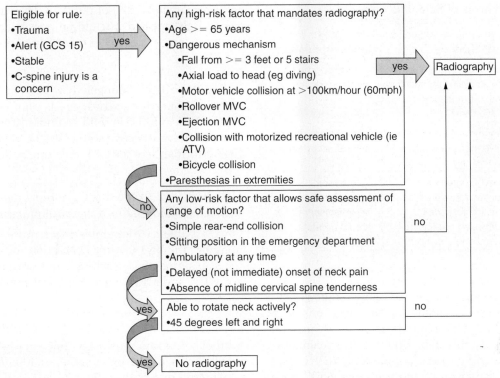

Figure 3-23. **The Canadian Cervical Spine Rule.** *GCS*, Glasgow Coma Score; *MVC*, motor vehicle collision.

Box 3-5 The Canadian Cervical Spine Rule

- **Prospective**
- **10 centers**
- **8924 patients**
- **Stable vital signs**
- **Glasgow Coma Scale = 15**
- **Blunt head and neck trauma**
  - 151 injuries (1.7%)
- **Derived rule for cervical radiography**
  - Sensitivity = 100%
  - Specificity = 42.5%
  - Reduces x-ray by 41.8%

Box 3-6 The Canadian Cervical Spine Rule versus the National Emergency X-radiography Utilization Study

- **Prospective**
- **9 Canadian centers**
- **8283 patients**
- **Cervical spine injuries**
  - 169 injuries (2%)
  - 845 (10.2%) could not be analyzed (no range of motion performed)
- **Sensitivity = 99.4% (CCR) vs. 90.7% (NEXUS) ($p < 0.001$)**
- **Specificity = 45.1% (CCR) vs. 36.8% (NEXUS) ($p < 0.001$)**
- **Radiography = 55.9% (CCR) vs. (NEXUS) 66.6% ($p < 0.001$)**
- **CCR misses 1 of 169 injuries**
- **NEXUS misses 16 of 169 injuries**

---

would be. It is possible that mixing the two rules would decrease the specificity of both, resulting in a rule that, although quite sensitive, did not diminish use to the extent achieved by either rule alone. More research is needed to determine whether a combined rule would have better diagnostic performance.

Do the Rules Apply to Geriatric Patients?

Geriatric patients raise special concerns for cervical spine imaging. Do NEXUS and the CCR apply to these populations? NEXUS included 2943 patients age 65 or older, accounting for 8.6% of the study group. Cervical spine injuries occurred in 4.59% of this group, a rate more than twice that in younger patients. Notably, 20% of injuries were odontoid fractures, compared with only 5% in younger patients.[5] Certainly elderly patients in this study were a high-risk group—could the NEXUS CDR actually reduce use in this group? While popular conception might hold that it would be fruitless to apply a CDR to geriatric patients, in actuality a greater percentage of the elderly met the NEXUS low-risk criteria and avoided imaging: 14% of geriatric patients compared

TABLE 3-3. Levels of Scientific Evidence

Class of Literature	Type of Study	Level of Recommendation
I	Randomized clinical studies using prospective data (or meta-analysis of the same)	A—high degree of clinical certainty
II	Nonrandomized trials or retrospective or case-control data	B—moderate degree of clinical certainty
III	Expert opinion or consensus; data from smaller, less well-controlled studies or case series; or both	C—guarded, inconclusive, or preliminary recommendations

with 12.5% of younger patients. Following the NEXUS rule, only two cervical spine injuries were missed in older patients, both fitting into the predefined "insignificant" category. By this definition, NEXUS maintained 100% sensitivity in a geriatric population. When considering geriatric patients with blunt trauma, NEXUS can be applied safely. However, many elderly patients will require cervical CT, if they require any form of imaging, due to inadequate or abnormal x-rays demonstrating degenerative changes.

The CCR found age of 65 years or older to be a high-risk factor mandating imaging in its derivation set,[7] and this was maintained as a mandatory criterion for cervical spine imaging in the multiple validation studies that have followed. Thus, for geriatric patients, application of NEXUS results in imaging of fewer patients than does the CCR.

Do the Rules Apply to Pediatric Patients?

NEXUS provides us with limited information about the pediatric population. In it, 3065 patients, 9% of the total NEXUS population, were younger than 18 years. However, only 88 children were younger than 2 years, 817 between the ages of 2 and 8, and 2160 children between the ages of 8 and 17. Only 30 patients under the age of 18 (0.98%) sustained any cervical spine injury, resulting in very wide confidence intervals (CIs) for the study results. Only 4 of the 30 injured children were under the age of 9, and no injured patient was younger than 2 years, so the study results should not be applied to children in these age-groups. Overall, the decision rule correctly identified all pediatric cervical spine injuries with a sensitivity of 100%. The small total number of injuries results in a lower 95% CI of 88%. Investigators concluded that cervical spine injuries are rare among patients 8 years and younger and that the NEXUS rule performed well in children, with the ability to safely eliminate imaging

in approximately 20% of patients. The rule is probably very safely applied in children ages 8 and older, who form the largest portion of the study population.[9]

The derivation and validation studies for the CCR excluded patients younger than 16 years of age.[7] One small retrospective study suggests poor performance of the CCR and NEXUS in children under 10 years, but larger multicenter prospective studies are needed to determine the performance of the CCR in young patients.[7a]

How Sensitive Are X-ray, CT, and Magnetic Resonance Imaging for Cervical Spine Injury?

Once a patient is determined to require cervical spine imaging, the best test for evaluation must be selected. Let's examine the sensitivity and specificity of plain x-ray, CT, and MRI for acute cervical spine injury.

How Sensitive Is X-ray for Cervical Spine Injury?

Studies of x-ray sensitivity find markedly different results, depending on whether inadequate films are considered or whether these are excluded from analysis and only "adequate" x-rays are considered in calculating the false-negative rate. In addition, if x-rays are credited as "positive" for detecting any fracture, they appear to have relatively good sensitivity, whereas when x-ray sensitivity is discounted for second and third fractures found on CT, their sensitivity appears quite poor. The consensus among multiple studies is that cervical spine plain x-rays miss some fractures—with a pooled sensitivity of 52%, compared with 98% for CT, according to a meta-analysis of seven studies.[10] As a consequence, the ACR has now advocated CT as the initial screening test for suspected cervical spine injury in adult patients, in place of x-ray. The ACR endorses no cervical spine imaging in patients meeting either the NEXUS or the CCR low-risk criteria. Certainly when high clinical concern exists for fracture, CT should be performed, often as the initial imaging study rather than x-ray. In a low-pretest probability patient with a normal cervical spine plain x-ray series, the risk of fracture is very low. Let's examine some of the evidence behind these conclusions.

Holmes et al. performed a meta-analysis of cervical spine imaging studies to determine the sensitivity of plain x-ray and CT, and their results are largely the basis of the current ACR recommendation. The authors imposed fairly strict inclusion and exclusion criteria for studies (Table 3-4). Studies were considered if they were either a randomized, controlled trial comparing x-ray and CT or a cohort study of patients undergoing both x-ray and CT. Studies were excluded if the x-ray series did not include the AP, lateral, and open-mouth odontoid views; if the CT scan did not extend from the

TABLE 3-4. Criteria Used to Select Studies for Inclusion in Meta-analysis of Cervical Spine Imaging

Methodologic Quality	Criteria
I	Randomized controlled trials comparing CT with plain radiography
II	Nonrandomized studies, sample size > 50 subjects, with a representative sample and an independent gold standard
III	Nonrandomized studies, sample size < 50 subjects, minimal to moderate selection bias, or lacking an independent gold standard
IV	Nonrandomized studies, <50 subjects or severe selection bias

Holmes JF, Akkinepalli R. Computed tomography versus plain radiography to screen for cervical spine injury: A meta-analysis. *J Trauma* 58(5):902–905, 2005.

occiput to the superior aspect of the first thoracic vertebra; or if distance between CT scan slices exceeded 5 mm. The authors also assessed the methodologic quality of the studies, using the rating scale in Table 3-2. Among 712 studies identified by the authors in Medline, only 7 met the inclusion criteria, and none of those were rated as methodologic quality I or II. The authors used the published raw data from these 7 studies and calculated a pooled sensitivity of 52% for x-ray (95% CI = 47%-56%) and 98% for CT (95% CI = 96%-99%). The meta-analysis authors acknowledge the methodologic limitations of the available data and state that CT should be used as the primary tool for screening high-risk patients, although further study is needed to determine whether x-ray is adequate for evaluation of low-risk patients. Despite this, the ACR has adopted an all-or-none approach to cervical spine imaging in the adult acute trauma patient and does not differentiate between patients at higher and those at lower risk once the decision has been made to perform cervical imaging.

Before accepting the results of this meta-analysis, let's consider whether the authors' criteria are reasonable and achievable. First, for cervical spine injury, what independent gold standard test should be used to confirm or rule out an injury, outside of CT? Clinical follow-up could be used but would only be useful for identifying injuries resulting in neurologic sequelae or surgical interventions, because stable fractures might heal uneventfully and not be appreciated on clinical grounds. Other imaging tests, such as MRI, could be used, but it is not clear that their results are a stronger gold standard than CT. Nonetheless, demanding an independent gold standard is essential when comparing x-ray and CT, as CT would otherwise be guaranteed the apparent better result. None of the studies included in this meta-analysis used a gold

standard independent of CT results. Their use of CT as the gold standard represents incorporation bias and limits the validity of the studies and of the meta-analysis. Moreover, because no false-positive CT results are possible under this definition (because the CT result is considered correct in every instance), specificity and positive and negative likelihood ratios for CT cannot be determined. In addition to problems with the gold standard in the included studies, the studies suffer from spectrum bias as a consequence of inclusion of mostly badly injured patients at high risk of multilevel cervical spine injury. Holmes et al acknowledged these limitations and suggested that CT might not be necessary in all patients.

Were the authors too stringent in their inclusion criteria for studies to be considered? Note that the sentinel NEXUS and CCR studies, with more than 40,000 patients between them, were not included in this meta-analysis because neither study compared x-ray to CT scan in all patients. Both studies used a combination of imaging studies and clinical follow-up to determine if a patient had a clinically important cervical spine injury, rather than asking whether any fracture was present.

Let's examine several additional studies, including some of those included in the meta-analysis. In a single-center study of 936 trauma registry patients over a 9-month period, 58 patients with cervical spine injuries (6.2%) were found. A substantial number of inadequate plain x-rays occurred. When considering only those cases in which a technically adequate plain x-ray series (three views of the cervical spine) was obtained, three false negatives occurred, resulting in a sensitivity of 90.3% and a specificity of 96.3% for x-ray. The positive predictive value of an adequate three-view series was 54.9%, with a negative predictive value of 99.5%.[11] In a second retrospective single-center study of 3018 blunt trauma patients, 1199 patients underwent both x-ray and CT scan. In this study, 116 patients with injury were detected (9.5%), and 41 (3.2%) had false-negative x-rays. All required treatment—the authors concluded that CT rather than plain x-ray should be used to screen trauma patients.[12-13] However, two limits of this study bear consideration. First, the average Glasgow Coma Scale score in patients with missed injuries was 12 and the average injury severity score (Box 3-7) was 14.6 (on a 0- to 75-point scale), so this was a population of moderately injured patients with altered mental status, not a population of alert and otherwise uninjured patients, which is a common scenario in which cervical spine evaluation is required. In addition, as in many studies, CT scan was the gold standard for diagnosis, and it automatically was credited with a sensitivity of 100%.

In a third, prospective study of 1356 blunt trauma patients with altered mental status, 95 injuries from C0 (skull base) to C3 were found in 70 patients (5.2%).

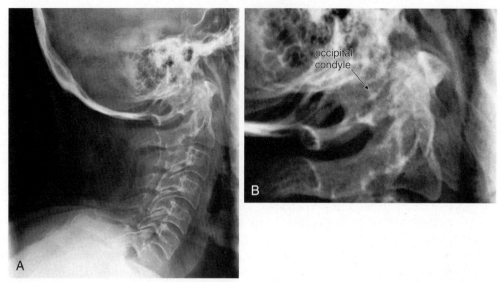

Figure 3-24. **Cranial–cervical junction x-ray: Occipital condyle fracture. A,** Lateral cervical spine x-ray. **B,** Close-up of atlanto-occipital junction. Fractures of the occipital condyle are extremely difficult to see or invisible on plain x-ray, as this lateral cervical spine x-ray illustrates. Computed tomography (CT) scan of the region clearly demonstrated a fracture (see Figure 3-25), but the complex overlap of multiple structures at the junction of the skull base and C1 vertebral body masks the pathology on x-ray. The cervical spine alignment appears normal. This patient also has a C2 fracture known from CT but not seen on this view.

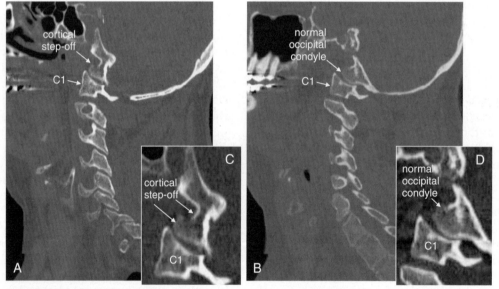

Figure 3-25. **Cranial–cervical junction CT: Occipital condyle fracture. A,** On this sagittal CT reconstruction, a fracture through the occipital condyle is seen, with a cortical defect and step-off. **B,** The normal opposite side for comparison. Both images are far lateral to the midline. **C, D,** Close-ups from **A** and **B,** respectively.

Box 3-7 Injury Severity Score Defined

Injury severity score values range from 0 to 75. Six body regions are considered, with the scores from the three most severely injured regions being squared and then summed.

From Baker SP, O'Neill B, Haddon W Jr, et al: The injury severity score: A method for describing patients with multiple injuries and evaluating emergency care. *J Trauma* 14(3):187–96, 1974

Plain x-ray found injuries in 38 patients (54%), while CT found injuries in 67 (96%).[14] The remaining 3 injuries (4%) not detected on CT were recognized by clinical neurologic deficits, and represented spinal cord injury without radiographic abnormality (SCIWORA) (see later discussion).

A fourth, prospective study of 324 blunt trauma patients compared two protocols for assessment of the cervical spine. By protocol, patients requiring head CT underwent a single lateral cervical spine x-ray and cervical CT

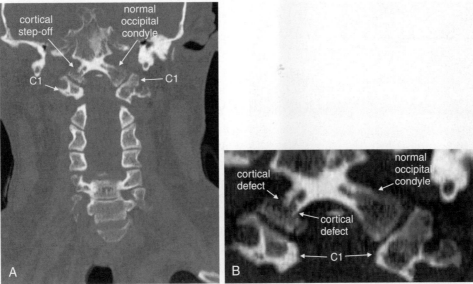

Figure 3-26. **Cranial–cervical junction CT: Occipital condyle fracture. A,** On this coronal CT image, a fracture through the right occipital condyle is seen, with a cortical defect and step-off. Compare with the normal opposite side. **B,** Close-up showing this fracture in detail.

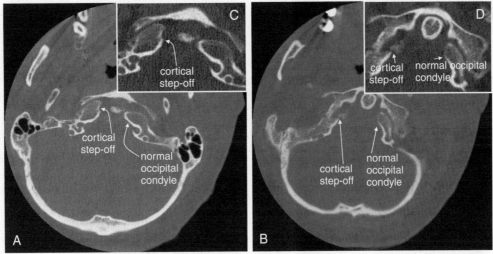

Figure 3-27. **Cranial–cervical junction CT: Occipital condyle fracture. A, B,** On these axial views, a fracture through the right occipital condyle is seen, with a cortical defect and step-off. Compare with the normal left occipital condyle. **C, D,** Close-ups from **A** and **B,** respectively, show this fracture in detail. Although this step-off is subtle, it should not be confused with a reconstruction artifact. Note that other bony cortices in horizontal alignment with the fracture appear intact. If reconstruction artifact were at fault, cortices would appear disrupted in a horizontal line spanning the entire image.

scan. If head CT was not clinically indicated, three views of the cervical spine were performed, with selective CT performed to evaluate areas not well seen on plain x-ray. Fifteen patients (4.6%) had cervical spine injuries, and x-ray had only 54% sensitivity compared with the gold standard of CT.[15] The authors concluded that CT is the appropriate initial cervical imaging test in patients undergoing head CT.

Contrary to these studies is the largest dedicated prospective study of cervical spine injury and imaging—NEXUS. This study of 34,069 patients included 818 patients with injuries (2.4%). The gold standard in this study was review of all final radiology reports, including CT and MRI when available, and clinical follow-up. X-ray revealed 932 injuries in 498 patients and missed

564 injuries in 320 patients. But 436 missed injuries in 237 patients occurred in the context of an inadequate plain x-ray, or an x-ray that was in fact abnormal and revealed at least one cervical spine injury, though not all of the injuries that were ultimately discovered. When the definition of a false-negative x-ray was limited to a normal and adequate x-ray in the presence of cervical spine injury, 23 patients with 35 injuries were found, including three unstable cervical injuries. By this more limited definition of false negatives, x-ray had a sensitivity of 97%. The authors concluded that (1) inadequate x-rays mandate additional imaging and (2) rarely, normal x-rays miss injury.[16]

Should we accept the NEXUS authors' definitions and believe their conclusions, or are they manipulating the

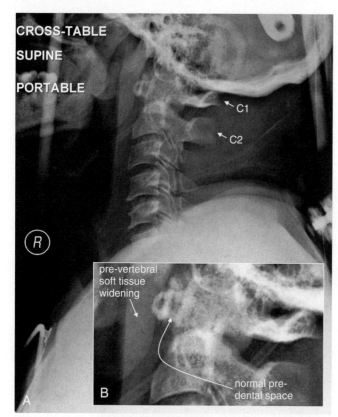

CROSS-TABLE

SUPINE

PORTABLE

C1

C2

R

pre-vertebral
soft tissue
widening

normal pre-
dental space

A   B

Figure 3-28. C1 Jefferson burst fracture. A, Lateral cervical spine x-ray. **B,** Close-up. C1 burst fractures (also called Jefferson fractures) result from axial force applied to the cervical spine, crushing the ring of C1 between the skull base and the body of C2. A common mechanism is diving into a pool and striking the head on the pool bottom. The resulting fragments of the C1 ring typically spread radially, and plain x-ray findings include a widened predental space (visible on a lateral x-ray), or laterally displaced margins of the C1 ring on an open-mouth odontoid x-ray. However, even a badly comminuted fracture can be difficult to detect on plain x-ray. Computed tomography (CT) is so widely used in the evaluation of potential cervical spine injuries that plain x-rays of this injury are becoming increasingly rare. In this patient, CT revealed a C1 fracture (Figures 3-29 through 3-31). This lateral x-ray with the patient in a halo device does not reveal the fracture directly, although the prevertebral soft tissues are slightly widened—the normal measurement being 7 mm or less. The predental space, which can be widened in burst fractures, is normal. This is not due to a failure of x-ray to detect an abnormality but rather due to the absence of predental widening in this patient, as shown on the patient's CT (Figures 3-29 through 3-31).

data to defend x-ray? From a practical clinical standpoint, an x-ray that shows one fracture but misses a second fracture is true positive, not false negative. This conclusion is based on the premise that all abnormal plain x-rays will be followed by CT, which presumably will detect the second injury. So, if the purpose of x-ray is to screen for the presence of one or more injuries, this definition is fair. Excluding inadequate plain x-rays from analysis also makes sense from a clinical perspective, because an indeterminate test should not be relied upon to exclude an important diagnosis. The NEXUS authors' take-home point is likely accurate—when normal and adequate x-rays are successfully obtained in a patient with a low pretest probability of injury, missed injuries are rare. The emergency physician should recognize

patients with a high pretest probability of injury and those in whom inadequate plain x-rays are likely to be obtained and should choose CT as the first imaging test. In addition, the emergency physician must reject inadequate plain x-rays, recognizing the high risk of missed injury, and perform additional imaging (usually with CT) when these occur.

What Constitutes an Adequate Plain X-ray Series? Are Five Views Better than Three?

Traditionally, five views of the cervical spine were performed at many medical centers: the standard three views (AP, lateral, and odontoid) and bilateral oblique views. Do these additional two views improve the sensitivity of x-ray? In a single-center study of 1006 blunt trauma patients with altered mental status, 116 patients with 172 injuries were enrolled. All underwent five views of the cervical spine followed by CT. The five-view plain x-ray series missed 52.3% of injuries in 56% of patients, including 93% of occipital fractures and 47.2% of fractures from C1 to C3. The overall sensitivity of the five-view series was only 44%, with 100% specificity. The positive predictive value was 100%, with negative predictive value of 99.7%. The authors concluded that five views offer inadequate sensitivity and that CT is more appropriate in patients with altered mental status.[6]

How Sensitive Is CT for Cervical Spine Injury?

CT scan is believed to be nearly 100% sensitive for bony abnormalities or dislocation, although this conclusion is limited by the lack of a clear alternative gold standard. Because CT is generally considered superior to plain x-ray and even MRI for evaluation of bony abnormalities, a finding on CT is considered to be real—CT is 100% sensitive for fractures. Missed injuries on CT are generally restricted to isolated soft-tissue injuries, included cervical spinal cord injuries without fractures or subluxations. These injuries are called spinal cord injury without radiographic abnormality (SCIWORA).

Spinal Cord Injury Without Radiographic Abnormality

It has long been recognized that some patients with cervical spinal cord injuries did not have visible fractures, subluxation, or soft-tissue injuries on plain x-ray or, in later years, on CT scan. These injuries can rarely be missed despite modern multiplanar CT. Originally, SCIWORA was believed to be an injury seen predominantly in children,[17-21] with the hypothesized reason being a more flexible cervical spine, one more prone to subluxation than to fracture. More recently, SCIWORA has been described in adults and may be as common in adults as in children—although it remains a rare injury pattern. NEXUS provides insight into the frequency of

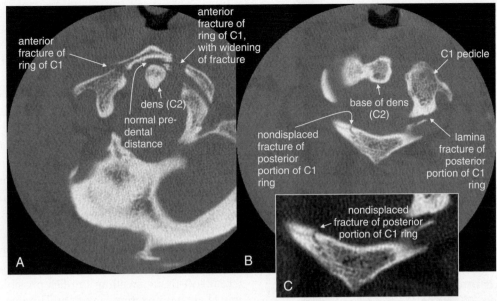

Figure 3-29. C1 Jefferson burst fracture: Cervical spine computed tomography (CT) without contrast, bone windows. Same patient as in Figure 3-28. In these axial views, the ring of C1 is clearly fractured in multiple locations, with some radial spread of fracture fragments. Two slices are shown to capture both the anterior **(A)** and the posterior **(B)** portions of the ring of C1, as the position of the patient in the CT scanner prevents the entire ring from being seen in a single slice. **C,** Close-up from **B.** Discriminating fractures from the normal appearance of vertebral bodies as they pass in and out of the image plane takes practice. The task is easier when using a complete digital stack of images than when looking at selected images, as in a textbook like this.

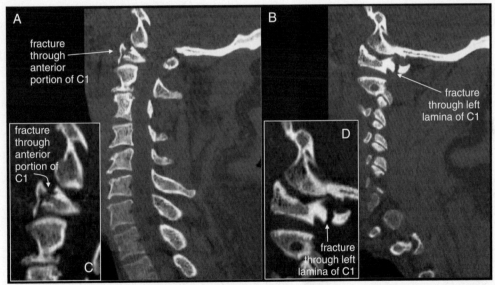

Figure 3-30. C1 Jefferson burst fracture, noncontrast CT, bone windows. Same patient as in Figure 3-28. **A, B,** Sagittal computed tomography (CT) reconstructions, with close-ups from the same slices (**C** and **D,** respectively). The optimal CT plane for detecting a fracture depends on the predominant direction of the fracture plane. In this patient, the sagittal reformations look nearly normal, as many of the C1 fractures are in a sagittal plane parallel to the sagittal plane of reconstruction. One fracture line through the anterior portion of C1 runs in a coronal plane and is therefore visible on the sagittal views. The left lamina fracture seen on the axial reconstructions is also in a coronal plane, intersects the sagittal plane, and is thus visible on the sagittal views.

SCIWORA. NEXUS defined SCIWORA as spinal cord injury on MRI with complete and technically adequate plain radiographic series showing no injury. Of 34,069 patients, and 818 (2.4%) with cervical injuries, only 27 (0.08%) had SCIWORA—all adults. NEXUS included 3000 children, with 30 (1%) having cervical injuries, but no instances of pediatric SCIWORA were observed. The most common MRI findings of SCIWORA are shown in Box 3-8.[22]

Other studies continue to suggest a relatively high incidence of this disease among children with cervical spine injuries. A 10-year review of the National Pediatric Trauma Registry including 75,172 children found 1098 (1.5%) with cervical spine injury, among whom 83% had bony injury and 17% had SCIWORA. Of the 35% with neurologic injury, 50% had SCIWORA. Nonetheless, 17% of 1.5% would mean an overall incidence of 0.255% of child victims of blunt trauma experience SCIWORA.

This study is also limited by a lack of CT data. Because CT results were not reported, it is possible that many of the cases of SCIWORA would have had abnormalities that could have been detected by CT.[23] Overall, SCIWORA appears exceedingly rare; occurs in adults, as well as in children; and might be more accurately renamed spinal cord injury with only abnormal MRI.

How commonly does CT miss spinal cord injuries? In one study of trauma patients with altered mental status, CT identified injuries in 67 of 70 patients with spinal injury (96%). The remaining 3 patients had neurologic deficits attributable to C0 to C3 spinal cord injury.[14] In a similar study of trauma patients with abnormal mental status, CT

Box 3-8 Most Common Magnetic Resonance Imaging Findings of Spinal Cord Injury Without Radiographic Abnormality

- ● **Central disc herniation**
- ● **Spinal stenosis**
- ● **Cord edema or contusion**
- ● **Central cord syndrome**
- ● **Ligamentous injury**

From Hendey GW, Wolfson AB, Mower WR, et al. Spinal cord injury without radiographic abnormality: results of the National Emergency X-Radiography Utilization Study in blunt cervical trauma. *J Trauma* 53(1):1–4, 2002.

---

sensitivity for cervical spine injury was 97.4% and specificity was 100%, with positive and negative predictive values of 100% and 99.7%, respectively. Again, by definition, CT only missed SCIWORA—in 2 of 116 patients (1.7%).[6]

Does a Normal CT Rule Out Soft-Tissue Injuries Such as Spinal Ligament Tears, Disc Protrusions, and, Most Importantly, Spinal Cord Injuries? Should Patients Remain Immobilized After a Normal Cervical Spine CT? Is Magnetic Resonance Imaging or Other Imaging, Such as Flexion–Extension X-rays, Required to Rule Out Additional Injuries?

CT scan is extremely sensitive for cervical spine injuries such as fracture and subluxation. The presence of prevertebral soft-tissue swelling implies possible ligamentous injury, and subluxation of vertebral bodies virtually guarantees ligamentous injury, although the spinal ligaments themselves are not well seen on CT. When sufficient injury has occurred to tear spinal ligaments, associated hemorrhage and soft-tissue swelling are expected to occur, increasing the thickness of prevertebral soft tissues. On CT, the width of prevertebral soft tissues is easily measured. Theoretically, if this tissue thickness is normal, ligamentous injury is quite unlikely, even if the ligament itself cannot be visualized. MRI is the test of choice if ligamentous injury is highly suspected, because the injured tissue can be directly visualized. By adjusting the window level on cervical spine CT, other soft-tissue

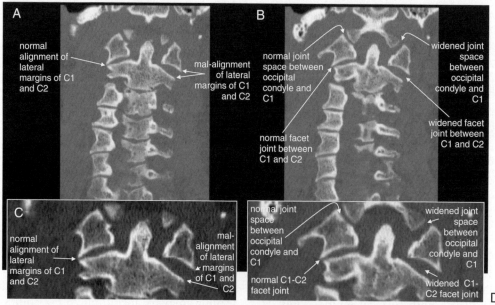

Figure 3-31. C1 Jefferson burst fracture, noncontrast CT, bone windows. Same patient as in Figure 3-28. A burst fracture of C1 is often recognized on plain x-ray using the open-mouth odontoid view (see normal odontoid image, Figure 3-16). **A, B,** Coronal planar CT reformations (with close-ups in **C** and **D,** respectively) mimic the odontoid x-ray view. The fractures in this patient are not directly visible, as they lie predominantly in the coronal plane, parallel to the plane of reconstruction. However, the radial dispersion of the fracture fragments has caused a classic abnormality, malalignment of the lateral masses of C1 with the margins of the C2 vertebral body. As a result of the fractures, the left-hand portion of the C1 ring is freely mobile and has shifted laterally with respect to C2. In addition, the facet joint between C1 and C2 is widened, as is the joint space between the occipital condyle and C1.

detail such as spinal epidural hematomas and disc protrusions can sometimes be seen, although MRI remains the gold standard.

When no fractures, subluxations, or soft-tissue injuries are seen on CT scan, are soft-tissue injuries ruled out, or is MRI needed, as has been the standard for the past decade? Two common clinical scenarios may raise this issue in emergency medicine practice. First, in the obtunded or sedated trauma patient, in whom a reliable neurologic examination cannot be performed, is MRI required to rule out cervical soft-tissue injuries? While this is an important question, for most emergency physicians this is a decision deferred to trauma teams following admission. Several recent studies have addressed this question, and their results may help us to

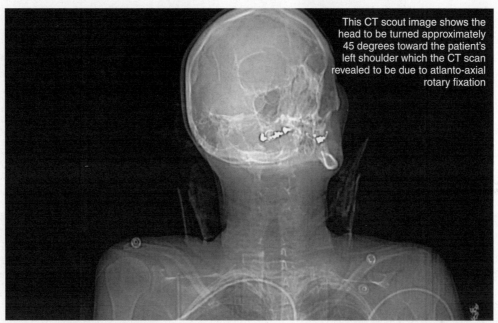

This CT scout image shows the head to be turned approximately 45 degrees toward the patient's left shoulder which the CT scan revealed to be due to atlanto-axial rotary fixation

Figure 3-32. C1-2: Atlantoaxial rotary fixation. Rotation of C1 on C2 is a normal joint motion—within limits. Excessive rotation at this level can result in facet dislocation ("jumped facet"), locking the joint in a malaligned position and preventing the head from assuming a midline position. This patient was in an altercation in which her assailant violently twisted her head. This computed tomography scout image shows the head to be turned approximately 45 degrees toward the patient's left shoulder. Figures 3-33 and 3-34 evaluate this injury in more detail.

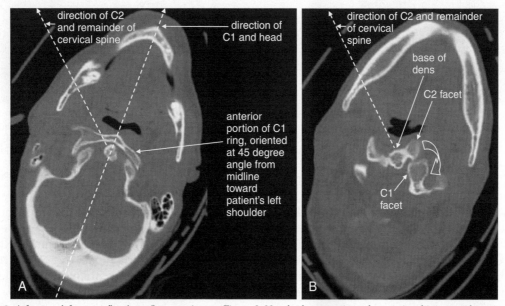

Figure 3-33. C1-2: Atlantoaxial rotary fixation. Same patient as Figure 3-32, who has experienced a rotational injury to the spine. **A,** The skull and C1 moved as a unit, rotating toward the patient's left shoulder relative to C2 and the remainder of the cervical spine. **B,** C2 and the remainder of the cervical spine are pointed toward the patient's right shoulder. The facet joints of C1 and C2 are both visible, having rotated relative to one another. The C1 facet has subluxed completely posterior to the C2 facet. Normally, the two facets cannot be seen in the same axial image, as one is directly cephalad to the other.

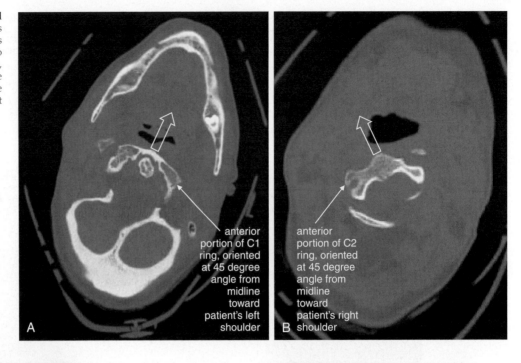

Figure 3-34. **C1-2: Atlantoaxial rotary fixation.** Same patient as Figures 3-32 and 3-33, who has experienced a rotational injury to the spine. On these axial images, note how the head and C1 are facing the left shoulder **(A)**, while C2 is directed toward the right shoulder **(B)**.

anterior portion of C1 ring, oriented at 45 degree angle from midline toward patient's left shoulder

anterior portion of C2 ring, oriented at 45 degree angle from midline toward patient's right shoulder

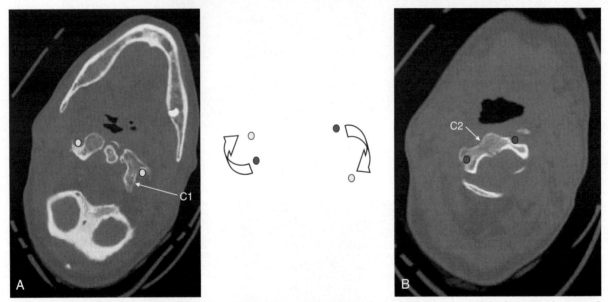

Figure 3-35. **C1-2: Atlantoaxial rotary fixation.** Same patient as Figures 3-32 to 3-34, who has experienced a rotational injury to the spine. On these axial images, note how the rotation of C1 on C2 has changed the normal position of the canals housing the vertebral arteries (transverse foramen). Because of the patient's rotated position, none of canals is seen completely on these images. Circular markers have been added to this figure to indicate the position of the vertebral arteries in the canals. In the center, they have been superimposed to show how rotation of this type could crimp or tear the vessels. This type of rotational injury can result in vertebral artery dissection or even transection. The patient underwent a computed tomography (CT) angiogram of the neck that showed no arterial injury. CT angiography for evaluation of cervical arterial injuries is discussed in Chapter 4.

understand the second common clinical scenario, that of the awake and alert emergency department patient who continues to complain of neck pain following a normal cervical spine CT. Does this patient require further imaging, either with MRI or with flexion–extension x-rays, to assess for ligamentous injury? Let's examine the results of some recent studies that may shed light on this topic.

Menaker et al.[24] reviewed the Maryland trauma registry and identified 234 obtunded blunt trauma patients with

normal cervical spine CT who underwent MRI for further assessment, following a clinical guideline. Of these patients, 18 (8.9%) had an abnormal MRI, including 2 who required surgical repair and 14 in whom extended cervical collar use was employed.

Stelfox et al.[25] retrospectively studied 140 consecutive intubated patients before and 75 consecutive intubated patients after a change in protocol for cervical spine clearance in obtunded trauma patients at Massachusetts

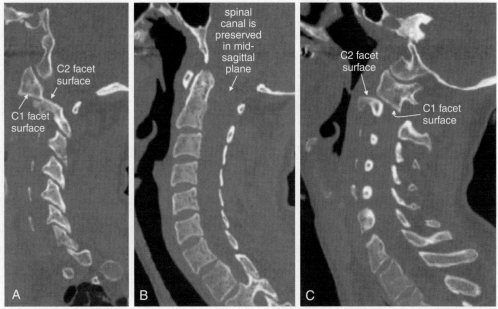

Figure 3-36. C1-2: Atlantoaxial rotary fixation. Same patient as Figures 3-32 to 3-35, who has experienced a rotational injury to the spine. On these sagittal CT images, alignment looks surprisingly normal when viewing a nearly midsagittal image (**B**). However, sagittal images through far right lateral positions (**A**) and far left lateral positions (**C**) reveal that the C1-2 facet joints are completely subluxed. The mid-sagittal image looks normally aligned because the rotation occurred about a midsagittal pivot point. The central spinal canal is preserved in this rotational injury, and the patient had no neurologic deficits. This type of injury can severely injure the vertebral arteries, although fortunately, no injury occurred in this case.

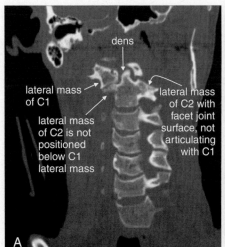

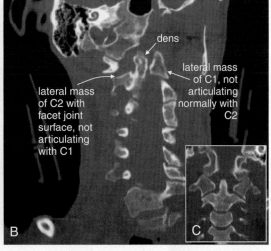

Figure 3-37. C1-2: Atlantoaxial rotary fixation. Same patient as Figures 3-32 to 3-38, who has experienced a rotational injury to the spine. On these coronal CT images, the usual open-mouth odontoid appearance with a midline dens flanked by the lateral masses of C1 cannot be found, due to rotation of C1 on C2. **A,** Instead, the right lateral mass of C1 is visible, but not positioned normally above the C2 lateral mass. **B,** The left lateral mass of C1 is visible, but again the lateral mass of C2 is not in normal position below it. **C,** A normal coronal section for comparison.

General Hospital. Before the protocol change, cervical spine immobilization in these patients was discontinued after normal findings on cervical spine CT with multiplanar reconstructions and one of the following: a reliable normal clinical neurologic examination (implying normalization of mental status), normal passive flexion–extension x-rays (which have been criticized because of risk of injury when the cervical spine of an obtunded patient is moved by a physician), or normal cervical spine MRI within 48 hours of admission. After the protocol change, normal CT findings alone were considered sufficient for cervical spine clearance. A normal CT was defined as one with no evidence of fracture, dislocation, subluxation, or indirect signs such as soft-tissue edema, inappropriate lordosis, or widening of the atlantodental distance. The study authors concluded that no missed cervical spine injuries were documented in either group. Does this prove that no injuries were present? No; in many of these patients, the neurologic examination may have remained uninterpretable because of concurrent injuries, such as traumatic intracranial injuries or anoxic brain injury. Cervical spine injuries could have been present but not recognized, and cervical spinal cord injuries resulting from discontinuation of cervical spine immobilization could have occurred but not been recognized or documented in the patient medical record. A stronger gold standard would have been helpful in proving that discontinuing cervical spine immobilization on the basis of CT findings alone is a safe practice. Assume for a moment that the authors are correct that no injuries were missed in the second group, of whom 70 had cervical spine clearance before death or discharge. If no injuries were missed in this group, the upper 95% CI limit of the actual missed injury rate can be estimated as 3 of 70 (a well-described estimation method for series with zero outcomes), or 4%. This would mean that a normal CT in this scenario predicts better than 96% chance of no cervical spine injury. We should be careful in accepting the authors' contention, however. The possibility of

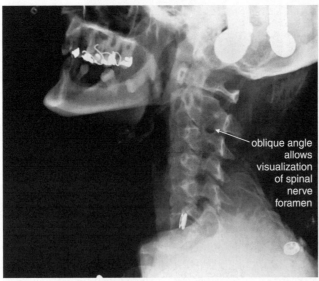

Figure 3-38. C1-2: Atlantoaxial rotary fixation. Same patient as Figures 3-32 to 3-37, who has experienced a rotational injury to the spine. This lateral plain x-ray appears more like a standard oblique view due to the rotational injury. Oblique x-ray views are discussed in more detail in the text. In some institutions, they are part of the standard x-ray series.

unrecognized missed injuries casts doubt on the results of this study.

A third, similar study examined the results of cervical spine MRI performed in obtunded trauma patients following a normal cervical spine CT with a 16-slice scanner. Como et al.[26] prospectively studied 115 obtunded blunt trauma patients at MetroHealth Medical Center in Cleveland, Ohio. They found that 6 of 115 patients (5.2%) had acute injuries identified on MRI that had not been recognized on CT, including microtrabecular bony injuries, intraspinous ligament injuries, a spinal cord signal abnormality, and a cervical spine epidural hematoma. The authors contend that none of these injuries changed patient management or required continued spine immobilization, though they admit limitations, including lack of long-term follow-up.[19] The authors did not report the lower limit of their 95% CI, but using their reported data, the negative predictive value of CT could be as low as 89%. Tomycz et al.[27] studied a similar population of 180 patients with normal cervical CT and found that 21.1% had abnormalities on MRI, none of which was unstable or required surgery. Similar limitations apply.

Sekula et al.[28] reviewed the charts of 6558 patients admitted for blunt trauma. They identified 447 patients with cervical fractures. Among the remaining 6111 patients without fracture, they identified only 12 (0.2%) with injuries requiring surgical fixation or halo placement. The authors contend that all were diagnosable by findings on multidetector CT, although interestingly, 3 of

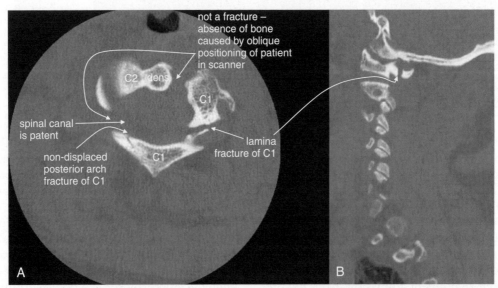

Figure 3-39. C1 posterior arch fracture, noncontrast CT, bone windows. This patient sustained a Jefferson burst fracture of C1. Among the multiple fractures were posterior arch fractures, seen on these axial **(A)** and sagittal **(B)** views. These injuries can occur in isolation or with a comminuted burst pattern. As a result of the ring shape of C1, solitary fractures are rare, and two or more fractures are usually seen. Axial computed tomography images often cause confusion in novice readers, because the irregular three-dimensional shape of the vertebral bodies and asymmetrical positioning of the patient in the scanner often conspire to create the appearance of fracture when none exists. When an apparent defect in bone is found, always look through adjacent images in the digital stack to ensure that you are not seeing an artifact caused as the vertebral body passes out of the image plane. Although ring fractures of C1 can create fracture fragments that impinge upon the spinal cord, in this case, the spinal canal is patent.

12 patients had injuries not recognized prospectively before MRI. The authors discount these as "misinterpretations" of CT. A more strict methodology would require that these 3 cases be counted as false-negative results, giving a sensitivity of only 75% (9 of 12) for CT in detection of unstable nonfracture injuries requiring stabilization. Moreover, the authors note that they had no follow-up on discharged patients who may have developed neurologic symptoms because of missed injuries.

Hogan et al.[29] retrospectively reviewed the records of 366 obtunded patients at Maryland's R. Adams Cowley Shock Trauma Center who had undergone normal cervical CT followed by MRI. MRI identified seven cervical cord contusions, four ligamentous injuries, and three intervertebral disc contusions. In this study, CT with a 4- or 16-slice scanner had a negative predictive value of 98.9% for ligamentous injury and 100% for unstable cervical spine injury. Although negative

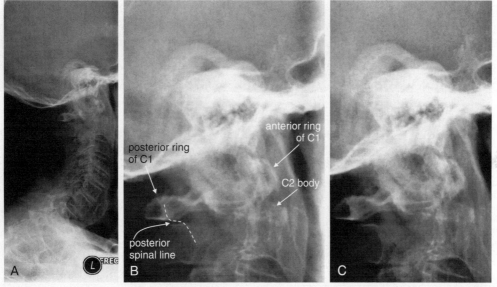

Figure 3-40. C2 dens fracture, type II. A, Lateral cervical spine x-ray. **B,** Close-up from **A. C,** The same image without labels. Fractures of the odontoid process or dens may be visible on the lateral cervical spine plain x-ray. Findings may include widening of the predental space or prevertebral soft tissues or actual cortical defects of the dens itself. The C1 ring may be intact but displaced posteriorly as well. The open-mouth odontoid plain x-ray view is also helpful for detecting this injury, although computed tomography is more sensitive and specific. In this patient, a cortical defect is present and the dens appears retropulsed. The anterior portion of the C1 ring is directly cephalad to the C2 body, instead of anterior to C2, which would be normal. The posterior ring of C1 is posteriorly displaced, so the posterior spinal line (also called posterior longitudinal ligament line) is disrupted. The dens itself is difficult to recognize. The prevertebral soft tissues are also widened, exceeding 7 mm at C2. Compare with the CT [in Figure 3-41].

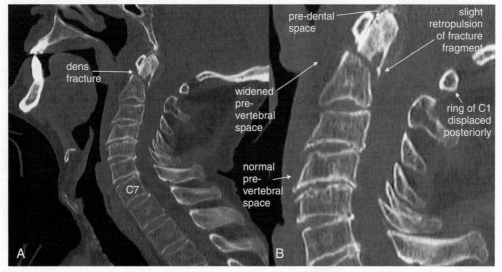

Figure 3-41. C2 dens fracture, type II. Same patient as in Figure 3-40. **A,** In this midsagittal computed tomography image, a type II dens fracture is seen. The fractured dens is slightly retropulsed into the spinal canal, though no significant stenosis has resulted. The predental space is not wide. The prevertebral soft tissues anterior to C1 and C2 are somewhat widened, likely indicating hematoma. **B,** Close-up. Look again at the lateral cervical spine x-ray in Figure 3-40 for comparison. As in that figure, the C1 ring here is attached to the dens by the transverse ligament and has moved posteriorly with the dens. This fracture is nearly parallel to the axial plane and is more difficult to identify on the standard axial images in Figure 3-42.

Figure 3-42. C2 dens fracture, type II, noncontrast CT, bone windows. Same patient as in Figures 3-40 and 3-41, axial images (A, B). This type II dens fracture is nearly parallel to the axial plane and is therefore almost undetectable on the axial images. At the posterior aspect of the base of the dens, a fracture line extends horizontally, and small fracture fragments have been slightly retropulsed into the spinal canal. Look at the sagittal images in Figure 3-41 for comparison.

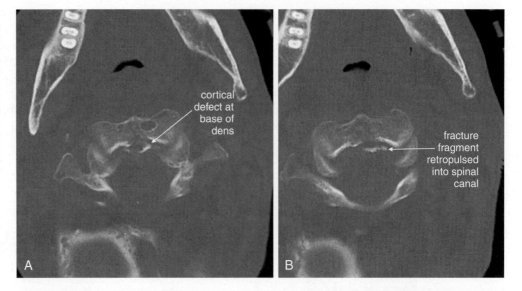

Figure 3-43. C2 dens fracture, type II. Same patient as in Figures 3-40 through 3-42. A, In this coronal CT reconstruction, a transverse fracture line is seen extending across the base of the dens. An open-mouth odontoid x-ray would give a similar view of this fracture, though one was never obtained in this patient. B, Close-up.

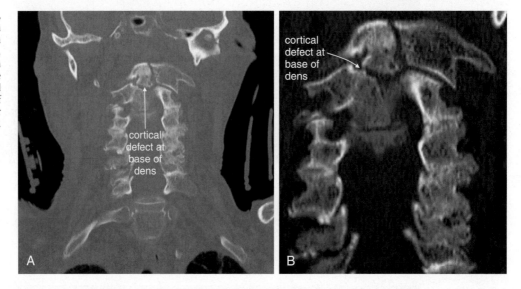

predictive values are generally discouraged as a means of presenting study results, as they are subject to change depending on the prevalence of injury in the population, these figures are impressive given the high-risk population in this study. The study did not report CT sensitivity, as the denominator of all patients with cervical spine injuries was not studied, only those with negative CT.

Smaller studies provide conflicting results. Stassen et al.[30] found that up to 30% of patients had cervical spine ligamentous injuries on MRI, when no fractures were detected on eight-slice cervical CT. The significance of these injuries is uncertain. Adams et al.[31] found no additional cervical spine injuries in 20 obtunded patients with normal CT.

How do these studies affect the management of the awake and alert patient with continued neck pain after a normal cervical CT? In general, these studies imply a very low rate of unstable cervical spine injury following a normal cervical spine CT scan. The populations studied are very high risk for injury, as the patients are intubated and obtunded, multiply injured patients at level I trauma centers. It is likely that cervical spine clearance following a normal CT would be even safer in an awake and alert patient with no other significant injuries. The current practice of immobilization until resolution of symptoms or clearance with flexion–extension x-rays has little evidence basis, although it carries the weight of long-held practice. Future higher-quality studies with strict gold standards (CT and MRI in all patients) and adequate follow-up would bolster the evidence at hand. Ideally, these studies would report sensitivity and specificity for CT by including in the studies not just patients with normal CT but all patients being evaluated with CT and MRI for cervical spine injury.

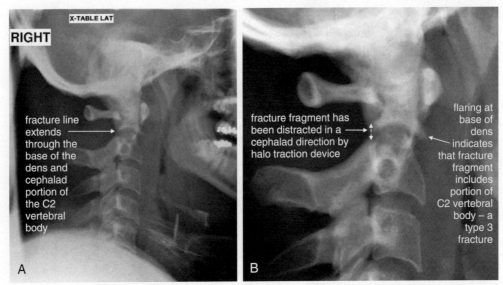

Figure 3-44. C2 dens fracture, type III. A, Lateral cervical spine x-ray. **B,** Close-up. In a type III dens fracture, the fracture line extends into the body of the C2 vertebra. This patient was noted to have a type III dens fracture on CT scan. A lateral cervical spine x-ray was subsequently obtained after the patient was placed in a halo traction device. A fracture line through the dens and cephalad portion of the body of C2 is seen, with the dens fracture fragment distracted in a cephalad direction by the traction device. Figures 3-45 through 3-47 demonstrate this fracture in more detail in CT images.

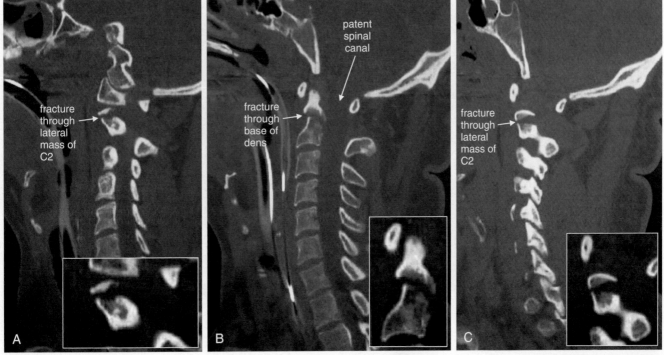

Figure 3-45. C2 dens fracture, type III. Same patient as in Figure 3-44. Sagittal CT images with close-ups. These sagittal CT views delineate the fracture from Figure 3-44 in more detail. In a nearly midsagittal plane **(B)**, this fracture resembles a type II dens fracture, with the fracture line running near the base of the dens. However, in more lateral parasagittal views **(A,** right parasagittal, and **C,** left parasagittal), the fracture line is seen running through the lateral masses of C2, consistent with a type III fracture. Importantly, there is no significant retropulsion of fracture fragments into the spinal canal.

The studies we have discussed do demonstrate that rarely CT misses soft-tissue cervical spine injuries. Consequently, patients who complain of neurologic abnormalities such as weakness, numbness, or parethesias after a normal CT scan should continue to be evaluated with MRI.

What Is the Value of Flexion–Extension Views of the Cervical Spine? Do They Assist in Identifying Ligamentous Instability?

Flexion–extension views (see Figure 3-18) historically have been performed to evaluate for ligamentous instability once fracture has been "ruled out" by x-ray or

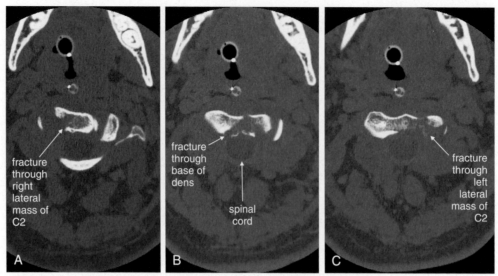

Figure 3-46. C2 dens fracture, type III. Same patient as in Figures 3-44 and 3-45. These axial computed tomography (CT) views delineate the fracture in more detail. **A,** The fracture line extends from the central vertebral body of C2 toward the right lateral mass. **B,** The fracture shows a greater degree of comminution than is evident from the lateral x-ray (Figure 3-44). **C,** The fracture continues through the left lateral mass of C2. In all of these views, the spinal canal appears patent, and the spinal cord is faintly visible as a dark gray ellipse (because of its low density) on these bone window views.

Figure 3-47. C2 dens fracture, type III. Same patient as in Figure 3-44 to 3-46. **A, B,** These coronal computed tomography (CT) views delineate the fracture in more detail. The fracture extends across the body of C2, completely separating the dens. The fracture continues laterally into the left lateral mass of C2. **C,** The fracture fragment shows mild craniocaudal diastasis, with the fragment having moved cranially relative to the body of C2 (close-up from **A**). Compare this with the plain x-ray in Figure 3-44. The close-up helps to illustrate what might be seen on an open-mouth odontoid plain x-ray of this injury, had one been obtained.

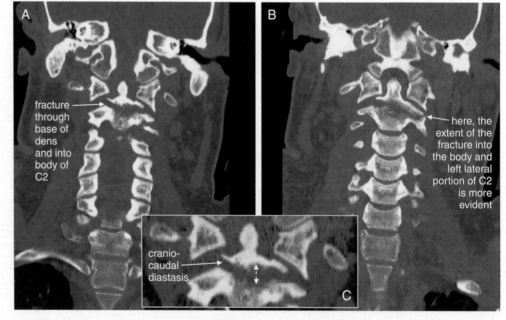

CT. *Flexion–extension views are contraindicated when an unstable fracture pattern or subluxation is evident on prior imaging (plain x-ray or CT), or when a patient has neurologic signs or symptoms, as motion of an unstable cervical spine may result in cervical spinal cord injury.* Flexion-extension views consist of lateral x-rays of the patient's cervical spine in active flexion and active extension. *Active* in this case means the patient must *consciously* and *without assistance* flex and extend the cervical spine. It is assumed that the patient will not worsen spinal cord injury, because increasing pain or neurologic symptoms will be warning signs to the patient to halt further flexion or extension. *Passive* flexion and extension, in

which the patient's cervical spine is physically manipulated into flexion and extension by a second person, should *never* be used; this may cause cervical spinal cord injury, because warning signs of pain or neurologic dysfunction might not be heeded quickly enough by the manipulator.

How might flexion–extension views detect ligamentous injuries? The spinal ligaments are not visible on plain x-ray, but torn, avulsed, or stretched spinal ligaments would presumably allow an abnormal degree of subluxation of one vertebral body relative to adjacent bodies. The acceptable degree of normal subluxation may

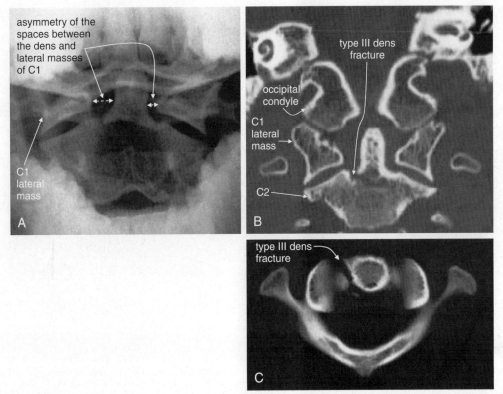

Figure 3-48. C2 dens fracture, type III, noncontrast CT. A 17-year-old male with neck pain after falling off a bicycle. The patient had a normal neurologic examination with cervical spine tenderness to palpation. **A,** The odontoid x-ray shows asymmetry of the spaces between the dens and lateral masses of C1. The space on the patient's right is wider than the space on the patient's left. Although no fracture is visible, this finding is concerning for dens fracture or for C1 burst fracture. Compare with the normal odontoid x-ray in Figure 3-16. **B,** A coronal computed tomography (CT) slice not only shows asymmetry but also confirms fracture—a type III dens fracture as it extends from the base of the dens to the body of C2. **C,** An axial CT image again confirms fracture. The patient was treated with halo fixation.

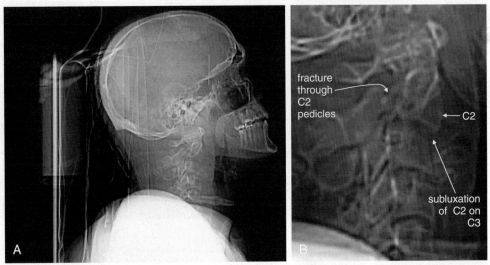

Figure 3-49. Hangman's fracture of C2. A, Lateral computed tomography (CT) scout image. **B,** Close-up. Scout images are usually used not for diagnosis but for selecting the region for the detailed CT scan. In this case, however, the scout images are diagnostic and give us an example of what might have been seen on lateral cervical spine x-ray, had one been obtained. This patient has a hangman's fracture of C2. The lateral scout image from the CT scan resembles a lateral cervical spine x-ray and shows typical findings, including subluxation of the body of C2 on C3. The body of C2 appears tipped slightly anteriorly. Fractures through the pedicles of C2 are faintly visible. The fracture is explored in detail in Figures 3-50 through 3-52.

vary with the age of the patient. In children under age 8, pseudosubluxation of up to 40% occurs in up to 40% of patients at the C2-3 level and in up to 14% of patients at the C3-4 level.[32-33] Pseudosubluxation should be visible in flexion but should resolve or diminish in extension views. Subluxation in extension likely represents real pathology. Swischuk's line, a line from the anterior portion of the C1 spinous process to the same point on the C3 spinous process, can assist with differentiation of pseudosubluxation from subluxation.[33] The anterior portion

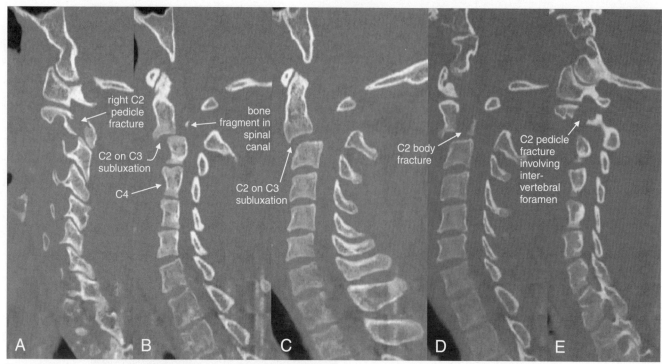

Figure 3-50. Hangman's fracture of C2. Same patient as in Figure 3-49. In this series of parasagittal CT images traversing from the patient's right to left (**A** to **E**), a hangman's fracture is demonstrated. **A,** The right pedicle is fractured. **B,** Just right of midline, the body of C2 is seen subluxed anteriorly on C3. C4 is labeled to assist in orientation. A tiny bone fragment is seen in the spinal canal. **C,** Subluxation of C2 on C3 of 6 mm is seen. **D,** The body of C2 is also fractured. **E,** The left pedicle is fractured, with the fracture involving the intervertebral foramen.

Figure 3-51. Hangman's fracture of C2. Same patient as in Figures 3-49 and 3-50. In this series of axial CT images (**A** to **C**), a hangman's fracture of C2 is visible. This involves the left and right pedicles, as well as the body of C2. Fracture fragments have been retropulsed into the spinal canal. Although on plain x-ray this type of fracture often appears simple, computed tomography frequently reveals a badly comminuted fracture.

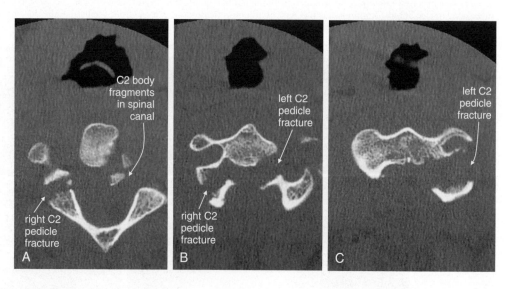

of the C2 spinous process should be within 2 mm of this line. In addition, no significant prevertebral soft-tissue swelling should be seen with pseudosubluxation.

In an adequate normal flexion–extension series, the patient flexes and extends and no abnormal subluxation is seen. Normally, the disc spaces should widen by no more than 1.7 mm, and the vertebral bodies should not translate by more than 1 mm. The inferior endplates of two adjacent vertebral bodies should not display greater than 11 degrees of angulation. If abnormal subluxation

is noted or if neurologic symptoms develop, MRI is indicated (Box 3-9). If pain prevents adequate flexion and extension, MRI may be performed, or the patient may be left immobilized in a cervical collar for several days, with flexion–extension views repeated when the patient's pain has subsided to a sufficient degree. Caution should be exercised when obtaining flexion–extension views long after the injury; theoretically, it would be possible for the pain and swelling of an unstable ligamentous injury to have resolved completely, and the patient could experience a dangerous degree of

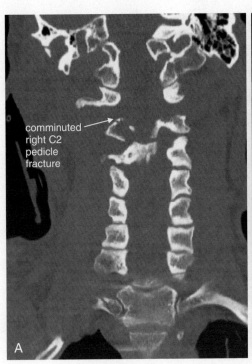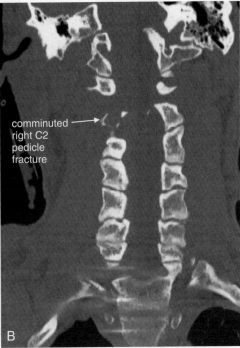

comminuted
right C2
pedicle
fracture

comminuted
right C2
pedicle
fracture

A

B

Figure 3-52. Hangman's fracture of C2. Same patient as in Figures 3-49 through 3-50. In these coronal CT images **(A, B),** the comminuted fracture through the right C2 pedicle is visible. The remaining fractures are difficult to see because they lie predominantly in a coronal plane, parallel to the plane of these computed tomography images. This emphasizes the importance of inspecting multiple image planes to detect fractures. Fractures are usually seen in images perpendicular to the fracture plane, while images in a parallel plane may disguise fractures. Fractures in an oblique plane may be visible in axial, sagittal, and coronal planes.

Box 3-9 Who Needs Magnetic Resonance Imaging after a Normal-Appearing Cervical Spine CT?

● **Patients with neurologic complaints or deficits require MRI**
● **Patients with altered mental status and normal CT have traditionally remained immobilized until MRI or exam rules out ligamentous, spinal cord, and other soft-tissue injuries—although recent studies question the necessity of this practice**

---

subluxation during flexion–extension imaging, resulting in spinal cord injury.

Does evidence support the practice of obtaining flexion–extension views? Subgroup analysis from NEXUS found that flexion–extension x-rays revealed only two stable fractures and four subluxations in 86 patients undergoing these additional views. The subluxation injuries were found in patients with other abnormalities already noted on neutrally positioned x-ray. The authors concluded that flexion–extension x-rays add little to the standard three views of the cervical spine—although this subgroup analysis includes too few patients to provide strong evidence.[34]

A retrospective review of 106 consecutive, awake, blunt trauma patients evaluated with flexion–extension

x-rays found that 32 patients (30%) had nondiagnostic studies due to inadequate flexion and extension and 4 of these patients (12.5%) had cervical spine injuries subsequently diagnosed by CT or MRI. In contrast, only 5 of the 74 patients (6.75%) achieving adequate range of motion on flexion–extension views were found to have cervical injuries, all detected with flexion–extension. This study is quite limited by its small numbers and the lack of a uniform gold standard. Although the authors asserted that adequate flexion–extension x-rays missed no injuries, many patients did not undergo further definitive imaging, a methodologic flaw called workup or verification bias.[35] The authors suggested that limited ability to perform flexion and extension on physical examination should indicate that flexion–extension x-rays not be performed, as they are likely to be nondiagnostic. They also concluded that additional cross-sectional imaging with either CT or MRI should be performed in patients who cannot perform flexion and extension after normal neutral x-rays, because this may be a marker of undetected injuries. Larger studies are required to confirm or refute this recommendation. The ACR states that the limited sensitivity and specificity of flexion-extension x-rays and the rarity of technically adequate x-rays make them almost useless in trauma patients. The ACR does suggest a role for flexion-extension x-rays in evaluation of potential ligamentous injury in patients with equivocal MRI, with abnormal ligament signal but no clear disruption.[1] As described earlier in the discussion of CT for cervical spine clearance, flexion–extension x-rays are also likely unnecessary after a completely normal cervical CT with no soft tissue abnormalities noted.

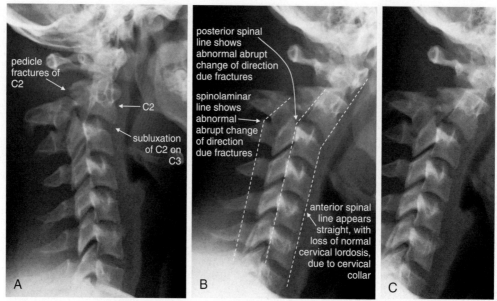

Figure 3-53. Hangman's fracture of C2. Two lateral x-ray views of another patient with a C2 hangman's fracture (**A, B; C** same as **B** without labels). Compare these images with the scout computed tomography image and sagittal CT images in the prior case (Figures 3-49 and 3-50). Subluxation of C2 on C3 is visible. In addition, displaced fractures through the pedicles of C2 are visible. Look at the normal rhomboid appearance of the pedicles and lamina of the lower vertebrae, and the loss of that normal appearance at C2 as a consequence of fracture. The cervical spine appears quite straight with loss of the normal cervical lordosis due to the cervical collar on the patient. Notice that the anterior and posterior spinal lines (also called anterior and posterior longitudinal ligament lines) and spinolaminar line are all disrupted by the fracture. Make a habit of inspecting these lines, which can draw your attention to fractures.

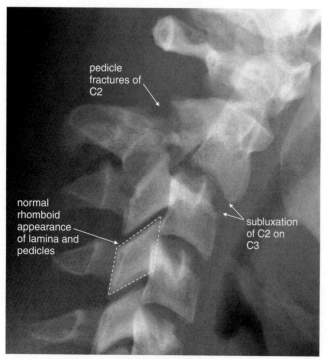

Figure 3-54. Hangman's fracture of C2. Close-up of the same C2 hangman's fracture as Figure 3-53. Compare this image with the scout CT image and sagittal images in the prior case (Figures 3-49 and 3-50). Subluxation of C2 on C3 is visible. In addition, displaced fractures through the pedicles of C2 are visible. Look at the normal rhomboid appearance of the pedicles and lamina of the lower vertebrae—which is disrupted in C2 due to the fracture. The anterior and posterior spinal lines and spinolaminar line are all disrupted, as seen in Figure 3-53.

Is There a Role for Fluoroscopy in Assessing for Unstable Cervical Spine Injuries?

Fluoroscopy has been suggested as a means of detecting ligamentous injury of the cervical spine in patients with altered mental status,[36] but critics *strongly discourage the use of fluoroscopy for this purpose. Passive manipulation of the cervical spine during fluoroscopy can result in cervical spine cord injury and should never be used.* In a study of 301 obtunded trauma patients, only 2 patients (0.7%) had ligamentous injury detected by fluoroscopy, and 1 patient developed quadriplegia.[37] Fluoroscopy shows bones but not soft tissues. It can detect ligamentous instability by revealing subluxation in real time, giving indirect evidence of ligamentous injury. Unfortunately, as the ligamentous injury is revealed on fluoroscopy, cervical spinal cord injury may be occurring, because the obtunded patient cannot complain of neurologic symptoms or pain. MRI should be used to evaluate for ligamentous injuries, because it does not carry this risk.

Do Cervical Spine Injuries Predict Arterial Injury? When Should Imaging of Cervical Arteries Be Performed, Following Detection of Cervical Spine Injury?

Sometimes cervical CT demonstrates fractures involving the transverse foramen, the bony channels housing the vertebral arteries. In other instances, subluxations or rotatory injuries of the cervical spine may shear or

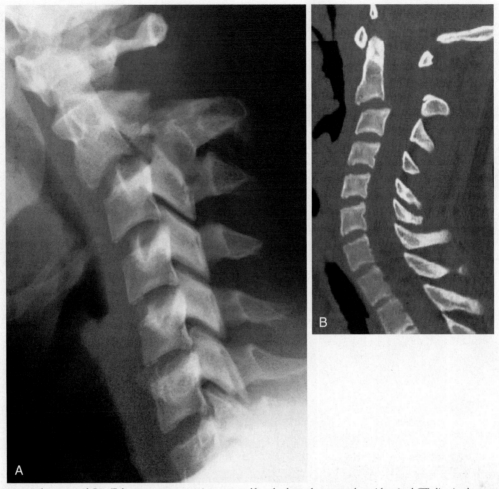

Figure 3-55. Hangman's fracture of C2. Take a moment to orient yourself to the lateral x-ray and a midsagittal CT slice in the same patient. In Figure 3-56, we focus on the region of C1 through C3, and explore the sagittal sections from the patient's right to left, to understand this fracture in depth. **A,** The lateral x-ray compresses lots of information into a single plane—not all the fractures present are actually in the midline, which explains the relative lack of abnormalities on the midsagittal CT **(B).** Most of the fractures are through lateral structures of the C2 vertebra.

stretch these vessels, potentially causing vascular tears. Do these injuries predict an increased risk of arterial injury? In a retrospective study, 92 of 605 patients (15%) evaluated with angiography for cervical arterial injury after blunt trauma were found to have arterial injuries. Of these 92 patients, 71 (77%) had an associated cervical spine injury. Of these spine injuries, 55% were subluxations, and 26% were fractures involving the transverse foramen. Most of the remaining spinal injuries associated with cervical arterial injury were injuries to C1 through C3. Does this study indicate that all high cervical spine fractures, subluxations of the cervical spine, or transverse foramen fractures should be followed with evaluation of cervical arteries? Blunt vertebral artery dissection is associated with stroke, which is perhaps prevented by anticoagulation therapy. When these types of cervical spine injury are present, arterial imaging appears warranted based on current evidence.[38] Arterial injuries are discussed in more detail in Chapter 4.

When Should CT Be the Initial Cervical Spine Imaging Modality, Rather Than X-ray?

The ACR now recommends a CT-first strategy in all adult patients with suspected cervical spine injury, as discussed earlier. If a technically adequate x-ray series can be obtained in a low-risk patient, x-ray can be used to screen for fracture, as it has been used for the past century. CT is the clear preferred first-line imaging technique in patients with high likelihood of cervical spine injury, in patients with multiple other injuries requiring CT for evaluation, in patients in whom rapid cervical spine clearance is especially desirable (e.g., to allow unusual positioning in the operating suite for treatment of other injuries), and in patients with a low likelihood of adequate plain x-ray, such as the elderly, obese patients, and patients with short necks, extensive cervical spine degenerative joint disease, prior injuries to the cervical spine that might be confused with acute injuries on plain film, and bone disorders such as ankylosing spondylitis (see Box 3-2).

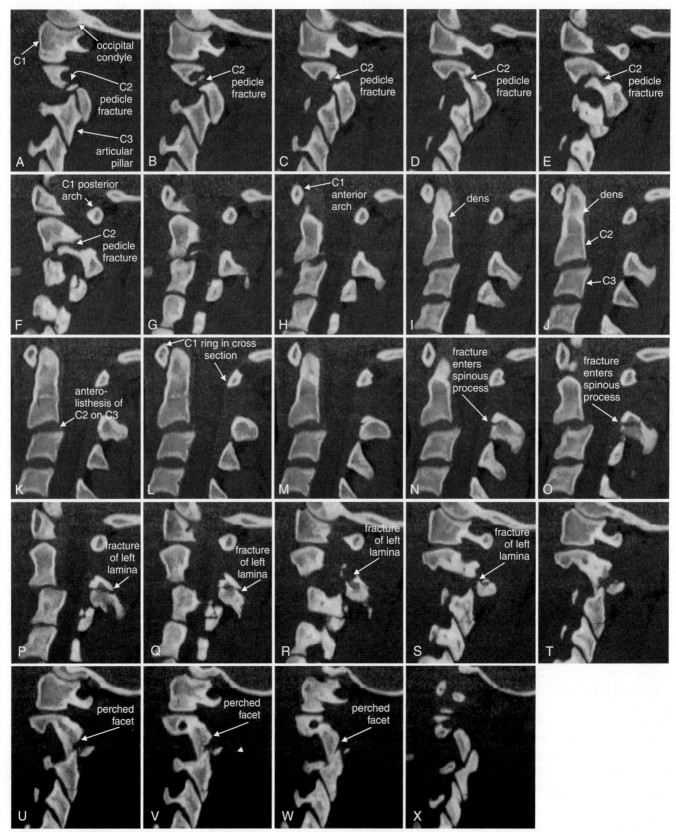

Figure 3-56. Hangman's fracture of C2. Sagittal computed tomography images from the same patient as in Figures 3-53 through 3-57 illustrate in more detail the abnormalities seen on the lateral plain x-ray. The sections shown are displayed from far right parasagittal **(A),** through the midline **(K),** and to far left sagittal **(X).** Take a moment to get oriented by looking at slice **K,** which shows the midline with the dens clearly demonstrated. In the far right slices starting at **A,** the facet joint is demonstrated. A fracture line runs through the right pedicle of C2, just anterior to the articular pillar. In the slices near the midline, the C2 body can be seen with anterior subluxation relative to C3, widening the spinal canal. In the slices approaching a left lateral position **(O to U),** a fracture is seen through the base of emergency spinous process and extending into the left lamina as you continue toward the patient's left in the series. The result of the bilateral fractures is complete separation of the posterior elements of the vertebral body from the anterior elements, an unstable fracture. A perched facet (articular pillar) is seen in **T** to **X;** this injury is explored in more detail in a later figure, as it is not technically part of the hangman's fracture pattern.

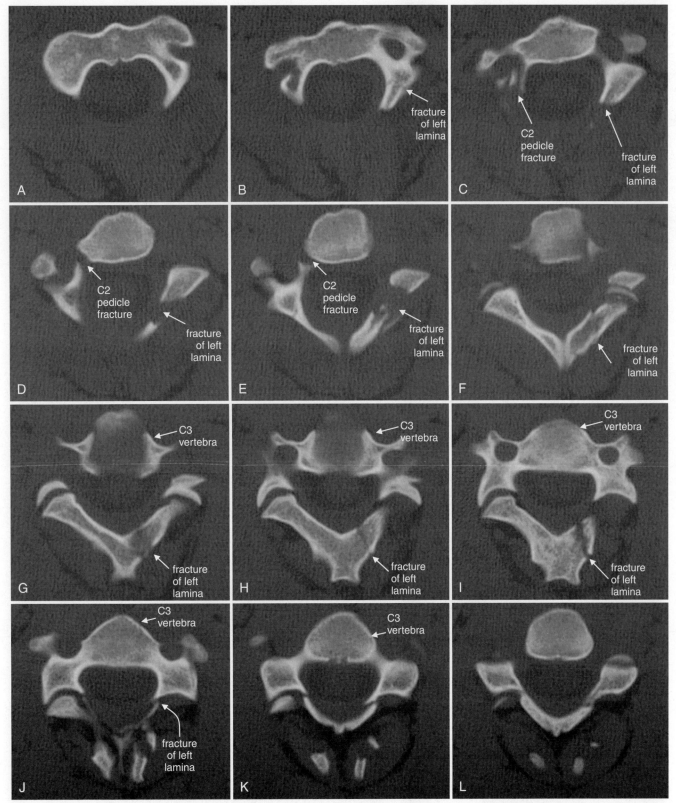

Figure 3-57. Hangman's fracture of C2. Same patient as in Figures 3-53 through 3-56. Axial views of the C2 vertebra again show a hangman's fracture, with fractures of the right pedicle and left lamina, as illustrated in the sagittal slices in Figure 3-56. Follow the series cephalad to caudad from **A** (just below the junction of the dens with the body of C2) through the base of the C2 vertebral body **(F).** Because the vertebrae do not lie in a perfect axial plane, images **G** to **L** actually show more than one vertebra: the anterior structures are the vertebral body and appendages of C3, while the posterior structures are the posterior elements of C2. This may confuse novices, but is a feature common to axial imaging of the cervical spine. This patient also has a jumped left C2-3 facet joint, which is explored in more detail in a subsequent figure.

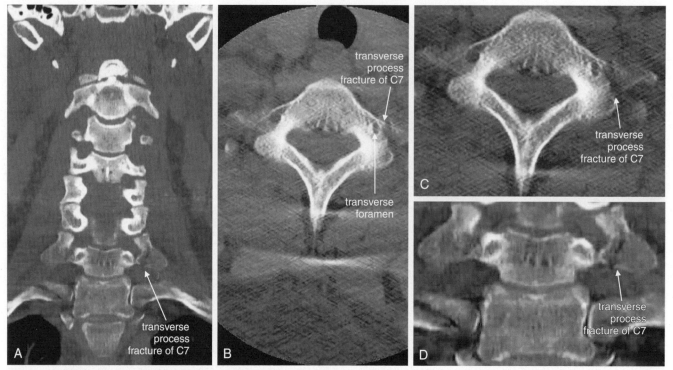

Figure 3-58. Transverse process fracture, noncontrast CT, bone windows. Spinous process fractures are frequently noted on plain x-ray and computed tomography (CT), though they usually have little clinical significance. In these images, a transverse process fracture of C7 is seen. Because the fracture line is oriented in a nearly sagittal plane, it is invisible on the sagittal CT images (not shown). **A,** A coronal view shows the sagittal fracture. **B,** The fracture line narrowly misses the transverse foramen housing the vertebral artery. **C, D,** Close-ups from **B** and **A,** respectively. The three-dimensional structure of the cervical spine is sometimes difficult to appreciate in the two dimensions of a single CT slice. **A,** The transverse processes of the more cephalad vertebral bodies are not well seen because of the normal cervical lordosis, which places the transverse processes of those vertebrae anterior to the coronal plane through the transverse processes of C7.

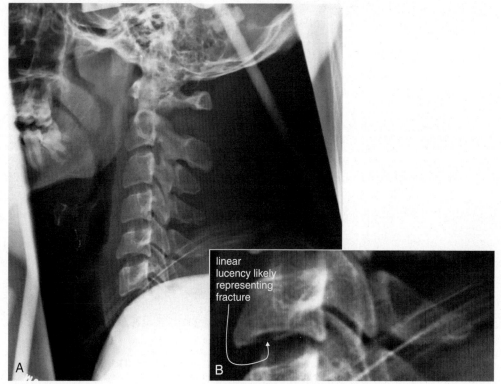

Figure 3-59. Cervical burst compression fracture, lateral cervical spine x-ray. This patient has a C5 burst compression fracture, first noted on computed tomography (CT) scan. **A,** This lateral cervical spine x-ray was obtained after CT scan was performed and the patient had been placed in a halo traction device. The x-ray is technically inadequate, as it does not show C7 and T1. However, a subtle linear lucency through the inferior cortex of C5 may correspond to fractures seen on CT. The x-ray is otherwise quite normal, with normal alignment of the vertebral bodies. The prevertebral soft tissues are also normal. **B,** Close-up.

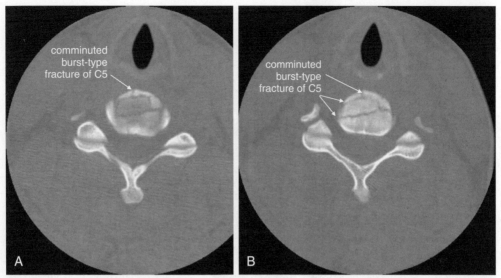

Figure 3-60. Cervical burst compression fracture, CT. Same patient as in Figure 3-59. This patient has a C5 burst compression fracture. These fractures are inherently unstable, as they involve all three spinal columns (discussed in the text). Despite a highly comminuted fracture, no fracture fragments have become displaced into the spinal canal. **A, B,** Two adjacent axial slices.

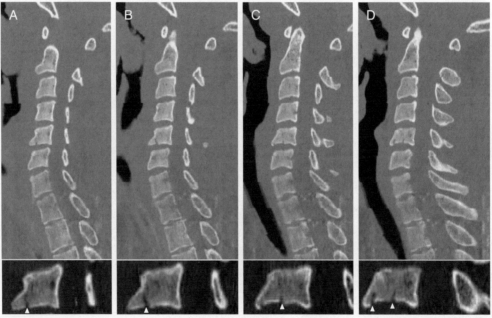

Figure 3-61. Cervical burst compression fracture. Same patient as in Figures 3-59 and 3-60. In these parasagittal CT views (**A** to **D**), compression burst fractures of the C5 vertebral body are visible, although not as evident in the axial views in Figure 3-60. Fractures are visible where they violate the bony cortex and cross through the sagittal plane. Note that the spinal canal appears patent, with no retropulsed fracture fragments. The lower panels are close-ups of C5 from the corresponding upper panels, with fractures marked by arrowheads.

Can Computed Tomography Detect Spinal Cord Injury and Nontraumatic Spinal Cord Abnormalities?

MRI, not CT, is considered the test of choice for spinal cord injury. CT shows secondary findings suggesting cord impingement, such as narrowing of the spinal canal from fracture fragments or subluxation of vertebral bodies. In some cases, the cord can be seen, but its tissue density is similar to that of cerebrospinal fluid, making detailed inspection difficult. A special technique called CT myelography (CT myelogram) is an alternative to MRI for visualization of the spinal cord. In CT myelography, contrast material is injected into the spinal canal through a spinal needle in a technique similar to diagnostic lumbar puncture. CT is then performed, and the spinal cord and nerve roots can be seen in relief against the contrast material outlining them. This technique is not commonly used but can be used in patients with contraindications to MRI. CT myelography provides information about spinal cord compression but does not provide information about intrinsic spinal cord pathology such as transverse myelitis, spinal cord infarction or edema, and multiple sclerosis. This type of pathology requires the soft tissue contrast of MRI.

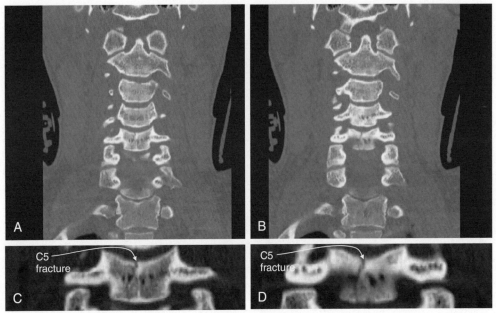

Figure 3-62. Cervical burst compression fracture. Same patient as in Figures 3-59 through 3-61. On these coronal views **(A, B)**, a C5 burst compression fracture is visible. A sagittally oriented fracture nearly bisects the vertebral body. **C, D,** Close-ups from **A** and **B,** respectively.

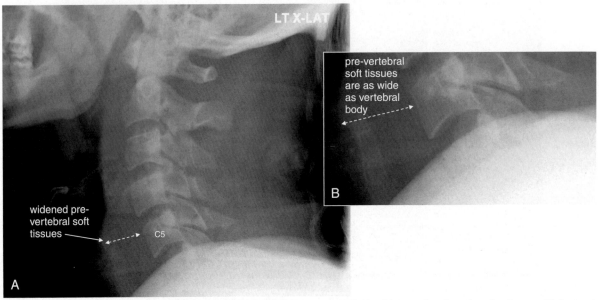

Figure 3-63. C6 flexion teardrop fracture. A, This lateral cervical spine x-ray was obtained in a patient later found to have a C6 flexion teardrop fracture by computed tomography. **B,** Close-up. Several important points are illustrated by this x-ray. First, an adequate lateral cervical spine x-ray must include C1 through T1. This x-ray visualized only through C5, with C6 being obscured by soft tissues of the shoulder. Ironically, this was the level of injury. Nonetheless, subtle signs of injury are present. The prevertebral soft tissues are prominent, a finding that can be due to prevertebral hemorrhage in the presence of a fracture. In addition, the distance between the C5 and the C6 (only partially visualized) spinous processes appears wide, indicating possible injury. The teardrop fragment was not noted but in retrospect may be visible. Compare with the CT in Figures 3-64 through 3-66.

How Long Does Cervical Computed Tomography Take to Perform? Which Is Faster, X-ray or Computed Tomography?

CT is the most time-efficient method of imaging the cervical spine. Daffner[39] measured the time required to perform six views of the cervical spine (AP, lateral, open-mouth odontoid, bilateral obliques, and swimmer's view) and found the average to be 22 minutes (range of 5 to 46 minutes). Many patients required at least one view to be repeated to achieve a satisfactory image. In the same study, and again in a separate study, Daffner measured the time required for cervical spine CT and found the average to be between 11 and 12 minutes (range of 3 to 35 minutes), depending on whether the cervical CT was performed in conjunction with a head

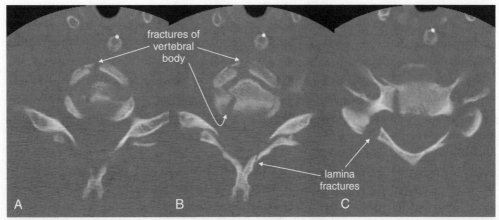

Figure 3-64. Flexion teardrop fracture. Same patient as in Figure 3-63. These adjacent axial computed tomography (CT) images **(A** to **C)** demonstrate perhaps the most surprising feature of a flexion teardrop fracture—the degree of comminution. Lateral cervical spine x-rays and midsagittal CT reconstructions often suggest a simple fracture with a single anterior "teardrop"-shaped fragment. Instead, the axial views reveal a badly comminuted fracture of the C6 vertebral body, as well as fractures of the lamina.

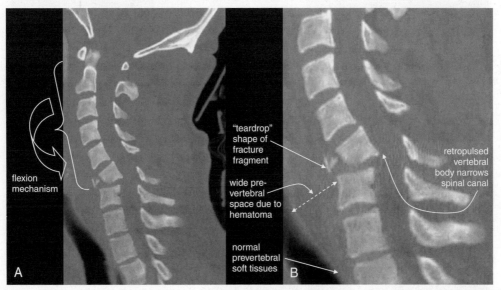

Figure 3-65. C6 flexion teardrop fracture. Same patient as in Figures 3-63 and 3-64. **A,** A midsagittal computed tomography reconstruction demonstrates the classic "teardrop"-shaped fracture fragment, the flexion mechanism of injury, and the potential for narrowing of the spinal canal and spinal cord injury. **B,** Close-up. The degree of comminution of the vertebral body is less evident here than on the axial views in Figure 3-64. The prevertebral soft-tissue swelling evident on the lateral x-ray (Figure 3-63) is seen well here. This patient developed complete paraplegia as a result of this injury.

CT.[39-40] These results were achieved using a 4-slice scanner, and imaging times with newer scanners are even faster. A 64-slice CT can perform sixty-four 0.625-mm slices per second, meaning that in each second of scanning, a territory 40 mm (64 × 0.625 mm) in length can be imaged. If the cervical spine is 20 cm (200 mm) in length, CT could be completed in 5 seconds. In addition, CT has the advantage of performing cervical spine imaging in the same location that diagnostic imaging for other injuries is being performed. Even if only three x-ray views of the cervical spine were performed, halving the time for x-ray, CT is faster with modern scanners.

Radiation

The radiation doses for cervical spine x-rays and CT differ by an order of magnitude.

A three-view cervical x-ray series (consisting of an AP, a lateral, and an open-mouth odontoid view) generates about 0.1 mSv, although the dose may rise if additional views or repeated attempts at the same view are needed to obtain diagnostic-quality x-rays. CT of the skull base and upper cervical spine for odontoid evaluation creates an effective dose of about 4.4 mSv using a single-slice scanner and about 2.3 mSv using a 16-slice scanner. CT of C0 to C3 and the cervicothoracic junction creates a dose of about 7.1 mSv using a single-slice scanner and 4.3 mSv for a 16-slice scanner. CT of the entire cervical spine generates a dose of 8.2 mSv using a single-slice scanner and 5.4 mSv for a 16-slice scanner.[54] Substantial thyroid radiation exposures occur with cervical spine CT. Estimates of lifetime attributable mortality from complete cervical CT are in the range of 1 in 2400 for

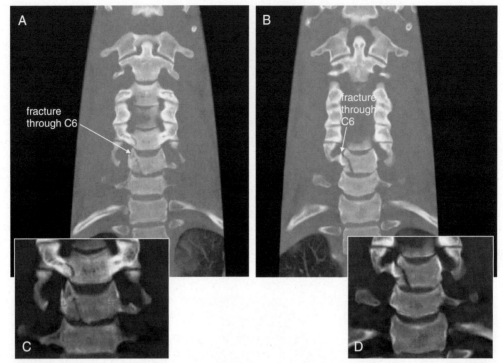

Figure 3-66. C6 flexion teardrop fracture. Same patient as in Figures 3-63 through 3-65. These coronal computed tomography reconstructions (**A, B,** with close-ups in **C** and **D,** respectively) reveal an oblique, vertical fracture through the C6 vertebral body, as well as the C5 body.

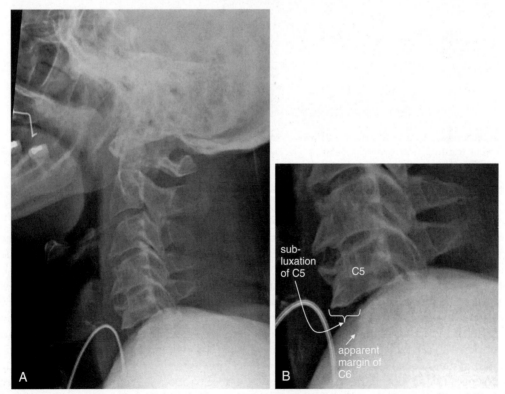

Figure 3-67. Bilateral facet dislocation (jumped facets). This pattern of injury is most often seen between C3 and T1. **A,** This lateral x-ray demonstrates the importance of visualizing the entire cervical spine from C1 to T1 in an adequate lateral x-ray. **B,** Close-up. In this case, the C6 vertebral body is partially obscured by soft tissues of the shoulder. C7 and T1 are not seen. Despite this, anterior subluxation of C5 on C6 is evident, with a ledge of C5 protruding by almost 50% of the width of the vertebral body. This degree of anterolisthesis is concerning for bilateral perched facets, which were confirmed on computed tomography scan (Figures 3-68 through 3-71).

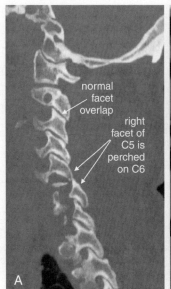

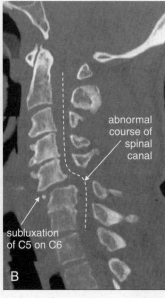

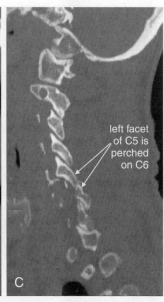

normal facet overlap

right facet of C5 is perched on C6

A

abnormal course of spinal canal

subluxation of C5 on C6

B

left facet of C5 is perched on C6

C

Figure 3-68. Bilateral facet dislocation (jumped facets). Same patient as in Figure 3-67. This series of sagittal CT reconstructions spans from the patient's right (A), through the midsagittal plane (B), and to the patient's left (C). Bilateral perched facets are present. Compare the "perched" position with the normal appearance of facet joints, which demonstrate overlap like shingles on a roof. B, The anterior subluxation of C5 seen on the lateral x-ray (Figure 3-67) is readily evident. As a result, the spinal canal has a zigzag appearance, and the spinal cord is impinged upon (see MRI in Figures 3-70 and 3-71).

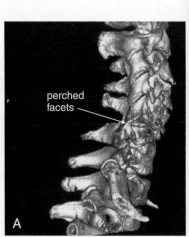

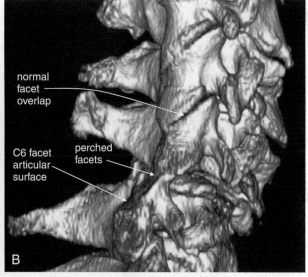

perched facets

A

normal facet overlap

C6 facet articular surface

perched facets

perched facets

B

Figure 3-69. Bilateral facet dislocation (jumped facets): Three-dimensional reconstruction. Same patient as in Figures 3-67 and 3-68. A, This three-dimensional reconstruction from the patient's computed tomography scan depicts the facet dislocation. B, Close-up. Viewed from the patient's right side, the C5-6 facet joint is seen to be perched. The C6 facet articular surface is completely exposed, as the entire cervical spine cephalad to this level has moved anteriorly. Notice how the facet joints above this level overlap normally like shingles on a roof.

a single-slice scanner and 1 in 3700 using a 16-slice CT scanner. Attributable mortality estimates may vary with age at exposure, with younger patients incurring greater risk. Improvements in CT will likely reduce the effective dose, but significant radiation doses will likely remain using CT.[41]

Cost of Cervical Imaging

Cost-effectiveness of cervical radiography and CT have been compared in models with estimates based on patient pretest probability of injury, assumptions about the cost of missed injuries and resulting health care costs to society, and the direct costs of imaging.[42-43] Blackmore[42] found that high- and moderate-risk patients

should be imaged with CT as the most cost-effective strategy. In low-risk patients, CT screening would be predicted to identify additional potentially unstable injuries, but the cost per quality-adjusted life-year would be greater than $80,000—making x-ray the more cost-effective strategy in this group. Like all cost-effectiveness analyses, this report may be subject to many inaccuracies due to potentially false assumptions about the sensitivity of x-ray and CT, the incidence of injury, the direct costs of imaging, and the costs associated with missed injuries. In a second cost-effectiveness analysis with similar suppositions about sensitivity, likelihood of injury, and costs, Grogan[43] found CT to be more cost-effective than x-ray. According to that analysis, CT

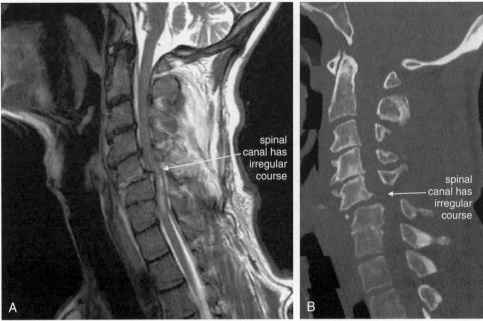

Figure 3-70. Bilateral facet dislocation (jumped facets). Same patient as in Figures 3-67 through 3-69. **A,** A midsagittal T2-weighted magnetic resonance image shows narrowing of the spinal canal with cord impingement at the C5-6 level. **B,** The midsagittal computed tomography image for comparison. On T2-weighted images, fluid such as cerebrospinal fluid (CSF) appears white, while fat-containing soft tissues such as the spinal cord appear dark gray. Narrowing of the spinal canal has displaced the CSF that would normally surround the cord at the level of injury. Edema within the cord caused by spinal injury appears white on T2 images. The dura appears nearly black. An epidural spinal hematoma is visible, appearing white outside the dark dura. These findings are explored in detail in Figure 3-71.

Figure 3-71. Bilateral facet dislocation (jumped facets). Same patient as in Figures 3-67 through 3-70. **A,** A midsagittal T2-weighted magnetic resonance image shows narrowing of the spinal canal with cord impingement at the C5-6 level. **B,** Close-up.

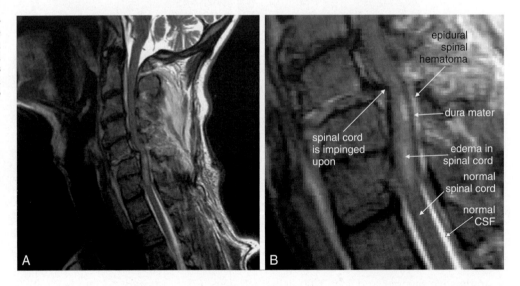

would have an institutional cost of $554 per patient, compared with $2142 per patient for x-ray, when the costs of missed injury settlements are included. Sensitivity analysis showed that x-ray could be more cost-effective if CT costs more than $1918 or if x-ray has a sensitivity greater than 90%.

Magnetic Resonance Imaging of Spinal Soft Tissue Injuries

MRI is the imaging modality of choice for patients with suspected spinal cord, nerve root, spinal ligament, or intervertebral disc injuries. MRI has outstanding soft-tissue contrast that allows direct visualization of these injuries. Ironically, MRI yields poor images of bone, as calcified bone has a paucity of protons to interact with the imposed magnetic field. MRI relies on the radiofrequency signal produced by protons subjected to a magnetic field. Tissues containing water and fat yield a strong MRI signal due to their high proton content. Bone contains little water or fat and consequently has poor proton content and MRI signal. Consequently, CT is an important complementary study to evaluate for spinal fractures. Typically, MRI sequences for traumatic injuries include transverse (axial) and sagittal

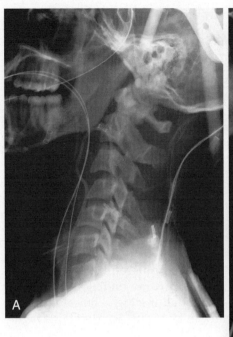

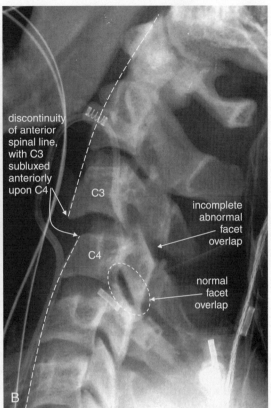

discontinuity of anterior spinal line, with C3 subluxed anteriorly upon C4

C3

C4

incomplete abnormal facet overlap

normal facet overlap

Figure 3-72. C3-4 unilateral facet dislocation. A, This lateral cervical spine x-ray shows a unilateral facet dislocation. **B,** Close-up. The normal curve of the anterior and posterior longitudinal spinal lines is disrupted, and C3 appears anteriorly subluxed relative to C4. Unlike the prior bilateral "perched" facet case, the pedicles and lamina show partial overlap, although the degree of overlap is not as great as usual.

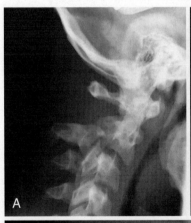

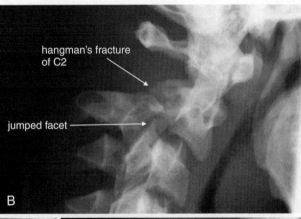

hangman's fracture of C2

jumped facet

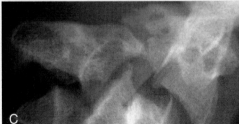

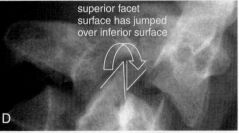

superior facet surface has jumped over inferior surface

Figure 3-73. C2-3 unilateral facet dislocation (jumped facet). In this patient, a hangman's fracture of C2 and a unilateral facet joint dislocation are both present. The lateral x-ray shows predominantly the hangman's fracture **(A),** although the anterior position of the jumped facet can be seen. **B** to **D,** Close-ups from **A.** Compare this appearance with the sagittal computed tomography images (Figure 3-75). Hangman's fractures are explored in more detail in other figures.

T1- and T2-weighted fast spin–echo sequences. Short T1 inversion recovery images may also be acquired. Gadolinium contrast is not needed for evaluation of acute traumatic injury. Boxes 3-10 and 3-11 summarize indications for spine MRI and pathology that can be detected.[28]

How Sensitive Is Magnetic Resonance Imaging for Detection of Soft-Tissue Injuries of the Spine?

Physics of MRI, common MRI sequences, and evidence for MRI are discussed in detail in Chapter 15. Good-quality studies of the sensitivity of MRI for detection of soft-tissue injuries require an independent gold standard. Because other imaging studies are felt to be inferior to MRI, these standards usually include either clinical follow-up or reports from pathology or autopsy findings. It may come as a surprise that when MRI is compared with a strong gold standard such as autopsy, it has poor sensitivity for soft-tissue injury. A study comparing MRI of 10 adult accident victims with autopsy thin sagittal sections showed that MRI detected only 11 of 28 spinal lesions (39%)—mostly soft-tissue injuries, including facet joint capsule injuries, ligamentous injuries, disk injuries, and spinal cord lesions. In the same study, x-ray identified only 4% of lesions.[44] Jonsson et al.[45] performed an autopsy study comparing x-ray to cryosectioned cervical spine and found that x-ray detected only 1 of 10 gross upper cervical spine ligamentous disruptions. The clinical significance of the missed findings is impossible to assess from autopsy,

and MRI is currently our best imaging modality for this purpose, as x-ray shows extremely low sensitivity in the same studies (Boxes 3-10 and 3-11).

IMAGING THE CERVICAL SPINE IN THE ABSENCE OF A HISTORY OF TRAUMA

Emergency imaging of the cervical spine is less commonly indicated in the absence of a history of trauma. However, when spinal cord compression is suspected in the absence of trauma, plain x-rays play a relatively minor role in the evaluation. They have limited sensitivity and specificity for the soft-tissue abnormalities typically at play, such as cervical disc herniation, syrinx, neoplastic mass, and cervical epidural abscess. X-rays may suggest a bony lesion, such as a metastatic lytic lesion or cervical stenosis, but soft-tissue abnormalities can occur without any x-ray findings, and further imaging is always required if a high clinical suspicion is present. CT scan can be useful, as it remains highly

---

Box 3-10 Pathology Identified by Magnetic Resonance Imaging

- Fractures (bones)—identified by marrow edema, as the cortex is invisible on MRI
- Dislocations and subluxation (ligaments)
- Soft tissues (nerves and discs)
- Fluid collections (hematomas, abscesses, and syrinx)
- Vascular injuries—when performed as magnetic resonance angiography of neck, a different study from spine MRI

Box 3-11 When Should I Order Spine Magnetic Resonance Imaging?

- Neurologic complaint following trauma
- Known or suspected spinal cord injury
- Cervical spine clearance in obtunded trauma patients, even following even normal CT—an area of controversy (see text)
- Neurologic abnormality localizing to the spinal cord in the absence of trauma

---

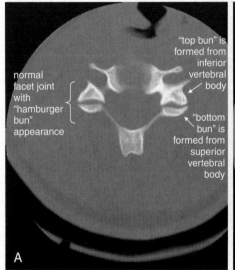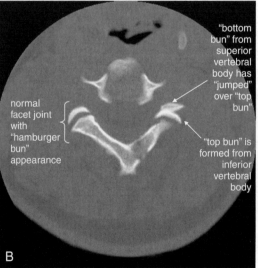

Figure 3-74. C2-3 unilateral facet dislocation (jumped facet). Same patient as in Figure 3-73. The normal appearance of a cervical facet joint on axial CT images is a "hamburger bun." The anterior (top) half of the "bun" is formed by the inferior cervical vertebra. The posterior (bottom) half of the "bun" is formed by the superior cervical vertebra. In a jumped facet, the superior articulating surface (bottom bun) jumps over the inferior articulating surface (top bun) and becomes anterior to it, reversing the normal configuration. **A,** A normal facet articulation bilaterally. **B,** The same patient, one cervical level higher. The patient's right facet joint has a normal hamburger bun appearance, while the left facet joint has jumped, assuming a reversed hamburger bun appearance.

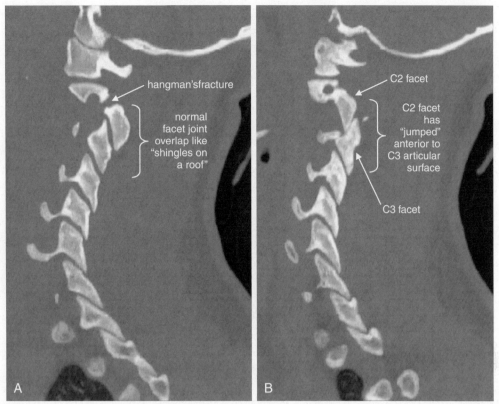

Figure 3-75. C2-3 unilateral facet dislocation (jumped facet). Same patient as Figure 3-73 and 3-74. Parasagittal CT images. **A,** The patient's right C2-3 facet joint is in normal position with appropriate overlap like shingles on a roof. **B,** A left unilateral jumped facet joint for comparison, with the superior articulating surface having moved anterior to the inferior articular surface. Injuries of this type require a substantial amount of force, and fractures often occur in association with jumped facets. This patient has a right hangman's type fracture of C2 as well. Hangman's fractures are explored in more detail in other figures. A jumped facet is more difficult to recognize on coronal views, which are not shown for this case.

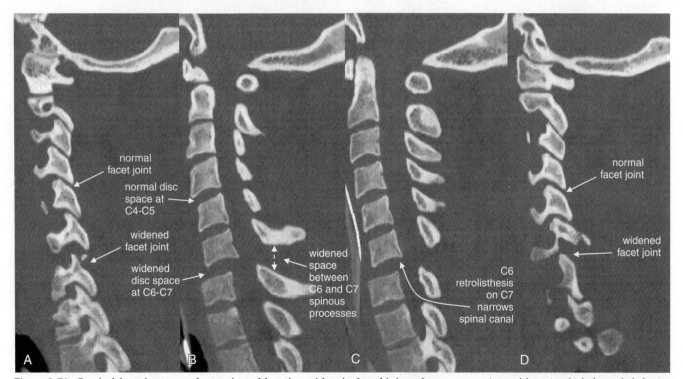

Figure 3-76. Cervical facet fracture and posterior subluxation with spinal cord injury. In contrast to a jumped facet, in which the cephalad spine subluxes anteriorly relative to the caudad spine, posterior subluxation may occur. This sagittal CT series progresses from the patient's right **(A)** to left **(D). A** and **D,** Note the widened facet joint at C6-7. **B,** The space between the spinous processes of C6 and C7 is also widened. **B** and **C** (a midline sagittal view), Posterior subluxation (retrolisthesis) of C6 on C7 is evident, narrowing the spinal canal. The distance between the C6 and the C7 vertebral bodies also appears wider than normal. Compare with the MRI in Figure 3-77.

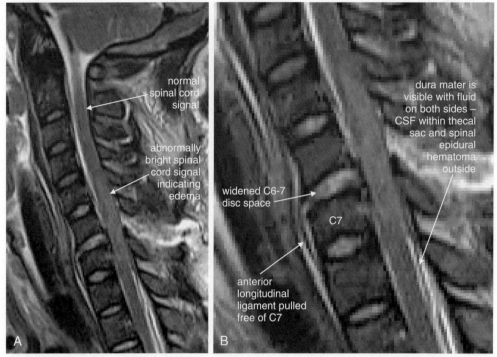

Figure 3-77. Cervical facet fracture and posterior subluxation with spinal cord injury. A, This T2-weighted magnetic resonance image from the same patient as in Figure 3-76 demonstrates disruption of the posterior longitudinal ligament with widening of the C6-7 disc space. The anterior longitudinal ligament remains attached to the anteroinferior corner of C6 but has been stripped from the ventral surface of C7. **B,** Close-up. There is an abnormal spinal cord signal from C4-5 through C7-T1 levels, with mild spinal cord expansion. In addition, there appears to be large extramedullary fluid collection posterior to the spinal cord from the C7 level through below the field of view, displacing the thoracic spinal cord ventrally against the posterior longitudinal ligament. The dura is outlined by fluid signal intensity on both sides. *CSF,* Cerebrospinal fluid.

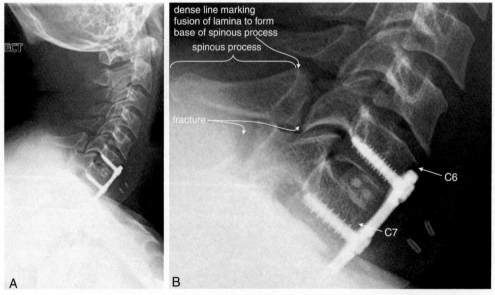

Figure 3-78. C6 and C7 laminar fractures. A, This lateral x-ray reveals fractures through the lamina of C6 and C7. **B,** Close-up. Look carefully at the images—the fracture line through C6 clearly runs anterior to the dense line marking the junction of the lamina with the spinous process. Fractures anterior to this line are lamina fractures, not spinous process fractures. Do not confuse lamina fractures, which can threaten the spinal cord, with spinous process fractures, which typically have little clinical consequence. The fracture line through C7 disrupts the dense line marking the anterior border of the spinous process. The x-ray is technically inadequate, because it shows the bottom margin of C7 but does not reveal the relationship with T1. The patient has hardware from a previous anterior spinal fusion. Compare with the CT in Figures 3-79 and 3-80.

sensitive for bony abnormalities, but *often MRI is the first and only test required in the absence of trauma.* MRI of the cervical spine is performed with gadolinium contrast when possible to evaluate the cervical spinal cord, discs, and surrounding epidural space. Gadolinium assists in detection and characterization of inflammatory, infectious, and neoplastic processes. However, cord compression can be identified without gadolinium if the patient has contraindications to gadolinium, such as poor renal function.

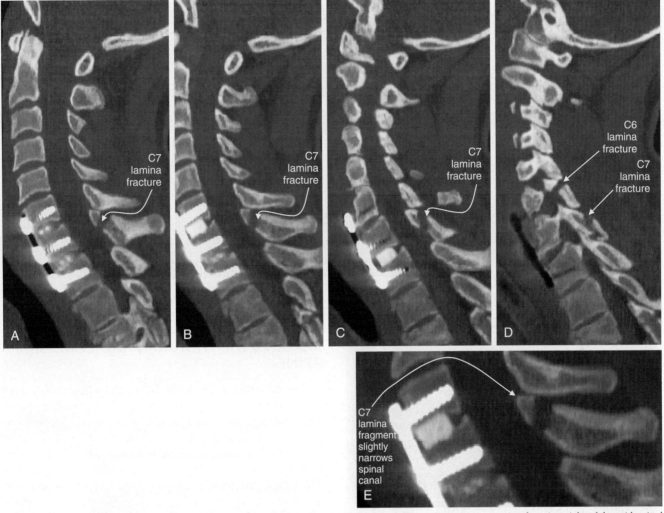

Figure 3-79. C6 and C7 laminar fractures. Same patient as in Figure 3-78. These sagittal CT reconstructions—moving from just right of the midsagittal plane **(A)** toward the patient's left **(D)**—demonstrate fractures through the C6 and C7 lamina. A fragment has drifted anteriorly into the spinal canal, slightly narrowing it at the C7 level. The patient has preexisting spinal fusion screws through C6, C7, and T1, which provide convenient landmarks. **E,** Close-up from **B.**

Cervical Spine Infections and Metastatic Disease

Unlike the case in traumatic cervical spine injuries, no clear CDRs exist, although some risk stratification can be performed. Because acutely dangerous spontaneous cervical spine pathology such as spinal cord compression from epidural abscess or hematoma or spinal and epidural metastases is relatively rare, typically many patients will require screening to identify a single case. Early identification of a lesion—before significant neurologic deficits have occurred—is extremely important, because neurologic deficits are often irreversible once present.[46] Risk factors for cervical epidural abscess include preexisting minor spinal pathology such as spondylosis, degenerative joint disease, previous laminectomy, or nonpenetrating trauma from a fall or motor vehicle collision. Underlying diseases may predispose patients to develop cervical epidural abscess, including diabetes mellitus, alcoholism, cancer, chronic renal failure, and other compromised immune states. Injection drug use is a significant risk factor, and patients may not reveal a history of cervical injection in 50% of cases.[47-48] Cervical osteomyelitis has been reported as a complication of cervical injection.[49-50] Other recent infections, including distant sources such as urinary tract infection or skin abscesses, can lead to cervical epidural abscess by hematogenous inoculation. Any previous invasive spinal procedure, even several months before presentation, should increase the suspicion of cervical epidural abscess. Patients typically will not offer this information unless asked specifically. Several reviews suggest that almost 20% of patients will have no identifiable predisposing factors for cervical epidural abscess.[51-52] Fever may not be present—reviews on this topic suggest fever is noted in only 30% to 80% of patients on presentation.[53-55] The classic triad of localized spine tenderness, progressive neurologic deficits, and fever occurs in only 37% of patients with cervical epidural abscess.[56]

Figure 3-80. C6 and C7 lamina fractures. Same patient as in Figures 3-78 and 3-79. Axial computed tomography images demonstrate lamina fractures through C7 **(A, B)** and C6 **(C).** The C6 fractures are present at the junction of the lamina and pedicle. The C7 fractures intersect the middle portion of the lamina and then enter the base of the spinous process at their more cephalad extent.

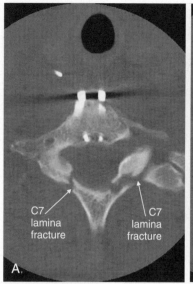
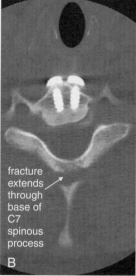
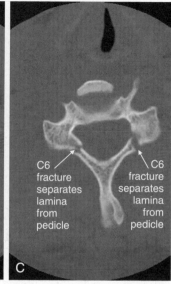

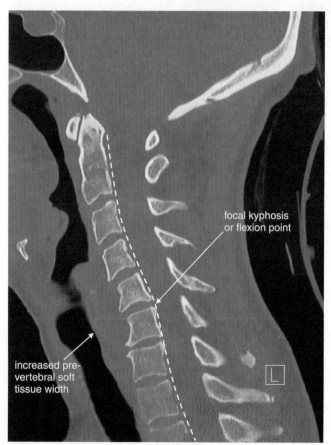

Figure 3-81. Acute cervical ligamentous injuries. This patient experienced syncope and fell from a standing position, striking her occiput. She complained of exquisite neck pain, and computed tomography (CT) was performed. On this midsagittal CT image, the normal cervical lordosis is lost, likely because of the cervical collar. In addition, a subtle focal kyphosis is now present at the C5-6 level, associated with an increased prevertebral soft-tissue space at this level. Just as on plain x-ray, the posterior longitudinal ligament line should be a smooth, continuous curve, but in this case the curve is interrupted by a flexion point. Also, as with plain x-ray, increased prevertebral soft tissue width can be a sign of prevertebral hematoma associated with an acute injury. No fractures were identified on CT. Magnetic resonance imaging (MRI) was performed to further evaluate (Figures 3-82 and 3-83).

IMAGING THE THORACIC AND LUMBAR SPINE

We now review epidemiology, decision rules, and imaging modalities for the thoracic and lumbar spine. Many of the same considerations discussed for cervical spine imaging apply. The ACR now recommends that CT of the thoracic and lumbar spine, rather than x-ray, be the initial screening test in blunt trauma patients requiring imaging of these regions. Images may be acquired from dedicated CT of these regions or from CT of the chest, abdomen, and pelvis obtained for evaluation of other injuries to these regions. The ACR recommends that the CT images include axial, sagittal, and coronal reformats,[1] because these improve detection of injuries in the axial plane, including fractures and subluxations. Because patients with low-energy trauma mechanisms may still be evaluated with plain x-ray, we will review both x-ray and CT interpretation.

Introduction to Thoracic and Lumbar Spine Injuries

Thoracic and lumbar spine injuries are common following high-energy blunt trauma. In motorcycle collisions, thoracic spine injuries actually outnumber cervical injuries, accounting for 54.8% of spinal injuries in one large study.[57] Overall, thoracic and lumbar spine injuries together account for more than half of all spinal injuries in car and motorcycle collisions, and multilevel injuries frequently occur. Falls from significant height account for another common presentation often requiring thoracic and lumbar spine imaging. Delays in diagnosis are common, occurring in as many as 19% of thoracolumbar injuries, implying a need for better clinical criteria to detect these injuries.[58]

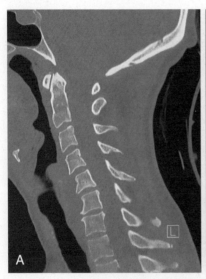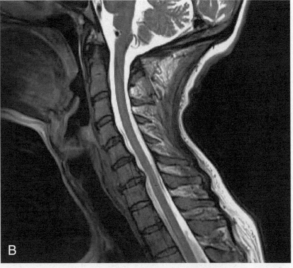

Figure 3-82. Acute cervical ligamentous injuries. Same patient as in Figure 3-81. A side-by-side comparison of results from sagittal computed tomography (CT) **(A)** and magnetic resonance imaging (MRI) **(B)** images. MRI gives excellent soft-tissue contrast, while CT provides high resolution for bone. On MRI, calcified bone gives only a signal void, because it has no free protons to resonate in the magnetic field and provide a radio signal. Differences between CT and MRI are described in Chapter 15.

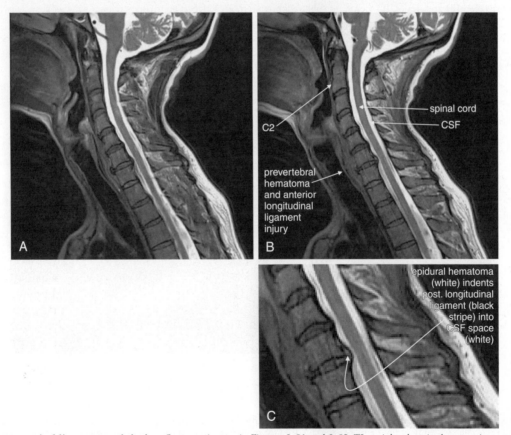

Figure 3-83. Acute cervical ligamentous injuries. Same patient as in Figures 3-81 and 3-82. T2-weighted sagittal magnetic resonance imaging of the cervical spine demonstrate an area of prevertebral soft-tissue injury from the inferior margin of C4 to the superior margin of T1. This corresponds to an acute injury of the anterior longitudinal ligament with hematoma formation. In addition, the thecal sac is indented at the C4-5, C5-6, and C6-7 levels. This is a result of to epidural hematoma formation, visible as a bright signal on T2-weighted images. On this image sequence, fluid (cerebrospinal fluid, or CSF, and acute hemorrhage) appears white, while the spinal cord is dark gray.

How Are X-rays of the Thoracolumbar Spine Interpreted?

X-rays of the lumbar and thoracic spine are interpreted with many of the same considerations as those for cervical spine radiographs. The standard views of the thoracic spine are AP and lateral, whereas the standard lumbar views are AP, lateral, and a spot view of L5 to S1 to allow adequate penetration while limiting radiation exposure.

On the AP view (see Figure 3-86), the thoracic spine should be assessed for alignment of adjacent vertebral

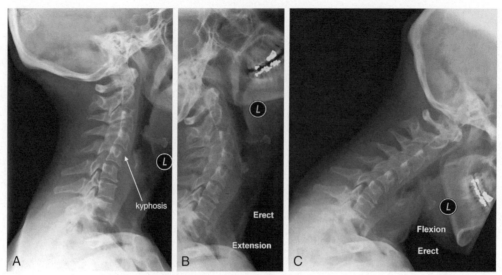

Figure 3-84. Acute cervical ligamentous injuries. Same patient as in Figures 3-81 through 3-83. Flexion–extension x-rays obtained 2 weeks after the acute injury in the same patient. The lateral x-ray in a neutral position **(A)** continues to show the focal kyphosis seen on the computed tomography. However, in the extension **(B)** and flexion **(C)** views, no subluxation is seen. Prevertebral soft tissues remain somewhat wide, which may indicate resolving hematoma.

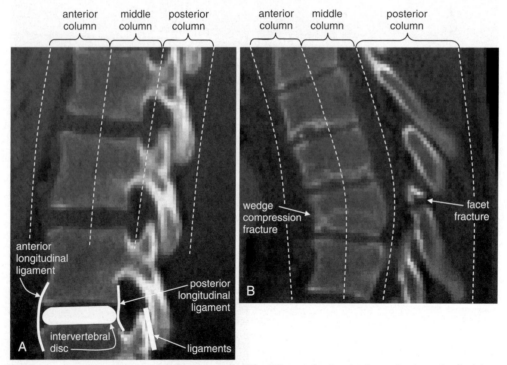

Figure 3-85. The three-column concept of thoracolumbar spine stability. When evaluating the thoracolumbar spine for injury, consider the spine to be composed of three columns, as depicted here. **A,** Sagittal CT image of lumbar spine. The anterior column is composed of the anterior half of the vertebral body and intervertebral disc, plus the anterior longitudinal ligament, which runs vertically along the anterior margin of each vertebral body. The middle column is composed of the posterior half of the vertebral body and intervertebral disc and the posterior longitudinal ligament, which runs vertically along the posterior margin of the vertebral bodies. The posterior column is composed of the facets with the strong ligaments joining these joints. When two of three columns are injured at a single spinal level, the spine is unstable. Injuries including subluxation, distraction, compression, and fracture may be sufficient to disrupt a column. **B,** Thoracic spine sagittal CT image, same patient. The anterior column has a compression injury, and the posterior column has a fracture. Only two of three columns need to be injured for the spine to be unstable.

bodies. The pedicles are usually visible like the "eyes of an owl," with the posterior spinous process present in the midline as the owl's beak. The posterior spinous processes may be displaced from the midline when fracture or subluxation is present. Pedicles may appear asymmetrical because of fracture or may be eroded by lytic processes such as spinal metastases and infection. The transverse processes should be inspected for fractures. Paraspinous soft-tissue masses or hematomas may be evident as asymmetrical densities, and their presence

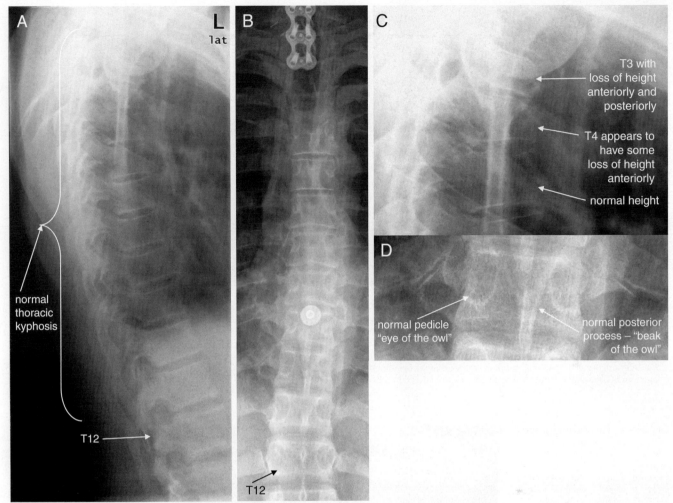

Figure 3-86. T2 corner avulsion fracture (extension teardrop) with T3 and T4 compression fracture. A, Lateral thoracic spine x-ray. **B,** Anterior–posterior thoracic spine x-ray. **C, D,** Close-ups from **A** and **B,** respectively. On a lateral view, each vertebral body should appear nearly rectangular, with similar height along its anterior and posterior borders. Anterior loss of height or "wedging" is common with compression fractures. Each body should appear similar in height to adjacent vertebra. The alignment of vertebral bodies should be assessed and should follow a slight thoracic kyphosis. Inspect carefully for any subluxation indicating injury. On the AP view, each vertebral body has two visible pedicles laterally (resembling the eyes of an owl) and a posterior spinous process in the midline (resembling an owl's beak). Fractures, dislocations, or malignant lytic lesions can disrupt this normal symmetrical radiographic anatomy. The alignment of vertebral bodies should be smooth, and the height of each body should be similar to that of the adjacent vertebrae. Fractures in the high thoracic spine can be extremely difficult to detect on x-ray because of the overlap with other thoracic structures, including scapula, ribs, soft tissues of the chest, and upper extremities. CT is more sensitive and is indicated when significant injuries are suspected. Low energy compression fractures such as from falls from standing may not require CT confirmation.

can suggest fracture, even when a fracture is not directly visualized. The heights of vertebral bodies should be equal on the AP projection, and the space between vertebral bodies should be even. Compression fractures of vertebral bodies can decrease their height, and disc injuries can decrease the space between adjacent bodies.

On the lateral x-ray (see Figure 3-86), the normal thoracic spine has a slight kyphosis, which should be a gradual and continuous curve. If the anterior margins of adjacent vertebral bodies do not align, subluxation is present; fractures may also be present. The upper thoracic spine is usually difficult to see on the lateral x-ray due to overlying shoulders. Swimmer's views can assist in revealing upper thoracic spine pathology. The spinal level involved can be determined by counting up from

the 12th rib on the AP projection. Children often have a normal variant that may be mistaken for an avulsion fracture on the lateral view. These are apophyses, small densities on the anterior superior and anterior inferior margins of adjacent vertebral bodies, which have the same appearance as anterior avulsion fractures in adults. Wedge compression fractures of the thoracic spine are common and result in decrease in the height of the anterior portion of a vertebral body relative to the posterior portion. Burst fractures can result in retropulsion of fragments into the spinal canal, and fragments may be seen on the lateral view posterior to the vertebral bodies.

The normal lumbar spine has a slight lordosis (see Figure 3-89), which should be smooth and continuous.

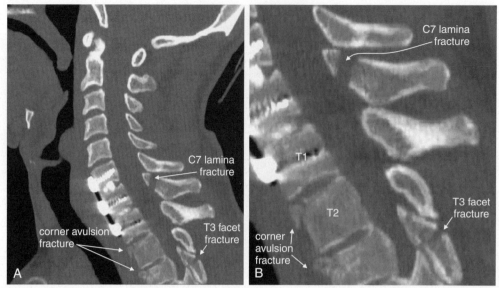

Figure 3-87. T2 corner avulsion fracture (extension teardrop). A, Sagittal CT image of the cervical spine in the same patient as in Figure 3-86 revealed anterior corner fractures of T2 and T3 (incompletely seen at the lower margin of the cervical spine CT). **B,** Close-up. He has previously undergone anterior fusion of C6, C7, and T1, perhaps contributing to this injury. The typical findings are triangular (teardrop) avulsion fragments, usually described as being due to the anterior longitudinal spinal ligament pulling away bone at its attachment points during hyperextension of the cervical spine. Whether this is the true mechanism is uncertain—in this patient, hyperflexion appears more likely, as the subsequent figures show the affected vertebrae to have findings of compression. More frequently, corner avulsion injuries occur in the cervical spine and result in teardrop fragments at the inferior corner of the vertebral body, rather than at the superior margin, as in this patient. Additional fractures are visible, including a T3 facet fracture and C7 lamina fracture. These are discussed in detail in other figures.

Figure 3-88. Thoracolumbar spine compression fracture. A, This patient has an L4 compression fracture, seen well on this lateral x-ray. **B,** Close-up. The anterior–posterior x-ray is less revealing (Figure 3-89). Computed tomography (CT) (Figures 3-90 through 3-92) revealed an unstable fracture. Note the normal L3 vertebra.

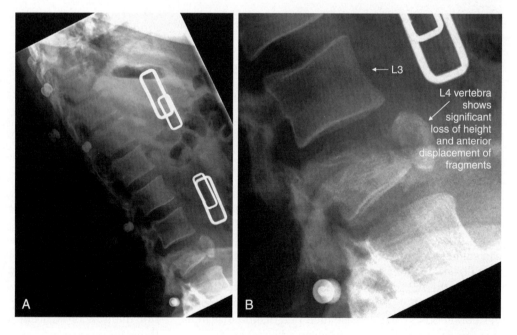

Other features of the lumbar spine are generally similar to those described earlier regarding the thoracic spine.

What Findings Suggest an Unstable Thoracolumbar Injury? What Is the Three-Column Concept?

Radiologists and spine surgeons (orthopedists and neurosurgeons) use a three-column concept to describe thoracolumbar spine injuries and to predict their stability.

Although described first for the thoracic and lumbar spine, the three-column system can also be applied to cervical spine injuries. For emergency physicians, it may often be sufficient to recognize that an injury is present. However, understanding the potential for an unstable fracture can be helpful in protecting the patient from neurologic injury, in ordering follow-up studies, and in engaging a consultant. Denis described a three-column system of classification in 1983, based on retrospective

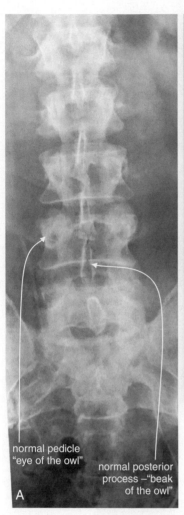

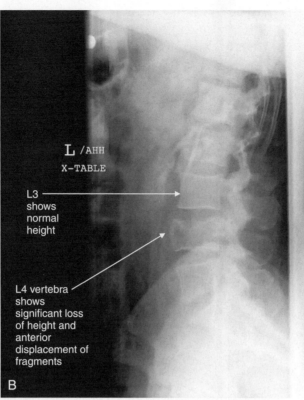

Figure 3-89. **Thoracolumbar spine compression fracture.** Same patient as in Figure 3-88. This patient has an L4 compression fracture, seen well on lateral x-ray (**B**). The anterior–posterior x-ray is less revealing (**A**). CT (Figures 3-90 through 3-92) revealed an unstable fracture.

review of 412 thoracolumbar injuries (see Figure 3-85). Previously, an anterior column (consisting of the anterior longitudinal ligament, marked on x-ray by the anterior borders of vertebral bodies) and a posterior column (consisting of posterior spinal ligaments) had been described. Denis[59] added a middle column, formed by the posterior border of the vertebral body, the posterior longitudinal ligament, and the posterior annulus fibrosis of the intervertebral disc. The same year, a CT description of the middle column was published, and CT findings have become the basis for operative treatment decisions, though these are outside the scope of this text.[60]

When two of three columns are disrupted, the spine is considered unstable. Whether reviewing x-ray or CT images, inspect the three columns for fractures or malalignment. Injuries to more than one column should be considered unstable; however, x-ray is relatively insensitive for thoracolumbar fracture (see later discussion) and spinal precautions should be maintained even when only one column appears injured on x-ray. CT should be obtained for further evaluation. Injuries to more than one column usually involve failure of the middle and anterior columns, the middle and posterior columns, or all three columns.[61] Injuries to anterior and posterior columns sparing the middle column are rare. Injuries to the anterior and posterior columns are often obvious. Middle-column injuries can be more subtle, but findings include widening of the pedicles, loss of posterior wall height greater than 25%, or obvious fracture of the cortex of the posterior vertebral body. For subluxation injuries without apparent fracture, translation greater than 3.5 mm or angulation greater than 11 degrees suggests column failure due to ligamentous injury.[61]

How Is Computed Tomography of the Thoracolumbar Spine Interpreted?

Interpretation of CT of the thoracolumbar spine follows the principles we described for cervical spine CT. Bone windows should be inspected in sagittal, coronal, and axial planes (see Table 3-2). Inspection of the sagittal images is extremely helpful for detection of anterior–posterior subluxation, as well as loss of height from compression fractures. The sagittal and axial images are useful for identifying retropulsion of fracture fragments into the

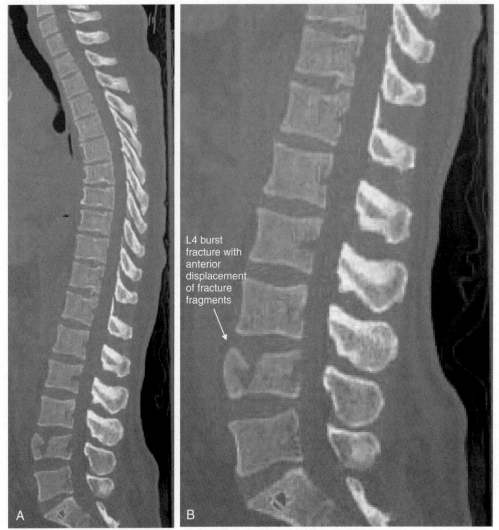

L4 burst fracture with anterior displacement of fracture fragments

Figure 3-90. Thoracolumbar spine compression–burst fracture. Same patient as in Figures 3-88 and 3-89. **A,** Sagittal CT shows L4 compression fracture, with loss of height of L4 vertebral body and slight radial spread of fragments. **B,** Close-up. The anterior margin of L4 is not aligned with the bodies above and below. The posterior margin is displaced slightly into the spinal canal.

spinal canal (see Figures 3-86 through 3-101). The coronal images are useful for assessing loss of height of vertebral bodies and disc spaces, lateral subluxation injuries, burst fractures with spread of fragments, and transverse process fractures. The sagittal images are particularly useful for assessing the three columns described earlier. All three series should be inspected to maximize detection of injuries, because fractures parallel to a given image plane will not be seen in that plane but are readily identified in images reconstructed in perpendicular planes. Anterior–posterior subluxation is best seen in sagittal images, whereas lateral subluxation is best seen in coronal views.

Who Needs Thoracic and Lumbar Imaging? Is There a Clinical Decision Rule for These Regions?

Unlike the case with injuries to the cervical spine, no single large study has produced a well-validated CDR for imaging of the thoracic and lumbar spine

that both detects all injuries and avoids unnecessary imaging. First, we lay out the best-evidence indications for imaging the thoracic and lumbar spine. Then, we examine the evidence behind these recommendations.

The ACR recommends thoracic and lumbar spine imaging for any of the following after major blunt trauma[1,62-63]:

- Back pain or midline tenderness
- Local exam findings of thoracolumbar injury (e.g., hematomas)
- Abnormal neurologic signs localizing to the thoracic or lumbar spine
- Cervical spine fracture
- Glasgow Coma Scale score of less than 15
- Major distracting injuries, particularly long-bone fractures
- Drug or alcohol intoxication

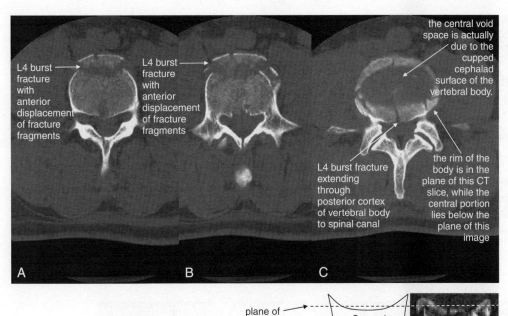

L4 burst fracture with anterior displacement of fracture fragments

L4 burst fracture with anterior displacement of fracture fragments

the central void space is actually due to the cupped cephalad surface of the vertebral body.

L4 burst fracture extending through posterior cortex of vertebral body to spinal canal

the rim of the body is in the plane of this CT slice, while the central portion lies below the plane of this image

A   B   C

plane of image C

Coronal view of L4

Figure 3-91. **Thoracolumbar spine burst–compression fracture.** Same patient as in Figures 3-88 through 3-90. Axial computed tomography views of the same lumbar (L4) burst fracture. Note the radial dispersion of the fracture fragments. **A** to **C** are arranged from caudad to cephalad. The central void in **C** is due to the cupped cephalad surface of the vertebral body (see diagram). The center of the vertebral body lies below the plane of **C,** while the raised rim lies in the plane of **C.** This is an unstable fracture because it involves all three columns of the spine.

Notice the similarity to NEXUS—the items are identical, with the addition of local examination findings and coexisting cervical spine fracture.

Several studies have contributed to these recommendations. A prospective study of 2404 patients evaluated seven high-risk criteria as a screening tool for identification of patients at risk for thoracolumbar injury.[64] The criteria included the five NEXUS criteria, with back pain and "severe mechanism of injury" as additional potential predictors of thoracolumbar fracture (Box 3-12). The authors also reported the predictive value of the presence of a cervical spine injury for detecting other spinal injuries, although this is not necessarily a data point available to the emergency physician at the initial assessment when many diagnostic imaging plans are formulated. The study identified 152 patients with spinal injuries. Use of the first six high-risk criteria resulted in 100% sensitivity (95% CI = 98%-100%) and 100% negative predictive value (95% CI = 97%-100%). Unfortunately, this rule is quite nonspecific (3.9%, 95% CI = 3.1%-4.8%) and has poor positive predictive value (6.6%, 95% CI = 97%-100%). As a result, application of this rule, while detecting all injuries, would result in imaging of virtually all major blunt trauma patients. Addition of "severe mechanism of injury" did not improve sensitivity (already 100%) but worsened specificity to only 2% (95% CI = 1.5%-2.7%). Of note, each of the first six high-risk predictors except intoxication was present as the sole predictor of injury in some cases—meaning that a simpler rule with fewer elements would miss injuries. Eliminating intoxication as a criterion would slightly improve specificity to 4.6% (95% CI = 3.7%-5.5%). The authors did calculate the sensitivity and specificity

---

Box 3-12 High-Risk Criteria for Thoracolumbar Injury*

- ● **Complaints of thoracolumbar pain**
- ● **Thoracolumbar spine tenderness on midline palpation**
- ● **Decreased level of consciousness**
- ● **Abnormal peripheral neurologic examination**
- ● **Distracting painful injury**
- ● **Evidence of intoxication with ethanol or drugs**
- ● **Severe mechanism of injury**
  - ○ Car collision with speed > 45 mph or rollover
  - ○ Car collision requiring extrication
  - ○ Ejection from a motor vehicle
  - ○ Motorcycle accident at speed > 20 mph
  - ○ Automobile versus pedestrian at speed > 5 mph
  - ○ Fall greater than 10 feet
  - ○ Cervical spine injury

---

*Studies suggest that the presence of even a single criterion indicates imaging. The first 6 criteria above are 100% sensitive, without inclusion of severe mechanism.

From Holmes JF, Panacek EA, Miller PQ, et al: Prospective evaluation of criteria for obtaining thoracolumbar radiographs in trauma patients, *J Emerg Med* 24(1): 1–7, 2003.

---

of other combinations of the high-risk elements, but minimal improvements in specificity were achieved at the price of loss of sensitivity. The presence of a cervical spine fracture was noted to have a stronger predictive value than any of the other risk factors assessed,

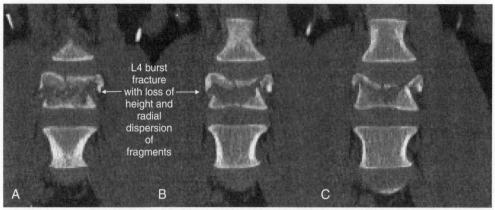

Figure 3-92. Thoracolumbar spine burst–compression fracture. Same patient as in Figures 3-88 through 3-91. These coronal CT views demonstrate the significant loss of height and comminution of L4.

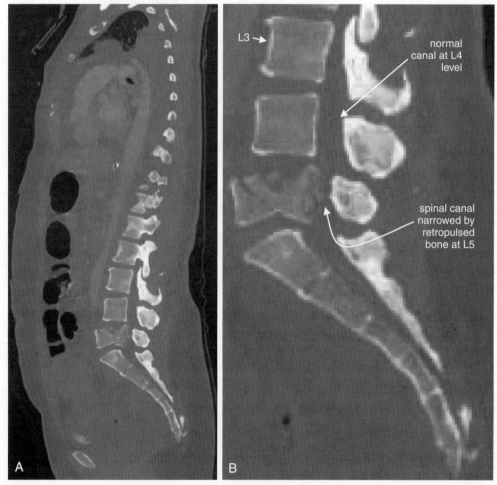

Figure 3-93. Thoracolumbar spine trauma: L5 burst fracture with cord compression. This 39-year-old female was ejected from a motor vehicle and sustained an L5 burst fracture. Due to retropulsion of bone fragments into the spinal canal, she had no motor function and minimal sensation after this injury. **A,** Sagittal CT view showing significant narrowing of the spinal canal at L5 due to retropulsion of fragments of the burst L5 vertebral body. **B,** Close-up. The L5 vertebral body is also shortened substantially compared with L3 and L4 due to a compression injury mechanism. Compare with the axial and coronal CT images in Figures 3-94 and 3-95.

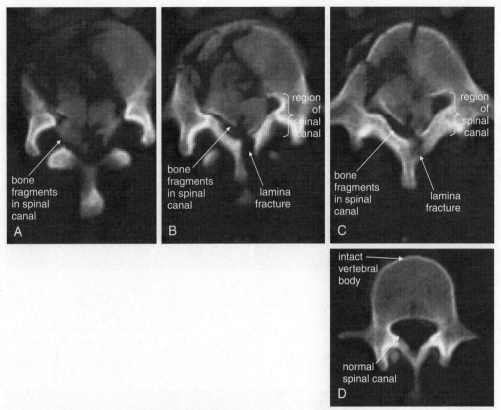

Figure 3-94. **Thoracolumbar spine trauma: L5 burst fracture with cord compression.** Same patient as in Figure 3-93. Axial CT views (**A,** cephalad portion of vertebral body, **B,** middle of vertebral body, **C,** caudad portion of vertebral body) show significant narrowing of the spinal canal at L5 due to retropulsion of fragments of the burst L5 vertebral body. **D,** The normal L4 vertebra for comparison.

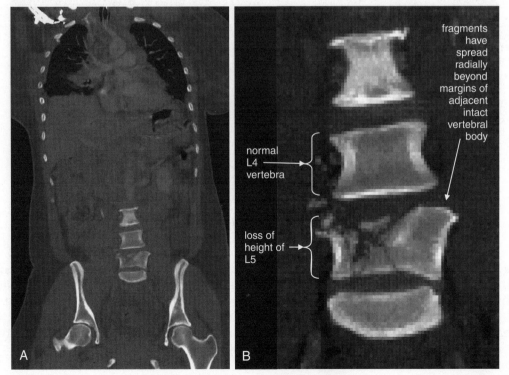

Figure 3-95. **Thoracolumbar spine trauma: L5 burst fracture with cord compression.** Same patient as in Figures 3-93 and 3-94. **A,** Coronal CT view shows radial spread of fracture fragments and loss of height of the L5 vertebral body. **B,** Close-up.

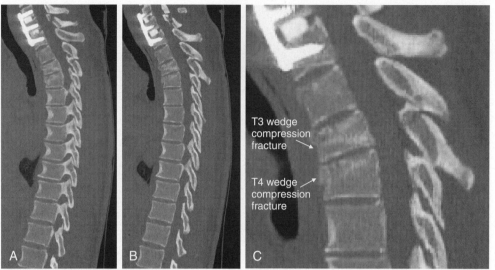

Figure 3-96. T2, T3, and T4 compression fractures. In this patient, thoracic spine CT shows spinal fixation screws at C6, C7, and T1, which provide convenient landmarks. **A** to **C,** Sagittal CT images (**C,** close-up from **B**) reveal significant loss of height of T3, consistent with a compression-type fracture. T4 also has loss of height and evidence of an anterior wedge compression fracture. T4 nicely demonstrates the "wedge" shape typical of flexion injuries of the thoracic and lumbar spine, with the anterior height being significantly less than the posterior height. T3, in comparison, has more uniform loss of height anteriorly and posteriorly. Compression fractures often lead to radial spread of fracture fragments, and retropulsion of fragments into the spinal canal can occur, leading to spinal cord injury. The spinal canal in this patient is preserved, with no retropulsion of fracture fragments.

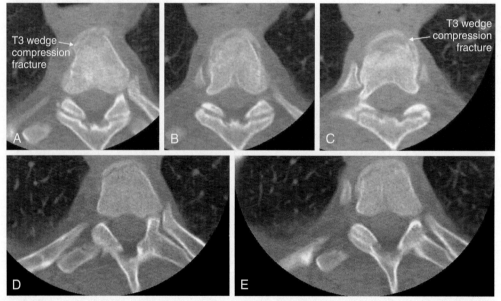

Figure 3-97. T2, T3, and T4 compression fractures. Same patient as in Figure 3-96. On these sequential axial CT images, the extent of comminution of the fractures becomes more apparent. The T3 vertebral body is seen with comminuted fragments of the anterior vertebral body.

increasing the risk of thoracolumbar injury by threefold when present. The authors recommended adding this to a CDR to enhance predictive value.

The same research group went on to delineate the types of distracting injuries most associated with thoracolumbar fractures. When "painful distracting injury" was the only high-risk predictor present, bony fractures were associated with thoracolumbar injury, while soft-tissue contusions, lacerations, head injuries, abrasions, visceral injuries, dental injuries, burns, ligamentous injuries,

amputations, and compartment syndrome were not. Although the investigators suggest that this data can be used to refine the screening definition of "painful distracting injury," only 13 thoracolumbar injuries were found in this group, limiting the ability to consider injury subtypes.[65]

Hsu et al.[62] conducted a retrospective chart review of 200 patients and reported the sensitivity of various physical exam findings for thoracolumbar fracture. In this study, a midline step-off was found to be poorly

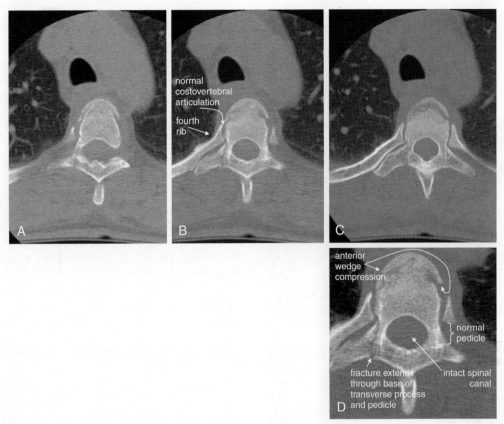

Figure 3-98. **T4 wedge compression fracture.** Same patient as in Figures 3-96 and 3-97. This wedge compression fracture of T4 extends through the right pedicle and base of the transverse process, but the spinal canal is not compromised. **A** to **C,** Sequential axial CT images. **D,** Close-up from **B.**

sensitive (13.8%) but highly specific (100%). Back bruising was only 6.9% sensitive but 98.6% specific. Back pain or midline tenderness had a sensitivity of 62.1% and a specificity of 91.5%. An abnormal neurologic examination was 41.4% sensitive and 95.8% specific.[62] This study is limited by its small size, resulting in wide CIs. In addition, the study faces significant methodologic problems. Physical examination findings were abstracted from the emergency department chart, and it is possible that examination findings may have been present but not written in the chart, resulting in inaccurate calculations of sensitivity and specificity. However, the apparent specificity of local findings such as bruising or step-offs has led to the recommendation by professional societies that these be criteria for thoracolumbar imaging.[1,63]

The case is less clear for low-energy mechanisms of trauma—for example, is any imaging required in the 30-year-old patient who complains of back pain after low-speed rear-end collision but is ambulatory in the emergency department? Thoracic and lumbar injuries are less common after minor trauma mechanisms, and many patients may require no imaging. Spectrum bias in studies such as those described earlier (biased toward moderately severely injured patients) may limit the application of these rules to less significantly injured patients.

What Is the Sensitivity of X-ray and Computed Tomography for Injuries of the Thoracolumbar Spine? Which Imaging Modality Should Be Used?

Studies comparing x-ray and CT for the diagnosis of thoracolumbar fracture suffer the same methodologic flaws as those for cervical spine injury, including the lack of a uniform and independent gold standard. The use of CT as the gold standard in studies is called incorporation bias and virtually guarantees that CT will appear to be the superior test. That said, CT is almost certainly far superior to x-ray for detection and characterization of fractures. Rhee et al.[66] reported the missed lumbar fracture rate for abdominal and pelvic CT to be 23.1%, versus 12.7% for AP and lateral x-ray. However, these figures are based on axial images from abdominal and pelvic CT viewed on bone windows without sagittal or coronal reformatted images, using a single-slice helical scan with slice thicknesses of 5 to 10 mm. Modern protocols routinely use thinner slices and incorporate multiplanar reformations, improving recognition of malalignment and fractures that may lie in the axial plane. In addition, this study had no uniform diagnostic standard, making the results uncertain. Multiple other studies have shown excellent test performance characteristics for images obtained from abdominal and pelvic CT, reformatted in the sagittal and coronal planes.[67-77] Some reports focused on use of

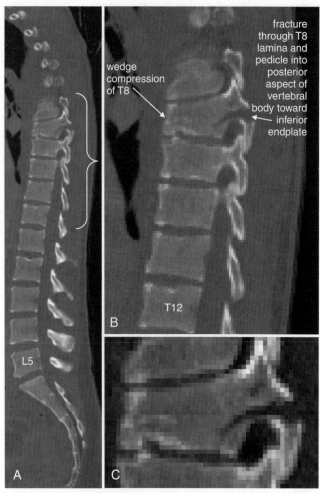

Figure 3-99. Thoracolumbar spine trauma: Chance fracture. A, Sagittal computed tomography image. **B, C,** Close-ups from **A.** A Chance fracture is a flexion injury, usually of the lower thoracic or upper lumbar spine. Unlike simple compression fractures, a Chance fracture involves fractures through the anterior, middle, and posterior columns of the spine. With lumbar Chance fractures, intraabdominal injuries are commonly found. A common mechanism is hyperflexion in a patient wearing a lap belt without a shoulder harness in a motor vehicle collision. This patient has a multilevel thoracic spine flexion injury, with wedge compression fractures of T7 and T8, as well as a fracture of T10. The T8 injury follows the Chance pattern, with a comminuted fracture through the pars, lamina, and spinous process and extending through the vertebral body, with an obliquely oriented fracture through the posterior third of the middle column extending to the inferior endplate. The posterior elements are splayed with 6 mm of craniocaudal distraction. This results in focal kyphosis at T8 and approximately 33% height loss of the anterior vertebral body. This fracture is explored in more detail in Figures 3-100 and 3-101.

axial CT images, supplemented by AP and lateral scout CT images. These were found to have sensitivity of 92% to 100% and specificity of 100% compared with AP and lateral lumbar spine x-ray.[68,78] A prospective study compared axial images from the chest–abdomen–pelvis CT with AP and lateral x-rays. The gold standard for the study was either separately acquired, dedicated thin-cut spine CT (1- to 2-mm cuts) or clinical exam of the patient once stable and awake. Axial images from the chest–abdomen–pelvis CT were found to have a sensitivity of 97% (95% CI = 86%-100%), with a specificity of

99% (95% CI = 96%-100%). In comparison, x-ray had a sensitivity of only 58% (95% CI = 41%-75%) and a specificity of 93% (95% CI = 89%-97%). From a methodology standpoint, this study suffers from its inconsistent gold standard (also called verification or workup bias) and a lack of blinding, as radiologists were aware of the results of other imaging studies when rendering their interpretation of the CT and x-rays.[69]

Sheridan et al.[75] prospectively investigated reformatted sagittal and coronal images obtained from chest--abdomen–pelvis CT–the technique used in most trauma centers today and advocated by the ACR. They reported 97% sensitivity and 95% specificity of CT for lumbar fractures, compared with 62% sensitivity and 86% specificity of x-ray. This study is limited by the lack of a uniform diagnostic standard; the final discharge diagnosis was considered to be correct, though not all patients underwent the same final workup. In addition, although the authors report that the CT and lumbar spine x-rays were generally read blinded, they admit that some were read by the same radiologist without blinding. This practice likely artificially inflates the sensitivity of x-ray, because findings on CT might lead to recognition of additional fractures. Theoretically, x-ray findings might also have led to recognition of CT abnormalities.[75]

Wintermark et al.[77] performed a prospective double-blinded study of 100 consecutive trauma patients undergoing both thoracolumbar x-ray and CT of the chest, abdomen, and pelvis with coronal and sagittal reformats. They reported the mean sensitivity for unstable fractures to be 97% for CT (95% CI = 85.5%-99.9%) and the mean sensitivity to be 33.3% for x-ray (95% CI = 21.7%-46.7%). In addition, the K value for interobserver agreement was 0.951 for CT, indicating near-perfect agreement of different interpreting radiologists, compared with poor agreement (K = 0.368) for x-ray.[77] For all fractures, including fractures predicted to be stable, agreement (K = 0.787), and sensitivity (78.1%) of CT were less perfect although arguably, stable fractures are less important to patient outcome. CT nonetheless was superior to x-ray in this category as well (sensitivity = 32%, K = 0.661). This study was well done, with its primary weakness being a mixed gold standard based on additional imaging, orthopedic interventions, and final discharge diagnosis or autopsy report.[77]

Who Needs Magnetic Resonance Imaging of the Thoracic and Lumbar Spine?

The ACR does not recommend MRI for evaluation of ligamentous injuries of the thoracolumbar spine when CT is normal. Unlike the case for the cervical spine, in which some controversy exists and MRI is commonly performed for evaluation of ligamentous injuries even

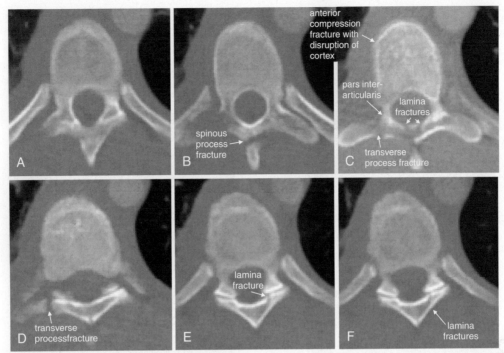

Figure 3-100. Thoracolumbar spine trauma: T8 Chance fracture. Same patient as Figure 3-99. Axial computed tomography (CT) reconstructions of the spine (**A** to **F**), performed from a dataset from CT of the chest, abdomen, and pelvis. The T8 vertebra shows a Chance fracture pattern, with injuries to the vertebral body including the lamina, pars interarticularis (a region at the junction of the pedicle and lamina), and vertebral body. The anterior body of T8 shows compression fracture findings.

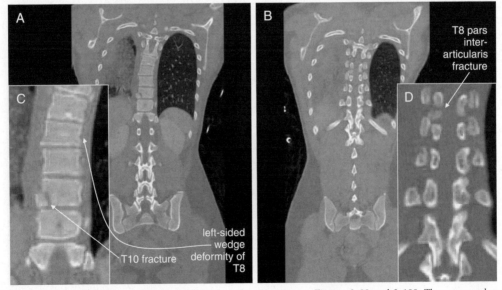

Figure 3-101. Thoracolumbar spine trauma: T8 Chance fracture. Same patient as Figures 3-99 and 3-100. These coronal reconstructions were created from the dataset from the computed tomography (CT) of the chest, abdomen, and pelvis performed for evaluation of visceral injury in this patient. They reveal a T8 Chance fracture, as well as injuries of T7 and T10. T8 and T7 have not only anterior wedge compression (seen best on the sagittal reconstructions in Figure 3-99) but also left-sided compression, creating a scoliosis toward the patient's left side. Spinal fractures often have complex patterns that do not strictly adhere to a single textbook description. **A,** Coronal view through the mid portion of the thoracic vertebral bodies. **B,** A more posterior coronal plane than **A,** showing the pars interarticularis. **C** and **D,** Close-ups from **A** and **B,** respectively.

in the presence of a normal CT scan (see earlier discussion), ligamentous injuries of the thoracolumbar spine almost never occur in the absence of CT findings. MRI is recommended solely for patients with neurologic deficits localizing to the thoracolumbar spine.[1]

Which Is Faster, X-ray or CT of the Thoracic and Lumbar Spine?

Wintermark et al.[77] reported thoracolumbar x-ray required a median of 23 minutes, while CT of the chest, abdomen, and pelvis required a median of 40 minutes,

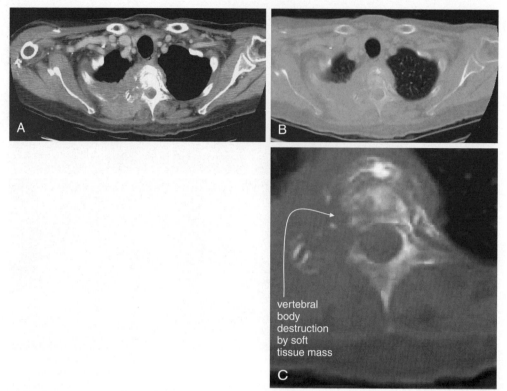

Figure 3-102. Thoracic spine metastases with cord compression. CT with IV contrast was performed due to concern for malignancy. In comparison, dedicated spinal CT for evaluation of trauma can be performed without IV contrast. In practice today, multisystem trauma patients usually have spinal CT images reconstructed from IV contrast enhanced CT datasets of the chest, abdomen and pelvis. IV contrast in that scenario is used to evaluate solid organ and vascular injuries, not spinal injuries. This patient has a right lung mass lesion that has now invaded the T2 thoracic vertebral body. The mass has eroded the vertebral body and extends posteriorly into the paravertebral musculature. The images show the same slice on soft tissue **(A)** and bone windows **(B).** A close-up shows erosion of the right pedicle of the vertebral body **(C).** Magnetic resonance imaging (MRI) demonstrates this lesion in greater detail in Figure 3-103.

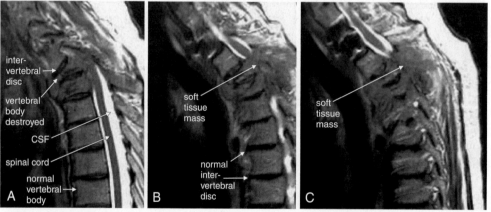

Figure 3-103. Thoracic spine metastases with cord compression. Same patient as in Figure 3-102. The intervertebral discs show abnormal alignment because of collapse of the vertebral body. **A** to **C,** The sagittal T2-weighted images (not to be confused with the T2 vertebral body) show a lesion obliterating the cerebrospinal fluid (CSF) space surrounding the spinal cord. With T2-weighted magnetic resonance imaging (MRI), fluid appears white and fat appears darker. The spinal cord appears gray due to its myelin (fat) content. The vertebral bodies are visible due to lipid-rich marrow. The bone of the vertebral bodies is black due to a lack of resonating protons to provide a radio signal. Computed tomography (CT) is generally better than MRI for evaluation of calcified bony pathology.

of which 7 minutes was required for postprocessing of images. In patients undergoing CT of the chest, abdomen, and pelvis for evaluation of other traumatic injuries, CT reformations are clearly the more rapid means of assessing the thoracolumbar spine.

What Is the Cost of X-ray and CT of the Thoracic and Lumbar Spine?

Wintermark et al.[77] reported costs of $145 per patient for x-ray and $880 for CT. They using reformats of the spine derived from chest–abdomen–pelvis CT. They

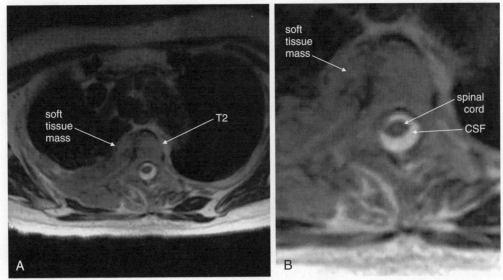

Figure 3-104. **Thoracic spine metastasis with cord compression. A,** In this T2-weighted axial magnetic resonance image from the same patient as Figures 3-102 and 3-103, a soft-tissue mass is seen involving the T2 vertebral body. **B,** Close-up. The spinal cord is visible, surrounded by cerebrospinal fluid (CSF). The cord is not impinged upon in this image.

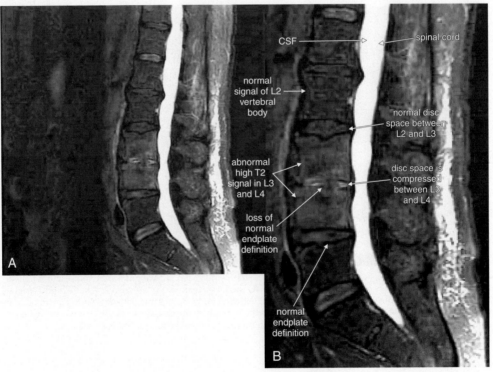

Figure 3-105. **Osteomyelitis and discitis of L3 and L4. A,** T2-weighted fast spin–echo magnetic resonance imaging without contrast demonstrates typical findings of vertebral osteomyelitis and discitis. **B,** Close-up. The inferior endplate of L3 and the superior endplate of L4 are abnormal and ill-defined. The L3 and L4 vertebral bodies show a high T2 signal, indicating an abnormally high fluid content. In comparison, L2 shows a normal marrow signal and appears dark gray due to a normal fat signal. CSF, cerebrospinal fluid.

discounted the cost of the CT spinal reformats, stating that these added nothing to the cost of CT. However, in some cases, additional fees for postprocessing may be charged to the patient. If the patient does not require chest, abdomen, and pelvis CT for evaluation of other injuries and dedicated spine CT is performed, CT is more costly, accounting for direct costs alone. Given the higher sensitivity of CT, economic models incorporating the cost of missed injuries would likely favor CT.

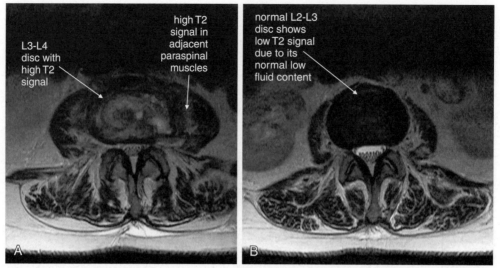

Figure 3-106. Discitis of L3 and L4. Same patient as in Figure 3-105. T2-weighted fast spin–echo magnetic resonance imaging without contrast demonstrates typical findings of vertebral discitis. **A,** The L3-4 disc is shown and has a high T2 signal, indicating elevated fluid content consistent with an inflammatory process. **B,** The normal L2-3 disc in the same patient is shown, with its normal dark appearance (a low T2 signal) due to low fluid content. **A, B,** A high T2 signal is seen in the paraspinal muscles, suggesting inflammation.

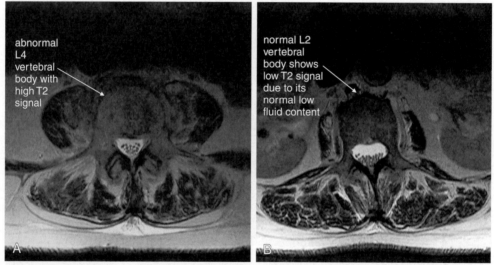

Figure 3-107. Osteomyelitis of L3 and L4. Same patient as in Figures 3-105 and 3-106. T2-weighted fast spin–echo magnetic resonance imaging without contrast demonstrates typical findings of vertebral osteomyelitis. **A,** The L4 vertebral body is shown and has a high T2 signal, indicating elevated fluid content consistent with an inflammatory process. **B,** The normal L2 vertebral body in the same patient is shown, with its normal dark appearance (a low T2 signal) due to low fluid content. **A, B,** A high T2 signal is seen in the paraspinal muscles, suggesting inflammation. Compare Figure 3-107B and Figure 3-106B. Normal intervertebral discs are darker in appearance than normal vertebral bodies on this MRI sequence.

What Is the Radiation Exposure of Thoracolumbar X-ray and CT?

Wintermark et al.[77] reported mean effective radiation dose from thoracolumbar x-ray to be 6.36 mSv, compared with 19.42 mSv for CT reformations of the spine derived from chest–abdomen–pelvis CT. They note that the reformations do not require any additional imaging or radiation exposure, compared with CT of the chest, abdomen, and pelvis alone. Consequently, if the patient requires CT of these regions for evaluation of other traumatic injuries, use of CT reformations allows a reduction of 6.36 mSv (by eliminating the additional radiation exposure from x-ray), nearly 25% of the entire dose required to perform both abdominal CT and x-rays of the spine.[77] However, if the patient does not require visceral CT of the chest, abdomen, and pelvis for trauma evaluation, dedicated CT of the spine would result in a significant increase in radiation exposure compared with x-ray.

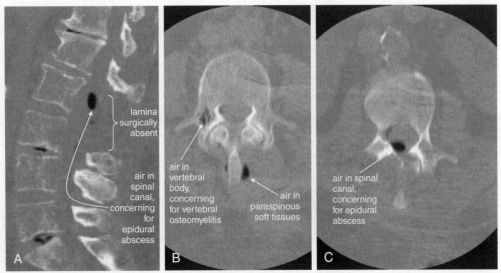

Figure 3-108. Spinal epidural abscess. This 67-year-old female presented with delirium and fever. Three months prior, she had undergone lumbar laminectomy, and her wound had been treated with a wound VAC dressing. Magnetic resonance imaging was not initially available, so noncontrast computed tomography (CT) was performed. Noncontrast CT is excellent at delineating air, which appears black on bone windows. **A,** The midsagittal view demonstrates air *(black)* in the spinal canal at the L2 and L3 levels. On the axial views **(B, C),** air is visible in the spinal canal, in paraspinal soft tissues, and within the vertebral body. These findings are concerning for a paraspinal infection that has developed into an epidural abscess with vertebral osteomyelitis. Compare with the MRI in Figure 3-109.

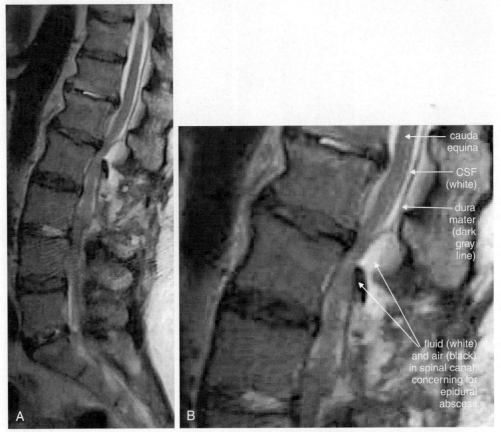

Figure 3-109. Spinal epidural abscess. Same patient as in Figure 3-108, in whom noncontrast computed tomography showed air in the spinal canal, concerning for epidural abscess. Magnetic resonance imaging (MRI) of the lumbar spine without contrast was performed, as the patient was in acute renal failure. **A,** This T2-weighted sagittal MR image provides useful information even without gadolinium contrast. **B,** Close-up. On T2-weighted MRI sequences, fluid including cerebrospinal fluid appears white. Fat-containing tissues such as bone marrow and the spinal cord or cauda equina appear dark gray. Calcified bone appears nearly black due to an absence of resonating protons. Air appears completely black for the same reason. The midline sagittal image shows the cauda equina to be impinged upon by an epidural fluid collection containing air—an epidural abscess. The dura mater is visible as a thin, dark gray line parallel to the spinal cord. It is indented in the region of the epidural abscess. Compare with the axial MRI images in Figure 3-110.

Figure 3-110. **Spinal epidural abscess.**
A, This axial image is taken at the same level as the air-fluid collection shown in the last figure. The air–fluid collection comprising the epidural abscess is seen posterior to the thecal sac (dura mater), which contains small, dark-gray circles representing a cross-section through the nerve roots of the cauda equina. These nerve roots are surrounded by white cerebrospinal fluid within the thecal sac. **B,** In another patient, the nerve roots of the cauda equina are more widely separated and are seen as discrete bundles with circular axial cross-sections.

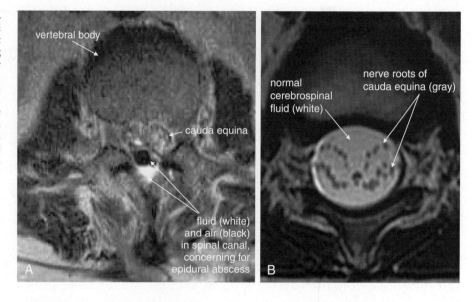

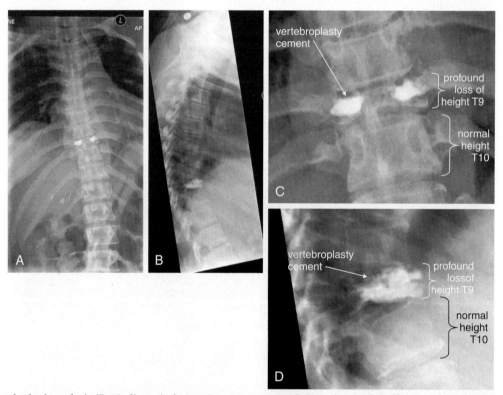

Figure 3-111. **Vertebral tuberculosis (Pott's disease). A,** Anterior–posterior x-ray. **B,** Lateral x-ray. **C, D,** Close-ups from **A** and **B,** respectively. This patient with known tuberculosis and medication noncompliance presented with worsening back pain and lower extremity weakness. Plain x-rays show extreme loss of height of the T9 vertebral body. The high-density material is cement from an earlier vertebroplasty intended to arrest loss of height of the vertebral body. Cultures from the vertebral body confirmed mycobacterium tuberculosis. Compare with the CT and MR images in Figures 3-112 through 3-116.

Should Minor Trauma Patients Undergo Lumbar CT or X-ray?

Most of the published studies comparing CT and x-ray involve patients with high trauma mechanisms and significant associated injuries. In these patients, CT is more sensitive, faster, more cost effective, and more radiation efficient than x-ray, because CT images of the spine can be reformatted from CT acquired for evaluation of other injuries to the chest, abdomen, and pelvis. Less clear is the best workup for patients with more minor trauma mechanisms. Some of these patients likely do not require CT evaluation of the chest, abdomen, and pelvis. For example, many blunt trauma

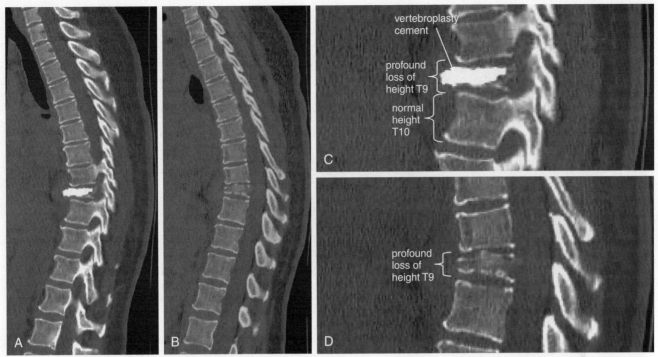

Figure 3-112. Vertebral tuberculosis (Pott's disease). Same patient as in Figure 3-111. Sagittal computed tomography reconstructions show extreme loss of height of the T9 vertebral body as a result of vertebral tuberculosis infection. Compression of the T9 body has resulted in kyphosis at this level. The high-density material is vertebroplasty cement from a prior procedure. **A,** A parasagittal section slightly to the right of midline. **B,** A more midline sagittal section. **C, D,** Close-ups from **A** and **B,** respectively.

patients with relatively low-energy mechanisms are probably not at risk for aortic trauma, a high-energy injury that is the strongest indication for chest CT. Despite this, CT is often ordered in this circumstance because of its value in imaging the thoracolumbar spine. Probably, patients with a low pretest probability of both major torso organ injury and thoracolumbar spinal injury should undergo thoracolumbar x-ray instead of CT. The ACR rates x-ray as less appropriate (three on a nine-point scale) than CT (nine on the same scale) for "blunt trauma meeting criteria for thoracic or lumbar imaging."[1] However, given the lower incidence of thoracolumbar injuries in very-low-energy trauma, such as falls from standing, CT appears inappropriate given its cost and radiation exposure.[1] If evaluation of the chest or abdomen is anticipated, it is clearly more efficient to order chest–abdomen–pelvis CT with spine reformats as the initial imaging study, rather than potentially subjecting the patient to two CTs: a dedicated spine CT followed later by CT of the chest, abdomen, and pelvis.

Which Patients Require Thoracolumbar Imaging for Low Back Pain? Are So-Called Red Flags Useful?

Red flags, or clinical features suggesting serious causes of back pain, are frequently cited in medical texts as indications for imaging. A number of national guidelines have been published with recommendations for

TABLE 3-5. Red Flags for Lumbar Vertebral Fracture

Clinical Feature	Positive Likelihood Ratio	Negative Likelihood Ratio
Age > 50 years	2.2	0.34
Female gender	2.3	0.67
History of major trauma	12.8	0.37
Pain and tenderness	6.7	0.44
Painful distracting injury	1.7	0.78

imaging only when red flags are present. Are these based on expert opinion or on high-quality research? A systematic review of Medline, the Cumulative Index to Nursing and Allied Health Literature, and Embase found 12 studies meeting sound methodologic quality criteria and investigating 51 clinical "red flags." Five clinical features were identified as useful in raising or lowering the probability of vertebral fracture (Table 3-5).[79] Likelihood ratios for each finding are presented. A likelihood ratio represents a multiplier used to modify pretest probability of disease, based on a "test," which in this case may be a clinical exam maneuver or historical feature. Of note, a positive likelihood ratio greater than or equal to 10, or a negative likelihood ratio less than or equal to 0.1, is generally accepted as having substantial value in clinical practice. Less extreme

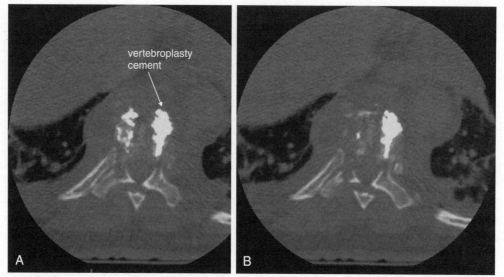

Figure 3-113. Vertebral tuberculosis (Pott's disease). Same patient as in Figures 3-111 and 3-112. Two axial computed tomography reconstructions **(A, B)** show nearly complete erosion of the T9 vertebral body as a result of vertebral tuberculosis infection. The high-density material is vertebroplasty cement from a prior procedure. Residual bone shows a moth-eaten appearance.

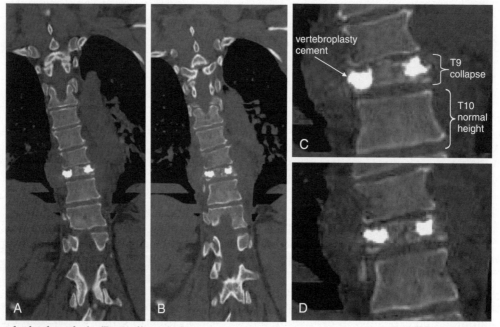

Figure 3-114. Vertebral tuberculosis (Pott's disease). Same patient as in Figures 3-111 through 3-113. Two coronal computed tomography reconstructions **(A, B)** show nearly complete erosion of the T9 vertebral body as a result of vertebral tuberculosis infection. The high-density material is vertebroplasty cement from a prior procedure. Residual bone shows a moth-eaten appearance. **C, D,** Close-ups from **A** and **B,** respectively.

likelihood ratio values do not alter pretest probability to an extent that is likely to assist in clinical decisions. Even the five "best" red flags identified in this review generally fall short of these criteria. The authors intentionally set a lower threshold, choosing features for which the upper 95% CI of the likelihood ratio was substantially below 1.0 or for which the lower 95% CI of the likelihood ratio was substantially above 1.0. This is because a likelihood ratio approaching 1.0 results in no mathematical change in pretest probability.

SUMMARY

Imaging of the spine is often indicated following trauma or for evaluation of neurologic complaints. CDRs exist to limit imaging in low-risk trauma patients. X-ray may be appropriate for screening of low-risk patients who require imaging, but the ACR recommends CT due to its higher sensitivity. The high costs and radiation exposures associated with CT make application of CDRs particularly important MRI is necessary when serious concern exists for spinal cord pathology.

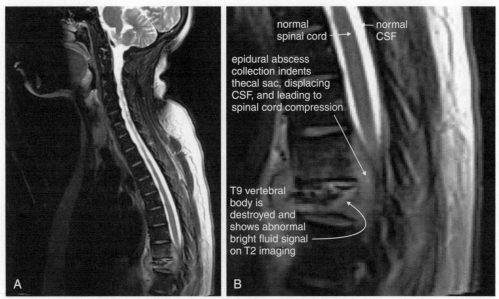

Figure 3-115. **Vertebral tuberculosis (Pott's disease) with epidural abscess. A,** Same patient as in Figures 3-111 through 3-114. Sagittal T2-weighted magnetic resonance reconstructions show nearly complete erosion of the T9 vertebral body as a result of vertebral tuberculosis infection. **B,** Close-up. The spinal cord is compressed from an epidural fluid collection. *CSF,* Cerebrospinal fluid.

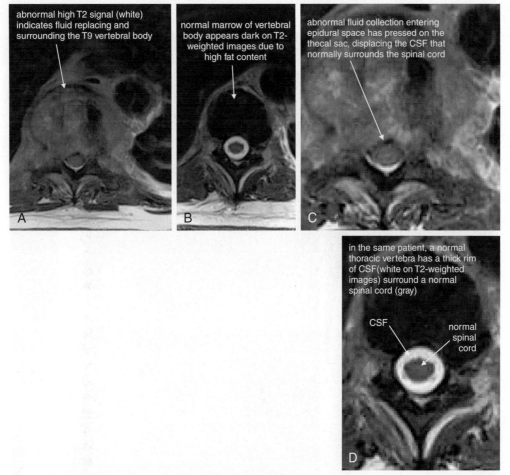

Figure 3-116. **Vertebral tuberculosis (Pott's disease) with epidural abscess.** Same patient as in Figures 3-111 through 3-115. **A,** Axial T2-weighted magnetic resonance (MR) images show nearly complete erosion of the T9 vertebral body as a result of vertebral tuberculosis infection. The region normally occupied by the T9 vertebral body shows a high T2 signal (white), indicating the presence of abnormal fluid (which appears white on T2-weighted MRI). The cerebrospinal fluid (CSF) that normally surrounds the spinal cord at this level has been displaced. **B,** A normal adjacent vertebral body and spinal cord from the same patient for comparison. **C, D,** Close-ups from **A** and **B,** respectively.

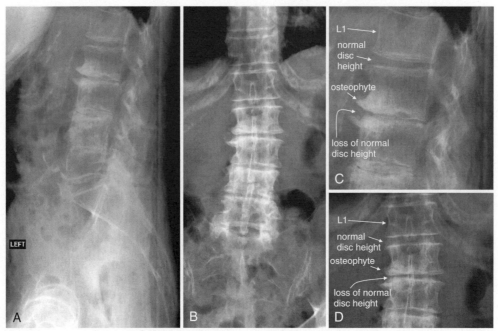

Figure 3-117. Degenerative joint disease and lumbar disc herniation. This patient has extensive degenerative joint disease of the lumbar spine. Note the normal spacing between the L1 and the L2 vertebral bodies and the loss of normal disc height at the L2-3, L3-4, and L4-5 levels. **A,** Lateral x-ray. **B,** Anterior–posterior x-ray. **C, D,** Close-ups from **A** and **B,** respectively. Compare with the MRI from the same patient in Figure 3-118 through 120.

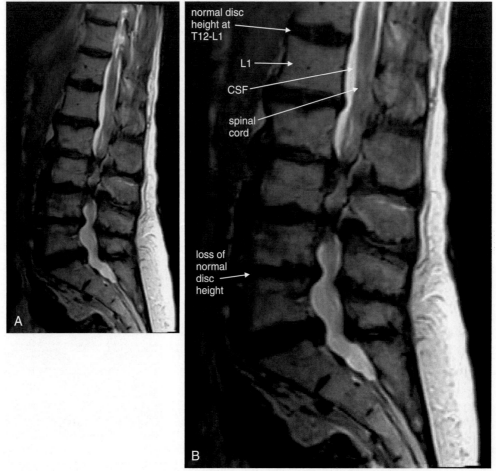

Figure 3-118. Degenerative joint disease and lumbar disc herniation: Magnetic resonance without contrast, T2-weighted image. Same patient in Figure 3-117. **A,** Sagittal reconstruction. **B,** Close-up. This patient has extensive degenerative joint disease of the lumbar spine. At the T12-L1 level, note the normal disc space. The spinal canal is patent, with cerebrospinal fluid (CSF) (white) surrounding the cord (gray). At the L2-3 level, the intervertebral disc is compressed and indents the thecal sac into the spinal canal, displacing the normal rim of CSF and resulting in severe spinal stenosis.

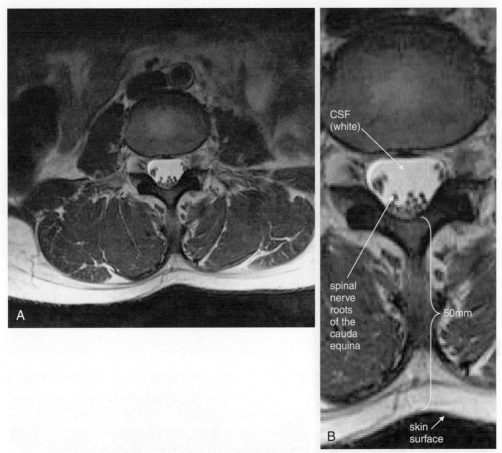

Figure 3-119. Normal cauda equina. Same patient in Figures 3-117 and 118. **A,** This axial T2-weighted magnetic resonance image is taken through the L3-4 region. It illustrates that the spinal cord has given way to the cauda equina, with individual nerve roots visible in cross section *(black circles)*. **B,** Close-up. Incidentally, the distance from the skin surface to the thecal sac (cerebrospinal fluid space) is 50 mm, so lumbar puncture at this level would be feasible.

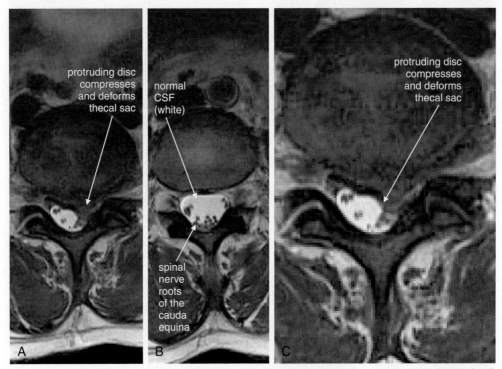

Figure 3-120. Disk herniation resulting in cauda equina compression: Magnetic resonance imaging (MRI) lumbar spine without contrast. Same patient as Figure 3-119, but at a lower spinal level. **A,** This axial T2-weighted MRI image is taken through the L4-5 disc region. A paracentral disc herniation is compressing the thecal sac on the patient's left, narrowing the left neural foramen. The spinal cord has already given way to the nerve roots of the cauda equina at this level. **B,** A normal section above the level of the disc herniation for comparison—note the triangular shape of the normal thecal sac at this level. **C,** Close-up from **A.**

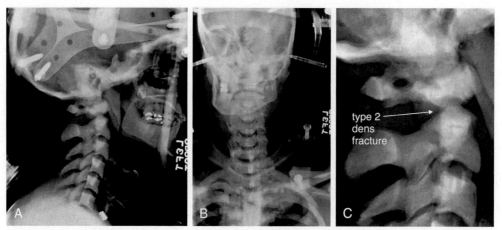

Figure 3-121. **Osteopetrosis with type II dens fracture. A,** Lateral x-ray. **B,** Anterior–posterior x-ray. **C,** Close-up from **A.** Osteopetrosis is a pathologic condition of increased bone density but high predisposition to fracture. Note this patient's high bone density, which is not simply a function of the exposure. This patient has a type II dens fracture. Compare with the CT in Figure 3-122.

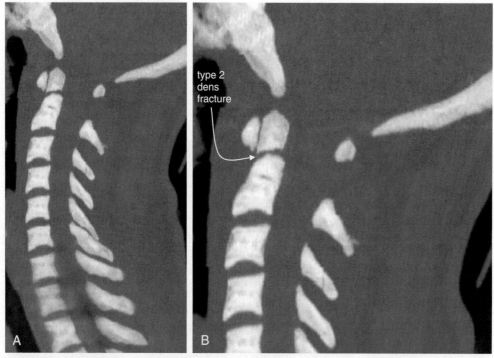

Figure 3-122. **Osteopetrosis with type II dens fracture.** Same patient as in Figure 3-121. **A,** Midsagittal computed tomography (CT) slice. **B,** Close-up. Note this patient's high bone density. This is not simply a function of the window level, which is set to "bone," as with most of the other CT images in this chapter. This patient has a type II dens fracture, with slight craniocaudal distraction of the fracture fragments. The dens is not retropulsed into the spinal canal.

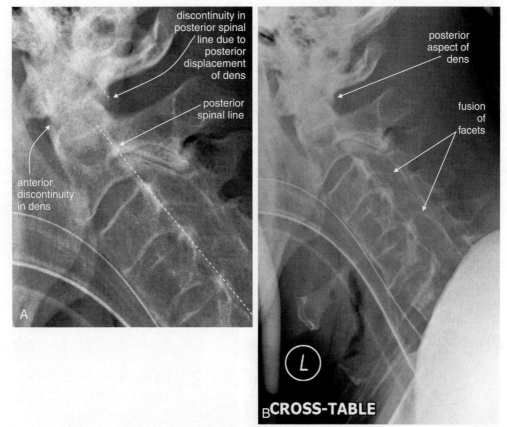

Figure 3-123. Ankylosing spondylitis with type II dens fracture. A, This lateral x-ray (**B,** broader view) shows typical features of ankylosing spondylitis with fusion of facet joints, straightening of the cervical spine, and diffuse osteopenia. A dens fracture is present with retropulsion of the dens into the spinal canal. The posterior longitudinal ligament line would intersect the dens rather than passing posterior to it. The patient's computed tomography scan is explored in Figures 3-124 through 3-126.

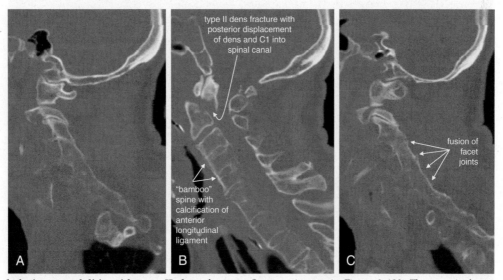

Figure 3-124. Ankylosing spondylitis with type II dens fracture. Same patient as in Figure 3-123. These sagittal computed tomography reconstructions show fusion of facets bilaterally (**A,** right, and **C,** left) and "bamboo" spine in the midline sagittal section **(B).** The spine shows diffuse osteopenia that is also typical of ankylosing spondylitis. The cervical spine is straightened, not due to the cervical collar but due to fusion of vertebrae. Worse still, the patient has a type II dens fracture. The dens and C1 vertebra are bound together by the transverse ligament and have moved posteriorly as a unit, intruding into the spinal canal and narrowing it by more than 50%.

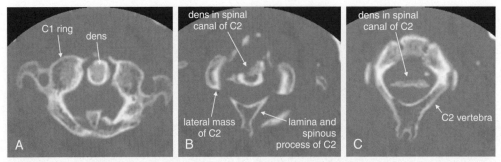

Figure 3-125. Ankylosing spondylitis with type II dens fracture. Same patient as in Figures 3-123 and 3-124. These axial computed tomography views may appear confusing at first. In the most cephalad slice **(A)**, the dens is normally positioned relative to the ring of C1. This is because the dens has remained attached to the anterior ring of C1 by the transverse ligament. However, a few slices caudad **(B)**, a cross section through the dens shows it to be in the center of the spinal canal of the C2 vertebra, not positioned anteriorly. Further caudad **(C)**, the bottom of the dens fragment is still seen in the spinal canal. Bone in the spinal canal threatens the spinal cord (as seen in magnetic resonance imaging in Figure 3-127).

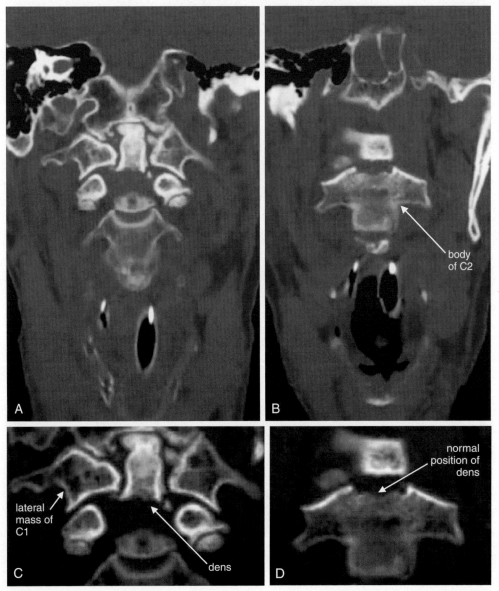

Figure 3-126. Ankylosing spondylitis with type II dens fracture. Same patient as in Figures 3-123 through 3-125. This badly displaced type II dens fracture is depicted in coronal CT views. Because the dens has been displaced significantly from the body of C2, the two are not seen in the same coronal view. These two views are separated by 10 mm in an anterior–posterior direction. The dens remains in its normal position relative to C1. **C, D,** Close-ups from **A** and **B,** respectively.

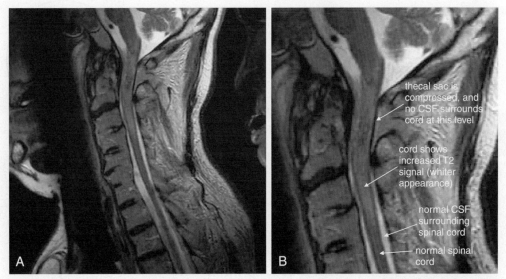

Figure 3-127.   **Ankylosing spondylitis with type II dens fracture: Cervical magnetic resonance imaging (MRI) without contrast.** Same patient as in Figures 3-123 through 3-126. **A,** In this T2-weighted midsagittal MRI, a dens fracture with retropulsion of the dens into the spinal canal has compressed the spinal cord. **B,** Close-up. Several features are evident. First, the thecal sac has been indented, displacing the rim of cerebrospinal fluid (CSF) that normally surrounds the spinal cord. In addition, the spinal cord shows an increased T2 signal, indicating traumatic edema of the cord. Compare this abnormal, whiter appearance of the cord with the normal, darker gray appearance of the cord above and below the level of injury.

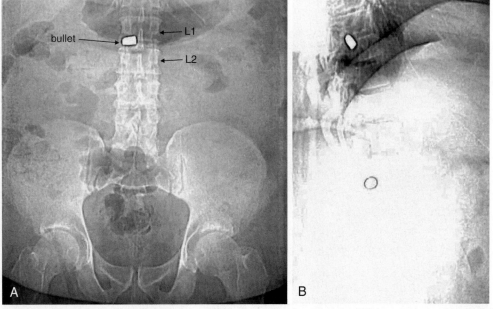

Figure 3-128.   **Penetrating spinal trauma: Bullet in spinal canal.** Scout computed tomography (CT) images show a bullet overlying the L1-2 disc space on both frontal **(A)** and lateral **(B)** reconstructions. Multiplanar CT reconstructions of the spine were performed (Figures 3-129 through 3-131).

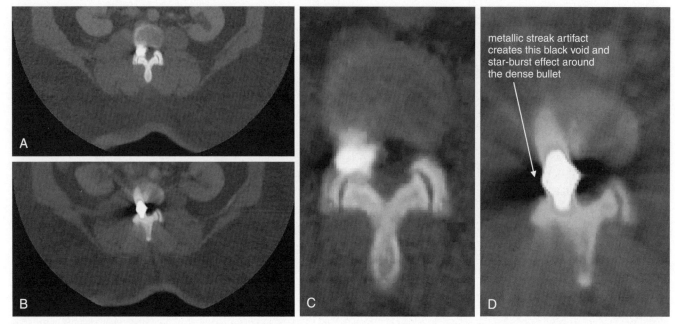

Figure 3-129. Penetrating spinal trauma: Bullet in spinal canal. Same patient as in Figure 3-128. **A, B,** Axial computed tomography (CT) slices. **C, D,** Close-ups from **A** and **B,** respectively. Axial CT reconstructions show a bullet located in the right lateral aspect of the disc space, neural foramina, and central canal at the L1-2 level. Metallic streak artifact limits detection of fractures in this CT. The patient is also morbidly obese, limiting the image quality.

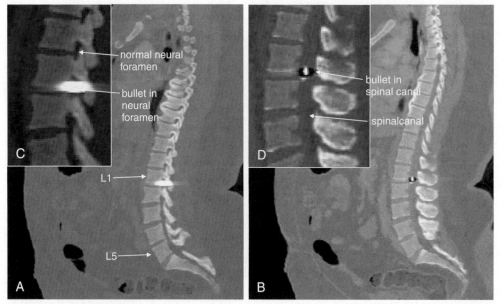

Figure 3-130. Penetrating spinal trauma: Bullet in spinal canal. Same patient as in Figures 3-128 and 3-129. **A, B,** Sagittal computed tomography (CT) slices. **C, D,** Close-ups from **A** and **B,** respectively. Sagittal reconstructions show the bullet in the right neural foramen and central spinal canal. Streak artifact makes it impossible to discern the exact margins of the bullet.

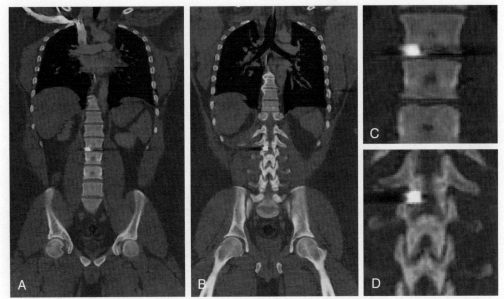

Figure 3-131. **Penetrating spinal trauma: Bullet in spinal canal.** Same patient as in Figures 3-128 through 3-130. These coronal CT reconstructions show the bullet to lie just inferior to L1, in the L1-2 interspace. Again, streak artifact makes finding the bullet margins and recognizing adjacent fractures impossible. **A,** Coronal view through the midportion of the affected vertebral bodies. **B,** A more posterior coronal plane shows posterior facets. **C** and **D,** Close-ups from **A** and **B,** respectively.

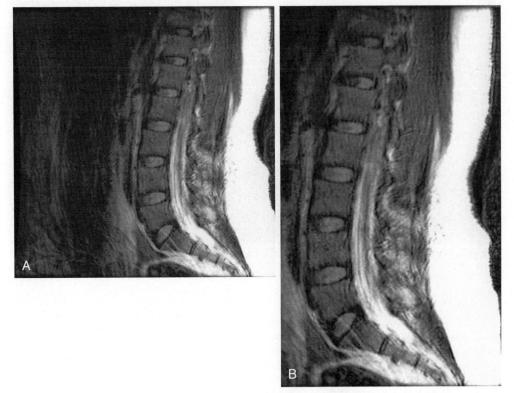

Figure 3-132. **Epidural hematoma after lumbar puncture with motion artifact. A,** T2-weighted sagittal image. **B,** Close-up. This patient underwent magnetic resonance imaging (MRI) to assess for epidural hematoma after a lumbar puncture. The patient had difficulty remaining still during the exam, which lasted approximately 45 minutes. As a result, significant motion artifact limits the diagnostic quality of the MRI.

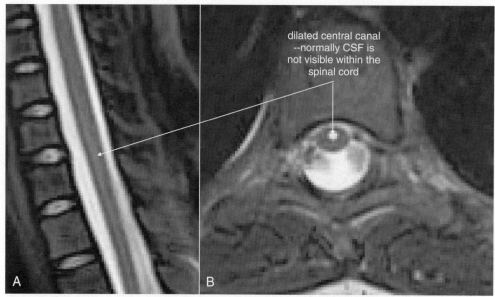

Figure 3-133. Syrinx. A, Sagittal T2-weighted magnetic resonance image. **B,** Axial T2-weighted image. A syrinx occurs when spinal fluid dissects within the spinal cord. A risk factor is Chiari malformation, as this can increase the pressure of cerebrospinal fluid (CSF) within the spinal cord. In this 10-year-old female presenting with leg numbness, a dilated cervical central canal gave way to a small syrinx at the T7 level.

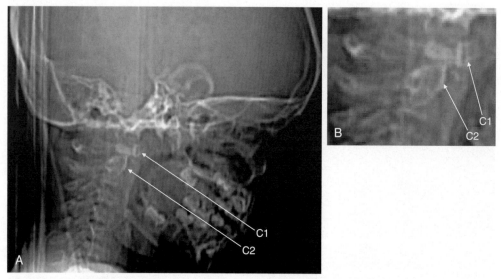

Figure 3-134. Pseudosubluxation. A, Lateral CT scout image. **B,** Close-up. This 3-year-old male presented with torticollis and was suspected of having a retropharyngeal abscess. The computed tomography (CT) was normal, but it demonstrates some important pediatric findings that can be mistaken for pathology by an inexperienced reader, especially one more accustomed to adult CT. The scout CT shows pseudosubluxation of C1 on C2.

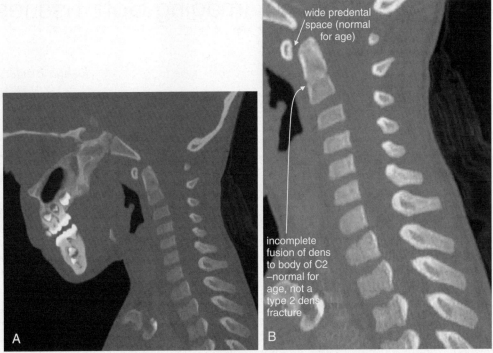

Figure 3-135. Pseudosubluxation. Same patient as in Figure 3-134. **A,** Sagittal computed tomography (CT) slice. **B,** Close-up. This 3-year-old male wmistaken for pathology by an inexperienced reader. The midsagittal view shows a slightly widened predental space (normal for age) and incomplete fusion of the dens to the body of C2 (normal for age), which should not be confused with type II dens fracture.

CHAPTER 4 Imaging Soft Tissues of the Neck

Joshua Broder, MD, FACEP

Imaging of soft tissues of the neck can be essential in the evaluation of patients with a variety of chief complaints, including neck trauma, ingested or aspirated foreign body, nontraumatic neck pain and swelling, dysphagia and voice change, visible or palpable mass, and central nervous system complaints with possible vascular causes. The neck contains vascular, nerve, airway, gastrointestinal, and bony structures, any of which may be the source of pain. Remember that referred pain from other regions of the body may present with neck pain, so a broad differential diagnosis should be entertained in formulating an imaging plan. Fascial planes connect compartments of the neck with the mediastinum and thoracic prevertebral spaces, posing a risk of spread of infection from the neck to these regions. Imaging of the neck often is performed with imaging of the head or chest, as structures passing through the neck extend into these adjacent body regions. In this chapter, we explore the modalities available for soft-tissue cervical imaging, discuss clinical indications for imaging in a variety of chief complaints, and review some characteristic findings of important pathology, using the figures throughout the chapter. Imaging of the soft tissues of the cervical spinal cord and ligaments are discussed in Chapter 3.

Who Needs Soft-Tissue Imaging? Which Imaging Modality Should Be Used?

Given the range of potential pathology discussed earlier, it should come as little surprise that no single clinical decision rule can be used to inform decisions for soft-tissue neck imaging. Instead, the differential diagnosis under consideration should drive the imaging decision, based on expected features of the pathology and the capabilities of each modality. Dilemmas for the practitioner include whether imaging is required and, if so, whether to screen with a limited test such as x-ray, rather than incurring the additional cost and radiation exposure of computed tomography (CT). Some soft-tissue neck abnormalities are best assessed with neither x-ray nor CT but rather with ultrasound, magnetic resonance imaging (MRI), fluoroscopy, or techniques such as bronchoscopy and esophagoscopy. First we consider some general principles regarding the available imaging modalities: x-ray, CT, ultrasound, and MRI. Fluoroscopy is discussed later with regard to esophageal pathology.

SOFT-TISSUE X-RAY OF THE NECK

Plain x-ray (Figures 4-1 and 4-2) provides limited information about the soft tissues of the neck. X-ray relies on differentiation of adjacent structures using four basic tissue densities: air, fat, water (which includes soft tissues, both solid organs such as muscle and fluids such as blood), and bone (sometimes called *metal density*). As we discuss in detail in Chapter 5 with regard to chest x-ray, two adjacent structures with the same basic tissue density are indistinguishable on x-ray; no border is seen separating them. When two tissues of different density abut one another, the transition is clear. For this reason, x-rays can demonstrate abnormal soft-tissue air (Figures 4-3 to 4-5), deviation or compression of normal air-filled structures (the trachea particularly) (Figures 4-3 and 4-6 to 4-10), air–fluid levels suggesting abscess, and radiopaque foreign bodies (Figures 4-11 to 4-15), as all of these involve a contrast between two key tissue densities. Unfortunately, many of the soft-tissue abnormalities of interest to us as emergency physicians may not involve such a contrast. Instead, one soft-tissue structure may abut a second soft-tissue structure, and these are indistinguishable on x-ray. This leaves an array of potentially devastating forms of neck pathology that are poorly assessed with x-ray. Examples include vascular dissections, abscesses, and subtle soft-tissue masses that may not be seen on x-ray.

What Information Can Be Gleaned from a Portable Soft-Tissue Neck X-ray? How Should It Be Interpreted?

Portable anterior–posterior (AP) and lateral soft-tissue neck x-rays provide basic information about the airway, as described earlier. Like a focused assessment with sonography for trauma (FAST), the soft-tissue neck film should be assessed by the emergency physician with several specific clinically relevant questions in mind. As you interpret an x-ray, ask yourself each of these questions, rather than simply looking at the x-ray, and assess the x-ray for relevant findings.

On the AP x-ray:
1. Is the airway deviated laterally or narrowed, suggesting an extrinsic mass?
2. Is the airway narrowed by concentric inflammation, producing a "steeple sign" characteristic of croup (see Figure 4-8)?

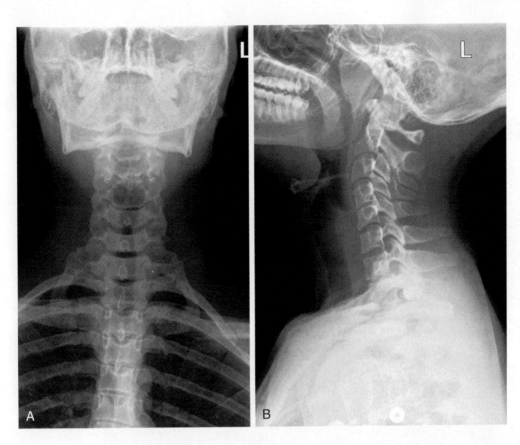

Figure 4-1. **Normal soft-tissue neck x-ray.** A soft-tissue neck series consists of an anterior–posterior (AP) **(A)** and a lateral **(B)** x-ray of the neck. Compared with a cervical spine x-ray, the images are intentionally underexposed to allow soft tissues to be examined. Figure 4-2 examines close-ups from these images.

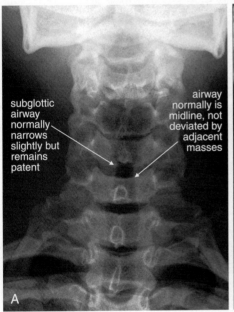

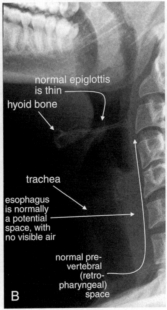

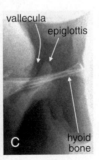

vallecula

epiglottis

hyoid bone

Figure 4-2. **Normal soft-tissue neck x-ray. A,** Anterior–posterior view. **B,** Lateral view. **C,** Close-up focusing on epiglottis. Compare with later figures showing pathology. This young adult has a normal x-ray. Note the normal epiglottis and vallecula, the position of the hyoid, and the thickness of the normal retropharyngeal (prevertebral) spaces. These become abnormal in disease states such as croup, epiglottitis, and retropharyngeal abscess.

Figure A labels:

subglottic airway normally narrows slightly but remains patent

airway normally is midline, not deviated by adjacent masses

Figure B labels:

normal epiglottis is thin

hyoid bone

trachea

esophagus is normally a potential space, with no visible air

normal prevertebral (retropharyngeal) space

3. Is air visible in the soft tissues of the neck, indicating potential pneumomediastinum, prevertebral air, esophageal or tracheal perforation, or retropharyngeal abscess?

4. Is a radiopaque foreign body visible (see Figures 4-11 and 4-14)?

On the lateral x-ray:

1. Is the airway deviated or narrowed in the AP direction? If so, why? Is an anterior neck mass compressing the trachea, or is a retropharyngeal process exerting a mass effect (see Figure 4-6)?

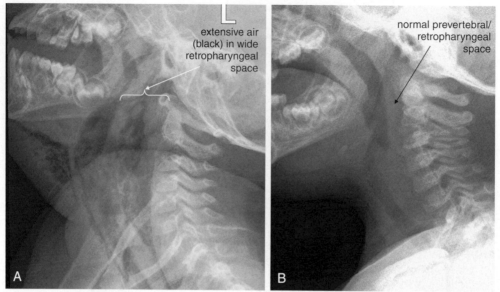

Figure 4-3. Retropharyngeal abscess with retropharyngeal air. This 22-month-old boy presented with drooling and hyperextension of the neck. He had been seen days earlier and diagnosed with a likely viral pharyngitis. **A,** Lateral soft-tissue x-ray of the neck shows extensive air (black) dissecting into tissue planes of the deep spaces of the neck, as well as the submental area. The retropharyngeal space is dramatically wide with visible air and is deviating the airway forward. Classically, soft-tissue x-ray in the setting of retropharyngeal abscess may also reveal an air–fluid level in the retropharyngeal space—a finding not present in this image. **B,** Normal soft-tissue x-ray is shown for comparison. The next figure demonstrates the computed tomography images from this patient. The patient was intubated and ultimately taken to the operating room for surgical drainage, which confirmed abscess.

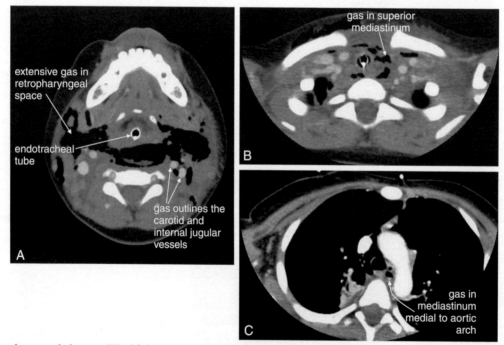

Figure 4-4. Retropharyngeal abscess: CT with intravenous (IV) contrast, soft-tissue windows. Same patient as Figure 4-3. Dramatic dissection of gas *(black)* is seen in the retropharyngeal space. **A,** The endotracheal tube is visible. Air outlines the carotid and internal jugular vessels. **B,** Air is seen dissecting into the superior mediastinum. **C,** Gas is seen medial to the aortic arch. This case highlights the dangers of retropharyngeal processes, as infections in this location can readily extend to the mediastinum. Interestingly, the patient's infection was caused by yeast, and the extensive gas collection may have been carbon dioxide produced by the *Candida* species.

2. Are the soft tissues directly behind the trachea in the retropharyngeal and prevertebral spaces thickened? If so, do they impinge upon the airway (see Figures 4-3, 4-5, and 4-6)? The normal thickness of prevertebral spaces has been reported in several studies, using both x-ray and CT (Table 4-1).[1-2]

3. Is an air–fluid level present posterior to the trachea, representing an abscess that could rupture into the airway or extrinsically compress it?

4. Is the epiglottis enlarged, threatening supraglottic airway obstruction from epiglottitis (see Figures 4-9 and 4-10)?

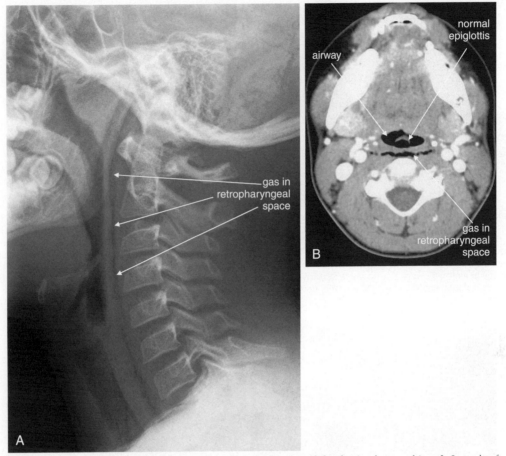

Figure 4-5. Retropharyngeal air. This 10-year-old boy complained of chest pain and dysphagia after coughing. **A,** Lateral soft-tissue neck x-ray reveals a thin stripe of air in the retropharyngeal space, extending from the skull base to the chest. Given the clinical history, the airway or lungs were the likely source of the air leak. Compare with the normal soft-tissue x-ray in a Figure 4-1, B. The patient underwent computed tomography (CT) of the neck and chest with intravenous contrast but the source of the air was not explicitly identified. **B,** Neck CT (shown on soft-tissue windows) shows a thin stripe of retropharyngeal air, correlating with the soft-tissue x-ray. Noncontrast CT could have revealed this finding, although contrast was given because of the possibility of an infectious source that might enhance with contrast.

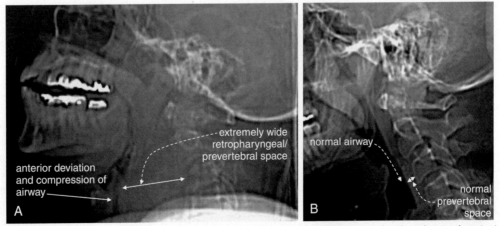

Figure 4-6. Retropharyngeal hematoma with airway compromise. This 67-year-old woman presented with neck pain after tripping, falling forward, and striking her nose against a windowsill. Although she did not lose consciousness, she reported a popping sound from her neck as hyperextension occurred. During computed tomography (CT) scan of the head and cervical spine, the patient developed stridor and was immediately removed from the CT scanner. Within 1 minute, she experienced a respiratory arrest and was intubated with difficulty. CT scans before and after her intubation are shown in the next figure. In this figure, lateral computed tomography (CT) scout images are shown, as these approximate the findings from a lateral x-ray, had one been performed. **A,** Scout CT image performed before the patient complained of dyspnea shows an extremely wide retropharyngeal space and airway compression. **B,** Normal scout film is shown for comparison. Beware of placing a patient supine for CT, because this can worsen airway compromise.

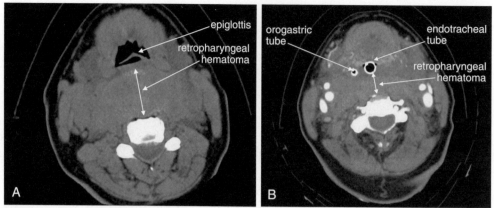

Figure 4-7. Retropharyngeal hematoma with airway compromise. Same patient as Figure 4-6. CT scans before and after her intubation are shown. **A,** The caudadmost slice of her noncontrast facial CT shows a dramatic retropharyngeal hematoma displacing the airway forward *(double arrow)*. The normal retropharyngeal space is less than 6 to 8 mm at C1-3 and 18 mm at C6 or C7, while this patient's hematoma was more than 40 mm in thickness. **B,** After intubation, the patient underwent repeat CT with intravenous contrast to assess for active hemorrhage—none was found. The retropharyngeal hematoma is still visible, 20 mm in thickness at this level posterior to the endotracheal tube *(double arrow)*. But for the presence of the endotracheal tube, the hematoma completely obscures the airway. The hematoma extended caudad into the mediastinum. The patient had no spinal injury detected, and coagulation studies on the patient were normal.

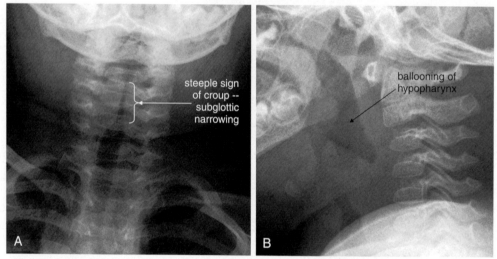

Figure 4-8. Croup. This 19-month-old, fully immunized boy presented with acute onset of stridor without fever. The patient's mother was uncertain whether he might have ingested a foreign body, and x-rays of the soft tissues of the neck and chest were obtained. **A,** The anterior–posterior neck x-ray shows a classic example of the long-segment subglottic narrowing typical of croup, called the "steeple sign" for its resemblance to a traditional peaked church steeple. **B,** The prevertebral soft tissues are normal, and the epiglottis appears normal on lateral x-ray. The hypopharynx appears ballooned, which is common in croup. X-rays are not needed routinely to confirm croup when a typical history and physical is present. The primary purpose of x-rays in this setting is to rule out other etiologies, such as foreign body aspiration or epiglottitis.

5. Is abnormal air visible in the neck, indicating potential pneumomediastinum, prevertebral air, esophageal or tracheal perforation, or retropharyngeal abscess (see Figures 4-3 and 4-5)?
6. Is a radiopaque foreign body visible (see Figures 4-11 and 4-13 to 4-15)?

SOFT-TISSUE NECK CT

CT is clearly superior to x-ray, as it is able to distinguish a subtler spectrum of tissue densities. CT scan readily distinguishes air, fat, fluid, solid soft tissues of muscle density, and bone. The window setting on CT (discussed in detail later) can be adjusted to highlight a particular tissue density, but on all window settings these tissues are color coded from black (lowest density) to white (highest density). On soft-tissue windows, which are key in our evaluation of neck soft-tissue pathology, air is black, fat is a dark gray (nearly black), fluids such as blood or pus are an intermediate gray, solid tissues are a slightly lighter gray, and high-density material such as bone or metal are white. Lung window settings are sometimes used to evaluate the neck, as air becomes quite evident (black) against all other tissue densities, which appear white on this window setting. Bone windows also highlight air (black) in contrast to all other tissues. Nonstandard window settings can be selected to highlight pathology. The precise density of a tissue can also be measured on CT scan on most picture archiving and communication systems (PACSs) (the name given to a digital diagnostic imaging

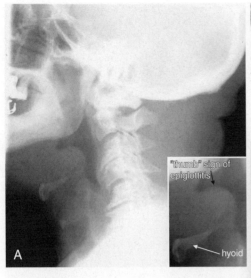

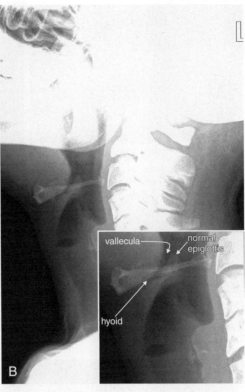

Figure 4-9. Epiglottitis. **A,** Lateral cervical soft-tissue x-ray showing epiglottitis in a 64-year-old man. The epiglottis is thickened, showing a classic "thumb sign." **B,** Normal soft-tissue x-ray for comparison. The brightness and contrast have been increased to point out the normal thin epiglottis, which is partially hidden behind the hyoid bone. The vallecula is seen as a narrow space anterior to the epiglottis. An anterior–posterior (AP) x-ray is not shown for this case, because the AP view is not usually diagnostic in cases of epiglottitis.

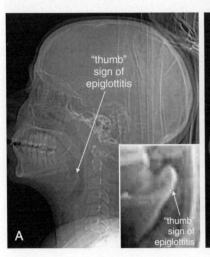

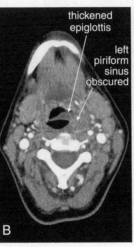

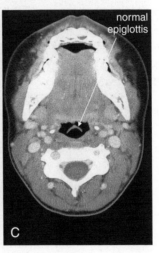

Figure 4-10. **Epiglottitis, seen on CT with IV contrast, soft tissue windows.** While a patient with suspected impending airway occlusion should not be placed supine in a CT scanner, CT can be a valuable tool for diagnosis of airway and retropharyngeal pathology. In this patient with epiglottitis, the CT scout image **(A)** demonstrates a thumb sign similar to the plain film findings in Figure 4-9. The axial image **(B)** also demonstrates an enlarged epiglottis, with an obscured left piriform sinus. A normal epiglottis in another patient is shown for comparison **(C).** The normal epiglottis is a thin crescent.

interface). The computer cursor can be placed over a single pixel or a broader region of interest, and the density of the tissue in Hounsfield units (HU) is reported. On the Hounsfield scale (Figure 000), water has a density of 0 HU, air has a density of −1000 HU, and the highest-density bone has a density of +1000 HU. Nonbiological high-density substances such as metal foreign bodies have densities exceeding +1000 HU. Fat is less dense than water and has a lower density, around −50 HU. Soft tissues such as muscle are denser than water and have a higher Hounsfield value, around 30–50 HU. Liquid blood has a density slightly greater than water, due to its cellular content; the density may vary with factors such as hematocrit and volume status. CT allows ready identification of a tissue abnormality such as abscess based on density

differences. An abscess (Figures 4-16 and 4-17) filled with liquid pus appears darker than denser surrounding soft tissues viewed on soft-tissue windows.

Structures with identical (or nearly identical) density are indistinguishable on CT without contrast, with several clinically important examples. Because pus is similar in density to surrounding normal soft tissues, IV contrast can assist in identifying an abscess. Normal soft tissues are highly vascular and enhance (increase in density) following administration of IV contrast. Pus within an abscess does not enhance with IV contrast, so the difference in density between abscess and normal surrounding tissues increases following IV contrast administration, increasing the conspicuity of the abscess. Similarly a

Figure 4-11. **Penetrating neck trauma.** This 30-year-old man was wounded with a shotgun. The patient ducked his head at the moment of the blast, and most of the shot impacted superficially in his scalp. However, one pellet entered the mental vertex of his mandible and lodged in the anterolateral neck. **A,** Anterior–posterior view shows the pellet to be in the lateral left neck, in the region of the carotid artery. **B,** The lateral x-ray combined with the AP view shows the pellet is not superficial. Computed tomography was performed to assess the carotid artery and adjacent structures Figure 4-12.

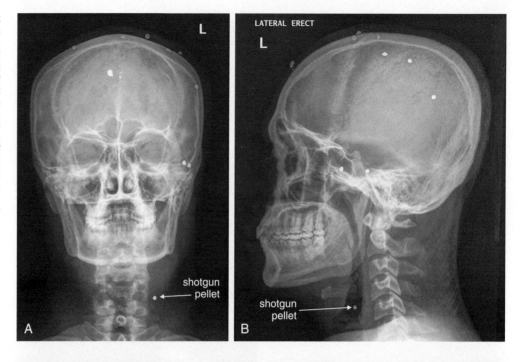

Figure 4-12. **Penetrating neck trauma.** Same patient as Figure 4-11. Computed tomography with intravenous contrast was performed to assess the carotid artery and adjacent structures. **A,** Soft-tissue windows. **B,** Bone windows. The pellet creates extensive metallic streak artifact, which completely obscures the vessels of interest. Conventional angiography could be performed in circumstances such as these, because it is free of this type of artifact.

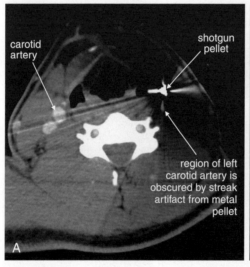

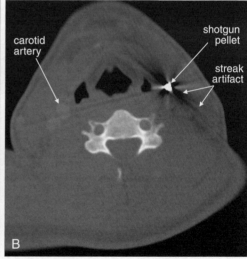

vascular dissection (Figures 4-18 to 4-20) would be difficult or impossible to recognize without contrast, because blood in the true and false lumen share the same density, and the thin intimal flap separating them is of nearly identical density. Administration of intravenous (IV) contrast changes this relationship by providing high-density (contrast) material flowing on both sides of the intimal flap. The low-density flap becomes visible against this background. Partially thrombosed vascular segments (Figures 4-21 to 4-22), which are common in dissections of the relatively small-caliber vessels of the neck, are also made visible by this same principle: high-density contrast flows through the patent lumen of the vessel, making low-density thrombus visible. Without contrast, liquid blood and thrombus share nearly identical densities and are nearly indistinguishable. Contrast also aids in detecting soft-tissue masses. Normal muscle and a muscle tumor

such as sarcoma (Figures 4-23 to 4-25) may share the same tissue density without contrast. However, a highly vascular neoplasm receives differentially more parenterally administered contrast and has a higher density when imaged with contrast. CT does not perfectly distinguish benign and malignant mass lesions, so biopsy is necessary for confirmation. Even when an abscess is not present, inflamed or infected soft tissues also have increased blood flow and enhance with IV contrast (Figure 4-26; see also Figures 4-16, 4-17, and 4-26). Without any contrast administration, CT is excellent for airway assessment, as very low-density air within the airway provides outstanding intrinsic contrast against surrounding soft tissues. (Figure 4-27; see also Figures 4-7, 4-10, 4-16, 4-17, 4-24, and 4-25). However, extreme caution should be applied in sending patients with suspected airway pathology to CT, as airway obstruction can be worsened by supine positioning for CT.

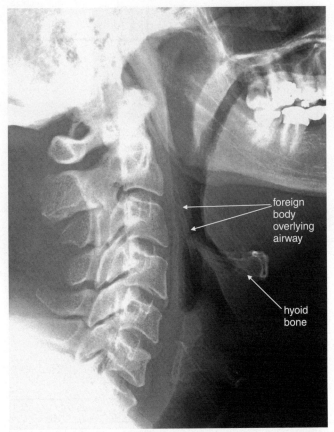

Figure 4-13. Airway foreign body: Chicken bone. This 47-year-old man was unable to speak after eating chicken. The patient pointed to his larynx, indicating a foreign body sensation. Lateral neck x-ray shows a foreign body superior to the larynx, perpendicular to the hyoid bone. Remember that you must look at both the anterior–posterior (AP) and the lateral view to localize an object; in this case, however, the object was not visible on the AP view, because it overlay the spine. Smaller foreign bodies such as fish bones may not be visible on plain film but may be identified on computed tomography. In this case, the patient was taken to the operating room for removal of the object, which was found to be a 4-cm chicken bone in the right piriform sinus.

Focus on CT Window Settings: What Is a Window?

A window setting (Figure 4-28) is a method of distributing the available gray shades on CT to emphasize a particular tissue. A window is defined by two Hounsfield density values: a center value (also called "window level," the tissue density that receives the middle gray shade in the available spectrum) and a width that defines the upper and lower tissue densities (which are colored white and black, respectively). Any tissue with a density lower than the lower limit of the window appears black. Any tissue with a density higher than the upper limit of the window appears white. The available gray shades from pure black to pure white are then evenly distributed among the densities within the window width. As a consequence, a narrow window setting allows fine differentiation of density differences surrounding the "center" value, but the ability to distinguish tissues above or below the window width is lost. Some typical window settings are shown in Table 4-2. Standard window settings optimized for evaluation of soft tissues, lung, bone, or vascular abnormalities are often preset on a digital PACS, although the user can vary the window settings or even save personalized settings.

What Is the CT Technique for Soft-Tissue Evaluation? Does It Differ from Cervical Spine CT?

CT for evaluation of soft tissues of the neck differs from CT for evaluation of the cervical spine. Cervical spine CT is performed without IV contrast, as bony injury can be seen without contrast material. For soft-tissue evaluation, IV contrast is given, as it reveals vascular abnormalities such as intimal tears or active bleeding (marked by

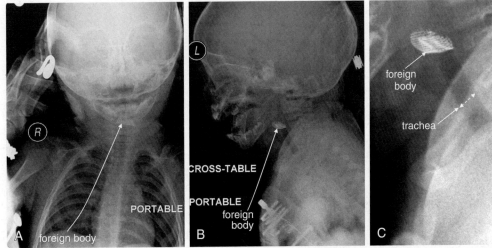

Figure 4-14. Airway foreign body: Metal mesh. The role of plain films in evaluation of soft tissues of the neck is limited, but when the patient's airway is threatened, plain film may offer the only safe imaging modality. Portable plain films with the patient in a "position of comfort" may offer some diagnostic information. CT in a supine position may further compromise airway patency. In this toddler, parents reported sudden stridor but did not witness an ingestion or aspiration. Portable x-ray revealed a radiopaque mesh object in the airway. The patient was taken emergently to the operating room for removal. Plastic or organic material may not be visible on plain x-ray. **A,** Anterior–posterior view. **B,** Lateral view. **C,** Close-up from **B.**

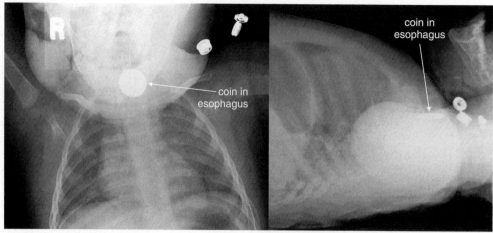

Figure 4-15. Esophageal foreign bodies. This 11-month-old presented with drooling after being witnessed to place a penny in his mouth. X-ray confirms a circular object apparently lodged in the esophagus. **A,** Anterior–posterior (AP). **B,** Lateral. Coins lodged in the esophagus tend to assume an "en face" position, with a circular appearance on the AP view (think British *oesophagus* for the O appearance of an esophageal coin). Coins lodged in the trachea tend to assume an "edge-on" linear appearance on the AP view, apparently directed to that position by the incomplete tracheal rings. This patient was taken to the operating suite for removal of the coin, which was found to be lodged in the esophagus at the level of the cricopharyngeus.

contrast extravasation). In addition, infectious processes such as abscess and inflammatory or neoplastic conditions enhance with IV contrast, improving their detection and characterization. If IV contrast is contraindicated because of renal insufficiency or allergy, noncontrast CT can still provide important information, but evaluation of vascular pathology such as dissection and subtle infectious or neoplastic process will be insensitive. In this case, other modalities such as ultrasound may be needed.

The cephalad–caudad scope and field of view of soft-tissue neck CT also differ from those of cervical spine CT. Typically, cervical spine CT is performed from the skull base to the bottom of the T1 vertebral body. This usually captures the lung apices, although the reconstructed image is usually "coned in" so that only the spine, not the full diameter of the neck and chest, is seen. Usually, soft-tissue neck CT spans from the skull base to the top of the aortic arch to capture the carotid and vertebral arteries as they emerge from the aortic arch. This also allows assessment of prevertebral space abnormalities as they extend into the chest. The exact cephalad–caudad scope may vary from institution to institution and based on clinical indication—for example, the CT protocol for soft-tissue infection assessment may be different from the protocol for vascular assessment in some institutions. The field of view for soft tissue neck CT is usually broader than that for cervical spine CT, as the image is not "coned in." Instead, soft tissue neck CT encompasses the entire diameter of the neck and any included regions of the chest.

Is Soft-Tissue Neck CT the Same as CT Cervical Angiography?

Cervical CT angiography overlaps substantially with other soft-tissue applications—at some institutions, the same CT protocol may be used. In cervical CT

TABLE 4-1. Normal Prevertebral Soft-Tissue Thickness

Imaging Modality and Location	Thickness
X-ray	
Retrocricoid soft-tissue thickness (x-ray)	0.7× diameter of C5 vertebral body
Retrotracheal soft-tissue thickness (x-ray)	1.0× diameter of C5 vertebral body
CT	
C1	8.5 mm
C2	6 mm
C3	7 mm
C4-5	Not determined because of variable position of esophagus and larynx
C6	18 mm
C7	18 mm

From Chen MY, Bohrer SP. Radiographic measurement of prevertebral soft tissue thickness on lateral radiographs of the neck. *Skeletal Radiol* 1999;28(8):444-6; Rojas CA, Vermess D, Bertozzi JC, et al. Normal thickness and appearance of the prevertebral soft tissues on multidetector CT. *AJNR Am J Neuroradiol* 30(1):136-41, 2009.

angiography, as with other CT angiography applications, a high-quality diagnostic study requires a rapid bolus of injected contrast material, properly timed with the CT acquisition to ensure that the bolus reaches the vascular bed of interest at the moment of image capture. For cervical CT angiography, this generally means a bolus of between 60 and 150 mL of iodinated contrast, administered at a rate of 4 mL per second. Automated bolus tracking software allows the CT technician to measure the enhancement of vessels such as the aortic

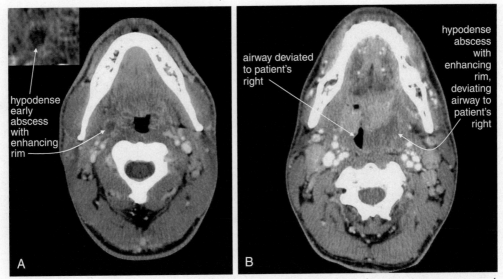

Figure 4-16. Peritonsillar abscess. A classic peritonsillar abscess requires no imaging, as it has a characteristic appearance on physical examination, with a deviated uvula and peritonsillar mass. In reality, some patients present with early abscesses that are not visible, and others experience too much trismus to allow a complete exam. If more information is needed and the airway appears sufficiently patent for the patient to lie supine safely, intravenous (IV) contrast-enhanced computed tomography can provide excellent diagnostic information. IV contrast leads to "ring enhancement," an increase in the density on the periphery of an abscess caused by increased blood flow. **A,** A small peritonsillar abscess is beginning to form, visible as a hypodense area with slight surrounding enhancement. **B,** A larger hypodense abscess has formed and is deviating the airway.

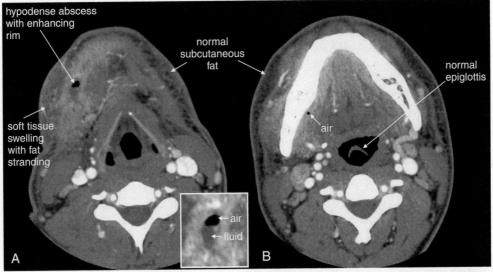

Figure 4-17. Anterior neck abscess, possibly arising from a dental infection. In this soft-tissue neck computed tomography with intravenous contrast viewed on soft tissue windows, a hypodense abscess containing fluid (*dark gray*) and air (*black*) is present in the patient's right neck in a submandibular position. **A,** Soft-tissue changes including swelling and inflammatory stranding (*smoky appearance*) of subcutaneous fat are present (compare with opposite side). **B,** A tiny fleck of air is visible just medial to the mandible, suggesting that infection may have arisen from a mandibular tooth.

arch (which leads directly to the cervical arteries) using a small test bolus. The necessary time delay from contrast injection until CT scan is then calculated. This time delay allows the contrast to transit from the peripheral vein, where it is injected; through the superior vena cava, right heart, and pulmonary vessels; and then to the left heart, where it is ejected through the aorta to the cervical vessels. Thin CT slices are obtained, and reconstructions in multiple planes are then used to inspect the vessels. Review of axial slices alone can be quite useful. CT venography of the neck uses the same technique as CT arteriography, but image acquisition is timed to coincide with the arrival of contrast in neck veins. By chance, often the image acquisition may occur when both arteries and veins are opacified with contrast. If evaluation of neck veins is the primary indication for imaging, ultrasound may be a better first choice, as it does not require radiation exposure or contrast administration. Soft-tissue cervical CT can be performed with a slower contrast bolus for evaluation of soft-tissue masses and infections, as the diagnosis is less reliant on dense opacification of blood vessels.

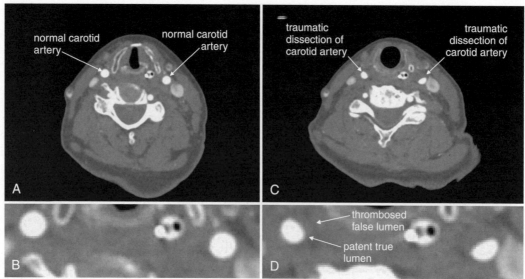

Figure 4-18. Vascular dissections (carotid artery). This 75-year-old woman presented after a motor vehicle collision. The patient was noted to have an ecchymotic seat belt mark across her left neck. The patient had multiple other injuries, including a diaphragm injury diagnosed by chest x-ray, so CT angiography of the neck was prospectively planned (for assessment of cervical vascular injury) to be performed at the time of chest and abdominal CT to avoid repeating the intravenous contrast bolus. **A,** The normal carotid arteries below the level of the injury. Note the rounded appearance and bright filling with contrast **B,** a close-up view from **A. C,** Bilateral carotid artery dissections at the level of injury. The normal round appearance is replaced by a three-quarter moon appearance. The false lumen has thrombosed bilaterally, so an intimal flap is not seen (compare with aortic dissection in Chapter 7). **D,** a close-up view from **C.** In some cases, irregularity of the contour of the artery may be the only abnormal finding. The dissection has resulted in significant stenosis, approximately 30% to 40% on the left, and 20% to 30% on the right.

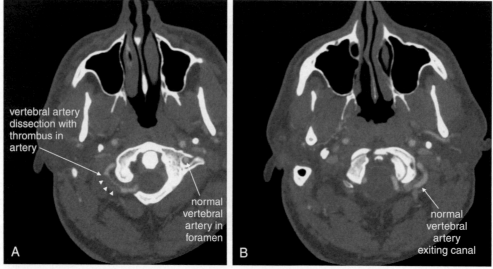

Figure 4-19. Vascular dissections (vertebral artery dissection): CT with IV contrast, viewed on vascular windows. Spontaneous dissection of the vertebral artery is a relatively rare event but is thought to be one of the most common causes of stroke in young patients. Computed tomography (CT) angiography and magnetic resonance angiography are the most common methods of assessment today, with catheter-based angiography usually reserved for patients with CT or magnetic resonance abnormalities. Remember that the vertebral arteries exit their canals at the C1 level, curve medially, pass through the ring of C1, and then merge to form the basilar artery. In these axial CT images, IV contrast has been administered to the patient. The window level is set to an intermediate value between bone and soft-tissue settings. You can recognize this from the subcutaneous fat, which is not nearly black, and bone, which is too bright to allow its internal structure to be easily recognized. **A,** The left vertebral artery is seen within its canal. The curving right vertebral artery is seen with a filling defect representing a thrombosed region of dissection. **B,** The normal left vertebral artery is seen filled with contrast.

Approach to Interpretation of Soft-Tissue Neck CT

The large number of anatomic structures visible on soft-tissue neck CT makes a systematic approach to interpretation both essential and difficult. For most emergency applications, a soft-tissue window setting is appropriate, with exceptions pointed out in the figures. A simple approach is to select a structure with suspected pathology, such as a carotid artery, and follow that single structure from the cephalad to caudad limits of the scan, inspecting for abnormalities. The opposite side often provides an excellent normal example for comparison, as the neck is usually bilaterally symmetrical until the intersection

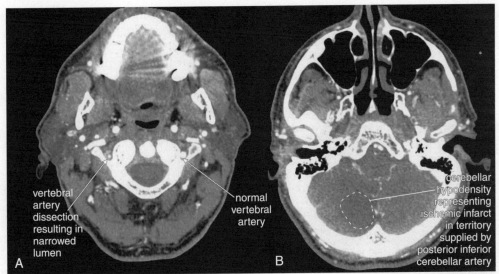

Figure 4-20. Vertebral artery dissection from C4 to C1 with posterior inferior cerebellar artery (PICA) territory infarct after cough. This patient presented with vertigo after paroxysmal cough, and a cervical computed tomography angiogram was performed to evaluate for vertebral artery dissection. **A,** The left vertebral artery is of normal caliber. The right vertebral artery is narrowed to a fraction of the normal size. Is this a normal variant or acute disease? In congenital hypoplasia of the vertebral artery, the bony canal also is smaller than normal, whereas in this patient the canal is of normal size, indicating that the artery has an acute abnormality. **B,** A corresponding acute ischemic infarct is seen in the cerebellum in a region supplied by the PICA. Magnetic resonance imaging or magnetic resonance angiography could be used to provide similar information.

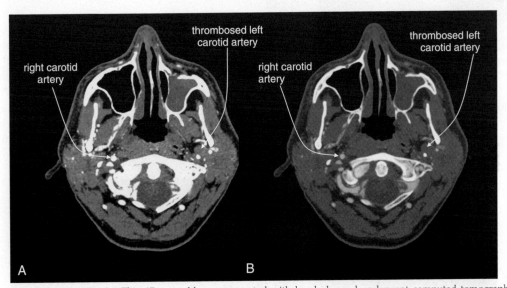

Figure 4-21. Carotid artery thrombosis. This 47-year-old man presented with headache and underwent computed tomography venography of the head and neck to assess for venous sinus thrombosis. Instead, complete occlusion of the left internal carotid artery was discovered. **A,** Soft-tissue windows. **B,** A window setting similar to bone windows often used for assessment of vascular structures. The benefit of this window setting is that the internal structure of blood vessels, such as intimal tears, irregularity, or thrombosis is more evident. On typical soft-tissue windows **(A),** contrast in the vessel is so bright that internal structural detail is often less visible. In this particular case, the pathology is subtle for a different reason—you must recognize the absence of a normal structure in the image. Use expected symmetry to help you. The right carotid artery is well opacified with intravenous contrast. The left carotid artery is devoid of contrast because it has completely thrombosed. On a picture archiving and communication system, follow blood vessels through multiple slices to inspect them. Incidentally, the patient's left maxillary sinus is opacified, suggesting sinusitis (see Chapter 2 for more information).

of cervical vascular structures with great vessels in the chest. As is our habit for a FAST examination, apply a structured clinical question: Is a dissection of the carotid artery present? Is the airway narrowed? Is the palpable mass on examination an abscess? Often, CT is ordered by the emergency physician with a binary question of this type in mind. For the radiologist, the task is more difficult, as all structures in the field of view must be inspected. For the emergency physician, a targeted inspection based on the differential diagnosis usually provides the immediately clinically relevant information. In cases of trauma or when a particularly broad differential diagnosis is being entertained, systematic inspection of all cervical structures, rather than selective inspection, is crucial.

CERVICAL SOFT-TISSUE ULTRASOUND

Ultrasound is excellent for distinguishing soft-tissue and fluid densities. Its utility in imaging soft tissues of the neck is limited by several factors. Sound waves are chaotically dispersed by air, disrupting the image;

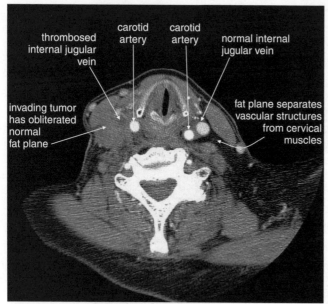

Figure 4-22. Internal jugular vein occlusion, CT with IV contrast, soft tissue windows. This patient with an aggressive esophageal tumor has cervical adenopathy resulting from tumor metastases. The enlarging tumor burden has created local mass effect on the right internal jugular vein, which has become thrombosed as a result. The internal jugular contains dark thrombus on the right, compared with the bright contrast–filled left internal jugular vein. The cervical fat planes on the right have become obscured by invading tumor.

for this reason, air-filled structures in the neck (trachea and, to a lesser degree, esophagus) obstruct imaging of deeper structures. In addition, bone is sufficiently dense that it reflects or absorbs essentially all sound waves, preventing imaging of deeper structures. As a consequence, ultrasound can be valuable for imaging relatively superficial neck structures and differentiating solid and cystic masses. It is advantageous in that it does not involve ionizing radiation or contrast administration.

Ultrasound can detect vascular dissections and stenoses of the carotid arteries and thrombosis of cervical venous structures (Figures 4-29 to 4-31). The vertebral arteries, partially hidden in the bony transverse foramina of the vertebral bodies (see Chapter 3), cannot be completely imaged with ultrasound, although portions can be assessed—in general, CT angiography or magnetic resonance angiography (MRA) is a better choice for evaluation of suspected vertebral artery pathology. Ultrasound is also limited in imaging the carotid arteries and cervical veins once those structures enter the skull base or chest; CT is not limited in this way.

Another appropriate use for ultrasound is in the evaluation of a palpable neck mass (Figures 4-32 to 4-34). Ultrasound can distinguish solid masses, which may suggest adenopathy or neoplasm, from fluid-filled structures such as cysts, abscesses, hematomas, and vascular anomalies. Examples of typical pathology of this type include thyroglossal duct cysts (see Figure 4-34), branchial cleft cysts, and goiters (see Figure 4-32). Ultrasound does

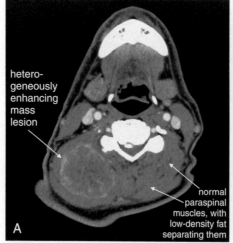
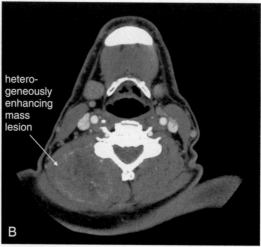

Figure 4-23. Neck mass. This 70-year-old patient presented with progressive right posterior neck swelling over a period of 1 month following a dental procedure. Asymmetry and a palpable mass were present on exam. Computed tomography (CT) with intravenous contrast was performed to assess for abscess or mass. A heterogeneously enhancing mass is visible in the right posterior paraspinous muscles, measuring approximately 5.2 by 4.2 cm in axial dimension. The mass does not have the appearance of an abscess, which most often would have a lower density (fluid density, darker gray) center. Note how the mass has obliterated the normal planes separating paraspinal muscles—compare this with the patient's left side, which is normal. Without contrast, these asymmetrical features and the overall size of the mass would be appreciated, but the discrete margins of the mass would not be seen without enhancement because the mass shares the same density with normal muscle. CT does not identify the exact etiology of the mass, although the differential diagnosis for a muscle-density mass lesion includes sarcoma. Biopsy or excision would be needed to prove the diagnosis. Interestingly, the patient underwent fine-needle aspiration that showed gram-negative rods and spindle-shaped cells initially thought to represent reactive myositis or fasciitis—possibly an infection caused by the reported dental procedure. Unfortunately, surgical pathology showed an undifferentiated sarcoma.

not always distinguish reliably between benign and malignant lesions, so additional workup with biopsy is prudent.

Doppler ultrasound can be used to assess for flow in fluid-filled structures. Ultrasound can detect air in cervical soft tissues, because the ultrasound image is unexpectedly disrupted by air interfering with sound transmission. When the pathology of concern would be expected to lie deep to air-filled or bony structures, or when evaluation of the cephalad and caudad extent of

the pathology would require cranial or chest imaging, CT is generally a better imaging choice. Ultrasound remains a good alternative in young patients because of radiation concerns.

SOFT-TISSUE NECK MAGNETIC RESONANCE IMAGING

MRI remains the test of choice for imaging of the cervical spinal cord, as well as ligaments and intervertebral discs of the cervical spine. This indication is discussed in more

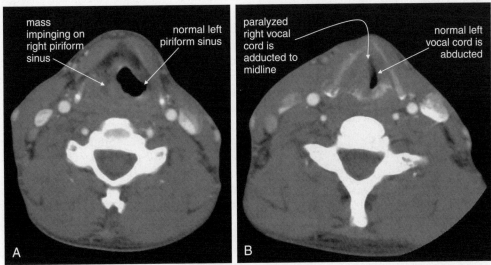

Figure 4-24. Neck masses: Laryngeal cancer with vocal cord paralysis, CT with intravenous contrast. This patient has a laryngeal mass with complete paralysis of the right vocal cord. **A,** The mass occupies and obscures the left piriform sinus. Without a history of cancer, this appearance could be similar to a soft-tissue infection adjacent to the airway. **B,** The right vocal cord is completely paralyzed and is therefore is passively adducted to the midline. The left vocal cord is not paralyzed and is thus abducted normally.

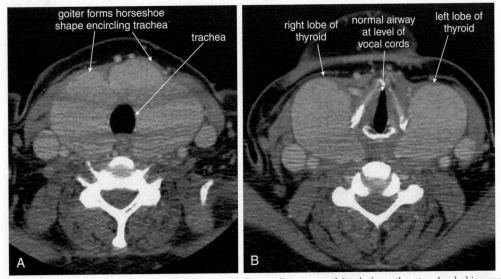

Figure 4-25. Goiter in Grave's disease. This 44-year-old woman with Graves disease complained of sore throat and a choking sensation. Computed tomography (CT) with intravenous (IV) contrast was performed. A large goiter surrounds the patient's trachea but does not impinge upon it **(A, B).** CT is useful in the evaluation of thyroid masses, because it can simultaneously evaluate for airway impingement and mediastinal extension of a thyroid mass. In cases of thyroid malignancy, local invasion and metastatic disease can be detected. Rarely, IV contrast agents such as iodixanol (Visipaque) have been reported to precipitate thyroid storm in patients with hyperthyroidism. In addition, iodixanol may interfere with thyroid function determination by altering serum protein–bound iodine concentrations for up to 16 days. Therefore blood for thyroid function tests should be obtained before contrast administration.

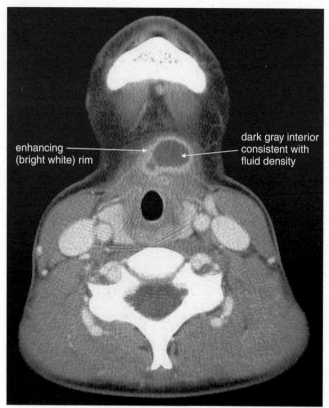

enhancing (bright white) rim

dark gray interior consistent with fluid density

Figure 4-26. Thyroglossal duct cyst: Computed tomography (CT) with intravenous contrast, soft-tissue windows. This patient presented with midline anterior cervical swelling, redness, and pain. Exam suggested an infected thyroglossal duct cyst, confirmed by the CT. The CT reveals a well-demarcated, rounded cystic structure with rim enhancement. The midline position is typical of a thyroglossal duct cyst, an anatomic remnant that can become superinfected and rapidly enlarge. Treatment is usually with antibiotics, followed by definitive surgical excision. Rim enhancement is typical of an inflammatory or infectious process. The dark gray internal appearance is consistent with fluid density. The sharp margins of this structure are more consistent with a preexisting cyst than with an infectious abscess.

detail in Chapter 3, whereas other applications of MRI of the neck are discussed here. MRI provides exceptional soft-tissue contrast and comparable resolution of vascular pathology to CT. It can be used to image thoracic and cranial structures, making it particularly useful when vascular dissections originating from the aortic arch and resulting in ischemic stroke are suspected. CT provides similar information in this setting, although MRI is more definitive for early brain ischemic changes and infarcts. MRI is relatively rarely used in the emergency department for cervical imaging because it is less readily available, more expensive, and more time consuming than CT, which provides similar information for most clinical purposes. MRI does not involve ionizing radiation, an advantage over CT, which does. In the past, MRI was recommended for patients with renal insufficiency due to concerns about contrast nephropathy from iodinated contrast used in CT. However, recently described gadolinium-associated nephrogenic systemic fibrosis in patients with renal insufficiency has limited the use of MRI in this population. Nephrogenic systemic fibrosis

is described in more detail in Chapter 15. MRI remains a good alternative in patients with iodine allergy who require cervical soft-tissue imaging with contrast.

A few principles of MRI bear emphasis here. MRI relies on the presence of protons to resonate in an applied magnetic field, providing a signal that is used to generate an image. Calcified bone does not have free protons to resonate in this way, so bone cortex lacks signal and appears black on all magnetic resonance sequences. For this reason, cortical bone fractures are not seen directly with MRI, although their presence is often inferred from associated soft tissue changes. Consequently, CT is the preferred modality for detection of cervical spine fracture. In contrast, bone marrow contains fat and is proton rich, providing a signal for detecting pathologic processes such as osteomyelitis and bone tumors. Air also lacks protons and does not generate a signal, although the absence of signal can be used to detect pathologic air in areas that would normally generate a soft-tissue signal. Even without the administration of gadolinium contrast, MRI thus often provides more information about soft tissues than does unenhanced CT scan, which cannot distinguish tissues that share the same physical density. CT with IV contrast can distinguish soft tissues with differing blood flow and enhancement characteristics, as described earlier in this chapter. MRI can readily detect differences in soft tissues based on differing signal characteristics from fat and water-containing soft tissues, both of which are rich in protons. MRI can be manipulated in different pulse sequences to allow differentiation of tissue types and forms of pathology. MRI pulse sequences are discussed in detail in Chapter 15. MR angiography (MRA) for assessment of vascular pathology is discussed later in this chapter, in comparison with CT angiography.

What Is the Best Strategy for Imaging of Airway Threats? Is Three-Dimensional CT Useful for Evaluation of Potential Penetrating Tracheal Injury?

Some general safety considerations guide soft-tissue neck imaging. Be extremely cautious in imaging of any patient with a threatened airway. This is obvious to us as emergency physicians, yet patients are frequently sent out of the emergency department for soft-tissue imaging when dyspnea or stridor is part of the clinical presentation. Soft-tissue x-rays may be useful in the setting of the endangered airway, as they can be performed portably with the patient in a position of comfort (see Figures 4-1 to 4-3, 4-5, 4-8 to 4-9, 4-11, and 4-13 to 4-15). In contrast, CT scan requires transportation of the patient out of the emergency department and supine positioning for the duration of the scan, which can compromise an already threatened airway (see Figures 4-6 and 4-7). Throughout this chapter, we see examples of pathology on x-ray

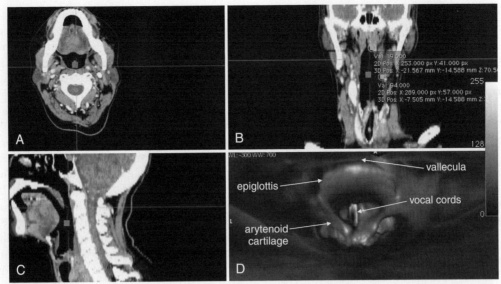

Figure 4-27. Computed tomography (CT) virtual laryngoscopy or bronchoscopy. Modern thin-slice multidetector CT can be used to assess the airway in axial **(A)**, coronal **(B)**, sagittal **(C)**, or three-dimensional **(D)** reconstructions. These images show a patient's airway from several supraglottic views. The crosshairs in **A** through **C** indicate the planes displayed in the other two-dimensional images. For example, the horizontal line in **A** indicates the coronal plane displayed in **B**. The horizontal line in **C** indicates the axial plane displayed in **A**. The vertical line in **B** indicates the sagittal plane shown in **C**. **D** is a three-dimensional view of the epiglottis, arytenoid cartilages, and vocal cords seen from the point of view of an observer located at the square in the other images. Software packages synchronize the four views so that changes made in one image are reflected in the other views. Renderings of this type can provide information similar to laryngoscopy or bronchoscopy, but beware of airway collapse while the patient is positioned supine for CT. CT also provides no therapeutic option.

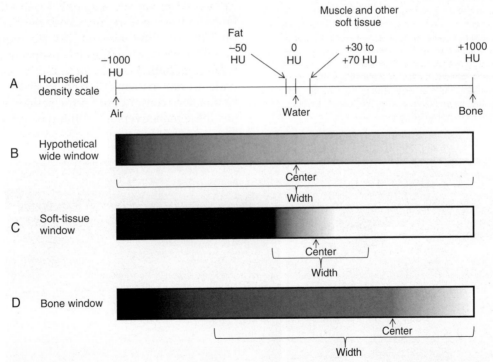

Figure 4-28. The Hounsfield CT density scale and CT windows. A, Each tissue has a fixed density on the Hounsfield scale, measured in Hounsfield units (HU). Air is defined as −1000HU. Water is defined as 0 HU. Densest bone is defined as +1000HU. Other tissues fall on the scale according to their relative densities. Although the density of a tissue is a fixed physical property, the appearance on CT depends on the window setting, which can be adjusted to accentuate a given range of densities. A window is defined by a center value, the density that is assigned the central gray shade in the available spectrum, and a width, which defines the densities on each side of the center that are assigned pure black and pure white. **B,** Hypothetical window centered on water density and distributing gray shades across the entire Hounsfield scale. On this setting, fine differences in density among body tissues from fat to water to muscle would be impossible to recognize, as all would be intermediate gray colors. **C,** Soft-tissue window centered on a soft tissue density around 50HU and distributing gray shades more narrowly, focusing on the range of densities representing most body soft tissues. On this window setting, fine differences in soft-tissue densities can be seen, but subtleties in very low density and very high density tissues are completely lost. **D,** Bone window centered on a density around 500HU and distributing gray shades across the range of densities representing bone. On this window setting, fine differences in bone densities can be seen. Soft tissues cannot be distinguished, as all share a dark gray color. Air can be distinguished from soft tissues on this window, as it appears completely black.

and CT that could seriously endanger a patient who has not been intubated orally, nasally, or by means of a surgical airway. If serious impairment of the airway is considered, think about protecting the airway before imaging. Bronchoscopic airway evaluation can provide key information about intrinsic airway edema, obstruction, or foreign bodies, as well as narrowing from extrinsic compression. Moreover, bronchoscopy may provide a therapeutic solution by fiberoptic intubation, whereas diagnostic imaging does not. Three-dimensional CT "virtual bronchoscopy" (see Figure 4-27) can be performed with excellent resolution—but at the expense of radiation exposure and without the ability to remove a foreign body, stent a stenotic

airway, or obtain cultures or pathologic samples—all possible with real bronchoscopy. The role of three-dimensional CT in airway imaging remains to be defined. In patients with a low pretest probability of pathology, the cost and radiation exposure of CT may not be warranted. In patients with a high probability of pathology, bronchoscopy may be the more appropriate test. Particularly in the case of suspected pediatric foreign body aspiration, CT has been described as a sensitive and specific imaging modality, but radiation concerns may make bronchoscopy the better choice. The risks of sedation for bronchoscopy must be weighed against the radiation effect of CT. Recent case series and case reports have reported the utility of three-dimensional CT virtual bronchoscopy for detection of tracheal injuries and foreign bodies.[3-7] However, the sensitivity of this technique is not yet well-established. Larger studies are required to validate the safety of this technique to replace diagnostic bronchoscopy.

TABLE 4.2. Window Settings for CT

Brain	42	155
Bone	570	3077
Lung	−498	1465
Soft tissue (used for most neck structures, also used for chest and abdomen)	56	342

Tissues with a density matching the center value are assigned the middle gray hue in the available range. The window width defines the tissue densities that will be assigned pure black and pure white. The center value plus one-half the width is assigned pure white. All tissues with this density or greater appear white. The center value minus one-half the width is assigned pure black. All tissues with this density or less appear black. The available gray shades are evenly distributed among tissues between these two extremes. Window settings can be adjusted by users, and no standards exist. The precise values used may vary among institutions and even among different CT readers. The values in this table are from the author's institution.

How Can CT Be Made More Specific for Airway Abnormalities?

It can be frustrating to obtain a CT scan in a patient with a potential airway problem only to have the CT interpretation indicate uncertainty about the airway structures. Multiple dynamic air contrast techniques have been described for stenting the airway open during CT, using humming, puffed cheeks, or valsalva maneuvers by the patient. Some patients with acute airway problems may be unable to comply, but for the patient who can cooperate, these maneuvers may eliminate artifacts created by

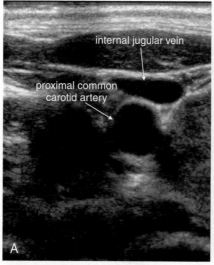
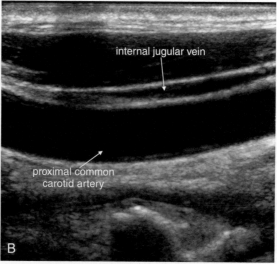

Figure 4-29. Normal carotid artery ultrasound. Ultrasound is useful in assessment of the carotid arteries and internal jugular veins. It can detect carotid stenosis with high sensitivity and can be used to assess for vascular dissection. Thrombosis of the internal jugular veins or carotid arteries can also be detected. Ultrasound has become a standard tool in the placement of internal jugular central venous catheters—the figures above illustrate why ultrasound can be invaluable in preventing accidentally puncture of the carotid artery. Anatomy textbooks show the carotid artery lying medial to the internal jugular vein. In this patient, however, the internal jugular vein lies superficial to the carotid artery, not medial to it. The internal jugular vein is compressible and often appears elliptic or even polygonal in short-axis cross section. The carotid artery is far less compressible and has a circular short-axis cross section. **A,** Short-axis (transverse) view. **B,** Long-axis (longitudinal) view.

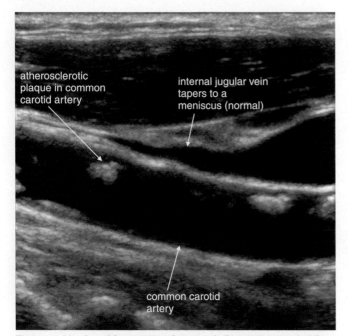

Figure 4-30. Carotid stenosis ultrasound (long-axis view). Ultrasound can reveal carotid stenosis. Plaques can be directly visualized, and flow velocity can be measured to allow quantitative assessment of the degree of stenosis. Here, plaques are visible in the common carotid artery. The internal jugular vein is also visible and appears to taper to a point at its cephalad end, as the patient does not have elevated right heart pressures that would result in jugular venous distension. The distance from the sternal notch to the point of tapering of the internal jugular vein has also been described as a method of assessing such distension in obese patients.

normal partial airway collapse in the supine position. True obstructing airway anomalies such as masses or abscesses would presumably remain, while physiologic collapse or "kissing" of airway mucosal surfaces would be prevented.[8] A discussion with the radiologist and CT technicians regarding your differential diagnosis can assist in selection of the optimal technique.

When Should X-ray Be Performed? Should All Patients Undergo X-ray Before CT? When Is CT the Best Initial Test?

As discussed earlier, x-ray relies on the juxtaposition of tissues of differing density for diagnosis. When present, these findings can indicate pathology. When absent, they may not reliably exclude pathology. The pretest probability and differential diagnosis should be carefully considered. X-ray may be the appropriate initial test for unstable patients and possibly the only test if positive. If an ingested or aspirated radiopaque foreign body is the primary concern, x-ray may be the appropriate first (and possibly sole) test. In patients with a low pretest probability of disease, x-ray is potentially the only test needed, although arguably no testing may be required in this group. If a negative x-ray would not be trusted to rule out disease as a result of high pretest probability, or if additional imaging would be required to delineate pathology found on x-ray, consider skipping x-ray and

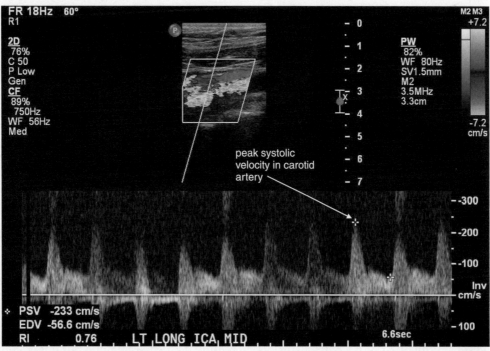

Figure 4-31. Severe carotid stenosis. Quantitative ultrasound measurement of flow in the carotid artery allows assessment of degree of stenosis. As blood flows past a stenotic region, the velocity actually increases, measured as the peak systolic velocity (PSV). The patient's measured value is compared to known normal and abnormal tabulated values to yield an estimate of stenosis. Here, the patient's PSV is 233 cm/sec, which corresponds to stenosis of greater than 70%. The caption at the bottom of the figure was added by the ultrasonographer to indicate that this image is of the midportion of the left internal carotid artery, taken in long-axis cross section. Computed tomography angiography and magnetic resonance angiography can also provide quantitative values of stenosis based on vessel short-axis cross-sectional measurements.

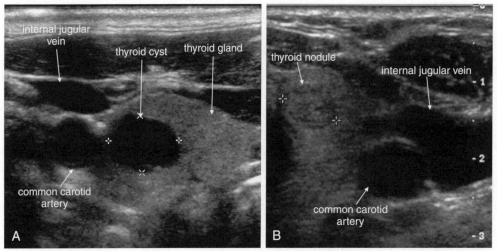

Figure 4-32. Thyroid cysts and nodules on ultrasound (short-axis view). Ultrasound is useful in assessment of superficial neck masses. It readily distinguishes cystic and solid lesions. Common examples are thyroid cysts **(A)** and nodules **(B).** The thyroid is seen medial to the carotid artery and internal jugular vein. Cysts and blood vessels may appear similar in short-axis cross section, but cysts remain round in long-axis cross section while blood vessels appear tubular. In addition, cysts have no flow using Doppler ultrasound.

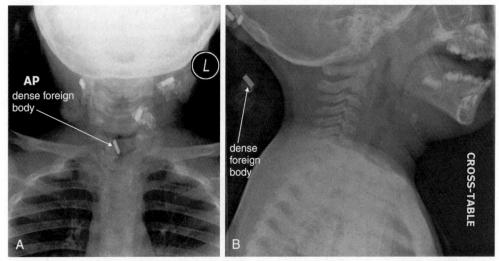

Figure 4-33. Foreign body or external object? This healthy 2-year-old girl presented to the emergency department with a "lump" in the anterior neck for 2 days. On examination, a midline, 2-cm mass overlying the thyroid cartilage was noted. This was mobile with swallowing and elevated with tongue projection. It was minimally tender with slight erythema. This examination finding and the history of sudden appearance are consistent with an infected thyroglossal duct cyst. X-rays are not usually required, nor are they diagnostic, and ultrasound can be used to confirm the cystic nature of the mass (see Figure 4-33). In this case, x-rays were obtained, which serve two educational purposes. On the anterior–posterior (AP) view **(A),** dense objects are seen, one of which appears to overlie the airway. Is this an aspirated foreign body? On the lateral x-ray **(B),** this is seen to lie outside of the patient, behind the neck—a hair clip. In other words, these are normal pediatric soft-tissue neck x-rays. Always remove radiodense material from the patient before x-ray to avoid confusion and artifact. Review both AP and lateral projections to identify the location of objects.

obtaining CT as the initial imaging test. CT is also the appropriate first test, rather than x-ray, when the differential diagnosis includes pathology difficult or impossible to detect by x-ray, such as vascular dissection or soft-tissue mass.

If X-ray Is Negative, Should CT Be Performed?

Given the limited sensitivity of x-ray, if a high suspicion of a structural abnormality exists, additional imaging may be required after a normal x-ray. If the patient's airway is thought to be safe, CT scan can be performed to assess with higher sensitivity and anatomic detail. If the

pretest probability of disease is low, no further imaging may be required following a normal x-ray.

Does CT Scan Necessarily Need to Be Performed for Further Evaluation of All X-ray Abnormalities?

Not all abnormalities on x-ray require further imaging with CT. For example, airway foreign bodies may require no further imaging but rather endoscopic extraction. Metallic foreign bodies often create streak artifact on CT, limiting the additional value of CT (see Figure 4-12). Epiglottitis identified by x-ray (see Figure 4-9) generally does not require further delineation with CT scan

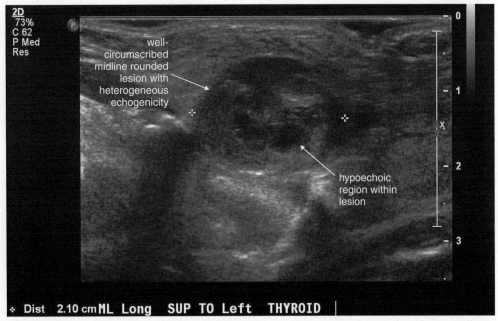

Figure 4-34. Infected thyroglossal duct cyst on ultrasound. Same patient as Figure 4-33. Ultrasound confirms a well-circumscribed, midline, rounded structure. An uninfected thyroglossal duct cyst typically appears as a simple cyst, which on ultrasound has a uniform hypoechoic (black) center. This lesion has internal septations and is only partially hypoechoic, with a heterogeneous appearance. This is typical of infection. The patient underwent surgical excision that confirmed the diagnosis.

(see Figure 4-10), and the patient may be endangered by supine positioning in CT. Treatment decisions for this condition do not require information from CT. Linear soft-tissue air may indicate pneumomediastinum, paratracheal or paraesophageal air, or air in the prevertebral space (see Figure 4-5). The clinical setting and suspected source of the air strongly determine the need for further imaging. For example, air in cervical soft tissues following cough or sneeze would generally not require CT for evaluation due to a predictably benign clinical course without intervention. Chest x-ray may be appropriate for evaluation of possible associated pneumothorax, but the anatomic detail provided by CT is quite unlikely to alter management. In contrast, soft-tissue air following vomiting could indicate esophageal perforation (Figure 4-35), and additional imaging to evaluate the esophagus may be appropriate. Fluoroscopy may be more useful than CT in this setting, though both can detect esophageal perforation as discussed later in this chapter.

How Sensitive Is X-ray to Rule Out Important Cervical Infections Such as Epiglottitis and Retropharyngeal Abscess? How Sensitive Is CT?

Classic x-ray findings of epiglottitis are quite specific but relatively insensitive. Therefore an abnormal x-ray rules in disease, but a normal x-ray may not rule out serious infection (Table 4-3). CT is sensitive and can identify complications such as local abscess formation, although supine positioning of the patient for CT can be hazardous. The patient should be carefully monitored if CT is performed.

Lateral neck x-ray has a reported sensitivity of only about 80% for retropharyngeal abscess, while in some studies CT is reported to be 100% sensitive for soft-tissue abnormalities associated with retropharyngeal cellulitis and abscess.[9-10] Other studies suggest that although CT identifies soft-tissue abnormalities, it is less useful in discriminating true abscess from soft-tissue infections that might resolve without surgical intervention. Compared with a criterion standard of surgical findings, CT was between 68% and 73.5% sensitive and 56% specific for abscess.[11-12]

Which Is Better for Detection of Retained Cervical Foreign Bodies, X-ray or CT?

X-ray is likely highly sensitive for retained metallic foreign body. However, less dense materials are variably detected by x-ray. In studies in which fish bones were placed into cadavers, providing a reliable criterion standard (as the number and location of foreign bodies were known), CT had a sensitivity of around 90%, compared with 39% for x-ray.[13-14] Newer-generation CT scanners with thinner slice thickness may be even more sensitive and specific.

How Should Soft-Tissue Air from a Suspected Gastrointestinal Source Be Further Evaluated? Is CT or Fluoroscopy the Best Test? What Test Is Better for Esophageal Foreign Body?

If cervical soft-tissue air is seen following forceful vomiting, the patient may require evaluation for an esophageal tear—usually imaged with a fluoroscopic swallowing

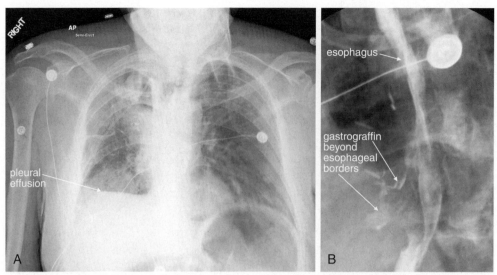

Figure 4-35. Esophageal perforation. This 55-year-old patient with metastatic colon cancer and a history of mediastinal radiation therapy underwent esophageal stent placement and subsequent removal for treatment of a stricture. He presented to the emergency department with persistent coughing and emesis. **A,** The chest x-ray reveals a pleural effusion and possible right middle lobe infiltrate. **B,** An esophagram was performed because of concern for esophageal perforation. Gastrografin extravasation beyond the borders of esophagus proves esophageal perforation. In esophageal perforation, chest x-ray may show infiltrate, pleural effusions, pneumothorax, pneumomediastinum, or subcutaneous emphysema. Although less sensitive than barium swallow, Gastrografin swallow is the preferred initial study to confirm the diagnosis, because Gastrografin is less reactive than barium if leaked into the pleural space or mediastinum. If high suspicion remains despite a normal Gastrografin study, barium swallow or contrast-enhanced CT scan can be diagnostic.

TABLE 4-3. X-ray Findings of Epiglottitis in Adults

X-ray Finding	Sensitivity (%)	Specificity (%)
Epiglottis width to AP width of C4 >0.33	96	100
Prevertebral soft tissue–to–C4 ratio >0.5	37	100
Width of hypopharyngeal airway to width of C4 >1.5	44	87
Aryepiglottic fold enlargement	85	100
Arytenoid swelling	70	100

From Nemzek WR, Katzberg RW, Van Slyke MA, et al. A reappraisal of the radiologic findings of acute inflammation of the epiglottis and supraglottic structures in adults. *AJNR Am J Neuroradiol* 16(3): 495–502, 1995.

study (see Figure 4-35). CT can demonstrate esophageal thickening suggestive of esophagitis, and it may even demonstrate orally ingested contrast outside of the esophagus or a frank mediastinal infectious process.[15-16] The decision to perform CT in this circumstance should be made after consideration of the differential diagnosis. If mediastinitis potentially requiring surgical intervention is considered, CT may be particularly useful. However, CT is a static study and does not demonstrate esophageal motility. Unlike CT of airway anatomy, virtual CT endoscopy of the esophagus is not generally useful because the esophagus is most often a potential space, not filled with air. Fluoroscopy can demonstrate detail of the mucosal folds of the esophagus and residual

contrast left in partial- or full-thickness esophageal tears. Esophagram should be performed first with Gastrografin contrast material, as this material is less toxic to the mediastinal tissues if extravasation occurs. Gastrografin has low viscosity and may not cling to partial-thickness injuries. A normal Gastrografin study is usually followed by a fluoroscopic barium swallow study, because the more viscous material may demonstrate subtle injury. Fluoroscopy can also demonstrate retained esophageal foreign bodies and esophageal strictures (Figures 4-36 and 4-37).

Is X-ray Useful in the Setting of Soft-Tissue Neck Trauma?

We discuss cervical spine imaging for trauma in detail in Chapter 3. Soft-tissue neck x-rays are generally not useful in blunt trauma patients with soft-tissue neck injuries, and the same cautions about airway protection discussed earlier apply. Most often, if serious soft-tissue injury from blunt trauma is suspected, CT scan is the most appropriate imaging test, as it can demonstrate even subtle cervical vascular injuries and abnormalities in prevertebral soft tissues. Esophageal injuries from blunt trauma are quite uncommon. Blunt traumatic airway injuries are more frequently directly examined with bronchoscopy, although as described earlier, CT is gaining an increasing foothold given the ability to perform multiplanar reconstructions and even three-dimensional virtual bronchoscopy (see Figure 4-27).

After penetrating trauma to the neck, x-rays are sometimes used for screening purposes if the patient is to go

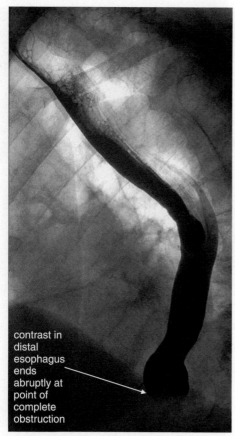

Figure 4-36. Esophageal steak foreign body, seen with fluoroscopy. This 82-year-old patient with Crohn's disease and a history of prior esophageal strictures presented with dysphagia after eating a steak 24 hours previously. He reported inability to swallow solids or liquids. A Gastrograffin swallow study was performed under fluoroscopy. An abrupt cutoff of contrast is seen in the distal esophagus, corresponding to complete obstruction. No contrast passes into the stomach. This fluoroscopic image does not reveal the cause of the obstruction, which could be due to a mass, stricture, or impacted food bolus. The patient underwent endoscopy that revealed a piece of steak lodged at the site of his prior strictures.

directly to the operating room for surgical exploration. X-ray in this case provides limited information about soft-tissue foreign bodies and extrinsic airway compression, as well as bony injury. In cases in which penetrating injury is thought to be superficial, x-rays sometimes demonstrate deep foreign bodies, indicating deep neck penetration requiring further evaluation, often with CT (see Figures 4-11 and 4-12).

How Does the Region of the Neck Injured Affect Imaging Strategy in Penetrating Trauma?

The neck is divided into three zones for purposes of evaluation following penetrating trauma, beginning with zone 1 inferiorly and progressing to zone 3 superiorly (Figure 4-38). Zone 1 extends from the thoracic inlet to the cricoid cartilage. It includes thoracic structures such as great vessels of the chest and neck, as well as the lung apices, trachea, esophagus, and cervical spine. Zone 2 extends from the cricoid cartilage to the angle of the

mandible. It includes the carotid and vertebral arteries, jugular veins, larynx, pharynx, trachea, esophagus, thyroid gland, and cervical spine. Zone 3 extends from the angle of the mandible to the skull base. It includes the salivary and parotid glands, esophagus, trachea, vertebral bodies, jugular veins, carotid arteries, and major nerves (including cranial nerves IX through XII).

The imaging approach to the three neck zones was traditionally structured based on both the range of possible injuries and the ease of direct surgical exploration. Zone 1 injuries would require thoracotomy for complete surgical evaluation, so imaging traditionally played a significant role, including chest x-ray, aortography, esophagoscopy, and bronchoscopy. Zone 3 injuries are surgically difficult to access, because the mandible obscures structures as they approach the skull base. The traditional imaging approach included angiography, as well as endoscopic evaluation. Zone 2 injuries were more frequently directly explored, as surgical access was technically feasible and important injuries such as carotid artery injury were common.

Today, the diagnostic approach is simplified by CT. In unstable patients with obvious injuries, immediate operative intervention is often required and CT may be foregone in favor of surgical exploration. Examples would include a patient with a zone 1, 2, or 3 gunshot wound and hemodynamic instability. In the stable patient, CT can provide comprehensive evaluation including assessment of vascular, airway, and digestive tract injuries. A normal CT scan may eliminate the need for surgery or other imaging maneuvers, although this remains an area of controversy. CT abnormalities may require operative investigation or further imaging or direct visualization with endoscopy. We discussed CT of airway anomalies earlier in the chapter. Next we consider the performance of CT for evaluation of vascular pathology and esophageal injuries.

CT EVALUATION OF CERVICAL VASCULAR INJURIES OR SPONTANEOUS VASCULAR DISSECTIONS

Spontaneous cervical artery (carotid and vertebral) dissection is thought to be a rare event yet is the most common cause of ischemic stroke in young adults, with 70% of cases occurring in patients in their 20s and 40s.[17] Presenting symptoms include sudden, severe, and persistent neck pain, sometimes accompanied by headache. Neck pain alone occurs in about 25% of patients.[18] Clinically, carotid and vertebral dissection may be indistinguishable unless an ischemic stroke results. Carotid artery dissections result in anterior circulation stroke symptoms, while vertebral artery dissection results in posterior circulation stroke. Both conditions can be evaluated by CT angiography or MRA. Carotid disease can

Figure 4-37. **Food foreign body fluoroscopy.** This 38-year-old patient with no prior medical history complained of dysphagia and odynophagia since lunch the previous day. **A** and **B,** A barium swallow study under fluoroscopy was performed. It reveals a well-circumscribed foreign body in the distal esophagus measuring approximately 2 × 2 cm and having a quadrilateral shape. Some contrast does flow past the foreign body into the stomach. Distal to the foreign body is a narrow stream of contrast, suggesting a region of stricture or achalasia—likely the reason for the food impaction. Endoscopy did not reveal any lesions at this location. Incidentally, the patient also has a small hiatal hernia.

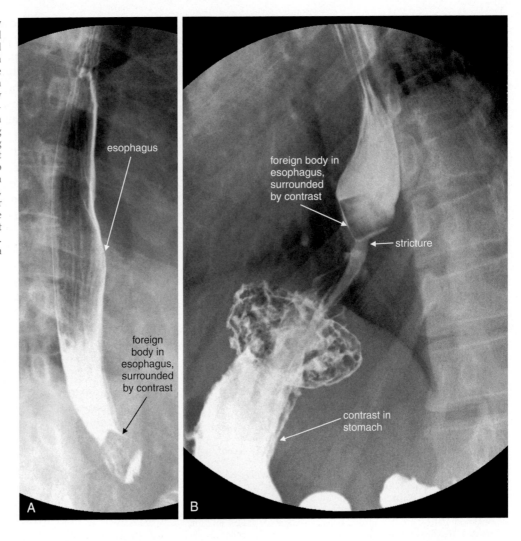

Figure 4-38. **Neck zones.** The neck is divided into three anatomic zones, which traditionally have directed diagnostic and therapeutic planning in penetrating neck trauma. Today, stable patients may be evaluated with computed tomography (CT) in many institutions, regardless of the zone injured. CT can detect vascular, airway, and esophageal injuries, though no high-quality prospective studies have evaluated CT against a criterion standard of endoscopic and surgical findings.

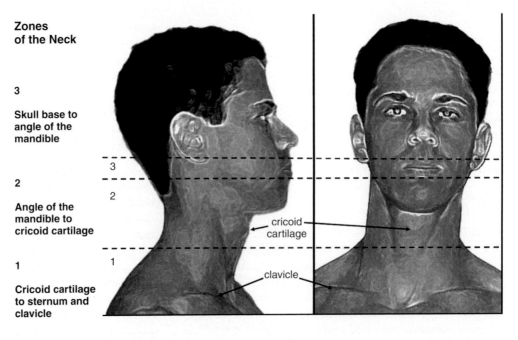

Zones of the Neck

3

Skull base to angle of the mandible

2

Angle of the mandible to cricoid cartilage

1

Cricoid cartilage to sternum and clavicle

also be evaluated by ultrasound, whereas the vertebral arteries are hidden within the transverse foramina of the cervical vertebrae and are not seen well with ultrasound. Blunt cervical arterial dissections can occur after major trauma, with the leading indications for imaging being known cervical spine fractures (especially high cervical injuries, subluxation, and fractures involving the transverse foramen; see Chapter 3) and neck hematomas or seat belt marks. Penetrating neck injuries, particularly zone 2 injuries, can result in carotid artery injuries. Some "spontaneous" cervical artery dissections may actually be the result of minimal trauma, such as cough, sexual activity, sporting activities, defecation, and chiropractic manipulation. In one series, 16% of "spontaneous" dissections occurred after chiropractic treatment.[19] True spontaneous dissections with no apparent trauma are also described in the literature.[19-27] Other risk factors include hypertension, tobacco use, connective tissue disorders, vasculitides, and migraines—the last being particularly unfortunate because of the potential overlap between symptoms of typical migraine and those of cervical artery dissection.

What History and Physical Examination Findings Suggest Cervical Artery Dissection? Can Physical Examination Rule Out a Vascular Problem?

Cervical artery dissections often present with headache, neck pain, or both, sometimes associated with ischemic symptoms developing hours or even days after the onset of neck pain. Delayed neurologic symptoms likely are the result of eventual thrombosis of the dissected segment, causing obstruction of flow, or embolization of thrombus from the dissected segment to intracranial arteries, resulting in stroke. An incomplete Horner's syndrome (ptosis and miosis without anhydrosis) occurs in about 36% to 58% of patients, and lower cranial nerve palsies occur in less than 15%.[17] In addition to headache or neck pain, vertebral artery dissection can present with posterior circulation stroke symptoms such as nausea or vomiting (53%), vertigo (57%), unilateral facial numbness (46%), gait disturbance (42%), diplopia (23%), dysphagia (11%), dysarthria (15%), or extremity paresthesias or weakness (11%).[18] Symptoms can be transient, and neurologic deficits can be absent upon emergency department presentation, as transient ischemic attack may occur rather than frank stroke.

How Sensitive Is CT for Cervical Artery Dissection? How Does MRA Compare?

Cervical CT angiography (as described earlier) is the diagnostic test of choice for suspected cervical artery dissection in the emergency department. It is nearly 100% sensitive and specific when compared with conventional angiography; is widely available, rapid, and noninvasive; and can evaluate alternative diagnoses. Alternative diagnostic techniques include digital fluoroscopic cervical angiography (78% to 84% sensitive), vascular ultrasound, or MRI or MRA of the head and neck, which is more than 95% sensitive. CT angiography is subject to rare false-positive and false-negative results, sometimes for technical reasons such as poor contrast bolus, patient movement, failure to include the entire artery in question, or metallic streak artifacts in the image field. If significant suspicion for this diagnosis remains despite a normal CT angiogram (e.g., in the patient with neurologic deficits and a history of cervical trauma), consider further evaluation with MRA or formal angiography.[28]

How Large an Intravenous Catheter Is Needed for CT Cervical Angiography? Does It Matter Where It Is Placed? Can Central Venous Catheters Be Used?

Two issues limit the size, location, and type of IV catheter used for cervical CT angiography (and other CT angiography applications). First, the catheter must allow a rapid contrast bolus for a diagnostically adequate study. Second, the catheter must resist contrast extravasation or catheter embolization. Cervical CT angiography requires a rapid contrast bolus for a high-quality diagnostic study to be obtained. Within seconds, enough contrast has to be injected to opacify the cervical arteries, allowing a luminal defect within the vessel to be accurately characterized as a dissection, or for a stenotic region to be recognized. If the contrast bolus is too slow, the cervical arteries may be poorly opacified. This can lead to both false positives (an apparent filling defect, which is just normal fluid blood within the cervical arteries) and false negatives (actual dissections or other anomalies attributed to poor contrast bolus and unopacified blood). The protocol for cervical angiography studies may vary a bit from institution to institution, but published protocols call for injection rates of 4 to 5 mL per second. What are the flow tolerances of peripheral angiocatheters, the color-coded IV catheters used in most emergency departments? Take a look at the packaging during your next shift, and you will see the flow rate marked on the package. From physics, you will recall that the rate of flow is inversely proportional to the resistance; high resistance means low flow. The resistance is directly proportional to the length of the catheter, so a long catheter means high resistance and low flow. More importantly, the resistance is inversely proportional to the radius of the catheter, raised to the fourth power! So a small increase in radius means a substantial decrease in resistance and increase in flow. Translation: For fast flow, use the shortest, fattest catheter available. Some sample flow rates for a common vendor are shown in Table 4-4.

These numbers reflect gravity flow rates, not flow through pressure injectors used for CT angiography. A phantom study using 14- through 24-gauge catheters

TABLE 4-4. Flow Rates Through Common Angiocatheters

Catheter Size and Color	Rated Flow per Minute (mL)	Flow per Second (mL)
24 g, 25 mm long (yellow)	17	0.28
22 g, 25 mm long (blue)	28	0.46
20 g, 48 mm long (pink)	42	0.7
18 g, 48 mm long (green)	79	1.3
16 g, 48 mm long (gray)	147	2.45
14 g, 48 mm long (orange)	277	4.6

*Manufacturer's Web site, Becton Dickinson (BD) peripheral IV.

showed adequate flow rates of 5 mL per second using 14-, 16-, 18-, and 20-gauge catheters. The 22-gauge catheters did not allow adequate flow because the safe pressure limit of 325 psi was reached at a lower flow rate. The 24-gauge catheter became disconnected because of high pressures.[29]

Recommended catheter location is driven by both flow rate and safety concerns. Generally, more peripheral placement of catheters may result in slower flow. Safety concerns exist for power injection through catheters placed in the neck (external jugular vein catheters), as contrast extravasation in this location can be particularly dangerous. Extravasated contrast can cause tissue necrosis, and in the neck it might pose threats to the airway, as well as critical vascular structures.

Triple lumen central venous catheters face the same issues described above as peripheral catheters—most have a single 16-gauge and two 18-gauge lumens, but the added length of the catheter means greater resistance and lower flow rates. Rare cases of central venous catheter fracture and embolization during injection exist, although most occur in the setting of long-term tunneled subclavian catheters, which may be pinched by bony structures.[30-32] Some newer permanent and emergency devices are designed for high-pressure rapid infusion. Examples include PowerPort and PowerLine (Bard Access Systems) which can tolerate 300 psi with a maximum infusion rate of 5 mL per second (information from the manufacturer's Web site).

Is CT Useful for Evaluation of Possible Esophageal and Tracheal Injury Following Penetrating Neck Trauma?

Given the utility of CT for evaluating potential vascular injuries following neck trauma, it would be particularly valuable if CT also offered adequate evaluation of the airway and esophagus. Traditionally, penetrating neck injuries often required multimodal evaluation with angiography, fluoroscopic swallow studies, and often both fiberoptic esophagoscopy and bronchoscopy. A study of 42 penetrating zone 2 neck trauma patients (including both stab and gunshot wounds) undergoing soft-tissue CT scan, esophagoscopy, and open neck exploration found that CT was equivalent to esophagoscopy for detection of esophageal stab wounds, but only 50% sensitive compared with surgical exploration. Patients received 250 mL of oral contrast before the CT exam, as well as IV contrast. CT detected four of seven internal jugular vein injuries (57%) identified during operative exploration. The authors concluded that CT is insensitive and added little to the evaluation of patients in whom neck exploration is planned. However, this study has several limitations. First, the confidence intervals on all results are limited by small numbers—only four esophageal injuries were found, and no carotid or airway injuries were present in the study group. Second, the study spans a period from 1997 to 2001 and used 5-mm CT slices. It is possible that more modern CT scanners with thinner slices would provide higher sensitivity.[33] In addition, the more important clinical question may be, Can a negative CT be used to avoid neck exploration in lower-risk patients? Can it eliminate the need for endoscopic evaluation and swallow studies? Unfortunately, the small studies of this topic do not fully answer our questions. CT findings of esophageal perforation have been described, including periesophageal air, periesophageal fluid, esophageal wall thickening, esophageal wall laceration, and extravasation of oral contrast. The sensitivity and specificity of these findings are not well known.[15,16,34] Despite a paucity of good evidence, many trauma centers are beginning to rely on CT to exclude injuries and to defer additional studies in selected patients.

What Considerations Should Be Made in Selecting Patients for CT Evaluation of Suspected Neck Infection?

CT can be valuable in ruling out significant causes of neck pain, but unfortunately no clear clinical decision rules guide the need for cervical CT. Given the radiation exposure, CT should not be used to screen patients with a benign history and examination, although as we review later, many exam findings are insensitive. The emergency physician should carefully consider the differential diagnosis of the patient with neck pain to identify patients for whom CT should be employed. When cervical epidural abscess, diskitis, or osteomyelitis is considered, MRI is the test of choice, as discussed in Chapter 3.

A variety of significant infections within the skull base and neck may present with neck pain. These include peritonsillar, parapharyngeal, and retropharyngeal abscesses; epiglottitis; Ludwig's angina; osteomyelitis; diskitis; and cervical epidural abscesses. Infections of congenital structures such as thyroglossal duct and branchial cleft cysts may occur. Infectious thrombophlebitis of the internal jugular vein (Lemierre's syndrome) may present with neck pain and has high mortality if not aggressively treated. Deep cervical infections can spread to the mediastinum along fascial planes, resulting in mediastinitis with mortality as high as 60%.[35]

Although epiglottitis is rare in pediatric patients since the introduction of the *Haemophilus influenzae* vaccine in the 1990s, it continues to occur in adults at rates similar to those in the prevaccine era.[36-37] Adult cases now outnumber pediatric cases by nearly five to one.[38] Rarely, *H. influenzae*–related epiglottitis affects fully vaccinated children. A 10-year retrospective study identified 19 pediatric epiglottitis cases in a single children's hospital, 6 positive for *H. influenzae,* and 5 of those 6 in fully vaccinated children.[39] Epigottitis can be diagnosed by x-ray and CT (see Figures 4-9 and 4-10), although direct visualization with nasopharyngoscopy may be a better choice.

Injection drug users are at risk for cervical venous thrombosis and deep neck abscesses, including epidural spinal abscess. Retained needle fragments may be present and can result in abscess or pseudoaneurysm. Patients may not reveal cervical injection in 50% of cases,[40-41] and cervical osteomyelitis is another complication of this practice (see Chapter 3).[42-43] Ingested foreign bodies, including bone fragments and other sharp objects, may also cause deep space infection. Neck pain with neurologic complaints localizing to the cervical spine may indicate cervical epidural abscess. Distant infectious sources such as skin abscesses and urinary tract infection can spread hematogenously, resulting in deep cervical infections that include cervical epidural abscess. Minor preexisting abnormalities of the cervical spine may increase the risk for hematogenous seeding. Immune compromise from diseases such as diabetes mellitus, alcoholism, cancer, chronic renal failure, organ transplantation, and acquired immunodeficiency syndrome increases the risk of cervical epidural abscess. Prior invasive spinal procedures, even several months before presentation, should increase the suspicion of cervical epidural abscess. No identified risk factors are present in about 18% of cases.[44-45]

Are History and Physical Examination Reliable in Excluding Deep Neck Infection, Eliminating the Need for Imaging?

Unfortunately, physical examination and history are only moderately sensitive for deep neck infection. In a retrospective review comparing physical examination findings and symptoms with CT diagnosis of deep neck infection, the physical examination for deep cervical infections was insensitive, approaching 70%. Signs and symptoms suggesting deep infection were present with the following frequency: pain (89.2%), odynophagia (63.1%), dysphagia (47.7%), neck swelling (84.6%), fever (75.4%), local erythema (66.7%), and localized increase in temperature (55.4%).[46] In epiglottitis, drooling occurs in only 15% of patients and stridor or dyspnea in only about 9%. Although "hot potato" voice may suggest epiglottitis,[39] one study suggested that a muffled voice occurs in only about 50% of patients.[47] Fever is an insensitive finding, occurring in between 30% and 80% of patients with cervical epidural abscess.[44,48-49] The classic triad of fever, localized spinal tenderness, and progressive neurologic deficits occurs in only 37% of patients with cervical epidural abscess.[50]

Do Laboratory Tests Assist in the Diagnosis of Deep Space Cervical Infections, Identifying Patients Who Require Imaging?

In cervical epidural abscess, leukocytosis is present in only about 60% of patients.[48] An elevated sedimentation rate is present in 95% of cases, although the mean value is only about 50 mm per hour. Because many conditions may elevate the sedimentation rate, reliance on this test may lead to unnecessary cervical imaging.[48,51] Immune compromise may limit changes in white blood cell count and sedimentation rate, and their sensitivity in immunocompromised patients is not well studied.

When Should Imaging Be Considered for a Possible Cervical Mass?

Neck pain or swelling may be an indication of a cervical mass, including malignant (see Figures 4-23 and 4-24) and benign neoplasms (see Figure 4-25). Congenital abnormalities include thyroglossal duct cysts (see Figures 4-26 and 4-34) in the midline, and branchial cleft cysts in the lateral neck. Both can be occult until infection occurs, at which time pain, swelling, and erythema may develop. Malignancy should be suspected and imaging should be performed when weight loss, hoarseness, odynophagia or dysphagia, or neurologic symptoms such as ptosis are present. Some neoplasms such as lymphomas occur in younger patients, so young age should not provide false reassurance. However, cervical neoplasms increase in incidence with age, and imaging of older patients should be strongly considered. Metastatic squamous cell carcinoma occurs in up to 23.5% of patients over the age of 40 with solitary, benign-appearing cervical cysts.[52] Alcohol use and cigarette smoking are risk factors.[53] Not all imaging for possible malignancy need occur in the emergency department. If the airway is not threatened, the patient is able to tolerate oral food and drink, and other factors in history and physical examination do not suggest an infectious cause, outpatient follow-up for imaging may be appropriate.

Can History and Physical Examination Rule Out a Serious Neck Mass, Eliminating the Need for Imaging?

Unfortunately, history and examination findings have shown poor positive and negative predictive values for malignancy, between 60% and 80%.[53] Factors such as progressive worsening over weeks or months and increasing number and size of lesions should raise suspicion.

Inspect the oropharynx for lesions, as oral cancers may spread locally or metastasize within the neck. Check the neck for asymmetry, and palpate the neck for anterior and posterior lymph nodes and abnormalities of the thyroid gland. Ask the patient about changes in voice, and listen for hoarseness. Although hoarseness can result from a benign diagnosis such as laryngitis, malignant involvement of the larynx and recurrent laryngeal nerve can also cause change in voice. Check the eyelid position and pupillary size and reactivity. Ptosis, miosis, and anhydrosis (Horner's syndrome) can occur from malignant or benign compression of sympathetic nerves innervating the face. In the end, the insensitivity of history and exam for masses means that patients with a normal examination may require imaging for further diagnosis. However, this can occur if symptoms persist at follow-up, rather than in the emergency department.

Is Soft-Tissue Neck X-ray Useful in Evaluation for Neck Masses? What Other Imaging Can Be Helpful?

X-rays of the neck are insensitive for masses and not generally useful. If a mass is considered, CT with IV contrast has excellent sensitivity. CT delineates the extent of a mass, its density and vascular enhancement pattern, its mass effect on adjacent structures, and local invasion and metastasis. If the patient has contraindications to iodinated contrast, MRI may be used. Ultrasound can differentiate cystic from solid masses.[54]

SUMMARY

Imaging of soft tissues of the neck requires careful consideration of the differential diagnosis to avoid unnecessary imaging in low-risk patients or imaging that does not positively influence management decisions. The broad list of soft-tissue pathology defies a simple clinical decision rule. CT is highly sensitive and specific for much of the important emergency pathology, but it carries a high radiation and economic cost and should not be ubiquitously applied. X-ray is insensitive and plays a limited role. Specialized tests such as contrast esophagram are indicated in selected patients.

CHAPTER 5 Imaging the Chest: The Chest Radiograph

Joshua Broder, MD, FACEP

Chest radiograph or x-ray is one of the most commonly performed imaging tests. It is a high-yield test, providing significant clinical information rapidly, at low cost, and with low radiation exposure, but many examinations are nonetheless unnecessary. In this chapter, we discuss the indications for chest x-ray, features of the chest x-ray technique and their effect on the resulting image, basic principles of chest x-ray interpretation, and a systematic algorithm for image interpretation. Following this, we present extensive figures with chest x-ray images depicting a spectrum of emergency findings. When available, corresponding computed tomography (CT) images are shown. These clarify chest x-ray findings, demonstrate the limitations of plain chest radiography, and illustrate the occasional need for advanced imaging for further delineation of pathology. This chapter focuses on chest x-ray in the nontrauma patient, although the principles also apply to patients with traumatic injuries, discussed in detail in Chapter 6.

Chest CT, ventilation–perfusion (VQ) scan, and thoracic ultrasound are discussed in detail in additional chapters focused on chest trauma (see Chapter 6), pulmonary embolism and aortic disease (see Chapter 7), and cardiac imaging (see Chapter 8).

CHEST IMAGING MODALITIES

Modalities for thoracic imaging include chest radiograph (x-ray), CT, VQ scan, echocardiography, magnetic resonance (MR), fluoroscopy (used for pulmonary angiography, aortography, and upper gastrointestinal imaging), and positron emission tomography (PET). MR has a limited role in the emergency department currently, largely because of issues of cost and availability, but is used in selected patients in diagnosis of conditions such as pulmonary embolism and aortic disease. PET scanning is used primarily in detection of metabolically active neoplastic disease and is therefore not routinely used in the emergency department. Characteristics of these imaging modalities are shown in Table 5-1. Issues related to CT and MR such as iodinated contrast nephropathy and allergy, radiation, and gadolinium-associated nephrogenic systemic fibrosis are discussed in Chapters 6, 7, 8, and 15.

Cost of Chest X-ray

Chest x-ray is one of the most cost-effective imaging examinations, with the cost to patients being between $50 and $220 in many medical systems.[1] However, charges for chest x-ray vary considerably, even in the same geographic region. According to data provided by health care facilities, the U.S. national average cost of chest x-ray was $370 in 2010.[2] Evidence-based guidelines for imaging should be followed when available and applicable, as the total cost of common, individually inexpensive tests such as chest radiography to the U.S. medical system is enormous.

Radiation Exposure From Chest X-ray

Chest x-ray provides minimal radiation exposure, around 0.01 to 0.02 mSv.[3] This is the equivalent of approximately a single day's background radiation exposure at most locations on the Earth. It equals the additional radiation exposure incurred by taking a commercial airline flight at 35,000 feet from New York to Los Angeles. The radiation exposure is focused and is quite safe in pregnant patients, with negligible scatter radiation to the abdomen and pelvis. Abdominal shielding has not been shown to be necessary to reduce fetal exposure substantially, though it remains a recommended action for the psychological well-being of the pregnant patient.[4-5] Radiation exposures from chest CT are far greater, by as much as 500 fold, and are discussed in detail in Chapters 7 and 8.

Are Health Care Workers at Risk From Chest X-ray Radiation Exposure?

The exposure to health care workers from portable chest x-rays is very low if simple precautions are taken; at a distance of 15 inches from the x-ray beam, the scatter radiation exposure is minimal (around 0.0008 mSv), requiring exposure to more than 1200 radiographs to equal annual background radiation exposure.[6] Multiple other studies suggest trivial exposures to health care workers using simple precautions to distance themselves from the x-ray source.[6-9] If an appropriate safe distance cannot be achieved because of patient care requirements, simple shielding devices such as thyroid and torso aprons should be used.

TABLE 5-1. Common Thoracic Imaging Modalities

Modality	Applications	Radiation Exposure	Cost	Contraindications
X-ray (radiograph)	Broad utility in chest pain, dyspnea, fever, hemopty-sis, pneumoperitoneum, foreign body, trauma	0.01-0.02 mSv (~1 day of background radiation on Earth)	$50-$200	None. X-ray is safe in pregnancy, with or without abdominal shielding.
Computed Tomography (CT)	Pulmonary embolism, aortic disease, coronary artery disease, trauma, abscesses, malignancy, further delineation of chest x-ray abnormalities	8-20 mSv, depending on factors such as electrocardiogram gating (see Chapter 8)	$1000-$2000	IV contrast used for CT angiography is contraindi-cated by renal insufficiency or allergy. Radiation dose is high, raising concerns in young patients and women due to breast exposure.
Ventilation-Perfusion (VQ) Scan, a nuclear scintigraphy technique	Pulmonary embolism; also used in nonemergent settings to evaluate lung ventilation	8 mSv	$1000-$2000	Use in pregnancy and non-pregnant women has been advocated as an alternative to CT, based on some studies showing lower radiation expo-sures from VQ. Use is con-traindicated in patients with extensive lung disease, e.g., COPD or asthma, due to high likelihood of nondiagnostic results in PE evaluation.
Echocardiography	Pericardial effusion, cardiac output, valvular abnor-malities, congenital heart disease, pulmonary embo-lism, cardiac arrest	None	$500; bedside echo by emergency physicians may or may not be billed depending on institution	None.
Magnetic reso-nance imaging (MRI)	Aortic disease, pulmonary embolism (not standard)	None	$3000-$4000	Pacemakers and other electronic devices are a contraindication, although some devices are safe (check device- and MRI machine–specific information). Gado-linium contrast used in many chest applications is con-traindicated in patients with severe renal disease.
Fluoroscopy	Pulmonary angiography, aortography, esophagography	4-20 mSv; high radiation exposure due to total duration of "beam on" time	Extremely variable; may exceed $10,000 for aortog-raphy or pulmonary angiography if used for diagnosis and treatment	Radiation exposure is a relative contraindication in young patients. Injected contrast agents are contraindicated by allergy or renal insufficiency.
Positron Emission Tomography (PET)	Detection of metabolically active neoplastic disease	Not routinely used in emergency department patients		

Clinical Indications for Chest X-ray

For reasons of time, cost, and radiation exposure as described earlier, best-evidence guidelines should be applied when possible to guide the use of chest x-ray. Chest x-ray is useful in evaluation of a multitude of patient presentations, including cough and fever, chest pain, dyspnea, hemoptysis, weight loss, hypoxia, suspected subdiaphragmatic pneumoperitoneum, even Horner's syndrome. Given the incredible range of possible patient presentations, no single clinical decision rule can govern chest x-ray use for all cases, and the emergency physician must make clinical decisions for radiography based on the individual patient presentation. However, the value of chest x-ray in common clinical scenarios has been reviewed extensively by the American College of Radiology (ACR) in its appropriateness criteria. These criteria, published on the ACR website, are expert consensus guidelines based on review of medical literature by radiologists and experts from other medical specialties. Summaries of ACR guidelines relevant to thoracic imaging are presented in Tables 5-2 and 5-3. The ACR rates imaging studies using a 1-to-9 scale, with 9 being "most appropriate" and 1 being "least appropriate." Although the use of plain chest radiography may appear "harmless" given its speed, relatively low cost and low radiation exposure, collective costs of unnecessary radiographs and other preoperative tests are believed to total in the billions of dollars in the United States annually.[10] Other potential harms from unnecessary radiography include delays in surgery prompted by the detection of incidental findings such as pulmonary nodules and costs and morbidity of additional diagnostic procedures triggered by chest x-ray findings. Consequently, chest x-ray should be ordered with attention to the evidence supporting its use for a given clinical presentation. Unfortunately, as we will review, high quality evidence to guide clinical decisions is lacking for many potential indications for chest x-ray.

Is a Chest X-ray Routinely Indicated for Chest Pain?

A multitude of causes can result in chest pain, including a number of abnormalities visible on chest x-ray. Pneumonia, pneumothorax, pneumomediastinum, neoplasms, rib fractures, and aortic dissection are just a few of the disease processes that can result in chest pain and that the chest x-ray may diagnose or suggest. Pulmonary embolism may have associated chest x-ray abnormalities such as pleural effusion or pulmonary infarct, although sensitivity and specificity of chest x-ray are too poor for clinical diagnosis of this entity. The ACR recommends chest radiography as the initial imaging study for patients with chest pain and a low probability of cardiac ischemia, given the range of possible diagnoses and the low cost and radiation exposure of chest x-ray.[11] The American College of Emergency Physicians (ACEP) recommended chest x-ray for many scenarios described in its 1995 "Clinical Policy for the Initial Approach to Adults Presenting With a Chief Complaint of Chest Pain, With No History of Trauma," which has since been retired (all ACEP clinical policies are subject to retirement if a new review of the literature is not conducted within a prescribed time frame).[12] Systematic prospective studies on the value of chest x-ray in undifferentiated chest pain are limited. In a retrospective study of 5000 portable or posterior–anterior (PA) and lateral chest radiographs performed on emergency department patients, Buenger et al.[13] discovered that "serious disease" was found in 35% of those with chest symptoms, based on the x-ray requisition. Requisition information may not reliably characterize a patient's symptoms, so the validity of this study remains in doubt.

Is a Chest X-ray Routinely Indicated for Stroke?

Sagar et al.[14] performed a retrospective review of 435 patients admitted with a diagnosis of acute stroke. They found that 86% had an admission chest x-ray performed and 77.5% of radiographs were technically inadequate, mostly because of poor patient positioning and poor inspiratory effort. Radiographic abnormalities were seen in 61 patients (16.4% of those undergoing radiography), and clinical management appeared to have been altered in 14 patients (3.8% of those undergoing radiography). The authors conclude that chest radiography is not routinely indicated for patients with acute stroke in the absence of suggestive clinical findings or complaints. As with many other clinical presentations, prospective studies for chest x-ray in stroke are lacking, and little evidence exists regarding the role of chest x-ray in presentations such as altered mental status (rather than obvious stroke syndromes such as hemiparesis).

Is a Chest X-ray Routinely Indicated for Gastrointestinal Bleeding?

Tobin et al.[15] reviewed 202 adult patients admitted to intensive care units for gastrointestinal hemorrhage. They found that 161 (80%) underwent admission chest x-ray. Review of radiographs by a radiologist blinded to the study purpose found 14.3% with minor radiographic abnormalities, none of which resulted in a therapeutic or diagnostic intervention. Major radiographic abnormalities were found in 13% of patients, with an intervention in only 5.6% of patients. Predictors of major abnormalities included history of lung disease and abnormal lung physical examination at presentation (sensitivity = 79%, negative predictive value = 96%). These variables also predicted major radiographic abnormalities associated with interventions (sensitivity 89%, negative predictive value = 99%). The authors found that selective radiography based on these criteria would have reduced the charges from chest radiography by more than $500 per major abnormality detected and by more than $1000 per major abnormality associated with an intervention. These findings have not been externally validated in a separate population but do suggest that routine chest x-ray is unnecessary for this clinical presentation.

Is a Chest X-ray Routinely Indicated for Acute Respiratory Illness With Features Such as Productive Cough?

Acute respiratory illness is defined by the presence of one or more factors, including cough, sputum production, chest pain, and dyspnea, with or without fever. A multitude of studies have examined the role of chest x-ray, examining varying populations including healthy hosts, immunocompromised patients, the elderly, and patients with asthma and chronic obstructive pulmonary

TABLE 5-2. American College of Radiology Appropriateness Criteria for Chest X-ray or Computed Tomography in Common Clinical Scenarios

Clinical Scenario	ACR Rating for X-ray Chest	ACR Rating for CT Chest
Acute chest pain		
• Low probability of coronary artery disease	9	CTA chest (noncoronary): 6—Useful in ruling out other causes of chest pain such as aortic dissection, pulmonary embolism, pneumothorax, pneumonia.
• Suspected aortic dissection	9—Should be performed if readily available at the bedside and does not cause delay in obtaining a CT or MRI. Alternative causes of chest pain may be discovered. Not the definitive test for aortic dissection.	CTA chest and abdomen: 9—Recommended as the definitive test in most patients with suspicion of aortic dissection.
• Suspected pulmonary embolism	9—to exclude other causes of chest pain	CTA chest (noncoronary): 9—Current standard of care for detection of PE.
Chronic chest pain		
• High probability of coronary artery disease	3—Usual initial imaging study in cardiac patients. Although used frequently, chest radiographs can neither establish nor exclude chronic ischemic heart disease. Insensitive for detecting coronary arterial calcification. Limited value in patients with high risk of CAD.	CTA coronary arteries: 7—Very good accuracy and negative predictive value in low to intermediate risk groups. However, may have false negatives in high-risk group, and negative studies may still require further diagnostic testing. Coronary calcification often found in older high-risk patients (especially males) can limit coronary luminal assessment.
• Low to intermediate probability of coronary artery disease	9	CTA chest (noncoronary) with contrast: 8— Important examination for pulmonary embolism and thoracic aortic aneurysm/dissection. To rule out PE and evaluate lung pathology. Appropriate for chronic anginal chest pain. CTA coronary arteries with contrast: 8—Can be used to assess for coronary atherosclerosis, anomalous coronary artery, and pericardial disease. High negative predictive value will exclude coronary artery disease and allow triage management to focus on more likely diagnoses. To eliminate unnecessary catheterizations.
CHF		
• Symptomatic, new onset or recurrent	9	2—readily diagnosed on CT obtained for other indications
• Known CHF, stable or asymptomatic	4	
Dyspnea—suspected cardiac origin	8	CTA coronary arteries: 6 CTA coronary arteries with advanced low dose techniques: 6 CTA chest (noncoronary): 6
Suspected bacterial endocarditis	9	CT heart function and morphology with contrast: 6—Multidetector with maximal temporal and spatial resolution. Probably indicated to rule out paravalvular abscess and/or psedoaneurysm. Emerging technology.
Known or Suspected congenital heart disease in the adult	7	CT heart function and morphology with contrast: 7. May be alternative to MRI and TTE/TEE. High spatial resolution to evaluate small and tortuous vessels. For evaluation of airway. CTA coronary arteries with contrast: 6. When there is a high index of suspicion for fistula or anomalous coronaries. CTA coronary arteries with contrast with advanced low dose techniques: 6. Important in young to middle-age adults because of reduced radiation dose.
Acute respiratory illness	Varies—see Table 5-3	Varies
Acute respiratory illness in HIV-positive patients	9	CT chest without contrast: 8—When negative, equivocal, or nonspecific chest radiograph.

TABLE 5-2. American College of Radiology Appropriateness Criteria for Chest X-ray or Computed Tomography in Common Clinical Scenarios—cont'd

Clinical Scenario	ACR Rating for X-ray Chest	ACR Rating for CT Chest
Chronic dyspnea—suspected pulmonary origin	8-9—depends on age and examination	Any age, nonrevealing or nondiagnostic clinical, standard radiography, and laboratory studies. In the setting of chronic dyspnea, the most appropriate imaging study is a thin section high resolution chest CT: 9. If a patient has dyspnea not clearly of pulmonary origin, other entities such as chronic or acute pulmonary embolism may need to be excluded. In that setting, a thin section chest CT with intravenous contrast is appropriate. See the ACR Appropriateness Criteria® topic on "Acute Chest Pain–Suspected Pulmonary Embolism".
Hemoptysis, Two risk factors (>40 years old and >40 pack-year history)	9	without contrast: 6 (useful for patients with renal failure or contrast allergy.); with contrast: 8 (optimal study shows enhancement of the systemic arteries.)
Rib fractures, adult < 65 years of age	8—PA view. Rib views are given a rating of 2.	2—with or without contrast
Routine admission and preoperative chest radiography		NA
• Asymptomatic, history and physical unremarkable	2 (preoperative or routine)	
• Acute cardiopulmonary findings by history or physical	9 (preoperative or routine)	
• Chronic cardiopulmonary disease in the elderly (>age 70), previous chest radiograph within 6 months available	6 (preoperative), 4 (routine admission)	
• Chronic cardiopulmonary disease in the elderly (>age 70), previous chest radiograph within 6 months not available	8 (preoperative or routine)	
Routine chest radiographs in uncomplicated hypertension (asymptomatic)		NA
• Mild hypertension—diastolic pressure 90-104 mm Hg	1	NA
• Moderate or severe hypertension—diastolic pressure 105-114 or ≥115 mm Hg	5	NA
Screening for pulmonary metastases	8-9—depends on malignancy type	7-9—depends on malignancy type; noncontrast CT
Solitary pulmonary nodule	NA—chest x-ray presumably already performed, demonstrating lesion	CT chest with contrast: 6 CT chest without contrast: 8
Staging of bronchogenic carcinoma	NA—chest x-ray presumably already performed, demonstrating lesion 8 or 9—if no baseline chest x-ray available	CT chest with or without contrast (including upper abdomen): 9—CT with contrast is preferred if there are no strong contraindications.
Blunt chest trauma—suspected aortic injury	9	CTA chest (noncoronary): 9 CT chest without contrast: 6—Useful to detect mediastinal hematoma when contrast contraindicated.

Rating scale: 1, 2, 3: Usually not appropriate; 4, 5, 6: may be appropriate; 7, 8, 9: Usually appropriate.

TABLE 5-3. American College of Radiology Appropriateness Criteria: Acute Respiratory Illness*†

Clinical Variant	ACR Rating for X-ray Chest
>Age 40	8
Dementia, any age	8
<Age 40, negative physical exam, and no other signs, symptoms, or risk factors	4
<Age 40, positive physical exam or other risk factors	9
Complicated pneumonia	9
Suspected severe acute respiratory syndrome	9
Suspected anthrax	9
Febrile, neutropenic	9
Acute asthma	
• Uncomplicated	4
• Suspected pneumonia or pneumothorax	9
Acute exacerbation of COPD	
• "Uncomplicated," with no history of CAD or CHF and no leukocytosis, fever, or chest pain	4
• With one or more of the following: leukocytosis, pain, history of CAD or CHF	9

American College of Radiology: ACR Appropriateness Criteria: Acute Respiratory Illness. Available at: http://www.acr.org/SecondaryMainMenu-Categories/quality_safety/app_criteria/pdf/ExpertPanelonThoracicImaging/AcuteRespiratoryIllnessDoc1.aspx. Accessed 3-21-2011.
Rating Scale: 1,2,3 Usually not appropriate; 4,5,6 May be appropriate; 7,8,9 Usually appropriate
* This is a truncated version of the full ACR Appropriateness Criteria, which also includes ratings for chest CT in each of the Clinical Variants. Reprinted with permission of the American College of Radiology, Reston, VA. No other representation of this material is authorized without expressed, written permission from the American College of Radiology. Refer to the ACR website at www.acr.org/ac for the most current and complete version of the ACR Appropriateness Criteria.
†Acute respiratory illness is defined by the presence of one or more factors including cough, sputum production, chest pain, and dyspnea, with or without fever.

disease (COPD). The ACR divides its recommendations based on these and other patient factors as shown in Table 5-3.[17] Benacerraf et al.[16] studied 1102 outpatients with acute respiratory illness and found that in patients below 40 years 96% of chest radiographs had no acute abnormalities. Limiting radiography in patients below age 40 to those with abnormal physical examination or hemoptysis would have reduced radiography by 58% and missed only 2.3% of acute abnormalities. *Fever, cough, and the presence of even purulent sputum were not predictive of chest x-ray abnormalities in patients under the age of 40.*[16-17] Patients above the age of 40 and

immunocompromised patients, such as those with HIV or neutropenia, represent higher risk groups for which radiography is recommended by the ACR for signs and symptoms of acute respiratory illness.[17] The emergency physician should incorporate other factors into the decision to obtain radiography and to treat the patient, including access to care, contacts with high-risk (immunocompromised) patients, endemic or epidemic disease, and risk factors for tuberculosis or undiagnosed HIV.

Is a Chest X-ray Routinely Indicated for Suspected Pneumonia?

When the emergency physician specifically suspects pneumonia, is radiography warranted? As discussed earlier, patients below the age of 40 with normal physical examination and no hemoptysis have a very low rate of radiographic abnormalities and should not routinely undergo chest x-ray. Does this mean that patients not meeting these "low risk" criteria must undergo chest x-ray? The ACR points out in its appropriateness criteria for acute respiratory illness some important disparities between clinical practice and professional society recommendations in the diagnosis of pneumonia. The Infectious Diseases Society of America and the American Thoracic Society recommend that chest radiography be obtained when pneumonia is suspected in adults to assist in distinguishing community-acquired pneumonia from other common causes of cough and fever, such as acute bronchitis. However, some clinicians may choose to treat patients empirically for pneumonia, without obtaining radiography, when a high clinical suspicion exists. This is an appropriate evidence-based strategy, as a negative chest x-ray does not rule out pneumonia. When a high pretest probability exists, a negative chest x-ray is inadequate to exclude pneumonia and should not be used as the sole basis to determine management.[17]

Is a Chest X-ray Routinely Indicated for Asthma?

In patients with asthma without features suggesting complications such as pneumonia or pneumothorax, x-ray likely has little role.[17] Findley and Sahn[18] studied 90 adult patients with asthma undergoing chest radiograph and found only 1 patient with an acute infiltrate; normal (55%), hyperinflation (37%), and unchanged minimal interstitial infiltrates (7%) were common patterns. Chest x-ray interpretation did not correlate with admission, suggesting that radiographs in asthma play little role in management. Gershel et al.[19] studied 371 consecutive children over the age of 1 year with first-time wheezing and found that 94.3% had x-ray findings compatible with uncomplicated asthma (negative). Of the 371 patients studied, 21 (5.7%) had positive chest x-ray findings, including atelectasis and pneumonia in 7, segmental atelectasis in 6, pneumonia in 5, multiple areas of subsegmental atelectasis in 2, and pneumomediastinum in 1. Although the authors call this 5.7% "positive," it is not clear that findings of atelectasis or even pneumomediastinum alter management in a clinically beneficial way, as no specific therapy is required for these abnormalities. When only pneumonia is considered a positive finding, only 3.9% of first-time wheezing children had positive chest x-rays. The authors found that 95% of abnormal x-rays could be predicted based on the presence of tachypnea greater than 60 breaths per minute, pulse greater than 160 beats per minute, and localized rales or diminished breath sounds, before or after treatment—suggesting that even in first-time pediatric wheezing, routine x-ray may not be necessary. Aronson et al.[20] reported on 125 consecutive adult asthma admissions and found no chest x-ray abnormalities in 81 patients characterized as uncomplicated, defined as having a prior history of asthma, presenting with dyspnea and wheezing, and having no history of fever or chills, immunosuppression, cancer, intravenous (IV) drug abuse, prior thoracic surgery, cardiac disease, or pulmonary disease such as COPD or granulomatous disease.

Is a Chest X-ray Routinely Indicated for Chronic Obstructive Pulmonary Disease?

In COPD, the ACR recommendations are somewhat at odds with work published in the emergency medicine literature. According to the ACR, in COPD patients without fever, leukocytosis, chest pain, or history of congestive heart failure (CHF) or coronary artery disease (CAD), chest x-ray has a low diagnostic utility, with an appropriateness rating of four out of nine.[17] These recommendations are concordant with the work of Sherman et al., who retrospectively reviewed 242 patients with admission chest x-rays for COPD. Although 14% had radiographic abnormalities, the authors concluded that only 4.5% had appropriate and clinically important management changes resulting from chest x-ray findings. They found that leukocytosis (white blood cell count $>15 \times 10^9$ per liter and neutrophil count $>8 \times 10^9$ per liter), history of CHF or CAD, chest pain, and extremity edema were a "high risk" criteria predictive of important acute radiographic abnormalities.

Emerman and Cydulka[21] attempted to validate these high-risk criteria in a retrospective series of 685 emergency department visits for acute COPD in which a chest x-ray was performed. In this series, 16% of patients had significant chest x-ray abnormalities: 88 with new infiltrates, 2 with new lung masses, 1 with pneumothorax, and 20 with evidence of pulmonary edema. Abnormalities were associated with history of CHF, fever, rales, pedal edema, and jugular venous distension. In contrast, white blood cell count, temperature in the emergency department, history of CAD, and complaints of chest pain or sputum production were not associated with chest x-ray abnormalities. The sensitivity of the high-risk criteria was only 76%, with a specificity of only 41%. The authors recommended routine x-ray in patients with apparent acute COPD.

Is a Chest X-ray Routinely Indicated for Asymptomatic Hypertension?

According to the ACR reviews, patients with asymptomatic hypertension should not routinely undergo chest x-ray, although debate remains about the value of radiography with rising levels of hypertension. In theory, chest x-ray might be of value in patients with asymptomatic hypertension by revealing cardiomegaly or left ventricular hypertrophy, aortic enlargement or coarctation, or pulmonary vascular congestion. Although a number of authors have suggested these benefits, others have argued that the management of hypertension is not positively influenced by chest x-ray findings; regardless of the presence or absence of chest x-ray abnormalities, blood pressure control should be attempted. Moreover, studies indicate that chest x-ray is insensitive and nonspecific for detection of left ventricular hypertrophy, which is better assessed with echocardiography.[22]

Is a Chest X-ray Routinely Indicated for Admitted Patients?

The ACR found that routine admission or preoperative chest x-ray is not indicated in the patient with no cardiopulmonary findings by history or physical examination, with an appropriateness of two out of nine.[10] In patients with acute cardiopulmonary findings by history or physical, chest x-ray is highly appropriate, with a rating of nine. Because of a lack of evidence against the use of routine chest x-ray, in elderly patients (70 years or older) with chronic cardiopulmonary disease, the ACR rates chest x-ray as appropriate (eight of nine), even in the absence of history or physical findings, when a chest x-ray has not been performed within the past 6 months. The value of chest x-ray is less clear in this asymptomatic group when a recent chest x-ray (within 6 months) is available for review (ACR rating four to six of nine).

What is the basis for the ACR recommendations in these cases? The ACR cites multiple studies addressing the utility of routine chest x-ray in patients admitted for gastrointestinal hemorrhage, acute stroke, and other conditions affecting the elderly. Gupta, Gibbins, and Sen[23] prospectively studied 1000 consecutive admissions to an acute geriatric ward and found that 35% to 50% of patients had no apparent indication for chest x-ray. In this group without chest x-ray indications, 5.5% had radiographic abnormalities but less than 1% had clinically important findings. In an exhaustive systematic review, Munro, Booth, and Nicholl[24] found that no randomized controlled trials of the effectiveness of routine preadmission or preoperative chest x-rays had been published, and most studies do not (or cannot, because of study design) assess the effect on clinical management of detected radiographic abnormalities. Estimates of the frequency of changes in clinical management suggest patient benefit in fewer than 5% of cases.[10]

We have discussed some common evidence-based indications for chest x-ray. Now we consider basic principles of chest x-ray technique relevant to emergency medicine and key principles of image interpretation. We finish with findings of specific pathology and a systematic approach to the interpretation of chest x-ray.

INTERPRETATION OF CHEST X-RAY: BASIC PRINCIPLES

Interpretation of chest x-ray requires several elements:
- An understanding of some basic principles and terminology of radiography
- A knowledge of the normal appearance of the chest x-ray
- A familiarity with the appearance of important pathologic findings
- A systematic approach to allow all key findings to be observed

We start with some basic principles. If you are already familiar with basic radiographic concepts and the normal appearance of the chest x-ray, move on to the section on pathology. But a few minutes familiarizing yourself with the ideas in this section can pay big dividends some day when you encounter an unfamiliar chest x-ray that does not fit any of the patterns of common pathology discussed in this chapter. Understanding basic principles may allow you to deduce the nature of the abnormality and avoid common pitfalls. A number of outstanding texts are devoted entirely to chest radiography.[25-26] We have drawn on numerous sources for the following discussion.

Chest X-ray Techniques and Effects on Resulting Images

Familiarity with the chest x-ray technique is important for the emergency physician because it can affect the appearance of important diagnostic findings and the sensitivity and specificity of a chest x-ray for these diagnoses. In some cases, a given chest x-ray technique may falsely simulate pathology; in other cases, the technique many hide important abnormalities. Here, we describe the most common chest x-ray techniques, along with pitfalls of each. The most common variations of the frontal chest x-ray used in the emergency department are the anterior–posterior (AP) view and the PA view. The AP view is commonly performed as a portable study in the patient's room, and it may be performed with the patient in a supine or upright position. The PA frontal view is performed in the radiology suite, and often a lateral projection PA chest x-ray is obtained at the same time.

Chest x-rays can be characterized by the following:
- The direction of the x-ray beam as it passes through the patient (posterior to anterior or anterior to posterior)
- The distances between the x-ray source, the patient, and the x-ray detector

- The position of the patient (upright, supine, lateral decubitus, lordotic, or oblique)
- The x-ray exposure

Each of these variables has important effects on the resulting image. In some cases, the technique is manipulated intentionally to achieve a desired diagnostic effect. In other cases, the patient's clinical condition limits the x-ray technique, and we are forced to accept a suboptimal diagnostic image. Understanding the effects of the x-ray technique on the resulting image is invaluable in helping the emergency physician to avoid misinterpretation of the image and misdiagnosis of the patient.

Direction of the X-ray Beam With Respect to the Detector: Posterior–Anterior Versus Anterior–Posterior Technique
When a frontal projection chest x-ray is obtained, the direction of the x-ray beam as it passes through the patient to the detector can be from patient posterior to anterior or from patient anterior to posterior (Figure 5-1). To restate this another way:

In the case of the PA x-ray, the patient is oriented with the x-ray film or detector in contact with the anterior surface of the thorax. The x-ray beam passes through the patient's posterior thorax to the detector. The patient faces toward the detector, away from the x-ray source (Figure 5-1).

In the case of the AP x-ray, the patient is oriented with the x-ray film or detector, in contact with the posterior surface of the thorax. The x-ray beam passes through the patient's anterior thorax to the detector. The patient faces toward the x-ray source, away from the detector.

Why does the direction of the x-ray beam through the patient to the x-ray detector matter? We return to this question in a moment, but first we describe a characteristic difference in the PA and AP x-ray techniques, which contributes to differences in the resulting image.

The PA chest x-ray is typically acquired in a radiology suite, with the x-ray source positioned 6 feet from the x-ray detector. In comparison, the AP chest x-ray is typically acquired as a portable examination, with only 3 feet separating the x-ray source and the detector.

Distance of the X-ray Beam With Respect to the Detector: Posterior–Anterior Versus Anterior–Posterior Technique
Why does the distance from the x-ray source to the detector matter? The answer becomes obvious if we consider the analogy of the children's game of creating shadows on a wall with a light source (Figures 5-2 and 5-3). You can try our example at home (use a light, not an x-ray) if it is unclear. Place a lamp 6 feet from a wall. Position your hand close to the lamp, and the shadow on the wall appears larger than the actual size of your hand, though

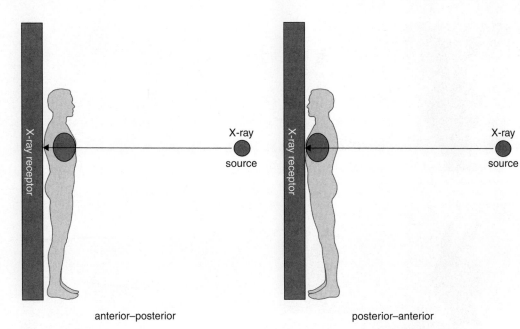

Figure 5-1. **Anterior–posterior and posterior–anterior chest x-rays.** The designation refers to the direction of passage of the x-ray beam through the patient to the receptor.

anterior–posterior   posterior–anterior

rather indistinct at its edges. Most people have used this trick for their amusement, making a hand appear as large as a head, for example. Without moving the lamp, move your hand closer to the wall; the resulting shadow becomes smaller (closer to its actual size), denser (darker), and sharper at its edges. We have now defined one of the two variables: with a light (or x-ray) source a fixed distance from a detector, positioning the object to be imaged close to the detector results in a sharper, truer image without false magnification. *Therefore, when performing medical imaging, we should place the body part to be imaged as close to the detector as possible to achieve a sharp, unmagnified image.* Now consider the same scenario, with a twist. Imagine that you cannot put your hand close to the wall because of furniture obstructing your path. How can you sharpen the image and reduce magnification? The answer is simple: move the lamp farther from your hand and the wall. Try this experiment, and you will find that the shadow of your hand becomes sharper and less magnified, truer to its actual size. Why would this scenario occur with medical imaging? Imagine placing your thorax against the wall; your ribs prevent you from moving your internal organs closer to the wall, although by facing toward or away from the wall you can position your heart (anterior in your chest) closer to the wall. However, you can easily control the distance of the light source from the wall to reduce magnification and improve the image sharpness. *Therefore, when performing medical imaging, we should position the x-ray source as far as possible (within reason) from the body part to be imaged, to improve sharpness and reduce magnification.*

Magnification: Asset or Artifact?

Although magnification may sound advantageous, it can introduce clinically deceptive artifacts if some body parts are magnified to a greater degree than others. The

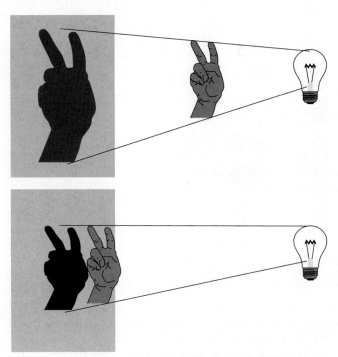

Figure 5-2. **A shadow experiment to illustrate principles of chest x-ray technique.** When the light source is a fixed distance from the wall, moving the hand closer to the wall results in a less magnified and sharper image.

most clinically accurate x-ray has no magnification. Why would we *not* want magnification? Wouldn't magnification potentially assist in identifying pathology? The problem again can be resolved by considering the shadow experiment. In medicine, we need an accurate estimate of the actual size of body parts and an accurate measure of their size relative to one another. Consider the example of the hand shadow and the shadow of the human head. Although it may be amusing to have your hand mimic a giant dog biting a head, this scenario of varying magnification is highly undesirable

Figure 5-3. **A shadow experiment to illustrate principles of chest x-ray technique.** When the hand is a fixed distance from the wall, moving the light source farther from the hand and wall results in a less magnified and sharper image.

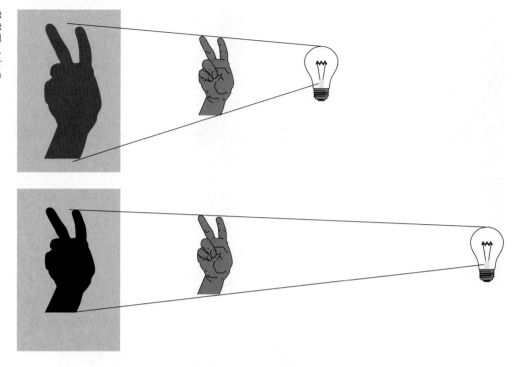

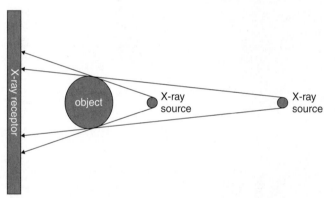

Figure 5-4. **Magnification and chest x-ray.** The degree of magnification is influenced by the distance of the x-ray source from the object being imaged. A more distant x-ray source results in a less magnified image.

in medical imaging. We need to know whether a mass has increased in size or if the heart and mediastinum are enlarged relative to the surrounding thoracic cavity. Our imaging technique must avoid false magnification, particularly when differential magnification of objects in the same image might occur.

Hopefully, we have convincingly demonstrated *how* the distances from the body part to the detector (assuming a fixed light source) and from the light source to the body part (assuming a fixed distance from body part to detector) affect the resulting images. Let's briefly consider *why* this is the case. Figures 5-4 through 5-6 illustrate the effect of distance on object magnification. The angle created between the x-ray source and an object's edges is determined by the distance from the x-ray source to the object. The shorter the distance from the x-ray source to the object, the greater the angle. Greater angles lead to

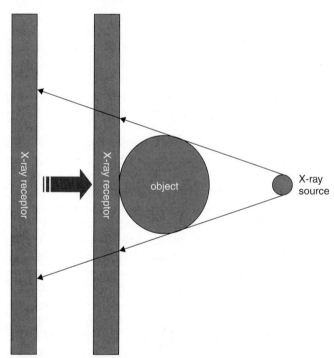

Figure 5-5. **Magnification and chest x-ray.** The degree of magnification is influenced by the distance of the x-ray receptor from the object being imaged. A more distant x-ray receptor results in a more magnified image. Moving the x-ray receptor closer to the object being imaged results in a less magnified image.

greater magnification; therefore, a shorter distance from the x-ray source to the imaged object leads to increased magnification. Although increased magnification may appear to be a benefit, in most clinical scenarios this can lead to a false appearance of cardiomegaly or a widened mediastinum. This is particularly a problem if very short distances are employed, as thoracic structures nearer to

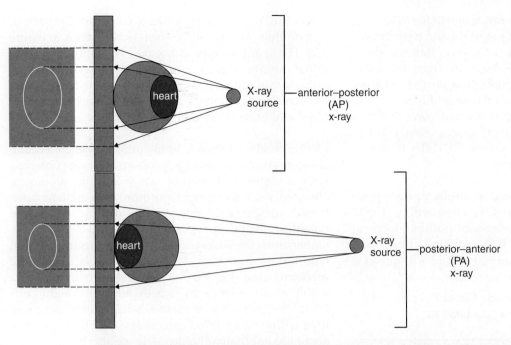

Figure 5-6. Chest x-ray technique and magnification. An anterior–posterior chest x-ray technique results in greater magnification of the heart. A posterior–anterior chest x-ray positions the x-ray source farther from the heart, and the x-ray receptor closer to the heart, resulting in less magnification of the cardiac silhouette relative to the thorax.

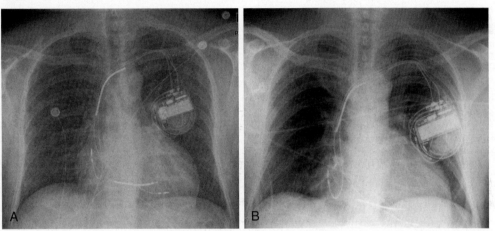

Figure 5-7. Differences between anterior–posterior (AP) and posterior–anterior (PA) chest x-rays and upright or supine positioning. As discussed in Figures 5-2 through 5-6, a PA chest x-ray results in a less magnified appearance of the heart, whereas an AP x-ray results in false magnification that can simulate or exaggerate cardiomegaly. Upright positioning typically results in better lung expansion. Supine positioning typically results in poorer lung expansion and clumping of pulmonary vessels in poorly expanded lungs, with an appearance that can simulate or exaggerate the appearance of pulmonary edema. Supine positioning also exaggerates the mediastinal width. **A,** An upright PA chest x-ray. **B,** A supine AP chest x-ray obtained a short time later in the same patient. The cardiac silhouette is enlarged in both but appears larger in **B.**

the x-ray source will be magnified to a greater degree than structures farther from the source. Positioning the x-ray source at a greater distance from the object to be imaged reduces this relative magnification, leading to a truer representation of the object. The AP portable examination places the x-ray source 3 feet from the patient, rather than the 6 feet usually used for a PA examination. Consequently, the AP portable chest x-ray examination typically has a greater degree of false magnification of the heart and mediastinum compared with the PA technique.

We asked earlier why the direction of the beam (AP vs. PA) matters to the resulting image. As we described in our shadow experiment earlier, sometimes we cannot fully control the location of objects relative to the x-ray detector. We cannot change the anterior location of the

heart in the chest; however, by positioning the detector on the anterior aspect of the chest, we bring the heart and the detector closer together, reducing magnification of the heart. Consequently, the PA x-ray technique results in less magnification of anterior structures compared with the AP technique. Remember this when viewing AP portable chest x-rays, which are more prone to false appearance of cardiomegaly or mediastinal widening (Figure 5-7).

Patient Positioning for Chest X-ray: Supine Versus Upright Technique

Now let's also consider the differences among a true upright, a supine, and an intermediate lordotic x-ray (Table 5-4). Although occasionally other positions of the patient are desirable in specific clinical scenarios, for most applications, a perfectly upright patient position is desirable during chest x-ray acquisition. When the patient is positioned perfectly upright and perpendicular to the direction of the x-ray source, thoracic structures are positioned equal distances from the x-ray source, ensuring equal magnification on the resulting x-ray image. In comparison, if the patient is positioned in a lordotic position with the upper and lower thorax at different distances from the x-ray source, the magnification of superior thoracic structures will differ from that of the lower thoracic structures.

When the patient is positioned in a fully upright position, fluid within structures of the chest will generally reside due to gravity in a dependent position, forming fluid levels. In comparison, if the patient is positioned supine, the horizontal plane in which fluid will spread is parallel to the x-ray film or detector beneath the patient, and no fluid levels will be seen. (see Chapter 6, Figure 6-2). The resulting appearance may be a diffuse increase in the density of the entire affected thorax, sometimes called a "veiling opacity." This may be mistaken for an increased parenchymal density, rather than being recognized as a broadly layered pleural effusion.

Pleural fluid and fluid within collections such as lung abscesses typically are not visible on an image obtained with a supine patient but are visible on an image obtained with an upright position. In a patient positioned upright, the upper surface of fluid within the potential pleural space usually forms a curved line, higher along the lateral chest wall than at its intersection with the mediastinum. This appearance is termed the **meniscus sign** (Figures 5-8 and 5-9). In contrast, fluid within an air-filled cavity usually forms a straight horizontal line without a lateral meniscus. Examples include fluid within an air-filled abscess cavity or fluid within a hemopneumothorax (Figure 5-10; see also Figure 5-8).

In an upright patient, air within the peritoneal cavity collects beneath the diaphragm, making it visible on x-ray because of the contrast between the density of air and diaphragmatic soft tissue. (Figures 5-11 through 5-14). In a supine patient, air within the peritoneal cavity may collect in the midline anterior abdomen rather than in a subdiaphragmatic position and in addition will spread in the same horizontal plane as the x-ray detector beneath the patient, preventing the air from being visible. An x-ray obtained with an upright patient position is therefore more sensitive for detection of pneumoperitoneum.

Another advantage of the upright chest x-ray is that the patient typically is able to accomplish a greater degree of inspiration. With greater inspiration, blood vessels

TABLE 5-4. Artifacts of Supine Chest X-ray Technique That Can Lead to Misdiagnosis

Supine Chest X-ray Finding	Possible Misdiagnosis
Heart appears large	Simulates cardiomegaly
Mediastinum appears wide	Simulates aortic or mediastinal abnormality
Increased vascular markings in upper lung zones	Simulates pulmonary edema
Poor inspiration	Simulates pulmonary edema and may hide small nodules
Layering of fluid in plane of x-ray detector	May prevent recognition of pleural fluid
Distribution of air to anterior chest and abdomen	May prevent recognition of pneumoperitoneum or pneumothorax

Figure 5-8. The meniscus sign. **A,** On an upright chest x-ray, fluid in the pleural space typically layers with gravity, forming a dependent collection. The upper surface of that collection usually forms a curve that is higher along the lateral chest wall than at its intersection with the mediastinum. This appearance is called the meniscus sign. **B,** In contrast, fluid within an air-filled cavity does not usually form a prominent meniscus and has a straight, horizontal upper surface. Examples include fluid within a pneumothorax and fluid within a lung abscess.

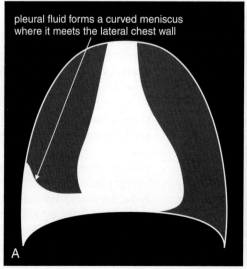

pleural fluid forms a curved meniscus where it meets the lateral chest wall

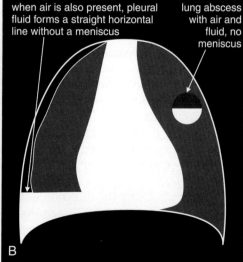

when air is also present, pleural fluid forms a straight horizontal line without a meniscus

lung abscess with air and fluid, no meniscus

become more widely spaced, allowing other abnormalities to be recognized. Radiologists have sometimes compared this with seeing a bird in a tree, which is more easily accomplished in a tree with widely spaced branches. Small lung masses can be more easily seen as a result. A well-expanded chest on an upright view also gives a truer estimate of the heart size. Rarely, a chest x-ray obtained at end-expiration provides diagnostic benefits, which we will review later.

In comparison, a supine chest x-ray is usually characterized by higher diaphragms, with poorer lung expansion

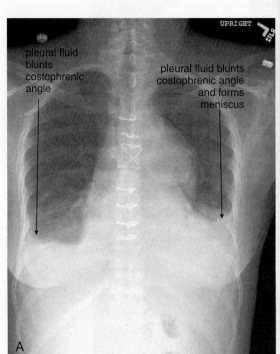

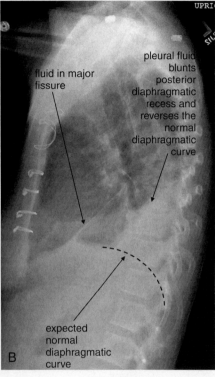

Figure 5-9. **Pleural effusions: Posterior–anterior (PA) and lateral upright views. A,** A PA upright view, where a pleural effusion is most evident on this patient's left side. Both costophrenic angles are blunted. The pleural effusion forms a meniscus against the left lateral chest wall. **B,** The lateral upright view shows two meniscus densities, suggesting bilateral pleural effusions. The posterior diaphragmatic recess is filled with pleural fluid, which forms a meniscus with the posterior chest wall. Compare with Figure 5-8 and 5-10.

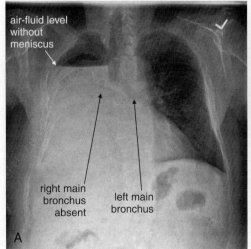

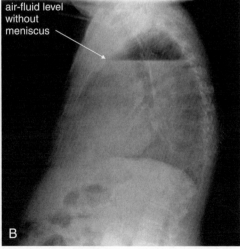

Figure 5-10. **Pleural effusion with air–fluid level. A,** Posterior-anterior (PA) upright x-ray. **B,** Lateral upright x-ray. This patient has a large fluid collection in the right pleural space following a pneumonectomy. The appearance is somewhat different from that of even a large typical pleural effusion because of the absence of a lung and the presence of air in the pleural space. Normally, an effusion collecting in the pleural space forms a meniscus with the lung margin, coming to a "beak" or sharp point along the lateral chest wall. No air–fluid level is seen in a typical pleural effusion, because the pleural space is a potential space that contains no air. An exception would be a hemopneumothorax, where blood and air would coexist in the pleural space. An air–fluid level might also be seen in an empyema, if gas-forming organisms are present. In this case, air was introduced into the pleural space during the pneumonectomy, and reactive pleural fluid has accumulated. The x-ray alone cannot rule out infection. **A,** Look carefully in the apex of the right thorax and note the absence of lung markings. Also note the absence of the right main bronchus, which has been surgically removed. Its silhouette is missing, whereas that of the left main bronchus remains. Another possible cause of an absent bronchus silhouette would be a bronchus filled with fluid or tumor, which are both of water density. Compare with Figure 5-8 and 5-9.

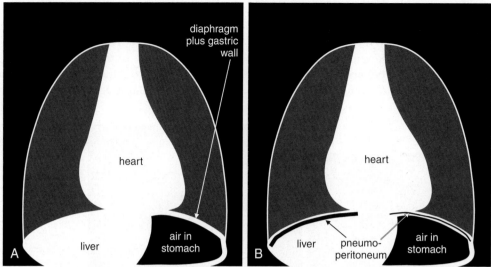

Figure 5-11. Free air (pneumoperitoneum). Free air (pneumoperitoneum) can be recognized on upright chest x-ray. This finding relies on the silhouette sign described later in this chapter (see Figure 5-26): air density is readily seen when in direct contact with water (soft-tissue) density. **A,** The normal appearance of the upright chest x-ray in the absence of pneumoperitoneum. **B,** The appearance of the upright chest x-ray in the presence of pneumoperitoneum. On an upright chest x-ray, normally the inferior surface of the right diaphragm is not seen, as the liver (water or soft-tissue density) is in direct contact with the inferior border of the diaphragm (also water density). When air is present within the peritoneal cavity, it may collect inferior to the right diaphragm, superior to the liver. This air may be recognized as a black line or collection, making the inferior border of the diaphragm visible. On the patient's left side, the normal gastric air bubble can simulate intraperitoneal air, as it is normal for the stomach to contain air. Fortunately, usually the gastric wall and adjacent diaphragm are thicker than the diaphragm alone would be, allowing the normal gastric bubble to be distinguished from subdiaphragmic pneumoperitoneum. In some cases, pneumoperitoneum may extend beneath the central diaphragm, in which case the inferior border of the heart may be partially visible. Normally, the heart, diaphragm, and liver are in contact, with no visible line separating them. Compare with Figures 5-12 through 5-14.

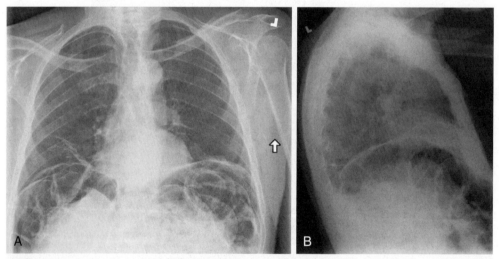

Figure 5-12. Free air. Pneumoperitoneum is a critical finding requiring recognition on chest x-ray. Occasionally, it may be an unanticipated finding on chest x-ray in a patient who cannot provide an adequate history. Remember that normally the inferior surface of the diaphragm cannot be seen, as it is contiguous with a solid organ sharing the same water density on chest x-ray: the liver on the right, the spleen on the left. On the left, the interior surface of the stomach may be shown in relief by air within it. It may be difficult to distinguish this inner surface of the stomach from the inferior surface of the diaphragm, although the diaphragm alone should be thinner than the combined thickness of diaphragm and stomach. Within the abdomen, the external surface of the bowel wall should not be seen, again because of its contiguity with other soft-tissue structures. Air within the bowel is readily seen and makes the internal surface of the bowel wall quite apparent. When pneumoperitoneum exists, the external surface of the bowel can be seen. A normal finding that may simulate this is the presence of two adjacent loops of bowel with their walls abutting. In this case, the internal surface of both walls may be seen, and it may appear that air is present on both sides of the wall of a single loop. In **A** (upright PA x-ray) and **B** (upright lateral x-ray), copious free air is present. **A,** Both diaphragms are outlined, and several bowel loops can be seen with air on both sides of their walls. **B,** The lateral x-ray also demonstrates this finding. Compare with the CT from the same patient in Figure 5-13.

and clumping of pulmonary vessels. In addition, blood flow to the upper lung is relatively increased by gravity, and the heart appears larger than on an upright x-ray. This is due to the portable AP technique but also because of the relatively unexpanded chest, which

makes the heart appear comparatively larger. In combination, these findings may mimic CHF (see Figure 5-7).

Supine and semilordotic views are often obtained in emergency department patients not by design but

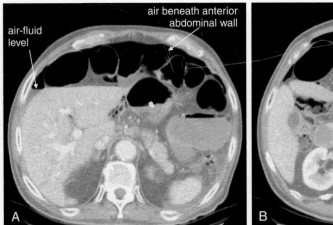
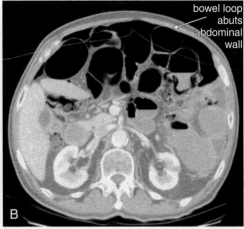

Figure 5-13. Free air, abdominal CT. Same patient as in Figure 5-12. **A** and **B** are shown on lung windows to highlight the contrast between air and other soft tissues. In these axial CT images, free air is seen outlining loops of bowel. Note how both sides of the bowel wall are clearly visible when contrasted with air. **B,** Notice that where a loop of bowel abuts the anterior abdominal wall, only the internal surface of the bowel wall is visible. This is because the bowel wall and the abdominal wall share the same soft-tissue density. On CT, air may accumulate along the anterior abdominal wall, as this is the highest point in the abdomen when the patient lies supine for CT. In contrast, in an upright patient undergoing chest x-ray, air accumulates under the diaphragm. Air is an outstanding contrast agent because of its much lower density than abdominal tissues, so no administered contrast agents are required to detect it.

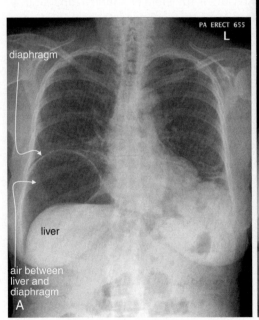
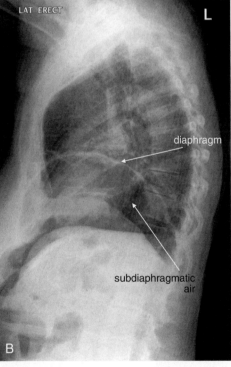

Figure 5-14. Free air. This patient presented with epigastric pain and has dramatic free air (pneumoperitoneum) visible under the right diaphragm on this upright chest x-ray. The inferior surface of the diaphragm is readily visible because of air separating it from the liver. Normally, these two structures are indistinguishable. In a more subtle case, the only clue to free air might be a thin black line separating the diaphragm and liver. On a supine x-ray, air might not collect in a subdiaphragmatic position and might not be visible. This patient was found to have a perforated gastric ulcer at laparotomy.

because patient condition prohibits the desired technique. Trauma patients, unstable medical patients, and intoxicated or neurologically disabled patients are just a few examples of patients who often undergo imaging in supine or semilordotic positions because of their inability to be positioned upright. The emergency physician must be aware of the limitations of these examinations and should recognize the patient position when interpreting the resulting images.

Lordotic and decubitus positions are sometimes obtained intentionally for specific diagnostic purposes, described later under "Additional Chest X-ray Views."

Normal Appearance of a Chest X-ray

Recognizing pathology requires a strong familiarity with the normal appearance of the chest x-ray. Classic abnormalities are often recognized by their distinct differences from the normal chest x-ray appearance. More subtle abnormalities may be missed by an inexperienced observer, but an experienced reader may immediately recognize that the chest x-ray differs from the norm even before characterizing and articulating the abnormality. Radiologists understand that recognizing familiar patterns of normal and abnormal requires constant exposure, much like recognizing a familiar relative. This pattern recognition approach has been dubbed the "Aunt Minnie" effect for this similarity. We briefly describe the appearance of a normal chest x-ray here. In the sections that follow, we present numerous examples of important pathology. Even with several examples of each type, you will only begin the exposure required to "recognize Aunt Minnie." Make a habit of looking at your patients' chest x-rays, even if the radiologist has already rendered an interpretation.

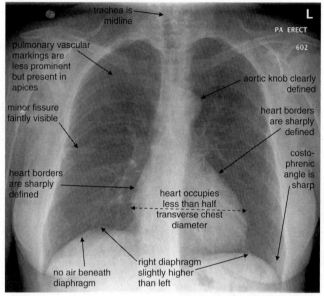

Figure 5-15. The normal frontal chest x-ray. Normal features of the posterior–anterior upright chest x-ray are demonstrated.

Frontal (Posterior–Anterior or Anterior–Posterior) Upright Chest X-ray View

The normal frontal upright chest x-ray (Figure 5-15) has the following features:

- The airway is midline.
- The bones show no fractures or lytic lesions.
- The cardiac silhouette occupies less than half of the transverse diameter of the thoracic cavity. The cardiac silhouette is crisp, with no adjacent pleural fluid or parenchymal opacities to disrupt the normal silhouette. The mediastinal width is less than 8 cm, and the aortic knob is well defined. The normal appearance of the aorta is described in detail in Chapters 6 and 7.
- The hemidiaphragms are visible as smooth curves bilaterally. No air is seen beneath them; the upper surface is not obscured by pleural effusion or infiltrates. The costophrenic angles are not blunted by pleural effusions. The right diaphragm is slightly higher than the left.
- The lung fields are clear, without opacities to suggest pleural effusion, parenchymal disease such as infectious infiltrate, or mass lesion. Lung vascular markings are visible to the periphery, without evidence of pneumothorax. Lung markings are less prominent in the lung apices because gravity diverts blood flow to the lung bases.
- The minor fissure is invisible or subtle in appearance, without significant thickening to suggest fluid accumulation in this potential space.

Lateral Upright Chest X-ray View: Retrosternal Space, Retrocardiac Space, and the Spine Sign

The lateral chest x-ray provides important diagnostic information. Unfortunately, this view is usually not obtained when a portable x-ray examination is performed—another good reason to send the patient to the radiology suite for imaging if the clinical condition permits this. The lateral view (Figure 5-16) reveals the

Figure 5-16. The normal appearance of the lateral chest x-ray. The normal lateral chest x-ray shows progressive lucency (darkening) of the thoracic spine as it approaches the diaphragm. This normal finding is called the "spine sign." Failure of the spine to become progressively more lucent as it approaches the diaphragm suggests an overlying opacity such as an infectious infiltrate or pleural effusion. The retrocardiac space should appear lucent (dark) as well, and the posterior diaphragmatic recess is dark and deep. The retrosternal space should be lucent (dark). **A,** A schematic representation. **B,** A patient with a normal spine sign and retrosternal and retrocardiac spaces.

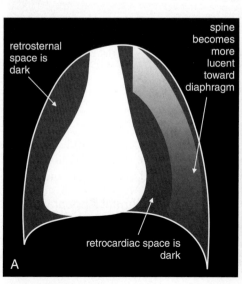

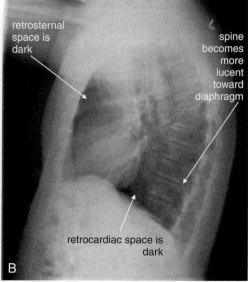

retrosternal space, which overlies the heart and mediastinum on a frontal projection. This space is usually quite lucent (black) because of the presence of a low-density epicardial fat pad and sometimes lung segments—but when occupied by a soft-tissue mass, this space may appear radiodense (white) (Figure 5-17). The lateral chest x-ray also reveals the retrocardiac space. This space normally should be quite lucent (black) (see Figure 5-16). Lower lobe pneumonias may be evident on the lateral view as an abnormally dense retrocardiac region (Figure 5-18). On the lateral view, the diaphragms usually form smooth curves descending from anterior to posterior. The space above the diaphragms is usually lucent (black), as it contains low-density lung tissue. Pleural effusions may be evident on lateral view as dense (white) layering

opacities replacing the normal curve of the diaphragm in this space (see Figure 5-9). Sometimes pleural effusions form a meniscus against the posterior wall of the thorax, actually reversing the normal curve of the diaphragm. In addition, air beneath the diaphragm (pneumoperitoneum) may be visible on the lateral view (see Figure 5-14).

The thoracic spine also is visible on a lateral chest x-ray. The normal appearance of the spine is a gradually more lucent (blacker) appearance moving from cephalad to caudad (see Figure 5-16). This is not a result of decreasing spinal density but rather is a normal artifact of the examination technique. When this progressively more lucent appearance is lost, it implies the presence of an abnormal density in the retrocardiac space. This

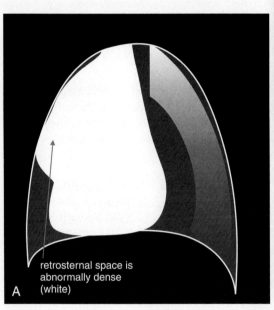

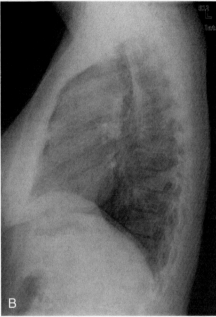

Figure 5-17. **Abnormal retrosternal space, suggesting anterior mediastinal mass.** The abnormal lateral chest x-ray shows loss of the normal lucent retrosternal space. This abnormality is easily missed but indicates soft-tissue density in the anterior mediastinum. The differential diagnosis includes the five terrible Ts: thyroid mass (goiter or malignancy), thymoma, teratoma, "terrible" lymphoma, and thoracic aortic aneurysm. **A,** A schematic representation. **B,** A patient with a retrosternal density, suggesting anterior mediastinal mass.

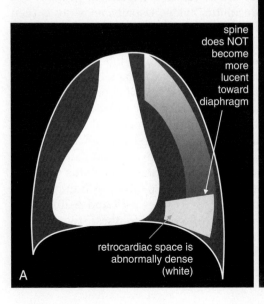

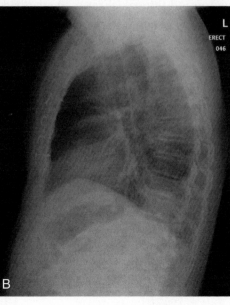

Figure 5-18. **The spine sign.** The abnormal lateral chest x-ray shows loss of the normal progressive lucency of the thoracic spine as it approaches the diaphragm, called the spine sign. In addition, the retrocardiac space may be less lucent than normal, and the posterior diaphragmatic recess may appear shallow or less lucent than usual, indicating pleural effusion or infiltrate. **A,** A schematic representation. **B,** A patient with a retrocardiac infiltrate, illustrating a pathologic spine sign.

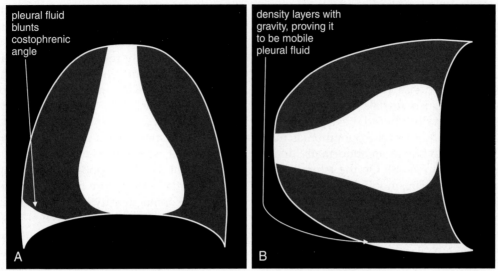

pleural fluid blunts costophrenic angle

density layers with gravity, proving it to be mobile pleural fluid

A

B

Figure 5-19. Lateral decubitus x-rays and pleural effusions. A density seen on an upright chest x-ray can be pleural fluid, atelectasis, or a parenchymal opacity. When these conditions cannot be differentiated on the upright view, a lateral decubitus x-ray can sometimes prove the opacity to be mobile pleural fluid, which layers with gravity. A parenchymal opacity, atelectatic lung segment, or loculated pleural fluid maintains its position and does not layer with gravity on a lateral decubitus view. **A,** Schematic upright chest x-ray. **B,** Schematic right lateral decubitus x-ray, showing mobile pleural fluid layering in a dependent position.

is called the **spine sign** and is a pathologic abnormality that can be a clue to disease. Remember that the increasing density has a differential diagnosis, including infectious infiltrate, pulmonary edema, pleural effusion, mass, and atelectasis. Other radiographic findings and the patient's clinical presentation must be used to sort through this differential diagnosis, and additional imaging may be necessary. Nonetheless, this finding can confirm a pneumonia not seen on the frontal projection x-ray. The lateral x-ray is often neglected but is a key additional view that should be obtained whenever possible and carefully reviewed.

Additional Chest X-ray Views

Early radiologists became extremely skilled at deducing clinically relevant information from additional chest x-ray views. The advent of cross-sectional imaging with CT scan has made some of these views less common, as CT imaging is able to determine the three-dimensional location of objects with high accuracy. However, in some cases, the detailed information provided by CT is unnecessary, and more limited information from x-ray may be sufficient for clinical action such as draining a pleural effusion. Although CT could be used in this scenario, the radiation dose from CT is approximately 500 times that of a single additional chest radiograph, and the cost is approximately 10 times higher. In addition, for chest angiography protocols, chest CT requires IV contrast administration, with risks of allergy or contrast nephropathy. X-ray avoids these issues. On an individual basis, the emergency physician should consider the information needed for clinical decision-making. If it is obvious that CT will be required for specific information, such as evaluation of pulmonary

embolism or aortic pathology, additional x-rays should generally not be obtained. However, if the information required can be provided by radiographs, these are a better choice for reasons of cost, radiation, and contrast exposure.

Lateral Decubitus Views. Lateral decubitus views allow assessment of radiographically visible mobile fluid collections and foreign bodies, as well as inferences about the presence of radiographically *invisible* foreign bodies. In a lateral decubitus view, the patient is positioned with one side of the thorax (right or left) in a dependent position (Figures 5-19 and 5-20). The view is labeled based on the side of the chest that is dependent. Thus an x-ray obtained with the patient positioned with the left side of the thorax in a dependent position is a "left lateral decubitus" view. Usually, an x-ray is then obtained using an AP projection, as described earlier.

Decubitus views can be useful in the following scenarios:
• *Differentiation of parenchymal consolidation from pleural effusion.* When opacities are visible on an upright or supine frontal projection (PA or AP), a lateral decubitus view can differentiate parenchymal consolidation from pleural effusion. A parenchymal opacity will not change in position relative to the patient when the patient is moved to a lateral decubitus position. A pleural fluid collection will layer with gravity if it is not loculated. (see Figures 5-19 and 5-20). Alternative means of differentiating these two entities include ultrasound, which readily identifies fluid as a hypoechoic collection, and CT.
• *Identification of loculated versus freely mobile pleural fluid collections.* When pleural fluid is seen on standard

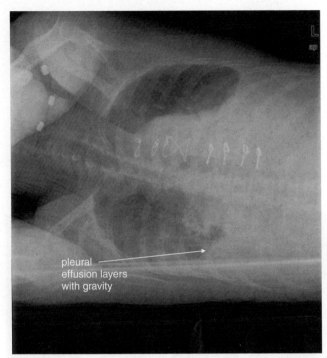

pleural
effusion layers
with gravity

Figure 5-20. Lateral decubitus x-rays and pleural effusions. Same patient as in Figure 5-9. In this patient with a pleural effusion, a decubitus view reveals the effusion to be mobile. A right lateral decubitus view (right side down) shows fluid to layer with gravity in the right chest, emphasizing the quantity and mobility of the right pleural fluid. If the density seen on the posterior–anterior upright x-ray had been a parenchymal infiltrate, atelectasis, or a loculated pleural effusion, it would not have moved with this change in the patient's position. Compare with Figure 5-9 and Figure 5-19, **A** and **B**.

radiographic views, decubitus views can reveal mobile collections which will maintain their position relative to the patient. Ultrasound and CT can also differentiate these.

• *Identification of mobile radiopaque foreign bodies.* In some cases, the location of a visible foreign body may be further delineated by repositioning the patient. Airway foreign bodies may shift from the midline, while foreign bodies within the esophagus will remain midline despite dependent positioning.

• *Identification of radiolucent (invisible) foreign bodies.* Some aspirated foreign bodies such as peanuts or plastic are too low in density to be visible on standard radiographs. Their presence can sometimes be deduced from their effect on pulmonary inflation. A foreign body lodged in an airway can occlude the airway in a ball-valve fashion, trapping air within a lung segment and causing relative hyperinflation. Normally, when a patient is placed in a lateral decubitus position, the dependent lung appears hypoinflated because of the weight of other thoracic structures resting upon it. In the case of an obstructing airway, foreign body, air trapped within a lung segment will make the affected lung remain fully inflated despite lateral decubitus positioning. Of course, a foreign body that does not create a ball-valve effect would not be detected by this method.

• *Identification of a pneumothorax in a patient who cannot tolerate an upright position.* Remember that a pneumothorax may not be visible on a supine x-ray, because air will collect in the anterior chest rather than near the thoracic inlet or lung apices. The patient should be placed in a decubitus position opposite to the side of the suspected pneumothorax (hemithorax with the suspected pneumothorax should be higher), allowing air within the pleural space to rise to the lateral chest wall. As a consequence, the pleural line and absence of lung markings typical of pneumothorax may then be more visible.

Lordotic Views. In a lordotic view, the patient is positioned in a semiupright position relative to the x-ray source. The resulting image provides more detail of upper thoracic structures by altering the position of upper ribs and clavicles relative to the upper lung. Normally, these bony structures obstruct the view of the upper lung; a lordotic position can allow assessment of upper lung masses, infiltrates, or apical abnormalities such as pneumothoraces. The ribs appear more horizontal on a lordotic view. Although lordotic positioning is sometimes used for intentional diagnostic benefit, often lordotic positioning is an undesired effect in an emergency department patient undergoing an AP portable chest x-ray. Artifacts of this technique include magnification of the heart and mediastinum, simulating cardiomegaly, mediastinal mass, or aortic aneurysm. In addition, lordotic positioning may increase the amount of soft tissue projected over the lower abdomen, resulting in increased apparent opacity at the lung bases. This may be mistaken for basilar infectious infiltrates, atelectasis, or pulmonary edema.

Oblique Views. Oblique views, though rarely used in the emergency department, use parallax to identify the location of objects or structures within the lung. Two structures that overlie each other on lateral or frontal projection views can be distinguished by an oblique view. More often in the emergency department, an oblique view is inadvertently obtained because of rotation of the patient. This commonly occurs when AP x-rays are obtained in patients with kyphosis, contractures, or neurologic deficits. Rotated or oblique views can introduce a number of artifacts. Among them, the mediastinum often appears artifactually widened, and the heart and mediastinum may appear shifted (Figure 5-21). Opacities in the lung bases may be hidden if the cardiac silhouette is projected over them because of rotation.

Phase of Respiration: Inspiratory and Expiratory Views. Normally, a chest x-ray is obtained at full inspiration, although in many cases patients may fail to inspire deeply because of chest pain or may be unable to hold their breath in this position because of dyspnea. The chest x-ray captures a frozen, static moment in time, but thoracic structures are actually in motion

Figure 5-21. Rotation. A good-quality chest x-ray should be obtained in a true frontal projection **(A),** free of rotation. An oblique film alters the apparent width and position of the mediastinum. Assess for this by checking the position of the clavicular heads, which should be symmetrically arrayed about the midline. Rotation of the patient shifts the position of the clavicular heads. Notice how the three-dimensional figures in the upper part of this diagram appear when rotated and then projected in two dimensions, as happens in a chest x-ray. The "heart" *(ellipse)* appears wider in the rotated views **(B** and **C).**

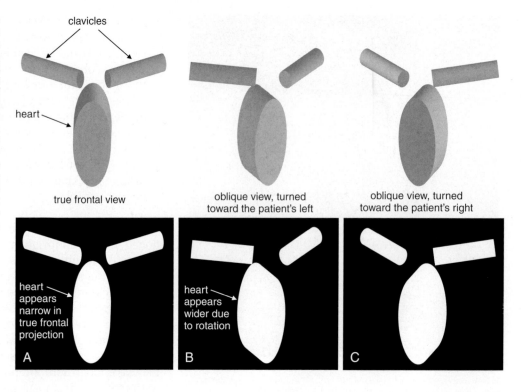

with patient respiration and cardiac activity. The apparent density of lung tissue varies with the phase of respiration. At end-expiration, lung volumes are very low, the diaphragms appear high, and lung tissue appears dense (whiter). Blood vessels in the lungs appear crowded together, contributing to the apparent density of lung tissue. If the phase of respiration is not considered, this appearance may be mistaken for pulmonary edema. In contrast, a chest x-ray obtained at end-inspiration shows well-inflated lungs, diaphragms that have descended fully, and widely spaced pulmonary vessels. Lung parenchyma under these conditions appears less dense. A clue to the phase of respiration is the number of ribs visible. A rule of thumb is that the diaphragm should lie at the level of the posterior 8th to 10th rib for an adequate respiratory effort in a good-quality chest x-ray. Abnormally dense lung parenchyma such as seen with pneumonia is more visible against the backdrop of fully inflated and lucent (black) lungs. Patients with COPD or asthma may have hyperexpanded lungs with low-density parenchyma and more than 10 ribs visible.

Occasionally, chest x-rays are intentionally obtained in other phases of respiration. Examples include:

1. Pneumothorax: An end-expiratory chest x-ray is sometimes used to exaggerate the appearance of a pneumothorax. At end-expiration, lung parenchyma is deflated and occupies a smaller percentage of the thorax. In contrast, air in the pleural space will not decrease in volume during expiration. As a consequence, a pneumothorax will appear to occupy a larger percentage of the thoracic cavity.

2. Foreign body. Low-density foreign bodies may be difficult to see on chest x-ray. However, they may exert a ball-valve effect by lodging in small airways. As a consequence, they may trap air within lung segments. During end-expiration, a normal lung will decrease in size. A lung with a partially obstructed bronchus due to a foreign body exerting a ball-valve effect may be unable to deflate during expiration. The abnormal lung or lung segment will therefore appear larger and more lucent than the normal side on an end-expiratory radiograph.

Chest X-ray Exposure (Penetration)

The exposure of chest x-ray is particularly critical, as the chest contains structures across a wide range of densities, from air to bone. A fully exposed x-ray film or detector results in a completely black image. For example, x-ray passes readily through air outside the patient, making the background around the patient appear black. Lungs are normally composed mostly of air, with a small density contribution from pulmonary blood vessels, and appear nearly black with a good exposure. A pneumothorax is even less dense, like air outside of the patient, and appears almost completely black. Metals and bones prevent transmission of much x-ray to the detector with a normal exposure; consequently, the detector is not exposed and the image appears white.

From these principles, we can extrapolate that an over-exposed chest x-ray will appear black (the entire detector is fully exposed). An underexposed chest x-ray will appear nearly white, as the detector is not exposed. Although the appearance of tissues can be adjusted

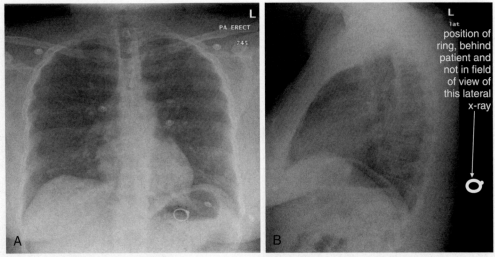

Figure 5-22. **Assessing for artifacts: Ring outside body. A,** Upright posterior-anterior (PA) x-ray. **B,** Upright lateral x-ray. This 39-year-old presented with shortness of breath. Chest x-ray was obtained and revealed an unexpected finding—a ring overlying the patient's gastric air bubble. The patient then reported having lost her wedding ring some days prior, after removing her shirt. Ingested foreign bodies are a frequent complaint in the emergency department. Plain x-rays can assist in localizing these, in identifying the ingested item, and in predicting the likelihood of passage and need for intervention. When an ingested foreign body is suspected, two orthogonal views (posterior–anterior or anterior–posterior and lateral) are needed to localize the object. In this case, the object was not seen on the lateral view, suggesting that it was not within the patient. On reexamination of the patient, the ring was found in a skin fold on the patient's back.

(brightness and contrast) on a digital picture archiving and communication system (PACS) display, no amount of image manipulation can overcome a badly over- or underexposed image. For example, in a badly overexposed image, the entire detector is fully exposed, and all pixels are completely black. Adjusting the contrast and brightness simply makes the entire image blacker or whiter, without revealing tissue detail. In a badly underexposed image, the entire detector fails to be exposed, and all pixels are completely white. Adjustment of brightness and contrast is not useful in this case, either. As the exposure level is increased above an "optimal exposure," lung tissue becomes "burned out" (black), and fine details of lung architecture, such as bulla, fissures, pulmonary vascularity, and pneumothorax, are lost. This loss comes with a gain in the visibility of bony detail, as x-ray can now penetrate through less dense regions of bone, including fracture zones. If exposure is lower than an "optimal level," detail of bone is lost, as no x-ray can penetrate through dense bone. At the same time, soft tissues become more visible, as the lower exposure prevents x-ray from fully exposing the detector behind them. Depending on the clinical presentation, overexposure- or underexposure may be intentionally performed to highlight either bone or soft-tissue detail.

Beware of some common scenarios in which poor exposure can simulate pathology:
- In the obese patient, underexposure is common. The detector is in effect "shielded" from the x-ray beam by overlying soft tissues. Consequently, the entire image, including lung tissues, appears brighter. This appearance can be mistaken for pulmonary edema if the overall image exposure is not considered.

- On a frontal projection, underexposure makes retrocardiac structures less visible, including the left lower lobe, which extends behind the heart.
- On a frontal projection, breast tissue can increase attenuation of the x-ray beam in the lower lung zones, resulting in relative underexposure of the lung in these regions. Consequently, the lower lung fields may appear brighter white, simulating bibasilar infiltrates, pulmonary edema, or atelectasis.
- In a patient with a unilateral mastectomy, an asymmetrical appearance of the lower lung zones can lead to false diagnosis of unilateral basilar pneumonia. Pay attention to this finding to avoid misdiagnosis. Use other x-ray findings such as the silhouette sign (described later) to assess for pathology in the lower lung fields.

Artifacts Outside of the Patient

Opacities and lucencies on the x-ray image may not originate within the patient (Figures 5-22 through 5-25). Overlying skin folds and clothing can create lines simulating pathology such as the pleural line of pneumothorax. Foreign bodies may appear to lie within the patient but may be discerned to be outside of the patient if a lateral view is obtained. Two orthogonal views are needed to confirm an object's location. Whenever possible, extraneous external foreign bodies should be removed before obtaining x-ray to prevent them from obscuring internal anatomy or being mistaken for objects within the patient. Sometimes surface anatomy such as nipples can simulate internal pathology such as lung nodules. When this is in doubt, marking the surface anatomy with a radiopaque tag can clarify the source of the chest x-ray finding.

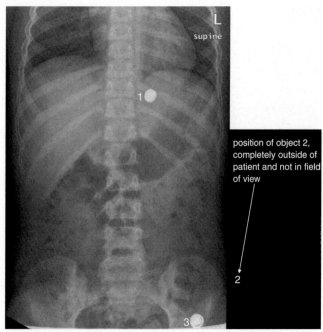

position of object 2, completely outside of patient and not in field of view

Figure 5-23. **Assessing for artifacts: Button battery ingestion.** This 7-year-old child was "washing" a button battery in her mouth in an effort to fix her electric toy when she reported accidentally swallowing the battery. Parents were uncertain whether any ingestion had occurred. When an ingested foreign body is suspected, two orthogonal views (PA or AP and lateral) are needed to localize the object. The anterior–posterior (AP) supine view shown here reveals two radiopaque objects, labeled 1 and 3 on this image. The lateral view (Figure 5-24) reveals 3 radiopaque objects, including an object not seen on this AP image but whose position is labeled 2. Did the patient ingest multiple batteries? Only object 1 is projected in a consistent location overlying the abdomen on both AP and lateral views and is intraabdominal. The other two objects are external to the patient. Object 3 on the lateral view (see Figure 5-24) corresponds to the caudad object on the AP view. Object 2 on the lateral view is so far lateral that it is not visible on the AP view. The patient underwent upper endoscopy, but the battery had moved beyond the pylorus and could not be retrieved. X-rays obtained 24 hours later confirmed passage of the battery.

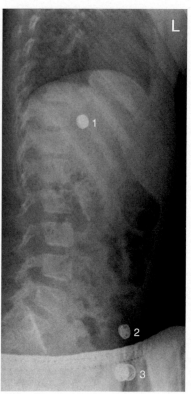

Figure 5-24. **Assessing for artifacts: Button battery ingestion.** Same patient as Figure 5-23. The lateral view shown here reveals the three radiopaque objects. (See also Figure 5-23.)

TISSUE DENSITIES AND CHEST X-RAY

On chest x-ray, only four basic tissue densities are present (Box 5-1): air, fat, water (typical of both fluids and most solid body organs, such as liver and muscle, which are more than 90% water), and metal. This includes calcium, which you will recall from chemistry class is actually a metal. Some texts distinguish bone from metal. A key principle of chest x-ray interpretation is that two tissues in direct physical contact with each other and sharing the same basic density are indistinguishable. For this reason, the diaphragm cannot normally be discerned from the abutting liver, because both are of water density. Similarly, blood (water density) cannot be seen within the heart (also water density). Pericardial fluid cannot be distinguished from myocardium, because both are of water density, but pericardial air can be distinguished from myocardium. A pleural effusion lying above the diaphragm shares the same density with the subjacent diaphragm and liver and cannot be directly distinguished.

Normal lung tissue (air density) can be distinguished readily from adjacent normal soft tissues (water density), because the two tissues do not share the same density. However, when normally air-filled alveoli become filled with water density, the border between that lung tissue and the adjacent heart disappears. The cause of the alveolar water density does not matter: pneumonia, hemorrhage, and aspirated material all have the same effect, increasing the density of the lung from air to water. Consequently, if the abnormal lung abuts another water density structure such as the heart or diaphragm, the junction between the two tissues cannot be discerned. A little anatomy illustrates the clinical utility of this fact. The right middle lobe abuts the lower right heart border, and the right lower lobe abuts the diaphragm. For this reason, a right middle lobe pneumonia obscures the lower right heart border, and a right lower lobe pneumonia obscures the diaphragm. On the left side, the lingula abuts the lower left heart border, and the left lower lobe abuts the diaphragm. Pneumonias in these areas obscure the left heart border and left diaphragm, respectively.

Silhouette Sign

As we have just discussed, two objects with the same basic chest x-ray density (air, fat, water, or metal/bone) abutting one another cannot be distinguished. The corollary of this is that when two structures of different basic density abut each other, their junction can be

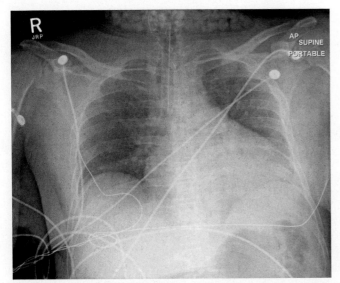

Figure 5-25. Assessing for artifacts. This adult male presented in cardiac arrest and was successfully resuscitated. Chest x-ray was obtained and shows popcorn-like densities in the neck and right axilla. Are they a sign of a disease process? Could these be calcifications in lymph nodes related to metastatic disease? No, they are due to ice in bags placed outside the patient for postresuscitation neuroprotective cooling. Densities on x-ray must be considered in clinical context. Not all opacities are caused by pathology within the patient.

discerned on x-ray. This is called the **silhouette sign** (Figure 5-26).[27] Loss of the normal silhouette sign along the heart borders or diaphragm is an important pathologic finding, though it does not always signify pneumonia, as we explore further. Any change that causes the abnormal juxtaposition of two tissues of the same density results in loss of the silhouette sign. Examples include a solid lung mass adjacent to the heart, a pleural effusion adjacent to the heart or diaphragm, dense pulmonary edema, or atelectasis of lung adjacent to the heart or diaphragm, in which case the "collapse" of lung tissue results in it taking on a solid organ density (water density). Box 5-2 outlines the differential diagnosis of increased lung parenchymal opacity.

In other cases, the pathologic change is not the *loss* of the silhouette sign but rather the *introduction* of a silhouette sign when one is not normally present. This occurs when a new, abnormal tissue density becomes interposed between two adjacent tissues that share the same density and normally are not distinguishable. For example, the junction between the liver and the diaphragm is not normally visible, as the two tissues are in direct physical contact and share the same density (water or soft-tissue density). If **pneumoperitoneum** develops, air can become interposed between the liver and the diaphragm, making this interface visible (see Figure 5-11). Air can also cause a pathologic silhouette sign when it is present within the pericardium (between the soft tissues of the heart and the pericardial sac) or in the abdomen when air is visible between two adjacent loops of bowel, making the external surface of the bowel wall visible.

Air Bronchograms: A Manifestation of the Silhouette Sign

The silhouette sign can sometimes be used to distinguish otherwise similar-appearing chest x-ray findings. For example, a pleural effusion and a dense pulmonary infiltrate may have similar appearances on upright chest x-ray. Because both conditions are water density and both may abut the heart and mediastinum, both may cause loss of the normal silhouette sign. However, a pleural effusion appears uniformly dense, whereas a pulmonary alveolar infiltrate may result in the appearance of a new, abnormal silhouette called an **air bronchogram** (Figure 5-27). Normally, bronchi within the lung parenchyma are not visible on chest x-ray. This is because the bronchi contain air and immediately abut alveoli, which also contain air. The bronchial wall itself is too thin to attenuate x-ray to a significant degree and is therefore invisible, except when it is seen end-on. In these cases, it may be visible as a small, circular density with a hollow, lucent (black) center. This normal scenario is disrupted when alveolar fluid is present—whether that fluid is pus (pneumonia), serous fluid (pulmonary edema), blood (pulmonary hemorrhage), or lunch (aspirated food material). Under these conditions, fluid-filled alveoli become visible as water density immediately adjacent to air-filled bronchi, and the silhouette of air-filled bronchi may be seen. At extremes of the conditions described, pus, pulmonary edema fluid, blood, or aspirated material may fill bronchi as well, in which case air bronchograms may not be seen. *When present, air bronchograms prove alveolar opacification.* When air bronchograms are absent, either pleural fluid or alveolar and bronchial fluid may be present.

Silhouette Sign and Lateral Chest X-ray

We discussed the lateral chest x-ray earlier in some detail in the section on x-ray technique and views. However, this topic is important enough to revisit in the context of the silhouette sign.

Retrosternal Space. The retrosternal space is invisible on the frontal chest x-ray, as it lies directly anterior to the soft tissues of the heart and upper mediastinum. On the lateral x-ray, this space is normally lucent (black) because of the presence of aerated lung tissue and epicardial fat; it forms a normal silhouette against the soft tissues of the heart and upper mediastinum. A

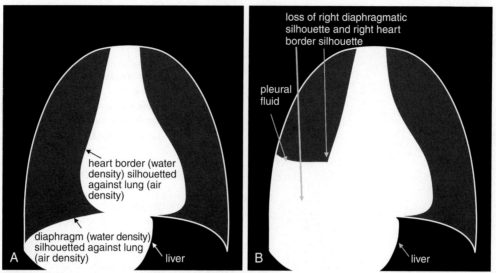

Figure 5-26. The silhouette sign. On chest x-ray, four densities are visible: air, fat, water (fluid, or soft tissues), and metal (bone). When two immediately adjacent organs or tissues share the same density, they cannot be distinguished. In contrast, when a tissue abuts another tissue of different density, it is silhouetted against the other tissue density. Loss of this normal silhouette, or the development of an unexpected silhouette at the interface of two tissues of similar density, is called the silhouette sign and indicates a pathologic change in tissue density. Normal examples of tissues that cannot be distinguished because they share the same density include the diaphragm and liver and the heart and intracardiac blood. Pathologic examples of the silhouette sign include the liver, the diaphragm and an adjacent subpulmonic pleural effusion; or a pleural effusion adjacent to the right heart. **A,** Normal chest. **B,** Pathologic chest with subpulmonic pleural effusion, which obscures the diaphragm and the right heart border.

Box 5-2: Causes of Apparent Lung Parenchymal Opacity, Leading to Loss of Normal Silhouette Sign

Normally, the heart and diaphragm (water density) abut low density lung tissue (air density) and thus are silhouetted against it. Loss of this silhouette implies that lung density has been replaced by water density. Causes include:
   Alveolar consolidation (pulmonary edema, infectious infiltrate, pulmonary hemorrhage, aspirated material)
   Atelectasis or lobar collapse
   Herniated abdominal solid organs
   Pleural fluid (effusion, empyema, or hemothorax)
   Solid mass pulmonary lesion

---

soft-tissue mass in this location abuts the soft tissues of the heart and mediastinum and thus is not discernible as a discrete structure, according to the principles of the silhouette sign discussed earlier. Thus loss of the normal lucent retrocardiac space and replacement with water density attenuation is evidence of an anterior mediastinal mass (see Figure 5-17). The differential diagnosis includes the five terrible "T"s (Box 5-3).

Retrocardiac Space. The normal retrocardiac space is lucent (black) on the lateral chest x-ray because of aerated lung in this location; it forms a normal silhouette with the soft tissues of the heart anteriorly, the diaphragm inferiorly, and the bones of the thoracic spine posteriorly. The space is hidden on the frontal projection by the presence of the heart. When tissue increases in density

in this area, the appearance is a brighter white—a possible indication of a retrocardiac infectious infiltrate or other cause of increased parenchymal or pleural opacity, such as mass or edema. Inspection of the retrocardiac space on the lateral chest x-ray is therefore an important step in assessing the x-ray. Loss of the normal silhouette sign in this location, or the presence of an abnormal density, is evidence of pneumonia, mass, pulmonary edema, or pleural effusion (see Figures 5-16 and 5-18).

FISSURES

The major and minor fissures can provide anatomic landmarks, revealing important disease when present (Figures 5-28 through 5-30). The fissures represent pleural boundaries and are actually a "sandwich" composed of the distinct pleura lining two adjacent pulmonary lobes and the potential space between. Thickening of a fissure on chest x-ray can be the result of thickening of the pleura itself, fluid accumulating in the potential space between the two pleural layers, or disease such as malignancy. The **minor fissure** (also called the transverse fissure) is usually visible as a thin horizontal line on both frontal (PA or AP) and lateral chest x-ray projections. It separates the upper and middle lobes of the right lung. The **major fissure** is not visible on the frontal chest x-ray projection. On the lateral projection, it is visible as a thin line running from the inferior portion of the anterior thorax to the superior aspect of the posterior thorax. It is actually composed of two fissures, superimposed on the lateral projection. On the left, it divides the upper and lower lobes of the left lung. On the right, it divides the upper and middle lobes from the lower lobe of the right lung.

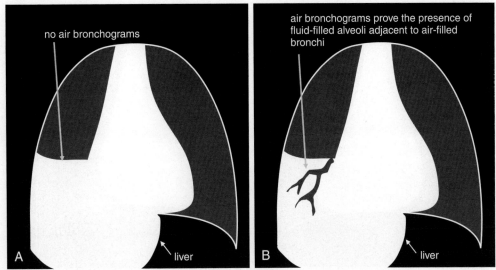

Figure 5-27. Air bronchograms prove the presence of air-space consolidation. Normally, air-filled bronchi are not visible because they are immediately adjacent to air-filled alveoli. The bronchial wall is too thin to be visible except when seen end-on. When alveoli fill with fluid (pus, edema, blood, or aspirated gastric material), they may silhouette the adjacent air-filled bronchi. **A,** The absence of air bronchograms is compatible with a pleural effusion or with both alveoli and adjacent bronchi having been filled with fluid, as may occur with massive aspiration or pulmonary hemorrhage, severe pneumonia, or extremes of pulmonary edema. In other words, when air bronchograms are absent in an opacified lung field, the explanation may be pleural fluid, infectious parenchymal infiltrate, aspiration, parenchymal hemorrhage, or pulmonary edema. **B,** When air bronchograms are present, they prove that alveolar fluid is present and that the adjacent bronchi remain air-filled. Thus a pleural effusion does not create an air bronchogram, which is by definition a finding of air-space disease. A differential diagnosis remains for air-space disease, including infectious infiltrate, aspiration, hemorrhage, and pulmonary edema. Therefore, air bronchograms are *not* pathognomonic for infection.

Box 5-3: Differential Diagnosis of Anterior Mediastinal Mass in Retrosternal Space on Lateral Chest X-ray

Five Terrible Ts
- **Thyroid mass (goiter or malignancy)**
- **Thymoma**
- **Teratoma**
- **"Terrible" lymphoma**
- **Thoracic aortic aneurysm**

Fissures can change rapidly in their appearance (Figures 5-31 through 5-34). Thickening of fissures can develop or disappear in a matter of hours, sometimes giving clues to the cause. Rapidly changing fissures generally indicate fluid within the fissure, rather than pleural thickening. Changes can be dramatic; fluid in the minor fissure can assume a rounded appearance mimicking a mass lesion but disappearing within days or hours. This has been called the "vanishing tumor" or "pseudotumor."

CHANGES IN VOLUME AND PRESSURE ON CHEST X-RAY

Changes in volume and pressure can be seen on frontal chest x-ray and can indicate immediately life-threatening pathology (Figure 5-35). Mediastinal shift is seen with both increased and decreased pressure and volume. Increased pressure and volume on the side with pathology *push* the mediastinum away from the abnormal side. Decreased pressure and volume *pull* the mediastinum toward the abnormal side. In both cases, tracheal deviation may be seen, in the same direction as the mediastinal shift.

Increased Pressure and Volume

Increased pressure and volume, as seen in a tension pneumothorax (Figure 5-36; see also Figure 5-35), result in the diaphragm on the abnormal side being pushed down. A tension pneumothorax on the right side may be notable for the right hemidiaphragm being lower than the left—a reversal of the normal pattern. Normally, the right hemidiaphragm is higher than the left because of the liver (right side) being larger than the spleen (left side) and displacing the diaphragm upward. In tension pneumothorax, a **deep sulcus sign** can be seen (see Figures 5-35 and 5-36), with the costophrenic angle on the affected side being deeper than on the unaffected side. In some extreme cases, the sulcus may be so deep that its inferior extent is not visible on the chest x-ray. Tension pneumothorax is discussed in detail in Chapter 6. We discuss pneumothoraces in more detail later, but naturally a pneumothorax is distinguished by an absence of lung markings on the affected side. Purists argue that tension pneumothorax is a clinical diagnosis, marked by hypotension and shock, and never to be found on chest x-ray. Nonetheless, chest x-rays sometimes record these findings, and an emergency physician must immediately recognize chest x-ray findings suggestive of tension pneumothorax and respond appropriately.

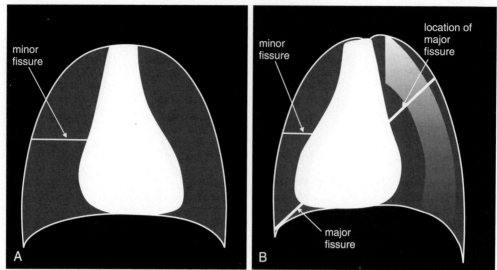

Figure 5-28. Fissures. The major and minor fissures are important landmarks on chest x-ray. They represent potential spaces that can fill with fluid in disease states such as pulmonary edema. They are anatomic boundaries that can bound pathologic processes such as pneumonias, masses, and infarctions. Deviations of the fissures from their normal positions can indicate changes in the volumes of lung segments. The minor fissure is visible as a horizontal line on both frontal **(A)** (posterior–anterior or anterior–posterior) and lateral **(B)** projections, as it lies in a transverse plane that is perpendicular to both chest x-ray projections. The major fissure is invisible on the frontal projection, as it lies in a plane oblique to that projection. It is visible on the lateral projection, as it lies perpendicular to this projection. In many normal cases, the major and minor fissures may be subtle or invisible.

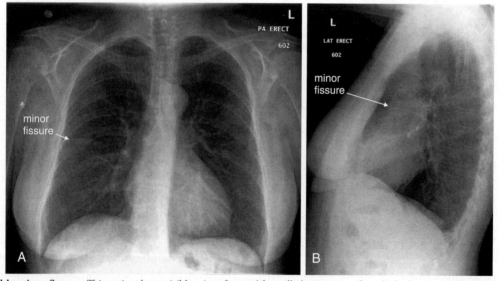

Figure 5-29. Visible minor fissure. This patient has a visible minor fissure (also called a *transverse fissure*), the horizontal fissure separating the upper and middle lobes of the right lung. Because it is perpendicular to the coronal plane and to the sagittal plane, the minor fissure is often visible on both the frontal chest x-ray **(A)** (whether posterior–anterior as in this case or anterior–posterior) and on the lateral chest x-ray **(B)**. When the fissure contains fluid or is thickened by pleural abnormalities, is appears as a thin horizontal line on the frontal chest x-ray and as a horizontal line curving inferiorly and posteriorly on the lateral x-ray. Why should an emergency physician care about the minor fissure? This is a landmark that can hint at other pathology. Movement of the minor fissure away from its normal position suggests lobar collapse—the fissure moves toward the collapsing lobe as volume is lost. In addition, infiltrates, pulmonary infarcts, and sometimes tumors abruptly stop above or below this fissure. Sometimes a large amount of fluid in the fissure may simulate a mass. During the remainder of this chapter, we give examples of abnormalities expressed through changes in the minor fissure. Compare with Figure 5-28.

Decreased Pressure and Volume

Decreased pressure and volume (see Figure 5-35) may result in the diaphragm appearing higher than usual—because of the absence of aerated lung pushing it down into its normal position. In addition, the normal position of the minor fissure may be changed on the frontal x-ray. The minor fissure is usually visible as a thin horizontal line roughly at the midpoint of the cephalad–caudad diameter of the thorax. When upper lobe collapse occurs, the minor fissure is elevated, whereas lower lobe collapse may result in the minor fissure assuming a lower-than-normal position. Think of lobar collapse as resulting in an accordion-like compression of the involved lung segment, with the minor fissure

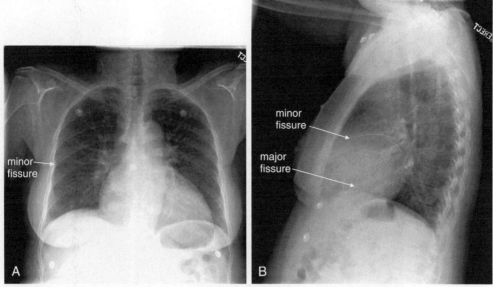

Figure 5-30. Prominent fissures. The major fissure is not visible on the frontal chest x-ray, as it lies in an oblique plane from anterior–inferior to posterior–superior. On the lateral chest x-ray, the major fissure is visible as a diagonal line from the anterior diaphragm to the posterior midthoracic spine. Like the minor fissure, the major fissure is not itself a sign of pathology, but knowing its usual appearance can help the emergency physician to recognize pathology impinging on the major fissure. In this patient, the minor and major fissures are visible on the lateral chest x-ray **(B)**. The minor fissure is faintly visible on the frontal chest x-ray **(A)**. Notice how the major fissure is not seen on the frontal x-ray because of its orientation. Compare with Figure 5-28.

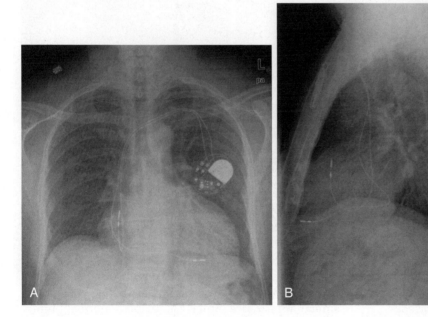

Figure 5-31. Fissures come and fissures go. In a normal patient, the minor and major fissures can be extremely subtle or even invisible. With the development of pleural fluid from any cause, the fissures can change dramatically in appearance in a short time frame. Consider this patient with heart failure. **A** and **B,** The patient has nearly invisible minor and major fissures. Follow the appearance of the fissures in the next three figures (Figures 5-32 through 5-34).

following in the direction of collapse and volume loss. In addition, the collapsed lobe may be visible as an increased density. If the collapsed lobe abuts the heart, abnormal loss of the silhouette sign may occur. Common scenarios leading to lobar collapse include basilar atelectasis (Figure 5-37), bronchial mucus plugging (Figure 5-38), iatrogenic right main bronchus intubation (Figure 5-39), obstructing endobronchial lesion (e.g., carcinoma), and extrinsic compression of a bronchus from a mass lesion. Patients who have undergone pneumonectomy also have significant volume loss (Figures 5-40 and 5-41).

SPECIFIC PATHOLOGIC DIAGNOSES

So far, we have reviewed many key principles of chest x-ray interpretation, with little discussion of the specific radiographic appearance of any acute pathology. With these basic principles in mind, we now discuss key findings of common and serious emergency medical conditions. The remainder of this chapter includes nearly 200 cases of key emergency diagnoses, with case descriptions and annotated figures displaying radiographic findings. To guide you through these figures, we have summarized the content of figures (Table 5-5).

Figure 5-32. **Fissures come and fissures go.** Same patient as Figure 5-31, now, with worsened heart failure. The fluid in the minor and major fissures is prominent, marking the locations of the previously invisible fissures. Also compare with Figures 5-33 and 5-34.

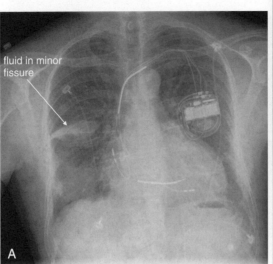

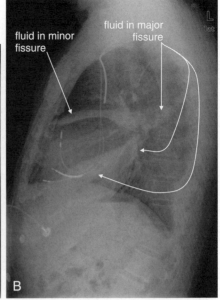

Figure 5-33. **Fissures come and fissures go.** Same patient as in Figures 5-31 and 5-32, now with progressively worsening heart failure. The fluid in the minor and major fissures is prominent and rounded, with a masslike appearance. Without prior and future chest x-rays to monitor the appearance, a mass cannot be excluded. Rapidly resolving fluid in the major and minor fissures has sometimes been termed "vanishing tumor" or "pseudotumor" because of this remarkable ability to simulate a mass lesion. Compare also with Figure 5-34.

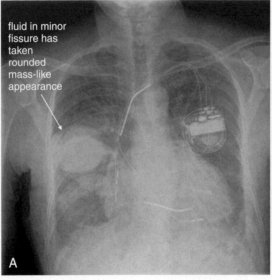

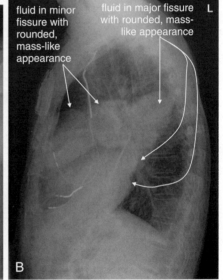

Findings of Common and Serious Emergency Pathology

Asthma and Chronic Obstructive Pulmonary Disease

Both asthma and COPD (Figures 5-42 and 5-43) are disease processes characterized by air trapping and lung hyperinflation. Consequently, they often share the findings of flattened diaphragms (because of hyperinflated lungs pushing the diaphragms down) and increased lung volumes, AP chest diameter, and retrosternal space. The lateral view is useful for assessment of the latter findings and may show the diaphragms to be flattened to a greater extent than was visible on the frontal projection. On the frontal view, the heart may appear small because of the hyperinflated lung fields. In patients with COPD, bullae (also called blebs) may develop (Figures 5-44 through 5-48). These regions are devoid of lung

markings and must be carefully distinguished from pneumothorax, as large peripheral bullae can have a similar appearance. Bullae can displace normal pulmonary blood vessels, sometimes crowding these vessels together. Patients with COPD and asthma can suffer barotrauma—spontaneously or because of mechanical ventilation. The chest x-ray should be inspected carefully for **pneumothorax** and **pneumopericardium**.

Other Forms of Chronic Lung Disease

Chronic lung diseases such as cystic fibrosis (Figure 5-49), idiopathic pulmonary fibrosis (Figure 5-50), and chronic injuries from smoke inhalation (Figure 5-51) have a similar appearance on chest x-ray. Dense interstitial markings may be seen, and air space disease may be chronically present. Bullae such as those seen in

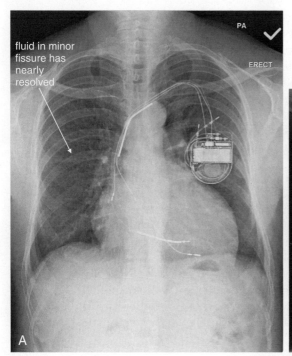

fluid in minor fissure has nearly resolved

PA

ERECT

A

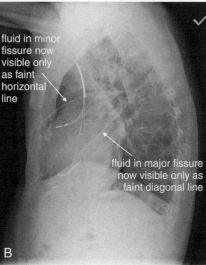

fluid in minor fissure now visible only as faint horizontal line

fluid in major fissure now visible only as faint diagonal line

B

Figure 5-34. **Fissures come and fissures go.** Same patient as in Figures 5-31 through 5-33, now after treatment for heart failure. The fluid in the minor and major fissures, which had previously assumed a rounded, masslike appearance, is nearly gone, in keeping with the term "vanishing tumor."

COPD may be present. Often, the appearance is quite abnormal, and comparison with prior chest x-rays is essential to distinguish new opacities suggesting acute infection from chronic disease. These diseases serve as an important reminder that chest x-ray findings should not be assumed to be acute and to explain new symptoms. Comparison with prior x-rays should always be performed when possible (Figure 5-52).

Pneumonia
Pneumonia can follow several common patterns on chest x-ray. First, air space opacification may be present, if alveolar fluid and cellular debris develops. This pattern is common in patients with "typical" bacterial infections such as *Streptococcus pneumoniae.* Air bronchograms (Figures 5-53 and 5-54; see also Figure 5-27) may be present, as described in earlier sections. Often, the increased density of lung parenchyma obscures the margins of adjacent solid organs such as the heart or diaphragm, resulting in a pathologic loss of the silhouette sign as described earlier. On a frontal projection, a right middle lobe pneumonia obscures the lower right heart border, and a right lower lobe pneumonia obscures the right diaphragm. A left lower lobe pneumonia obscures the left diaphragm, and an infiltrate in the lingula obscures the left heart border (remember that the left lung does not have a middle lobe). Upper lobe pneumonias may obscure the borders of the upper heart and mediastinum. On the lateral view, a pathologic spine sign (described earlier) may be seen, with increased density in the retrocardiac space and overlying the lower thoracic spine. A pleural effusion may be present with pneumonia. If infection is confined to

a lobe, the increased density may extend to, but not beyond, a fissure (described earlier) on the frontal or lateral views. **Volume loss** (described earlier) may occur if mucous plugging is present, with resulting findings including deviation of fissures, elevation of the diaphragm, or mediastinal and tracheal shift. Figures 5-55 through 5-85 depict pneumonias with air space disease in patients of varying ages, and with varying lung regions involved. Pneumonia remains a key diagnosis because of its mortality in patients at extremes of age. The appearance can be highly variable, and chest x-ray is not always diagnostic. Review the figures to gain perspective on the potential appearance of infiltrates.

A second common pattern of pneumonia is an interstitial pattern, often seen with "atypical" pathogens such as *Bordetella pertussis* (Figure 5-86), *Chlamydia pneumonia,* and *Mycoplasma.* In this circumstance, fluid becomes evident in the interstitial connective tissues of the lung, rather than within alveoli. Air bronchograms should *not* be seen as a result of an interstitial pneumonia. Peribronchial cuffing may be seen. **Peribronchial cuffing** (Figure 5-87) is a thickened appearance of bronchioles when viewed end-on on chest x-ray. Normal bronchioles are not visible when oriented in the plane of the x-ray but are visible as small black circles (air within the bronchiole) surrounded by a thin white line (the bronchial wall) when they are oriented perpendicular to the plane of the chest x-ray. With the development of interstitial edema, this thin white line thickens and is then called peribronchial cuffing. Peribronchial cuffing is not specific to bacterial infection and is seen in other disease states, including pulmonary edema, asthma, pneumocystis pneumonia (PCP), viral pneumonitis, and bronchiolitis such as that from respiratory syncytial virus. Other findings of interstitial pneumonia can include fluid in the minor and major fissures.

Pneumonia Differential Diagnosis. It is essential to remember that a differential diagnosis exists for increased lung parenchymal density (see Box 5-2). Any process that results in fluid and solid material accumulating within alveoli can have this x-ray appearance. This includes not only infectious pneumonitis (pneumonia) but also physical aspiration of noninfectious material (Figures 5-88 through 5-90), pulmonary hemorrhage, pulmonary infarction in the setting of pulmonary embolism (see Chapter 7) or sickle cell anemia acute chest syndrome (Figure 5-91), atelectasis, mucous plugging with segmental collapse, mass lesion, and pulmonary edema. A pleural effusion can resemble parenchymal opacity, with some differences as outlined in earlier sections. When a parenchymal opacity is seen, the emergency physician must resist the temptation to conclude that "the chest x-ray shows pneumonia." Instead, the physician must determine that "the chest x-ray shows increased parenchymal opacity." This finding should be considered with other clinical data to reach the correct diagnosis. In the words of a radiologist, clinical correlation is required.

Cavitary Lesions. Some pulmonary infections characteristically produce cavitary lesions on chest x-ray. These include tuberculosis and lung abscesses from pathogens such as *Staphylococcus aureus* or aspirated anaerobes. Necrotic neoplastic lung masses may cavitate. Bullae resulting from emphysema can become secondarily infected, sometimes with fungal pathogens. A typical cavitary lesion may have an air–fluid level on an upright chest x-ray. This may not be visible on a supine image, as fluid within the cavity layers in the same plane

Figure 5-35. **Changes in pressure and volume on chest x-ray. A,** The lungs and mediastinum under normal conditions of pressure and volume. The heart and airway are near the midline. The minor fissure is in normal position. The right diaphragm is usually slightly higher than the left, because of the larger size of the liver relative to the spleen. **B,** Increased pressure results in mediastinal shift and tracheal deviation to the opposite side. In the case of a right-sided tension pneumothorax, the right hemidiaphragm may be displaced in a caudad direction and may be lower than the left hemidiaphragm—the reverse of their normal positions. In addition, in any tension pneumothorax, the costophrenic angle may be extremely deep on the abnormal side due to a hyperinflated pleural space—the "deep sulcus sign." **C,** Decreased pressure and volume, such as is seen with lobar collapse, results in mediastinal and tracheal shift *toward* the affected side. The diaphragm may be elevated because of decreased lung volume. The minor fissure may move in the direction of the collapsed lobe. In addition, the collapsed lobe may be visible as an increased density. If the collapsed lobe abuts the heart, a pathological silhouette sign may be present.

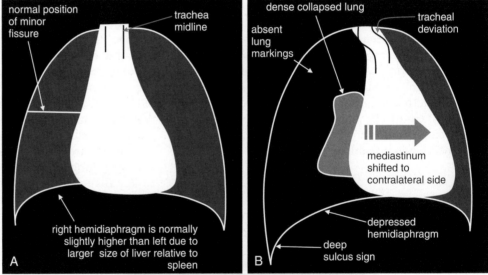

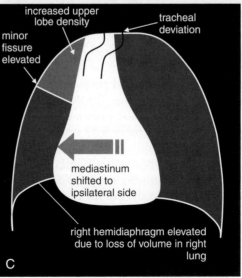

as the x-ray detector. As with other chest x-ray findings, a differential diagnosis should be considered based on appearance and other clinical data. Figures 5-92 through 5-101 show cavitary lesions worrisome for tuberculosis or abscess.

Embolic Pneumonia. In the case of endocarditis, septic emboli may be distributed throughout the lungs. The typical appearance is of numerous or innumerable nodules, often bilaterally distributed (Figures 5-102 and 5-103). The chest x-ray appearance is indistinguishable from metastatic disease.

Pulmonary Edema and Heart Failure

Chest x-ray findings of pulmonary edema follow a sequential pattern from early or mild findings to late or advanced findings (Table 5-6). A number of artifacts can simulate these findings and should be recognized to avoid misdiagnosis (Table 5-7). In general, early findings include pulmonary venous congestion, which is associated with cephalization, and cardiomegaly. **Cephalization** (Figures 5-104 and 5-105) refers to the redistribution of visible pulmonary vessels into the upper lung fields as pulmonary vascular volume and pressures increase. On a normal upright chest x-ray, the upper lung fields are relatively sparsely populated with visible pulmonary vessels compared to the lung bases because of the effect of gravity in preferentially filling dependent vascular beds. Remember that cephalization can be simulated by a supine chest x-ray, in which the upper pulmonary vessels are filled because of the patient's supine position. An underpenetrated (underexposed) chest x-ray may simulate this appearance as well, as all blood vessels and soft tissues appear more prominent. A poor inspiratory effort also increases the apparent density of lung tissue, simulating pulmonary edema. In a poorly expanded lung (because of poor inspiratory effort at the moment of the x-ray),

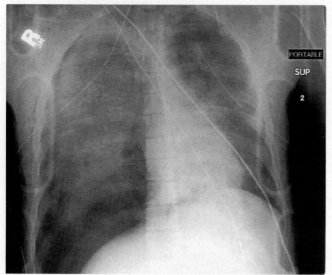

Figure 5-36. A case of increased pressure and volume: Tension pneumothorax. This example shows mediastinal shift to the patient's left, as well as depression of the right hemidiaphragm and a deep sulcus sign (the right costophrenic angle is pushed below the lower margin of the image). Absence of lung markings indicates the pneumothorax, whereas the lung shows increased density, likely from a combination of collapse and pulmonary contusion. In this particular case, bilateral chest tubes have already been placed without resolution of the pneumothorax, suggesting large airway disruption. The rate of air leak from the bronchus defect exceeds the rate at which air is being removed through the thoracostomy tube. Compare with Figure 5-35.

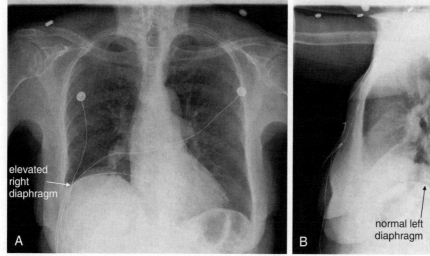

Figure 5-37. Atelectasis with elevated diaphragm: An example of volume loss. The right hemidiaphragm in this patient appears elevated on both the posterior–anterior **(A)** and the lateral **(B)** views. Is this the correct interpretation of the x-ray, and if so, what is the cause? Consider the alterative interpretations. A subpulmonic pleural effusion would appear similar, as it would have the same density as liver, heart, and diaphragm and would layer over the diaphragm with the patient upright. This appears less likely in that a meniscus might be seen along the lateral chest wall with a pleural effusion but is not present here. In addition, a pleural effusion occupies space and might be expected to push the heart to the left, whereas in this case the heart may be slightly deviated to the right. Atelectasis of the lower right lung would result in volume loss, pulling the heart and hemidiaphragm into the space normally occupied by lung. This is consistent with the observed features. An infiltrate in this location could explain the x-ray findings but appears less likely for similar reasons to those cited for effusion. Some simple maneuvers could narrow the differential diagnosis. Chest ultrasound, decubitus x-ray views, or CT could identify an effusion.

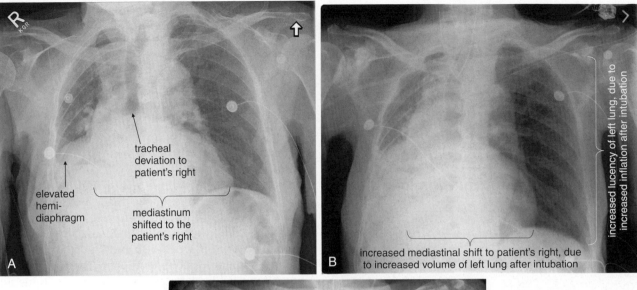

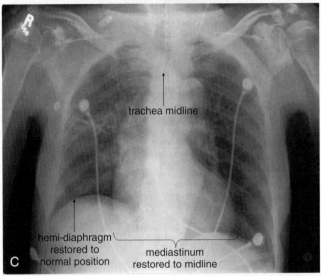

Figure 5-38. Lobar collapse and volume loss with mediastinal shift. This 70-year-old male presented with hypoxia, hypotension, and altered mental status. **A,** Initial chest x-ray before intubation. **B,** Chest x-ray after intubation was performed. The patient's vital signs did not improve. **C,** Chest x-ray minutes later, after an intervention was performed and the patient's vital signs improved. The initial chest x-ray **(A)** shows evidence of "volume loss." Volume loss refers to a decrease in the size of the contents of a portion of the thoracic cavity. In contrast to tension pneumothorax, where an *increase* in the volume of one hemithorax displaces the mediastinum *away* from the affected side, volume loss means *decrease* in volume and causes mediastinal shift *toward* the affected side. Three signs point to volume loss in this patient: the mediastinum is shifted toward the patient's right, tracheal deviation is present toward the patient's right, and the right hemidiaphragm is elevated. In this case, the patient had volume loss resulting from lobar collapse because of mucous plugging. Intubation initially worsened the patient's condition, because the normal (left) lung readily inflated under positive pressure. This increased the degree of mediastinal shift toward the patient's right **(B),** further compressing the left lung. Adjusting the ventilator to increase positive pressure ventilation and positive end-expiratory pressure resulted in reinflation of the collapsed lobe, resolving the chest x-ray abnormalities and improving the patient's clinical condition **(C).** In some patients, such as those with collapse because of an obstructing bronchial mass, this intervention might not be helpful. Bronchoscopy with stenting of the obstructed airway might be necessary to restore lobar inflation. Avoid mistaking volume loss for pleural effusion. A pleural effusion might appear similar to the elevated right hemidiaphragm, but pleural effusion occupies volume and thus should not cause mediastinal shift or tracheal deviation toward the affected side. Bedside ultrasound may help to discriminate between the two conditions. In this case, no effusion was present, and the patient's liver was visible on ultrasound, at the level of the nipple viewed through the right axilla. Compare with Figure 5-35.

pulmonary blood vessels appear more closely spaced and may be mistaken for edema.

Cardiomegaly (Figures 5-106 through 5-109; see also Figures 5-104 and 5-105) is another frequent finding in cases of pulmonary edema, though not all patients with heart failure will have an enlarged cardiac silhouette. Heart size is measured on chest x-ray using the **cardiothoracic ratio,** which equals the ratio of the transverse

heart to the greatest internal diameter of the thoracic cage. A normal value is less than or equal to 0.5 for adults, and cardiomegaly is radiographically defined by values exceeding this. Poor inspiration, supine positioning, or magnification from an AP portable x-ray all may falsely elevate the cardiothoracic ratio, simulating cardiomegaly. Figures 5-110 through 5-122 show cardiomegaly, often in association with other findings of pulmonary edema.

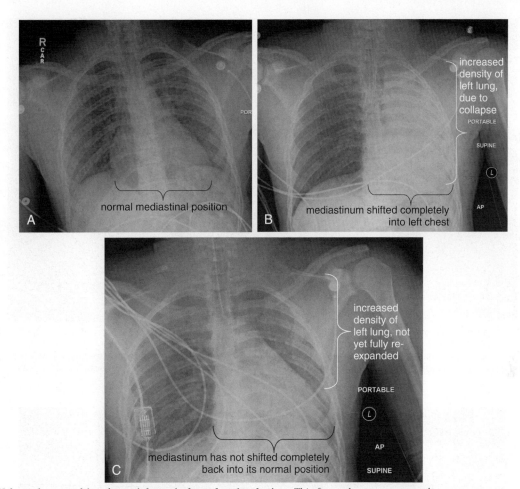

Figure 5-39. Volume loss resulting from right main bronchus intubation. This figure demonstrates another common cause of volume loss—iatrogenic right main bronchus intubation. **A,** The patient has not yet been intubated. **B,** The patient has been intubated and the left lung appears completely collapsed (opacified). One clue to volume loss here is that the entire mediastinum has shifted into the left chest and is not visible against the background of collapsed lung. This is an example of the pathologic silhouette sign. The scenario in **B** may present without the benefit of the comparison x-ray **A,** if the patient is intubated before a chest x-ray can be obtained. The emergency physician must recognize right main-stem intubation as a possible cause, rather than mistaking this for a left pleural effusion or dense pneumonia. **C,** The endotracheal tube has been repositioned at a shallower depth, and the left lung is partially reexpanded. The left lung parenchyma appears slightly denser than the right, as it has not yet fully reinflated. The mediastinum has not yet shifted back to its usual position because of hypoinflation of the left lung. The appearance in **B** can also be seen in a patient with a pneumonectomy, as mediastinal shift into the empty hemithorax occurs (see Figure 5-10, 5-40, 5-41). Compare also with Figures 5-35 and 5-38.

An enlarged cardiothoracic ratio may also occur with **pericardial effusion** (Figures 5-123 through 5-130). This can be indistinguishable from cardiomegaly on chest x-ray, though classically the appearance of a large pericardial effusion is described as a "water bottle" appearance on upright chest x-ray. Imagine the appearance of a full water balloon that is placed on a flat surface. The balloon sags, creating a broader inferior aspect. A large pericardial effusion may have a similar appearance when the heart and pericardium rest in an upright position on the diaphragm and solid liver beneath. Although chest x-ray may assist in this diagnosis, ultrasound (see Chapter 6) and CT scan are definitive and should be used to differentiate cardiomegaly from pericardial effusion when clinical concern exists. Figures 5-131 through 5-135 (see also Figures 5-123 through 5-130) show the similar chest x-ray appearance of cardiomegaly and pericardial effusion. Pericardial effusion may accompany cardiomegaly in severe heart failure.

Diagnostic imaging does not definitively determine the cause of a pericardial effusion, although associated findings such as lung opacities consistent with metastatic disease or primary lung neoplasms may suggest the cause.

Later in the course of heart failure or developing pulmonary edema, increased hydrostatic pressure results in the development of **interstitial edema.** This is manifested on chest x-ray as peribronchial cuffing (see Figure 5-119) described earlier in the section on interstitial pneumonia and Kerley B lines. Peribronchial cuffing is not specific to pulmonary edema and is seen in other states, including viral pneumonitis and bronchiolitis, such as that from respiratory syncitial virus. **Kerley B lines** are parallel, fine lines extending from the pleural surface into the subpleural lung, especially in lung bases, and thought to result from fluid accumulation in interlobular septa.

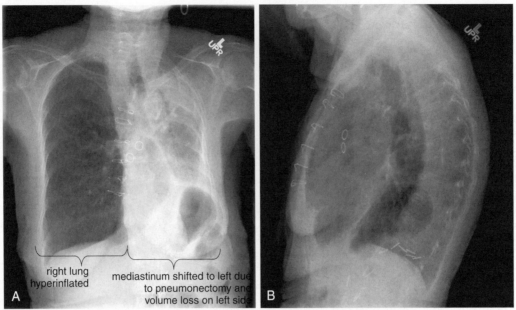

Figure 5-40. Pneumonectomy: Another cause of volume loss. A, Posterior-anterior (PA) upright chest x-ray. **B,** Lateral upright chest x-ray. This 86-year-old female has a history of lung cancer treated with left pneumonectomy. As a consequence, there is significant loss of volume in the left chest, and the heart, mediastinum, and trachea have shifted to the left to fill the void. The right lung appears hyperinflated, which is typical in cases of contralateral volume loss. This is due to the extra space created in the right thorax by shift of the heart and mediastinum to the left.

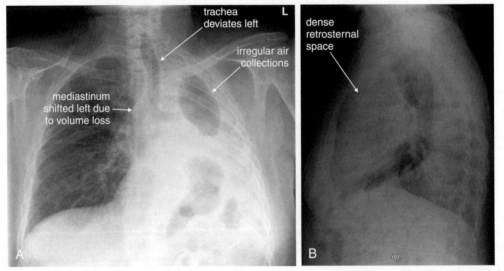

Figure 5-41. Pneumonectomy. A, Posterior-anterior (PA) chest x-ray. **B,** Lateral chest x-ray. This 60-year-old male underwent left pneumonectomy for non–small cell lung cancer months prior and presented with hypotension. **A,** His chest x-ray shows an irregular opacification of the left chest, with rounded air densities and fluid. The mediastinum has shifted into the left chest because of the expected volume loss from pneumonectomy. We have seen this appearance previously with lobar collapse. Notice how the trachea deviates left as well. This patient's chest x-ray appearance was unchanged from priors, but two additional diagnoses should have been considered if increased air had been seen. One is abscess with gas-producing organisms in the pleural space. The second is bronchopleural fistula, which would allow air to escape from the residual left bronchus. This would also pose a risk of infection, as nonsterile air would enter the poorly defended pleural space. **B,** The patient also has a dense retrosternal space, concerning for an anterior mediastinal mass.

Late in the course of pulmonary edema, hydrostatic pressure forces fluid into alveoli, usually first in the lung bases and then in the upper lung segments (see Figure 5-110, *B*). This is usually symmetrical, although asymmetrical pulmonary edema can occur. Before frank air space edema occurs, symmetrical perihilar "butterfly" or "bat wing" air space disease may be seen. As described earlier in the section on air bronchograms, fluid within alveoli arising from heart failure may create a silhouette against the adjacent air-filled bronchi—an air bronchogram. The presence of this finding proves the presence of alveolar fluid but does not distinguish edema from infection, hemorrhage, aspiration, or other fluid. If edema progresses further, fluid may fill bronchioles adjacent to alveoli, eliminating the silhouette of the air bronchogram.

TABLE 5-5. Arrangement of Figures

Figure content	Figure number	Figure content	Figure number
acute chest syndrome	91	lobar collapse	38, 39
air bronchograms	27, 53-54	lung abscess	97-101
aortic pathology	see Chapter 7	lung masses	159-175
aspiration pneumonitis	88-90	mediastinal widening	176-178
asthma	42	meniscus sign	8
atelectasis	37	nasogastric tube	189
cardiac CT	see Chapter 8	normal chest x-ray	15, 16
cardiomegaly	104-115, 131-135	pacemaker complications	190-197
cavitary lesions/tuberculosis	92-96	pericardial effusion	123-130
central venous catheter	188	pertussis	86-87
changes in pressure and volume	35	pleural effusions	9-10, 136-152
chest x-ray technique	1,2,3,4, 5, 6,7	pneumonectomy	40, 41
congestive heart failure/pulmonary edema	116-122	pneumonia	55-85
chronicity of chest x-ray findings	52	pneumopericardium	153-156
chronic obstructive pulmonary disease	43-48	pneumoperitoneum	11, 12, 13, 14
cystic fibrosis	49	pulmonary embolism	see Chapter 7
dextrocardia	198	retrosternal space	17
esophageal foreign body	187	right main bronchus intubation	39
esophageal rupture	157	rotation artifact on chest x-ray	21
external objects	22, 25	septic emboli	102-103
fissures	28, 29-34	silhouette sign	26
hiatal hernia	185-6	smoke inhalation	51
hilar adenopathy	183-184	spine sign	18
idiopathic pulmonary fibrosis	50	subcutaneous emphysema	158
internal foreign bodies	23, 24	superior vena cava syndrome	179-182
lateral decubitus x-ray	19, 20	tension pneumothorax	36
		traumatic injuries	see Chapter 6

Pleural effusions are another common finding in pulmonary edema, although they may occur from many other causes, including infection, malignancy, and pulmonary embolism. When a unilateral pleural effusion occurs in the setting of heart failure, a right-sided pleural effusion is more common. Figures 5-136 through 5-152 show a variety of pleural effusions, emphasizing their variable size and appearance by chest x-ray, ultrasound, and CT.

Pneumothorax

Pneumothorax is discussed in detail in Chapter 6. (See the extensive figures in that chapter.) Pneumothorax can occur outside of the setting of trauma. Spontaneous pneumothorax and iatrogenic injury from mechanical ventilation or procedural complications (e.g., during central venous catheter placement) may occur. Pneumothorax is characterized by an absence of normal lung vascular markings in the zone of pneumothorax.

The resulting lung field appears extremely lucent or dark. The pleural line of the injured lung is often visible on x-ray and should be carefully sought. This line must be distinguished from skin folds, objects outside of the patient, and the curved cortices of ribs, which may have a similar appearance. In each of these cases, and unlike the true pleural line of a pneumothorax, lung markings are visible beyond the suspect line. In addition, skin folds are usually a sharply defined line on one side but not on the other. In contrast, the pleural surface usually appears sharply defined on both sides. The medial border of the scapula should be identified explicitly to avoid confusing this line with the pleural line of a pneumothorax.

Subcutaneous air (Figure 5-153; see also Figure 5-158) can be associated with pneumothorax and should be sought as an additional clue. Subcutaneous air appears

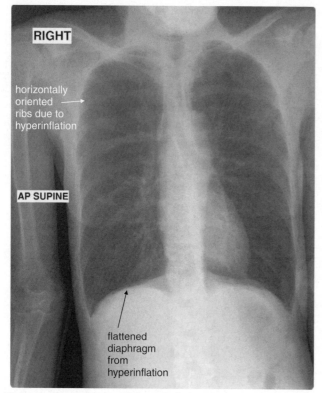

Figure 5-42. Asthma with hyperinflation. X-rays are not routinely needed for the evaluation of patients with asthma, although they should be considered if pneumonia or barotrauma such as pneumothorax is suspected. Common findings include hyperinflated and thus very lucent lung fields. Hyperinflation flattens the diaphragms as well. An overexpanded thorax often has ribs oriented more horizontally than usual. A good-quality inspiratory film in a normal patient should reveal lungs inflated to the 10th rib. This patient, a 46-year-old asthmatic with multiple prior intubations, has 11 visible ribs even on this supine x-ray. Supine position normally raises the diaphragm because of the pressure of abdominal contents, whereas upright position lowers the diaphragm by gravity.

more lucent (dark) than surrounding soft tissues. Air may track into the axilla and neck and sometimes outline skeletal muscle fibers in exquisite detail. Rib fractures may be seen, suggesting occult trauma or spontaneous fractures related to osteopenia, cough, or malignancy.

Changes suggesting increased volume and pressure on the affected side of the chest must be carefully sought, as these are evidence of developing tension pneumothorax (see Figures 5-35 and 5-36). Deviation of the trachea to the contralateral side, mediastinal deviation, depression of the diaphragm, and a deep sulcus sign (a deep costophrenic angle; see Chapter 6) are all radiographic findings suggesting tension pneumothorax. The clinical state of the patient is the most important factor, so the patient should be assessed for signs of obstructive shock such as hypotension and tachycardia. Difficulty ventilating an intubated patient is a clinical sign of tension pneumothorax.

As described in Chapter 6, ultrasound and CT are believed to be more sensitive for pneumothorax than is chest x-ray, although the clinical importance of a small pneumothorax found by these modalities is debated.

Pneumopericardium and Pneumomediastinum

Pneumopericardium and **pneumomediastinum** are described in detail in Chapter 6. The radiographic appearance of air in the pericardial sac or mediastinum is a thin black line outlining the heart, often extending into the superior mediastinum (Figures 5-154 through 5-156; see also Figure 5-153). Air may be visible on both the frontal and the lateral projections. On the lateral view, a black line may be seen separating the anterior

Figure 5-43. Chronic obstructive pulmonary disease (COPD). A, Posterior-anterior (PA) upright chest x-ray. **B,** Lateral upright chest x-ray. This 63-year-old male with a history of COPD presented with 2 weeks of worsening cough with yellow sputum and dyspnea. His oxygen saturation was 87% in the emergency department. As in Figure 5-42, this patient has evidence of hyperinflation, with flat diaphragms (particularly evident on the lateral x-ray, **B**). The patient also has a blunted right costophrenic angle with an apparent effusion and increased densities in both the right and the left lung base **(A)**. The lateral x-ray also shows increased density overlying the inferior thoracic spine, an abnormal spine sign. Findings of pleural effusions and pneumonia are discussed in detail in other figures.

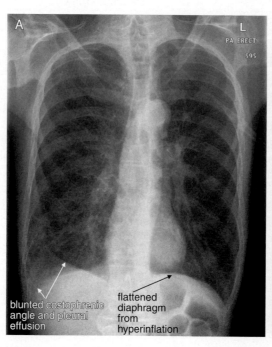

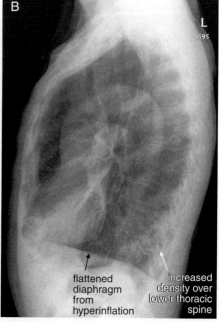

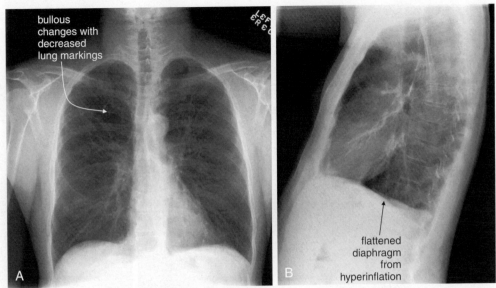

bullous changes with decreased lung markings

LEFT ERECT

flattened diaphragm from hyperinflation

Figure 5-44. Bullae in chronic obstructive pulmonary disease (COPD). A, Posterior-anterior (PA) upright chest x-ray. **B,** Lateral upright chest x-ray. In emphysema, destruction of alveoli results in formation of bullae, which may have an appearance similar to pneumothorax with a paucity of lung markings. Bullae may be single or multiple. As disease progresses, they may coalesce into a single, large bulla. Asymmetry from left to right and even within a single lung is common. This 46-year-old male with COPD presented with cough and increased shortness of breath over a 3-week period. **A,** His chest x-ray shows large bullae in the right upper lobe. **B,** His lateral x-ray also shows flattened diaphragms typical of COPD. See close-up from the same patient in Figure 5-45.

surface of the heart from fat in the retrosternal space. A **continuous diaphragm sign** may be seen (see Figures 5-154 through 5-156). This sign occurs when pericardial air is present beneath the heart. Normally, the upper surfaces of the right and left domes of the diaphragm (water density) are visible, silhouetted against the lung parenchyma (air density). The central surface of the diaphragm is not usually visible, as the diaphragm, pericardium, and myocardium are in physical contact and share the same density. When air is present within the pericardium, it is visible as a thin black line between the diaphragm and the inferior surface of the heart. This line of pericardial air visually connects the right and left diaphragms, creating the continuous diaphragm sign.

Outside of the setting of trauma, pneumopericardium and pneumomediastinum can occur with barotrauma from asthma or COPD, forceful cough, repeated vomiting, or forceful valsalva, sometimes seen with cocaine or marijuana use. An associated pneumothorax should be sought during the review of the chest x-ray. The clinical history is extremely important to determine the likely source of mediastinal or pericardial air: the respiratory or gastrointestinal tract. If the source is determined to be the respiratory tract, and no large pneumothorax or persistent air leak is found, no further evaluation or treatment may be needed. However, if the source of mediastinal air is the gastrointestinal tract, as with an esophageal tear from forceful vomiting (Figure 5-157), life-threatening mediastinal infection may result. A suspected gastrointestinal source of pneumomediastinum should be further evaluated using a contrast esophagram, discussed in more detail in Chapters 4 and 9.

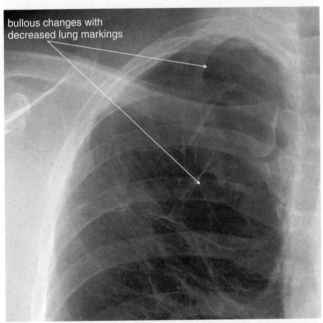

bullous changes with decreased lung markings

Figure 5-45. Bullae in chronic obstructive pulmonary disease. Close-up of bullous changes from the same patient as Figure 5-44. The walls of the large bullae are visible, and a paucity of lung markings makes these regions appear abnormally lucent (black).

Occasionally, pneumomediastinum, pneumopericardium, and pneumothorax may be the result of a persistent air leak from the lung or tracheobronchial tree. **Subcutaneous emphysema** (Figure 5-158) may be significant in these cases and may be the patient's presenting complaint. Increasing subcutaneous emphysema suggests a continued air leak. In the absence of trauma, air leaks of this type are often the

Figure 5-46. Bullae in chronic obstructive pulmonary disease (COPD). **A,** Posterior-anterior (PA) chest x-ray. **B,** Lateral chest x-ray. This 77-year-old female has severe COPD with extensive bullous changes of both upper lungs. **A,** Note how lucent (black) the upper lungs appear compared with the lower lungs. Figures 5-47 and 5-48 show a close-up of this finding and then a CT scan from the same patient.

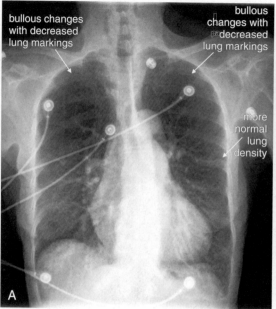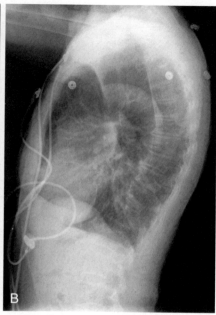

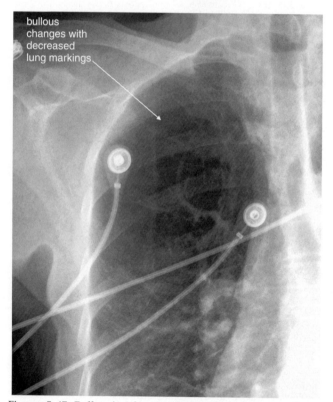

Figure 5-47. Bullae in chronic obstructive pulmonary disease (COPD). Same patient as Figure 5-46. In the lung apex, the normal lung has been replaced by large bullae, which are air-containing regions lacking the normal parenchymal supporting structures and blood vessels. Consequently, these areas do not attenuate the x-ray beam and look blacker than normal lung on chest x-ray. Compare with the CT scan from the same patient in Figure 5-48.

result of surgical procedures such as thorascopic lung resections. In the presence of large amounts of subcutaneous air, the underlying lung may be difficult to evaluate because of the overlying soft-tissue artifacts. CT is sometimes necessary and allows evaluation of deeper structures regardless of the presence of soft-tissue air.

Aortic Pathology

Aortic trauma is discussed in detail in Chapter 6. Nontraumatic aortic dissection and aortic aneurysm are discussed in Chapter 7. Please refer to these chapters for dedicated discussion and figures on x-ray and CT findings of these disease processes.

Pulmonary Embolism

Risk stratification and imaging of pulmonary embolism is discussed in detail in Chapter 7. Please see Chapter 7 for extensive figures on this topic.

Masses and Neoplastic Disease

Mass lesions on chest x-ray can have numerous appearances (Figures 5-159 through 5-175). Large mass lesions may appear spiculated or rounded (see Figures 5-159 through 5-162). Some mass lesions plug large airways to the affected lung segment, resulting in volume loss (see Figures 5-163 through 5-165). Masses can appear identical to consolidation from pneumonia, and as a consequence, radiologists typically recommend a repeat chest x-ray after clinical resolution of infectious symptoms to ensure that an underlying mass lesion is not present. Small primary masses or metastatic disease may appear as solitary or multiple nodular opacities (see Figures 5-166 through 5-175). Nipple shadows may simulate nodules; this problem can be resolved by adding external markers at the location of the nipples and obtaining a repeat chest x-ray. Aggressive malignancies may result in bony destruction of adjacent ribs or vertebral bodies. Pleural and pericardial effusions may be seen in association with masses. Masses may have associated mediastinal adenopathy.

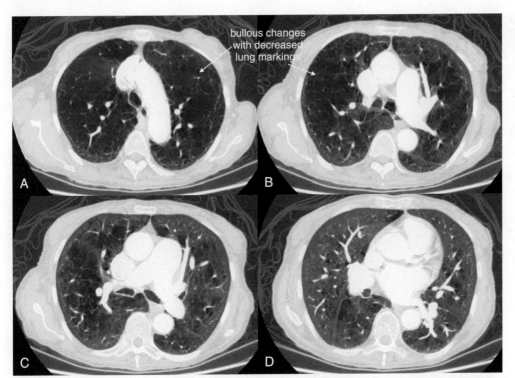

Figure 5-48. **Bullae in chronic obstructive pulmonary disease (COPD).** CT scan from the same patient as Figures 5-46 and 5-47, viewed on lung windows. Slice at the level of the aortic arch **(A)**, through the pulmonary artery **(B and C)**, and through the level of the left atrium **(D).** Note the severe bullous changes in the more cephalad slices. **D,** The lung parenchyma appears nearly normal in this more caudad slice.

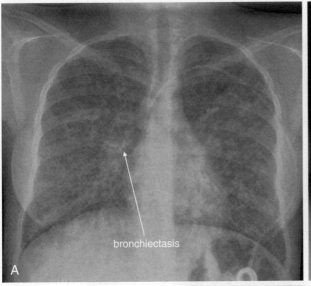

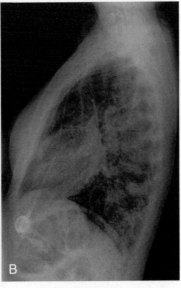

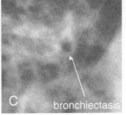

Figure 5-49. **Cystic fibrosis.** Cystic fibrosis is aptly named. Chest x-ray findings include increased interstitial density of fibrosis and cystic changes of lung parenchyma similar to chronic obstructive pulmonary disease. Bronchiectasis (dilatation of bronchi, potentially eroding into bronchial arteries and presenting with hemoptysis) may be visible on chest x-ray as large and thickened bronchioles, particularly when viewed in short axis (when bronchioles are oriented perpendicular to the frontal plane). This 15-year-old with cystic fibrosis presented with cough and dyspnea. Does she have pneumonia? Comparison with prior x-rays showed no changes. **A,** Posterior-anterior (PA) chest x-ray. **B,** Lateral chest x-ray. **C,** Close-up from **A** showing bronchiectasis.

Mediastinal Masses and Adenopathy. Mediastinal masses and adenopathy may widen the mediastinum on the frontal projection (Figures 5-176 through 5-178). On the lateral projection, the retrosternal space may be opacified, indicating a mass lesion (see Box 5-3) (Figures 5-179 through 5-182). Hilar adenopathy may be seen with malignancies, infections, and conditions such as sarcoidosis (Figures 5-183 and 5-184). CT scan may be necessary to distinguish a possible mediastinal mass from conditions as benign as hiatal hernia (Figures 5-185 and 5-186) or as life threatening as aortic aneurysm (discussed in detail in Chapter 7). Mediastinal masses

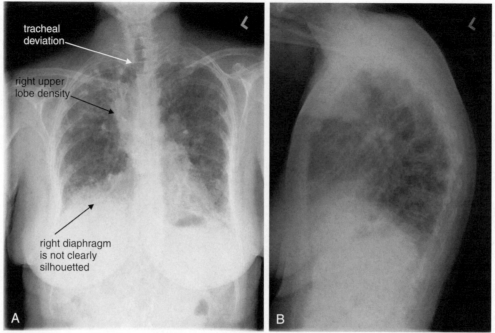

Figure 5-50. Idiopathic pulmonary fibrosis. This patient with idiopathic pulmonary fibrosis presented with increased dyspnea. The x-ray shows diffuse predominantly peripheral irregular and reticular opacities. The trachea is deviated to the right, suggesting volume loss on the right side, although a mediastinal mass such as adenopathy could also cause this deviation. Both diaphragmatic silhouettes are obscured—raising the possibility of bibasilar infiltrates or atelectasis. The right upper lobe appears dense along the right upper border of the mediastinum—with the possibility of a mass, lobar collapse, or an infectious infiltrate. Patients with such chronically abnormal chest x-rays can be difficult to evaluate. Comparison with prior x-rays to assess chronicity of findings is essential. **A,** Posterior–anterior view. **B,** Lateral view.

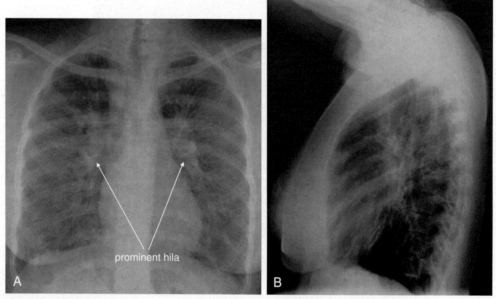

Figure 5-51. Chronic smoke inhalation. A, Posterior-anterior (PA) chest x-ray. **B,** Lateral chest x-ray. This 25-year-old female suffered a severe smoke inhalation injury when she was 12 years old and is oxygen dependent. She presented with increased dyspnea and an oxygen saturation of 81%. Her chest x-ray shows coarse reticular opacities throughout the lungs bilaterally. The hila are prominent bilaterally, suggesting possible secondary pulmonary hypertension from chronic hypoxia. Another cause of prominent hila is lymphadenopathy. Compare with the x-ray of cystic fibrosis in Figure 5-49 and that of idiopathic pulmonary fibrosis in Fiure 5-50. These chronic lung diseases share similar radiographic appearances and mandate comparison with prior x-rays whenever possible to determine the acuity of findings.

can result in superior vena cava syndrome (see Figures 5-179 through 5-182). Chest x-ray may detect the mass but does not evaluate compression or internal thrombosis of the superior vena cava, which is best assessed with CT with IV contrast.

Esophageal and Tracheal Foreign Bodies

Esophageal and tracheal foreign bodies are a common emergency department complaint, particularly in children. Dense foreign bodies composed of metal may be readily seen on chest x-ray. Other foreign

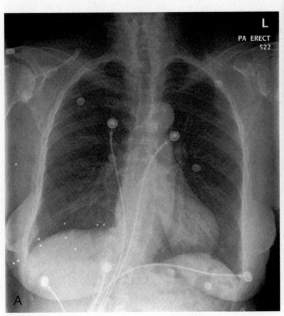

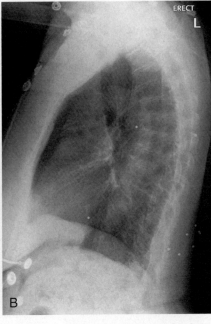

Figure 5-52. **Chronicity of chest x-ray findings. A,** Posterior-anterior (PA) upright chest x-ray. **B,** Lateral upright chest x-ray. This 80-year-old female presented with sudden dyspnea and syncope. Her workup revealed pulmonary embolism. Incidentally, her chest x-ray shows buckshot from a remote prior injury. Remember that chest x-ray findings are not necessarily acute and do not always explain acute symptoms. Comparison with prior x-rays can assist in determining chronicity.

bodies may be radiolucent and invisible on x-ray. In some cases, the presence of a foreign body may be deduced by its effect on lung inflation. An airway foreign body causing a ball–valve effect may cause unilateral hyperinflation, sometimes most visible on expiratory or lateral decubitus views (described earlier in dedicated sections on those specialized views). CT scan is accurate and can localize even low-density objects.

Esophageal foreign bodies often lodge at the thoracic inlet. If an esophageal foreign body is suspected but is not visible by chest x-ray, a barium swallow can be performed and can outline a nonradiopaque esophageal foreign body.

Tracheal foreign bodies may lodge at multiple levels depending on object size relative to the patient's airway. Coins are a commonly aspirated or ingested foreign body. Classically, a coin appears en face as an "O" on the frontal view when lodged in the esophagus (Figure 5-187). A mnemonic for this is the British spelling, *oesophagus*. A coin in the trachea typically is turned "edge on" and appears as a linear opacity on the frontal chest x-ray, coaxed into this position by the incomplete tracheal cartilages, which are open posteriorly.

Chest X-ray Findings of Traumatic Injury

Chest x-ray and adjunctive imaging evaluation of traumatic injury is discussed in detail in Chapter 6. Please see Chapter 6 for a discussion of pneumothorax, pulmonary contusion, diaphragm rupture (also discussed in Chapter 10), rib and sternal fractures, and aortic injury.

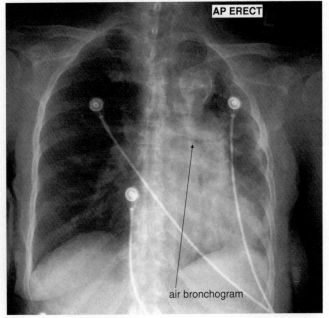

air bronchogram

Figure 5-53. **Air bronchograms.** Pulmonary alveolar fluid accumulation results in air bronchograms—the silhouetting of the air-filled (normal) bronchi by fluid-filled (abnormal) alveoli. Normally bronchi are not seen except when they are directly oriented perpendicular to the plane of the x-ray. The reason is simple; as described in the discussion of chest x-ray in the text, the borders of two tissues will not be seen on chest x-ray if they are immediately adjacent and share the same tissue density. Normally, bronchi (air density) and alveoli (air density) cannot be distinguished. The thin walls of bronchi do not attenuate the x-ray beam sufficiently to be visible unless a long segment is oriented perpendicular to the x-ray plane, which leads to the occasional appearance of a circular bronchiole. Compare with Figure 5-27.

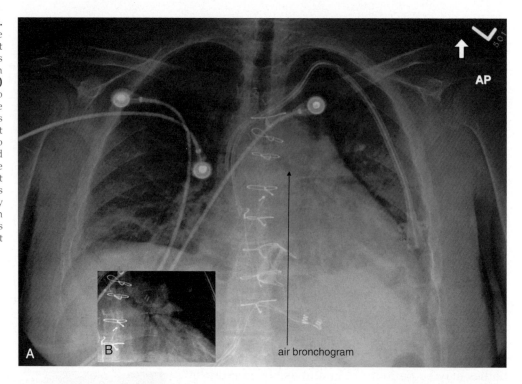

Figure 5-54. Air bronchograms. This patient again has a visible air bronchogram **(A)**, with the left main bronchus and its branches silhouetted like a tree turned on its side. The cropped view **(B)** has been contrast adjusted to make this even more evident. The appearance of air bronchograms is not specific for pneumonia but indicates that alveoli adjacent to an air-filled bronchus have filled with fluid, resulting in a difference in tissue density of two adjacent tissues. Look for air bronchograms in a dense chest, as these identify alveolar fluid. A pleural effusion would not give this appearance, as air-filled alveoli would persist next to the air-filled bronchi.

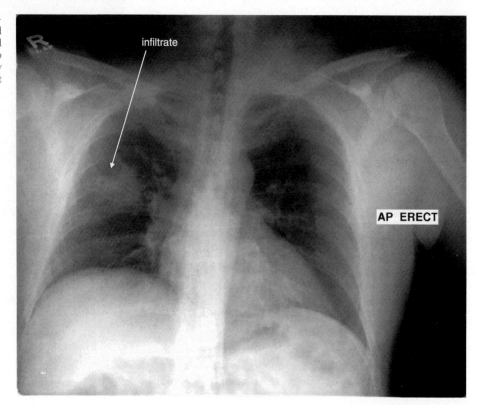

Figure 5-55. Pneumonia. This 37-year-old patient with Crohn's disease presented with fever, tachycardia, and increased abdominal pain. Abdominal CT showed no evidence of acute pathology, but chest x-ray showed a right midlung opacity consistent with pneumonia.

CHEST X-RAY EVALUATION OF MEDICAL DEVICES

Chest x-ray is commonly used to evaluate the location of medical devices within the chest, as well as complications of their insertion. Endotracheal tubes, nasogastric and orogastric tubes, central venous catheters, and thoracostomy tubes are discussed in detail in Chapter 6. Please see the description of their assessment in that chapter. The discussion here supplements but does not replace the discourse in Chapter 6.

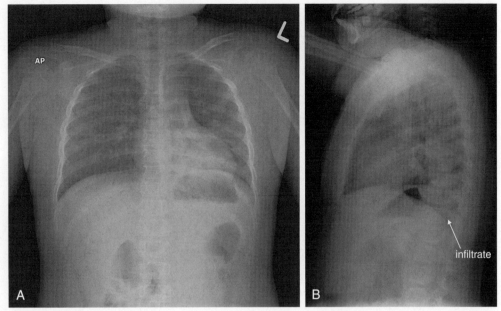

Figure 5-56. Pneumonia: Pediatric, left lower lobe. A, Anterior-posterior (AP) chest x-ray. **B,** Lateral chest x-ray. This 7-year-old presented with fever and 5 days of productive cough, now with orange sputum. **A,** Chest x-ray shows increased subtle density in the left lower lobe on the anterior–posterior (AP) x-ray. **B,** The lateral x-ray shows a definite increased density overlying the lower thoracic spine—a left lower lobe pneumonia. Recall that the thoracic spine normally appears progressively more lucent as it approaches the diaphragm, a finding called the spine sign. Lack of this progressive lucency suggests an overlying infiltrate. Returning to the AP x-ray, recall that a lingular pneumonia normally would obscure the left heart border because the lingula lies immediately adjacent to the lower heart. An upper lobe pneumonia would obscure the border of the upper left mediastinum, to which it is adjacent.

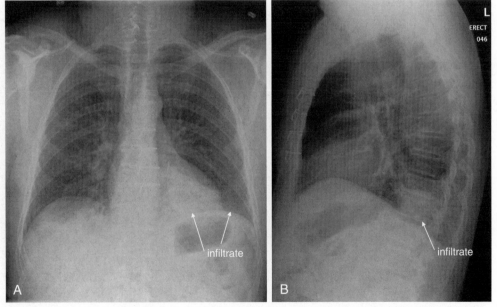

Figure 5-57. Pneumonia: Left lower lobe infiltrate with retrocardiac location. A, Posterior-anterior (PA) upright chest x-ray. **B,** Lateral upright chest x-ray. This 53-year-old male with a history of heart transplant presented with 1 week of fever, productive cough, dyspnea, and left-sided chest pain. He was febrile in the emergency department. **A,** His posterior–anterior (PA) chest x-ray appears fairly normal at first glance. Look at the lateral x-ray **(B),** however. A dense infiltrate overlies the thoracic spine in the retrocardiac space, interrupting the normal progressive lucency of the spine approaching the diaphragm. Looking back at the PA chest image, the heart appears quite dense in this location, and faint increased density is seen above the left diaphragm. This is a left lower lobe pneumonia.

Endotracheal Tubes

Chest x-ray is commonly obtained following endotracheal intubation to assess endotracheal tube position. *It is essential to recognize that chest x-ray assesses the depth of endotracheal tube insertion, not correct tracheal placement.* Because the esophagus lies deep to the trachea and both are midline structures, a frontal projection chest x-ray cannot distinguish tracheal from esophageal intubation. Other factors, including direct visualization of the endotracheal tube passing through the vocal cords during intubation, the presence of appropriate end-tidal carbon dioxide production, oxygen saturation, the presence of

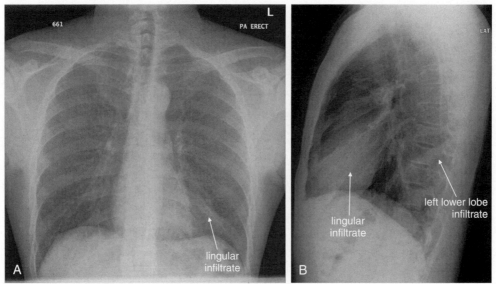

Figure 5-58. Pneumonia: Lingula and left lower lobe. A, Posterior-anterior (PA) upright chest x-ray. **B,** Lateral upright chest x-ray. This 27-year-old male presented with chills, nausea, and anterior inferior left chest pain. His chest x-ray shows a lingular and left lower lobe pneumonia. Remember that the lingula lies anterior and abuts the left heart border—an infiltrate is seen in this location on both the posterior–anterior (PA) **(A)** and lateral **(B)** views. Note how the left heart border is indistinct because of the infiltrate on the PA view. On the lateral view, the lingular infiltrate has the appearance of a dense wedge with discrete borders. Also on the lateral view, a second area of increased density is seen, indicating a left lower lobe infiltrate. It overlies the spine, again interrupting the normal increased lucency as the spine approaches the diaphragm. The importance of the lateral x-ray for diagnosing pneumonia cannot be overemphasized. Figure 5-59 shows the same patient 5 days later.

Figure 5-59. Pneumonia: Lingula and left lower lobe. A, Posterior-anterior (PA) upright chest x-ray. **B,** Lateral upright chest x-ray. Same patient as Figure 5-58, now 5 days later. The patient returned with worsened symptoms. **A,** Note how the lingular infiltrate has now significantly hidden the left heart border. **B,** The retrocardiac left lower lobe infiltrate persists.

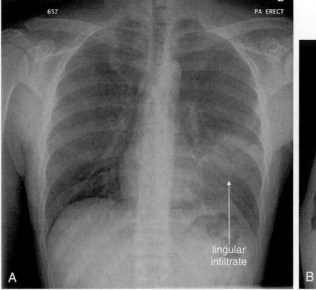

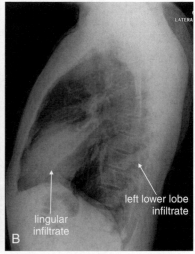

bilateral breath sounds, and the absence of gastric air sounds during ventilation, should be used in conjunction with the chest x-ray. Chest x-ray alone should never be used to confirm correct endotracheal positioning.

On chest x-ray, the distal tip of the endotracheal tube should be positioned no deeper than approximately 1 to 3 cm above the carina and no higher than the suprasternal notch. Deeper insertion may lead to right main bronchus intubation if the patient's neck becomes flexed or if the tube is advanced farther. Insertion to a depth shallower than the suprasternal notch risks accidental

extubation (withdrawal of the endotracheal tube to a supraglottic position) if the patient's neck is extended or if the tube is retracted farther.

Right main bronchus intubation (see Figure 5-39) is a common complication of endotracheal intubation and should be routinely suspected and assessed for on chest x-ray. Clinical assessment should also be performed for decreased breath sounds on the patient's left side. If not corrected rapidly, right main bronchus intubation can be followed by complete collapse of the left lung. Chest x-ray findings include volume loss in the left chest, with

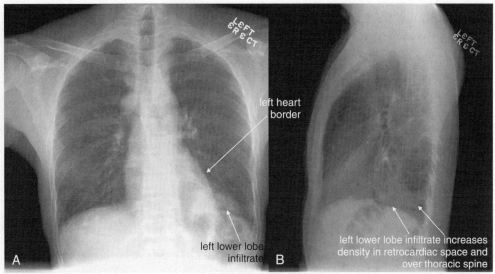

Figure 5-60. Pneumonia: Left lower lobe. This 35-year-old male with a history of renal transplantation presented with dyspnea, fever, and chest pain. His posterior–anterior (PA) upright chest x-ray **(A)** shows a left lower lobe density, also seen as a retrocardiac density on the lateral x-ray **(B)**. Note on the PA view how the left heart border can still be seen, as the infiltrate does not directly abut that border but rather lies posterior to it. Remember that the retrocardiac space is usually quite black, and the thoracic spine should be progressive more lucent (black) as it approaches the diaphragm on lateral chest x-ray. Both of these rules are violated in this case because of the left lower lobe infiltrate. Always inspect the lateral x-ray for these features. Also compare this lateral x-ray to the lateral x-ray in Figure 5-59, which showed a density in the lingula. The immediate retrocardiac space in that x-ray was clear.

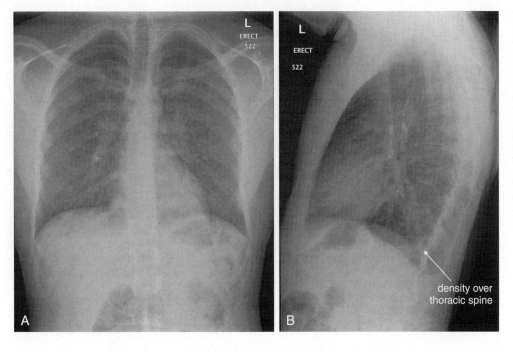

Figure 5-61. Pneumonia, visible on lateral x-ray. This 27-year-old male presented with 2 days of myalgias, fever, and productive cough. Look first at the posterior–anterior chest x-ray **(A)**. Do you see an infiltrate? The right and left heart borders and diaphragms are clear. The lung fields do not show an infiltrate. Now look at the lateral x-ray **(B)**. An abnormal density overlies the inferior thoracic spine, interrupting the normal progressive darkening as the spine approaches the diaphragm. This is the only sign of pneumonia. Always inspect the lateral chest x-ray for the spine sign.

tracheal and mediastinal shift to the left (see the section earlier in this chapter on volume loss). This is usually rapidly corrected with appropriate repositioning of the endotracheal tube. Sometimes right main bronchus intubation occludes large branches of the right bronchus, with segmental collapse, most often of the right upper lobe.

Central Venous Catheters

Chest x-ray can detect misplaced central venous catheters whose course does not follow the intended vascular anatomy (Figure 5-188). For example, a catheter inserted into the subclavian vein may be found to ascend the neck, suggesting an improper course into the internal jugular vein rather than descent into the superior vena cava. An internal jugular catheter may turn laterally toward the shoulder, rather than medially, suggesting accidental subclavian vein placement. It is essential to recognize that even these findings do not rule out the more serious complication, arterial catheterization. A catheter placed into the carotid artery and advanced into the subclavian artery would have a similar chest x-ray appearance. Though it is commonly requested

Figure 5-62. **Pneumonia: Pediatric.**
A, Posterior-anterior (PA) chest x-ray. **B,** Cross-table lateral chest x-ray. **C,** close-up from **A**. This 5-month-old was born at 27 weeks of gestation and presented with cough. **A,** The posterior–anterior chest x-ray shows increased density in the right upper lobe, consistent with pneumonia. In addition, an air bronchogram is visible along the right heart border (see **C,** close-up from **A**).

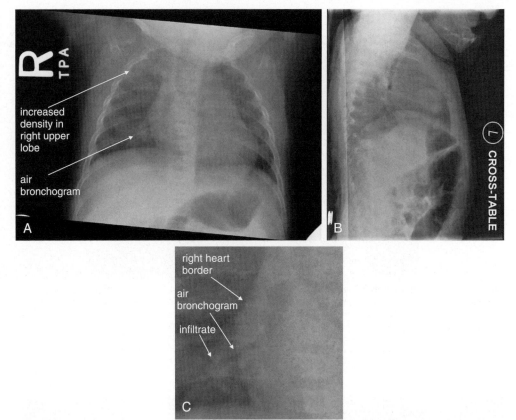

Figure 5-63. **Pneumonia: Right middle lobe. A,** Anterior-posterior (AP) chest x-ray. **B,** Lateral chest x-ray. This 73-year-old male presented with cough with yellow sputum, fever 39.3°C, tachycardia, and oxygen saturation of 93% on room air. His chest x-ray shows a classic right middle lobe pneumonia. **A,** This opacity obscures the right heart border, which lies immediately adjacent. **B,** On the lateral x-ray, this appears as a more circumscribed density overlying the heart.

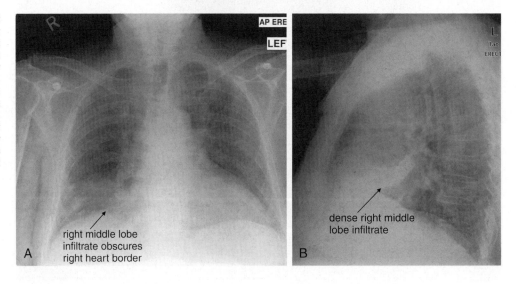

that a chest x-ray be performed before the use of a central venous catheter to confirm correct placement, chest x-ray does not confirm intravenous insertion. Other factors, including the absence of pulsatile blood suggesting arterial placement, the ease of infusion through the catheter, and ultrasound assessment of the catheter position, can be used with chest x-ray to assess catheter location. In cases of particular uncertainty, blood gas sampling or transduction of central venous pressure waveforms may be useful. The major functions of the chest x-ray are to determine the depth of insertion of the catheter and to evaluate for pneumothorax. A central venous catheter should terminate in the lower superior vena cava, above the right atrium.

Thoracostomy and gastric tubes are discussed in Chapter 6. An improperly placed gastric tube may be seen coiled in the hypopharynx or esophagus on chest x-ray. More subtle but critical misplacement in the trachea and bronchus may be seen as a gastric tube that deviates right or left from the midline at the level of the carina (Figure 5-189). Failure to recognize this can be fatal, if lavage fluids or feeding solutions are passed into the lung through the misplaced gastric tube.

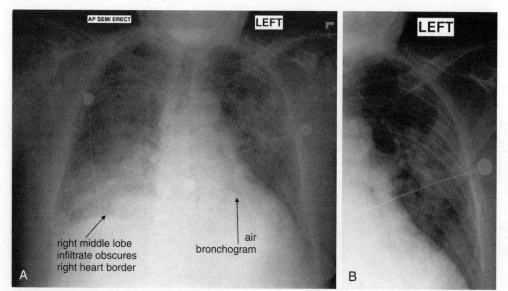

Figure 5-64. Pneumonia: Right middle lobe and left upper lobe. A, Anterior-posterior (AP) chest x-ray. **B,** Close-up from **A.** Same patient as Figure 5-63, where his initial chest x-ray showed a classic right middle lobe pneumonia. This x-ray was obtained one week later, with a progressive density appearing to involve the entire right middle lobe. **A,** The right heart border remains obscured, and the right diaphragm is also partially hidden, which may indicate right lower lobe involvement or an associated pleural effusion. Increased density is also seen in the bilateral upper lungs. **B,** An air bronchogram is faintly visible behind the left heart.

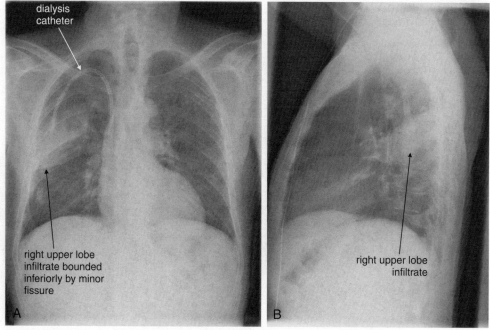

Figure 5-65. Pneumonia: Right upper lobe. A, Posterior-anterior (PA) chest x-ray. **B,** Lateral chest x-ray. This 46-year-old male with human immunodeficiency virus and end-stage renal disease presented with fever to 39.1°C, cough, and right chest pain. **A,** His PA chest x-ray shows a dense infiltrate in the right upper lobe, bounded inferiorly by the minor fissure. **B,** On the lateral x-ray, this appears bounded superiorly as well—this boundary identifies this as a right posterior segment upper lobe infiltrate, though this level of anatomic localization is not necessary to the emergency physician. **A,** The curved density in the right chest is the patient's dialysis catheter.

Automatic Implantable Cardioverter–Defibrillators and Implanted Pacemakers

Chest x-ray can be used to evaluate the integrity of automatic implantable cardioverter–defibrillator (AICD) and pacemaker electrical leads (Figures 5-190 through 5-192). The leads should be visible originating from the

pacemaker or AICD, tracking in a path corresponding to great veins returning to the superior vena cava and then to the right atria and right ventricle. The correct position of the leads depends on the specific device; for example, some devices pace both ventricles. The wires should not be kinked, have discontinuities, or terminate in a location outside the atria or ventricles. Rarely, patients with Twiddler's syndrome may be found to have wound the electrical leads completely around the pacemaker or AICD by rotating the device inside its subcutaneous pocket.[28]

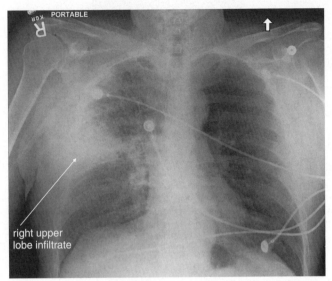

Figure 5-66. Pneumonia: Right upper lobe. This 71-year-old male with a history of prostate cancer presented with dyspnea, hemoptysis, and right-sided chest pain. His chest x-ray shows a wedge-shaped right upper lobe infiltrate, consistent with pneumonia. The patient grew *Haemophilus influenza* from blood cultures. This radiographic appearance can also be seen with pulmonary infarction from pulmonary embolism. Computed tomography was performed because of the patient's history of cancer and hemoptysis but was negative for pulmonary embolism.

Transvenous Pacemakers

Transvenous pacemakers placed in the emergency department should be assessed after placement using chest x-ray (Figures 5-193 through 5-197). Chest x-ray in this scenario performs several functions. First, it assesses for pneumothorax resulting from the insertion of the vascular catheter through which the pacemaker electrodes have been introduced. Second, it assesses the depth of insertion of the pacemaker electrode. Typically, this is a single electrical wire, terminating in the right ventricle to allow ventricular pacing. Ideally, the electrode should not be coiled or kinked. If extra loops of wire are present in the atria or ventricle, they may become a nidus for thrombus formation and may also induce premature ventricular contractions or other dysrhythmias from mechanical irritation of the ventricle. In some cases, the electrode may be found to have passed from the superior vena cava, through the right atrium, and into the inferior vena cava, rather than entering the right ventricle. Typically, this scenario would have been suspected from the failure of the transvenous pacemaker to achieve electrical capture of the ventricle. Although chest x-ray is important to assess for complications of the procedure, remember that the function of the transvenous pacemaker is more important than cosmetic considerations on chest x-ray. Resist the urge to reposition a coiled but functioning pacemaker electrode until the patient has been stabilized. Repositioning a coiled electrode may disturb the contact of the electrode with the ventricle and could result in failure to capture.

Figure 5-67. Pneumonia: Right upper lobe on computed tomography (CT) with IV contrast. Same patient as Figure 5-66. CT images show the extent of parenchymal opacification. Lung windows are shown; the soft-tissue windows were negative for pulmonary embolism. **A,** Axial CT lung window image. **B** and **C,** Coronal CT lung window images.

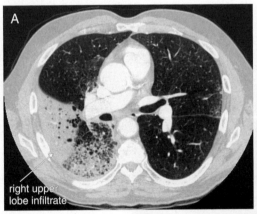
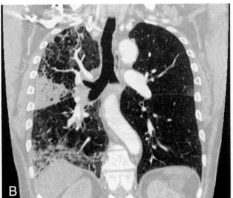
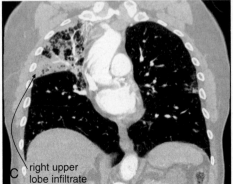

STRUCTURED AND SYSTEMATIC APPROACH TO CHEST X-RAY IMAGE INTERPRETATION

Now that we've reviewed basic principles of chest x-ray imaging, and features of pathologic conditions, we are ready to interpret the chest x-ray in a systematic fashion (Tables 5-8 and 5-9).

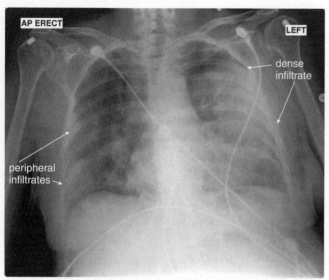

Figure 5-68. Pneumonia: Bilateral *(Streptococcus pneumoniae)*. This 58-year-old female with a history of multiple myeloma presented with back pain and dyspnea, as well as a temperature of 38.5°C and tachycardia to 150 beats per minute. Her chest x-ray shows bilateral infiltrates, including nearly complete opacification of the left chest with an obscured left heart border. Pulmonary embolism was suspected, as the patient had just returned from a long flight, but renal insufficiency allowed only noncontrast computed tomography (Figure 5-69), which cannot rule out thromboembolic disease. Her urine antigen test was positive for *S. pneumoniae,* which also grew from blood cultures. The patient died of septic shock.

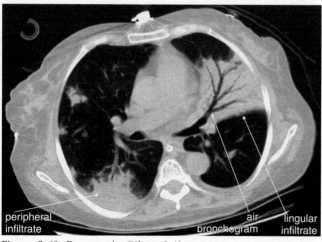

Figure 5-69. Pneumonia: Bilateral *(Streptococcus pneumoniae)* on computed tomography (CT) lung windows. Same patient as Figure 5-68. On lung windows, dense infiltrates are seen in the right posterior lung and lingula. Note how, even on CT, a lingular infiltrate hides the left heart border. A clear air bronchogram with a treelike form is seen because of adjacent alveoli filled with fluid. See how the lingular infiltrate is tightly circumscribed along its posterior border by a pleural boundary.

Whenever possible, view the chest x-ray using low ambient light conditions. Radiologists have the benefit of dark-adapting for long periods and viewing x-rays under low-light conditions. Emergency physicians more often view x-rays in fully lit rooms or immediately after dimming the room lights, compromising the eye's ability to adapt optimally. Nonetheless, using low light conditions can improve your ability to recognize subtle findings.

Assessing Chest X-ray Image Quality and Technique

Before beginning a systematic search of the chest x-ray image, look at the image as a whole to gain a general sense of the patient's anatomy and positioning. Consider the patient's age and gender, as these create a context and differential diagnosis for any imaging findings. This step is particularly important for a radiologist, who generally has not met or examined the patient. For the emergency physician, this step has generally occurred already during the history and physical examination, but taking a moment to refocus on these questions can be valuable.

Follow these basic steps to avoid errors in diagnosis (see Table 5-8). First, confirm that the image belongs to the patient in question. Second, confirm that the date of the image being viewed corresponds to the current or the desired date. Third, note the examination technique (e.g., PA or AP and supine or upright). As you have already discovered, a PA image gives a more accurate and less magnified view of the heart, so understanding which type of image you are viewing will help you to accurately assess heart size and mediastinal width. As discussed earlier, a supine film may not display air–fluid levels and may be less sensitive for detection of subdiaphragmatic air, so the patient's position at the time of the examination is important to assess. Assess for lordotic versus fully upright positioning. Lordotic positioning (positioning of the patient in only a semiupright position, with the upper thorax leaning backward) results in more horizontal appearance of the upper ribs compared with the fully upright technique.

Next, confirm left and right orientation (Figure 5-198). The conventional orientation of the image is with the patient's right side displayed on the left side of the screen or printed image, as if the examiner is facing the patient. The patient's position and left–right orientation are usually identified by radiopaque markers placed on the x-ray detector at the time of image acquisition. Although left–right orientation may appear obvious because of the usual orientation of the heart within the chest, rare cases of dextrocardia may occur. In these cases, without skin markers to indicate orientation, the image might be falsely assumed to be reversed, potentially leading to patient injury—for example, by erroneous placement of a thoracostomy tube on the wrong side of the patient. A more common human error may occur; an image may be loaded incorrectly into the digital radiography system, and erroneous labeling of the image is probably more likely than dextrocardia. Nonetheless, leave nothing to chance if questions exist about the patient's anatomy. If necessary, repeat a chest x-ray to confirm the heart's position.

Next, assess patient rotation. Rotation can create artifacts, such as apparent tracheal deviation or mediastinal shift. In addition, rotation of the patient artifactually widens the mediastinum, simulating pathology. Occasionally, rotation (an oblique view of the chest) is intentionally used for diagnostic purposes, but this is rarely done in the emergency department. Rotation may be assessed by examining the position of the medial heads

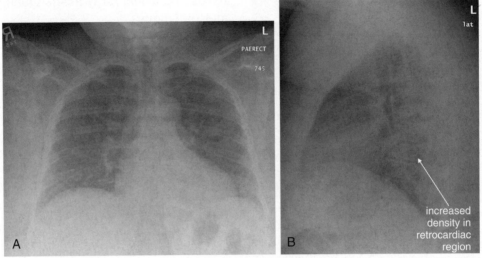

Figure 5-70. Pneumonia: Left lower lobe. A, Posterior-anterior (PA) chest x-ray. **B,** Lateral chest x-ray. This 41-year-old female presented with productive cough, dyspnea, subjective fever, and chills for 2 days. **A,** Her posterior–anterior chest x-ray appears essentially normal, although breast tissue overlies the lower lung fields, increasing their density. The heart and diaphragm borders are clear. **B,** On the lateral x-ray, increased density is seen in the retrocardiac region, consistent with left lower lobe pneumonia. The lateral chest x-ray may hold the only clues to diagnosis in some cases. Obtain a lateral x-ray when possible, and always inspect it carefully. The thoracic spine should become progressively more lucent as it approaches the diagram. Absence of this normal finding should suggest an infiltrate.

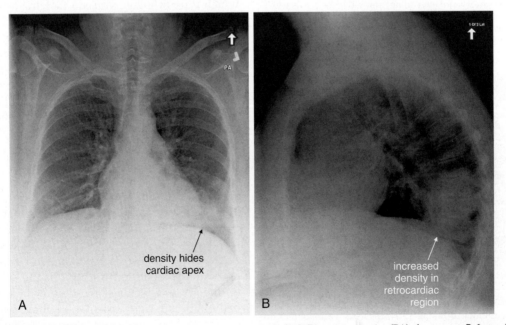

Figure 5-71. Pneumonia: Left lower lobe infiltrate (*Streptococcus pneumoniae*). A, Posterior-anterior (PA) chest x-ray. **B,** Lateral chest x-ray. This 51-year-old female with a history of chronic obstructive pulmonary disease presented with 2 days of cough with yellow sputum, fever (38.0°C), and chills. Her chest x-ray shows a density in the left lower lung. **A,** On posterior–anterior chest x-ray, all but the most inferior heart border (apex) is visible, with clear diaphragms. **B,** The lateral chest x-ray unequivocally shows a density in the retrocardiac space overlying the thoracic spine. The thoracic spine should become progressively more lucent as it approaches the diagram. Absence of this normal finding should suggest an infiltrate. The patient tested positive for *S. pneumoniae* by urine antigen and blood cultures.

of the clavicles relative to one another. If the patient is rotated, the more anterior clavicle will appear medially displaced (see Figure 5-21). To simulate this effect, sit in a swiveling chair and place your fingertips on your sternoclavicular joints. Sit facing fully forward, and then rotate right and left. Imagine the change in the position of your clavicular heads if a chest x-ray were performed with you in these positions. In addition to shifting the position of the clavicular heads, the distance between

the clavicular heads appears to narrow with an increasing degree of rotation from a true frontal position. The apparent width of the mediastinum may also change with this adjustment in position.

Assess the adequacy of lung expansion–inspiratory effort, as this can affect the apparent density of lung tissues and the size of pneumothoraces, as described earlier. Ideally, the patient should have 10 visible ribs above the diaphragm.

As described earlier, the chest x-ray exposure should be assessed. An overexposed film appears excessively black, as the detector or x-ray film has been fully exposed by excess radiation. An overexposed film loses most soft-tissue detail, but bony structures may be preserved, as these dense objects prevent through transmission of some radiation. An underexposed film appears excessively white, as not enough radiation has been applied to the patient to be transmitted through to the detector or film to change the color from white to black. Modern PACS displays allow adjustment of brightness and contrast, to some degree alleviating these issues, but no amount of adjustment of brightness and contrast can eliminate problems from substantial overexposure or underexposure.

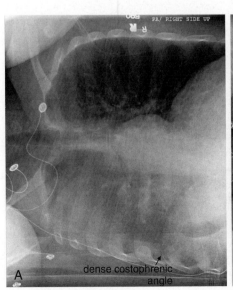

Figure 5-72. Pneumonia: Left upper lobe. This 41-year-old male with a history of hypertension and asthma failed outpatient pneumonia therapy. He presented with 6 days of fever, chills, and dyspnea with a rising white blood cell count to 31,000 per cubic millimeter despite oral azithromycin. His left chest appears almost completely opacified. The left heart border cannot be seen, although the left diaphragm is still faintly visible. A dense infiltrate or possible pleural effusion was considered. In the upright position, a pleural effusion would be expected to hide the diaphragm, as pleural fluid shares the same density with the diaphragm. Additional imaging was performed to evaluate further (Figures 5-73 and 5-74).

A final key step in interpretation of chest x-rays and other diagnostic imaging is to compare the current examination with previous images from the same patient. In some cases, a glaring abnormality on the current examination may be found to be unchanged or even improved from prior examinations and therefore not the likely cause of current acute symptoms. Unnecessary diagnostic testing and therapeutic interventions may be prevented by such comparison. In other cases, a subtle abnormality on the current examination may prove to

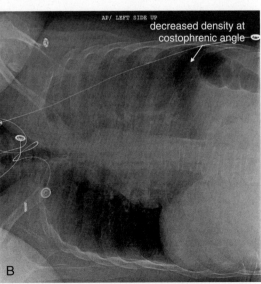

Figure 5-73. Pneumonia: Left upper lobe. Same patient as in Figure 5-72. **A,** Left lateral decubitus x-ray. **B,** Right lateral decubitus x-ray. Decubitus views were obtained in an attempt to identify an effusion if present. No significant change is seen in the density of the left lung with these positional changes. The left costophrenic angle appears slightly more lucent when the left chest is positioned higher, suggesting that a small effusion may have contributed to its density when the left chest is down. Computed tomography was performed to further evaluate this (Figure 5-74).

be new compared with prior images and thus cause for concern, with further diagnostic testing or treatments being indicated.

Systematic Search of the Chest X-ray

After assessing the chest x-ray image, conduct a systematic search of all regions of the image, rather than gazing at the image center and relying on peripheral vision to reveal abnormalities. Because the maximum image resolution is obtained by centering an image on the fovea of your eye, centering your vision on each region of the chest x-ray in turn is necessary, in addition to taking an overall view of the image.

Many algorithms have been proposed for the systematic review of the chest x-ray. All share a common feature: they force the reader to analyze all major elements of the image comprehensively, rather than allowing an unstructured image review that may be prematurely terminated when an abnormality is seen. We have described in detail already the normal and pathologic appearance of many thoracic structures. Inspect each structure or region sequentially, using the mnemonic **ABCDEFFL** (Table 5-9). Do not allow yourself to complete your interpretation until you have visited each letter of the mnemonic and performed an appropriate review of the findings.

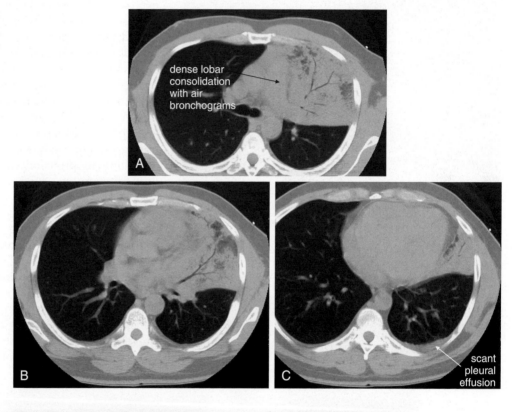

Figure 5-74. Pneumonia: Left upper lobe on computed tomography (CT) lung windows. CT demonstrated dense consolidation of the left upper lobe and lingula with air bronchograms. Only trace pleural fluid was seen. **A,** An axial slice at the level of the superior mediastinum. **B,** A slice through the middle of the heart. **C,** A slice through the lower heart.

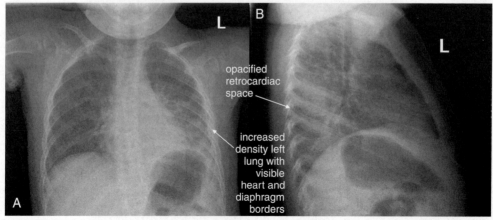

Figure 5-75. Pneumonia: Left lower lobe infiltrate. A, Posterior-anterior (PA) chest x-ray. **B,** Lateral chest x-ray. This previously healthy 2-year-old presented with increased work of breathing. **A,** His chest x-ray shows increased density in the left chest, although the diaphragm and left heart border remain visible on the posterior–anterior x-ray. This suggests a left lower lobe pneumonia. This is confirmed by the lateral x-ray **(B),** which shows dense opacification in the entire retrocardiac space. The thoracic spine is completely hidden by this opacity.

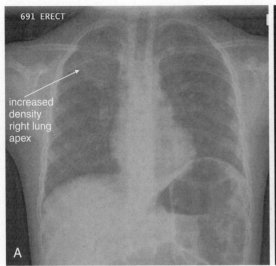

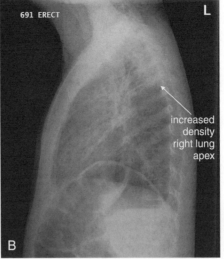

Figure 5-76. Pneumonia: Pediatric, right upper lobe. This 9-year-old female presented with fever to 39.0°C and 4 days of cough with tachypnea. Her posterior–anterior chest x-ray **(A)** shows increased density in the right upper lobe, more impressive on the lateral view **(B)**.

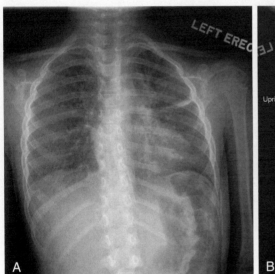

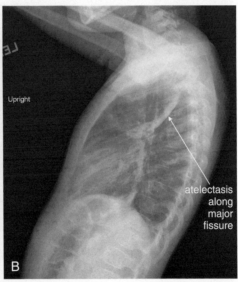

Figure 5-77. Pneumonia: Pediatric, bilateral versus asthma. A, Posterior-anterior (PA) chest x-ray. **B,** Lateral chest x-ray. This 6-year-old female with a history of asthma had been admitted recently for an asthma exacerbation and returned with hypoxia to 80% on room air. **B,** Her lateral chest x-ray shows an area of increased density along the major fissure, interpreted by the radiologist as atelectasis. She has other streaky opacities on posterior–anterior x-ray **(A)**. She improved with albuterol and steroids and was not treated with antibiotics, so presumably this was not a case of bacterial pneumonia.

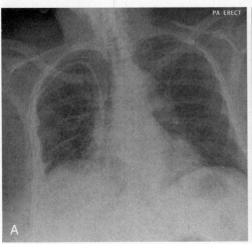

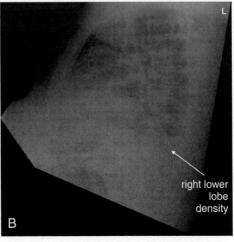

Figure 5-78. Pneumonia: Right lower lobe. A, Posterior-anterior (PA) chest x-ray. **B,** Lateral chest x-ray. This 66-year-old female with end-stage renal disease presented with fever and right upper abdominal pain. Her chest x-ray shows a right lower lobe opacity, best seen on the lateral x-ray as a density in the retrocardiac space. Is this real? A CT scan (Figure 5-79) confirmed the finding. Does it represent pneumonia or atelectasis? We lack an independent gold standard. The patient's blood cultures grew *Staphylococcus aureus*, and she improved with antibiotic therapy.

Figure 5-79. Pneumonia: Right lower lobe on CT lung windows. Same patient as Figure 5-78. CT was performed because of concern for abscess, as the patient had abdominal pain and an indwelling dialysis catheter that could be a source for bacteremia. On lung windows, an area of increased density is visible in the right lower lobe, corresponding to the area of increased density on her lateral chest x-ray (Figure 5-78). This is likely pneumonia—the patient's blood cultures grew *Staphylococcus aureus*. **A,** Axial view. **B,** Coronal view.

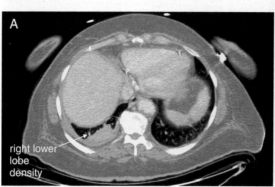
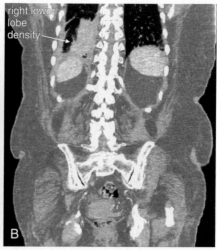

Figure 5-80. Pneumonia: Pediatric, right middle lobe. **A,** Anterior-posterior (AP) chest x-ray. **B,** Lateral chest x-ray. This 12-month-old was born at 31 weeks and presented with cough, tachypnea, and hypoxia to 85% when sleeping. The chest x-ray shows an irregular right heart border, likely indicating an infiltrate in this region. **A,** On frontal projection, the right middle lobe abuts the heart, and an infiltrate in this location obscures the right heart border. Incidentally, the left diaphragm appears elevated, with the possibility of herniated abdominal contents. This is also seen on the lateral view **(B).**

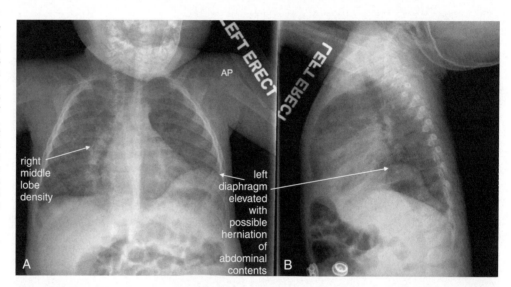

Figure 5-81. Pneumonia: Right middle lobe. This 39-year-old presented with right-sided chest pain, fever, chills, and a productive cough. **A,** Her posterior–anterior chest x-ray shows a right middle lobe opacity, even more impressive on the lateral view **(B)** as a dense, wedge-shaped opacity overlying the heart. This is a right middle lobe pneumonia. Notice how on the PA view this might be mistaken for a breast shadow, but the lateral view confirms the abnormality.

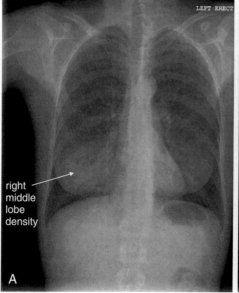
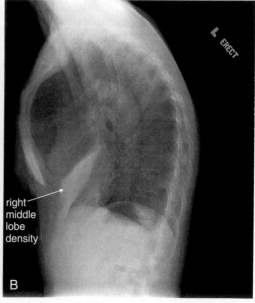

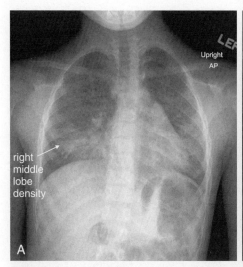
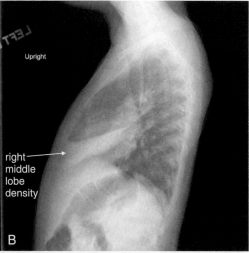

Figure 5-82. Pneumonia: Pediatric, right middle lobe. This 4-year-old female presented with 3 days of cough and upper abdominal pain. She was febrile and tachypneic in the emergency department. Her chest x-ray shows bilateral densities. **A,** On the anterior–posterior view, the right heart border is obscured by a right middle lobe opacity, and air bronchograms are visible just right of the thoracic spine. **B,** On the lateral view, the right middle lobe infiltrate is evident as a wedge-shaped density overlying the heart.

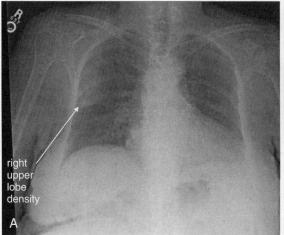
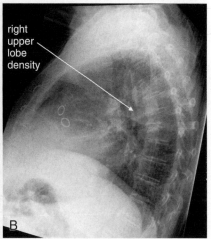

Figure 5-83. Pneumonia: Right upper lobe. This 87-year-old female presented for placement of a peripherally inserted central catheter (PICC) for treatment of a resistant *Escherichia coli* urinary tract infection. The patient had dementia and denied any complaints. Her chest x-ray, performed to assess the position of the PICC, showed a right upper lobe opacity, bounded inferiorly by the minor fissure. This is visible on both the frontal projection **(A)** and the lateral **(B)** x-rays.

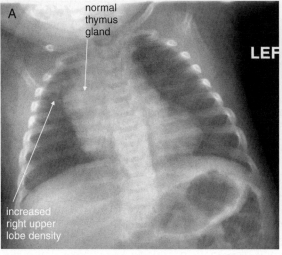
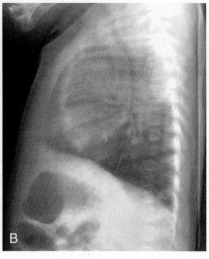

Figure 5-84. Pneumonia: Pediatric, right upper lobe. **A,** Frontal projection chest x-ray. **B,** Lateral chest x-ray. This 5-month-old female was born at 23 weeks. She presented with respiratory distress and hypoxia to 84% on room air. Her x-ray shows increased density in the right lung apex. Conservatively, this was interpreted and treated as pneumonia. The interpretation is made more complex by the normal broad mediastinum of young infants, which is due to the residual thymus. The increased density in the upper lobe may indicate upper lobe collapse as well. Note the increased upper chest density on the lateral x-ray.

PEARLS AND PITFALLS OF CHEST X-RAY INTERPRETATION

Emergency physicians typically differ from radiologists in their interpretation approach. Emergency physicians ask a specific question when viewing a radiograph or other test, and they may stop their interpretation prematurely once that question has been answered. For example, the emergency physician may ask, "Does this patient have pneumonia?" Once inspection of the lung parenchyma is completed, the emergency physician may fail to note subdiaphragmatic air—a surgical emergency.

Figure 5-85. **Pneumonia: Pedia-tric, right upper lobe. A,** Frontal projection chest x-ray. **B,** Lateral chest x-ray. Same patient as Figure 5-84. Follow-up x-rays the next day showed increased density along the right heart border, suggesting progression of pneumonia. Note the increased upper chest density on the lateral x-ray as well. On the lateral view, the retrosternal space appears dense because of the presence of the normal thymus.

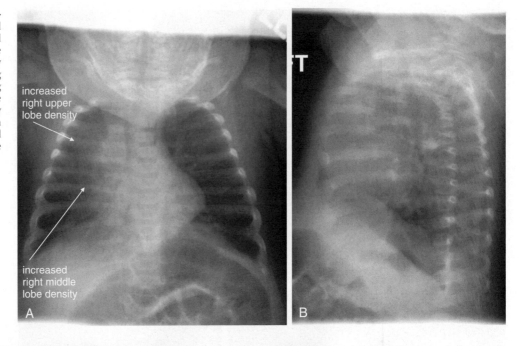

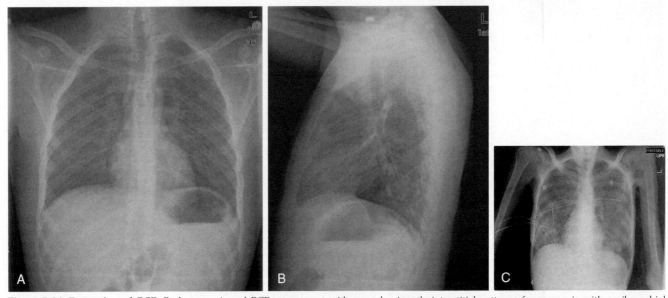

Figure 5-86. **Pertussis and PCP.** Both pertussis and PCP can present with a predominantly interstitial pattern of pneumonia with peribronchial cuffing. **A** and **B,** PA and lateral chest x-rays in a patient with pertussis. This 19-year-old male with sickle cell trait and short gut syndrome presented with cough and emesis. He had been seen multiple times in the emergency department over the past 3 weeks for moderately productive cough, diagnosed with bronchitis, and treated with azithromycin. His current presentation included 5 days of post-tussive emesis. His chest x-ray showed peribronchial cuffing and prominent interstitial markings but otherwise was near normal. His polymerase chain reaction test and cultures were positive for *Bordetella pertussis*, which does not typically cause a focal infiltrate on chest x-ray. Perhaps the most important point is to consider pertussis even with normal imaging findings when the clinical history is suggestive. Peribronchial cuffing is discussed in more detail in Figure 5-87. **C,** This 30 year old male with advanced AIDS presented with nonproductive cough and hypoxia. His chest x-ray shows a bilateral mixed alveolar and intertitial infiltrate pattern classic for PCP. Unfortunately, even a normal chest x-ray cannot exclude PCP.

Emergency physicians are thus subject to several important interpretation pitfalls that can be anticipated and avoided by self-conscious application of a series of questions (Table 5-10).

SUMMARY

The chest x-ray is an inexpensive, rapid, and low-radiation tool in emergency medicine, rich in diagnostic information. Evidence-based guidelines can assist in appropriate use. Understanding basic principles of chest x-ray technique and interpretation can assist the emergency physician in making the correct diagnosis, avoiding pitfalls, and recognizing when more advanced imaging such as CT is needed. A systematic approach to interpreting the chest x-ray image is essential to avoid misdiagnosis.

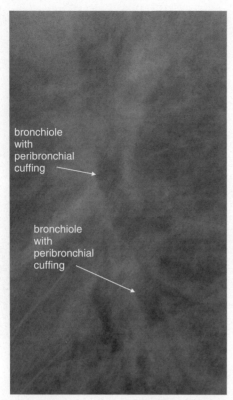

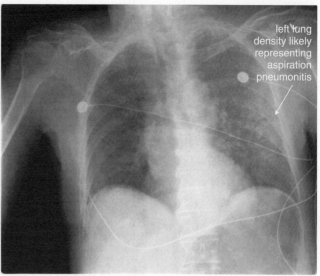

Figure 5-88. Aspiration pneumonitis: Reuben sandwich. This elderly male patient was eating a Reuben sandwich when he had sudden respiratory distress. Friends attempted cardiopulmonary resuscitation and the Heimlich maneuver and called 911. On emergency department arrival, the patient was in extremis. A Magill forceps was used to withdraw a large piece of roast beef from the patient's airway, with immediate improvement in the patient's cyanosis and mental status. However, the patient remained hypoxic. His chest x-ray shows an infiltrate, which is undoubtedly aspirated material, not an infectious process this soon after his event. Does aspiration have a unique appearance on chest x-ray? No, as we have discussed throughout this chapter, the appearance of tissues on x-ray is a function of density. Aspirated food material usually has soft-tissue density (fluid or water density), and the inflammatory response results in fluid and white blood cells moving into affected alveolar air spaces. The appearance ultimately is no different from that of a bacterial infection of the same lung segment. Classically, gravity leads aspiration to affect the right lower lobe when it occurs in the upright position and the posterior segments of upper lobes and superior segments of lower lobes if the patient is supine. Aspiration in the prone position involves the right upper lobe—a classic feature in patients with severe alcohol intoxication. In reality, any lobe can be affected.

Figure 5-87. Pertussis and peribronchial cuffing. Close-up from Figure 5-86, **B.** What is peribronchial cuffing? Peribronchial cuffing is edema of bronchioles, resulting from diverse causes including asthma, viral illnesses, heart failure, and pertussis. The bronchial wall becomes thickened and denser from edema fluid. Like an air bronchogram, this creates contrast with the air-filled bronchiole lumen, making it more visible. Normally, bronchioles are visible only when they are oriented perpendicular to the image plane. They are thin-walled and appear as discrete circles in short-axis cross section. When edema is present, the bronchiolar wall is thickened in cross section, and bronchioles may be seen in other orientations, such as long-axis cross section, because of their increased density. Look at the close-up of the hilum, taken from the lateral x-ray in the prior figure. You will see one bronchiole in short-axis cross section and several others in long-axis cross section. The density surrounding the air-filled lumen is the edematous bronchial wall.

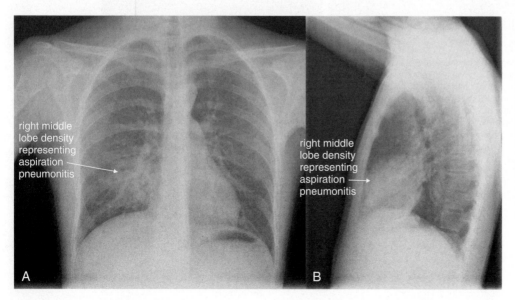

Figure 5-89. Aspiration: Gasoline. A, Posterior-anterior (PA) chest x-ray. **B,** Lateral chest x-ray. This 23-year-old male was siphoning gasoline by mouth when he swallowed a mouthful of gasoline with some inhalation. He coughed for approximately 1 minute afterward and presented with right-sided chest pain. His chest x-ray shows a right middle lobe opacity that obscures the right heart border on the posterior–anterior view **(A).** On the lateral x-ray **(B),** some increased density overlies the heart. Figure 5-90 shows progression on chest x-ray 24 hours later.

Figure 5-90. Aspiration: Gasoline. Same patient as Figure 5-89. In a chest x-ray obtained 24 hours after presentation, his right middle lobe infiltrate has progressed. **A,** Posterior-anterior (PA) chest x-ray. **B,** Lateral chest x-ray.

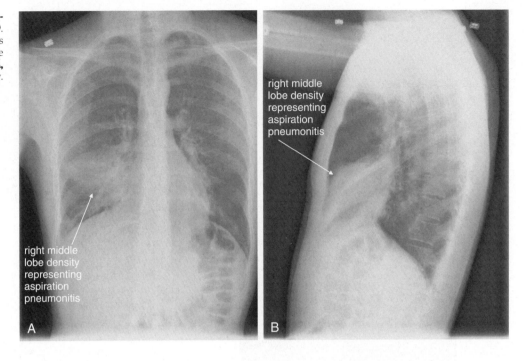

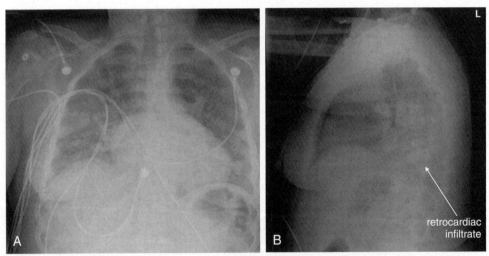

Figure 5-91. Acute chest syndrome: Sickle cell anemia. Acute chest syndrome of sickle cell anemia does not have a single pathognomonic appearance on chest x-ray. The condition is caused by microvascular sludging of sickled red blood cells, resulting in infarction of the lung from small vessel occlusion. In the face of parenchymal necrosis, fluid accumulates within alveoli, increasing the density of lung tissue from air density to soft-tissue density (fluid density). The radiographic appearance is indistinguishable from that of other pneumonias. Because the infarction occurs in small vessels, the distribution of infarction is not in the territory of a large vessel as might be seen with pulmonary embolism, where infarction of an entire lung segment distal to the point of thrombotic occlusion may be seen. Thus the distribution of lung infiltrates in acute chest syndrome may be patchy or may follow a lobar distribution. Because alveoli fill with fluid, air bronchograms may be seen, as in bacterial pneumonia. Making the diagnosis even more indistinct, patients with sickle cell anemia may have bacterial pneumonia with negative blood and sputum cultures, so a pulmonary infection may be wrongly labeled as acute chest syndrome. With these caveats, this x-ray is from a 24-year-old male with sickle cell anemia disease, presenting with fever and an oxygen saturation of 60% on room air. He improved with oxygen, fluids, and antibiotic administration, although antigen testing for *Streptococcus pneumoniae, Legionella,* and influenza were negative, as were cultures. **A,** The posterior-anterior (PA) chest x-ray demonstrates patchy bilateral infiltrates. The right lower lobe shows particular density, and increased density is seen in the retrocardiac space on the lateral x-ray **(B)**—note the absence of the usual decrease in density toward the diaphragm (see text introduction to chest x-ray and text section on the spine sign).

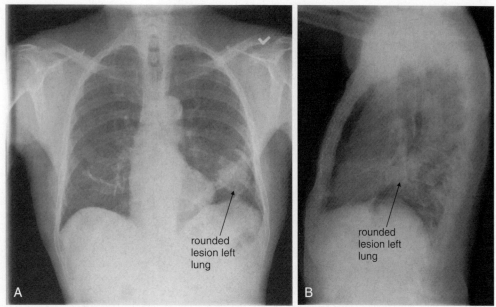

Figure 5-92. Possible tuberculosis or cavitary lesion. A, Posterior-anterior (PA) chest x-ray. **B,** Lateral chest x-ray. This 72-year-old male with a history of heart transplant presented with cough and 30-pound weight loss. His chest x-ray shows a rounded lesion in his left lung on posterior–anterior view **(A).** On the lateral view **(B),** this appears as increased density near the hilum. Given his immunosuppressed status, the differential diagnosis included tuberculosis, lung abscess, neoplasm, and fungal infection. He was readmitted for video-assisted thorascopic surgery and left upper lobe wedge resection. Pathology revealed only an organizing hematoma. Compare this x-ray with his CT in Figure 5-93.

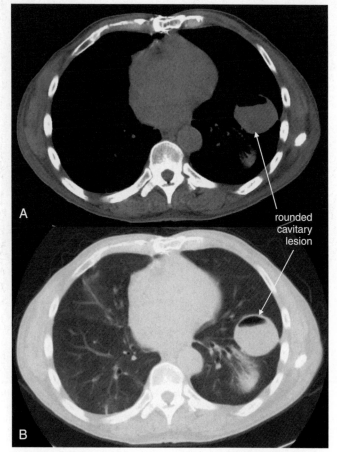

Figure 5-93. Tuberculosis or cavitary lesion. Chest CT without IV contrast from the same patient as Figure 5-92. Soft-tissue **(A)** and lung **(B)** windows show a well-circumscribed rounded lesion 4 cm in diameter with an air–fluid level. Given his immunosuppressed status, the differential diagnosis included tuberculosis, lung abscess, neoplasm, and fungal infection. He was readmitted for video-assisted thorascopic surgery and left upper lobe wedge resection. Pathology revealed only an organizing hematoma.

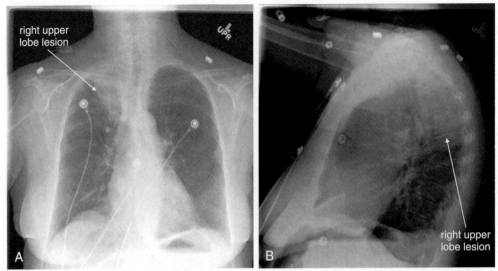

Figure 5-94. **Tuberculosis or cavitary lesion. A,** Posterior-anterior (PA) chest x-ray. **B,** Lateral chest x-ray. This 63-year-old female presented with weakness and hypotension. Her chest x-ray shows a right upper lobe infiltrate or mass—suspicious for malignancy or tuberculosis. The patient underwent bronchoscopy, but initial acid-fast bacilli (AFB) cultures and cytology were negative. She refused further workup and was lost to follow-up.

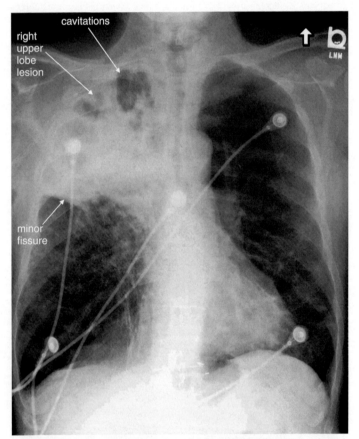

Figure 5-95. **Tuberculosis or cavitary lesion.** This 70-year-old male with chronic obstructive pulmonary disease presented with increasing dyspnea and cough with sputum production. He had a history of incarceration 15 years prior. His chest x-ray shows a dense right upper lobe infiltrate with areas of cavitation, concerning for abscess, tuberculosis, or malignancy. Note how the lesion stops sharply at the minor fissure inferiorly. Computed tomography was performed (Figure 5-96). The patient's purified protein derivative test and acid-fast bacilli (AFB) cultures were negative.

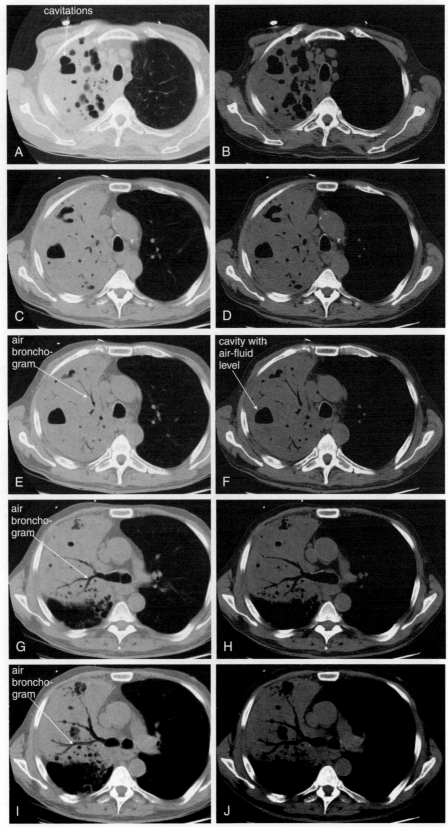

Figure 5-96. Tuberculosis or cavitary lesion. Same patient as Figure 5-95. Chest CT without IV contrast shows dense consolidation of the right upper lobe, with air bronchograms and multiple cavitary regions with air–fluid levels. These may represent infected bullae, areas of necrotizing pneumonia and abscess formation, or tuberculous cavitation. CT cannot discriminate among these causes. Left column **(A, C, E, G, I)**, axial slices viewed on lung windows, progressing from cephalad to caudad. Right column **(B, D, F, H, J)**, axial slices at the same anatomic levels as **A, C, E, G,** and **I** viewed on soft tissue windows.

Figure 5-97. Lung abscess. A, Posterior-anterior (PA) chest x-ray. **B,** Lateral chest x-ray. This 58-year-old male complained of 2 weeks of abdominal pain and fever. He noted pleuritic back pain with deep inspiration. **A,** His posterior–anterior chest x-ray appears normal, and once again the lateral x-ray provides important information. **B,** On the lateral view, a rounded density overlies the lower thoracic spine. The patient also grew methicillin sensitive *Staphylococcus aureus* from blood cultures, and chest computed tomography was performed to further evaluate the lesion (Figure 5-98).

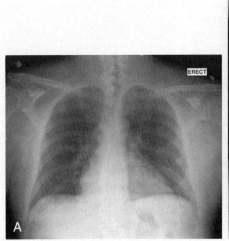

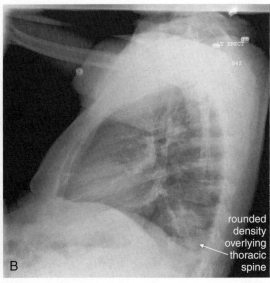

Figure 5-98. Lung abscess. Same patient as Figure 5-97. Chest CT with intravenous contrast shows a lung abscess located immediately right of the thoracic spine. The thick rim enhances with contrast, giving it a brighter white appearance. The center of the abscess contains fluid density *(dark gray)* with a tiny focus of air. This abscess corresponds to the retrocardiac density seen on the patient's chest x-ray. No air–fluid level was seen on chest x-ray because the abscess contains only small gas bubbles. **A,** Axial slice viewed on soft-tissue windows. **B,** The same slice viewed on lung windows. **C,** Close-up from **A.**

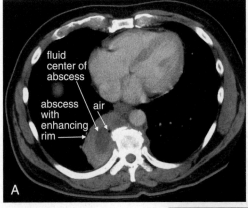

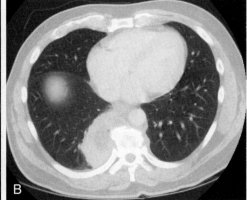

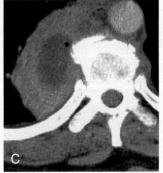

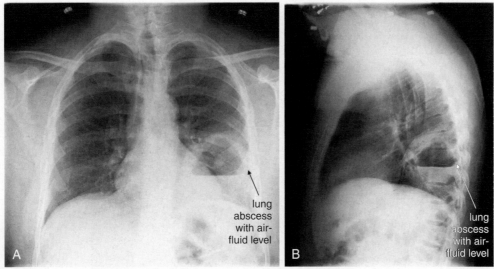

Figure 5-99. Lung abscess. A, Posterior-anterior (PA) upright chest x-ray. **B,** Lateral upright chest x-ray. This 39-year-old patient presented with cough, fever, and left-sided chest pain for the past 3 days, despite 5 days of antibiotic therapy for pneumonia. He admitted to daily alcohol use. His chest x-ray shows a definite left lung cavitary lesion with an air–fluid level, consistent with lung abscess. He underwent computed tomography (Figure 5-100) to further characterize this lesion. The patient was found to be human immunodeficiency virus positive with a CD4 count of 800. Two weeks after this presentation, the abscess began to drain spontaneously, with the patient coughing up grossly purulent material. Testing for tuberculosis was negative.

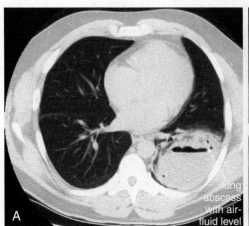

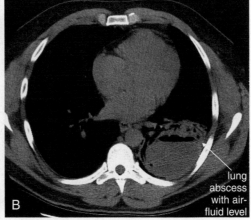

Figure 5-100. Lung abscess. Same patient as Figure 5-99. Chest CT without IV contrast. **A,** Lung windows. **B,** Same slice viewed on soft-tissue windows. This 9-cm left lung abscess has a thick rind and an air–fluid level. The patient was treated with antibiotics and 2 weeks later began to cough up grossly purulent sputum. Repeat CT showed a decreased air–fluid level suggesting spontaneous drainage of the abscess (Figure 5-101).

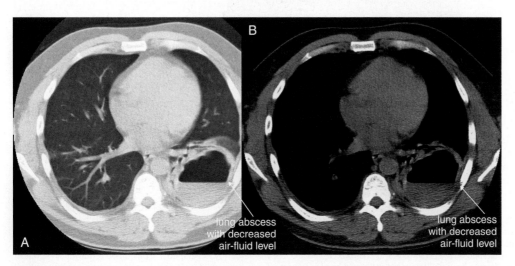

Figure 5-101. Lung abscess. Same patient as Figures 5-99 and 5-100. Chest CT without IV contrast. **A,** Lung windows, **B,** Soft-tissue windows. This chest CT was performed after 2 weeks of antibiotic therapy and showed a decreased air–fluid level suggesting spontaneous drainage of the abscess (compare with prior figure).

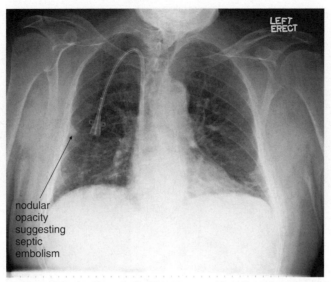

Figure 5-102. Septic emboli. This 72-year-old male with end-stage renal disease requiring hemodialysis presented with fever and 3 days of right axillary chest pain. A rounded nodular opacity is seen near the periphery of the right lung. Endocarditis with septic emboli was suspected, and chest computed tomography was performed (Figure 5-103).

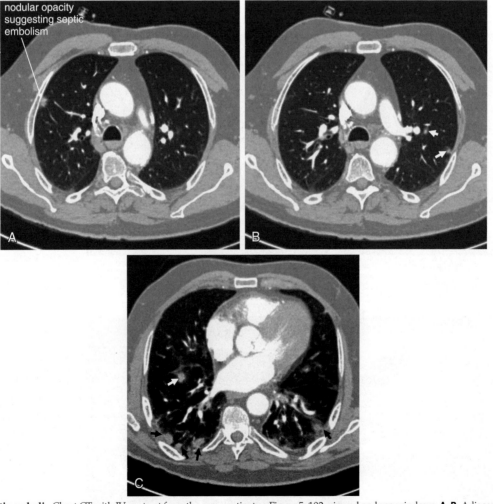

Figure 5-103. Septic emboli. Chest CT with IV contrast from the same patient as Figure 5-102, viewed on lung windows. **A, B,** Adjacent axial slices at the level of the proximal aorta and pulmonary artery. **C,** A more caudad slice through the heart. Multiple peripheral nodules are seen in the slices shown, labeled with *small arrows*. This is consistent with septic emboli, although metastatic disease could have the same appearance and cannot be differentiated on CT. However, the patient had no known primary malignancy, and his clinic course suggests that these were indeed septic emboli. The patient's blood cultures became positive for coagulase-negative *Staphylococcus epidermidis* and *Enterococcus faecalis*. He subsequently developed a septic ankle requiring washout in the operating room. His echocardiogram showed no valvular vegetations, and his dialysis catheter was removed, as it was the suspected source of infection.

TABLE 5-6. Chest X-ray Findings of Pulmonary Edema

Finding	Description
Cephalization	Pulmonary vascular markings are redistributed to upper lung zones on an upright x-ray.
Cardiomegaly	The ratio of the heart to the greatest transverse rib cage has a diameter >0.5.
Pericardial effusion	This may simulate cardiomegaly, but a water-bottle appearance is classically present.
Interstitial edema	Fluid appears in interstitial regions of the lung.
• Peribronchial cuffing	Thickening of the walls of bronchioles is seen when viewed end-on, perpendicular to the chest x-ray plane.
• Kerley B lines	Parallel fine lines extend from the pleural surface into the subpleural lung, especially in lung bases, thought to result from thickened interlobular septa.
Alveolar fluid with or without air bronchograms	Air bronchograms prove the presence of alveolar fluid. Their absence does not disprove the presence of alveolar fluid. Air bronchograms do not result from pleural effusion alone.
Pleural effusion, including fluid within lung fissures	Right-sided pleural fluid is more common than left when a unilateral effusion occurs from heart failure.

TABLE 5-7. Chest X-ray Techniques and Artifacts
That May Simulate Pulmonary Edema

Technique or Artifact	Effect
Supine technique	Mimics cephalization and cardiomegaly
AP technique	Mimics cardiomegaly
Poor inspiratory effort or hypoinflated lungs	Mimics interstitial edema and prominent pulmonary vascularity
Underexposure, e.g., in the obese patient	Mimics interstitial edema and pulmonary vascular congestion

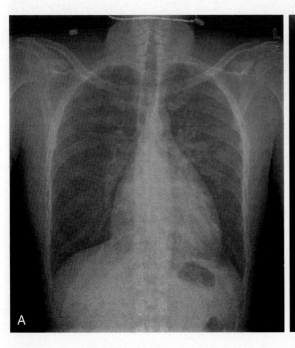

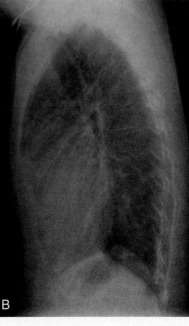

Figure 5-104. **Cardiomegaly. A,** Posterior-anterior (PA) chest x-ray. **B,** Lateral chest x-ray. This previously healthy 40-year-old male presented with 2 weeks of cough, sputum production, subjective fever, and mild dyspnea. His chest x-ray was interpreted by the radiologist as showing borderline cardiomegaly, mild left suprahilar opacity, and questionable retrocardiac opacity. He was treated with moxifloxacin and discharged home. Is this chest x-ray remarkable? Is cardiomegaly really present? The heart occupies slightly more than half of the right-to-left diameter of the chest on posterior–anterior view. Compare with Figures 5-105 through 5-109. When available, always compare the chest x-ray with prior images to detect subtle changes.

Figure 5-105. Cardiomegaly with cephalization. Same patient as Figure 5-104. **A,** Posterior-anterior (PA) chest x-ray. **B,** Lateral chest x-ray. The patient returned to the emergency department for similar symptoms 13 days after his initial visit. He was diagnosed by the emergency physician with bronchitis and discharged. The radiology report notes stable cardiomegaly and mild pulmonary edema. Is the heart size really unchanged? Notice how the pulmonary vascular markings are prominent in the upper lung fields. This redistribution of vascular markings is called cephalization and is an early finding of pulmonary edema.

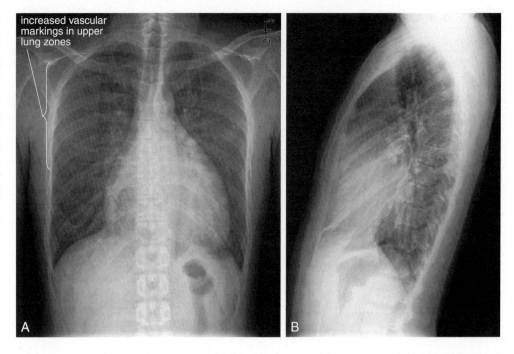

Figure 5-106. Cardiomegaly. Same patient as Figures 5-104 and 5-105. **A,** Posterior-anterior (PA) chest x-ray. **B,** Lateral chest x-ray. The patient returned again 7 days later (20 days after his initial presentation). He continued to complain of cough, and his vital signs were notable for tachycardia to 130 and a temperature of 38.3°C. An interval increase in heart size was noted by the emergency physician, and a viral cardiomyopathy was suspected. The x-ray shows increased cardiomegaly with some increased vascular markings, suggesting mild pulmonary edema with cephvalization.

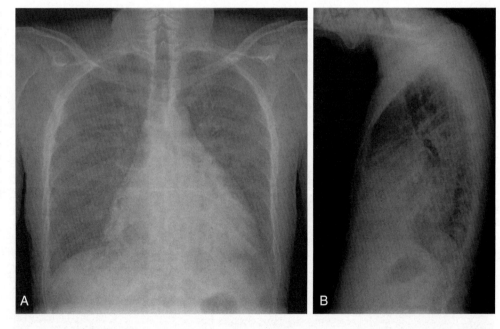

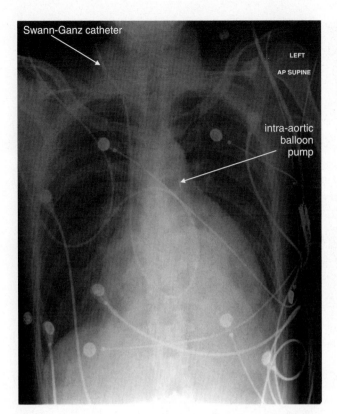

Swann-Ganz catheter

LEFT
AP SUPINE

intra-aortic balloon pump

Figure 5-107. Cardiomegaly. Two days after Figure 5-106, the patient is in the cardiac intensive care unit. The heart appears slightly larger on this view, although the supine anterior–posterior technique may exaggerate any difference. Notably, the patient has a right internal jugular catheter that curls into the right pulmonary artery—a Swann-Ganz catheter for measurement of pulmonary capillary wedge pressures. In addition, a radiopaque marker below the aortic knob marks an intra-aortic balloon pump.

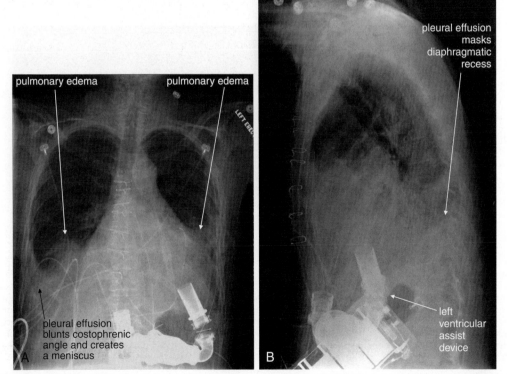

pulmonary edema   pulmonary edema

LEFT ERE...

pleural effusion blunts costophrenic angle and creates a meniscus

A

pleural effusion masks diaphragmatic recess

left ventricular assist device

B

Figure 5-108. Cardiomegaly. Same patient as Figure 5-107, 6 days later. **A,** Frontal projection chest x-ray. **B,** Lateral chest x-ray. The patient now has a left ventricular assist device implanted in the abdomen. This device pumps blood from the left ventricle to the ascending aorta. Bilateral pleural effusions are present, masking the diaphragms. Infiltrates representing edema are also present. Remarkably, the patient received a heart transplant 6 weeks later and did well. Review Figure 5-109.

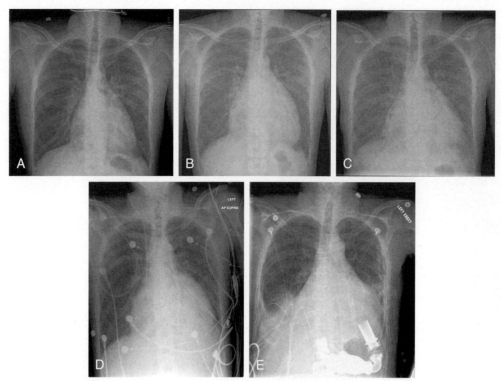

Figure 5-109. Cardiomegaly progression. This series illustrates the progression of cardiomegaly in the same patient as Figures 5-104 through 5-108 over a period of 30 days. Notice the increase in heart size over this period, the increased cephalization of vascular markings, and the development of bilateral effusions and frank pulmonary edema as you move from **A** to **E.** When interpreting a chest x-ray, always compare with prior x-rays if available. A finding on the most recent x-ray may turn out to be old and thus unlikely to be the cause of acute symptoms. Or a subtle finding on the current x-ray may represent a significant change from prior x-rays and thus be important.

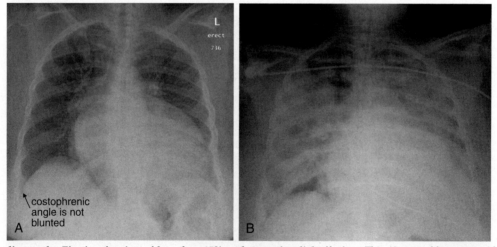

Figure 5-110. Cardiomegaly: Ejection fraction of less than 15% and no pericardial effusion. This 40-year-old woman with a known dilated cardiomyopathy and an ejection fraction of less than 15% presented with 1 week of fatigue and orthopnea. **A,** Her chest x-ray on the day of her emergency department presentation. The heart is massively enlarged, occupying more than two thirds of the lateral diameter of the chest. Her lung fields appear relatively clear. Her right costophrenic angle is not blunted, though her left is difficult to evaluate because of the overlying heart. Does she have a pericardial effusion? Chest x-ray cannot firmly discriminate cardiomegaly from pericardial effusion, but none was seen on echocardiogram the same day. **B,** Days later, the patient was intubated in the cardiac intensive care unit with gross pulmonary edema. The chest x-ray shows diffuse bilateral opacities. Notice how the left and right heart borders, as well as both hemidiaphragms, are obscured. During this hospitalization, the patient required placement of a left ventricular assist device.

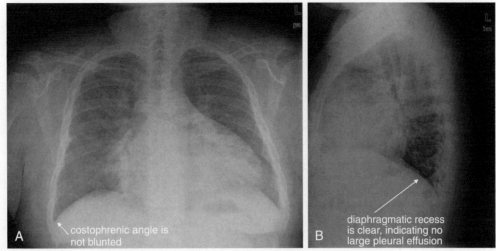

Figure 5-111. Cardiomegaly: Mild pulmonary edema. A, Posterior-anterior (PA) chest x-ray. **B,** Lateral chest x-ray. This 25-year-old male with end-stage renal disease presented with mild dyspnea. His chest x-ray shows a markedly enlarged cardiac silhouette. No significant pulmonary edema is present—notice that the costophrenic angles are not blunted and the heart borders are fairly clear. Some densities at the right lung base may be atelectasis or mild edema. Notice how these intermittently mask the right heart border in **A.** Echocardiogram the same day showed moderate left ventricular hypertrophy, no pericardial effusion, and an ejection fraction greater than 55%. An enlarged cardiac silhouette on chest x-ray can be compatible with cardiomegaly, pericardial effusion, or a combination of both. Because pericardial fluid, myocardium, and blood within the heart share the same fluid density on x-ray, they cannot be distinguished. Sometimes pericardial fluid gives the heart a globular "water bottle" appearance, but this is unreliable. Echocardiography can reliably identify pericardial fluid. In addition, an enlarged heart on chest x-ray does not always correlate with a depressed ejection fraction on echocardiogram, as was the case with this patient.

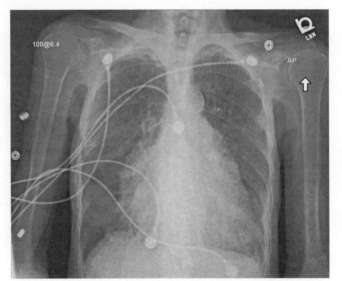

Figure 5-112. Cardiomegaly: Bilateral atrial enlargement and ejection fraction greater than 55%. This 89-year-old female with a history of heart failure and atrial fibrillation presented with 2 weeks of increasing dyspnea and orthopnea. She reported sitting up to sleep. Her chest x-ray shows significant cardiomegaly, with enlargement of the left atrium and appendage and right atrium. Her heart size was not increased compared with prior x-rays, and her chest x-ray actually shows less edema than in the past. Notice how the right diaphragm is quite clear, with no blunting of the costophrenic angle. The left costophrenic angle is less clear because of the overlying heart, but the diaphragm can still be seen. An echocardiogram the same day showed biatrial enlargement, an ejection fraction greater than 55%, and no pericardial effusion. Although this is a very abnormal chest x-ray, another cause for her acute dyspnea should be considered.

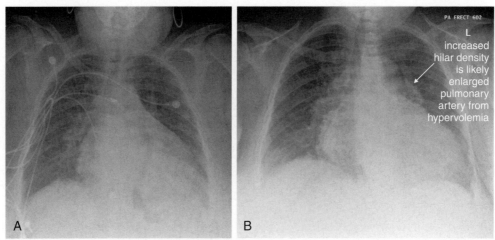

Figure 5-113. Cardiomegaly: Mild pulmonary edema, mild pericardial effusion, and ejection fraction greater than 55%. This 50-year-old with human immunodeficiency virus, chronic obstructive pulmonary disease, and end-stage renal disease presented with 2 days of dyspnea **(A).** She reported missing dialysis for a week. Her chest x-ray shows significant cardiomegaly —or is this a pericardial effusion? Chest x-ray cannot reliably discriminate the enlarged cardiac silhouette of cardiomegaly from pericardial effusion. Increased densities at the right and left lung bases appear consistent with mild pulmonary edema, although overlying soft tissue may be a contributor. Her echocardiogram on this date showed left ventricular hypertrophy, an ejection fraction greater than 55%, and a mild pericardial effusion. A year later, the patient was seen for a similar complaint **(B).** The heart size is unchanged, although increased fullness of the hilum bilaterally suggests a greater degree of volume overload. Notice how the heart borders are clearer in **A** than in **B.** In both cases, the patient felt better after dialysis.

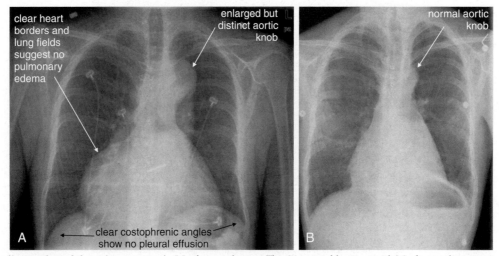

Figure 5-114. Cardiomegaly and thoracic aneurysm in Marfan syndrome. This 24-year-old patient with Marfan syndrome presented with dyspnea **(A).** His heart appears markedly dilated, as does his aortic root and arch. His ejection fraction at this time was estimated at 10% by magnetic resonance imaging. No effusion was seen, despite the globular heart shape. This is a dilated cardiomyopathy. His lung fields, heart borders, and hemidiaphragms appear clear, without evidence of pulmonary edema. **B,** Three years earlier. Compare the heart size and aortic contour at this time, before progression of his disease. Sternotomy wires are visible, as the patient had already undergone mitral valve repair.

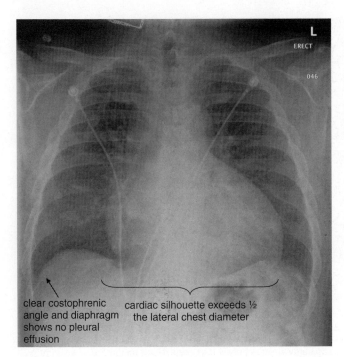

clear costophrenic angle and diaphragm shows no pleural effusion

cardiac silhouette exceeds ½ the lateral chest diameter

Figure 5-115. **Congestive heart failure: Ejection fraction of less than 15% and mild pericardial effusion.** This 45-year-old male with a history of hypertension reported chronic dyspnea, worse in the last week. His blood pressure was 190 systolic with bilateral lower extremity edema. Although his cardiac silhouette is enlarged, his diaphragm and heart borders are clear without evidence of pleural effusions. His superior pulmonary vascular markings are increased, a finding called cephalization that is an early marker of increased pulmonary vascular volume and heart failure. An echocardiogram was preformed, showing global hypokinesis with an ejection fraction of less than 15%—decreased from 45% on echocardiogram 3 years prior. Only a mild pericardial effusion was seen, indicating that the majority of the increased heart size seen on x-ray is due to true cardiomegaly.

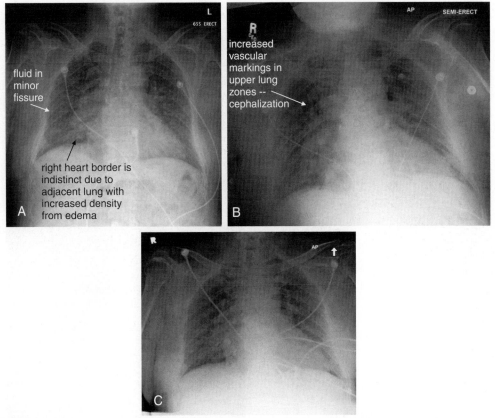

fluid in minor fissure

right heart border is indistinct due to adjacent lung with increased density from edema

increased vascular markings in upper lung zones -- cephalization

Figure 5-116. **Congestive heart failure: Mild left ventricular hypertrophy with restricted filling, ejection fraction greater than 55%, and no pericardial effusion.** This 63-year-old male with coronary artery disease, chronic renal sufficiency, and diastolic heart failure (ejection fraction greater than 55%) presented multiple times for dyspnea **A, B,** and **C,** first through third clinical presentation. Each of these three x-rays shows signs of moderate pulmonary edema. The diaphragms and costophrenic angles are clear, suggesting no pleural effusion. The right heart border in all three images is indistinct because of interstitial edema in these locations. Portions of the left heart border are also indistinct. The upper lung fields have a hazy appearance indicating mild edema. Fluid is visible in the minor fissure on all three images. Does the similarity of these x-rays mean that edema is not the cause of the patient's dyspnea? No, he simply presented with pulmonary edema on all three occasions.

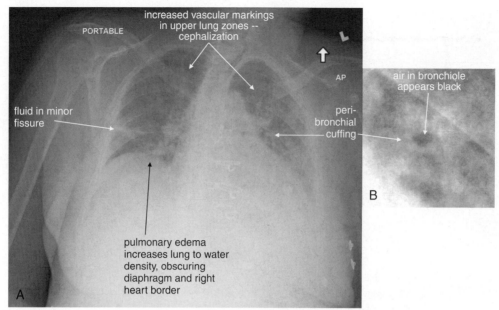

Figure 5-117. Pulmonary edema. A, Anterior-posterior (AP) chest x-ray. **B,** Close-up from **A.** This 53-year-old female with end-stage renal disease missed dialysis and presented to the emergency department. Her examination demonstrated bilateral rales. Her x-ray shows mild cardiomegaly, bilateral interstitial opacities, and cephalization of the pulmonary vascular markings. The minor fissure appears thickened. These findings are consistent with pulmonary edema. In addition, peribronchial cuffing is present. As discussed elsewhere, this is a nonspecific thickening of the bronchial wall that can occur from edema in the setting of heart failure, asthma, viral illness, or even infections such as pertussis. The thickened wall appears white, whereas the air-filled bronchiole appears black and has a circular short-axis cross section.

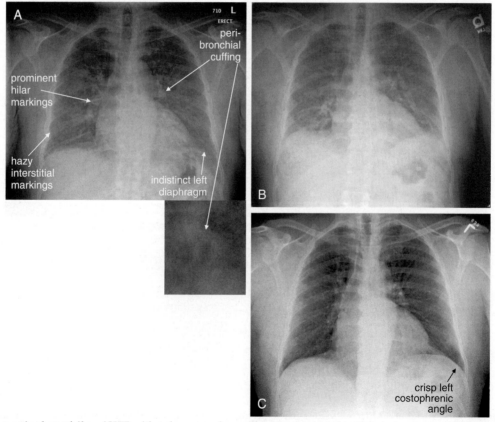

Figure 5-118. Congestive heart failure (CHF) with pulmonary edema. This 56-year-old male with hypertension and CHF presented with 2 weeks of dyspnea, orthopnea, paroxysmal nocturnal dyspnea, and diaphoresis. His blood pressure was 200/90 with an oxygen saturation of 98% on room air when upright but 90% when supine. **A,** On emergency department presentation, the patient had evidence of pulmonary edema with prominent hilar markings, indicating full main pulmonary arteries. Streaky lower lung interstitial markings and peribronchial cuffing (small panel, close-up from **A**) are present. **B,** Two days later, these appear slightly worse. **C,** One month later, the patient has improved and has crisper diaphragms, clearer lung fields, and less prominent hilar fullness.

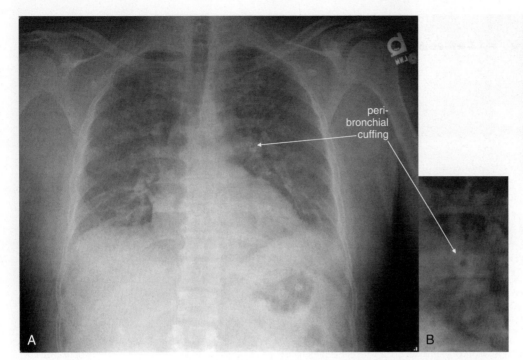

peri-
bronchial
cuffing

A   B

Figure 5-119. **Pulmonary edema.** Same patient as in Figure 5-118. **A,** Frontal projection chest x-ray. **B,** Close-up from **A.** Pulmonary edema is an important finding to recognize, so take a moment with this x-ray. Note the hazy upper lung fields, the dense lower lungs with prominent interstitial markings, and the indistinct hemidiaphragms and heart borders. **B,** Peribronchial cuffing is also present.

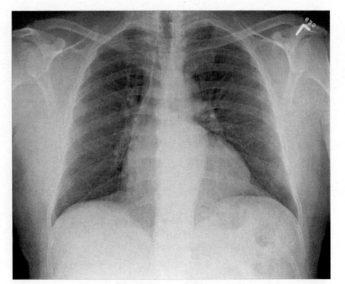

Figure 5-120. **Pulmonary edema, resolved.** Same patient as Figure 5-119, 1 month later. Note the clear diaphragms and heart borders, the decrease in vascular markings in the upper lungs, and the resolution of lower lung interstitial markings and peribronchial cuffing.

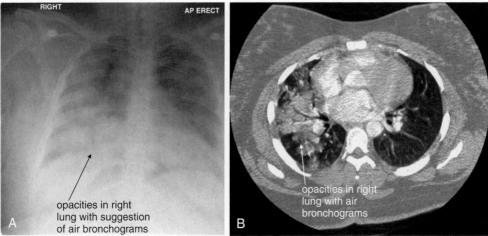

Figure 5-121. **Postpartum congestive heart failure or community-acquired pneumonia?** This 31-year-old female was 3 days postpartum and presented with acute dyspnea and inspiratory chest pain with a nonproductive cough. She was tachypneic and tachycardic, with an oxygen saturation of 90% on room air. Postpartum cardiomyopathy, pneumonia, and pulmonary embolism were each considered. A chest computed tomography (CT) scan was performed and was negative for pulmonary embolism. An echocardiogram showed an ejection fraction greater than 55% with no pericardial effusion. **A,** Her anterior-posterior (AP) upright chest x-ray shows diffuse opacities in the right mid-thorax and lower thorax, which mask the right heart border and diaphragm. She has a more normal-appearing left lung. Compare this with the chest CT image **(B),** viewed on lung windows. On the CT image, air bronchograms are present, with opacification of alveoli surrounding the bronchi. A suggestion of this is seen on chest x-ray. Can frank pulmonary edema be discerned from infectious infiltrate on chest x-ray or CT? Both processes lead to fluid accumulation in alveoli, resulting in similar fluid density on either imaging modality. Air bronchograms can occur with either pulmonary edema or infection, as these are the result of fluid in alveoli, regardless of the causes. In this case, the marked asymmetry is more suggestive of infection, as the left lung appears quite normal on CT. The patient improved with antibiotic therapy.

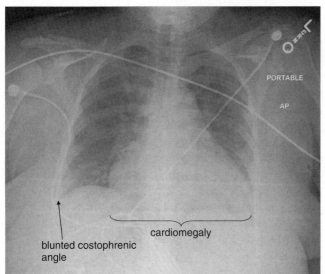

Figure 5-122. **Congestive heart failure, postpartum: Ejection fraction of less than 15%, no pericardial effusion.** This 33-year-old female was brought to the emergency department after being found unresponsive. Her chest x-ray shows cardiomegaly, with the possibility of a pericardial effusion. Both costophrenic angles appear slightly blunted, suggesting at least small pleural effusions. The right lung base appears somewhat dense, possibly indicating edema; the left base is hidden behind the heart. Vascular markings are prominent in the upper lung fields. Sadly, the patient was found to have a postpartum cardiomyopathy. Her echocardiogram showed an ejection fraction of less than 15% with no pericardial effusion. She had left ventricular thrombus—the source of a large ischemic stroke that caused her unresponsive state.

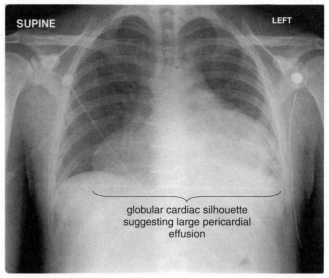

Figure 5-123. **Massive pericardial effusion and tamponade.** This 23-year-old male has a history of aortic valve replacement for infective endocarditis. He presented with increased chest pain and dyspnea. His chest x-ray shows a globular cardiac silhouette, suggesting a large pericardial effusion. The lung fields and right costophrenic angle appear clear, although the left costophrenic angle is hidden behind the heart and cannot be assessed. The patient underwent chest computed tomography to evaluate his aorta, as he complained of severe interscapular pain as well (see Figure 5-125). Also see Figure 5-124, which compares his pre- and post-operative chest x-rays.

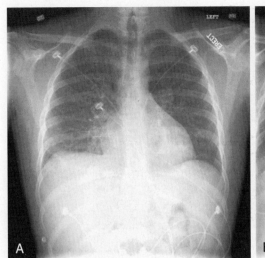
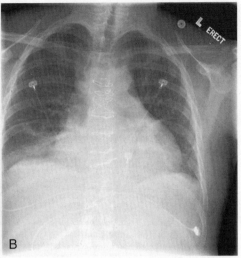

Figure 5-124. **Massive pericardial effusion and tamponade.** Same patient as Figure 5-123. His preoperative **(A)** and postoperative **(B)** chest x-rays are shown from his aortic valve replacement. These preceded his presentation in Figure 5-123.

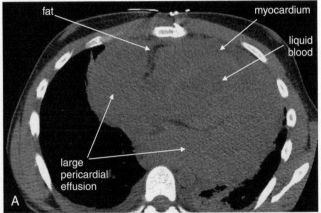
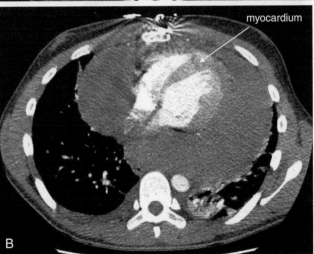

Figure 5-125. **Massive pericardial effusion.** Same patient as Figures 5-123 and 5-124. The patient underwent chest computed tomography (CT) without **(A)** and then with **(B)** intravenous contrast to evaluate his aorta, which was normal. However, the CT confirmed a massive pericardial effusion surrounding a normal-appearing heart. Without contrast, note that fluid blood within the chambers of the heart has a slightly lower density than the pericardial effusion, which has a density more similar to that of myocardium. When contrast is administered, the ventricular chambers fill completely, and the myocardium enhances and becomes somewhat brighter than the surrounding pericardial effusion. The heart itself is outlined by a thin stripe of fat, which appears nearly black on soft-tissue windows. The patient developed hypotension, suggesting cardiac tamponade, and pericardial window was performed for drainage of the effusion. In the operating room, the effusion was found to be coagulated blood.

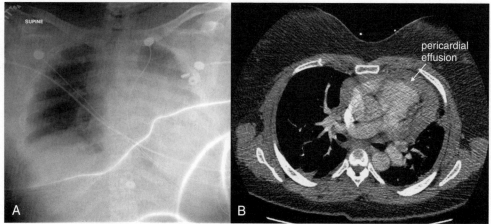

Figure 5-126. Massive pericardial effusion and tamponade. This 35-year-old female with a history of pulmonary fibrosis treated with cyclophosphamide was brought to the emergency department by emergency medical services with a systolic blood pressure of 60mm Hg and a heart rate of 178 beats per minute. She complained of dyspnea. Her chest x-ray **(A)** showed an enlarged and indistinct heart, with the suggestion of a pleural effusion given the hazy appearance of the left hemithorax. The emergency physician suspected pulmonary embolism given her tachycardia and hypotension. **B,** CT with IV contrast was performed, showing no pulmonary embolism but a large pericardial effusion, which was causing cardiac tamponade. Interestingly, echocardiogram 2 hours before the CT scan was read as showing "trivial pericardial fluid." However, based on the CT, the patient underwent left anterior thoracotomy, pericardial window, drainage of hemopericardium, and evacuation of intrapericardial fibrin clots. Her symptoms resolved. Echocardiogram is the usual modality for assessment of pericardial fluid. The patient's body habitus likely interfered with an accurate transthoracic echocardiogram.

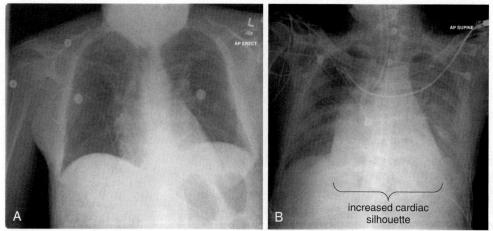

Figure 5-127. Pericardial effusion and tamponade (patient underwent pericardial window). This 58-year-old lung transplant patient presented with 1 day of gradual dyspnea and cough. The patient had recently been admitted with *Pseudomonas* bacteremia and pulmonary embolism, was treated simultaneously with ciprofloxacin and coumadin, and had an INR of 2.5. Initial chest x-ray **(A)** was read as normal. Chest computed tomography (Figure 5-128) was negative for pulmonary embolism but showed a moderate pericardial effusion. The patient was admitted but then developed increased pericardial fluid **(B)** with pericardial tamponade requiring pericardial window. Remember that pericardial tamponade does not require a large volume pericardial effusion. Chest x-ray can be relatively insensitive for pericardial fluid. Consider bedside echocardiogram to assess for pericardial fluid in patients with dyspnea, chest pain, or hypotension.

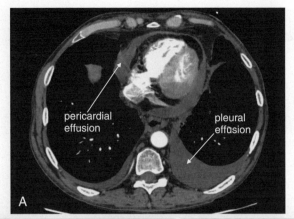

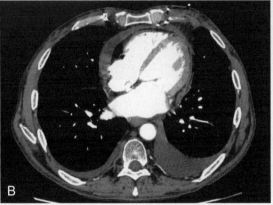

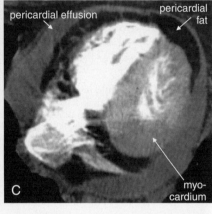

Figure 5-128. Pericardial effusion and tamponade. Same patient as Figure 5-127. The patient's chest CT with IV contrast shows a moderate pericardial effusion. On soft-tissue windows, unenhancing fluid such as pericardial or pleural effusions appears as an intermediate gray. The pericardial effusion surrounds a nearly black band, which is pericardial fat (fat is nearly black on soft-tissue windows). Within this lies the heart itself—the myocardium enhances with contrast and appears somewhat brighter than the effusion. **A, B,** Axial slices through the heart viewed on soft-tissue windows. **C,** Close-up from **A.**

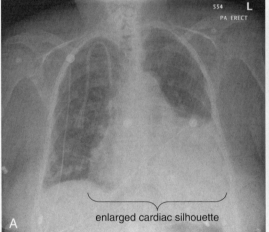

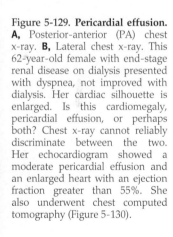

Figure 5-129. Pericardial effusion. A, Posterior-anterior (PA) chest x-ray. **B,** Lateral chest x-ray. This 62-year-old female with end-stage renal disease on dialysis presented with dyspnea, not improved with dialysis. Her cardiac silhouette is enlarged. Is this cardiomegaly, pericardial effusion, or perhaps both? Chest x-ray cannot reliably discriminate between the two. Her echocardiogram showed a moderate pericardial effusion and an enlarged heart with an ejection fraction greater than 55%. She also underwent chest computed tomography (Figure 5-130).

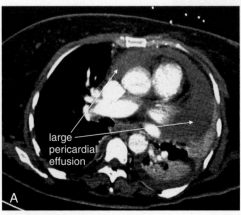

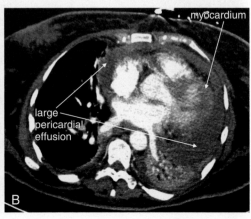

Figure 5-130. Pericardial effusion and tamponade. Same patient as Figure 5-129. Chest CT with IV contrast. The patient has a large pericardial effusion. **A,** Axial CT slice just below the aortic arch, viewed on soft-tissue windows. **B,** A more caudad slice.

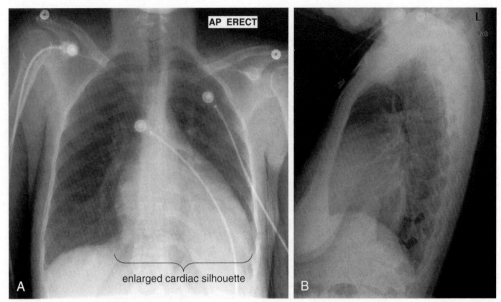

Figure 5-131. **Cardiomegaly: Ejection fraction of 35% and mild pericardial effusion. A,** Anterior-posterior (AP) chest x-ray. **B,** Lateral chest x-ray. This 32-year-old female presented with right chest pain and dyspnea for the past few hours. She reported a history of mitral valve prolapse and had recently returned from a long car ride, greater than 16 hours. Does her x-ray give any hint of these abnormalities? Her heart appears enlarged, though chest x-ray cannot determine whether this is cardiomegaly or pericardial effusion. Chest computed tomography was performed to rule out pulmonary embolism (Figure 5-132) and discriminates these two findings. On bedside echocardiogram by the emergency physician, she was found to have a mild pericardial effusion and severe mitral regurgitation. Her ejection fraction was estimated at 35%. The patient was admitted and underwent mitral valve replacement.

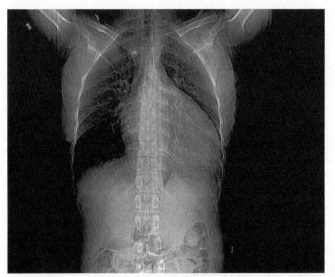

Figure 5-132. **Cardiomegaly or pericardial effusion?** Computed tomography scout image from the same patient as Figures 5-131 and 5-133 again shows an enlarged cardiac silhouette. It is not clear from this view whether cardiomegaly or pericardial effusion is at play.

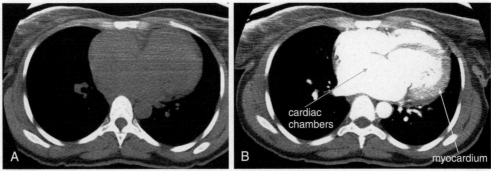

Figure 5-133. Cardiomegaly. Chest CT from the same patient as Figures 5-131 and 5-132, without **(A)** and with **(B)** contrast. In these images, the heart appears significantly enlarged without a pericardial effusion. Without contrast, blood within the chambers of the heart are difficult to distinguish from myocardium. When contrast is injected, the chambers become an intense white, whereas the myocardium enhances somewhat.

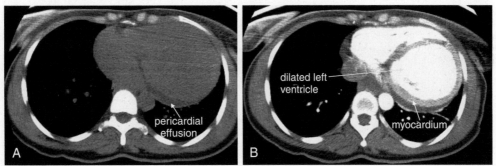

Figure 5-134. Pericardial effusion and cardiomegaly. Same patient as in Figure 5-133. Here, a small pericardial effusion is visible in a dependent position deep to the left ventricle. The ventricle appears quite dilated as well. The pericardial fluid is dark gray and does not enhance with intravenous contrast (compare **A,** without contrast, and **B,** with contrast). The myocardial wall does enhance and becomes visible in **B.**

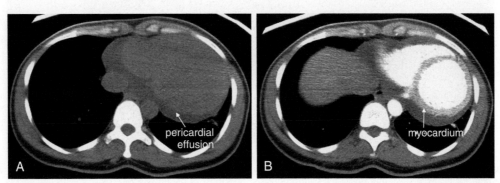

Figure 5-135. Pericardial effusion and cardiomegaly. Same patient as in Figure 5-134. Lower in the chest, the pericardial effusion appears larger. The pericardial fluid is dark gray and does not enhance with intravenous contrast (compare **A,** without contrast, and **B,** with contrast). The myocardial wall does enhance and becomes visible in **B.**

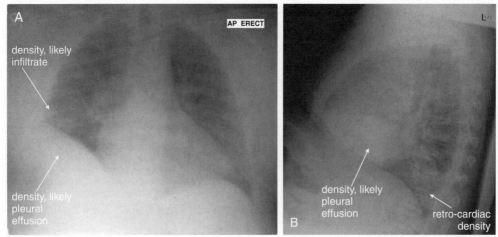

Figure 5-136. Pleural effusions or elevated hemidiaphragm? A, Anterior-posterior (AP) upright chest x-ray. **B,** Lateral upright chest x-ray. This 52-year-old male with renal insufficiency and heart failure presented with increasing lower extremity edema and dyspnea. The patient was also febrile on emergency department arrival. His chest x-ray shows a density overlying the right lower chest. Remember that for diagnostic imaging findings, a differential diagnosis exists. On the anterior–posterior x-ray, this density is fluid density—it is indistinguishable from the appearance of the liver and diaphragm. It may be an elevated diaphragm, a subpulmonic pleural effusion, or a dense right lower lobe infiltrate. It appears to form a meniscus with the lateral chest wall, which supports pleural effusion. On lateral x-ray, the density is again seen and has a sharp and horizontally oriented upper margin. This suggests pleural fluid, although the minor fissure also represents a horizontal boundary in this location. This differential diagnosis can easily be explored with bedside ultrasound, which could confirm pleural effusion, or with decubitus x-rays that may show layering fluid. Superior to the density we described is a second less discrete density, which may represent an infiltrate. Increased density is also seen on the lateral x-ray behind the heart and overlying the lower thoracic spine.

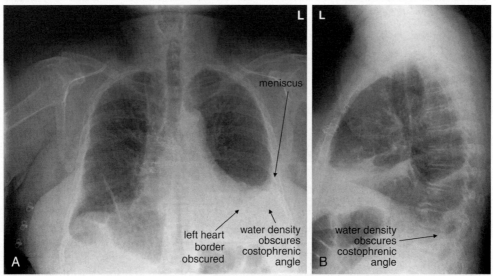

Figure 5-137. Pleural effusions. A, Frontal projection upright chest x-ray. **B,** Lateral upright chest x-ray. This 59-year-old female recently underwent aortic valve replacement for bicuspid valve and presented with progressive shortness of breath and fever. Her chest x-ray shows a large left pleural effusion that obscures the left heart border and diaphragm on frontal view. It forms a meniscus with the lateral chest wall, another common feature of pleural effusions. On lateral chest x-ray, the posterior costophrenic angle is blunted, and a fluid meniscus is seen posteriorly.

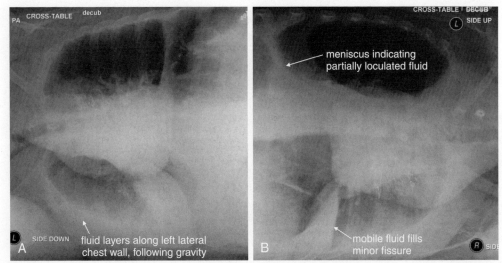

Figure 5-138. Pleural effusions. Same patient as in Figure 5-137. The patient underwent decubitus x-rays to further delineate her pleural effusions. **A,** Left lateral decubitus chest x-ray. **B,** Right lateral decubitus chest x-ray. Decubitus views are named for the side positioned down. An x-ray obtained with the right side down is a right decubitus view. In the case of this patient, the left pleural effusion is seen to layer along the lateral chest wall in the left decubitus view—compare with the upright view in Figure 5-137, which shows the upper lateral left chest to be clear. On the right decubitus view, fluid fills the minor fissure, indicating that fluid is also mobile in the right pleural space. A meniscus remains visible in the left thorax on the right decubitus view, suggesting partial loculation of the left pleural effusion. Note that the lung in the nondependent position looks more lucent in these examples as fluid drains to a dependent position. The nondependent lung also is better aerated, with less atelectasis and less overlying soft tissue.

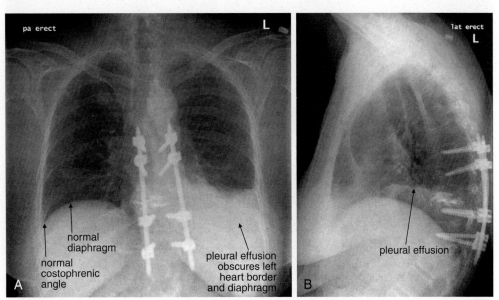

Figure 5-139. Pleural effusions. A, Posterior-anterior (PA) upright chest x-ray. **B,** Lateral upright chest x-ray. This 62-year-old female with metastatic non–small cell lung cancer presented with 2 weeks of increasing dyspnea. Her chest x-ray shows a large left pleural effusion, which obscures the left heart border and diaphragm on the posterior–anterior view **(A).** On the lateral view **(B),** a fluid level is visible. Remember that pleural effusion can accompany many other disease processes. For this patient, malignant effusion, infection, heart failure, and effusion related to pulmonary embolism should be considered. Chest x-ray cannot directly differentiate these. The right chest has no effusion and provides a good comparison of a normal diaphragm and costophrenic angle.

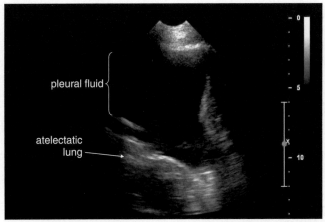

Figure 5-140. Pleural effusions. Same patient as in Figure 5-139. An ultrasound of the chest was performed in preparation for thoracentesis. The large black region is pleural fluid. Lung tissue is seen deep to this and has echo characteristics similar to abdominal solid organs because it is atelectatic because of the pleural effusion. Thoracentesis should be possible here with little risk of pneumothorax, because 10 cm of pleural fluid separates the chest wall and lung in this location.

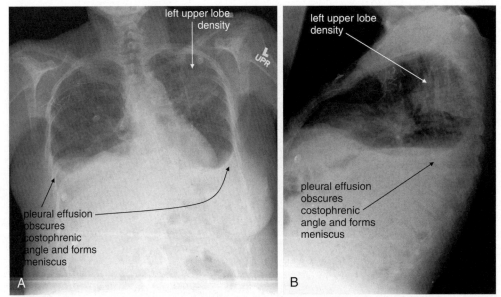

Figure 5-141. Pleural effusions. A, Upright frontal projection chest x-ray. **B,** Upright lateral chest x-ray. This 49-year-old female with a history of breast cancer metastatic to bone and liver presented with shortness of breath and left-sided pleuritic chest pain. Her chest x-ray shows several findings, including a left upper lung opacity and bilateral large pleural effusions. The pleural effusions blunt the costophrenic angles and form meniscuses with the lateral chest walls on the posterior–anterior view. On the lateral view, pleural fluid fills the posterior recess. The infiltrate is also visible on the lateral x-ray. Given the clinical history, many causes for the pleural effusions must be considered, including malignant effusion, pulmonary embolism, heart failure, and infection. The infiltrate also may represent infection, metastatic disease, or pulmonary infarction. This is a reminder to consider the differential diagnosis for chest x-ray findings.

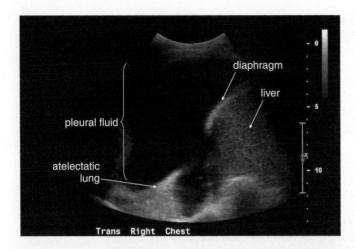

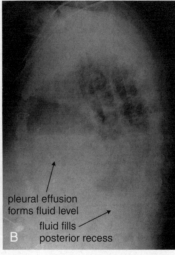

Figure 5-142. Pleural effusions. Chest ultrasound was performed before thoracentesis. The black collection is pleural fluid. The white echogenic curve is the diaphragm, and beneath that lies the liver. An atelectatic lung is visible as well, 10 cm deep to the chest wall. Thoracentesis should be performed with little danger of pneumothorax.

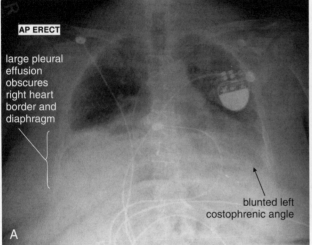

Figure 5-143. Pleural effusions. A, Anterior-posterior (AP) upright chest x-ray. **B,** Lateral upright chest x-ray. This 71-year-old female presented with dyspnea on exertion and had a history of sick sinus syndrome and ischemic heart failure. A large right pleural effusion hides the right heart border and diaphragm on the anterior–posterior view. The left costophrenic angle is also hidden, although it is impossible to determine the size of the left pleural effusion as the left heart also overlies this area. On the lateral chest x-ray, a fluid level is visible overlying the heart, corresponding to the pleural effusions seen on the AP view. The posterior diaphragmatic recess is also filled with fluid.

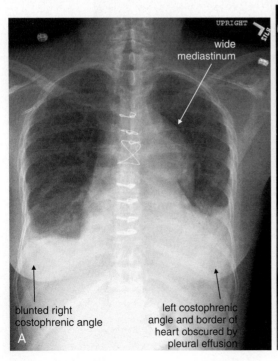

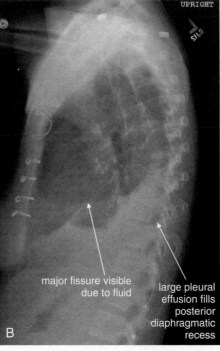

Figure 5-144. Pleural effusions. A, Posterior-anterior (PA) chest x-ray. **B,** Lateral chest x-ray. This 48-year-old female with end-stage renal disease and a history or aortic dissection repair presented to the emergency department from clinic for transfusion. She denied chest pain or increased dyspnea. Her chest x-ray shows slight blunting of the right costophrenic angle, with a large left pleural effusion visible on the posterior–anterior x-ray. The left-sided effusion forms a classic meniscus with the lateral chest wall. The lateral x-ray shows a large pleural effusion. In addition, the major fissure is readily visible because of fluid tracking within it. The mediastinum has an abnormal contour and is widened. Abnormalities of the aorta and mediastinum are discussed in detail elsewhere.

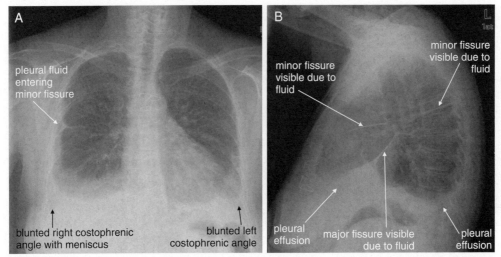

Figure 5-145. Pleural effusions. A, Posterior-anterior (PA) upright chest x-ray. **B,** Lateral upright chest x-ray. This 54-year-old female presented with sudden onset right upper abdominal pain while exercising. Her chest x-ray shows bilateral pleural effusions on the posterior–anterior (PA) view, with the right forming a classic meniscus with the right chest wall. Fluid is also seen in the minor fissure on both the PA and the lateral views. On the lateral x-ray, fluid is also seen entering the major fissure. Is the pleural effusion the cause of the patient's pain? What is the cause of the effusion? Chest x-ray does not answer these questions, and a careful differential diagnosis is required based on the history and physical examination. Premature closure based on the chest x-ray findings could lead to failure to diagnosis an underlying cause, such as pulmonary embolism, malignancy, heart failure, or abdominal pathology with sympathetic pleural effusion.

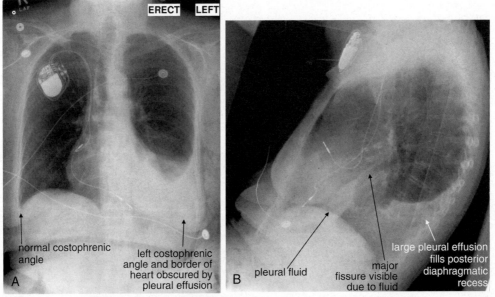

Figure 5-146. Pleural effusions. This 71-year-old female with a history of atrial fibrillation presented with generalized weakness. Her primary care physician had also noted decreased breath sounds on the left. **A,** Her upright frontal projection chest x-ray shows a normal right chest with a clear costophrenic angle and right heart border. The left heart border and diaphragm are hidden by pleural effusion, which shares the same water density on x-ray. Note the classic meniscus formed between the pleural effusion and the left chest wall. **B,** On the lateral x-ray, pleural fluid is seen tracking into the major fissure and filling the posterior diaphragmatic recess. The effusion was aspirated but grew no organisms and had negative cytology.

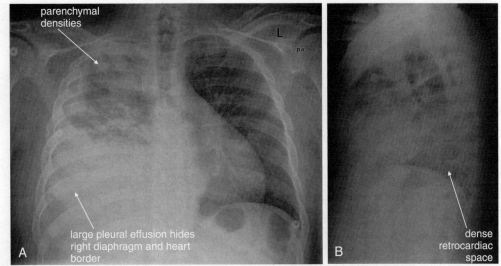

Figure 5-147. Pleural effusions. A, Posterior-anterior (PA) chest x-ray. **B,** Lateral chest x-ray. This 30-year-old male with lung cancer presented with fever, dyspnea, and right chest pain. His chest x-ray shows a large right pleural effusion, as well as opacities of the upper lung that may indicate lymphangitic spread of tumor or superimposed infiltrate. How can pleural effusion be discriminated from dense pneumonia in the lower lung? Again, decubitus x-rays could demonstrate shifting fluid, or ultrasound could be used to evaluate. Computed tomography can discriminate pleural fluid from infiltrated lung as well. On x-ray, the presence of air bronchograms would indicate that the alveoli surrounding air-filled bronchi were opacified. A pleural effusion does not create air bronchograms. The absence of air bronchograms does not prove that this is a pleural effusion, because fluid or tumor infiltration of bronchi can eliminate air bronchograms even when alveolar opacification is present.

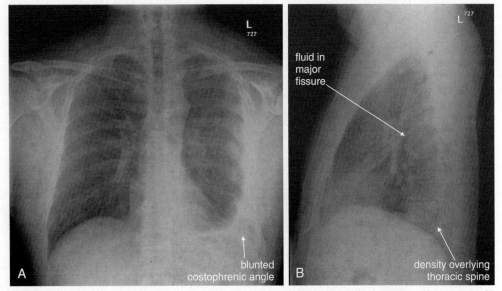

Figure 5-148. Pleural effusions. A, Posterior-anterior (PA) upright chest x-ray. **B,** Lateral upright chest x-ray. This 44-year-old male presents with 2 weeks of cough, left chest pain, and dyspnea on exertion. Five months earlier, he had sustained a pneumothorax and several left-sided rib fractures. His chest x-ray shows a blunted left costophrenic angle with a meniscus along the left chest wall on posterior–anterior view. On the lateral x-ray, a meniscus and increased density are visible in the retrocardiac region overlying the lower thoracic spine. Some fluid is visible in the major fissure as well. Though the most likely cause may be residual hemothorax from his trauma, the patient was a heavy smoker and computed tomography was performed to exclude an underlying mass (Figure 5-149). Pulmonary embolism was also considered.

Figure 5-149. Pleural effusions. Same patient as Figure 5-148. **A,** CT with IV contrast, axial slice viewed on soft-tissue windows. **B,** Same slice viewed with lung windows. A moderate left pleural effusion is seen. Computed tomography (CT) cannot discriminate the cause of a pleural effusion, other than by excluding parenchymal masses and pulmonary emboli. The density of pleural fluid can be measured on CT, but this is relatively nonspecific, as blood, serous fluid, and infected pleural fluid can have overlapping densities. Aspiration of pleural fluid for cytology, cultures, and chemical testing is necessary to further delineate the cause. No pulmonary emboli or masses were found on the patient's CT.

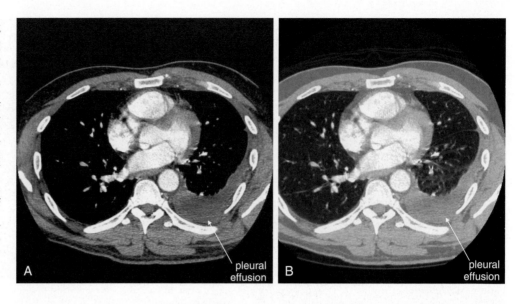

Figure 5-150. Pleural effusions. **A,** Anterior-posterior (AP) upright chest x-ray. **B,** Lateral upright chest x-ray. This 85-year-old male presented with new right facial weakness and slurring of speech. His chest x-ray shows a large right pleural effusion that obscures the right heart border and diaphragm. This is visible on the lateral chest x-ray as well. The patient has taken a very small inspiration—notice how high the diaphragm is on the left on the AP view and on the lateral x-ray. Low lung volumes make the lungs look denser because of the crowding together of blood vessels.

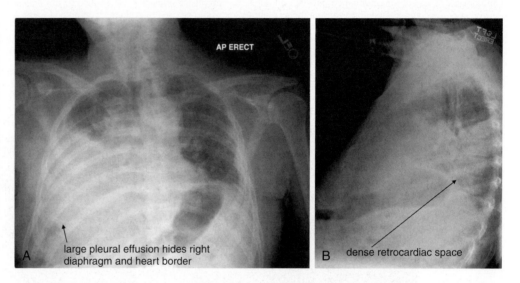

Figure 5-151. Pleural effusions. **A,** Frontal projection upright chest x-ray. **B,** Lateral upright chest x-ray. This 60-year-old female presented with chest pain and dyspnea. She had undergone coronary artery bypass and grafting 2 weeks prior and had noted some swelling of her leg near the site of her saphenous vein harvest. Her chest x-ray shows a left pleural effusion with blunting of the costophrenic angle and a meniscus. Computed tomography was performed because of concern for possible pulmonary embolism (Figure 5-152).

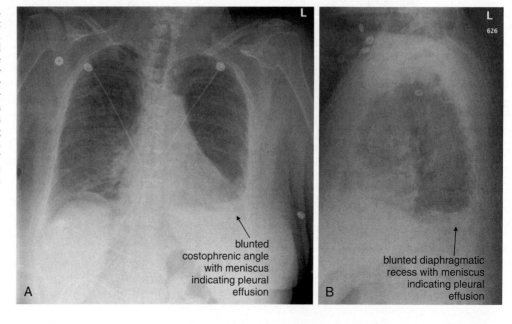

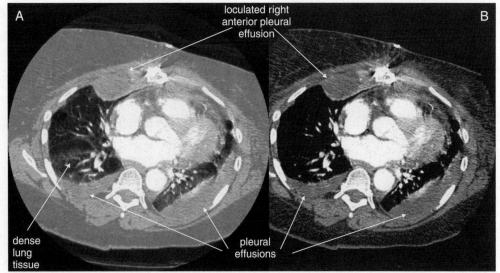

Figure 5-152. Pleural effusions. Same patient as Figure 5-151. CT with IV contrast was negative for pulmonary embolism but showed bilateral pleural effusions, including a loculated right anterior effusion that did not move with gravity. **A,** Lung windows. **B,** Same slice viewed on soft-tissue settings. On lung windows, the dependent lung appears denser—this is likely due to compressive atelectasis from the adjacent pleural effusions.

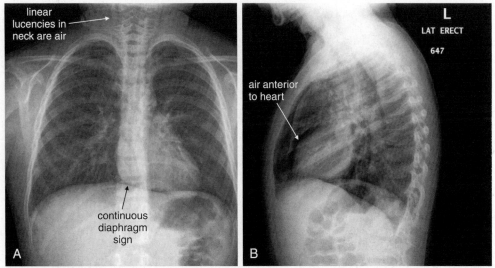

Figure 5-153. Pneumopericardium. A, Posterior-anterior (PA) chest x-ray. **B,** Lateral chest x-ray. This 8-year-old female presented with acute onset of coughing the previous night. She was hypoxic to 90% on room air. Her chest x-ray shows evidence of pneumopericardium. Look carefully at the diaphragm on the posterior–anterior view. Normally, the diaphragm cannot be seen beneath the heart, because both structures are water density on chest x-ray. In this case, the diaphragm can be seen because a thin stripe of air in the pericardial sac separates the heart and the diaphragm. This is called the continuous diaphragm sign. A fine ribbon of lucent air also outlines the left heart border. On the lateral view, a thin stripe of air is visible as a linear lucency anterior to the heart. Linear lucencies in the neck are subcutaneous emphysema originating in the mediastinum. What happened to this patient? She likely has asthma exacerbated by a viral infection, given the hyperinflated anterior–posterior diameter of her chest on x-ray and the streaky opacities around her hilum. Coughing or bronchospasm against a closed glottis can force air into the mediastinum and pericardium.

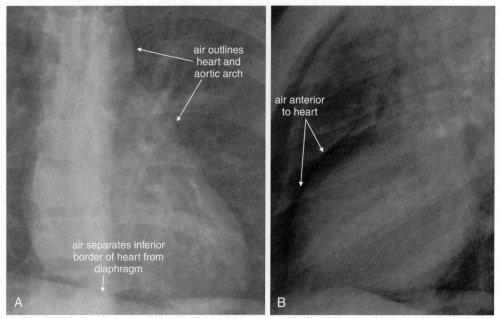

Figure 5-154. Pneumopericardium and pneumomediastinum: Close-up views from Figure 5-153. A, PA view. **B,** Lateral view. **A,** Air is visible between the inferior wall of the heart and the diaphragm, two structures that are normally indistinguishable on x-ray because they share the same density. This is called the continuous diaphragm sign. **B,** Air is also visible anterior to the heart on the lateral image.

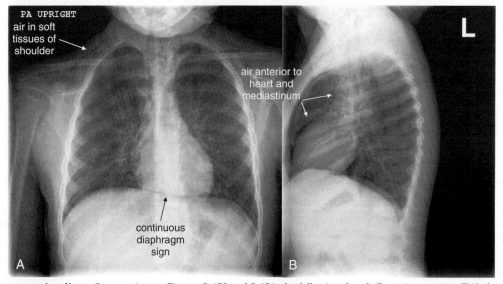

Figure 5-155. Pneumopericardium. Same patient as Figures 5-153 and 5-154, the following day. **A,** Posterior-anterior (PA) chest x-ray. **B,** Lateral chest x-ray. The continuous diaphragm sign is still present, because of air creating contrast between the otherwise similar densities of the soft tissues of the heart and the diaphragm. Air is visible in the soft tissues of the shoulders. On the lateral x-ray, air is clearly visible anterior to the heart and along the anterior aspect of the great vessels of the mediastinum.

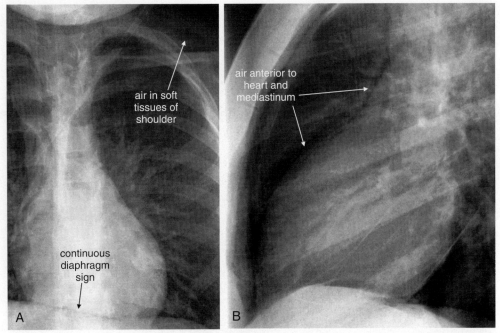

Figure 5-156. Pneumopericardium. Close-ups from Figure 5-155. **A,** PA view. **B,** Lateral view. The continuous diaphragm sign and air in the anterior mediastinum are present. Subcutaneous air is visible within the soft tissues of the left shoulder.

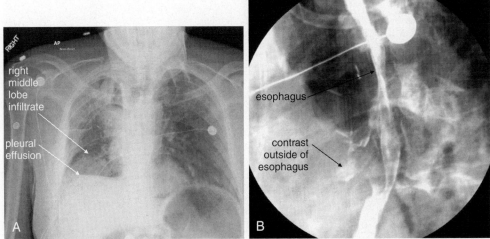

Figure 5-157. Esophageal rupture: Boerhaave's syndrome. This 55-year-old male has metastatic colon cancer, for which he had undergone mediastinal irradiation. The patient had an esophageal stent placed and subsequently removed 4 weeks ago for a stricture because of a metastatic lesion. He now presents with persistent coughing and emesis, tachycardia to 118, and hypoxia (pulse oximetry 83% on room air). Chest x-ray **(A)** demonstrates a right middle lobe infiltrate and right-sided pleural effusion. These findings are nonspecific but should be recognized in this clinical setting as potential findings of esophageal perforation, not simply pneumonia with associated pleural effusion. Unrecognized esophageal perforation may lead to mediastinitis and death. Consider the diagnosis of esophageal perforation in a patient with a history of forceful coughing or emesis, or a history of instrumentation of the esophagus. Chest x-ray may be normal or may show infiltrate, pleural effusions, pneumothorax, pneumomediastinum, or subcutaneous emphysema. A Gastrografin swallow study **(B)** shows contrast beyond the borders of the esophagus *(arrowheads)*, indicating an esophageal perforation. Although less sensitive than barium swallow, Gastrografin swallow is the preferred initial study to confirm the diagnosis, as Gastrografin is less reactive than barium if leaked into the pleural space or mediastinum. If high suspicion remains after a negative Gastrografin study, barium swallow or contrast-enhanced computed tomography scan should be ordered. Broad-spectrum antibiotics and early cardiothoracic surgery consult are the mainstays of initial treatment for esophageal perforation; nonoperative therapy with tube drainage of fluid collections is an emerging therapy. The patient underwent pigtail catheter thoracostomy and esophageal stent placement in the operating room with subsequent recovery.

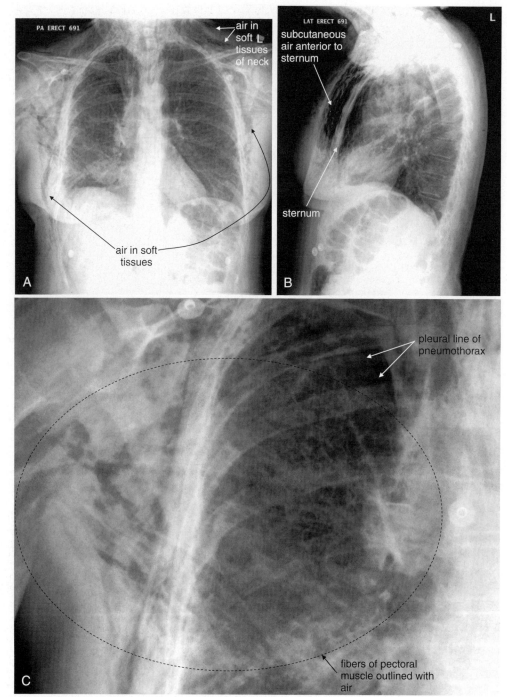

Figure 5-158. Subcutaneous emphysema. Figure 5-156 showed subtle subcutaneous emphysema in the context of pneumopericardium. This patient presented with massive and increasing subcutaneous emphysema after a right thoracoscopic upper lobectomy for a stage I non–small cell lung cancer. Increasing subcutaneous emphysema after a procedure suggests an ongoing air leak from the respiratory tract and should prompt a search for a pneumothorax. This patient was treated with a chest tube for a right apical pneumothorax, visible in **C. A,** Posterior–anterior view. Air is visible in the chest wall, including the axilla, and in the subcutaneous tissues of the neck. **B,** Lateral view, showing dramatic subcutaneous air anterior to the sternum. **C,** Close-up from **A** shows air dissecting between fibers of the pectoral muscles. The pleural line associated with a right-sided pneumothorax is also faintly visible.

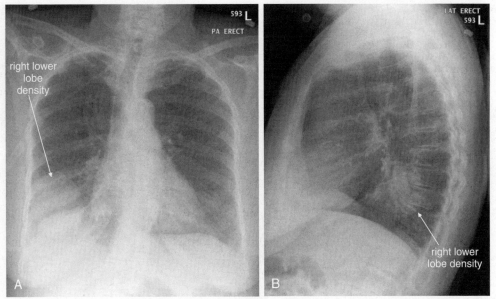

Figure 5-159. **Lung mass presenting with hemoptysis. A,** Posterior-anterior (PA) chest x-ray. **B,** Lateral chest x-ray. This 83-year-old female presented with hemoptysis of a quarter-sized clot. Her posterior–anterior chest x-ray shows a rounded right lower lobe density. On the lateral view, this is visible in the retrocardiac space. This density measures 7.6 cm in diameter. Pneumonia, neoplasm, or abscess could have this appearance on chest x-ray. Computed tomography was performed to further delineate the pathology (Figure 5-160).

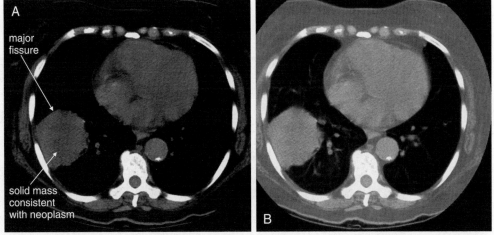

Figure 5-160. **Lung mass presenting with hemoptysis.** Same patient as in Figure 5-159. Noncontrast computed tomography was performed (contrast was withheld as a consequence of the patient's renal dysfunction) and shows a 6 by 6 cm round lesion abutting the oblique fissure (also called the major fissure) and lateral chest wall. **A,** Soft-tissue windows. **B,** Lung windows. On soft tissues windows, the center appears slightly darker, indicating lower density that may represent central necrosis. If IV contrast had been given, an area of necrosis would have failed to enhance. Infection or infarction is technically possible, but a pulmonary neoplasm is the most likely explanation for this lesion. Biopsy showed this to be a moderately differentiated squamous cell carcinoma.

Figure 5-161. Lung mass. This 48-year-old with asthma and human immunodeficiency virus was brought to the emergency department by emergency medical services with dyspnea, fever, productive cough, and wheezing. Her chest x-ray shows opacities in the bilateral lower lung fields, partially obscuring the right diaphragm, compatible with pneumonia. Apparently incidentally, along the margin of the left mediastinum and aortic knob is a rounded left upper lobe opacity, concerning for a mass. The patient was treated with ceftriaxone and azithromycin for pneumonia, with resolution of her lower lung opacities, but the mass persisted. Testing for pneumocystis pneumonia and tuberculosis was negative. The mass was biopsied and was found to be adenocarcinoma.

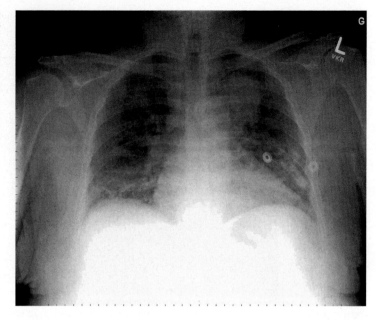

Figure 5-162. Lung mass. Same patient as Figure 5-161. Computed tomography was performed the same day; images are shown with lung windows. Two separate processes are present here. **A,** Evidence of pneumonia is present, with a "tree in bud" appearance (**C,** close-up). The opacities have a ground-glass appearance with lobular sparing, which in an immunocompromised host could suggest *Pneumocystis carinii.* (now called *Pneumocystis jirovecii*) This patient actually was found to have a CD4 count of 1667, essentially ruling out opportunistic infection. **B,** A lobulated mass is seen in the left upper lobe, consistent with neoplasm.

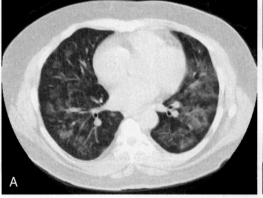

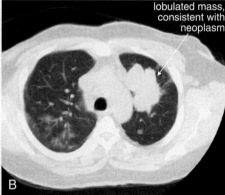

lobulated mass, consistent with neoplasm

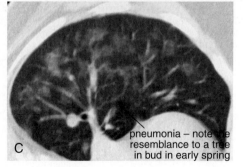

pneumonia – note the resemblance to a tree in bud in early spring

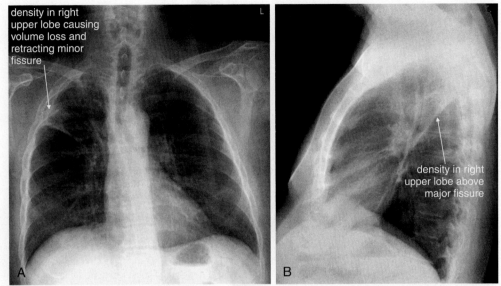

Figure 5-163. Lung mass. A, Posterior-anterior (PA) chest x-ray. **B,** Lateral chest x-ray. This 59-year-old male with stage IIIB non–small cell lung cancer presented with an episode of hemoptysis during which he expectorated approximately ½ mL of blood mixed with sputum. On the posterior–anterior view, the patient's mass is present just above the minor fissure and has caused volume loss in the right upper lobe. Retraction of the right upper lobe like an accordion has pulled the minor fissure cephalad (remember, the minor fissure should be a thin horizontal line on the frontal chest x-ray). On the lateral view, the mass extends to the major fissure. Although technically an upper lobe pneumonia could be associated with mucous plugging and atelectasis with volume loss, these findings should suggest an associated mass. If the clinical history suggests pneumonia, with fever, cough, and sputum production, treat for possible postobstructive pneumonia—but arrange follow-up imaging to evaluate for an underlying mass. See additional chest x-rays from this patient, Figures 5-164 and 5-165.

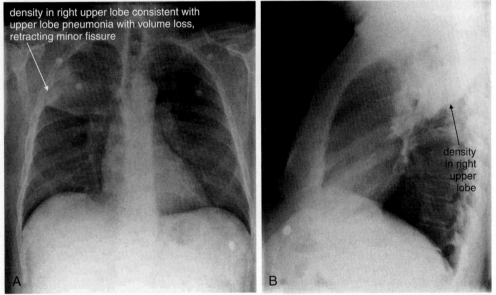

Figure 5-164. Lung mass presenting with hemoptysis. Same patient as Figure 5-163. **A,** Posterior-anterior (PA) chest x-ray. **B,** Lateral chest x-ray. This chest x-ray preceded his cancer diagnosis. On this occasion, he presented with chest pain and was diagnosed with a right upper lobe pneumonia. Note the volume loss, indicated by elevation of the minor fissure on the posterior–anterior view. On the lateral view, the density is bounded inferiorly by the major fissure. The radiologist diagnosed right upper lobe pneumonia but appropriately recommended "radiographic follow-up to complete resolution." The lesion failed to resolve completely, leading to the diagnosis of lung cancer.

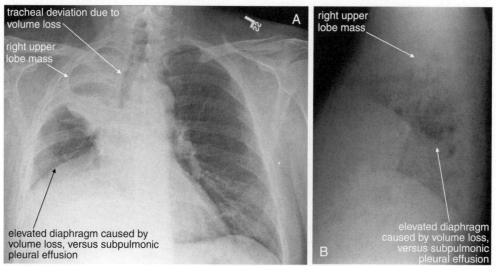

Figure 5-165. Lung mass. Same patient as Figures 5-163 and 5-164. **A,** Posterior-anterior (PA) chest x-ray. **B,** Lateral chest x-ray. Two years later, the patient has progression of his cancer and has continued chest pain. The lesion has caused more volume loss in the right upper lobe. Not only is the minor fissure pulled cephalad, but the trachea is also deviated to the right. The right diaphragm is now elevated as well because of right lung volume loss. A subpulmonic effusion is also possible.

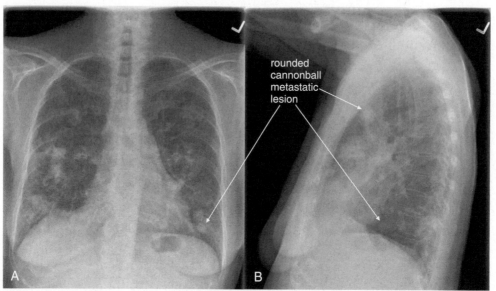

Figure 5-166. Metastatic disease with cannonball emboli. A, Posterior-anterior (PA) chest x-ray. **B,** Lateral chest x-ray. Any neoplasm with hematogenous spread to lung can form so-called cannonball emboli. These are small tumor emboli that shower the lungs, implant, and then grow in situ. The characteristic appearance is of scattered, rounded, bilateral lung opacities. Septic emboli from endocarditis could have a similar appearance. The primary neoplasm cannot be determined from the radiographic appearance. As these lesions grow, they can become confluent and lose their rounded shape. This 66-year-old female with metastatic non–small cell lung cancer and rectal carcinoma presented with right upper back pain and upper extremity paresthesias. Review her CT images in Figure 5-167.

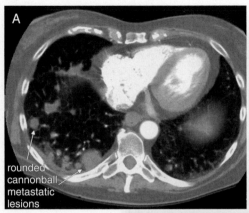

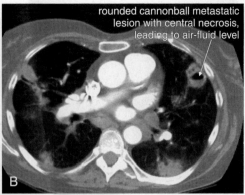

rounded cannonball metastatic lesion with central necrosis, leading to air-fluid level

rounded cannonball metastatic lesions

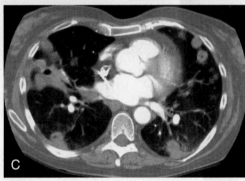

Figure 5-167. **Metastatic disease with cannonball emboli.** Same patient as Figure 5-166. CT with IV contrast, viewed on lung windows. A, B, and C are axial slices at various levels through the chest, depicting the extent of metastatic disease. Some of the lesions have undergone central necrosis and have air–fluid levels (remember, air is black on lung windows). Septic emboli from endocarditis could result in small lung abscesses with an identical appearance.

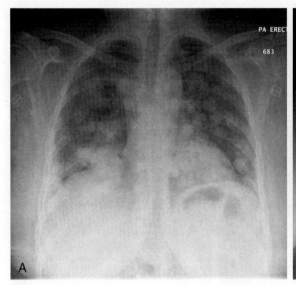

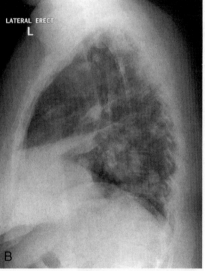

Figure 5-168. **Metastatic disease with cannonball emboli. A,** Posterior-anterior (PA) chest x-ray. **B,** Lateral chest x-ray. This 46-year-old female with metastatic cervical cancer presented with lower extremity weakness and gait difficulty. Her x-ray shows the same pattern of scattered, rounded, bilateral, fluffy densities as in the previous patient, a hallmark of metastatic tumor emboli.

Figure 5-169. Metastatic disease with cannonball emboli. Same patient as Figure 5-168. The patient's chest CT with IV contrast shows numerous rounded lung densities consistent with diffuse metastatic disease. Some have lower density centers (darker gray on lung windows), consistent with central necrosis. **A, B,** and **C,** axial slices at various levels through the chest depicting the extent of metastatic disease, viewed on lung windows.

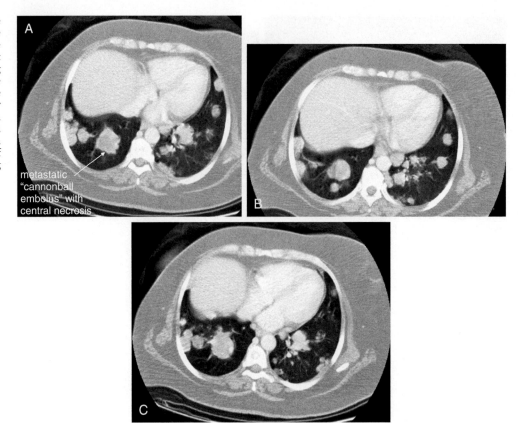

Figure 5-170. Metastatic disease with cannonball emboli. A, Posterior-anterior (PA) chest x-ray. **B,** Lateral chest x-ray. This 27-year-old female with metastatic pancreatic cancer presented with fever. Her fever workup included a chest x-ray that shows metastatic disease in the same pattern as the previous figures, with multiple scattered, rounded, bilateral lung densities.

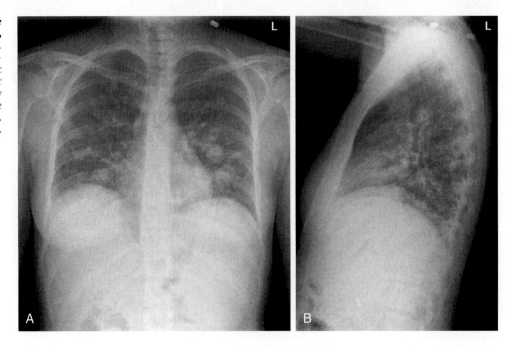

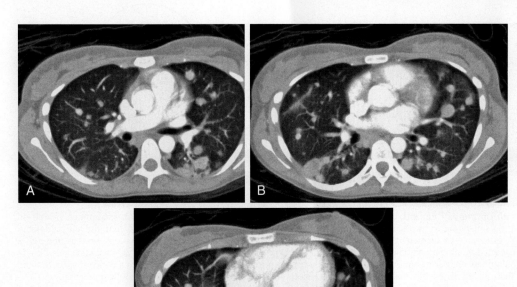

Figure 5-171. Metastatic disease with cannonball emboli. Same patient as Figure 5-170. The patient's chest CT with IV contrast shows the same pattern of scattered bilateral rounded lung lesions, characteristic of metastatic tumor emboli. Tiny emboli shower the lungs, implant, and grow. Some have lower-density centers, suggesting central necrosis. The rounded appearance occurs from concentric growth of a clone of tumor cells. **A-C,** Axial slices viewed on lung windows, progressing from cephalad to caudad.

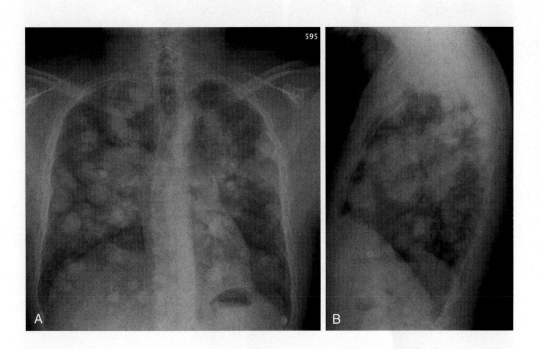

Figure 5-172. Metastatic disease with cannonball emboli. A, Posterior-anterior (PA) chest x-ray. **B,** Lateral chest x-ray. This patient with metastatic osteosarcoma has the classic appearance of pulmonary metastatic disease, with innumerable rounded, bilateral nodules. These occur as tumor cells are carried hematogenously to the lungs, implant, and grow. Nodules of different sizes may have seeded at different times.

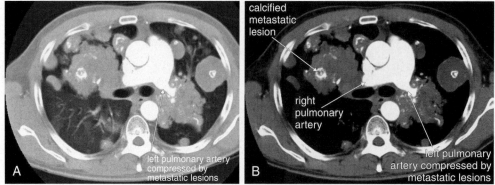

Figure 5-173. Metastatic disease with cannonball emboli. Same patient as Figure 5-172. **A,** Chest CT with IV contrast, axial image viewed on lung windows. **B,** Same image viewed on soft-tissue windows. Here, confluent metastatic lesions are creating a unique problem: the left pulmonary artery is surrounded and compressed. Compare the diameter of the right and left pulmonary arteries. Consider if this patient were to undergo a ventilation–perfusion (VQ) scan for suspected pulmonary embolism. Extrinsic compression of a pulmonary artery can create VQ mismatch, resulting in a false-positive result for thrombotic pulmonary embolism. Another feature of these lesions is internal calcifications, although a noncontrast computed tomography would demonstrate this more clearly. The white markings within the lesions are calcium deposits, not injected contrast material.

Figure 5-174. Metastatic disease with cannonball emboli. Same patient as Figure 5-172 and 5-173. The right pulmonary artery remains patent despite encroaching metastatic lesions. **A,** Chest CT with IV contrast, axial image viewed on lung windows. **B,** Same image viewed on soft-tissue windows.

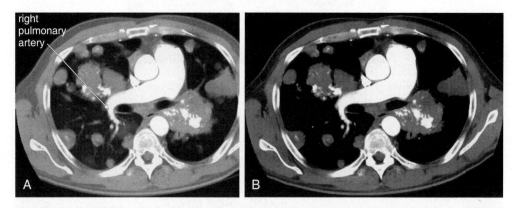

Figure 5-175. Metastatic disease with cannonball emboli: Testicular cancer. Previously healthy 22-year-old male presenting in respiratory distress. **A,** Anterior-posterior (AP) chest x-ray showed diffuse cannon-ball emboli. These are so extensive that they are becoming confluent. On examination, he was noted to have a previously undiagnosed testicular mass. **B,** Posterior-anterior (PA) chest x-ray obtained months later, the patient has shown a response to chemotherapy, albeit incomplete.

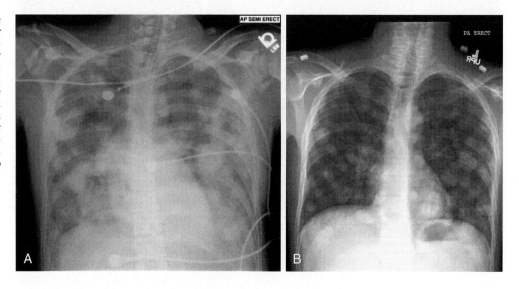

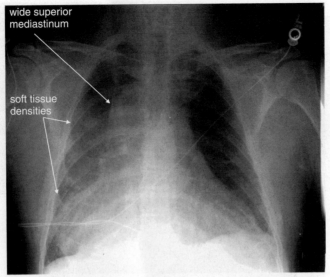

Figure 5-176. Wide mediastinum. This 64-year-old male presented with interscapular back pain, chest pain, and neck pain. Chest x-ray shows a wide mediastinum with an indistinct right heart border and medial right diaphragm, corresponding to possible infiltrates in the right middle and lower lobes. Is this a pleural effusion? The right costophrenic angle is not blunted. What is your interpretation? Compare this with the posterior–anterior and lateral chest x-ray in Figure 5-177 and the CT in Figure 5-178.

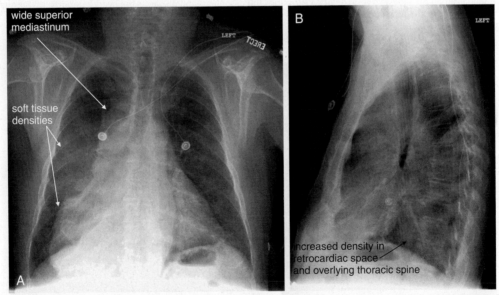

Figure 5-177. Wide mediastinum. Same patient as Figure 5-176. **A,** Posterior-anterior (PA) chest x-ray. **B,** Lateral chest x-ray. The PA chest x-ray shows a bizarre mediastinal contour, wide at the top and even more so near the diaphragm. Without other clinical information, an appropriate interpretation could be densities overlying the right heart border and right medial diaphragm, corresponding to the right middle and lower lobes. On the lateral view, the retrocardiac space appears dense, without the normal increase in lucency of the thoracic spine approaching the diaphragm (the spine sign). Computed tomography was performed for evaluation of the aorta and mediastinum (Figure 5-178).

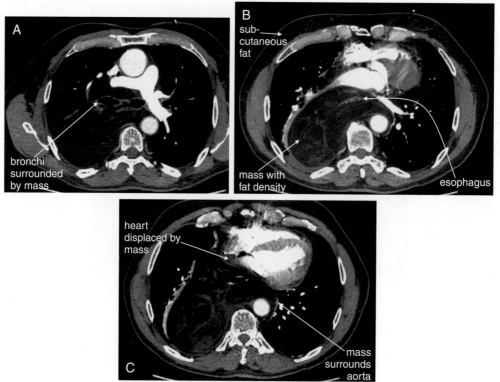

Figure 5-178. Liposarcoma of mediastinum. Same patient as Figures 5-176 and 5-177. His chest x-ray showed a wide mediastinum. **A-C,** Chest CT with IV contrast, axial images viewed on soft-tissue windows. **A** through **C** progress from cephalad to caudad. His CT showed a normal aorta—a wide mediastinum is not synonymous with aortic pathology. Instead, a large mediastinal mass surrounding the aorta was found. This mass is fat density—compare with subcutaneous fat on the same images. The mass surrounds the esophagus and displaces the heart anteriorly. It also surrounds the trachea and esophagus and displaces the main bronchi. Look back at the chest x-rays in the prior two figures. The mediastinal silhouette is more understandable with the CT findings in mind.

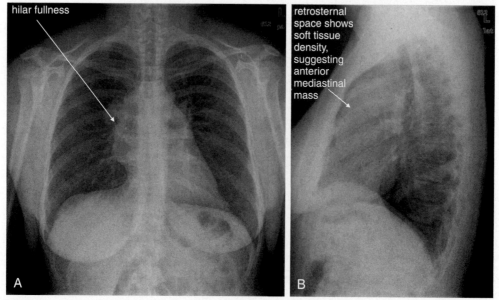

Figure 5-179. Mediastinal mass with superior vena cava syndrome. A, Posterior-anterior (PA) chest x-ray. **B,** Lateral chest x-ray. This 39-year-old healthy female presented with 1 week of bilateral neck pain, shortness of breath, and lightheadedness. She also noted enlarging neck veins a few days prior. Her chest x-ray shows prominence in both hila on the posterior–anterior view. The lateral view shows soft-tissue density in the retrosternal space anterior to the heart—suspicious for an anterior mediastinal mass. Compare this with Figures 5-16 and 5-17, which show both normal and abnormal retrosternal spaces. Also compare with Figure 5-183, where hilar masses are present on the frontal projection, but the lateral x-ray shows a clear retrosternal space. The clinical presentation suggests either superior vena cava syndrome or a pericardial effusion. The heart size is normal on this chest x-ray, and the other findings suggest an anterior mediastinal mass with superior vena cava syndrome. Chest CT from the patient is shown in Figure 5-180.

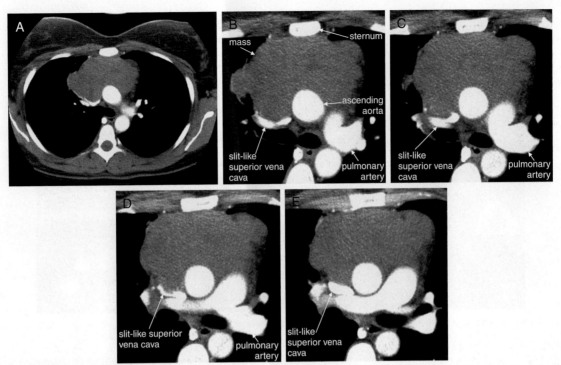

Figure 5-180. Mediastinal mass with superior vena cava (SVC) syndrome because of extrinsic compression. As suggested by the chest x-ray in Figure 5-179, this patient has an anterior mediastinal mass. Chest CT with IV contrast, viewed on soft-tissue windows. **A,** A single complete axial slice is shown for context. The remaining slices have been cropped to focus on the mass and great vessels. **B** through **E** progress from cephalad to caudad. Between the sternum and the ascending aorta lies a large soft-tissue mass. This is extrinsically compressing the SVC to a slit, explaining the patient's dilated neck veins. Compare with the next case, which shows internal thrombosis of the SVC, also causing SVC syndrome. Biopsy here confirmed diffuse large B cell lymphoma, primary mediastinal.

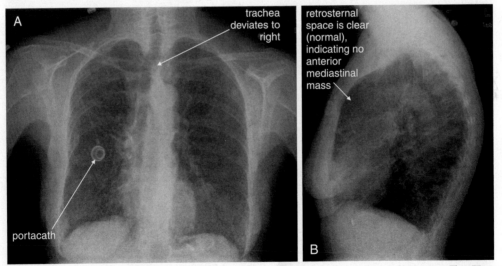

Figure 5-181. Superior vena cava (SVC) syndrome. A, Posterior-anterior (PA) chest x-ray. **B,** Lateral chest x-ray. This 75-year-old female with *Mycobacterium avium* and subsequent bronchiectasis presented with 2 days of increasing swelling in the face and dilatation of her neck veins. The presentation suggests SVC syndrome or large pericardial effusion impairing venous return to the chest. However, on her chest x-ray, the heart size appears normal and the mediastinum appears normal in size, making mediastinal mass less likely. The trachea does appear deviated on the posterior–anterior view, which can be a sign of a mediastinal mass. On the lateral view, the retrosternal space is clear, making anterior mediastinal mass unlikely. The patient has a portacath in the right chest. A chest CT was performed to assess further (Figure 5-182).

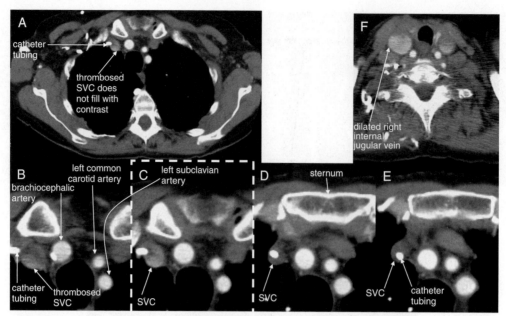

Figure 5-182. Superior vena cava (SVC) syndrome from internal thrombosis of the SVC. Same patient as in Figure 5-181. Chest CT with IV contrast, viewed on soft-tissue windows. **A,** Single full axial slice is shown for context. **C,** The image outlined in a dashed line is a cropped view from the full slice **(A).** The other views are cropped and enlarged to focus on the great vessels. **B** through **E** progress from cephalad to caudad. Her CT shows thrombosis of the SVC at the point at which her portacath tubing enters from the right subclavian vein—note the absence of contrast within the SVC. The portacath tubing is visible as a bright white circle, surrounded by thrombus. **F,** Cephalad to the entry of the catheter, the internal jugular veins are patent and contrast filled—in fact, dilated because of the obstructed SVC. Not shown, the SVC becomes visible again below the level of thrombosis and is filled with contrast. Compare this case with the prior case of SVC syndrome from extrinsic compression (Figures 5-179 and 5-180).

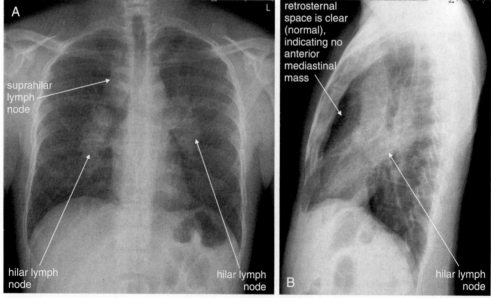

Figure 5-183. Lymphoma versus sarcoidosis. A, Posterior-anterior (PA) chest x-ray. **B,** Lateral chest x-ray. This 31-year-old male presented with hematuria, suprapubic abdominal pain, nausea and vomiting, and nonproductive cough. Chest x-ray showed bilateral hilar and suprahilar lymph nodes. On the posterior–anterior and lateral views, these are seen as densities outlining the trachea and main bronchi. The anterior mediastinum does not appear to be involved, as a normal lucency persists anterior to the heart on the lateral x-ray. The differential diagnosis includes sarcoidosis and lymphoma. Computed tomography was performed (Figure 5-184). The patient's workup was consistent with sarcoidosis.

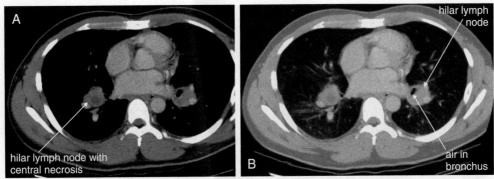

Figure 5-184. **Lymphoma versus sarcoidosis.** Same patient as Figure 5-183, where chest x-ray shows bilateral hilar lymphadenopathy. **A,** Soft-tissue windows. **B,** Lung windows. The patient's chest CT without IV contrast shows soft-tissue densities consistent with lymph nodes near both hila. The right lymph node has a central area of decreased (fluid) density, consistent with necrosis. The air collection adjacent to the left lymph node can be tracked through adjacent CT slices and is actually a branch of the left main bronchus, not an air–fluid level in the lymph node. Importantly, no other mediastinal nodes are seen, and the remainder of the patient's CT of the chest and abdomen was negative for other adenopathy. His workup was consistent with sarcoidosis, not lymphoma.

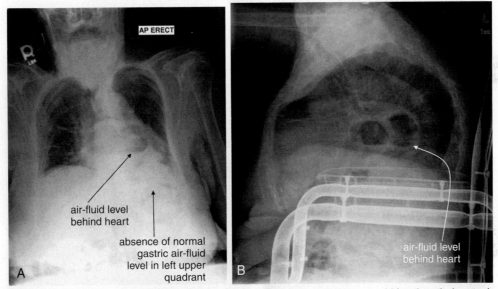

Figure 5-185. **Hiatal hernia. A,** Anterior-posterior (AP) chest x-ray. **B,** Lateral chest x-ray. This 82-year-old female with chronic obstructive pulmonary disease presented with 10 days of cough and dyspnea. Her heart rate was 129 with a temperature of 38.2°C and an oxygen saturation of 92% on room air. Her chest x-ray shows an air–fluid level overlying the heart on the anterior–posterior view and behind the heart on the lateral view. The patient is severely kyphotic. Consider the normal mediastinal anatomy. The esophagus lies in the posterior mediastinum behind the heart and anterior to the aorta. Note the absence of a gastric air bubble in the left upper quadrant. The mass with the air–fluid level in this case is a hiatal hernia. CT was performed to rule out a pulmonary abscess, given the patient's fever and respiratory symptoms (Figure 5-186). A gastric volvulus could have a similar appearance and could be evaluated with barium swallow.

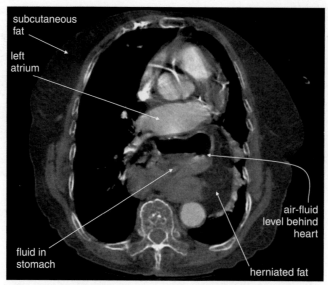

Figure 5-186. Hiatal hernia. CT with IV contrast, viewed on soft-tissue windows. Compare with the chest x-ray from the same patient in Figure 5-185. This image is taken at the level of the left atrium, which lies just anterior to the air- and fluid-containing structure—a hiatal hernia. Just left of the stomach is herniated fat (compare with subcutaneous fat).

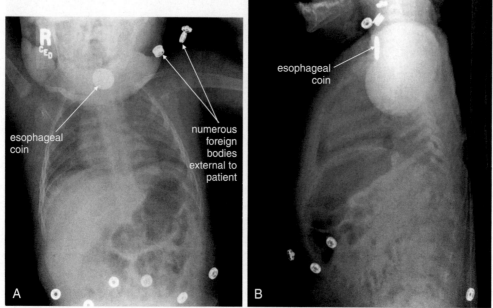

Figure 5-187. Esophageal foreign bodies (coin). A, Frontal projection chest x-ray. **B,** Lateral chest x-ray. This 11-month-old child developed cough and irregular breathing and was thought to have ingested a foreign body. Chest x-ray shows a disc-shaped object with the classic appearance of an esophageal coin. This had the dimensions of a nickel and was removed with a coin forceps under general anesthesia. Typically, coins in the esophagus orient themselves en face in the frontal plane so that they appear circular like an "O" on frontal chest x-ray (think of the British spelling *oesophagus*). Naturally, they appear linear on lateral x-ray. Tracheal coins tend to orient themselves in a midsagittal plane, apparently because of the incomplete cartilaginous tracheal rings, which are open posteriorly. Remember also the risk of esophageal perforation from an ingested watch battery, which can have a similar appearance to coins. An example is shown in the abdominal imaging chapter (Chapter 9). Learn one more lesson from the images here: when searching for an ingested foreign body, undress the patient and remove any unnecessary external radiopaque foreign bodies to avoid confusion.

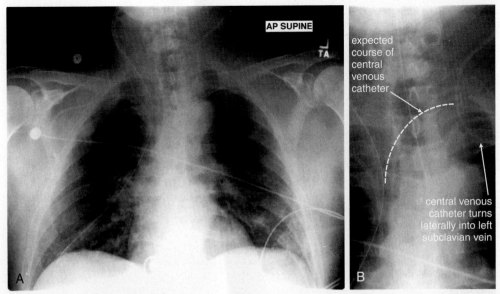

Figure 5-188. Misplaced central venous catheter. Chest x-rays are routinely obtained to assess the position of medical devices such as central venous catheters and to identify complications such as pneumothorax. Routine parts of the process of image review should be to locate foreign bodies, assess their identity, and determine whether they are correctly positioned. This patient has multiple foreign bodies visible. The left internal jugular catheter does not take the expected course toward the superior vena cava on the patient's right. Instead, it turns laterally into the left subclavian vein. **A,** Anterior-posterior (AP) supine chest x-ray. **B,** Close-up from **A.**

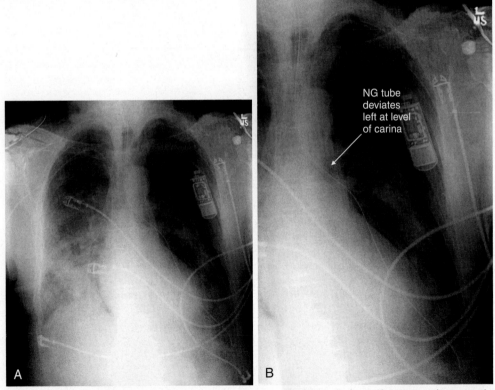

Figure 5-189. Misplaced nasogastric tube. Always assess the chest x-ray image for foreign bodies and attempt to determine their locations. In this patient, a nasogastric tube has been placed. The tube unexpectedly leaves the midline and courses through the left chest before terminating as expected in the left upper quadrant of the abdomen. This unusual path makes it unlikely that the tube is within the esophagus, which is usually a midline structure until it crosses the diaphragm and reaches the stomach. Instead, the nasogastric tube appears to diverge left at the level of the carina—meaning that it has been erroneously placed into the trachea and then the left main bronchus. Had the patient been fed or received lavage through this tube, the results could have been disastrous. **A,** Frontal projection chest x-ray. **B,** Close-up from **A.**

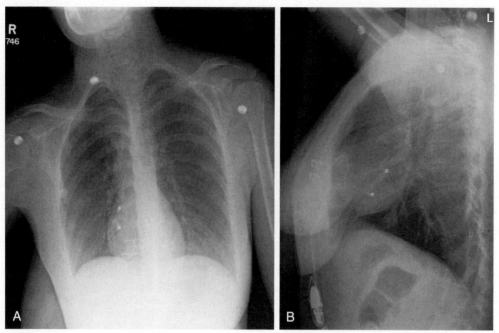

Figure 5-190. **Pacemaker wire not attached. A,** Frontal projection chest x-ray. **B,** Lateral chest x-ray. This 25-year-old female recently underwent thoracic pacemaker replacement with an abdominal pacemaker because of local site irritation. She presented with lightheadedness. The inferior epicardial pacemaker wire does not connect to the pacemaker (see the close-up in Figure 5-191). When a pacemaker problem is suspected, always inspect the course of the wires for kinks or discontinuities.

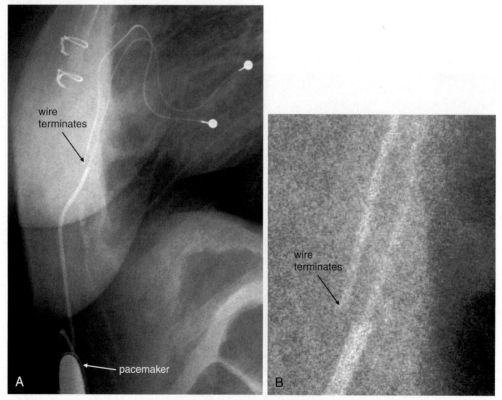

Figure 5-191. **Pacemaker wire not attached.** Same patient as in Figure 5-190. **A,** Close-up from lateral chest x-ray. **B,** A very enlarged view from **A** with the contrast and brightness adjusted to visualize the disconnected pacemaker wire.

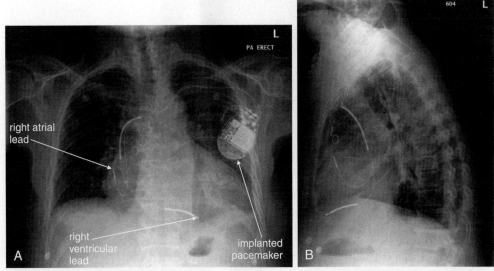

Figure 5-192. Pacemaker wires. A, Posterior-anterior (PA) chest x-ray. **B,** Lateral chest x-ray. This 58-year-old male with a history of coronary artery disease, heart failure, and renal insufficiency presented with increasing dyspnea and edema to the lower abdomen. His chest x-ray shows the normal configuration of an implanted pacemaker with right atrial and ventricular leads. The wires connect to the pacemaker appropriately and show no kinks or breaks. The tips are in the expected positions overlying the right atrium and ventricle. An electrocardiogram and pulse examination are needed to assess whether the pacemaker is firing appropriately and achieving capture.

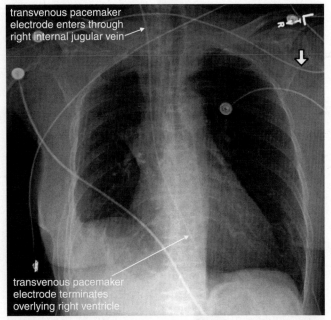

Figure 5-193. Transvenous pacemaker wire. Frontal projection chest x-ray. This 77-year-old female, recently discharged after admission for rapid atrial flutter, had increased her calcium channel and beta-blocker doses. Today, her husband noted the patient felt "sick." Emergency medical services found the patient to be diaphoretic, hypotensive, and bradycardic. In the emergency department, the patient had an unmeasurable blood pressure with a heart rate of 35. Her electrocardiogram showed atrial flutter with third-degree heart block and a junctional escape rhythm. She did not respond to medications and a transvenous pacemaker was placed by a right internal jugular vein approach by an emergency physician using ultrasound guidance. Note the relatively straight course of the catheter from this entry point, which makes this the preferred approach. Physical examination for pulses and electrocardiogram are needed to confirm that the pacemaker is achieving capture.

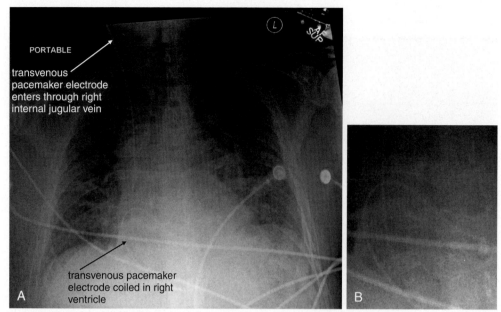

Figure 5-194. Transvenous pacemaker wire. This 58-year-old male with a history of paroxysmal atrial fibrillation and sick sinus syndrome underwent an atrioventricular nodal ablation 2 days earlier. He presented with syncope and was unable to stand. His electrocardiogram showed no P waves and a junctional rhythm. No blood pressure could be obtained, and the patient remained lightheaded, bradycardic, and dyspneic despite medications. A transvenous pacemaker was placed by a right internal jugular vein approach. The electrode is coiled in a position overlying the right ventricle. Despite this, it achieved capture and the patient was stabilized. Notice the heterogeneous opacities consistent with pulmonary edema—this patient was in cardiogenic shock because of his bradycardia. **A,** Anterior-posterior (AP) supine chest x-ray. **B,** Close-up from **A** to demonstrate the coiled electrode.

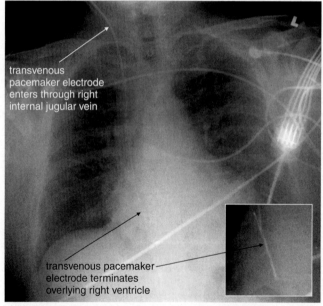

Figure 5-195. Transvenous pacemaker wire. Same patient as Figure 5-194. The pacing electrode has been repositioned and is no longer coiled. The patient's lung fields appear clearer than in the previous x-ray, indicating resolution of his pulmonary edema now that his pacemaker is functioning and his heart rate is appropriate. Small panel is an enlarged view from the AP chest x-ray, with contrast adjusted to accentuate the pacemaker wire.

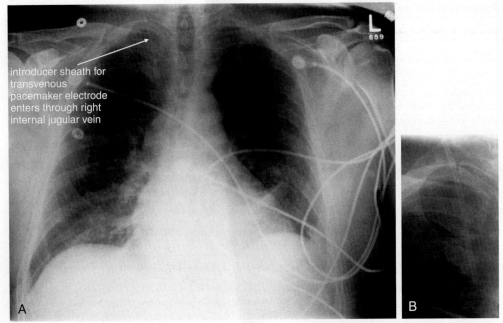

Figure 5-196. Transvenous pacemaker wire. Same patient as Figure 5-195, the following day. The pacemaker has been removed, as the patient had returned to normal sinus rhythm. The introducer catheter is still present through the right internal jugular vein. **A,** Anterior-posterior (AP) chest x-ray. **B,** Close-up from **A,** focused on the internal jugular catheter.

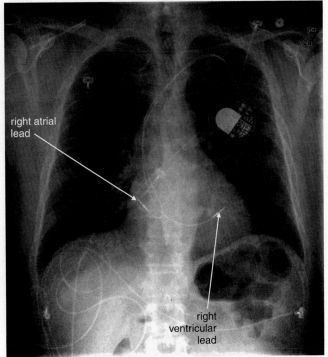

Figure 5-197. Permanent implanted pacemaker. Same patient as Figures 5-194 through 5-196. The patient presented again with syncope and bradycardia. A permanent pacemaker was placed with right atrial and ventricular leads.

TABLE 5-8. Assessment of a Chest X-ray Technique in Preparation for Interpretation

Action	Error Prevented
Lower the room lights	Improves contrast resolution, making low-contrast lesions more visible.
Confirm that the image belongs to the patient in question	Prevents "wrong patient" error.
Confirm that the date of the image being viewed corresponds to the current or desired date	Prevents erroneous action based on previous radiograph.
Note the exam technique (e.g., PA, AP, supine, upright, or lordotic)	Reminds the physician of diagnostic limitations and artifacts associated with specific x-ray techniques.
Assess for lordotic positioning	May cause asymmetrical magnification of mediastinum and heart.
Confirm right–left orientation	Prevents "wrong site" error.
Assess for patient rotation	Prevents false appearance of mediastinal widening, mediastinal shift, or tracheal deviation due to rotation.
Assess adequacy of lung expansion–inspiratory effort	Checks for poor inspiratory effort, which can simulate pulmonary edema.
Assess chest x-ray exposure	Checks for underexposure, which can simulate pulmonary edema, and overexposure, which can hide lung field details such as pneumothorax.
Compare the current exam with previous images from the same patient	May reveal an abnormality on the current examination to be unchanged from prior examinations and therefore not the likely cause of current acute symptoms. Unnecessary diagnostic testing and therapeutic interventions may be prevented by such a comparison. In other cases, a subtle abnormality on the current exam may prove to be new compared with prior images and thus cause for concern, with further diagnostic testing or treatments being indicated.

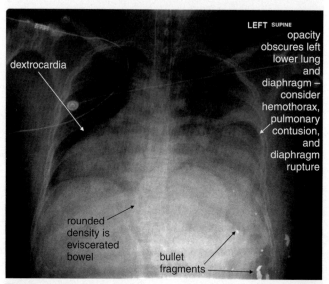

Figure 5-198. Situs inversus or dextrocardia with gunshot wound. This 34-year-old male presented with gunshot wounds to the left upper abdomen and lower chest. On examination, small bowel was noted to be protruding from center of the anterior chest. Clearly, the patient requires operative exploration, and imaging plays a limited role. However, chest x-ray in this case shows several important findings. The heart lies completely in the right chest. From this x-ray, it is not clear if this is isolated dextrocardia or situs inversus. In the operating room, the patient was found to have situs inversus with left upper quadrant liver injury from the gunshot wound. The left diaphragm is obscured on this chest x-ray. As we discussed earlier, in the supine position this may indicate pleural fluid (hemothorax), pulmonary contusion, or diaphragm injury with herniation of abdominal contents into the chest. If a chest tube is placed, special care must be taken to avoid injury to any herniated abdominal contents. The eviscerated bowel is visible as a density in the central abdomen. Bullet fragments are also seen. No pneumothorax was visible, although a chest tube was placed because of obvious concern for this.

TABLE 5-9. Mnemonic for Systematic Interpretation of Chest X-ray

A	**Airway** • Review the airway, inspecting the trachea and main-stem bronchi and looking for deviation or evidence of luminal obstruction. • Is the trachea deviated, suggesting tension pneumothorax, lobar collapse, or other mass effect?

B	**Bones and Breast Shadows**
	• Inspect the bones for radiographic density, fractures, lytic lesions, or deformity.
	   • Are lytic lesions present?
	   • Are fractures evident from cortical disruptions?
	   • Is the medial scapula visible? Do not mistake this for the pleural line of a pneumothorax.
	• Note breast shadows to avoid mistaking these for lower chest pathology such as infiltrate or effusion.

C	**Cardiac Silhouette** • Assess the cardiac and mediastinal silhouette for general size and contour. • Note an enlarged cardiac silhouette, suggesting cardiomegaly or pericardial effusion. • Inspect for pericardial air, air in the soft tissues of the neck, or a continuous diaphragm sign. • Inspect the borders of the heart and mediastinum. If the margins are not easily discerned, this may indicate the pathologic silhouette sign of an adjacent infiltrate or effusion. • Note the width of the mediastinum. • A wide mediastinum may be due to patient position or x-ray technique, a mediastinal mass, or aortic pathology.

D	**Diaphragm**
	• Assess the diaphragm, with attention to the contour and costophrenic angle, bilaterally.
	• Look for blunted costophrenic angles, suggesting pleural fluid.
	• Note a deep sulcus sign, suggesting tension pneumothorax.
	• Look for an elevated or irregular diaphragm.
	   • Are both diaphragms distinct? If the margin of the diaphragm is indistinct, consider an adjacent infiltrate or effusion.
	   • Is one diaphragm higher than the other? (Right normally is higher than left.) The appearance of an elevated diaphragm may indicate volume loss, pleural effusion, infiltrate, diaphragmatic paralysis, or diaphragmatic hernia.
	   • Are abdominal organs or nasogastric tubes visible in the chest, suggesting diaphragmatic hernia or diaphragm rupture?
	• Is a black line visible beneath the diaphragm, indicating pneumoperitoneum?
	• Is a continuous diaphragm sign visible, indicating pneumopericardium?

E	**Everything Else** • Review everything else around the lung fields, including the subcutaneous soft tissues and pleural boundaries.

F	**Lung Fields**
	• Review the lung fields themselves, looking for evidence of pneumonia, pulmonary edema, parenchymal mass, pleural effusion, or pneumothorax.
	• Is a pneumothorax present?
	   • Do lung markings extend to the periphery?
	   • Is a pleural line visible?
	   • Is subcutaneous air visible?
	• Is a pleural effusion present?
	   • Is the density of one hemithorax different from the other?
	   • Is a meniscus visible?
	• Is a parenchymal opacity visible?
	   • Are air bronchograms present, confirming airspace consolidation?
	   • Is cephalization present, suggesting pulmonary edema?
	• Are cavitary lesions present, suggesting abscess or tuberculosis?

F	**Foreign Bodies or Devices**
	• Are foreign bodies present? Are two orthogonal views available to confirm the location (within or external to the patient)?
	• Are medical devices properly positioned?
	   • Endotracheal tube: Terminates 1 cm above the carina and below the suprasternal notch
	   • Central venous catheters: Follow the expected course of the target vessel
	   • Thoracostomy tubes: all fenestrations are within pleural space
	   • Nasogastric and orogastric tubes: Should not deviate from midline above diaphragm
	   • Pacemaker and AICD wires: Not kinked or discontinuous

L	**Lateral View** • Have you inspected the lateral view, if one is available?

Adapted from Crausman RS: The ABCs of chest X-ray film interpretation. *Chest,* 113:256-257, 1998.

TABLE 5-10. Pitfalls and Pearls in Interpretation of the Chest X-ray

Pitfall	Example	Pearl
Failure to interpret the image for findings other than those relevant to the clinical presentation	Failure to note a lung mass in a patient presenting with fever and cough	Establish a clinical question, but recognize and perform a systematic review of the entire image as outlined in Table 5-9.
Distraction by obvious abnormalities	Not noting a small pneumothorax in a patient with significant cardiomegaly	Follow a systematic search pattern, as outlined in Table 5-9. After completing the image review, ask yourself the following: • Do additional abnormalities exist that I have overlooked due to my focus on the obvious?
Failure to notice second (third, fourth, etc.) abnormalities once a single abnormality is found	Failure to observe pneumoperitoneum in a patient with a pleural effusion	Follow a systematic search pattern, as outlined in Table 5-9. After completing the image review, ask yourself the following: • Did I answer the clinical question? • Did I review all important features of the x-ray systematically?
Failure to consider the differential diagnosis of an abnormality due to use of simple pattern recognition	Interpretation of all parenchymal opacities as infectious infiltrates, forgetting that pulmonary infarction can have a similar appearance; thus, a patient with pulmonary embolism might be misdiagnosed with pneumonia	Consider the differential diagnosis of all imaging abnormalities. Ask yourself the following: • Am I certain that the image abnormality represents the diagnosis I have ascribed to it? • Could other disease processes explain the radiographic appearance?
Failure to confirm that the image being evaluated is from the correct patient	Chest tube placed in the wrong patient	Confirm the patient's name on the imaging study.
Failure to confirm that the image being evaluated is from the correct date	Chest tube placed in the correct patient but for a pneumothorax that was present on an x-ray from the prior year	Confirm the image date.
Failure to confirm that the image being evaluated has the correct image orientation	Chest tube placed on the wrong side	Confirm the image's left–right orientation.
Failure to recognize limitations due to the radiographic technique	Inability of a supine x-ray to identify subdiaphragmatic air	Note the radiographic technique. Consciously ask the following: • Does this technique have diagnostic limitations in evaluating certain disease processes?

Diagnostic imaging plays a critical role in the evaluation of many patients with blunt and penetrating chest trauma. In this chapter, we discuss the indications for imaging with chest x-ray, ultrasound, and computed tomography (CT). We review a systematic approach to interpretation of chest x-ray and CT. We also discuss and compare imaging findings of key thoracic injuries using chest x-ray, CT, and ultrasound in those cases where it is commonly applied. Our discussion highlights current controversies in imaging of thoracic trauma.

THORACIC IMAGING MODALITIES

The major diagnostic imaging modalities for blunt and penetrating chest trauma are chest x-ray, ultrasound, and chest CT with intravenous (IV) contrast. Aortography is more rarely used, most often following an abnormal chest x-ray or CT result. We review these modalities here, including a detailed discussion of the indications for and interpretation of each imaging technique.

In this chapter, figures are clustered by patient to illustrate injuries using multiple modalities. As a consequence, the order of reference to figures in the chapter is not always sequential.

CHEST X-RAY

Chest x-ray is the most commonly used diagnostic modality for all forms of chest trauma. Benefits of chest x-ray include portability (allowing it to be used in the resuscitation bay without moving an unstable patient), speed of acquisition (seconds) and image availability (minutes), low expense (approximately $50 to $100), and low radiation exposure (0.01 mSv, equivalent to 1 day's background exposure on Earth) (Table 6-1).

Clinical Decision Rules: Which Patients Require Chest X-ray?

Chest x-ray historically has been routinely recommended following blunt or penetrating chest trauma.[1] However, a number of studies have examined the sensitivity of history and physical examination in detection of thoracic injury in children and adults. These studies suggest that in stable and alert blunt trauma patients, injuries are extremely rare with a normal thorax examination and the absence of chest complaints.

Bokhari et al.[2] performed a prospective study of 523 stable patients with blunt trauma and 153 stable patients with penetrating trauma (Box 6-1). Before chest x-ray, patients were interviewed and examined for signs and symptoms of hemo- and/or pneumothorax, including chest pain or tenderness, tachypnea (greater than 20 breaths per minute), and abnormalities of bilateral lung sounds. Distracting injuries such as fractures or peritonitis were also noted.[2] The authors found auscultation to be 100% sensitive for detection of hemo- and/or pneumothorax following blunt trauma. Chest pain and tenderness and tachypnea were insensitive (57% and 43%, respectively) but had negative predictive values of 99%. In the set of patients with penetrating chest trauma, history and examination were insufficient to exclude hemo- and/or pneumothorax. The authors conclude that stable blunt trauma patients with normal lung sounds and no chest pain, tenderness, or dyspnea do not require chest x-ray to evaluate for hemo- and/or pneumothorax. This study suffers from nonconsecutive enrollment with potential selection bias. Moreover, the rate of hemo- and/or pneumothorax in this population of blunt trauma patients was only 1.3% (7 of 523 patients), so negative predictive values provide a distorted view of the clinical value of history and physical exam. In a population with a higher rate of hemopneumothorax, the same sensitivity and specificity values would result in inadequate negative predictive values. Moreover, this study assessed the sensitivity of examination for hemo- and/or pneumothorax but did not assess for other important thoracic injuries such as mediastinal injury. In patients with a high-energy blunt injury mechanism suggesting possible mediastinal injury, the value of physical examination and history in excluding injury is uncertain. Nonetheless, in patients with a low-energy blunt trauma mechanism from which mediastinal injury is unlikely, a normal thoracic physical exam, and no complaints of chest pain, chest x-ray does not appear routinely necessary.

In children with blunt thoracic trauma (Box 6-2), Holmes et al.[3] performed a prospective study of 986 patients below the age of 16 years to derive a clinical decision rule for detection of pulmonary contusion, hemothorax, pneumothorax, pneumomediastinum, tracheal–bronchial disruption, aortic injury, hemopericardium, pneumopericardium, blunt cardiac injury, rib fracture, sternal fracture, or any injury to the diaphragm. Of their population, 8.1% sustained a thoracic injury. The following

TABLE 6-1. Comparison of Portability, Speed, Costs, Radiation Exposure, and Information Provided for Common Chest Imaging Modalities for Trauma

	X-ray	Ultrasound	CT
Portable	Yes	Yes	No
Speed	Seconds to acquire, minutes to view	Instantaneous acquisition, simultaneous viewing	Seconds to acquire, minutes to view
Expense	$50-$100	Depends on local institution; is usually performed by emergency physician; and may be billed separately as a procedure at some institutions	Approximately $1000 charge to patient, around $100 institutional cost
Radiation exposure	0.01 mSv, 1 day on Earth	None	4-20 mSv, several years on Earth
Information provided	• Pneumothorax • Hemothorax • Pericardial effusion • Possibly mediastinal injury • Pulmonary contusion • Fractures • Diaphragmatic injury • Pneumoperitoneum	• Pericardial effusion (traditionally performed as part of FAST exam) • Pneumothorax • Hemothorax	Detailed information about • Pneumothorax • Hemothorax • Pericardial effusion • Mediastinal injury, including specific information about aortic injury • Pulmonary contusion • Fractures • Diaphragmatic injury • Pneumoperitoneum

From Renton J, Kincaid S, Ehrlich PF: Should helical CT scanning of the thoracic cavity replace the conventional chest x-ray as a primary assessment tool in pediatric trauma? An efficacy and cost analysis. *J Pediatr Surg* 2003;38(5):793-797, 2003.

Box 6-1: Indications for Chest X-ray Following Chest Trauma

Blunt Trauma
Chest x-ray may not be routinely indicated in stable, alert patients with normal thoracic physical examination and no complaints of chest pain or dyspnea.

Penetrating Trauma
Chest x-ray is routinely required for injuries penetrating the dermis.

Adapted from Bokhari F, Brakenridge S, Nagy K, et al: Prospective evaluation of the sensitivity of physical examination in chest trauma. *J Trauma* 53(6):1135-1138, 2002.

Box 6-2: Clinical Decision Rule for Chest X-ray in Pediatric Blunt Trauma Patients

Chest x-ray is not required in the absence of these criteria:
● **Low age-adjusted systolic blood pressure**
● **Elevated age-adjusted respiratory rate**
● **Abnormal results of thorax exam**
● **Abnormal chest auscultation**
● **Femur fracture**
● **Glasgow Coma Scale score <15**
Sensitivity 98%, negative predictive value 99.4%

Adapted from Holmes JF, Sokolove PE, Brant WE, et al: A clinical decision rule for identifying children with thoracic injuries after blunt torso trauma. *Ann Emerg Med* 39(5):492-499, 2002.

---

features identified thoracic injuries: low age-adjusted systolic blood pressure, elevated age-adjusted respiratory rate, abnormal results of thorax exam, abnormal chest auscultation, femur fracture, and Glasgow Coma Scale score less than 15. Sensitivity was 98% with a 95% confidence interval (CI) of 91% to 100%, with a negative predictive value of 99.4% (95% CI = 97.9%-99.9%).[3]

Chest X-ray Technique and Limitations

For acute trauma patients, a portable chest x-ray is often the initial imaging test. The portable chest x-ray is performed as a supine or upright anterior–posterior (AP) examination (Figure 6-1). The supine examination is most commonly used in blunt trauma resulting from concern about possible coexisting spine trauma that would contraindicate an upright chest x-ray. On a chest x-ray obtained in the supine position, important diagnostic findings, such as subdiaphragmatic air indicating pneumoperitoneum or the layering fluid level of a hemothorax, may not be appreciated (Figures 6-2 through 6-10). Moreover, a supine portable chest x-ray exaggerates the apparent width of the heart and mediastinum, simulating cardiomegaly and potential mediastinal

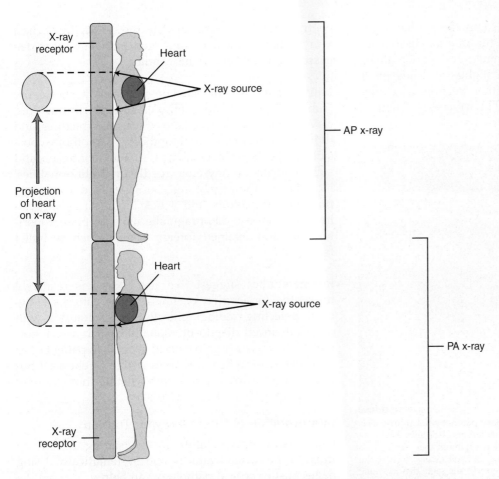

Figure 6-1. **Differences between anterior–posterior (AP) and posterior–anterior (PA) chest x-rays.** The designation refers to the direction of passage of the x-ray beam through the patient to the receptor. The PA chest x-ray positions the x-ray source farther from the heart, and the x-ray receptor closer to the heart, than does the AP x-ray, resulting in less magnification of the cardiac silhouette relative to the thorax. This is explored in more detail in Chapter 5.

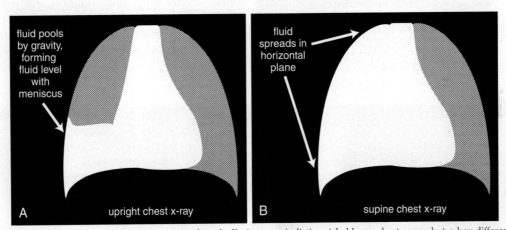

Figure 6-2. **Hemothorax.** Hemothorax and nontraumatic pleural effusions are indistinguishable on chest x-ray, but a key difference in appearance may occur resulting from the use of supine chest x-ray in immobilized trauma patients. In the supine position, pleural fluid (blood or other pleural effusion) layers in the plane of the x-ray, providing a diffuse hazy appearance rather than the fluid level typical on an upright chest x-ray. A small amount of hemothorax may be difficult to appreciate, whereas a large hemothorax makes the affected side appear denser than the unaffected side. A diffuse pulmonary contusion could have a similar appearance. If an upright chest x-ray is obtained, the fluid layers and provides the same diagnostic appearance as a pleural effusion, with blunting of the costophrenic angle, and a meniscus sign at the interface with the chest wall. **A, B,** Schematic of how the same hemothorax could appear quite different depending on the patient's position.

injury (see Figure 6-1). For all of these reasons, when possible, an upright chest x-ray should be performed. Particularly in penetrating chest or abdominal trauma, where spinal injury is less likely, an upright chest x-ray should be obtained to maximize detection of *hemothorax* (see Figures 6-2 through 6-10) and *pneumoperitoneum*

(Figure 6-11). In patients who are completely stable hemodynamically and in whom a low suspicion for mediastinal injury exists based on factors such as low-energy trauma mechanism, a posterior–anterior (PA) and lateral chest x-ray should be obtained if a widened mediastinum on portable chest x-ray raises suspicion of mediastinal injury. In some cases, the mechanism of injury (e.g., a blow with fists to the anterior chest) is not consistent with mediastinal injury, and minor abnormalities on chest x-ray (e.g., a slightly widened mediastinum) may not require further imaging. If a high suspicion exists for mediastinal injury, chest CT with IV contrast should be performed, as the sensitivity of chest x-ray is inadequate to exclude mediastinal injury, as discussed in detail later in this chapter.

Injuries that can be detected or suggested by chest x-ray (Table 6-2) include bony injuries such as rib fractures, clavicle fractures or dislocations, scapular fractures, and thoracic spinal injury; pneumothorax, hemothorax, possible tracheobronchial injury, pulmonary contusion, and subcutaneous emphysema; mediastinal abnormalities, including cardiomegaly suggesting pericardial effusion, pneumopericardium, and a host of findings suggesting aortic injury; diaphragmatic injuries; pneumoperitoneum; and retained foreign bodies, such as bullet fragments.

Recent studies suggest that chest x-ray is relatively insensitive for a variety of clinical injury patterns. However, detecting radiographically occult injuries with more advanced diagnostic modalities such as CT scan may not always result in clinical benefits to patients. For example, when a hemothorax is visible on chest CT but not on chest x-ray, it is uncertain whether thoracostomy tube drainage is routinely necessary.

Interpretation of Chest X-ray for Trauma

Chest x-ray interpretation in the setting of trauma must be performed rapidly and systematically. Using a checklist of critical pathology can help you avoid the pitfall of stopping interpretation after recognition of a single abnormality. We review a few important points about the AP portable chest x-ray technique relevant to interpretation, and then we proceed with systematic interpretation.

Figure 6-3. Hemothorax and pulmonary parenchymal injury. This gunshot wound victim has a large hemothorax—despite having a thoracostomy tube in place. The patient is supine in this x-ray, so no layering fluid level is seen. Because blood and soft tissues, such as the heart, diaphragm, and spleen, share essentially the same density, none of the margins of these structures can be discerned where they abut one another. The most cephalad portion of the patient's left thorax appears slightly less dense resulting from the presence of some aerated lung in this region. The two irregular radiopaque structures on the patient's left are bullet fragments. Compare with the CT scan in Figure 6-4. Understand that not all hemothoraces require CT for management but we examine corresponding CT images to clarify chest x-ray findings.

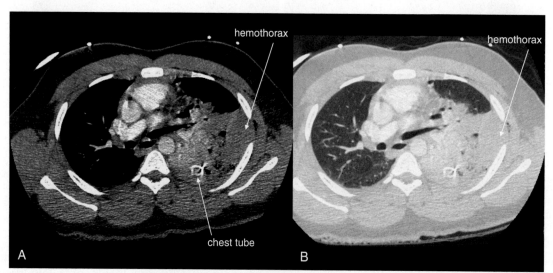

Figure 6-4. Hemothorax. Same patient as Figure 6-3. This CT with IV contrast clarifies the findings on the chest x-ray. **A,** Soft tissue window. **B,** Lung window. The anterior portion of the left lung appears fairly normal (compare with the normal right lung). The posterior left thorax contains two separate denser substances: hemothorax and contused and atelectatic lung. On both the soft-tissue **(A)** and the lung **(B)** windows, the hemothorax is visible as a homogeneous collection along the inner aspect of the ribs. The injured lung has been compressed medially by the hemothorax and appears somewhat more heterogeneous resulting from the presence of both air and contrast-filled pulmonary vessels. The hemothorax is causing mass effect upon the heart, deviating it to the patient's right. The chest tube is visible in cross-section as a bright ring.

The usual technique for acquisition of chest x-ray in blunt trauma is a supine AP portable chest x-ray. This technique allows maintenance of spinal precautions in patients with possible spine trauma, and it is appropriate for unconscious patients who are unable to sit or stand. The AP supine technique has several consequences:

- *The heart and mediastinum appear enlarged, relative to an erect PA x-ray* (see Figure 6-1). This results from the shortened distance from x-ray tube to film or digital media (3 feet, compared with 6 feet for a typical PA x-ray), and from the increased distance between the heart (an anterior chest structure) and the detector. The consequence is apparent cardiomegaly and a wide mediastinum in some patients, which may purely be artifacts of the x-ray technique. Unfortunately, these findings can simulate important pathology such as traumatic pericardial effusion or aortic injury. In one study, 38% of blunt trauma patients demonstrated a wide mediastinum on supine x-ray but a normal mediastinum on an upright view.[4] When a high suspicion for mediastinal injury exists, chest x-ray abnormalities should be further evaluated by more definitive imaging, such as ultrasound (for pericardial effusion) or CT (for aortic injury or pericardial fluid). When a low suspicion exists—for example, in the stable, alert, and minimally symptomatic patient—an upright PA x-ray can be performed and is often normal enough to provide reassurance of the absence of injury.
- *Pleural fluid and air tend to layer in the plane of the x-ray* (see Figure 6-2). This often makes them less apparent. Blunting of the costophrenic angles by pleural fluid is often absent in a supine x-ray, even with large hemothorax. Even a large hemo- or pneumothorax may be invisible. Sometimes a subtle and diffuse density difference between the right and the left chest indicates an abnormality such as a hemothorax layered horizontally in the plane of the x-ray (see Figures 6-2 through 6-10). An upright chest x-ray may reveal layering of pleural fluid (hemothorax) with a more familiar meniscus sign (see Figures 6-6 and 6-7). Ultrasound or CT may also reveal findings not recognized on chest x-ray.
- *The diaphragms are usually higher than in an upright x-ray.* This is caused by the weight of abdominal contents pushing against the diaphragm. It results in a lesser degree of lung inflation, with denser-appearing lung parenchyma.
- *Pneumoperitoneum may not be apparent.* Air may not collect in a subdiaphragmatic location in a supine patient; instead, it may collect preferentially at the highest point in the midline abdomen. If free abdominal air is suspected (rare in blunt trauma but common in penetrating trauma), an upright AP or PA x-ray should be obtained whenever possible (see Figure 6-11).

In penetrating trauma, an upright chest x-ray is often obtained in stable patients, increasing the sensitivity for pneumoperitoneum and hemothorax. However, the AP portable technique still results in an enlarged cardiac and mediastinal silhouette, as described earlier. With these features in mind, we review a systematic approach to interpretation of the chest radiograph. Many approaches have been described, and any approach that allows

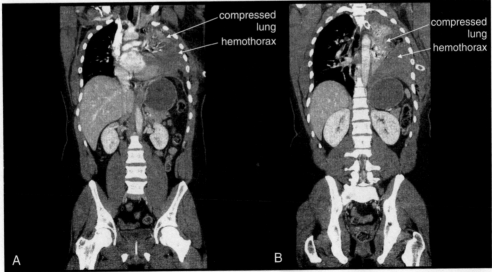

Figure 6-5. Hemothorax, CT with IV contrast. Same patient as Figure 6-4. These coronal reconstructions were performed for evaluation of the spine, but they provide an interesting perspective on the extent of the hemothorax. Remember that although these images suggest a standing patient, they were acquired with the patient in a supine position. **A,** A somewhat more anterior plane than **B.** In both slices, the large hemothorax is seen, and the remaining lung tissue is compressed like an accordion in a medial and cephalad direction. Compare with the patient's chest x-ray in Figure 6-3, also taken in a supine position. Now the dense left hemithorax makes sense, including the decreasing density in the upper lung field resulting from partially aerated lung. The left lung tissue is dense from a combination of compressive atelectasis and probable contusion from the patient's gunshot wound—which are indistinguishable on CT, because both increase the density of lung tissue to a variable extent. Here, we know atelectasis plays a role, because the lung occupies a smaller-than-normal volume.

rapid but comprehensive assessment is appropriate. Table 6-3 reviews a common mnemonic for interpretation of chest x-ray, which we introduced in Chapter 5.

Pneumothorax and Tension Pneumothorax

A **pneumothorax** is evident on chest x-ray as an area of increased lucency at the periphery of the lung. The normal lung markings are absent, giving the region of pneumothorax an unusually black appearance compared with the normal appearance (Figures 6-12 through 6-23). Comparison with the contralateral side is

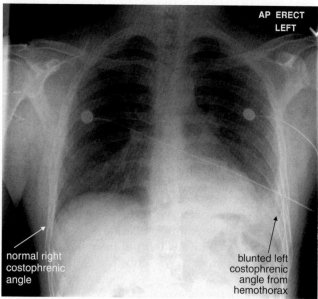

Figure 6-6. Hemothorax: Upright chest x-ray. This 21-year-old male was stabbed in the left posterior thorax and had an oxygen saturation of 94%. This upright chest x-ray shows a blunted left costophrenic angle—compare with the normal right side. The diaphragm and heart border cannot be clearly identified, because blood, heart, and diaphragm share the same x-ray density (fluid density). Compare with Figure 6-7.

useful, although bilateral pneumothoraces may be present. In some cases, the lung edge (visceral pleura) may be visible as a discrete line (see Figures 6-12, 6-13, 6-16, 6-20, and 6-21). The average distance from the ipsilateral thoracic cage to the pleural surface (based on three linear measurements) on upright chest x-ray has been described as predicting pneumothorax volume.[5]

A common pitfall is mistaking the medial border of the scapula for such a pleural line or, conversely, mistaking a pneumothorax for a scapular marking. In cases of very large pneumothorax, the lung may be seen as a density contracted medially toward the lung hilum. Although this is a dramatic and overt finding, to the inexperienced viewer, it may not be recognized without forewarning of this possibility (see Figure 6-13).

Large pneumothoraces can exert pressure effects, resulting in clinically important hemodynamic compromise. Medical dogma states that a tension pneumothorax should never be recorded on x-ray, as it should be treated empirically as soon as suspected. In reality, some large pneumothoraces are difficult to detect clinically, and some patients remain stable despite radiographic appearances suggesting tension pneumothorax. Classic findings of pressure effects associated with tension pneumothorax include the following (Figures 6-24 through 6-28):

- *A very lucent hemithorax,* nearly black compared with the contralateral side, caused by a large pneumothorax.
- *A collapsed lung* medially contracted toward the hilum.
- *The "deep sulcus sign,"* a particularly deep costophrenic angle, resulting from air under pressure in the pleural space pushing the affected diaphragm inferiorly.

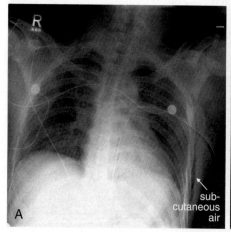
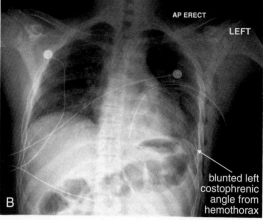

Figure 6-7. Hemothorax: Supine vs. upright chest x-ray. Same patient as Figure 6-6. **A,** A supine film just after placement of a left chest tube. The left costophrenic angle appears clearer (and was interpreted by the radiologist as demonstrating decreased pleural fluid), but don't be fooled. This x-ray was taken in a supine position; thus the fluid moved from its pooled dependent position in the costophrenic angle to a broadly distributed location in the horizontal, supine plane (as discussed in an earlier figure). How can we be sure that the chest tube had not resolved the fluid? **B,** An upright x-ray a few hours later. Again, the left costophrenic angle is obscured as the hemothorax collects in the dependent costophrenic angle. Incidentally, the thoracostomy tube in both figures takes a suboptimal course toward the diaphragm. Subcutaneous air is visible in the left chest wall from the chest tube placement.

Text continues on page 306

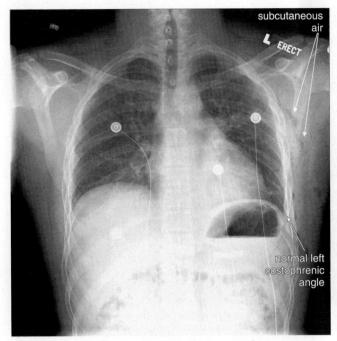

Figure 6-8. Hemothorax: Upright chest x-ray. Same patient as Figure 6-7. This chest x-ray was performed 36 hours after the first, after removal of a chest tube that had been placed for both presumed pneumothorax and treatment of the hemothorax. The left costophrenic angle is sharp and distinct resulting from resolution of the hemothorax. This is an upright chest x-ray, so this changed appearance is not simply a result of the patient's position. Subcutaneous air from the chest tube placement is visible as scattered black densities—compare the right and left chest walls. A few of these patches are labeled—try to identify more collections.

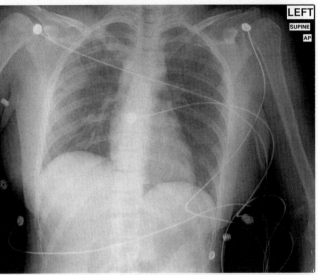

Figure 6-9. Hemothorax: Supine chest x-ray with a subtle density difference. This supine x-ray shows a subtle increase in density of the right hemithorax compared with the left, indicating a hemothorax. This subtle change is sometimes described as a "veiling opacity." Because of the supine position of the patient, the hemothorax does not pool in the costophrenic angle but rather distributes broadly across the entire right hemithorax. As a result, the costophrenic angle remains sharp. As you will see in the corresponding CT images in Figure 6-10, the total amount of fluid is relatively small, so the chest does not appear markedly denser. Can this appearance be distinguished from pulmonary contusion? The two may coexist, but an upright chest x-ray could confirm hemothorax by allowing fluid to become dependent, if the patient's spine has been cleared. Incidentally, the patient has a right clavicle fracture.

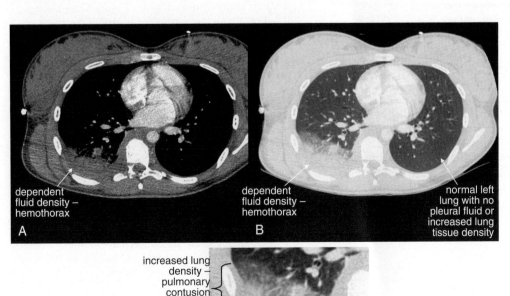

Figure 6-10. Hemothorax, CT with IV contrast. Same patient as Figure 6-9. **A,** Soft-tissue window. **B,** Lung window of the same slice. **C,** Close-up from **B.** Dependent fluid is seen layering in the posterior right thorax—a hemothorax. The immediately adjacent lung appears dense as well; it is impossible on CT to distinguish the increased density of compressive atelectasis resulting from the hemothorax vs. actual pulmonary contusion. Compare with the patient's normal left chest, where the lung is fully aerated even in the most posterior portion. Can we be sure that the increased density seen on the chest x-ray in the prior figure was a consequence of the hemothorax and not the dense lung? No; both contribute to the increased chest x-ray density.

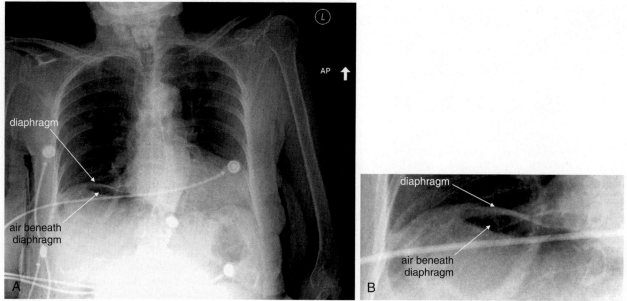

Figure 6-11. Pneumoperitoneum: Upright chest x-ray. A, Upright chest x-ray. **B,** Close-up. An upright chest x-ray is the preferred view for detection of subdiaphragmatic air (pneumoperitoneum). On the supine view commonly obtained in blunt trauma, free air may not be visible, because it may collect in the anterior abdomen, rather than beneath the diaphragm.

TABLE 6-2. Injuries Detected or Suggested by Chest X-ray[25,98,109]

Injury Type	Specific Injury or Finding	Sensitivity
Bony injuries	• Rib fractures • Clavicle fractures or dislocations • Scapular fractures • Thoracic spinal injury	Varies depending on degree of displacement.
Injuries to the lungs, pleura, or airways	• Pneumothorax • Hemothorax • Possible tracheobronchial injury • Pulmonary contusion • Subcutaneous emphysema	Varies depending on degree of injury. Controversy exists about the necessity for explicit diagnosis and treatment of subtle injuries not evident on chest x-ray. Chest x-ray has been reported to be only 45% sensitive for pneumothorax compared with CT, but the necessity for treatment of CT-only pneumothoraces is unclear.
Mediastinal and cardiac injuries	• Cardiomegaly, suggesting pericardial effusion • Pneumopericardium • Findings suggesting aortic injury	Around 86%-93% sensitive for aortic injury.
Diaphragmatic injuries	• Herniated bowel and solid organs in thorax	Around 60%.
Abdominal injuries	• Pneumoperitoneum	Varies with degree of pneumoperitoneum. Sensitivity is reportedly around 38% for any pneumoperitoneum but as low as zero in patients with minimal free air (1-mm air pockets) and as high as 100% in patients with ≥13-mm collections.
Foreign bodies	• Bullets • Shrapnel • Knives	Varies depending on size and density of object.

From Ball CG, Kirkpatrick AW, Laupland KB, et al. Factors related to the failure of radiographic recognition of occult posttraumatic pneumothoraces. *Am J Surg* 189(5):541-546, 2005; discussion 546; Smithers BM, O'Loughlin B, Strong RW. Diagnosis of ruptured diaphragm following blunt trauma: Results from 85 cases. *Aust N Z J Surg* 61(10):737-741, 1991; Stapakis JC, Thickman D. Diagnosis of pneumoperitoneum: Abdominal CT vs. upright chest film. *J Comput Assist Tomogr* 16(5):713-716, 1992.

TABLE 6-3. Mnemonic for Systematic Interpretation of Chest X-ray in Trauma[110]

A	**Airway** • Review the airway, inspecting the trachea and main-stem bronchi and looking for deviation or evidence of luminal obstruction. • Is the trachea deviated, suggesting tension pneumothorax or lobar collapse?

B	**Bones and Breast Shadows**
	• Inspect the bones for radiographic density, fractures, lytic lesions, or bony deformity. Note breast shadows to avoid mistaking these for chest pathology, such as pneumothorax or pulmonary contusion.
	  • Are rib fractures present?
	  • Is a flail segment present?
	  • Is the scapula, clavicle, sternum, or a combination of these fractured?
	  • Are spinal fractures present?
	  • Is the humerus fractured?
	  • Are the acromioclavicular, sternoclavicular, and glenohumeral joints properly located?

C	**Cardiac Silhouette**
	• Assess the cardiac silhouette for general size and contour.
	  • Note an enlarged cardiac silhouette, suggesting pericardial effusion.
	  • Inspect for pericardial air, air in the soft tissues of the neck, or a continuous diaphragm sign.
	  • Note the width of the mediastinum. Other abnormal mediastinal findings are reviewed in more detail in Table 6-4.

D	**Diaphragm**
	• Assess the diaphragm or diaphragms, with attention to the contour and costophrenic angle, bilaterally.
	  • Look for blunted costophrenic angles, suggesting pleural fluid (hemothorax).
	  • Note a deep sulcus sign, suggesting tension pneumothorax.
	  • Look for an elevated or irregular diaphragm, suggesting diaphragm rupture.
	  • Are both diaphragms distinct?
	  • Is one diaphragm higher than the other? (Right normally is higher than left.)
	  • Are abdominal organs or NG tubes visible in the chest?
	  • Is a black line visible beneath the diaphragm, indicating pneumoperitoneum?
	  • Is a continuous diaphragm sign visible, indicating pneumopericardium?

E	**Everything Else** • Review everything else around the lung fields, including the subcutaneous soft tissues and pleural boundaries.

F	**Lung Fields**
	• Review the lung fields themselves, looking for evidence of pneumothorax, pulmonary contusion, hemothorax, or herniated abdominal contents, suggesting diaphragm rupture.
	  • Is a pneumothorax present?
	    • Do lung markings extend to the periphery?
	    • Is a pleural line visible?
	    • Is subcutaneous air visible?
	  • Is a hemothorax present?
	    • Is the density of one hemithorax different from that of the other?
	    • Is a meniscus visible?
	  • Is a tension pneumothorax present?
	    • Is the mediastinum deviated?
	    • Is the diaphragm depressed?
	    • Is there a deep sulcus sign?
	    • Is the trachea deviated?
	  • Is a pulmonary contusion visible?
	    • Is the lung denser in some regions than in others?

F	**Foreign Bodies or Devices**
	• Are foreign bodies, such as shrapnel or knives, present? Are two orthogonal views available to confirm the location?
	• Are the following medical devices properly positioned?
	  • Endotracheal tube
	  • Central venous catheters
	  • Thoracostomy tubes
	  • NG and OG tubes

From Crausman RS. The ABCs of chest X-ray film interpretation. *Chest* 113:256-257, 1998.

TABLE 6-4. Chest X-ray Findings Suggesting Aortic Injury

Wide mediastinum	The mediastinum may appear wider than normal. An upper limit of 8 cm (measured from the left aortic arch to the right mediastinal margin) has been described, although lesser degrees of widening can occur with small mediastinal hematomas. Unfortunately, this finding is only about 90% sensitive and 10% specific. The supine AP chest x-ray often obtained following blunt trauma can simulate pathologic mediastinal widening from aortic injury.
Indistinct aortic knob	The aortic knob may lose its distinct and rounded appearance due to hematoma surrounding it. The margins may appear indistinct or irregular.
Loss of aortopulmonary window	A normal lucent region, the aortopulmonary window (formed by the intersection of the normal left pulmonary artery and the descending aorta) may be obscured by mediastinal hematoma.
Wide right paratracheal stripe	The right paratracheal stripe (PTS), which is normally a thin water-density stripe between the air column of the trachea and the adjacent lung on frontal projection chest x-ray, may become widened by the presence of mediastinal hematoma. The upper limit of normal is 4 mm, with 5 mm reliably being abnormal. In one study, no patient with PTS <5 mm had an aortic injury, while 22.9% of those with PTS ≥5 mm had a vascular injury.
Displaced left paraspinous line	The left paraspinous line may be displaced by mediastinal blood.
Apical pleural cap	An apical pleural cap may form as blood tracks into the superior mediastinum and over the pleura at the lung apex, creating a soft-tissue density in this location.
Pleural effusion	A pleural effusion may be present if blood has leaked from the mediastinum into the pleural space.
Displacement of mediastinal structures	Other structures passing through the mediastinum may be distorted or displaced by mediastinal hematoma. These include normal anatomic structures and medical devices commonly seen in trauma patients: • The trachea may be deviated to the patient's right. • The left main-stem bronchus may appear deflected in a caudad direction. • A NG or an OG tube within the esophagus may appear deviated to the left or right. • An endotracheal tube may appear deviated with the trachea.
Skeletal injuries	Other injuries such as first and second rib, scapula, or thoracic spine fractures may be present. These are not signs of aortic injury; rather, they suggest a high-energy trauma mechanism, compatible with aortic injury. Studies have refuted the traditional association between these injuries and aortic trauma.

From American College of Radiology. ACR appropriateness criteria: Blunt chest trauma—Suspected aortic injury. (Accessed at http://www.acr.org/SecondaryMainMenuCategories/quality_safety/app_criteria/pdf/Vascular/BluntChestTraumaSuspectedAorticInjuryDoc6.aspx.); Lee RB, Bass SM, Morris JA Jr, et al. Three or more rib fractures as an indicator for transfer to a level I trauma center: A population-based study. *J Trauma* 30(6):689-694, 1990; Lee J, Harris JH Jr, Duke JH Jr, et al. Noncorrelation between thoracic skeletal injuries and acute traumatic aortic tear. *J Trauma* 43(3):400-404, 1997; Savoca CJ, Austin JH, Goldberg HI. The right paratracheal stripe. *Radiology* 122(2):295-301, 1977; Savoca CJ, Brasch RC, Gooding CA, et al. The right paratracheal stripe in children. *Pediatr Radiol* 6(4):203-207, 1978; Ungar TC, Wolf SJ, Haukoos JS, et al. Derivation of a clinical decision rule to exclude thoracic aortic imaging in patients with blunt chest trauma after motor vehicle collisions. *J Trauma* 61(5):1150-1155, 2006; Woodring JH, Pulmano CM, Stevens RK. The right paratracheal stripe in blunt chest trauma. *Radiology* 143(3):605-608, 1982.

In some cases, the sulcus is so deep that the full extent is not visible on the caudad margin of the chest x-ray.

- *A depressed and flattened hemidiaphragm,* again resulting from the effect of pressurized air in the pleural space pushing on the diaphragm. In the case of a right-sided tension pneumothorax, the right hemidiaphragm may appear lower than the left, reversing their normal relationship. (Remember that normally the right diaphragm is higher than the left, because the liver is larger than the spleen.)
- *Mediastinal shift,* in which the heart and other mediastinal structures are pushed toward the opposite side of the thorax by the effect of pressurized air in the pleural space. In addition to the shift of the heart, the trachea and medical devices such as endotracheal tubes and nasogastric tubes may be shifted to the contralateral side. The superior vena cava may appear kinked on chest x-ray. This can restrict venous return of blood to the heart, which, along with high intrathoracic pressure from the tension pneumothorax, impairs cardiac filling and output, leading to hypotension and the physical examination finding of jugular venous distension.
- *Horizontally oriented ribs* on the affected side, caused by hyperinflation of the hemithorax. The normal oblique course of the ribs from posterior to anterior is lost on the frontal chest x-ray projection.

Tracheobronchial Injury

Tracheobronchial injury (see chest x-rays and related CTs, Figures 6-25 through 6-30) is a rare but life-threatening injury usually associated with large or

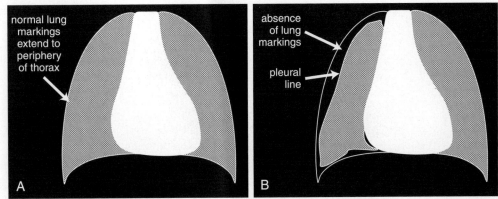

Figure 6-12. Pneumothorax. A, Schematic of normal lung. **B,** Schematic of pneumothorax. Pneumothoraces can range in size from tiny to massive—we examine some tension pneumothoraces in later figures. Because of the variability in their size and location, pneumothoraces can be difficult to detect on chest x-ray. For example, a pneumothorax that is anterior or posterior rather than lateral may be hidden on frontal chest x-ray, particularly one taken in the supine position. An upright chest x-ray should be obtained if possible. An expiratory film is thought to be more sensitive, because the lung and thorax decrease in size during expiration, but air trapped in the pleural space remains the same size and thus appears relatively larger. Subtle pneumothoraces may not be visible on chest x-ray. In some cases, subcutaneous air may be the only visible clue to underlying lung injury. CT is extremely sensitive for pneumothorax, although controversy remains over the proper management of pneumothoraces seen only on CT (see text). Ultrasound is also thought to be more sensitive than chest x-ray for detection of pneumothorax, although again, the management of pneumothorax seen only on ultrasound is uncertain, because this is a relatively newly described method of detection. The chest x-ray findings of pneumothorax include a lack of the normal lung markings, which should be visible to the periphery of the chest wall. Sometimes a line marking the boundary of the lung and visceral pleura is visible, although this can be confused with ribs and with the medial margin of the scapula. Depending on the degree of pneumothorax and lung collapse, the lung parenchyma may appear denser than the opposite side. In extreme cases of tension pneumothorax, the pressure exerted by the air in the pleural space may begin to displace other structures, including the diaphragm and mediastinum. In tension pneumothorax, the hyperinflated hemithorax may also have abnormally positioned ribs, with a position more horizontal than usual. Review the figures that follow for examples of varying degrees of pneumothorax. Subtle cases can be hard to reproduce in print.

tension pneumothorax and requiring surgical intervention. Clues to the presence of this injury include the persistence of a large or even tension pneumothorax despite the apparently appropriate placement of a thoracostomy tube.[6] This finding indicates that the rate of air leaking into the pleural space exceeds the rate at which it is being removed from that space by the thoracostomy tube. Two possibilities explain this scenario:

- *Malfunction of the thoracostomy tube,* which may be misplaced (outside of the pleural space), internally clogged with blood or debris, kinked or compressed within the chest cavity or external to the body, not connected to suction or to a pleural vacuum device, or placed so that one or more of its holes are external to the pleural space, allowing air to enter the thoracostomy tube and pleural space. See the later discussion about evaluation of thoracostomy tubes on chest x-ray.
- *A rapid rate of air leak into the chest from a tracheobronchial injury or large pulmonary laceration,* exceeding the thoracostomy tube capacity. When a large pneumothorax persists despite a large (e.g., 40-French) and properly functioning thoracostomy tube, a tracheobronchial injury is likely. In some cases this can be temporarily addressed by placement of additional thoracostomy tubes to allow faster egress of pleural air, but definitive surgical management will be necessary. In a stable patient, the injury can be confirmed with CT (Figures 6-29 and 6-30). In an unstable patient, immediate surgical intervention is necessary. Intentional selective intubation of the unaffected main bronchus

can prevent delivery of additional air into the affected pleural space.

A rarer but more specific sign of tracheobronchial injury is the **fallen lung sign,** in which the collapsed lung falls away from the mediastinum rather than being retracted medially toward the hilum as a consequence of bronchial transection (see Figure 6-30).[6]

Tracheobronchial and esophageal injuries are rare following blunt trauma (occurring in only about 1%) but may be suggested by CT.[7] In cases of tracheobronchial injury, chest x-ray may be nondiagnostic in 30%, whereas CT may show a defect in the wall of major airways. Air in the airway may be contiguous with that in the pleural space or mediastinum when viewed with CT lung windows.[8] In cases of esophageal injury, CT may show pneumomediastinum and esophageal thickening at the level of injury (see Figure 6-36). A Gastrografin swallow study followed by barium swallow can be diagnostic.[7] Imaging of the esophagus is discussed in more detail in Chapter 4. If aerodigestive injuries are suspected but the source of the air leak is unclear from diagnostic imaging, bronchoscopy and esophagoscopy can be used to differentiate the source.

Subcutaneous Air

Subcutaneous air, while itself almost never life-threatening, should be carefully sought because it can provide clues to other important injuries including pneumothorax. The appearance is increased lucency (black appearance) in soft tissues resulting from the presence of

Text continues on page 309

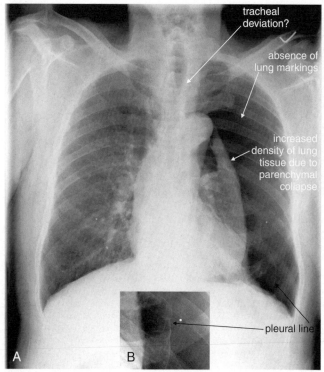

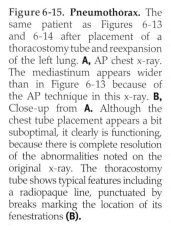

tracheal deviation?

absence of lung markings

increased density of lung tissue due to parenchymal collapse

pleural line

A

B

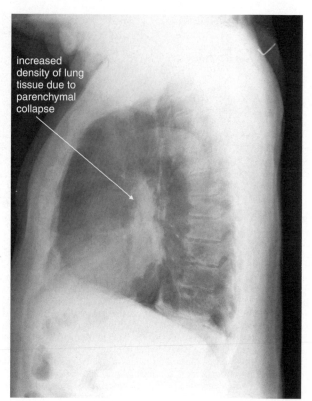

increased density of lung tissue due to parenchymal collapse

Figure 6-13. Pneumothorax. A, PA x-ray demonstrating a very large spontaneous pneumothorax. **B,** Close-up from **A.** This image demonstrates the classic features described in Figure 6-12 no lung markings to the periphery of the thorax, a visible visceral pleural line, and increased density of the lung parenchyma—resulting from the marked degree of collapse in this case. Is this a tension pneumothorax? Some would argue that the definition of tension pneumothorax is clinical, based on hypotension and exam findings such as jugular venous distension and tracheal deviation. On a radiographic basis, tension pneumothorax is marked by some combination of tracheal deviation, mediastinal deviation to the opposite side, depression of the diaphragm and a deep sulcus (costophrenic angle), and elevation of ribs to a more horizontal position. This patient may have slight tracheal deviation and a degree of mediastinal shift, but the diaphragm appears normal, there is no deep sulcus sign, and the ribs are oriented normally. The white dots seen on each side are nipple markers.

Figure 6-14. Pneumothorax. Same patient as Figure 6-13. The lateral chest x-ray is not usually diagnostic, even in dramatic cases such as this one, because the normal thorax is superimposed upon the abnormal. Here, a hint of the complete collapse of the left lung is seen, with increased density near the hilum, but the lateral x-ray is neither necessary nor particularly helpful in this case.

Figure 6-15. Pneumothorax. The same patient as Figures 6-13 and 6-14 after placement of a thoracostomy tube and reexpansion of the left lung. **A,** AP chest x-ray. The mediastinum appears wider than in Figure 6-13 because of the AP technique in this x-ray. **B,** Close-up from **A.** Although the chest tube placement appears a bit suboptimal, it clearly is functioning, because there is complete resolution of the abnormalities noted on the original x-ray. The thoracostomy tube shows typical features including a radiopaque line, punctuated by breaks marking the location of its fenestrations **(B).**

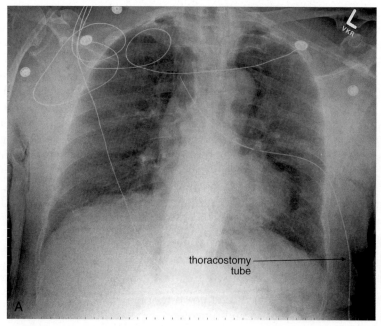

thoracostomy tube

A

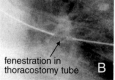

fenestration in thoracostomy tube

B

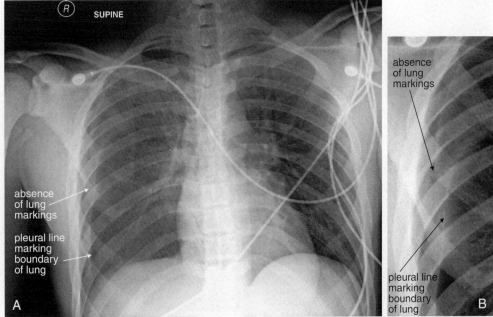

Figure 6-16. Pneumothorax. A, Supine portable chest x-ray. **B,** Close-up from **A.** This moderate pneumothorax is much subtler than in Figure 6-13 but demonstrates many of the same findings. A pleural line is faintly visible—beyond this line, no lung markings are visible. Compare this with the opposite side, where the fine markings of pulmonary blood vessels are seen to the periphery of the pleural space. Although the normal result of a pneumothorax is a more lucent hemithorax, the entire right thorax appears somewhat denser in this case; the CT from the same patient in Figure 6-18 illustrates why. It is a good practice to find and follow the scapular border and rib borders to avoid confusion of these lines with the pleural line of a pneumothorax. None of the findings of a tension pneumothorax are present in this chest x-ray. The right costophrenic angle and lateral diaphragm are somewhat indistinct. This, plus the density of the right hemithorax, should make you consider hemothorax or pulmonary contusion, in addition to the pneumothorax.

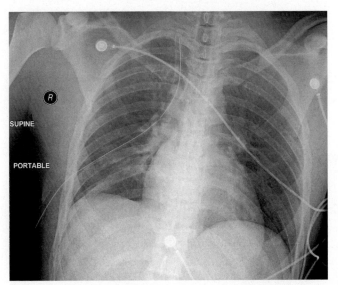

Figure 6-17. Pneumothorax. Same patient as Figure 6-16. A chest tube has been placed, and the previously seen pleural line and absence of lung markings have resolved. The right chest looks somewhat less dense than before.

low-density air. The appearance can be extremely subtle (see Figure 6-22) or grossly evident (see Figure 6-28), with air outlining muscle fibers and multiple tissue planes. The chest wall, axilla, and neck should be thoroughly inspected. Air within soft tissue can have several sources:

- *An external wound that has introduced air into soft tissues.* Common associated findings would be radiodense foreign bodies. The presence of an external wound and foreign bodies *do not* rule out the concurrent presence of a pneumothorax as the source of subcutaneous air.

- *A pneumothorax with leak of air from the pleural space into adjacent soft tissues* (see Figures 6-22 and 6-28). Common associated findings are rib fractures in either penetrating or blunt trauma or radiodense foreign bodies in the case of penetrating trauma. The associated pneumothorax may not be visible on chest x-ray in all cases.

- *An esophageal injury with air leak.* This is extremely rare in the case of blunt trauma and occurs rarely with penetrating trauma. Radiographic clues to this injury pattern include associated pneumomediastinum.

- *Valsalva maneuver against a closed glottis during blunt trauma.* Again, associated pneumothorax is likely but may be small or invisible on chest x-ray.

- *Barotrauma from mechanical ventilation.* An associated pneumothorax is not always seen on chest x-ray.

- *Necrotizing infections.* These can produce soft-tissue gas but would not be expected in the setting of acute trauma.

Hemothorax

Hemothorax may be subtle (see Figure 6-6) or gross (see Figure 6-3) on chest x-ray. Technically, chest x-ray reveals the presence of pleural fluid but does not prove it to be blood; a preexisting pleural effusion would have an identical radiographic appearance. The clinical

Text continues on page 312

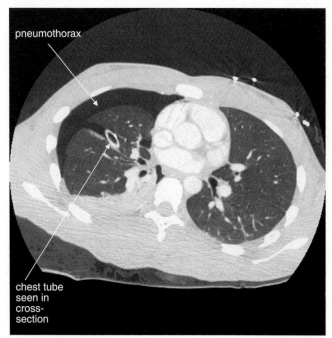

pneumothorax

chest tube seen in cross-section

Figure 6-18. Pneumothorax. This CT with IV contrast was performed for evaluation of the mediastinum. Chest CT is not routinely needed for evaluation of pneumothorax. Nonetheless, it reveals several interesting findings. First, despite the chest tube, a pneumothorax remains (remember, air is black on all CT windows), and this was not seen on the supine chest x-ray in Figure 6-17. Why not? The pneumothorax is anterior, so the lung tissue intervening between the x-ray tube and the detector plate prevented recognition of the pneumothorax. The posterior lung tissue is quite dense, and a tiny amount of pleural fluid is present—likely indicating pulmonary contusion and small hemothorax. Alternatively, the posterior lung tissue may be dense resulting from atelectasis. This seems less likely because the left lung does not demonstrate dependent atelectasis. Does the residual pneumothorax require treatment? It will likely resolve with continued use of the existing chest tube, though that chest tube should be examined for kinks and checked for the presence of a continued air leak. When a large pneumothorax persists despite a properly functioning thoracostomy tube, a large airway injury or pulmonary laceration should be suspected.

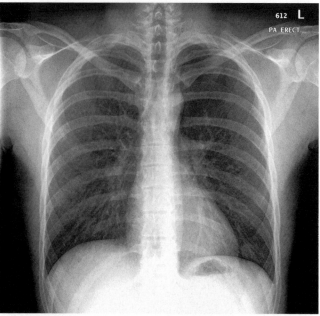

Figure 6-19. Pneumothorax. This young male suffered a spontaneous left pneumothorax. The x-ray demonstrates several features typical of pneumothorax and is subtle, though the pneumothorax is relatively large. This pneumothorax appears to be restricted to the left apical region on this upright chest x-ray. There is an absence of lung markings, and the apical thorax appears more lucent than usual resulting from the absence of lung parenchyma. A faint pleural line can be seen. A close-up (Figure 6-20) shows these findings better.

Figure 6-20. Pneumothorax. Same patient as Figure 6-19, spontaneous apical pneumothorax. The absence of lung markings is clear, and the pleural boundary can be seen.

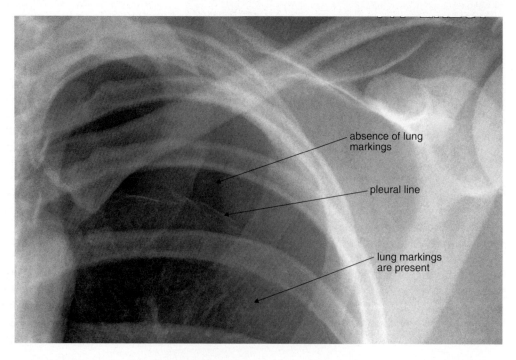

absence of lung markings

pleural line

lung markings are present

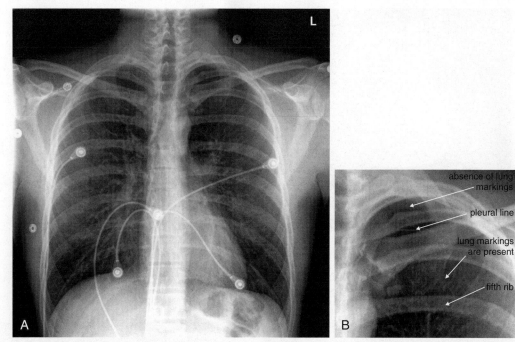

Figure 6-21. **Pneumothorax.** Same patient as Figures 6-19 and 6-20. **A,** Frontal chest x-ray. **B,** Close-up from **A.** Needle aspiration of the pneumothorax was performed, and this x-ray was obtained 6 hours later. A small residual pneumothorax is present **(B),** although lung markings are now visible above the fifth rib, where they were not previously.

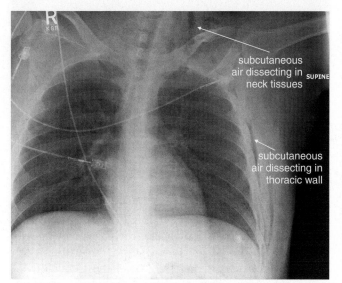

Figure 6-22. Pneumothorax with subcutaneous air on chest x-ray but no visible pneumothorax. This trauma patient has no visible pneumothorax, with lung markings seen to the periphery. However, subcutaneous air (black) in the lateral left chest wall and neck indicate some form of lung or airway injury, as the patient had no external wounds through which air might have been introduced. Subcutaneous air of this degree, while essentially proving the existence of some respiratory (or less likely, aerodigestive tract) injury, would not mandate CT. For example, in a patient with spontaneous chest pain after cough, CT should not be performed to hunt for associated pneumothorax, although a pneumothorax should be suspected. In this case, chest CT was performed to evaluate for possible thoracic spine injury but incidentally provided more information about the source of the subcutaneous air and is reviewed in Figure 6-23.

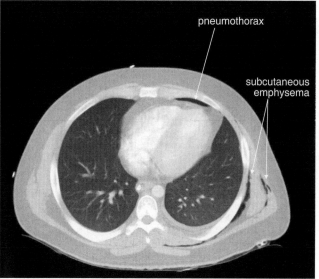

Figure 6-23. Small pneumothorax with subcutaneous air on CT with IV contrast. Same patient as Figure 6-22. A tiny anterior pneumothorax is visible, as well as some dependent pleural fluid, which is likely hemothorax in the setting of trauma. The subcutaneous air is readily visible on lung windows. How should small pneumothoraces seen only on chest CT be managed? Controversy exists (see text). In general, very small pneumothoraces such as this should not be treated. Some authors advocate prophylactic placement of a thoracostomy tube if the patient will be transported long distances, transported by air, or placed on positive-pressure ventilation, which could result in an enlarging pneumothorax. Small studies show a low risk of increasing pneumothorax with positive-pressure ventilation, though this is an obvious complication that must be anticipated.

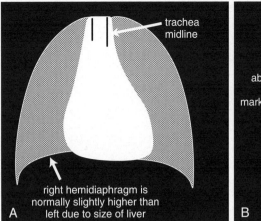
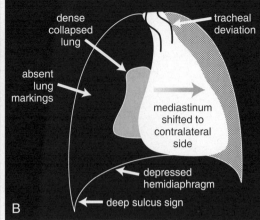

Figure 6-24. Tension pneumothorax on chest x-ray. A, The normal chest. **B,** Schematic of tension pneumothorax. In the case of a tension pneumothorax, a large pneumothorax is typically visible, with a dense-appearing, medially displaced, collapsed lung. Increased pressure results in mediastinal shift and tracheal deviation to the opposite side. The affected side has a depressed hemidiaphragm. If tension pneumothorax occurs on the right side, the right hemidiaphragm may be displaced in a caudad direction and may be lower than the left hemidiaphragm—the reverse of their normal positions. In addition, the costophrenic angle may be extremely deep on the abnormal side (the deep sulcus sign).

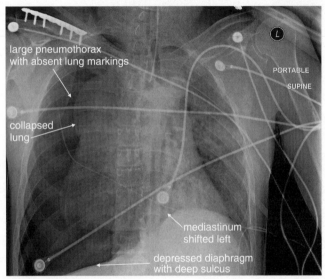
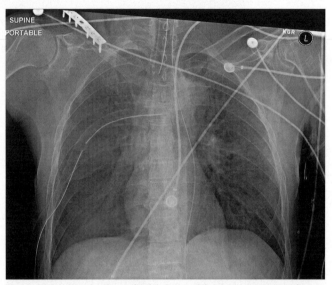

Figure 6-25. Tracheobronchial injury with tension pneumothorax. This 46-year-old male presented unresponsive after a motorcycle collision and was noted to have decreased breath sounds with tachycardia and a blood pressure of 120/80. The patient was intubated and chest x-ray was performed, showing findings concerning for tension pneumothorax. Findings included a large pneumothorax, a dense and medially contracted lung, a deep sulcus sign, a flattened diaphragm, and a shift of the mediastinum to the left. Figure 6-26 shows the patient's chest x-ray after thoracostomy tube placement. His CT (Figure 6-27) suggested a tracheobronchial injury. Bronchoscopy confirmed transection of the bronchus just distal to the takeoff of the right main bronchus. This was repaired operatively.

Figure 6-26. Tracheobronchial injury with tension pneumothorax. Same patient as in Figure 6-25. After placement of a right thoracostomy tube, the patient's findings of tension pneumothorax have resolved.

setting is essential to determining the course of action. As described earlier, the commonly used supine portable chest x-ray can compromise detection of hemothorax by causing fluid to layer in the plane of the horizontally positioned x-ray detector. Small amounts of hemothorax may be invisible on supine x-ray; on upright x-ray, these may appear as simple blunting of the costophrenic angles (see Figures 6-2 through 6-10). Large hemothoraces may give the entire thorax a denser (whiter) appearance relative to the normal side on supine x-ray, sometimes referred to as a "veiling opacity" (see Figure 6-9). On upright AP or PA chest x-ray, these may appear as obvious radiodense layered fluid collections with a curved meniscus where they meet the thoracic wall (see Figure 6-7). Other chest x-ray findings commonly associated with hemothorax include pneumothorax, rib fractures, pulmonary contusions, mediastinal injury, and spinal trauma. Large hemothoraces can obscure underlying pulmonary contusions. The diaphragm on the affected side may be obscured, and the possibility of concurrent diaphragmatic injury must be considered. Diaphragm injuries are discussed in more detail later in this chapter and in Chapter 10. Particularly in the case of penetrating trauma, the subdiaphragmatic area should be assessed for pneumoperitoneum.

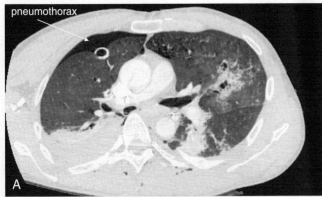

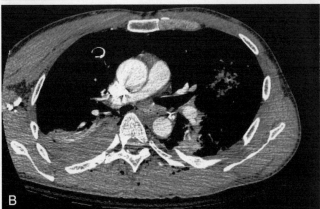

Figure 6-27. Tracheobronchial injury with tension pneumothorax. Same patient as in Figures 6-25 and 6-26. This CT with IV contrast suggests but does not prove a tracheobronchial injury. A moderate-size pneumothorax persists despite the right thoracostomy tube, implying that more air is leaking into the pleural space than can be removed by the chest tube. Explanations for this include a large airway injury, a significant pulmonary parenchymal laceration, or a malfunctioning chest tube that is kinked, is plugged, is not attached to suction, or does not have its fenestrations within the pneumothorax. The pneumothorax is visible on the lung window **(A)** but not on the soft-tissue window **(B)**. Other injuries are present but are discussed separately in other figures—return to this figure later and try to identify pleural fluid (hemothorax), pulmonary contusion, rib fractures, and subcutaneous emphysema. This patient was taken to the operating room, where a bronchial injury was confirmed by bronchoscopy.

Pulmonary Contusion and Laceration

Pulmonary contusion, laceration, and hematoma refer to pulmonary parenchymal injuries that result in hemorrhage into the alveolar space and into interstitial spaces. In blunt trauma, the term *contusion* is common; in penetrating trauma, the term *laceration* is more often used, though the chest x-ray appearance is the generally the same. The accumulation of blood, other fluid, and cellular debris increases the density of the normally air-filled alveolar space, making it appear white on chest x-ray (chest x-rays and related CTs, Figures 6-37 through 6-46).[9] The interstitial spaces also become more prominent. The affected lung tissue takes on the appearance of a solid organ or fluid. Much confusion exists about the appearance of pulmonary contusion on chest x-ray and the time course over which pulmonary contusion becomes radiographically apparent. Some authors have stated that pulmonary contusion may not be evident

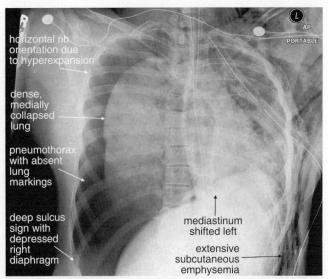

Figure 6-28. Tracheobronchial injury with tension pneumothorax. This 19-year-old female struck a telephone pole and was unresponsive at the accident scene. Emergency medical services providers attempted to decompress a suspected left tension pneumothorax. The patient arrested en route to the emergency department, and on arrival a left chest tube was placed, just before this x-ray. The x-ray shows classic findings of tension pneumothorax, with a deep sulcus sign (so deep that the complete sulcus is not visible on the x-ray). The mediastinum is deviated to the left. The right ribs have assumed an abnormally horizontal position resulting from hyperexpansion of the chest. A left chest tube is present, and extensive subcutaneous air is present (compare with the normal right chest wall). Compare these findings to the CT images in Figure 6-29.

for hours, but a more common sense explanation must be understood: *If sufficient hemorrhage and injury to lung has occurred to increase the density of the tissue, the injury is immediately apparent on chest x-ray.* If a lesser degree of injury is present such that the density of the tissue remains relatively normal, the injury may be invisible initially. If continued hemorrhage or fluid accumulation into the injured tissue occurs, the appearance may become more evident over hours. Pulmonary contusion has no pathognomonic features; the same increased density can occur with pneumonia, aspiration, or pulmonary infarction—all processes that can result in alveolar consolidation. The context of trauma defines the appearance as contusion rather than one of these other processes. It is impossible to distinguish an evolving pulmonary contusion on chest x-ray from a pneumonia developing in the region, because both become visible on chest x-ray by the same process of alveolar and interstitial fluid accumulation. Clinical factors such as the presence of fever are used to make the distinction, which may be impossible even on these grounds. Pulmonary contusion, aspiration, and pneumonia may occur simultaneously. Associated chest x-ray findings can include rib fractures, hemo- or pneumothorax, or radiodense foreign bodies in the setting of penetrating trauma. CT is more sensitive than x-ray and may predict the need for ventilatory support—although it is the clinical state of the patient, not imaging findings, that defines the need for intervention.[9]

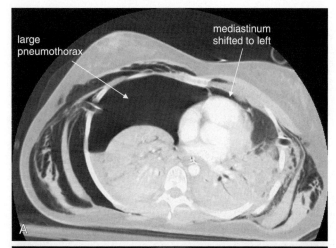

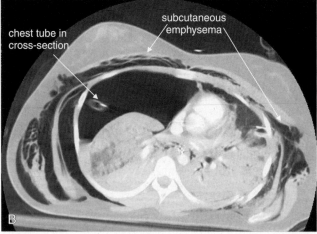

Figure 6-29. Tracheobronchial injury with tension pneumothorax: CT with IV contrast viewed with lung windows. A, B, Two sequential axial images. Same patient as in Figures 6-28 and 6-30. This CT is highly suggestive of tracheobronchial injury. A right chest tube has been placed and is clearly seen entering the right pleural space. Despite this, a large tension pneumothorax is still present. The mediastinum remains deviated to the left. The most likely explanation is a large airway injury, which would allow air to enter the pleural space faster than it can be removed by a large-bore chest tube. An alternative explanation would be complete occlusion of the chest tube by kinking or internal plugging. The patient is intubated and receiving positive pressure ventilation, increasing the risk that a bronchial injury would result in tension pneumothorax. Massive subcutaneous emphysema has accumulated bilaterally.

Lobar Collapse

Following trauma or as a consequence of endotracheal intubation, lobar collapse with volume loss can occur. Familiarity with the chest x-ray appearance is essential, because this condition can be mistaken for other serious abnormalities, including mediastinal trauma, tension pneumothorax, pulmonary contusion, hemothorax, and diaphragm rupture. Treatment includes maneuvers to reexpand the affected lung segment, sometimes including repositioning of an endotracheal tube or altering ventilator settings. A collapsed lung segment appears dense on chest x-ray (Figure 6-47 and CT Figure 6-48), similar in appearance to other parenchymal abnormalities, such as pulmonary contusion, or to pleural space abnormalities, such as hemothorax. However, because a collapsed lung segment occupies a smaller-than-normal volume, radiographic evidence of **volume loss** is present. Findings of volume loss include shift of structures toward the area of volume loss. This can include shift of the mediastinum, tracheal deviation, and elevation of the diaphragm on the affected side (see Figure 6-47). This is in stark contrast to tension pneumothorax, where structures are shifted *away from* the affected side. Nevertheless, to an inexperienced observer, the obvious shift of structures may be mistaken for tension pneumothorax. Elevation of the diaphragm can be mistaken for a diaphragmatic injury. If the area of lobar collapse abuts the mediastinum, the mediastinum may appear wide, simulating aortic trauma. In an intubated patient, the position of the endotracheal tube should be noted. Right main bronchus intubation commonly can result in left lung collapse or right upper lobe collapse (because the endotracheal tube may occlude the right upper lobe bronchus). Plugging of bronchi with blood, mucus, or aspirated material can also lead to lobar collapse.

Diaphragm Injury

Injury to the diaphragm is discussed in detail in Chapter 10. On chest x-ray, the appearance depends on the degree of injury. In cases of overt herniation of

Figure 6-30. Tracheobronchial injury with tension pneumothorax. CT with IV contrast, lung windows. **A,** Axial CT image. **B,** Close-up from **A.** Same patient as in Figures 6-28 and 6-29. The actual tracheobronchial injury is seen. The right main bronchus is seen in direct continuity with the large pneumothorax in right pleural space.

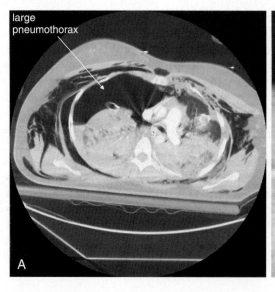

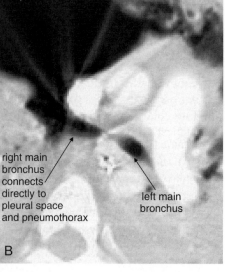

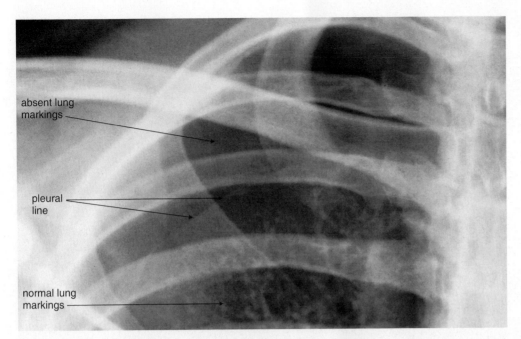

Figure 6-31. Pneumothorax, comparison of chest x-ray and ultrasound findings. This 19-year-old male had spontaneous right chest pain while playing soccer. This close-up from his chest x-ray shows a moderate apical right pneumothorax. Lung markings are absent at the right apex, and a pleural line is visible. Ultrasound images from the same patient are shown in Figures 6-32 through 6-34.

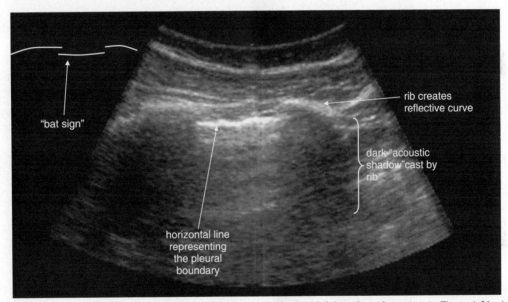

Figure 6-32. B mode ultrasound findings of normal lung and pleura. The normal left lung from the patient in Figure 6-31, viewed with B mode ultrasound. The anterior cortices of two adjacent ribs are visible as echogenic, horizontally oriented curves. Deep to these are acoustic shadows cast by the ribs. Between the ribs lies the horizontal pleural line, a bright white reflection at the interface between the parietal and the visceral pleura. Some authors have described the three lines formed by two adjacent ribs and the pleural line as the bat sign resulting from its resemblance to a stylized line drawing of a bat in flight (diagrammed in figure margin; try to identify this for yourself in the ultrasound image). When real-time ultrasound images are viewed, horizontal motion along the pleural line is normally seen—the sliding lung sign. In the presence of pneumothorax, movement along this line is not seen, as the visceral pleura is separated from the parietal pleura by a buffer of air.

intestinal contents into the chest, the appearance can be obvious. In subtle diaphragm tears without herniation of abdominal contents, no radiographic abnormalities may be seen on chest x-ray. Left diaphragmatic injuries are more common than right. In the case of left diaphragm rupture, the stomach (gastric air bubble) and loops of small bowel may be visible within the chest (Figures 6-49 through 6-55). If a nasogastric (NG) or an orogastric (OG) tube is present, it may be visible curled within the thorax (see Figure 6-49). Sometimes the appearance suggests only an elevated hemidiaphragm, but diaphragmatic injury must be suspected. When right diaphragm injury is present, the liver may appear to occupy an unusually cephalad position (see Figure 10-33). Overall, initial chest x-ray is thought to be only about 17% to 50% sensitive for detection of diaphragm rupture, and positive pressure ventilation is thought to reduce sensitivity, likely resulting from positive pressure pushing the affected diaphragm to a more normal caudad position.[10-11]

Figure 6-33. **M mode ultrasound findings of normal lung and pleura—seashore sign.** Figures 6-31 through 6-34 show images from the same case. Most ultrasound machines allow simultaneous acquisition of a B mode image (**A**) and an M mode image (**B**) that represents motion through the line in the B mode image. An M mode image of the normal left lung shows the seashore sign. Motionless tissues superficial to the pleural line have the appearance of a laminated series of horizontal lines, like wave fronts approaching a seashore. Deep to the pleural line, respiratory motion of normal lung gives a granular appearance—the "sand" on the sea shore.

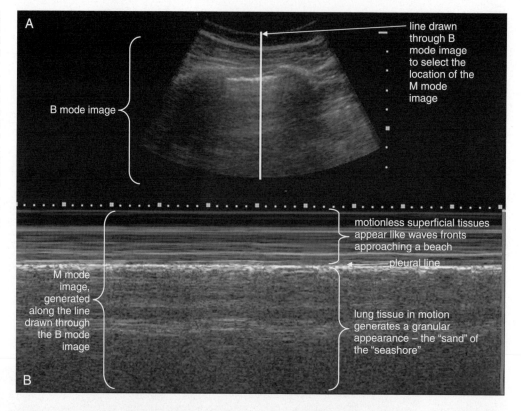

Figure 6-34. **M mode ultrasound findings of pneumothorax.** Figures 6-31 through 6-34 show images from the same case. Most ultrasound machines allow a split screen mode, showing B mode (typical two-dimensional images, **A**) and M mode (motion mode, **B**) on the same screen. In this figure, a B mode image of the chest wall is seen in the upper portion of the screen, **A.** An acoustic shadow from a rib is visible, just to the right of the vertical white line. This line has been drawn by the emergency ultrasonographer through the pleura between two ribs. Motion along this line is then depicted in the M mode image in **B.** The M mode image of the abnormal right lung shows the stratosphere sign, consistent with pneumothorax. Most ultrasound machines allow simultaneous acquisition of a B mode image (**A**) and an M mode image (**B**), representing motion through the line in the B mode image.

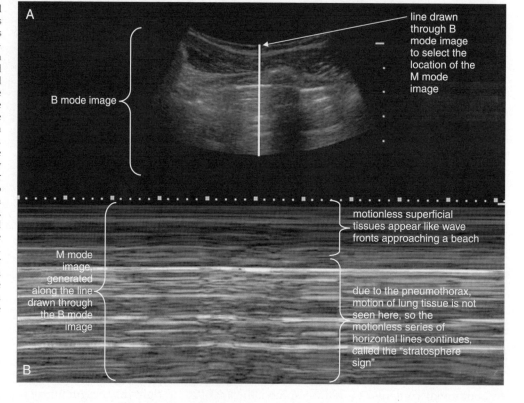

Mediastinal and Aortic Injuries

Life-threatening injury to the aorta and other mediastinal structures can occur with blunt or penetrating trauma. A variety of chest x-ray findings can provide clues to these injuries, as we describe later. Of paramount importance is understanding that an aortic injury may be present with a completely normal chest x-ray, albeit rarely. We discuss some controversies surrounding this rare event later in this chapter. Understanding the mechanisms behind aortic injuries can

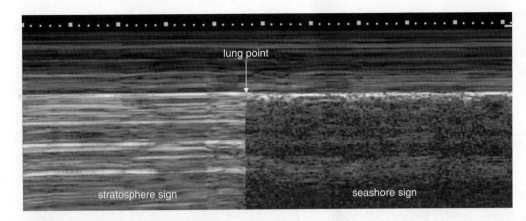

Figure 6-35. **Ultrasound findings of normal lung and pneumothorax.** A lung point sign is simulated in this figure. When an M mode image reveals a transition between the abnormal stratosphere sign and the normal seashore sign, this is called the lung point sign. It is an indication of a partial pneumothorax, with the lung surface intermittently contacting the thoracic wall. Compare with Figures 6-33 and 6-34.

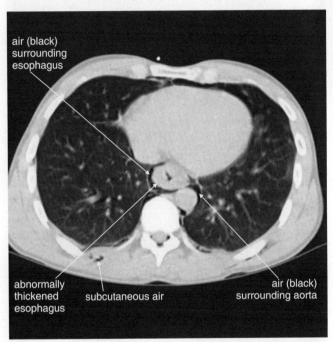

Figure 6-36. **Esophageal tear with pneumomediastinum.** CT can demonstrate esophageal injuries following trauma. These are extremely rare following blunt trauma but can occur with penetrating chest trauma. In the case of thoracic gunshot wounds, CT can demonstrate the missile trajectory, indicating its proximity to the esophagus and other mediastinal structures. In addition, focal thickening of the esophagus may be seen at a site of injury. Air leaking from an esophageal injury can create pneumomediastinum visible on CT. In this patient, who has an esophageal injury not from external trauma but from forceful vomiting, the esophagus appears thickened and air is visible surrounding the esophagus (pneumomediastinum). Lung windows reveal air and, in the case of trauma, can reveal a missile trajectory by demonstrating injured lung parenchyma.

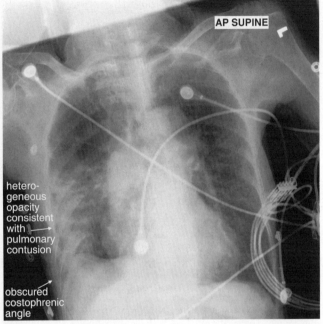

Figure 6-37. **Pulmonary contusion.** This 77-year-old female was in a car struck by a train. Her chest x-ray shows dense consolidation of the right mid- and lower lung. The costophrenic angle is blunted, and the lateral right diaphragm appears elevated and cannot be distinguished from the consolidation. From Chapter 5, recall the silhouette sign, the principle that two adjacent tissues of the same density cannot be distinguished on chest x-ray. Because the right lateral and lower lung cannot be distinguished from the diaphragm and liver in this patient, they must share the same soft-tissue (fluid) density. Figure 6-38 demonstrates CT images from this patient. Can pulmonary contusion be distinguished from aspiration or other pneumonia? Not based on the chest x-ray findings. Theoretically, this patient could have aspirated—or could have had pneumonia before her collision with the train.

assist both in recognizing the radiographic appearance and in determining when chest x-ray abnormalities require further imaging. Because of the importance of this injury, we have included numerous example figures to illustrate the range of findings (Figures 6-56 through 6-108).

Consider for a moment the events occurring with aortic injury. Aortic injury from blunt trauma is a deceleration injury, requiring significant energy to be imparted into the chest. Because the kinetic energy of an object is determined by $(1/2)mv^2$ (where m = mass and v = velocity), the dominant variable in determining the energy involved in trauma is usually velocity. Exceptions can occur when an extremely massive object is involved, but generally the energy transfer from blunt chest trauma with objects such as fists or baseball bats is not sufficient to result in aortic injury, as both the mass and

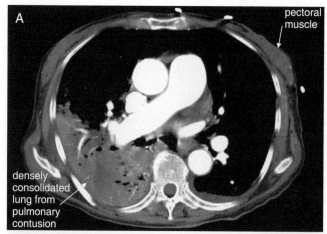

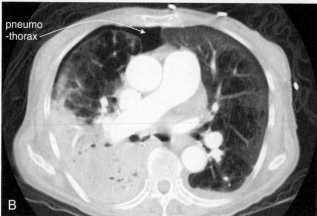

Figure 6-38. **Pulmonary contusion.** This 77-year-old female was in a car struck by a train. Compare these CT with IV contrast images with Figure 6-37 showing her chest x-ray. **A,** Soft-tissue window settings. **B,** Lung window settings. These images demonstrate that the injured right lung has taken on the same tissue density as muscle tissue—a remarkable transformation of lung to "solid organ." On soft-tissue window settings, the lung tissue and pectoral muscle appear nearly the same density. The contused lung parenchyma increased in density resulting from alveolar hemorrhage and fluid leaking from injured lung parenchymal cells. Compare with the fairly normal appearance of the left lung on lung windows. Note the different information provided by the two window settings. The lung window setting demonstrates a pneumothorax that is not visible on the soft-tissue window. Incidentally, the anterior right lung shows extensive bullous changes of emphysema, discussed in more detail in Chapter 5.

the velocity are low. Thus a mediastinal abnormality on chest x-ray in a patient who had been punched in the chest or who has fallen from a standing position to the ground is unlikely to represent a mediastinal injury, even if injuries such as rib fractures are present. As a consequence, incidental x-ray findings that hint at mediastinal pathology may not need to be pursued acutely in this setting.

In higher-velocity (higher energy) blunt trauma, the thorax is brought to a rapid stop by a collision with a static object. The aorta continues to move forward in the thorax until it is halted by reaching the end of its tether, the ligamentum arteriosum—the remnant of the embryonic ductus arteriosus. This structure attaches to the inferior surface of the aorta at a point near the origin of the

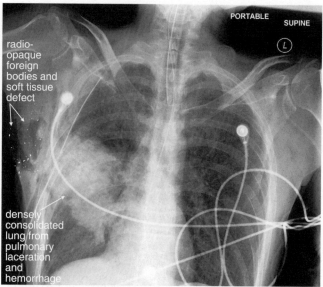

Figure 6-39. **Pulmonary laceration or hemorrhage.** Not all pulmonary injuries are contusions from blunt trauma. This 46-year-old male was shot in the right axilla by police. Bullet fragments are visible in the soft tissues of the right axilla, where a large soft-tissue defect is visible. The lung parenchyma is densely consolidated in the trajectory of the bullet—presumably from bleeding into the damaged tissue. The silhouette sign is again seen; the injured lung parenchyma of the right middle lobe is adjacent to the right heart border and shares the same soft-tissue (fluid) density. As a consequence, the right heart margin is obscured. A chest tube has been placed, and no hemopneumothorax is visible, although the supine position of this chest x-ray reduces its sensitivity for these, as described in an earlier figure.

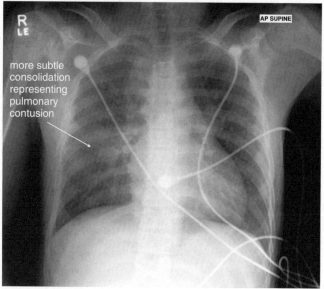

Figure 6-40. **Pulmonary contusion.** This 16-year-old male was a restrained passenger in a motor vehicle collision. He self-extricated and ambulated at the scene but complained of chest pain. His chest x-ray shows a subtle consolidation of the right mid lung. The flexible chest wall of pediatric patients may allow lung contusion without rib fracture.

descending aorta or distal aortic arch. The ligamentum arteriosum is attached inferiorly to the pulmonary artery and restricts anterior aortic motion. An aortic tear most often occurs at this location in blunt trauma, although other injury locations are possible. As you review the CT

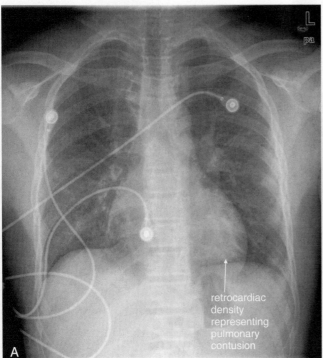

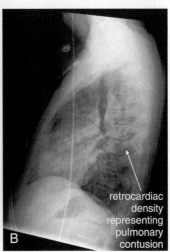

Figure 6-41. **Pulmonary contusion.** Same patient as in Figure 6-40. **A,** PA chest x-ray. **B,** Lateral chest x-ray. This chest x-ray was taken 7 hours after the first and shows an evolving pulmonary contusion. Compare with the CT in Figure 6-42.

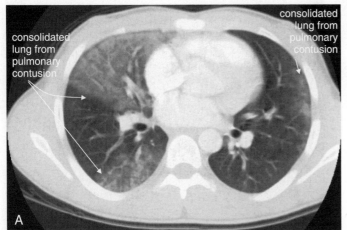

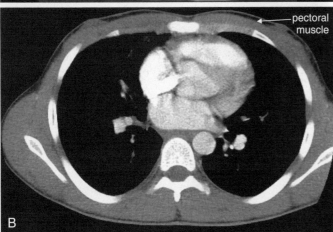

Figure 6-42. **Pulmonary contusion: CT with IV contrast.** Same patient as Figures 6-40 and 6-41. This patient has a subtler pulmonary contusion than does the victim of the car–train collision (Figures 6-37 and 6-38). In those figures, the lung tissue was so densely consolidated that it was easily visible on both chest x-ray and CT soft-tissue windows, with the same apparent density as pectoral muscle. The patient in this figure has less severe injury, with less dense lung tissue in the region of injury. Whereas the injured lung is readily visible on lung windows **(A),** it is invisible on soft-tissue windows **(B).** Bilateral pulmonary contusions are visible on CT, whereas the initial x-ray demonstrated only the right-sided contusion clearly.

Figure 6-43. Pulmonary contusion with pneumothorax. **A,** AP supine chest x-ray. **B,** Close-up from **A.** This 34-year-old male was an unrestrained driver who was thrown through his windshield. His chest x-ray shows a pulmonary contusion with density along the superior right heart border. Careful inspection also reveals a lateral right pneumothorax **(B)**. The width of the upper mediastinum cannot be determined because of the adjacent dense right lung apex. Therefore, CT was performed to evaluate for mediastinal hematoma and aortic injury (Figure 6-44).

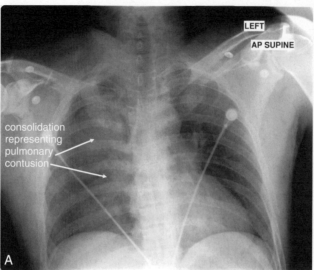
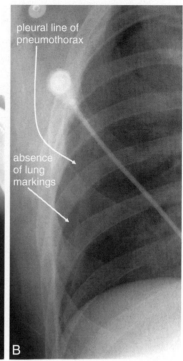

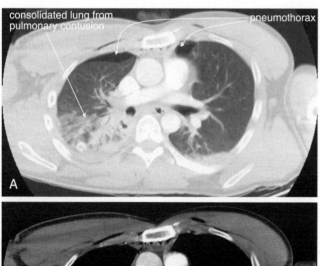
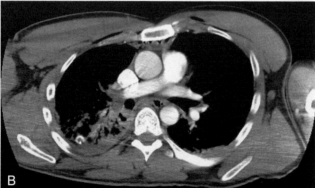

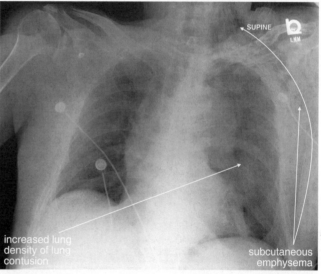

Figure 6-45. **Pulmonary contusion with pneumothorax.** This 89-year-old male was in a motor vehicle collision in which his airbags deployed. The patient's chest x-ray shows extensive subcutaneous emphysema of the left chest wall, extending to the left neck. His left lung appears denser than the right, suggesting pulmonary contusion. A small basilar left pneumothorax is difficult to see on this image but is the likely source of the subcutaneous air.

Figure 6-44. **Pulmonary contusion with pneumothorax.** Same patient as Figure 6-43. **A,** CT with IV contrast, axial slice viewed with lung windows. **B,** Same slice, viewed with soft-tissue windows. Some areas of injured lung are densely consolidated and are visible even on soft-tissue windows. Others are less dense, reflecting less alveolar hemorrhage and parenchymal injury—these are visible only on lung windows **(A)**. A small right anterior pneumothorax persists despite the presence of a chest tube, and a small left pneumothorax is present. The pneumothoraces are not visible on soft-tissue windows **(B)**.

and aortography images in this chapter, note this consistent location of aortic injuries.

Some aortic tears are full thickness, resulting in rapid exsanguination and death at the scene of injury. In other cases, the tear is either partial thickness (involving the aortic intima and muscularis but leaving the adventitia intact) or full thickness but limited by the formation of a **mediastinal hematoma,** allowing survival and transport to the emergency department. In these patients, the

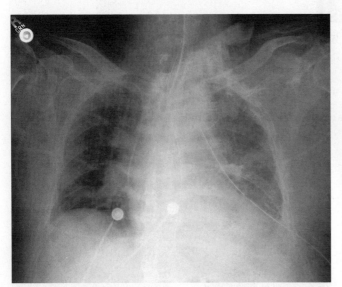

Figure 6-46. **Pulmonary contusion with pneumothorax.** Same patient as Figure 6-45, 2 days later. Does this x-ray show progression of pulmonary contusion? It is hard to be sure. The patient has a chest tube in place and may have a hemothorax contributing to increased left lung density. He is intubated, and a ventilator-associated pneumonia may be in progress as well. Upright portable chest x-ray cannot differentiate these causes of increased lung density.

aortic contour may appear abnormal, and the silhouette on the AP or PA chest x-ray may be altered by the presence of mediastinal hematoma. Several classic chest x-ray findings can result from this mediastinal hematoma (Table 6-4) (see Figures 6-56, 6-58, 6-60, 6-63, 6-66, 6-69, 6-73, 6-77, 6-81, 6-85, 6-86, 6-90, 6-93, 6-99, 6-105, and 6-107):

- The mediastinum may appear wider than normal. An upper limit of 8 cm (measured from the left aortic arch to the right mediastinal margin) has been described, although lesser degrees of widening can occur with small mediastinal hematomas. Unfortunately, because this finding depends on the size of the mediastinal hematoma, it is only about 90% sensitive and 10% specific.[12] The supine AP chest x-ray often obtained following blunt trauma can simulate pathologic mediastinal widening from aortic injury as described earlier.
- The aortic knob may lose its distinct and rounded appearance resulting from hematoma surrounding it. The margins may appear indistinct or irregular.
- A normal lucent region, the aortopulmonary window (located at the intersection of the normal left pulmonary artery and the descending aorta) may be obscured by mediastinal hematoma.
- The right **paratracheal stripe,** which is normally a thin water-density stripe between the air column of the trachea and the adjacent lung on frontal projection chest x-ray, may become widened by the presence of mediastinal hematoma. The upper limit of normal is 4 mm, with 5 mm reliably being abnormal.[13-15]
- The left paraspinous line may be displaced by mediastinal blood[16]

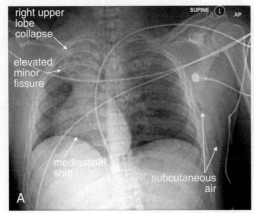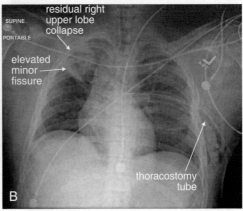

Figure 6-47. **Lobar collapse with mediastinal shift resulting from volume loss.** This 38-year-old male was ejected from his vehicle after rolling the car at high speed. **(A)** His initial chest x-ray shows dramatic mediastinal shift to the right, which in the setting of trauma might first bring to mind left tension pneumothorax. However, mediastinal shift can occur from the "push" of high pressure on the contralateral side (e.g., tension pneumothorax) or from the "pull" of low volume on the ipsilateral side. In this case, the patient has collapse of the right upper lobe, seen as a density in the right lung apex. The minor fissure has tilted diagonally from the accordion-like collapse of the upper lobe, rather than having its normal horizontal configuration. Collapse of the right upper lobe results in volume loss on the right, and the mediastinum shifts right to occupy the resulting space. Was the right upper lobe collapse a traumatic injury? More likely, it represents plugging of the right upper lobe bronchus with mucous or blood. The CT depicting this finding is seen in Figure 6-48. **(B)** Same patient 2 hours later. The right upper lobe has reexpanded, although density representing atelectasis or possible pulmonary contusion remains. The mediastinum has shifted back toward its normal position. A left chest tube has been placed, as CT did demonstrate a small left pneumothorax—clearly not the cause of the mediastinal shift.

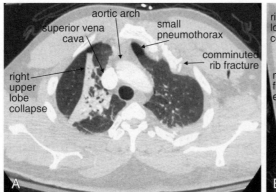
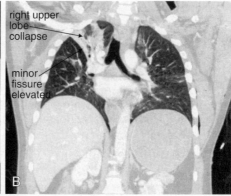

Figure 6-48. Lobar collapse with mediastinal shift resulting from volume loss. CT with IV contrast viewed on lung windows to best illustrate lobar collapse. Same patient as Figure 6-47, in which his initial chest x-ray shows dramatic mediastinal shift to the right. This is due not to left-sided tension pneumothorax but to significant collapse of the right upper lobe. This results in volume loss on the right, and the mediastinum shifts right to occupy the resulting space. **A,** An axial slice through the upper chest shows a triangular cross section through the collapsed lung segment. The upper mediastinum has shifted right, and the aortic arch has a nearly right–left transverse orientation rather than an anterior–posterior orientation. A small left pneumothorax is visible as air *(black)* with no lung markings. **B,** A coronal view, in which the upper lobe collapse is again visible. The heart and trachea appear shifted right. The left lung does not show any evidence of pneumothorax in this view, though other images show a small pneumothorax. Certainly, a tension pneumothorax was not present and was not the cause of the mediastinal shift.

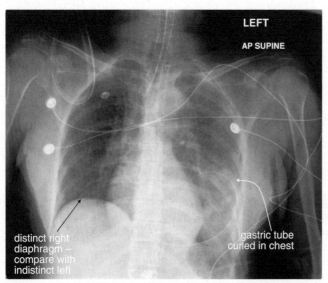

Figure 6-49. Diaphragm injury. This 68-year-old female was ejected from a vehicle. Her chest x-ray shows several classic features of diaphragmatic rupture. The right diaphragm is normal in appearance, whereas the left diaphragm is not identified. The patient has an orogastric tube in place, which is coiled in the stomach—in the left lower to midthorax. This is consistent with herniation of the stomach through a diaphragmatic injury into the left thorax. Not specific to diaphragm rupture, the patient also has an indistinct aortic arch, concerning for traumatic aortic injury. The left thorax also appears denser than the right, possibly indicating hemothorax or diffuse pulmonary contusion. Compare with the patient's CT in Figures 6-50 and 6-51.

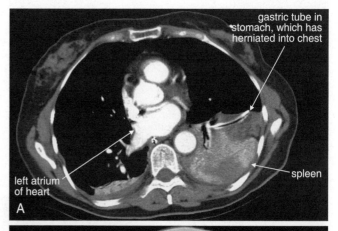
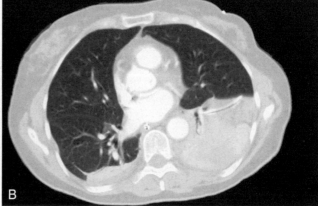

Figure 6-50. Diaphragm injury, CT with IV contrast. CT images from the same patient as Figure 6-49 show the stomach and spleen to be present in the left chest, consistent with a diaphragm rupture. These two images show the same slice, at the level of the left atrium in the chest, on soft-tissue **(A)** and lung **(B)** windows. An orogastric tube is seen in the stomach. A portion of the spleen is also seen. On lung windows, no pneumothorax is identified.

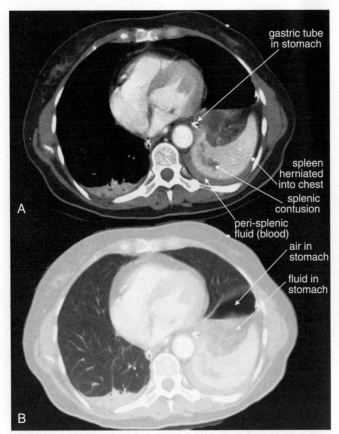

Figure 6-51. Diaphragm injury, CT. CT images from the same patient as Figures 6-49 and 6-50. These two images show the same slice through the chest, on soft-tissue **(A)** and lung **(B)** windows. An orogastric tube is seen in the stomach, with an air–fluid level representing gastric contents. The spleen is also seen herniated into the chest with an area of parenchymal contusion. Perisplenic fluid is also seen. On lung windows, no pneumothorax is identified—the area of air is within the stomach.

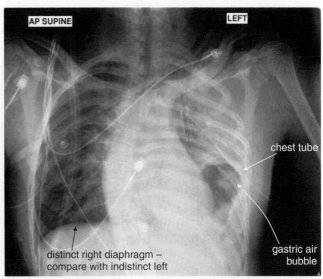

Figure 6-52. Diaphragmatic rupture. This 21-year-old male was a rear-seat passenger in a head-on collision with dump truck. Two other passengers were killed at the scene. The patient was noted to have decreased oxygen saturations and no breath sounds. Needle decompression was performed by emergency medical services. This chest x-ray, taken in the emergency department after placement of a chest tube, shows features of diaphragmatic rupture. The normal curvature of the left diaphragm is not seen. The gastric air bubble is seen in the left chest. Note how closely the chest tube passes to the gastric air bubble, a reminder that care should always be taken to assess for solid organs in the chest when placing a chest tube. Not specific to diaphragm rupture, the patient also has opacification of the left hemithorax, which could represent pulmonary contusion or hemothorax on this supine film. In addition, herniation of abdominal contents into the chest can compress lung tissue, giving it this appearance. Compare this x-ray with the CT findings in Figures 6-53 through 6-55. Incidentally, the patient has a severe dextroscoliosis that is not a result of trauma.

- An **apical pleural cap** may form as blood tracks into the superior mediastinum and over the pleura at the lung apex, creating a soft-tissue density in this location.
- A pleural effusion may be present if blood has leaked from the mediastinum into the pleural space.
- Other structures passing through the mediastinum may be distorted or displaced by mediastinal hematoma. These include normal anatomic structures and medical devices commonly seen in trauma patients:
  - The trachea may be deviated to the patient's right.
  - The left main-stem bronchus may appear deflected in a caudad direction.
  - A NG or OG tube within the esophagus may appear deviated to the left or right.
  - An endotracheal tube may appear deviated with the trachea.
- Other injuries such as first and second rib, scapula, or thoracic spine fractures may be present. These are not signs of aortic injury; rather, they suggest a high-energy trauma mechanism, compatible with aortic injury. Studies have refuted the traditional association between these injuries and aortic trauma.[17-18]

In effect, most of the chest x-ray findings of aortic injury are secondary signs of mediastinal hematoma, which can be present in the absence of aortic injury or absent in the presence of aortic injury.[12,19] Because the size of the hematoma and the degree of aortic injury vary from patient to patient, the severity and prominence of these findings varies. Some patients with aortic injuries have all of these findings; others have only a few. Rarely, the aortic injury is so subtle that the chest x-ray, which gives only the silhouette of superimposed mediastinal structures, appears normal. More commonly, the chest x-ray suggests possible aortic injury when none is present. For example, mediastinal widening may occur resulting from supine position, preexisting and intact thoracic aortic aneurysm, mediastinal lymphadenopathy unrelated to trauma, a tortuous course of the aorta, goiter extending to the mediastinum, or venous hematomas from sources other than the aorta, including spinal injuries with prevertebral hematomas. For this reason, an abnormal chest x-ray with findings of mediastinal hematoma is not specific for aortic injury. Overall, chest x-ray is normal in only about 7% of traumatic aortic injuries,[20] and the negative predictive value of chest x-ray has been reported as 95%, due in large part to the rarity of aortic injury.[21]

Direct evidence of aortic injury may also be seen on chest x-ray: a change in aortic contour may be a direct result of the aortic tear and potential aortic pseudoaneurysm formation. Table 6-5 shows the frequency of various chest x-ray findings in cases of aortic injury.

Pneumomediastinum and Pneumopericardium

Pneumomediastinum and **pneumopericardium** can be seen on chest x-ray in blunt and penetrating trauma, and they occur periodically without any history of trauma, sometimes following forceful vomiting or cough. The significance of these findings varies substantially with the history and clinical context. For example, following vomiting, pneumomediastinum is concerning for esophageal rupture with threat of consequent mediastinitis, whereas the same chest x-ray finding following cough usually is due to a microscopic leak of air from the lung or airway and results in a benign clinical course without any intervention. In the setting of blunt trauma, pneumomediastinum and pneumopericardium should raise suspicion of accompanying pneumothorax or tracheobronchial injury. The chest x-ray should be scrutinized for evidence of these, and depending on the degree of suspicion, additional imaging may be warranted—for evaluation of the source of the air, not for specific

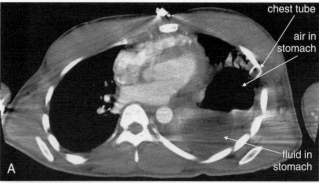

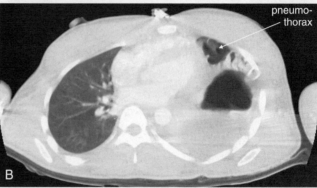

Figure 6-54. Diaphragmatic rupture. These CT images are from the same patient as Figures 6-52, 6-53, and 6-55. **A,** Soft-tissue windows. **B,** The same slice viewed on lung windows. Here, the stomach is seen in the left chest adjacent to the heart. The air–fluid level represents gastric contents. Note how close to the stomach the thoracostomy tube passes—a reminder to consider diaphragm rupture and to perform a finger sweep when placing a thoracostomy tube for trauma.

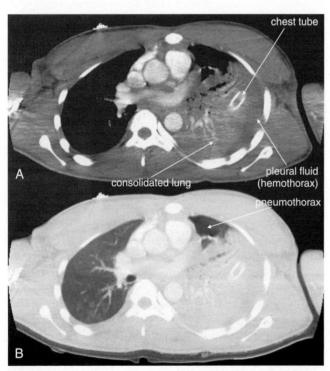

Figure 6-53. Diaphragmatic rupture, CT with IV contrast. Figures 6-52 through 6-55 show images from the same case. **A,** Soft-tissue windows. **B,** The same slice viewed on lung windows. In these images near the lung apex, the thoracostomy tube is seen passing into consolidated lung parenchyma. From these images, it is not possible to determine whether this increased density of lung tissue represents contused lung from the original blunt injury or compressive atelectasis from the pressure exerted by herniated abdominal contents. A small anterior pneumothorax is seen on lung windows, despite the chest tube. Fluid density is seen surrounding the lung parenchyma on soft-tissue windows, representing hemothorax.

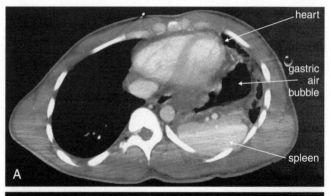

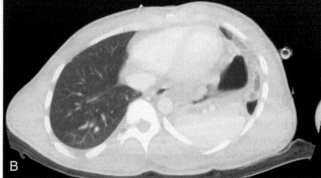

Figure 6-55. Diaphragmatic rupture, CT with IV contrast. Figures 6-52 through 6-55 show images from the same case. **A,** Soft-tissue windows. **B,** The same slice viewed on lung windows. Here, the spleen and gastric air bubble are seen adjacent to the heart in the left chest. The right chest appears normal.

treatment of the pneumopericardium or pneumomediastinum. In penetrating chest trauma, these findings again can suggest injury to the lung or tracheobronchial tree, but an esophageal injury should also be considered as a potential source.

Air in the pericardium or mediastinum appears black on chest x-ray (Figures 6-109 through 6-113). The

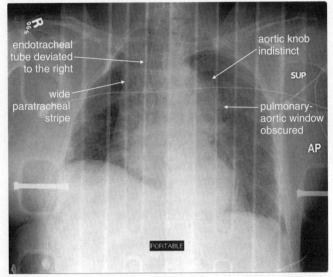

Figure 6-56. Thoracic aortic injury. This patient has a classically abnormal chest x-ray for aortic injury. The mediastinum is wide, the aortic knob and aortopulmonary window are obscured, the trachea and endotracheal tube are deviated by mediastinal hematoma, and the right paratracheal stripe is extremely wide. The patient's CT is shown in Figure 6-57.

finding can be extremely subtle, but the cardiac silhouette should be scrutinized on the frontal projection (and the lateral view, if available) for a thin black line on either the interior of or the exterior of the pericardium. Normally, the pericardium is in contact with a thin lubricating layer of pericardial fluid that in turn is in contact with the epicardial surface of the heart. Because these all share the same density, the internal surface of the pericardium is not normally visible. When air is present within the pericardium, it provides contrast between the pericardium and the cardiac surface, allowing the inner pericardial surface to be seen. An additional finding sometimes seen is called the **continuous diaphragm sign,** which occurs when air is visible along the caudad surface of the heart (see Chapter 5). Normally, the cephalad surface of each hemidiaphragm is visible resulting from low-density lung abutting this surface. The central surfaces of the diaphragm are not normally visible, as the heart and pericardium abut the diaphragm centrally and share its density. Therefore the normal appearance of the diaphragm when traced from the patient's right to left is discontinuous, with the upper surface becoming invisible at the center of the chest and then reappearing to the left of the heart. When air is present within the pericardium, the superior diaphragmatic surface is visible as an apparently continuous line from the patient's right to left. Air in the upper mediastinum may outline structures extending into the neck, so fine linear lucencies should be sought outlining the trachea, great vessels, and muscles extending into the cervical region (see Figure 6-109).

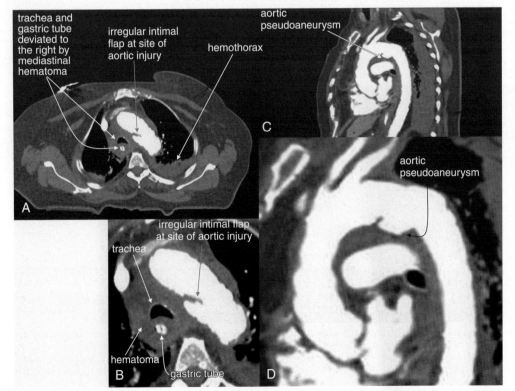

Figure 6-57. Thoracic aortic injury, CT with IV contrast, viewed with soft-tissue windows. Same patient as Figure 6-56. **A,** Axial CT image. **B,** Close-up from **A. C,** Sagittal CT image. **D,** Close-up from **C.** The CT confirms aortic injury with mediastinal hematoma as the cause of the abnormal chest x-ray findings. The mediastinal hematoma surrounds the trachea and esophagus and deviates these to the patient's right, at the same time creating a wide mediastinum. An aortic intimal injury and pseudoaneurysm are present at the classic location–the insertion site of the ligamentum arteriosum

Pericardial Effusion and Hemopericardium

On chest x-ray, water, blood, other fluids, and soft tissues such as the myocardium share the same density. Two structures in direct contact and sharing the same density cannot be distinguished from one another on chest x-ray (see Chapter 5 for more discussion of the **silhouette sign**). Consider, for example, the normal radiographic appearance of the heart; the solid (soft tissue) myocardium cannot be distinguished from the liquid blood within its chambers. Fluid within the

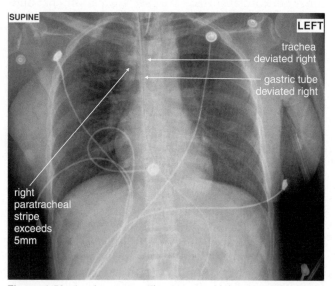

Figure 6-58. Aortic trauma. This 29-year-old female was struck by a car and was found unresponsive. Her mediastinum appears wide, and her trachea and orogastric tube are deviated to the right, relative to her thoracic spine. The aortic knob is not clearly seen, and the aortopulmonary window is not seen. These abnormalities can be the result of the mass effect of periaortic hematoma from aortic trauma. The radiology report stated that in this case they likely were resulting from the supine anterior–posterior technique, but CT confirmed aortic injury (Figure 6-59).

pericardium outside of the heart also cannot be distinguished from the myocardium. With a moderate to large pericardial effusion, the appearance on a supine AP chest x-ray usually demonstrates an enlarged cardiac silhouette—though this appearance may be simulated even in the absence of a pericardial effusion resulting from the supine AP technique (as described earlier in this chapter; see Figure 6-1). Cardiomegaly would be expected to have a similar appearance and cannot be formally distinguished with chest x-ray. Ultrasound and CT can readily differentiate the two conditions. If an upright chest x-ray is obtained, a pericardial effusion may take on the classic "water bottle" shape resulting from pooling of fluid in the dependent pericardium (see Chapter 5). However, this appearance is most prominent when a large pericardial effusion is present. In many cases of blunt and penetrating trauma, the amount of pericardial blood is less significant than in more slowly accumulating pericardial effusions from uremia or malignancy, and the radiographic appearance may be subtler with mild apparent cardiomegaly. Even a small quantity of rapidly accumulated pericardial fluid can result in hemodynamic compromise, because the pericardium itself has not been stretched over time, as is sometimes seen in nontraumatic pericardial effusions. Consequently, even subtle traumatic pericardial effusions suspected by chest x-ray or confirmed by ultrasound or CT may be clinically significant.

Pneumoperitoneum

Pneumoperitoneum is infrequently seen in blunt trauma but can be seen with either blunt or penetrating trauma. Stab wounds and gunshot wounds to the chest can traverse the diaphragm and injure bowel. Sometimes air from thoracic sources such as pneumothorax can cross the diaphragm into the abdomen, resulting in

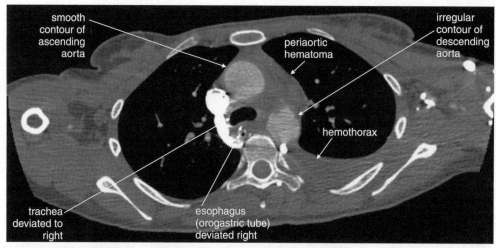

Figure 6-59. Aortic trauma, CT with IV contrast viewed with a variation on soft-tissue windows. Same patient as Figure 6-58. This aortic injury is subtle but definite. Note the irregular contour of the descending aorta, compared with the smooth contour of the ascending aorta. Blood has escaped into the mediastinum, deviating the trachea and esophagus (marked by the orogastric tube) to the patient's right. The periaortic hematoma also widens the mediastinum. A left hemothorax is present, possibly extending from the aorta. No active extravasation of injected contrast is seen. This is typical of survivors, because patients whose hemorrhage is not initially self-limited often die before reaching the emergency department.

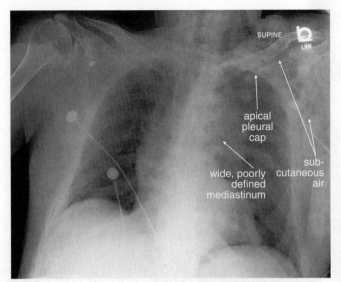

Figure 6-60. Aortic trauma or spontaneous aortic dissection? This 89-year-old male was in a motor vehicle collision. His chest x-ray is concerning for aortic injury on several accounts. His mediastinum is widened, and the aorta is poorly defined. A left apical pleural cap, an indication of blood escaping from the superior mediastinum, is present (compare with the right lung apex, which appears normal). Although not specific for aortic injury, subcutaneous emphysema is seen in the patient's left chest wall and neck. His CT is reviewed in Figure 6-61.

pneumoperitoneum, so the finding of intraperitoneal air is not pathognomonic for bowel perforation.[22-23] On an upright chest x-ray, the expected finding is a lucent (black) collection beneath the diaphragm (see Figure 6-11). Air beneath the left diaphragm may be mistaken for the gastric air bubble, or vice versa. Air beneath the right diaphragm is almost always true pneumoperitoneum, although colonic interposition (positioning of the colon between the liver and the diaphragm) can rarely simulate free air. The supine AP portable chest x-ray most often used in blunt trauma may fail to detect pneumoperitoneum, because air in a supine patient may collect in the midline anterior abdomen rather than in a subdiaphragmatic position.[24] When possible, an upright chest x-ray should be obtained to maximize detection of free peritoneal air. Alternatively, CT of the abdomen can be performed, as this is extremely sensitive for even minute quantities of pneumoperitoneum.[25]

Foreign Bodies

Chest x-ray can detect and assist in the localization of radiopaque foreign bodies, including metal, glass, and stone. Organic fragments such as wood may be invisible on x-ray. When assessing the position of a radiopaque foreign body using x-ray, two orthogonal views (x-rays

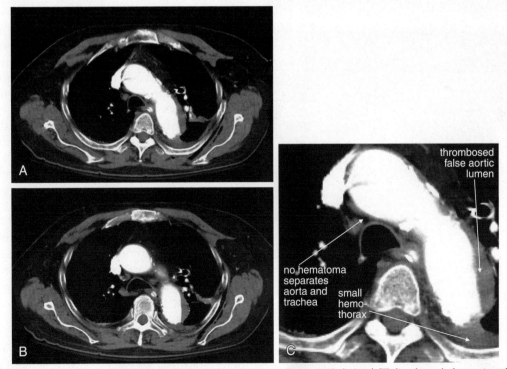

Figure 6-61. Aortic trauma or spontaneous aortic dissection? Same patient as Figure 6-60. **A,** Axial CT slice through the aortic arch, viewed on soft-tissue windows. **B,** Axial slice slightly caudad to **A,** through the ascending and descending aorta. **C,** Close-up from **A.** The patient's CT with IV contrast shows an abnormal aorta, but findings are more typical of a spontaneous aortic dissection than of aortic trauma. Did the patient have an aortic dissection leading to his car collision? We will never know—the patient was moribund on emergency department arrival. He certainly sustained trauma, with other injuries including splenic lacerations and rib fractures. Unlike the aortic traumatic injury in the previous case, there is no periaortic hematoma between the aorta and the trachea. Spontaneous aortic dissections often do not lead to blood loss from the aorta, because the injury involves the intima. The small hemothorax here may emanate from rib fractures.

Figure 6-62. Aortic trauma or spontaneous aortic dissection? Same patient as Figures 6-60 and 6-61. CT with IV contrast viewed with soft-tissue windows. The descending aorta has an intimal flap, more typical of spontaneous aortic dissection than of traumatic aortic injury. **A,** At the level of the pulmonary artery, the descending aorta shows thrombosis of the false lumen. **B,** Farther caudad, contrast is seen in both the true and the false lumen. **C,** Close-up from **B**.

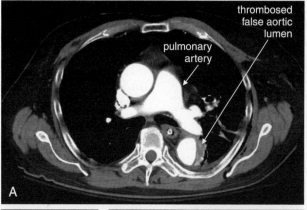

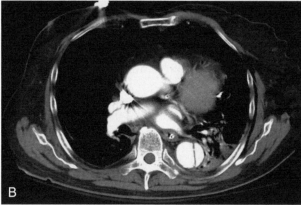

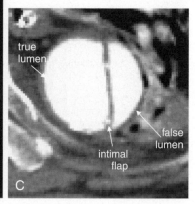

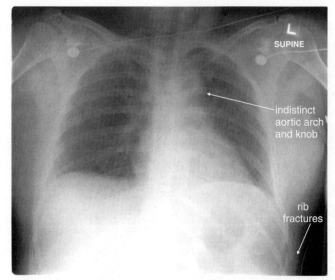

Figure 6-63. **Aortic trauma.** This 36-year-old female was a restrained passenger in a head-on collision. She had multiple evident injuries on emergency department arrival, including tibial plateau fractures and a pulseless right foot. Her chest x-ray shows an indistinct and somewhat broadened mediastinal contour, although the latter was attributed to the supine anterior–posterior technique. Rib fractures are also visible. Compare with the CT images in Figures 6-64 and 6-65.

obtained at 90 degrees to each other) are essential. A single view provides no information about the depth of the object in the plane of the x-ray. For example, an object that appears to be internal to the patient on the frontal projection (AP or PA view) may be in front of, within, or behind the patient. Comparison with the lateral view can clarify the location (see Figures 6-114 through 6-120). Chest x-ray reveals the relative positions of chest organs and foreign bodies at an instant in time, but these organs are in motion resulting from respiration and cardiac activity. Because the frontal and lateral x-ray projections are not obtained at the same moment, they can reflect different phases of respiration and cardiac contraction. Consequently, the precise position of a foreign body can occasionally be misrepresented by chest x-ray (see Figure 6-117). For example, an object may appear to overlie a structure such as the heart when it has been superimposed transiently by respiratory motion. CT is more definitive, as three-dimensional relationships are clarified (see Figures 6-116, 6-119, and 6-120). Modern CT scanners acquire image data so rapidly that motion artifact is minimal. One exception is that dense metallic objects can create streak or starburst artifacts that can make precise localization difficult (see Figure 6-108).

Bones

Chest x-ray can provide useful initial information about bony injuries, including fractures and dislocations. CT is more sensitive, but for many injury patterns, an injury does not require definitive visualization for adequate treatment, and CT may not alter management. For example, nondisplaced rib fractures may be invisible on x-ray but usually require only supportive care

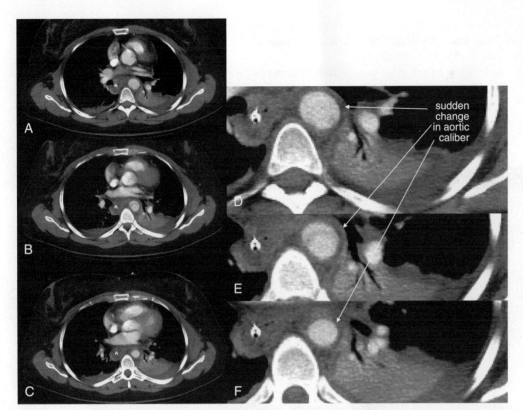

Figure 6-64. **Aortic trauma, CT with IV contrast.** Same patient as Figures 6-63 and 6-65. A sudden change in aortic caliber is seen on these images, indicating a traumatic aortic injury. Figure 6-65 shows sagittal and three-dimensional reconstructions, demonstrating a pseudoaneurysm. **A** through **C**, Consecutive axial CT slices viewed on soft-tissue windows, progressing from cephalad to caudad. **D** through **F**, Close-ups from **A, B,** and **C,** respectively.

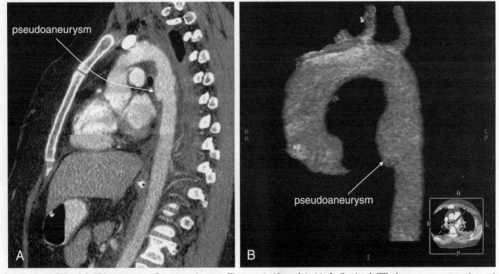

Figure 6-65. **Aortic trauma, CT with IV contrast.** Same patient as Figures 6-63 and 6-64. **A,** Sagittal CT planar reconstruction, viewed on soft-tissue windows, depicting the aorta from its root through the arch and into the descending aorta. **B,** Three-dimensional reconstruction of the same region, with other thoracic structures digitally removed. The tiny image in the right lower corner of panel **B** is an axial cross-section inserted automatically by 3D software for orientation purposes. A, R, L, and P in that image indicate anterior, right, left, and posterior. These reformats are not necessary to make the diagnosis of traumatic aortic pseudoaneurysm but do help indicate the extent and assist with surgical planning. The patient underwent endovascular repair.

with analgesics. Dedicated rib x-rays can be obtained to improve sensitivity, but these are generally unnecessary, as standard chest x-ray provides the more clinically important information—namely, the presence of underlying injuries such as pneumothorax or pulmonary contusion. Bones visible on standard frontal (AP or PA) chest x-ray include ribs, sternum, scapula, proximal humerus, clavicles, thoracic spine, and portions of the cervical and lumbar spine. Joints visible on chest x-ray include the sternoclavicular, acromioclavicular (AC), and glenohumeral joints, as well as the articulations of ribs with spinal facets. These joints should be inspected for dislocation or subluxation. Dislocations of the sternoclavicular joints are discussed in this chapter, whereas acromioclavicular and glenohumeral joint dislocations are discussed in Chapter 14.

Fractures

Fractures can be subtle on chest x-ray. When specific bony fractures are suspected clinically or abnormalities are seen on chest x-ray, dedicated views of the affected region may be needed, depending on the specific injury. On x-ray, the contours of bones should be inspected for cortical step-offs. Comparison with structures on the contralateral side should be used to reveal subtle abnormalities.

Rib Fractures. Rib fractures are the most common thoracic injury and are a frequent finding on chest x-ray after trauma (Figures 6-121 through 6-124).[26] Rib films are not typically indicated to assess for rib fracture, as it is the underlying parenchymal injury or the clinical status of the patient that most often drives management.[26] The x-ray should be inspected for associated pneumothoraces, pleural effusions (hemothorax), and pulmonary contusions. CT is also not routinely indicated to pursue rib fractures, unless other important thoracic injuries are suspected.

Ribs should be traced from their articulation with the facets of the thoracic spine, through their course, to the sternum. Displaced fractures are usually readily apparent and should not distract from a separate thorough search for associated pneumothorax, hemothorax, or pulmonary contusion as described earlier. Subtle cortical defects can be harder to recognize. The overlap of ribs can create confusing intersecting lines that may be mistaken for or may disguise fractures. Solitary rib fractures may occur, but as with other ring structures in the body, ribs often fracture in multiple locations or become displaced at articulations with other structures, so detection of a rib fracture should prompt a search for additional fractures or dislocations. If two or more adjacent ribs are fractured in two or more places, a "flail segment" is present, which may significantly interfere with respiratory mechanics. Patients with flail segments are at increased risk for respiratory failure requiring mechanical ventilation with either continuous positive airway

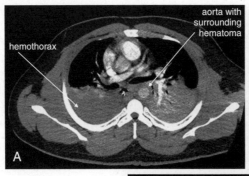

Figure 6-66. Aortic trauma. This 18-year-old man was involved in a severe motor vehicle collision. Among his many injuries were an open-book pelvis fracture and shock bowel. His chest x-ray shows an elevated left hemidiaphragm consistent with diaphragm rupture. His mediastinum is indistinct and shifted to the right, worrisome for aortic injury—which was confirmed on CT (Figures 6-67 and 6-68). Look carefully at the position of the endotracheal tube and gastric tube—both are shifted to the right. The right paratracheal stripe is also wide. These features are concerning for mediastinal hematoma, possibly from aortic injury. The patient developed multiorgan failure and died on hospital day 2.

Figure 6-67. Aortic trauma, CT with IV contrast, axial images viewed with soft-tissue windows. Same patient as Figures 6-66 and 6-68. Moving from cephalad **(A)** to caudad **(C),** note the change in aortic caliber. The enlarged region in **B** is a pseudoaneurysm. The patient has multiple other chest injuries, including a diaphragm rupture with the stomach in the left chest and a large right hemothorax.

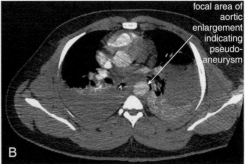

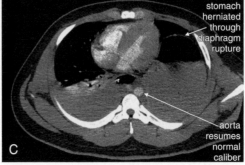

pressure or endotracheal intubation.[27] Fractures of the first and second ribs historically have been associated with high-energy mechanisms of trauma and with aortic trauma. However, several studies suggest no increased risk for aortic injury with upper rib, sternal, scapular, or thoracic spine fractures.[17,18,26,28] Lee et al.[17,18] found that the rate of thoracic aortic injury increased in a statistically significant but not a clinically meaningful degree in patients with rib fractures.[17,18]

Stawicki et al.[29] noted an increase in mortality associated with rising numbers of rib fractures, particularly in the elderly. Overall, it is likely that rib fractures are a marker of high-energy trauma and morbidity from other injuries (including extrathoracic injuries), although in this study multiple rib fractures were independent predictors of mortality. Lee et al.[18,30] suggested that three or more rib fractures were an indication for transfer to a trauma center, because of increased mortality, mean injury severity score, mean hospital stay, mean number of intensive care unit days, and rates of liver and spleen injuries. Other studies have shown that pain from rib fractures is a significant cause of disability, with pain persisting well beyond 30 days in some cases.[31]

Sternum Fractures. Sternal fractures are a marker of significant force to the thorax (see Figures 6-125 through 6-129). Associated injuries such as blunt cardiac injury, mediastinal injury, and pneumothorax should be considered. Sternal x-rays are not routinely performed, because they yield relatively little clinically important information. If associated injuries to the aorta are strongly considered, chest CT can evaluate these while allowing examination of the sternum using bone windows.

Sternal fractures are often not seen on the frontal chest x-ray. In some cases, they can be recognized by a subtle area of lucency or increased density, depending on the fracture pattern. A lateral chest x-ray or sternal view can depict the degree of AP displacement (see Figure 6-126). CT reveals more definition of the degree of fracture (see Figures 6-126, 6-128, and 6-129) but is generally more important for revealing associated injuries such as mediastinal trauma, as sternal fractures themselves require primarily supportive care with analgesics.[32] A sternal fracture should prompt careful attention for possible sternoclavicular dislocation (Figures 6-130 through 6-135), as described later. A separate careful assessment of the mediastinum should be performed, as described earlier.

Scapular Fractures. Scapular fractures are also discussed in Chapter 14. Here, we briefly describe these injuries, because they may be noted on x-ray obtained for chest trauma. Scapular fracture can be subtle on frontal chest x-ray. The entire perimeter of the scapula should be traced to assess for cortical step-offs. The medial border of the scapula can be mistaken for the pleural line of a pneumothorax, and vice versa, so a separate careful search for pneumothorax should be performed as described earlier. The scapular spine and the cup of the glenoid fossa should be inspected for discontinuities. If scapular fracture is suspected, CT provides detailed three-dimensional information. Scapula fractures have been associated with high-energy trauma and to a lesser degree with aortic injury, so careful evaluation of the mediastinum should also be performed when scapular fracture is detected. Scapular injuries can occur in

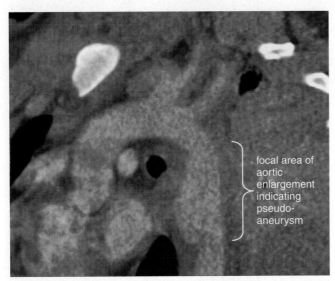

Figure 6-68. Aortic trauma, CT with IV contrast. Figures 6-66 and 6-67 show images from the same case. This reconstruction in a parasagittal plane shows an area of traumatic pseudoaneurysmal dilatation. This can be recognized on the axial images (Figure 6-67) as a sudden change in aortic diameter.

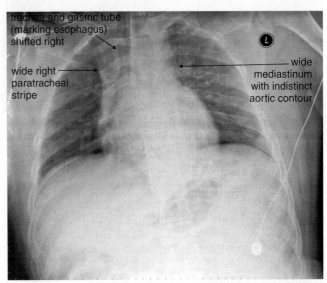

Figure 6-69. Aortic trauma. This 20-year-old male struck a tree with his car and was hypotensive during emergency transport. His chest x-ray shows the now-familiar findings of a widened mediastinum, wide right paratracheal stripe, deviated trachea and gastric tube, indistinct aortic knob, and lack of the normal pulmonary artery window, consistent with traumatic aortic injury. See CT images, Figures 6-70 and 6-71, and aortogram, Figure 6-72.

Figure 6-70. Aortic trauma, CT with IV contrast, axial image viewed with soft-tissue window. Same patient as Figure 6-69. The aortic injury itself is not seen, but periaortic hematoma is present, deviating the trachea and gastric tube (within the esophagus) to the right, just as was seen on chest x-ray. Figure 6-71 shows the aortic injury.

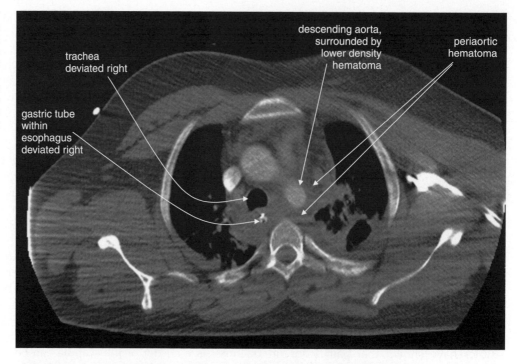

Figure 6-71. Aortic trauma, CT with IV contrast. Figures 6-69 through 6-72 depict the same case. **A,** Axial CT slice viewed with soft-tissue windows. **B,** Close-up from **A.** More caudad, the descending aorta has an irregular contour and internal filling defects, indicating both an internal tear and a pseudoaneurysm formation. Compare with the angiogram from the same patient in Figure 6-72.

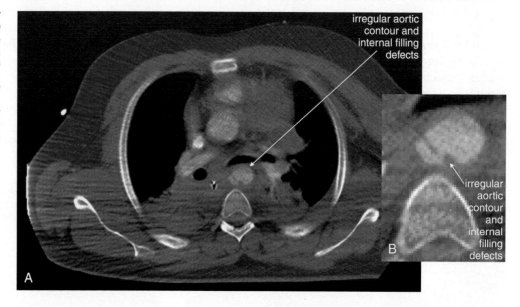

patients without other chest trauma, so aortic imaging is not mandatory in a stable, alert patient with no signs or symptoms of aortic injury on examination or chest x-ray.

Humerus Fractures. The proximal humerus is visible on frontal chest x-ray and should be inspected for fractures, which are discussed in detail in Chapter 14.

Clavicular Fractures. Clavicular fractures are common following falls, bicycle accidents, and motor vehicle collisions. These fractures are discussed in more detail in Chapter 14. The clavicle should be inspected for cortical defects from its articulation with the sternum (discussed later in this chapter) to the AC joints

(see Chapter 14). A clavicle fracture should prompt careful reexamination of the AC and the sternoclavicular joints, which may be dislocated or separated by a fracture. The degree of displacement and impaction or overriding should be noted. Most clavicular fractures are treated nonoperatively, but severely displaced fractures may be fixed surgically. Careful examination of the underlying lung for pneumothorax should be performed as described earlier.

Spine. The thoracic spine and portions of the cervical and lumbar spine are visible on frontal and lateral chest x-ray. When spine injury is suspected clinically, dedicated imaging of these regions is mandatory and is

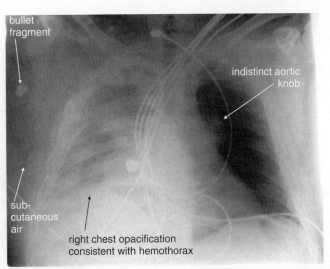

Figure 6-73. **Aortic trauma.** A 26-year-old male was shot just left of the sternum. The bullet crossed the midline, coming to rest in the right axilla. This chest x-ray demonstrates complete opacification of the right chest, consistent with a large hemothorax, as well as possible underlying pulmonary contusion. Subcutaneous air is visible in the right chest wall. The aortic knob is not clearly defined, raising the question of a mediastinal injury. The patient underwent CT (Figures 6-74 and 6-75).

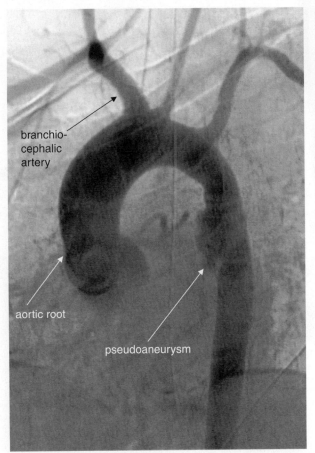

Figure 6-72. **Aortic trauma.** Figures 6-69 through 6-72 show images from the same case. The patient underwent an aortogram, confirming an aortic pseudoaneurysm. Note the similarity to the appearance on CT reconstructions from the prior cases. No active extravasation of contrast is seen. The patient's injury was repaired using endovascular stents.

described in detail in Chapter 3. Gross deformity of the spine should be assessed for on chest x-ray.

Dislocations

Sternoclavicular Joints. Sternoclavicular dislocation can be a radiographically subtle but life-threatening injury. Posterior dislocation of these joints can result from deceleration mechanisms such as motor vehicle collisions and falls. This can lead to impingement of the clavicular head upon the aortic arch and its major branches, the brachiocephalic, innominate, and subclavian arteries (see Figures 6-130 through 6-135), sometimes requiring operative reduction or closed reduction in the operating room.[33] The normal appearance of the sternoclavicular joints is the bilaterally symmetrical location of the clavicular heads on each side of the upper sternum. Rotation of the patient can cause apparent asymmetry, simulating sternoclavicular dislocation. In true dislocation, one clavicular head usually appears superior or inferior to the other and may appear medially or laterally displaced. A lateral chest x-ray or sternal view can confirm sternoclavicular dislocation but does not depict associated vascular injury. CT is useful

to further characterize the degree of dislocation and the location of the clavicle relative to the great vessels. CT also depicts mediastinal hematoma or overt vascular injury resulting from sternoclavicular dislocation.[32]

Acromioclavicular Joints. AC joint injuries are discussed in more detail in Chapter 14. The AC joints are visible on frontal chest x-ray. The normal AC joints are bilaterally symmetrical, so comparison of the left and the right AC joints should be a routine part of your evaluation. A normal AC joint is generally no more than 4 mm in width, though variation occurs and comparison with the opposite side may be more useful than a fixed measurement.[34]

Glenohumeral Joints. Glenohumeral joint injuries are discussed in more detail in Chapter 14. The humeral head is visible on frontal chest x-ray and should be located within the cup of the glenoid fossa. The glenohumeral joints should be bilaterally symmetrical, so always compare the left and the right. Theoretically, posterior or anterior dislocation of the humeral head could be missed on a single frontal projection, because this view does not indicate the AP position of the humerus relative to the glenoid fossa. If glenohumeral dislocation is suspected clinically or if an abnormality is seen on chest x-ray, a dedicated shoulder series should be obtained.

ASSESSING MEDICAL DEVICES

The AP or PA chest x-ray is used to assess a number of medical devices in trauma patients. Common devices include endotracheal tubes, NG or OG tubes, central

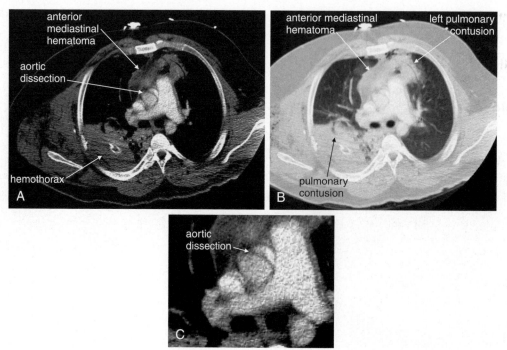

Figure 6-74. Aortic trauma CT with IV contrast. Figures 6-73 through 6-76 depict other images from the same case. **A,** Axial CT slice, viewed with soft-tissue windows. **B,** The same slice, viewed with lung windows. **C,** Close-up from **A.** The bullet has tracked across the anterior mediastinum, resulting in a left anterior pulmonary contusion, an anterior mediastinal hematoma, and apparent dissection of the ascending aorta with an intimal flap. The left pulmonary contusion, anterior mediastinal hematoma, and right posterior pulmonary contusion all contribute to the appearance of the wide mediastinum and obscured aortic knob on chest x-ray. The patient underwent thoracotomy and intraoperative ultrasound, in which the intimal flap seen on CT was thought to represent artifact. No aortic repair was performed. The ascending aorta is subject to motion artifacts on CT that can simulate aortic dissection. Electrocardiogram-gated CT can eliminate this motion artifact to allow more accurate evaluation.

Figure 6-75. Aortic trauma, CT with IV contrast. Same patient as Figures 6-73, 6-74, and 6-76. **A,** Axial CT slice, viewed with soft-tissue windows. **B,** The same slice, viewed with lung windows. Note how different window settings reveal different information from the same anatomic region.

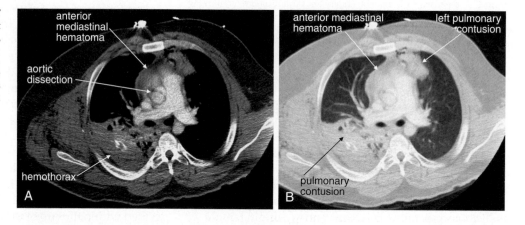

venous catheters, and thoracostomy tubes. A common misconception is that chest x-ray "confirms" device placement. The frontal chest x-ray provides information about the depth of insertion of devices but does not reveal the AP depth of these structures, as described earlier in the section on foreign bodies. While in some cases an abnormal position of a device may be readily apparent based on chest x-ray, in other cases a device can be catastrophically misplaced but appear in good position on chest x-ray. For example, AP chest x-ray can reveal the depth of insertion of an endotracheal tube, but a tube misplaced in the esophagus may not be recognized,

because the esophagus lies posterior to the trachea. Consequently, other methods of assessment of device placement should always be used, in addition to assessment with x-ray.

Endotracheal Tubes

Chest x-ray allows assessment of the depth of insertion of an endotracheal tube. The tube has radiopaque markers and should be seen to terminate below the thoracic inlet and approximately 1 to 2 cm above the carina in adults (see Figures 6-25, 6-26, and 6-39). This position is optimal, because it prevents extubation or right main

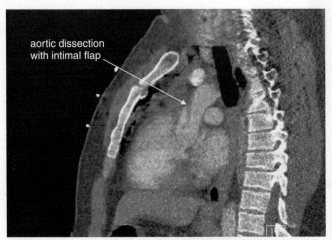

Figure 6-76. Aortic trauma. This sagittal CT reconstruction from the same patient as Figures 6-73 through 6-75 also appears to show an intimal flap of the ascending aorta. Intraoperative ultrasound was felt to be negative for dissection. Motion artifact at the aortic root can cause false positive findings. ECG gating (discussed in Chapter 8) can eliminate this artifact.

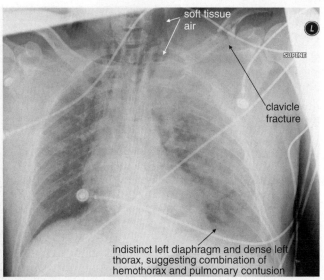

Figure 6-77. Aortic trauma. This 34-year-old male was riding a motorcycle when he was struck by an oncoming car. His chest x-ray demonstrates multiple abnormalities, including a left clavicle fracture and left first rib fracture, and increased density of both hemithoraces, suggesting possible pulmonary contusion. The left diaphragm is not clearly seen, which may indicate a layering hemothorax on this supine chest x-ray. Diaphragm rupture can also result in an indistinct diaphragm. Air is visible, tracking in the left neck and outlining the superior mediastinum. The heart and mediastinum appear slightly deviated to the right side. The aortic knob is not clearly seen. The patient's chest CT is reviewed in Figures 6-78 and 6-79.

bronchus intubation resulting from changes in patient position. Chest x-ray can reveal a tube to be inserted too deeply, resulting in right main bronchus intubation. Associated findings can include right upper lobar collapse or left lung collapse. In other cases, the tube may be inserted to a very shallow depth, terminating far above the sternoclavicular joints. This places the patient at risk for accidental extubation—for example, if the neck is extended during patient repositioning. *Remember that chest x-ray does not confirm the endotracheal tube to be correctly positioned within the trachea; a tube accidentally placed in the esophagus can have an identical midline position.* Other methods of assessment of endotracheal tube positioning, including auscultation, end-tidal carbon dioxide measurement, and pulse oximetry, are essential additions to chest x-ray assessment.

Nasogastric and Orogastric Tubes

OG and NG tubes are visible on chest x-ray. X-ray allows assessment of depth of insertion but in some cases does not confirm correct placement in the stomach. X-ray can reveal a tube to be curled in the esophagus, but inadvertant placement into the trachea can have a similar appearance to correct esophageal placement. An NG or OG tube that deviates slightly from the midline in the thorax can suggest the presence of a mediastinal hematoma from aortic injury, resulting in deviation of the esophagus, as discussed earlier. An NG or OG tube that deviates substantially from the midline within the thorax may indicate accidental placement within a bronchus (see Figure 5-189), so great care should be taken to check the position before any materials are instilled into the tube. A gastric tube should normally be seen curling in the stomach; if the tube position overlies the thorax, diaphragm rupture with herniation of the stomach into the chest should

be suspected (see Figure 6-49). Diaphragm injuries are discussed in more detail in Chapter 10.

Central Venous Catheters

Frontal chest x-ray should be rapidly performed following attempted internal jugular or subclavian central venous catheter placement—even following failed attempts. The primary purpose is to evaluate for accidental iatrogenic pneumothorax. Secondarily, chest x-ray reveals the depth of insertion. The central venous catheter should terminate in the superior vena cava, approximately at the level of the right tracheobronchial angle. Deeper insertion can result in irritation of the atrium or ventricle by the device, potentially increasing the risk for dysrhythmias and thrombus formation.[35-38] Chest x-ray can reveal abnormal placement, including catheters that incorrectly traverse to the contralateral subclavian vein or ascend the internal jugular vein (see Figure 5-188). A common misconception is that chest x-ray confirms correct placement within the intended venous structure. Because the carotid artery and subclavian artery share similar positions to the internal jugular vein and subclavian vein, respectively, inadvertent arterial catheterization may not be evident on chest x-ray. In some cases, this incorrect placement may be evident if the catheter tip overlies the aorta. However, other means of assessment for arterial catheterization, including visual inspection for pulsatile blood flow, use of ultrasound guidance or postplacement ultrasound assessment, transducing pressure waveforms from the

Figure6-78. **Aortictrauma.** Figures 6-77 through 6-80 depict the same case. **A,** Axial CT slice, viewed with soft-tissue windows. **B,** Close-up from **A.** On the patient's initial CT with IV contrast, only a single slice revealed a possible aortic injury. A transverse filling defect suggested an intimal flap where the aorta passes the pulmonary artery—the location of the ligamentum arteriosum. Coincidence? This was suspected to be artifact, and repeat CT with finer cuts was performed (Figure 6-79).

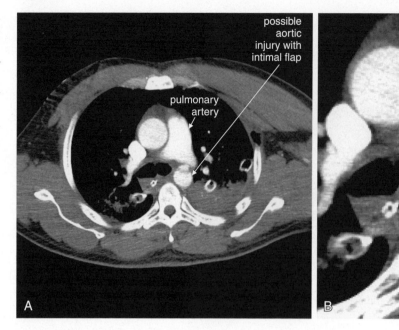

Figure 6-79. **Aortic trauma. A,** Axial CT slice, viewed with soft-tissue windows. **B,** Close-up from **A.** Repeat CT showed the same appearance of a transverse filling defect at precisely the same level as in Figure 6-78, proving an aortic injury. This injury is at the level of the ligamentum arteriosum, which once connected the pulmonary artery and aorta. Coronal and sagittal reconstructions are shown in Figure 6-80.

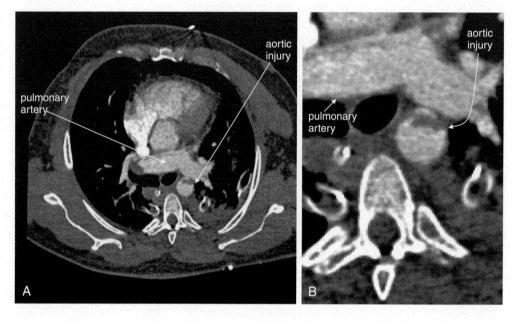

catheter to assess for venous or arterial waveforms, or blood gas analysis, should be considered.

Thoracostomy Tubes

Chest x-ray should be rapidly performed following placement of a thoracostomy tube. As with the other devices described earlier, chest x-ray can reveal grossly abnormal placement or can suggest correct placement, but other means of device assessment are essential. For example, a thoracostomy tube incorrectly placed into posterior subcutaneous tissues can appear to be correctly placed within the pleural space on frontal chest x-ray.

Several chest x-ray features should be assessed following thoracostomy tube placement. First, and critically, the tube should be placed to a sufficient depth that all fenestrations on the tube appear to overlie the pleural space (see Figs. 6-17, 6-26, 6-28, and 6-46). Fenestrations are marked as discontinuities in a radiopaque line along the length of the tube. If fenestrations are not within the pleural space (see Fig. 6-114), air may be entrained from outside of the patient, preventing evacuation of the pneumothorax. The tube should not intersect the mediastinum or cross the diaphragm. Second, the tube should not be kinked (see Figure 6-52) and should have

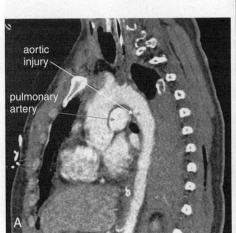

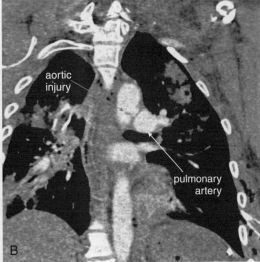

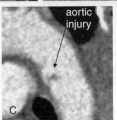

Figure 6-80. Aortic trauma, CT with IV contrast. Figures 6-77 through 6-80 depict the same case. **A,** Sagittal CT reconstruction, viewed with soft-tissue windows. **B,** Coronal CT reconstruction. **C,** Close-up from **A.** These reconstructions confirm an aortic injury at the level of the ligamentum arteriosum, which once connected the pulmonary artery and aorta. Endovascular repair was performed.

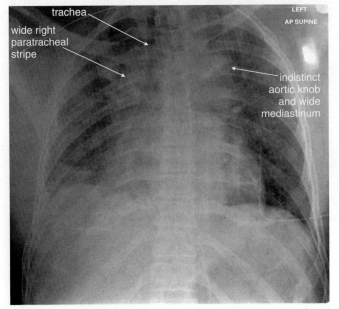

Figure 6-81. Aortic trauma. This 46-year-old male was found unconscious and hypothermic in a car that had crashed at an unknown time. His core temperature was 31°C. The patient was found in the passenger seat and was unrestrained. His chest x-ray shows a wide mediastinum with no distinct aortic knob. The right paratracheal stripe is wide. These findings could be the result of a mediastinal hematoma from aortic injury. CT was performed (Figure 6-82 and 6-83), followed by aortography (Figure 6-84).

an oblique position terminating near the apex of the lung on the side of insertion. These latter features are less important than tube function, and a properly functioning tube should not be removed solely because of suboptimal radiographic appearance.

If a pneumothorax was seen on chest x-ray before thoracostomy tube placement, it should be reduced in size following placement. A pneumothorax that remains large or increases in size following thoracostomy tube placement suggests one of several possibilities:

- Incorrect thoracostomy tube placement
- A correctly positioned but nonfunctional thoracostomy tube, resulting from factors such as failure of the external vacuum system, external kinking, or internal clogging of the tube
- An extremely rapid leak of air into the pleural space, as can be seen with a tracheobronchial injury

Further assessment of the function of the thoracostomy tube, including assessment for air leak, should be performed but is beyond the scope of this text.

ULTRASOUND

Ultrasound is useful in the evaluation of blunt and penetrating chest trauma, because it is portable, rapid to perform, uses no ionizing radiation, and adds little to the cost of patient care (see Table 6-1).

Bedside ultrasound has long been used to evaluate trauma patients for hemopericardium. Examination of the heart from a subdiaphragmatic location is a routine part of the focused assessment with sonography for trauma (FAST) exam. On ultrasound, fluid in the pericardial sac appears black (hypo- or anechoic)

Figure 6-82. Aortic trauma. A CT with IV contrast (axial image, soft-tissue window) from the same patient as Figure 6-81 demonstrates an irregular aortic contour and a small amount of periaortic hematoma just anterior to the aorta. Figure 6-83 shows two slightly oblique reconstructions that further define this injury.

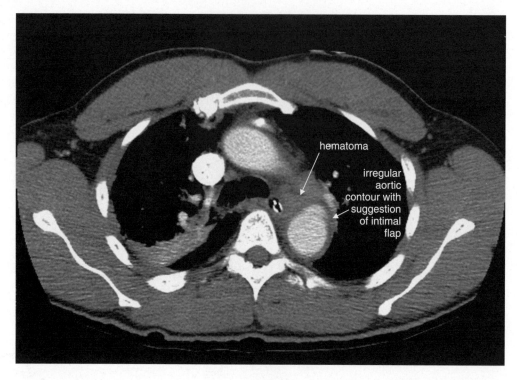

Figure 6-83. Aortic trauma, CT with IV contrast. Figures 6-81 through 6-84 explore the same case. **A,** Sagittal CT image, soft-tissue window. reconstruction from the same patient demonstrates an irregular aortic contour and a small amount of periaortic hematoma (dark gray, soft-tissue density on these soft-tissue windows) just anterior to the aorta. **B,** The area of injury begins with a narrowed region (pseudocoarctation) and progresses into a dilated area (pseudoaneurysm). Aortogram was performed (Figure 6-84).

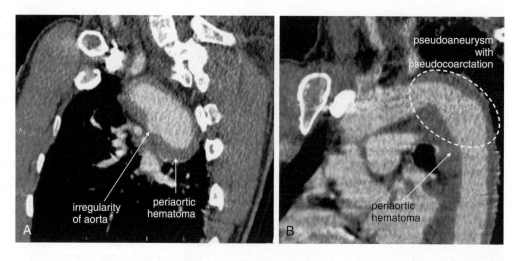

(Figures 6-136 and 6-137). In addition to determining the simple presence or absence of pericardial fluid, ultrasound can provide evidence of pericardial tamponade, as described later in the section on interpretation of ultrasound. Even a small traumatic pericardial effusion can compromise cardiac filling, resulting in pericardial tamponade. Ultrasound can be used to identify pneumothorax with high sensitivity,[39-41] exceeding that of supine chest x-ray.[42-44] However, as is the case for chest CT, it is not clear that detection of a pneumothorax by ultrasound when it is invisible on chest x-ray results in any clinical benefit to the patient. For example, a pneumothorax so small that it is undetectable by chest x-ray may not require thoracostomy even if it is detected by ultrasound. Arguably, detection of small pneumothoraces with ultrasound might be detrimental, because it might result in unnecessary procedures such as thoracostomy, extended clinical observation or admission, or repeat diagnostic imaging with increased costs and radiation exposures. The role of ultrasound in diagnosis of pneumothorax remains uncertain as a consequence of these concerns. Ultrasound also allows detection of fluid in the pleural space (compare x-ray Figure 6-139 and ultrasound Figure 6-140). Fluid in the pleural space appears black, and the lung may be seen floating or moving within the pleural fluid collection. Ultrasound to detect hemopneumothorax has been described as the "extended FAST exam."

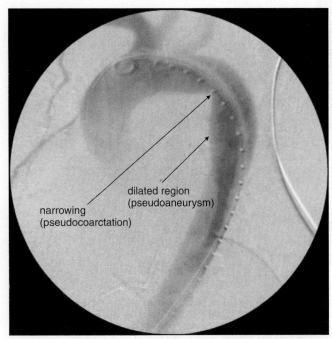

Figure 6-84. Aortic trauma. Figures 6-81 through 6-84 explore the same case. Aortogram from the patient demonstrates the same configuration of pseudocoarctation and pseudoaneurysm. An aortic stent graft was placed.

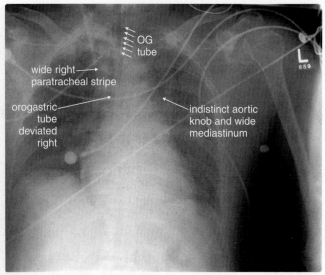

Figure 6-86. Aortic trauma. Same patient as Figure 6-85. The patient has now been intubated, and an orogastric tube has been placed. The orogastric tube is also deviated to the right, suggesting a mediastinal hematoma. The right paratracheal stripe is also wide. The patient's CT scan is reviewed in Figures 6-87 and 6-88.

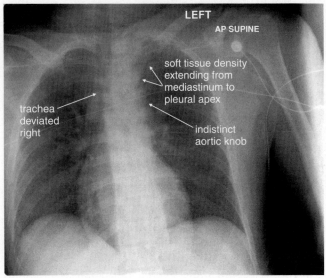

Figure 6-85. Aortic trauma. This 29-year-old male was an unrestrained driver in a high-speed motor vehicle collision. His injuries included a hip dislocation, femur fracture, and open tibia fracture. The patient's chest x-ray shows deviation of the trachea to the right, which we have seen can be the effect of a mediastinal hematoma from aortic injury. The mediastinum does not appear especially wide, but the aortic knob is indistinct. In addition, there is suggestion of an apical pleural cap. Some of these features may be a result of supine position and the patient's rotation to the right. The patient's chest x-ray after intubation supports the concern for mediastinal hematoma (Figure 6-86).

Acquisition and Interpretation of Ultrasound for Chest Trauma

Common views for cardiac ultrasound include subxiphoid, parasternal long axis, and apical four-chamber views. Any of these views can be used to assess for pericardial effusion, with patient body habitus dictating which view provides the best images. The *subxiphoid view* is obtained by placing the ultrasound probe below the xiphoid process in the upper abdomen, pointed cephalad toward the left shoulder. The liver is used as an acoustic window, and the inferior wall of the heart is usually seen, sometimes with views of all four cardiac chambers. The *parasternal long axis view* is obtained by placing the ultrasound probe left of the sternum in the third or fourth intercostal space, with its long axis parallel to that of the heart, pointed toward the left nipple. From this vantage, a portion of the right ventricle is seen in the proximal field. The left atrium and ventricle are seen in the far field of view, and a dependent pericardial effusion may be seen. The parasternal long-axis view is considered most accurate for detection of pericardial effusion, because the posterior pericardium is usually seen well, and fluid may preferentially accumulate in this dependent position.[55-56] An *apical four-chamber view* is obtained by placing the ultrasound probe below the left nipple, angled toward the sternal notch. As the name indicates, all four cardiac chambers are seen, with the ventricles in the near field of view.

The appropriate ultrasound probe for examination of the chest depends on the intended application. For examination of the pericardium, a cardiac or an abdominal probe is appropriate. Both probes provide adequate depth of penetration and resolution for detection of pericardial fluid (Table 6-6). When a subxiphoid view or an apical four-chamber view is acquired, either probe is satisfactory. If a parasternal view is used, the cardiac probe has the advantage of a smaller footprint on the chest wall, allowing it to be used to image between ribs.

Figure 6-87. **Aortic trauma, CT with IV contrast.** Same patient as in Figures 6-85 and 6-86. Consecutive axial CT images viewed with soft-tissue windows. **A** through **H** descend from cephalad to caudad. In **B**, a defect resembling an intimal flap is seen. **C** through **F**, An irregularity projects into the lumen from the posterior aortic wall.

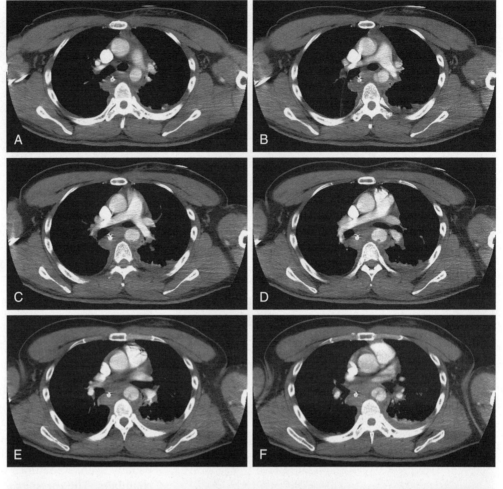

Figure 6-88. **Aortic trauma.** Same patient as in Figures 6-85 through 6-87. **A,** a defect resembling an intimal flap is seen. **B,** the aorta resumes its normal size and smooth internal contour.

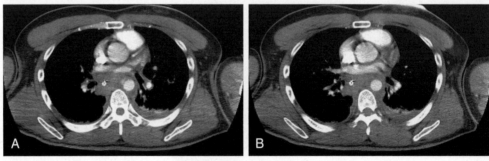

The abdominal probe has a larger footprint, usually resulting in rib shadows obscuring portions of the image. A linear high-frequency transducer is usually not used for examination of the heart, as its depth of penetration is generally limited—around 6 cm. For assessment of pleural fluid or pneumothorax, any of the probes (cardiac, abdominal, or linear high frequency) may be used, because the pleural surface is usually within 6 cm of the skin surface. In obese patients, the linear high-frequency probe may have inadequate depth of penetration.

Ultrasound Modes

Two ultrasound modes are useful in examination of the chest. **Brightness (B) mode** ultrasound refers to the common two-dimensional planar imaging mode familiar to most emergency physicians. **Motion (M) mode** provides a record of motion along a single line extending deep to the probe from the skin surface. In this mode, the user selects the line position on the two-dimensional B mode image, and then a graph of motion along this line is produced. In this chapter, all ultrasound applications refer to B mode imaging unless otherwise specified. M mode is specifically useful in detection of pneumothorax, as described later.

Ultrasound Findings of Pericardial Fluid (Hemopericardium)

Ultrasound has been used for diagnosis of pericardial fluid since the 1960s.[45-51] Thourani et al.[52] documented the replacement of pericardiocentesis with ultrasound for diagnosis of traumatic hemopericardium over a 22-year period in a large urban trauma center. In the

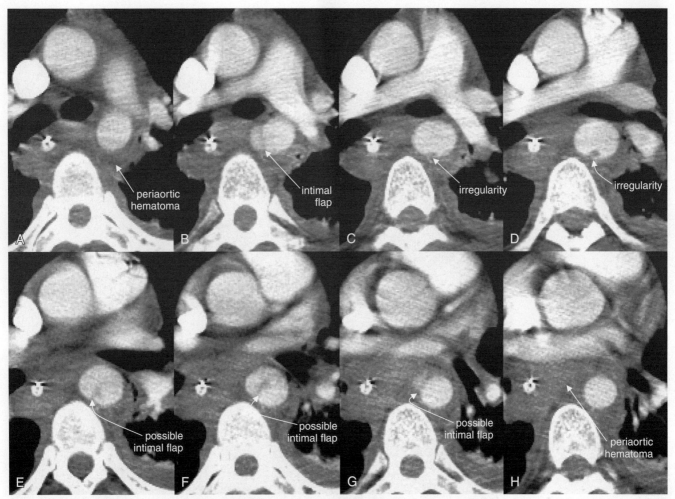

Figure 6-89. Aortic trauma, CT with IV contrast. Figures 6-85 through 6-89 explore the same case. **A** through **H** here are close-ups from panels **A** through **H** in Figures 6-87 and 6-88. They are taken from consecutive axial CT images through the region of the descending thoracic aorta, viewed with soft-tissue windows. **A** to **H** descend from cephalad to caudad. Periaortic hematoma and irregularities of the descending aorta are seen.

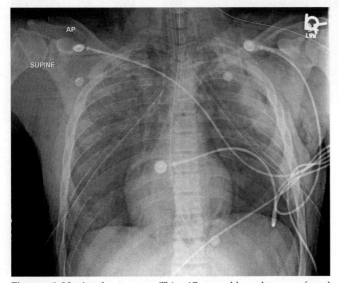

Figure 6-90. Aortic trauma. This 17-year-old male was found outside of his vehicle at 4:15 AM. In the emergency department, he was unresponsive, with fixed and dilated pupils and priapism. The patient is intubated and bilateral chest tubes have been placed. Both lungs show increased density, suggesting pulmonary contusion. The gastric tube is deviated to the right, and the aortic knob is indistinct. A black line surrounds the heart, suggesting pneumomediastinum. Fractures of the first and second ribs were also noted, although they are hard to see in this image. CT was performed (Figures 6-91, 6-92).

setting of penetrating chest trauma, bedside ultrasound by trauma surgeons as been shown to be accurate (sensitivity = 100%, specificity = 96.9%) and to be associated with rapid time to operation.[53] Immediate bedside echocardiography is associated with improved survival in patients with penetrating cardiac injury.[54]

The normal pericardium is a bright white line surrounding the ventricular and atrial chambers (see Figs. 6-136 and 6-137). In the presence of pericardial blood, a black stripe is seen within the confines of the pericardium, outside of the cardiac chambers. Even a relatively small pericardial effusion may interfere with ventricular filling, reducing cardiac output—if not causing frank cardiac tamponade. A pericardial fat pad may be present and may be hypo- or anechoic, simulating pericardial fluid.[56]

Pitfalls in Diagnosis of Pericardial Effusion by Ultrasound
Pericardial Fat Pad Simulating Pericardial Fluid. Blaivas, DeBehnke, and Phelan[56] documented a significant rate of potential misdiagnosis of pericardial effusion. In a study of emergency medicine residents and faculty, participants were asked to evaluate short video clips of subxiphoid cardiac ultrasound examinations for

Figure 6-91. Aortic trauma, CT with IV contrast. A through D, Consecutive axial CT slices through the thorax, viewed with soft-tissue windows. A through D descend from cephalad to caudad. E, Close-up from B. F, Close-up from C. A CT from the same patient as Figure 6-90 shows a focal defect in the posterior wall of the descending aorta, visible only on two consecutive slices. This is a traumatic pseudoaneurysm. Figure 6-92 shows this in sagittal reconstructions.

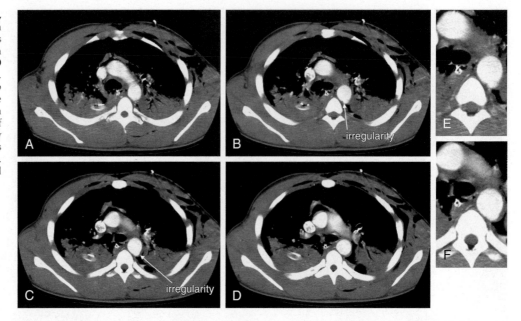

Figure 6-92. Aortic trauma, CT with IV contrast. A, Sagittal CT reconstruction from the same patient as in Figures 6-90 and 6-91 shows a focal defect in the posterior wall of the descending aorta. This is a traumatic pseudoaneurysm. B, Close-up from A. Both images are viewed with soft-tissue windows.

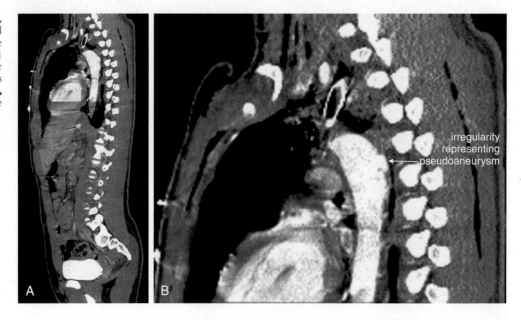

the presence of effusion and tamponade. Pericardial fat pads and true effusions were frequently confused, with poor sensitivity (73%) and specificity (44%) for effusion. The authors suggest two alternative views to avoid this confusion:

1. A parasternal long-axis view, to visualize dependent fluid posterior to the heart
2. A modified subxiphoid view, in which the probe is oriented perpendicular to the skin surface, allowing the following:
   a. Visualization of the inferior vena cava (IVC) entering the right atrium, with detection of pericardial fluid in this location.
   b. Detection of inferior vena collapse. Collapse of the IVC by at least 50% is normal with sudden inspiration. Lack of this degree of collapse can be associated with elevated central venous pressures seen in cardiac tamponade.[56]

Pericardial Laceration Decompressing Pericardial Fluid. Ball et al.[57] described a series of patients with stab wounds to the chest, resulting in penetrating cardiac injury and laceration of the pericardial sac. All had negative cardiac ultrasound findings, which the authors attribute to decompression of the pericardial space through the pericardial laceration into the thoracic cavity.

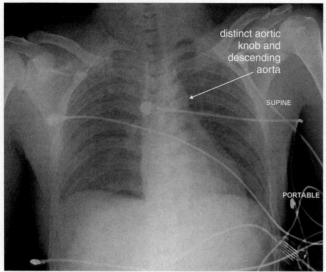

Figure 6-93. **Aortic trauma.** This 30-year-old male fell from a tower while doing electrical work—an estimated 20 to 50 feet. He complained of back and abdominal pain, as well as dyspnea. Notably, he had no palpable pulses in his lower extremities. His chest x-ray was interpreted as normal—the trachea is not deviated, the mediastinum is not wide for a supine x-ray, and the aortic knob and descending aorta are clearly visible. His CT is shown in Figures 6-94 through 6-98.

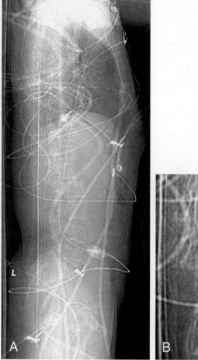

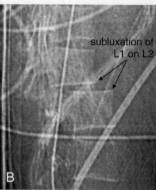

Figure 6-94. **Aortic trauma: Abdominal aorta. A,** The patient's scout CT image is telling—a significant step-off is visible at the L1-2 level. Remember that the abdominal aorta lies just anterior to the spinal column at this level. **B,** Close-up from **A.** Figure 6-95 examines axial CT slices.

Ultrasound Findings of Pericardial Tamponade

The presence of a pericardial effusion is necessary but not sufficient for the diagnosis of pericardial tamponade. Unfortunately, some small and localized but hemodynamically significant effusions may not be readily visible on transthoracic echocardiography. In the case of large pericardial effusions, the heart may swing like a pendulum within the pericardium, but this is not an indication of high pericardial pressures. As pericardial fluid pressure increases, it may exceed pressures in the right heart, resulting in collapse of the right atrium and ventricle. Right ventricular collapse during early diastole is insensitive (38% to 48%) but specific (84% to 100%) for pericardial tamponade. Right atrial collapse is too nonspecific (50% to 68%) and insensitive (55% to 60%) for clinical utility.[58] Pericardial tamponade results in increased central venous pressures, which prevent the normal collapse of the IVC with sudden inspiration (the "sniff test").[56,58]

If pericardial fluid is documented with ultrasound and cardiac tamponade develops, ultrasound-guided pericardiocentesis can reverse hemodynamic instability, at least as a temporizing measure. The procedure has a low complication rate, although pneumothorax, right ventricular laceration, intercostal vessel injury, and transient dysrhythmias may occur.[59]

Blunt myocardial injury (previously called myocardial contusion) may also be demonstrated by ultrasound, although controversy exists about the very definition. Pericardial fluid alone is not sufficient to make the diagnosis. Evidence of right ventricular dysfunction may be seen. No gold standard other than autopsy has been agreed upon, making sensitivity and specificity of ultrasound uncertain.[60]

Ultrasound Findings of Hemothorax

Fluid in the pleural space is readily seen on ultrasound. As with other ultrasound applications, fluid appears black (hypoechoic or anechoic). The lung parenchyma may be seen as a hyperechoic structure floating within pleural fluid. Because fluid layers with gravity, the dependent portions of the thorax should be inspected carefully. If the patient is able to be placed in an upright position, the sensitivity of ultrasound for detection of pleural fluid will be improved (Figure 6-140). Ma and Mateer[61] prospectively compared ultrasound with chest x-ray for the detection of traumatic hemothorax in 240 patients, using a gold standard of CT. Both modalities showed 96.2% sensitivity, 100% specificity, and 99.6% overall accuracy. Brooks et al.[62] showed similar performance of ultrasound (sensitivity = 92%, specificity = 100%) in a smaller cohort of 61 patients. In this study, four hemothoraces detected with ultrasound (25%) were not seen on initial chest x-ray. Whether small hemothoraces detected with ultrasound or CT alone require thoracostomy remains uncertain. Sharma, Hagler, and Oswanski[63] reported that delayed development of hemothorax

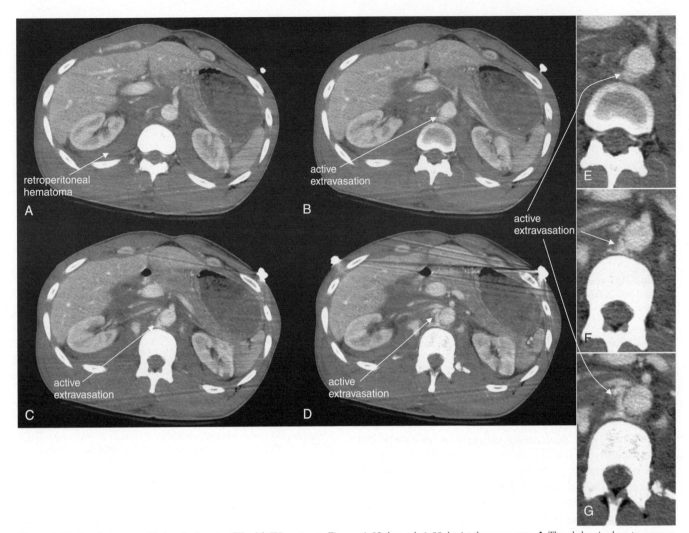

Figure 6-95. Aortic trauma: Abdominal aorta, CT with IV contrast. Figures 6-93 through 6-98 depict the same case. **A,** The abdominal aorta appears nearly normal, but already a very large bilateral retroperitoneal hematoma is visible (soft-tissue density, gray on these soft-tissue windows), extending posterior to both kidneys. This abnormality is seen in all of the slices shown but labeled only in **A. B** to **D,** A blush of contrast (white) indicating active extravasation of injected contrast is visible adjacent to the aorta. **E, F,** and **G** at right are close-ups from **B, C,** and **D,** respectively.

is rare after blunt trauma, occurring in only 5% of cases, but may occur in patients with rib fractures.

Ultrasound Findings of Pneumothorax

As early as 1987, ultrasound was described as a method of detecting pneumothorax.[64] Air in the pleural space (pneumothorax) can be detected using a cardiac, abdominal, or linear high-frequency probe. Even novice ultrasonographers have been shown to be capable of performing the ultrasound examination and recognizing abnormal findings with high sensitivity and specificity.[65-66] The degree of pneumothorax can also be recognized by ultrasound.[42,67] Wilkerson and Stone[68] performed a systematic review and identified four prospective studies comparing ultrasound and x-ray with a gold standard of CT. The sensitivity of ultrasound ranged from 86% to 98%, and the specificity ranged from 97% to 100%. The sensitivity of supine AP chest radiographs for the detection of pneumothorax ranged from 28% to 75%, with a specificity of 100%.

Before describing the appearance of pneumothorax, we review the normal appearance of the lung and pleura using B mode ultrasound. We then describe the appearance of pneumothorax using B mode. Finally, we compare the ultrasound appearance of normal lung and pleura to that of pneumothorax using M mode ultrasound.[69]

B Mode Ultrasound Findings

Normal Lung and Pleura

Normally, in the absence of pneumothorax, the pleural surfaces of the chest wall (parietal pleura) and lung (visceral pleura) are in close contact, separated only by a thin film of fluid. This interface is called the **pleural line** (see Figure 6-32; see also Fig. 6-31 for chest x-ray findings in same patient). An ultrasound probe placed on the chest wall in a longitudinal orientation shows the pleural line as a bright white, thin, horizontal line. Bounding the pleural line cephalad and caudad are two adjacent ribs, each indicated by a bright white curve (the superficial cortex of the rib) with posterior **acoustic shadowing.**

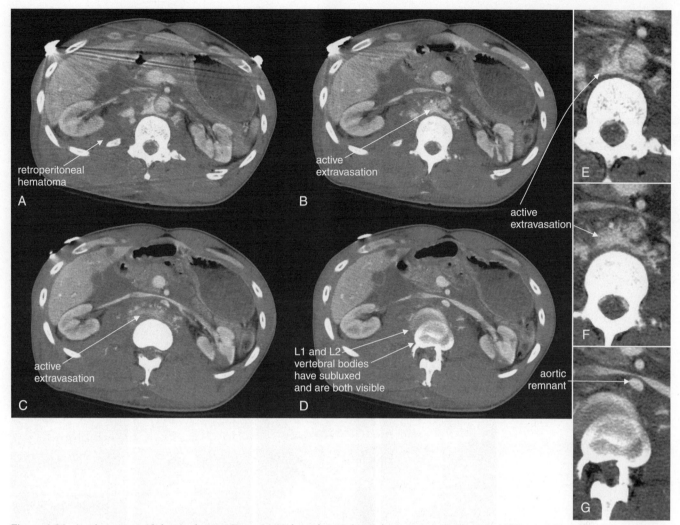

Figure 6-96. Aortic trauma: Abdominal aorta. Figures 6-93 through 6-98 depict the same case. Continuation of Figure 6-95. **A,** The abdominal aorta is identifiable, with active extravasation and a large retroperitoneal hematoma. Blood that had collected before CT appears soft-tissue density (gray), whereas actively extravasating blood is mixed with contrast and appears white. By **B** to **D,** the aorta is a tiny remnant vessel. **D,** The double image of the vertebral body is not artifact—this is the level of the subluxation of L1 on L2, and both vertebrae are seen. **E,** Close-up from **A. F,** Close-up from **B. G,** Close-up from **D.**

The superficial rib cortices are located about 0.5- to 1-cm superficial to the pleural line. The posterior acoustic shadows of ribs are created by the dense bone reflecting and absorbing the ultrasound beam, preventing through-transmission of sound. The pattern of a rib, followed by the pleural line, followed by an adjacent rib is sometimes described as the **bat sign** (see Figure 6-32) because of the resemblance to the wings and body of a flying bat. Deep to the pleural line, a series of horizontal lines is often seen—a repetition artifact called the **A line.** A lines are believed to arise from the interaction of the ultrasound beam with air; consequently, they are seen both with normal lung and in the presence of pneumothorax. On real-time ultrasound, lateral motion is seen at the pleural line as the parietal and visceral pleura slide relative to each other with respiration. This finding is sometimes called the **sliding lung sign.** Some ultrasound machines are equipped with automated software motion filters that can obscure this relatively subtle motion; these software filters should be turned off when assessing for this sign.

Comet tail artifacts (B lines) may be seen in normal cases (Table 6-7), and their absence can be a clue to the presence of pneumothorax. B lines must be distinguished from two other comet tail–like phenomena, which are described later. First, we define B lines, which have five mandatory features:

1. Are vertical and bright, arising from the pleural line and extending deep to the pleural line
2. Are well defined and narrow (sometimes described as "laser beam–like")
3. Spread to the deep edge of the screen (field of view) without fading
4. Erase A lines (horizontal repetition artifact lines that lie parallel and deep to the pleural lines)
5. Move with lung sliding

Figure 6-97. **Aortic trauma: Abdominal aorta, CT with IV contrast.** Figures 6-93 through 6-98 depict the same case. **A** to **H,** Sagittal CT reconstructions reveal both the spinal subluxation and the major aortic injury. Remarkably, the patient survived and was able to walk with a rolling walker despite some spinal cord injury.

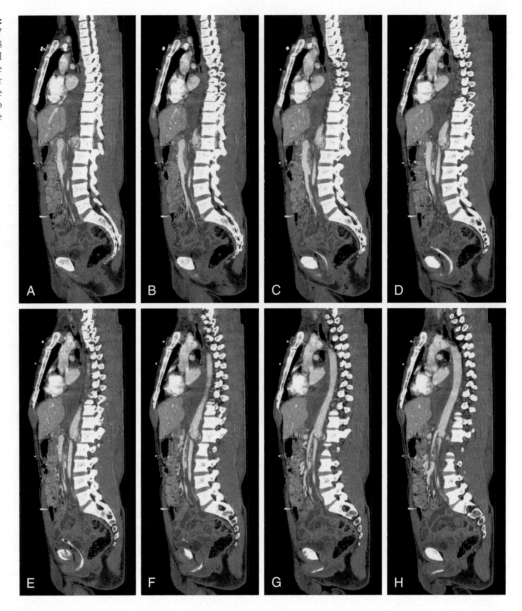

B lines are believed to arise from the ultrasound beam's interaction with the visceral pleura; consequently, they are absent in cases of pneumothorax.

Two other comet tail–like findings may be seen, neither of which reliably confirm the presence or absence of pneumothorax. The first, **Z lines,** do not distinguish between normal lung and pneumothorax, because they may be seen with both. Z lines have four features that differ from those of B lines:

1. Are ill-defined vertical lines arising from the pleural line and extending deep to it, in contrast to B lines, which are well defined
2. Fade after 2 to 5 cm of depth, in contrast to B lines, which continue without fading to the deep edge of the field of view
3. Do not erase A lines, in contrast to B lines, which do erase A lines

4. Are independent of lung sliding, in contrast to B lines, which move with lung sliding

Emphysema (E) lines are comet tails arising superficial to the pleural line and preventing its visualization. The bat sign is therefore not seen. These lines extend deep to their origin and do not fade. The source of E lines is subcutaneous emphysema, which may accompany pneumothorax. However, because the pleural line itself is obscured by the E line comet tail, motion at the pleural line cannot be assessed.

Pneumothorax

In the case of pneumothorax, air separates the parietal and visceral pleural surfaces. As a consequence, the sliding lung sign is not seen. In addition, B lines, which are generated by the ultrasound beam's interaction with the visceral pleura, are not seen resulting from the presence of air between the parietal and the visceral pleura.

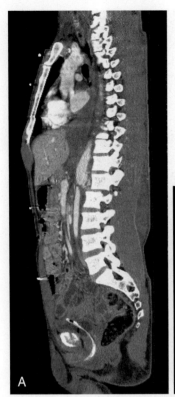

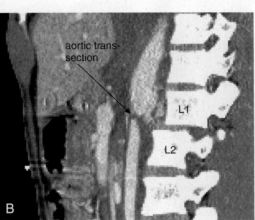

Figure 6-98. Aortic trauma: Abdominal aorta, CT with IV contrast. Other images from the same patient are shown in Figures 6-93 through 6-97. **A,** Sagittal reconstruction viewed with soft-tissue windows reveals both the spinal subluxation (L1 on L2) and the major aortic injury. The abdominal aorta reconstitutes below the level of transection but has a smaller diameter. **B,** Close-up from **A.** Remarkably, the patient survived and was able to walk with a rolling walker despite some spinal cord injury.

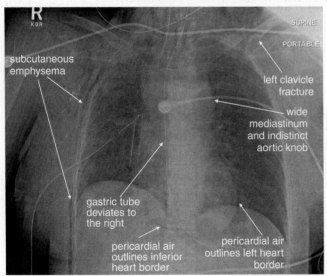

Figure 6-99. Aortic trauma. This 54-year-old female was an unrestrained passenger in a car that struck a tree. Her chest x-ray shows a wide mediastinum with deviation of the trachea. The gastric tube, which appears nearly midline at the top of the x-ray, deviates to the right upon entering the mediastinum, suggesting possible mediastinal hematoma. The aortic knob is not well defined. These findings could indicate aortic injury. Other trauma findings in this patient include a left clavicle fracture, multiple right rib fractures, a right chest tube with subcutaneous air in the right chest wall, and pneumopericardium. This last finding is indicated by the visible inferior and left heart borders. The inferior border of the heart is not normally seen, because it is fluid density and lies in direct contact with the diaphragm, also fluid density. In this case, air in the pericardial sac provides contrast. Compare with the CT (Figure 6-100).

Therefore loss of the sliding lung sign and absence of B line comet tails are signs of pneumothorax.[70] A lines may be seen despite pneumothorax, because they are an artifact arising from the air. The presence of A lines without any intersecting B lines is called the **A line sign** and is a highly sensitive but nonspecific indication of pneumothorax (sensitivity = 100%, specificity = 60%).[70-71]

M Mode Ultrasound Findings

As described earlier, M mode is an ultrasound setting that generates a graph of motion over time along a single line through the two-dimensional B mode image. Three important signs can distinguish between normal lung and pneumothorax using M mode.

In the absence of pneumothorax, tissues superficial to the pleural line do not move appreciably and thus generate a series of parallel horizontal lines on the M mode image, indicating no motion. Deep to the pleural line, moving lung tissue generates a homogeneous granular pattern. The combination of these findings is called the **seashore sign** resulting from its resemblance to wave fronts approaching a sandy beach (see Figure 6-33).

In the case of pneumothorax, air in the pleural space deep to the pleural line is also motionless, so the parallel horizontal lines seen in motionless superficial tissues continue throughout the M mode image. This appearance of parallel horizontal lines throughout the M mode image is called the **stratosphere sign** (see Figure 6-34).

Text continues on page 351

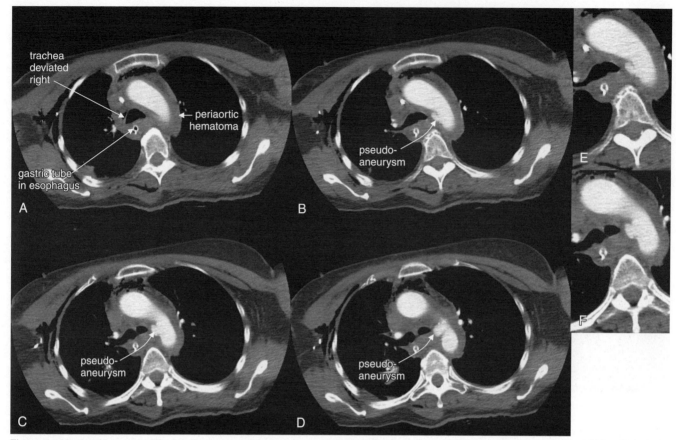

Figure 6-100. Aortic trauma, CT with IV contrast. Same patient as in Figure 6-99. Consecutive axial CT images viewed with soft-tissue windows, descending from **A** through **H.** The images show periaortic hematoma (soft-tissue density, gray) surrounding the aortic arch and deviating the trachea and esophagus to the patient's right. A focal defect in the distal aortic arch is visible—a traumatic pseudoaneurysm. **E,** Close-up from **B. F,** Close-up from **C.** Figure continues in Figure 6-101.

Figure 6-101. Aortic trauma. Additional images for the same patient are shown in Figures 6-99 through 6-104. **A-D,** The circumferential periaortic hematoma extends distally around the uninjured portion of the descending aorta. This hematoma continues to deviate the esophagus and gastric tube, as was seen on chest x-ray.

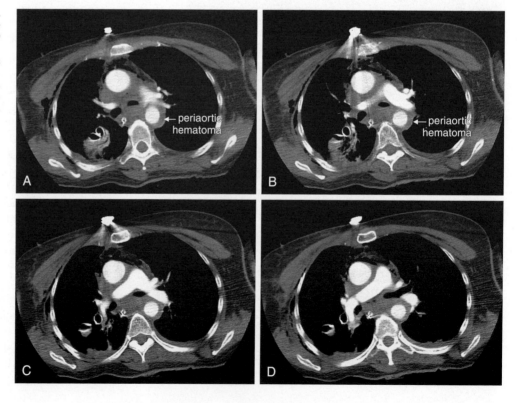

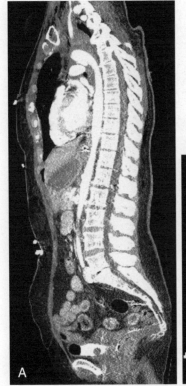

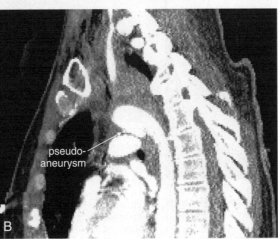

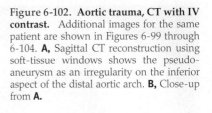

Figure 6-102. **Aortic trauma, CT with IV contrast.** Additional images for the same patient are shown in Figures 6-99 through 6-104. **A,** Sagittal CT reconstruction using soft-tissue windows shows the pseudo-aneurysm as an irregularity on the inferior aspect of the distal aortic arch. **B,** Close-up from **A.**

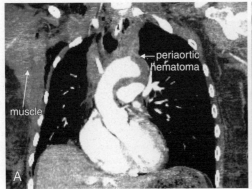

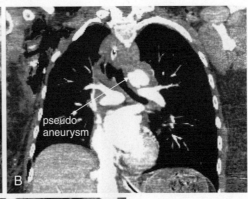

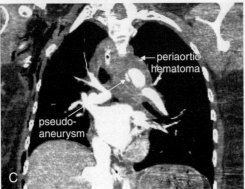

Figure 6-103. **Aortic trauma, CT with IV contrast.** Additional images for the same patient are shown in Figures 6-99 through 6-104. These coronal images show the periaortic hematoma and traumatic pseudoaneurysm. **A** to **C** move from anterior to posterior. **B, C,** The aorta does not have the normal smooth and rounded contour. In all three images, circumferential periaortic hematoma is present. On these soft-tissue windows, hematoma is gray, similar to skeletal muscle.

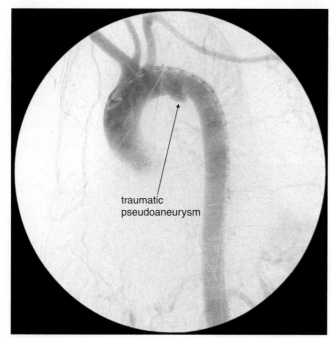

Figure 6-104. Aortic trauma. Additional images for the same patient are shown in Figures 6-99 through 6-104. This aortogram demonstrates the pseudoaneurysm. Although aortography has been the historical gold standard for this diagnosis, CT can give more three-dimensional information. This pseudoaneurysm appears relatively small in this image, because a portion of it extends posterior to the opacified aortic arch and is hidden in this projection. During aortography, usually several projections are obtained from different angles to overcome this limitation.

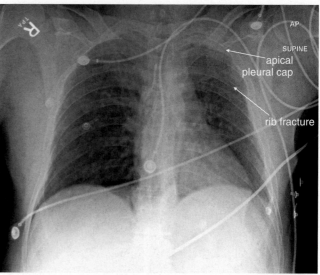

Figure 6-105. Apical pleural cap. An apical pleural cap is a finding associated with traumatic aortic injury. It is a soft-tissue (fluid) density at the lung apex, which can represent blood tracking out of the superior mediastinum and above the pleural surface of the lung apex. This 48-year-old male struck a car on his motorcycle. His chest x-ray shows an apical pleural cap on the left—compare with the normal right apex. He also has left-sided rib fractures. CT did not show an aortic injury; an apical pleural cap is a nonspecific finding, though it warrants further study with CT in the setting of significant trauma.

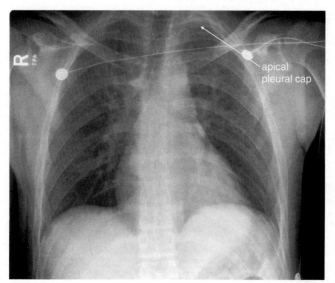

Figure 6-106. Apical pleural cap. This 25-year-old male rolled his car and was transported by emergency medical services. His chest x-ray shows a possible apical pleural cap, as well as a poorly defined aortic knob. Follow-up CT did not show an aortic injury.

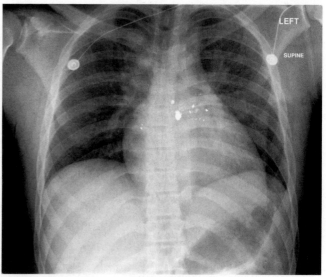

Figure 6-107. Gunshot wound to back with bullet adjacent to aorta. This 22-year-old male was shot in the posterior thorax just left of midline. He complained of back and abdominal pain. His supine chest x-ray shows radiopaque bullet fragments left of the thoracic spine. The x-ray is otherwise unremarkable. CT was performed to localize the bullet (Figure 6-108).

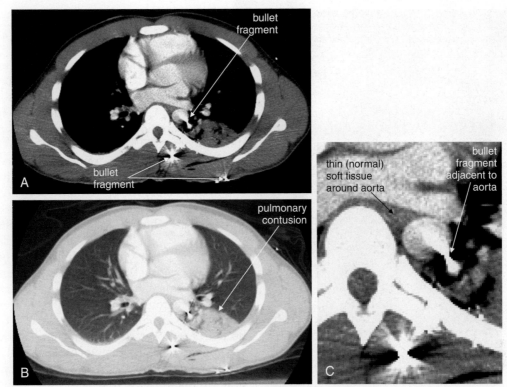

Figure 6-108. Gunshot wound to back with bullet adjacent to aorta, CT with IV contrast. A, Axial CT slice viewed with soft-tissue windows. **B,** The same slice, viewed with lung windows. **C,** Close-up from **A.** This CT from the same patient as in Figure 6-107 shows three bullet fragments, marked by metallic streak artifact. One lies immediately subcutaneously. The second is within paraspinal muscle exterior to the bony thorax. The third lies immediately adjacent to the aorta. Streak artifact makes complete evaluation of the aorta impossible, but no significant hematoma surrounds the aorta. The adjacent lung shows contusion but no hemopneumothorax. This patient was observed briefly and did not undergo further imaging to evaluate the aorta. However, aortography could have been used to assess this injury. Unlike CT, aortography is not subject to metallic streak artifact and could have identified irregularity of the aorta near the bullet fragment.

TABLE 6-5. Abnormal Chest X-ray Findings in Traumatic Aortic Injury

Finding	Frequency in Cases of Aortic Injury
Wide mediastinum	85%
Indistinct aortic knob	24%
Apical pleural cap	19%
Left pleural effusion	19%
First and/or second rib fracture	13%
Tracheal deviation	12%
NG tube deviation	11%

From Fabian TC, Richardson JD, Croce MA, et al. Prospective study of blunt aortic injury: Multicenter Trial of the American Association for the Surgery of Trauma. J Trauma 42(3):374-380, 1997; discussion 380-383.

The seashore sign is absent in this case, because air in the pleural space prevents through-transmission of the ultrasound beam to the lung deeper in the chest.

Another M mode finding of pneumothorax is the **lung point sign** (see Figure 6-35). This finding is present when the seashore sign and the stratosphere sign alternate rhythmically in concert with the patient's respiration.

The finding is thought to arise as the region of pneumothorax shifts with variations in the degree of lung inflation. When ventilated lung is in contact with the parietal pleura or chest wall, the seashore sign is present. When air from the pneumothorax separates the lung surface from the parietal pleura or chest wall, the stratosphere sign is seen.[70] The lung point sign has been reported to be highly specific though insensitive for pneumothorax (sensitivity = 66%, specificity = 100%).[72]

The reported sensitivity and specificity of various combinations of ultrasound findings are shown in Table 6-8. Chronic obstructive pulmonary disease has been reported to decrease the specificity of ultrasound.[73]

CHEST COMPUTED TOMOGRAPHY

Chest CT with IV contrast is the most definitive diagnostic imaging test for a variety of blunt and penetrating chest injuries. Two important indications for chest CT are definitive diagnosis of aortic injury, for which chest CT is clearly superior to chest x-ray, and detection of thoracic spinal injury.[20-21] As described in Chapter 3, multiplanar reformatted images derived from standard chest CT can also be used to evaluate for spinal trauma, with sensitivity far exceeding that of x-ray. Studies comparing chest

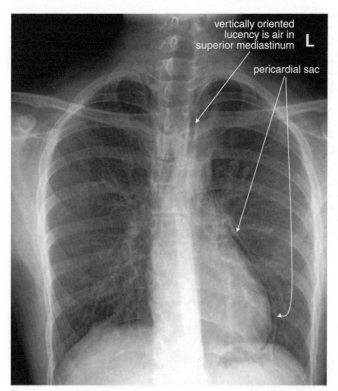

vertically oriented
lucency is air in
superior mediastinum
L

pericardial sac

Figure 6-109. Pneumomediastinum. This 18-year-old college student developed chest pain while lying in bed. He had no history of trauma, cough, or vomiting but had played basketball earlier in the day. His chest x-ray shows the typical subtle findings of pneumomediastinum. The white line paralleling the left heart border is the pericardium—the lucent region between the pericardium and the left heart border is air within the pericardial sac. Some vertically oriented lucent areas are seen in the upper mediastinum as well. The inferior border of the heart is not outlined with air in this case, although air may be seen in that location. What was the source of the air? No pneumothorax is seen, but perhaps the patient performed the Valsalva maneuver during his basketball game and forced air from the respiratory tree into the mediastinum. Compare with his lateral chest x-ray (Figures 6-110 and 6-111). His CT images are reviewed in Figures 6-112 and 6-113, although arguably CT was unnecessary. The patient recovered uneventfully.

CT to chest x-ray clearly demonstrate the higher sensitivity of chest CT for a variety of other injuries, including rib fractures, hemopneumothorax, subcutaneous air, diaphragmatic injuries, pneumopericardium, pneumomediastinum, and pneumoperitoneum. However, for many of these injuries, it is uncertain whether their detection with CT results in clinical benefit to patients. A classic example is the detection of a small pneumothorax on chest CT that was not visible on chest x-ray. A number of studies have examined the necessity for thoracostomy in this scenario, as described in detail at the end of this chapter. Thoracostomy does not appear to be routinely required for radiographically occult pneumothorax, even when the patient will be placed on positive pressure ventilation. For other injuries frequently detected on chest CT, including small hemothoraces, pulmonary contusions, rib fractures, transverse spinal process fractures, and pneumopericardium, no specific therapy is required. For example, regardless of whether rib fractures are confirmed with CT scan or simply suspected based on the patient's complaint of chest pain with inspiration, management is usually supportive, using analgesics and incentive spirometry. Rarely, multiple rib fractures are managed more aggressively with epidural anesthesia. Pulmonary contusions detected on chest CT require no specific therapy; it is the patient's clinical status, including hypoxia or increasing work of breathing, that determines the therapeutic intervention, not the radiographic appearance on CT scan.

Undoubtedly, the most important use of chest CT following trauma is in the detection of aortic injury. Before the clinical introduction of chest CT, suspected mediastinal injuries required formal angiography for evaluation.

Figure 6-110. Pneumomediastinum. Same patient as in Figures 6-109 and 6-111. **A,** The lateral chest x-ray shows some subtle findings of pneumomediastinum. **B,** Close-up from **A.** A faint black line (air) marks the anterior surface of the heart. In addition, normally no interface can be seen between the inferior heart border and the diaphragm, because they share the same x-ray density. However, a lucent line marks the inferior heart border here, indicating air in the pericardium.

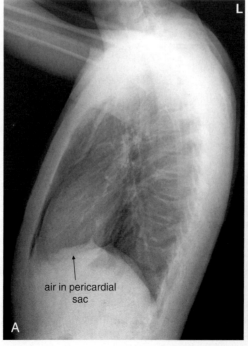

L

air in pericardial
sac

A

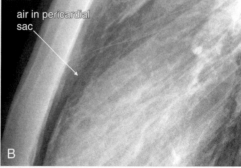

air in pericardial
sac

B

Angiography is resource intensive, requiring a team of specialized interventional radiologists; is time consuming; and has risks associated with femoral arterial catheterization. Modern chest CT is noninvasive, has excellent multiplanar spatial resolution, and is able to detect traumatic aortic injury with the level of detail sufficient for operative planning. Aortic branch vessel involvement can be readily detected. Modern studies suggest diagnostic sensitivity and specificity essentially equivalent to that of formal angiography. For patients with penetrating chest trauma, CT can sometimes provide critical information about the precise location of retained foreign bodies or about the path of transthoracic projectiles. This information sometimes dictates thoracotomy or eliminates concerns about mediastinal and cardiac injury (see Figures 6-115, 6-116, and 6-118 through 6-120).

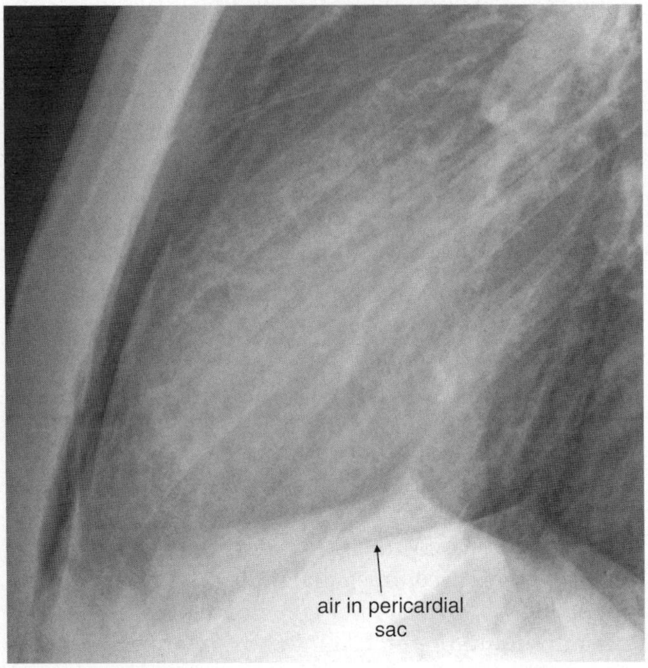

Controversy exists about the need for chest CT in trauma patients with a normal chest x-ray. Studies suggest that a completely normal chest x-ray is only approximately 92% to 93% sensitive for detection of aortic injury.[20,74,75] In addition, many findings suggestive of aortic injury are nonspecific, resulting in many normal CT scans following abnormal chest x-ray findings. If chest x-ray alone were used as the screening modality for aortic injury, as many as 1 in 12 patients with life-threatening aortic injury would be missed. However, this is an uncommon injury pattern overall, occurring in only 274 cases in 50 trauma centers over a 2.5-year period—a rate of only about 2 cases per year in major trauma centers.[20] As a consequence, the negative predictive value of a normal chest x-ray is excellent in all but the most high-risk patients. In pediatric patients, if chest CT were used ubiquitously as the initial screening test in place of x-ray (or following a normal chest x-ray), the number needed to treat to find a single case of aortic injury has been estimated to be more than 200.[76] Proponents of chest CT argue that the extreme morbidity and mortality (around 30% in those patients who survive to the emergency department) of aortic trauma necessitate definitive imaging with CT in all cases.[20,74] Opponents of

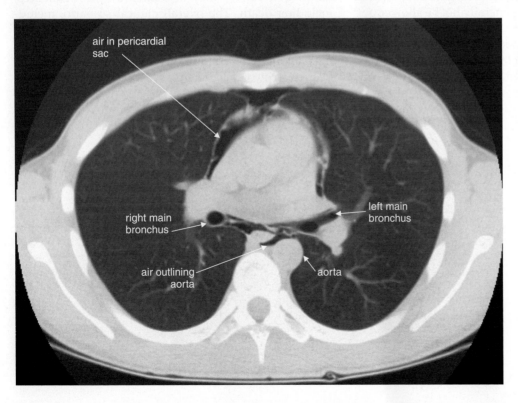

Figure 6-111. Pneumomediastinum. Figures 6-109 through 6-113 explore this case with x-ray and CT.

air in pericardial sac

Figure 6-112. Pneumomediastinum. Figures 6-109 through 6-113 explore this case with x-ray and CT. This CT image (lung windows) high in the mediastinum just inferior to the carina shows air outlining the heart anteriorly, as well as air posterior to the heart, including outlining the aorta.

air in pericardial sac

right main bronchus

left main bronchus

air outlining aorta

aorta

CT argue that the cost of CT, nephrotoxicity of contrast agents, and radiation exposure outweigh the benefits in low-risk trauma patients. The radiation exposure from chest CT is on the order of 400 times that of chest x-ray.[77] Many trauma patients are relatively young, compounding concerns about carcinogenesis. New studies suggest cancer risks associated with chest CT, ranging from a lifetime risk around 1 in 400 at age 20 to 1 in 1000 at age 60.[78-80] Trauma patients undergoing multiple CT scans have documented radiation exposures on the order of 40 mSv, the equivalent of more than 1000 chest x-rays.[81] These and other controversies in the use of chest CT for trauma are discussed at the end of this chapter. Radiation risks of chest CT are discussed in more detail in Chapters 7 and 8.

Performance of Chest CT for Trauma

Chest CT for evaluation of thoracic trauma requires the use of injected contrast whenever possible. Parenteral contrast allows detection of vascular abnormalities, particularly injury to the thoracic aorta, the primary indication for chest CT. A rapid contrast bolus is performed, with CT image acquisition immediately following to ensure arterial phase imaging of the aorta. Automated bolus tracking software helps ensure that the CT is performed at the moment of optimal aortic enhancement, as described in Chapter 7.

What Diagnostic Procedure Should Be Performed in Patients with Contraindications to Intravenous Contrast Used for Computed Tomography?

In patients who have contraindications to the use of iodinated contrast, including renal insufficiency or contrast allergy, delays should generally not be allowed for premedication such as steroid prep or N-acetylcysteine therapy if traumatic aortic injury is legitimately suspected. This injury can lead to rapid death if not immediately detected and treated. Among initial survivors of this injury, 30% die within 6 hours if diagnosis is not made and treatment initiated.[12] An individualized risk–benefit decision must be made for each patient. One option is immediate noncontrast chest CT. If this test is normal, with no evidence of mediastinal hematoma, the likelihood of aortic injury is very low; the American College of Radiology thus calls noncontrast CT useful to detect mediastinal hematoma when contrast is contraindicated.[12] Depending on the level of pretest probability of aortic injury, other diagnostic imaging modalities can be employed, including CT with IV contrast after appropriate premedication, transthoracic or transesophageal echocardiography, or magnetic resonance imaging. If immediate noncontrast chest CT is performed and is abnormal (e.g., demonstrating a large mediastinal hematoma), the decision may be made to proceed with formal aortography, with therapeutic options such as placement of an endovascular graft. By proceeding with formal angiography rather than with chest CT, the total exposure to iodinated contrast may be minimized. Another strategy would be to perform CT with IV contrast following an abnormal noncontrast chest CT, confirming or excluding aortic injury. The disadvantage to this approach would be that the patient might require a second dose of iodinated contrast if CT findings then prompt formal aortography.

A second approach to the patient with contraindications to injected contrast material is to proceed with immediate IV contrast after consideration of risks. This decision should not be taken lightly, because renal failure requiring dialysis or CT severe anaphylaxis and death may occur. However, the late diagnosis of traumatic aortic injury may also have dire consequences, including death. The overall clinical scenario, including the patient's hemodynamic stability, mechanism of the injury, complaints of chest pain, chest x-ray findings, and specific contraindications to injected contrast (e.g., severity of prior allergic reaction or degree of renal

Figure 6-113. Pneumomediastinum. Same patient as in Figures 6-109 through 6-112. Figures 6-109 through 6-113 explore this case with x-ray and CT. **A,** This computed tomography image (lung windows) lower in the mediastinum shows air (black) outlining the aorta and esophagus—areas where no air should be found. **B,** Close-up from **A.**

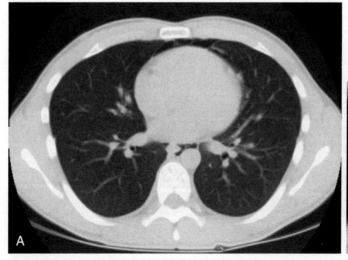

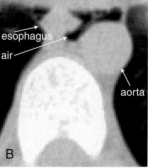

insufficiency), should be incorporated into this decision. When possible, informed consent from the patient or patient's representatives should be obtained if a decision to give IV contrast despite significant contraindications is made.

Approach to Interpretation of Chest CT

Here, we describe a general approach to the interpretation of chest CT for evaluation of thoracic trauma. Chest CT can be rapidly interpreted by the emergency physician in a matter of minutes. Axial images alone are sufficient for detection and delineation of most important injuries, although we illustrate some of these injury patterns using additional coronal and sagittal images to

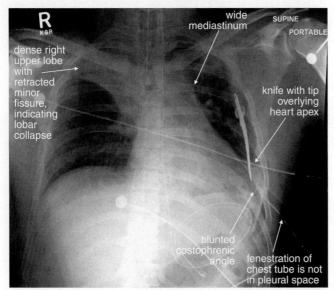

Figure 6-114. **Knife wound to chest.** This 33-year-old male presented with a self-inflicted stab wound to the left chest. His chest x-ray shows a wide mediastinum. The left costophrenic angle is blunted, suggesting hemothorax, despite a left thoracostomy tube. This tube is badly positioned, as one of the fenestrations is not in the pleural space. A knife overlies the heart apex, though a single x-ray view cannot determine whether it lies within the patient. Given the wide mediastinum, a cardiac injury with blood in the mediastinum is possible. The right upper lobe is dense with cephalad retraction of the minor fissure, indicating right upper lobe collapse. CT was performed (Figures 6-115 and 6-116)

assist you in visualizing the injury in three dimensions. We begin with a brief discussion of CT window settings.

CT windows are discussed in more detail in other chapters. In brief, windows allow the CT gray scale to be adjusted to accentuate detail of tissues of a particular density. A given CT image can be viewed on windows settings that accentuate soft tissue, lung, or bony detail. In general, the entire chest should be examined using first soft-tissue, then lung, and finally bone windows. Here, we review the findings that can be recognized on each of these three settings.

Soft-tissue windows

Soft-tissue windows (also called mediastinal, chest, vascular, or abdominal windows) are the key to detection of aortic injury. On this setting, the low-density lung parenchyma is invisible (black), and *pneumothorax cannot be recognized readily*. However, contrast-filled vascular structures including the aorta and its major branches are seen in detail (see Figure 6-4). Contrast appears white on this setting. Soft tissues including muscles and mediastinal soft tissues such as the heart or blood products (including mediastinal hematoma, or blood within the pleural space representing hemothorax) appear as an intermediate gray shade (see Figure 6-4). A pericardial effusion is also visible on this setting as an intermediate gray band surrounding the heart, whose chambers are generally filled with white contrast (see Figure 6-138).

On soft-tissue windows, inspect the entire aorta from the aortic root, cephalad through the arch, and caudad along the descending aorta to the diaphragm. Pay particular attention to the distal aortic arch and proximal descending aorta, the most common location of traumatic aortic injuries. A normal aorta has a well-defined, smooth margin. The ascending aorta and the descending aorta appear circular in axial cross section. The arch appears elliptic. The normal aorta should be uniformly filled with white vascular contrast, with no filling defects or visible intimal flaps. The branch vessels of the aorta, including

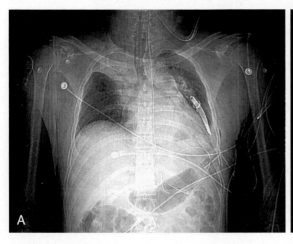
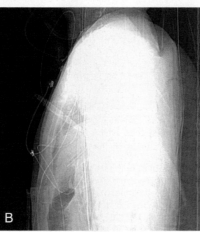

Figure 6-115. **Knife wound to chest.** CT scout images from the patient in Figures 6-114 and 6-116. Given both the frontal **(A)** and the lateral **(B)** scout images, the knife is buried to the handle in the patient's chest.

the subclavian, brachiocephalic, and innominate arteries, should be inspected for these same qualities. The position of the medial clavicular heads relative to these vessels should be noted, because posterior dislocation of the clavicle with impingement on great vessels can occur (see Figures 6-131 through 6-133).

Mediastinal Hematoma. Mediastinal hemorrhage is a potentially serious finding in major trauma—with the most concerning source being aortic injury. Periaortic hematoma is a sensitive finding of aortic injury, occurring in 91% of cases.[82-83] Other causes of mediastinal hematoma include venous hemorrhage and extension

Figure 6-116. Knife wound to chest, CT without IV contrast. Same patient as Figures 6-114 and 6-115. Lung windows. These CT images show the trajectory of the knife to skirt the pericardium. As a result of metal artifact, the precise location of the knife cannot be judged. No large pericardial effusion is seen. The CT was performed without intravenous contrast, so extravasation of contrast from the heart cannot be definitively ruled out. A small anterior pneumothorax is seen. Some dependent pleural fluid is visible. The patient underwent thorascopic surgery that showed no cardiac injury.

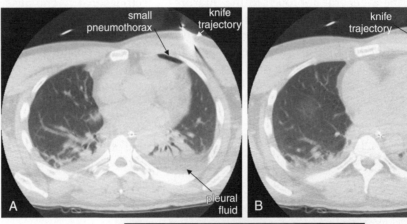

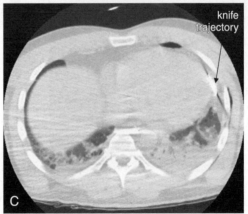

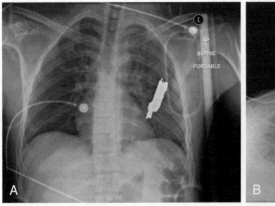

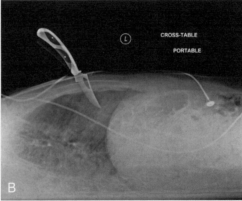

Figure 6-117. Knife wound to chest. This 23-year-old male presented with a self-inflicted stab wound to the left chest. He was hemodynamically stable and alert, with the knife in place in the left chest wall, on emergency department arrival. Bedside echocardiography did not demonstrate a pericardial effusion. A portable chest x-ray was obtained. This x-ray demonstrates the importance of two orthogonal views when determining the location of a foreign body. **A,** The anterior–posterior (AP) view shows the knife to overlie the left chest, although in theory the knife could be outside of the patient, either behind or in front of his torso. **B,** In the lateral projection, the depth of penetration of the knife is revealed, although the position of the knife is not certain—in theory, it could lie outside of the patient to the left or right of the thorax. **A,** The anterior–posterior (AP) view shows the location to overlie the left chest, although in theory the knife could be outside of the patient, either behind or in front of his torso. Together, these views confirm a deep central stab wound to the chest. On the AP view, the knife appears to contact the left heart border, but penetration of the pericardium or heart is uncertain. A CT was obtained to delineate the knife's position in greater detail (Figures 6-118 through 6-120). If the knife did not penetrate the pericardium, it could be removed at bedside, rather than requiring thoracotomy.

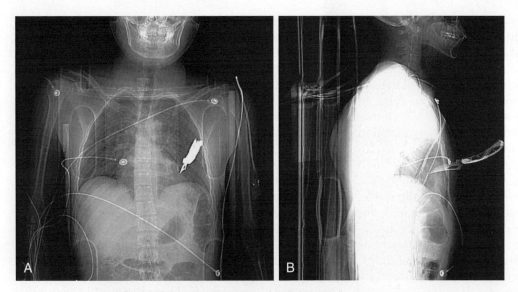

Figure 6-118. **Knife wound to chest.** Figures 6-117 through 6-120 explore this case using x-ray and CT. Scout images from the CT reveal the same information depicted on chest x-ray (Figure 6-117). **A,** Frontal scout image. **B,** Lateral scout image.

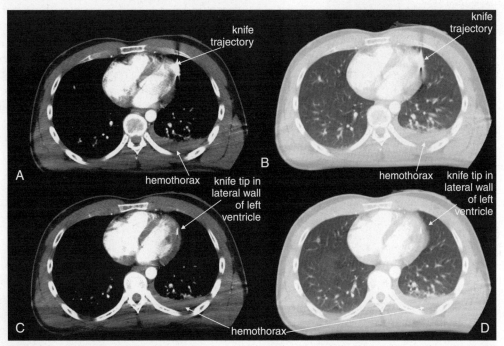

Figure 6-119. **Knife wound to chest, CT with IV contrast.** Figures 6-117 through 6-120 include additional images from this case. **A** and **C,** Consecutive axial soft-tissue windows. **B** and **D,** Lung windows of the same axial slices shown in **A** and **C,** respectively. Soft-tissue windows show the knife tip to lie within the lateral wall of the left ventricle. There is no pericardial effusion. Remarkably, lung windows show no pneumothorax, although a small hemothorax is seen. In this case, CT provided important clinical information that determined patient management. X-ray (Figure 6-117) suggested an injury tangential to the heart, which could possibly have been managed nonoperatively by removal of the knife in the trauma bay. CT prompted thoracotomy. Intraoperatively, the patient had brisk myocardial bleeding that could have resulted in pericardial tamponade if a pericardial window had not been created.

of prevertebral hematomas associated with cervical and thoracic spine injuries. When aortic injury is present, definitive therapy is essential, with endovascular grafting or open techniques applied depending on the location and type of injury. If no active bleeding or aortic injury is noted, most mediastinal hematomas require no specific therapy.

CT findings of hematoma include nonenhancing densities within the mediastinum, surrounding the aorta (see Figures 6-57 and 6-100). The density of hematoma is typically around 45 Hounsfield units, which appears an intermediate gray on CT soft-tissue windows. The hematoma may create mass effect, leading to a wide mediastinum and deviation of mediastinal structures including the trachea, endotracheal tube, and OG or NG tubes in the esophagus (see Figures 6-57).

Aortic Trauma. In aortic injury, irregularities in the normally smooth and circular aortic cross-sectional contour may be visible.[84-85] Active extravasation of injected contrast indicating active hemorrhage may be visible as white contrast material outside the lumen of the aorta and is an indication for immediate thoracotomy.[86] An intimal flap is visible in most cases—91% in one study.[83] Pseudoaneurysm, a focal bulge or diffuse enlargement of the aortic diameter, occurs in 97% of cases at the site where the ligamentum arteriosus tethers the aorta, in the distal aortic arch. Pseudoaneurysms differ from true aneurysms in that true aneurysms refer to dilatation involving all three layers of the aortic wall. In a pseudoaneurysm, a tear in the muscularis layer occurs, through which the intimal layer may protrude. Although a patient with a pseudoaneurysm may be initially stable, the thin-walled pseudoaneurysm is at high risk for rupture, leading to sudden decompensation or death. Mediastinal or periaortic hematoma may be present as described earlier.[83] Pericardial blood may be seen.[84-85]

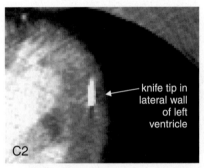

Figure 6-120. Knife wound to chest. Figures 6-117 through 6-119 include additional images from this case. The knife tip is seen in the lateral wall of the left ventricle on this close-up CT image. Contrast is not seen to escape the ventricle.

Figures 6-56 through 6-108 demonstrate multiple aortic injuries with chest x-ray, CT, and aortogram images.

When contrast cannot be given, rapid assessment of the aorta for traumatic injury can be performed with noncontrast CT—though the sensitivity of this technique has not been rigorously tested.[12] Because traumatic aortic injury differs from spontaneous aortic injury in the involvement of multiple layers of the aorta, mediastinal hematoma (which can be detected on noncontrast CT) usually accompanies this injury. Although details of the internal contour of the aorta cannot be recognized without contrast, the absence of mediastinal hematoma is strong evidence of the absence of traumatic aortic injury.[12] Noncontrast CT is not routinely performed for chest trauma. As a result, information on the sensitivity of noncontrasted findings is based largely on studies of contrasted CT, extrapolated based on the likelihood that some findings would be seen without contrast. Periaortic hematoma at the level of the diaphragm on abdominal CT has a reported sensitivity of 70% and specificity of 94% for thoracic aortic injury.[87] On chest CT, periaortic hematoma has a reported sensitivity of 91%, whereas pseudoaneurysm is reported to be 97% sensitive.[83] Clearly, contrast should be used if possible, given the importance of accurate diagnosis of aortic injury and the limited evidence for noncontrasted CT in this setting.

CT with IV contrast for evaluation of aortic trauma has sensitivity and specificity described as exceeding 99% based on a combination of surgical findings,

Figure 6-121. Rib fractures: Chest x-ray. This 27-year-old male crashed his motorcycle at an estimated speed of 100 mph. On emergency department arrival, he complained of difficulty breathing. His chest x-ray shows multiple right-sided rib fractures **(A)**, as demonstrated in the close-up **(B)**, which shows the disrupted cortex of several ribs. Perhaps more importantly, the patient has a moderate-sized pneumothorax and opacities that may represent pulmonary contusion. These other abnormalities are reviewed in more detail in Figures 6-122 through 6-124.

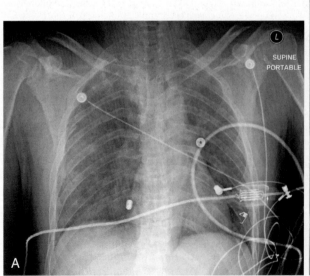
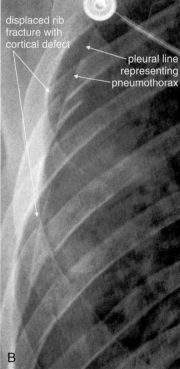

autopsy, and clinical follow-up.[21,88-90] Some studies have suggested CT to be more sensitive that traditional aortography.[91] As we have discussed in Chapter 7 with regard to chest CT for pulmonary embolism, the clinical outcome following negative chest CT may be more important than the reported test sensitivity. An outcome study of 278 consecutive trauma patients

evaluated with contrast-enhanced chest CT suggested no mortality from aortic injury among those with negative CT.[92]

Diaphragm Injury. Gross diaphragm injuries with herniation of abdominal contents into the chest are readily seen using soft-tissue windows. Subtler injuries

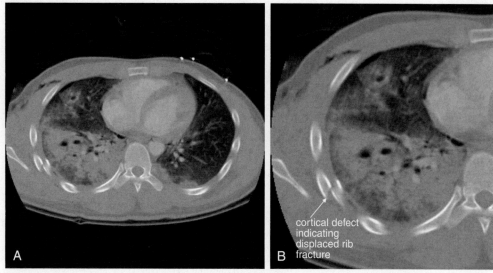

Figure 6-122. Rib fractures: CT with IV contrast. Figures 6-121 through 6-124 include images from this case. **A,** Axial CT image viewed with bone windows. **B,** Close-up from **A.** On CT scan, this patient has several findings, which demonstrates the importance of inspecting the chest using appropriate window settings for the suspected injury. Bone windows demonstrate a displaced right rib fracture. Although fractures may be visible on other window settings when badly displaced, bone windows are optimized for evaluation of the cortex and allow detection of even minimally displaced fractures. Other abnormalities are seen on this view, including a significant pulmonary contusion, but these would be better viewed on lung windows. IV contrast was given for evaluation of other injuries, although it is not needed for assessment of bone.

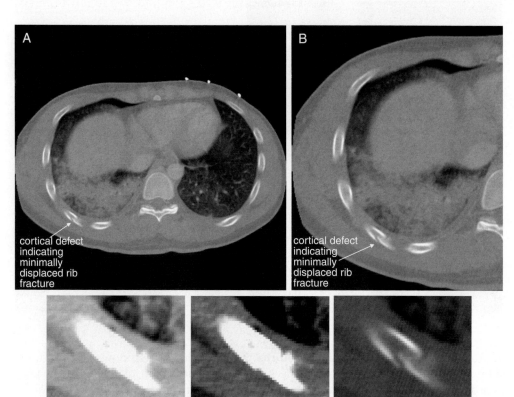

Figure 6-123. Rib fractures. Figures 6-121 through 6-124 include other images from this case. **A,** Axial CT slice viewed with bone windows. **B,** Close-up from **A.** A more posterior rib fracture is less displaced and thus subtler. Note how this rib fracture is not easily seen on lung or soft-tissue window settings, because bone is excessively bright on these settings. Compare the window settings in **C** (lung), **D** (soft tissue), and **E** (bone).

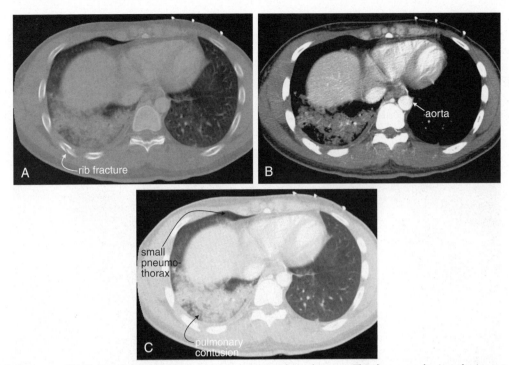

Figure 6-124. Rib fractures, CT. Figures 6-121 through 6-124 include images from this case. This figure emphasizes the importance of inspecting the chest for trauma using window settings appropriate to the suspected injury. Bony injuries are best evaluated on bone windows **(A).** The aorta and other mediastinal structures should be inspected on soft-tissue settings **(B)**. Lung parenchyma and pneumothoraces are best seen on lung windows **(C)**. The various injuries present in this single slice are highlighted by the three window settings. The small right pneumothorax is essentially invisible on soft-tissue windows but is visible on lung and bone windows. Is a pneumothorax present on the patient's left? Soft-tissue windows again offer no help, but the lung window image clearly rules this out. The rib fracture could easily be missed on soft-tissue or lung windows. The extent of the pulmonary contusion is best seen on lung windows—it appears smaller on soft-tissue windows, as only the densest central region is visible. The aorta is best inspected for defects on soft-tissue windows, which offer the best contrast with surrounding structures.

Figure 6-125. Sternal and manubrial fractures. A, Frontal chest x-ray. **B,** Close-up from **A.** This 92-year-old female was a restrained driver in a collision with a truck and complained of chest pain. Her chest x-ray is notable for a left pneumothorax. Because of her sternal tenderness, a lateral sternal x-ray was obtained, suggesting a fracture. CT of the chest did confirm a nondisplaced sternal fracture, though no specific therapy was needed. The typical frontal x-ray obtained in trauma is not sensitive for sternal fracture, and none was noted on the chest x-ray in this figure. Compare with the lateral sternal x-ray and CT images in Figure 6-126.

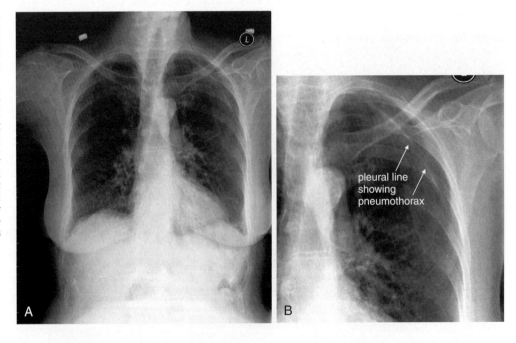

without overt visceral herniation are more difficult to recognize but are characterized by discontinuities of the diaphragm, which is visible as a thin, curved band on soft-tissue windows (see Figs. 6-49 through 6-55). These injuries are discussed in detail in Chapter 10.

Hemothorax. On soft-tissue windows, hemothorax is visible as a dependent region of intermediate gray opacity (around 45 Hounsfield units). Lung windows are needed to determine whether an associated pneumothorax is present, as normal lung parenchyma itself

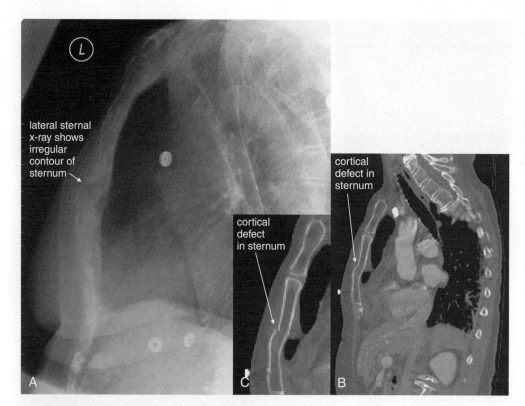

Figure 6-126. **Sternal and manu-brial fractures.** Same patient as in Figure 6-125. **A,** Lateral sternal x-ray. **B,** Sagittal CT image, viewed with bone windows. **C,** Close-up from **B.** Compare this with the sag-ittal reconstructions from her chest CT, which confirm a cortical defect of the sternum. No specific therapy was needed. Chest CT with IV con-trast in this case was indicated for evaluation of the aorta, more so than for sternal evaluation.

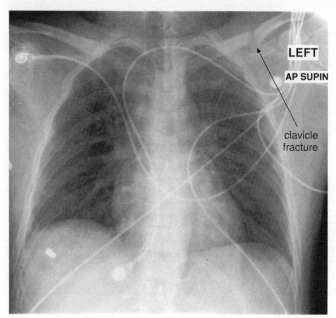

Figure 6-127. **Sternal and manubrial fractures.** This 30-year-old male crashed his car at 70 mph. His airbag deployed, and he was wearing a seat belt with a shoulder strap at the time of the collision. His chest x-ray shows a left clavicle fracture—a CT was performed to evaluate the aorta and incidentally showed a sternal fracture (Figure 6-128). Like most sternal fractures, this one is not visible on anterior–posterior chest x-ray.

is invisible on soft-tissue windows (see Figs. 6-4, 6-5, and 6-10).

Pericardial Effusion. CT with IV contrast read-ily identifies pericardial effusions, provides accurate size information, and can differentiate hemorrhagic effusions from serous effusions (see Fig. 6-138).[93] Blood has a density of approximately 45 Hounsfield units, depending on factors including hematocrit. Serous effu-sions have a density closer to that of water, 0 Hounsfield units. Whereas the size of a traumatic pericardial effu-sion (hemopericardium) can be assessed with CT, the hemodynamic effect is not as apparent—ultrasound is more definitive. Although CT can be used to generate electrocardiogram–gated movies of cardiac motion (see Chapter 8), typical trauma CT protocols do not use this capability, which results in a higher radiation exposure to the patient. Consequently, a static image of the heart is seen on trauma CT, and effects such as right ventricu-lar collapse signifying pericardial tamponade are not evident. Occasionally, CT may reveal findings of car-diac tamponade, including right ventricular collapse, if image acquisition happens to coincide with this event.[58]

Foreign Bodies. Foreign bodies can be precisely local-ized using CT. In penetrating trauma, CT can identify injuries to structures such as the heart, affecting man-agement decisions (see Figures 6-115, 6-116, and 6-118 through 6-120). Very dense foreign bodies can create metallic streak artifact, interfering with exact localiza-tion. Use of bone windows can minimize this effect. CT can identify some low-density foreign bodies that may be difficult to see on x-ray.

Lung Windows
Following review of soft-tissue windows for important injuries, review the entire chest again using lung win-dows to identify the injury types that follow.

Figure 6-128. **Sternal and manubrial fractures.** Same patient as Figure 6-127. **A,** Axial CT slice viewed with bone windows. **B,** Close-up from **A.** This 30-year-old male crashed his car at 70 mph. His airbag deployed and he was wearing a seat belt with a shoulder strap at the time of the collision. CT was performed to evaluate the aorta and incidentally showed a sternal fracture. On soft-tissue windows, this nondisplaced fracture would not be visible—not that any specific therapy would be required.

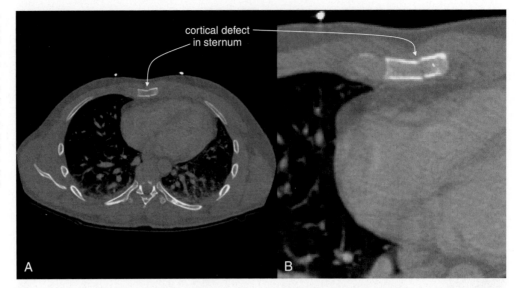

Figure 6-129. **Sternal and manubrial fractures. A,** Axial CT slice, bone windows. **B,** Close-up from **A.** This 51-year-old male collided head on with another vehicle. His chest x-ray was nondiagnostic, but CT showed a manubrial fracture. Again, the purpose of chest CT in this circumstance is to evaluate for associated mediastinal injury, not to evaluate for manubrium fracture, which is treated nonsurgically in almost every case.

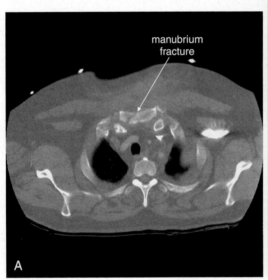
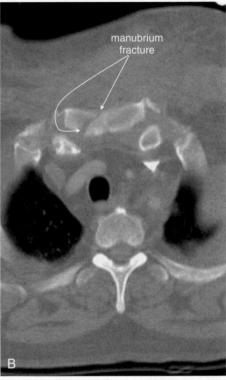

Pneumothorax. Lung windows allow detection of even small pneumothoraces. As with soft-tissue windows, the entire thorax should be inspected to confirm or exclude an injury. On this window setting, all soft tissues and denser structures, including contrast-filled vessels and bones, appear bright white. Air appears nearly black on this window setting. The lung parenchyma is readily visible as a fine latticework of air-filled alveoli, which appears an intermediate gray because of the small size of air-filled structures alternating with a matrix of solid tissue (see Figures 6-18, 6-27, 6-29, and 6-30). As a consequence, air within the pleural space (nearly black) can be readily distinguished from air within the lung parenchyma. On this window setting, **subcutaneous air** or pneumomediastinum may also be easily recognized (see Figures 6-29, 6-36, and 6-112).

Pneumomediastinum. Pneumomediastinum is readily visible on CT scan using lung windows. Often, air is visible tracking along the superior mediastinum and following great vessels as they extend into the neck. The source of pneumomediastinum may be apparent from CT. In the case of an esophageal source, thickening of the esophagus at the site of injury may be visible (see

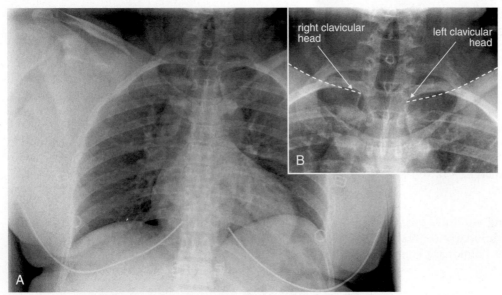

Figure 6-130. Sternoclavicular dislocation. Dislocations of the medial head of the clavicle can be life threatening yet subtle on x-ray. This 43-year-old female was a seat-belted driver struck on the driver's side by a second vehicle. Her chest x-ray was interpreted as normal by the radiologist, but she complained of severe pain near her sternal notch. Compare with the CT images in Figures 6-131 through 6-133. In retrospect, her left clavicular head appears slightly inferiorly displaced, although this could be a positional artifact. Resulting from the chest x-ray exposure, this is difficult to see, but if we carefully follow the superior border of each clavicle toward the midline, the asymmetry becomes apparent. **A,** Frontal chest x-ray. **B,** Close-up from **A.**

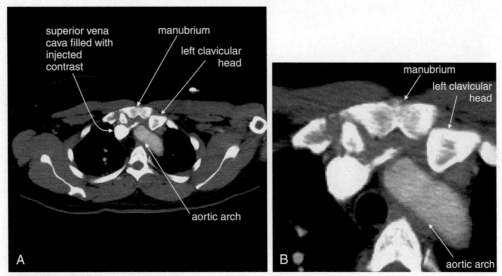

Figure 6-131. Sternoclavicular dislocation, CT with IV contrast. Same patient as in Figure 6-130. **A,** Axial CT image. **B,** Close-up from **A.** This computed tomography slice is a conventional image of the type most emergency physicians would have immediately available for viewing. The slice is viewed on soft-tissue windows to highlight the relationship of the left clavicle to the aortic arch. The left clavicular head is displaced posteriorly relative to the sternum, and it is close to the aortic arch. Compare with the reformatted images in Figures 6-132 and 6-133, which illustrate the dislocation even more clearly. This patient was taken to the operating room by the orthopedic service, and the chest was prepped for possible thoracotomy, with thoracic surgeons standing by. A closed reduction was performed without incident.

Figures 6-36, 6-112, and 6-113). In the case of a significant tracheobronchial injury, a discontinuity in the bronchial wall may be seen (see Figures 6-27, 6-29, and 6-30). In other cases, the source of mediastinal air may not be evident—an associated pneumothorax may suggest the cause, or pneumomediastinum may be present in isolation without an obvious source.

Ironically, although CT is exquisitely sensitive for detection of pneumomediastinum, it may not be the best imaging modality to pursue a suspected esophageal source. Typically, a fluoroscopic Gastrografin swallow study, followed by a fluoroscopic barium swallow study, is performed to assess for mucosal or full-thickness esophageal tears. Chest CT is performed without orally ingested contrast, and CT does not offer good assessment of the undistended esophagus. Without oral contrast, CT assessment for esophageal tears relies on secondary signs of injury such as esophageal thickening or surrounding air.

In a patient presenting late after chest trauma, pneumomediastinum may also be a sign of gas-forming organisms within the mediastinum from mediastinitis. Therefore when fever and a mechanism for mediastinal infection are present, pneumomediastinum is an ominous finding. It is a normal finding immediately after mediastinal surgery.

Hemothorax. Hemothorax is visible on lung and on soft-tissue windows (see Figures 6-4, 6-5, 6-10, and 6-18). The typical Hounsfield density is around 45 Hounsfield units, which appears an intermediate gray on soft-tissue windows.

Pulmonary Contusion. Lung windows are also useful for identification of **pulmonary contusion** (see Figures 6-38, 6-42, and 6-44). Pulmonary contusion is characterized by hemorrhage into the alveolar space, which increases the density from the normal air density (−1000 Hounsfield units, nearly black on lung windows) to fluid density (around 0 Hounsfield units, white on lung windows). An area of pulmonary contusion is also visible on soft-tissue windows. Because contused lung parenchyma has a higher density than normal lung tissue (near that of other soft tissues), it stands out as an intermediate gray on soft-tissue windows, surrounded by normal lung tissue, which appears black on this window setting.

CT is more sensitive than chest x-ray for pulmonary contusion even on initial examination because of its fine ability to discriminate tissue densities. A parenchymal density seen on initial chest CT indicates alveolar fluid—usually blood and serous fluid in the case of blunt or penetrating trauma. However, aspiration occurring during the patient's injury, during endotracheal intubation, or resulting from poor airway protection in an intoxicated or head-injured patient would have exactly the same appearance. Moreover, lung tissue may undergo compressive atelectasis resulting from adjacent hemopneumothorax, and this increases lung parenchymal density, giving the same radiographic appearance. The clinical context may differentiate contusion from these other conditions.

Atelectasis. Atelectasis is commonly seen in trauma patients. Usually, this appears as a bilaterally symmetrical band of increased density in the dependent lung fields (see Figures 6-10 and 6-48). Patients who have been immobilized for long periods on backboards or in bed before CT may have significant atelectasis seen on CT. This can usually be differentiated from pulmonary contusion by its dependent position and bilateral symmetry; pulmonary contusion, in contrast, may be present in any location and is often asymmetrical. Atelectasis, like pulmonary contusion, can be seen on soft-tissue or lung windows. The reported density of dependent atelectasis varies between −100 and +100 Hounsfield units.[94] In contrast, hemothorax and pulmonary contusion always

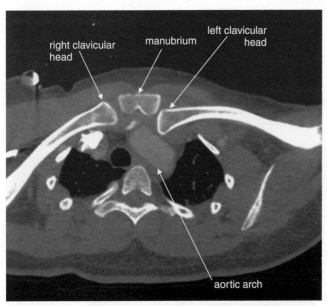

Figure 6-132. Sternoclavicular dislocation, CT with IV contrast. Figures 6-130 through 6-133 include images from this case. This Maximum Intensity Projection (MIP) reconstruction uses a thickened image slab to allow both clavicles and the sternum to be seen in the same plane. The left clavicle is clearly seen to be displaced posteriorly, touching the aortic arch. The patient underwent closed reduction in the operating room, with thoracic surgeons standing by.

Figure 6-133. Sternoclavicular dislocation. Figures 6-130 through 6-132 include images from this case. This three-dimensional reconstruction is viewed looking down upon the thoracic inlet. This is the opposite of the conventional orientation for axial computed tomography, where the point of view is that of an observer looking up from the patient's feet. The left clavicle is seen posteriorly displaced.

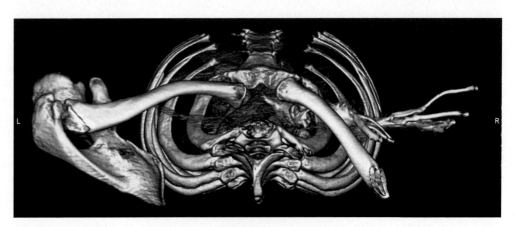

have a density greater than 0 Hounsfield units (water density), usually around 45 Hounsfield units.

Tracheobronchial Injuries. Tracheobronchial injuries can be identified on chest CT using lung windows (see Figures 6-27, 6-29, and 6-30). Typically, a large or even tension pneumothorax persists, regardless of the presence of thoracostomy tubes. Mediastinal shift may be present resulting from tension pneumothorax. A defect in the wall of major airways may be directly visible, connecting into the pleural space.[8]

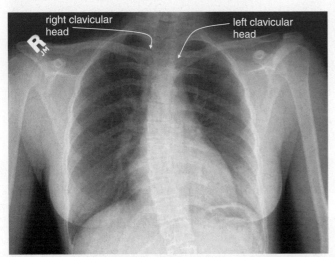

Figure 6-134. **Sternoclavicular dislocation.** This young woman has the same injury as the prior patient—a left sternoclavicular dislocation. Her chest x-ray more readily demonstrates the asymmetry of the clavicular heads at the sternoclavicular joints. Compare with the CT images in Figure 6-135.

Bone Windows

After reviewing soft-tissue and lung windows, inspect the chest a third time using bone windows. Bone windows allow detection of subtle, minimally displaced fractures. More gross and displaced fractures may be visible on lung or mediastinal windows, but the bright white appearance of bone on these window settings masks subtle injuries. In addition to the use of bone windows, special bone reconstruction algorithms are used to create thin sections of bones with minimal artifact. In many medical centers, these are routinely created from the CT dataset and are loaded into the digital picture archiving and communication system as an additional CT series. For most emergency purposes, use of bone windows from the body dataset is sufficient, and specific bone reconstruction views can be reviewed later to provide additional detail of detected injuries.

Although bony injuries are often less immediately dangerous than underlying soft-tissue chest injuries, some isolated bony injuries are quite important. Multiple adjacent rib fractures, particularly a flail segment, may compromise respiratory efficiency (see Figures 6-122 through 6-124). Fractures to the scapula, including intraarticular fractures involving the glenoid fossa, may be seen on bone windows. Thoracic spine fractures (discussed in detail in Chapter 3) can be seen using bone windows. Posterior dislocations of the sternoclavicular joints can threaten the great vessels and may be recognized on either bone or soft-tissue windows (see Figures 6-131 through 6-133).

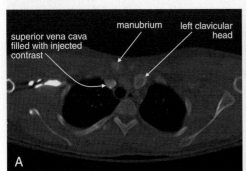
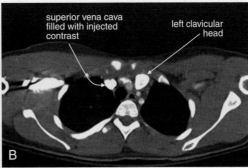
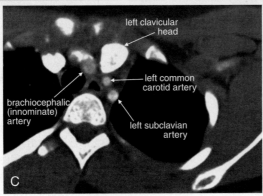

Figure 6-135. **Sternoclavicular dislocation.** CT images from the same patient as in Figure 6-134. **A,** Axial CT image, bone window. **B,** Same CT slice viewed with soft-tissue window. **C,** Close-up from **B.** The left clavicular head is posteriorly displaced and impinges upon the great vessels emerging from the aortic arch (brachiocephalic, left common carotid, and left subclavian). Like the patient in Figures 6-130 through 6-133, this patient underwent closed reduction in the operating room, with thoracic surgeons prepped for possible thoracotomy.

Figure 6-136. Pericardial effusion (hemopericardium). Bedside echocardiogram shows hypoechoic fluid in the pericardial sac. In the setting of trauma, this is likely blood. Care should be taken to differentiate fluid from a pericardial fat pad (see text).

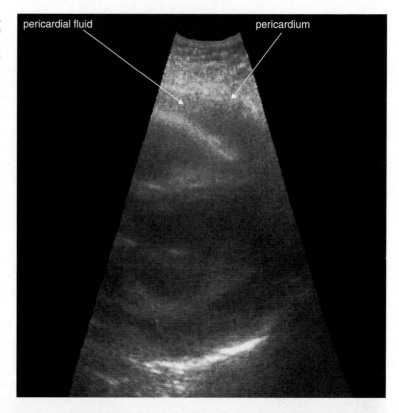

Figure 6-137. Pericardial effusion (hemopericardium). This 57-year-old man struck a utility pole on a bicycle. He was alert but hypotensive on emergency department arrival. His bedside echocardiogram shows pericardial fluid and bowing of the right ventricular free wall, suggesting cardiac tamponade. Compare with the CT findings in Figure 6-138.

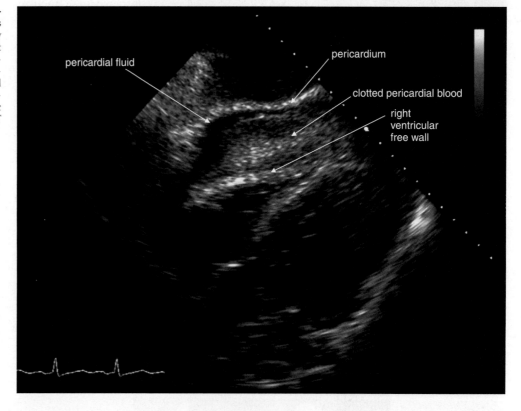

CONTROVERSIES IN THORACIC TRAUMA IMAGING

CT technology has become ubiquitous in the United States and much of the developed world, and a trend toward increasing use of CT for assessment of thoracic injury has occurred over the past decade. Questions remain about the clinical value to patients of this additional imaging, which carries with it both additional cost and radiation exposure with associated cancer risks.[81] The high sensitivity of CT for thoracic spine fracture and aortic injury is not in dispute; when

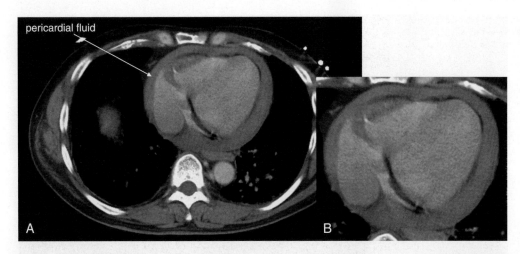

Figure 6-138. Pericardial effusion (hemopericardium), CT with IV contrast. Same patient as in Figure 6-137. The patient remained stable and underwent CT for evaluation of other injuries. His CT also shows a large pericardial effusion, which was treated in the operating room with pericardial window. **A,** Axial CT slice, variation on soft-tissue window. **B,** Close-up from **A.**

pericardial fluid

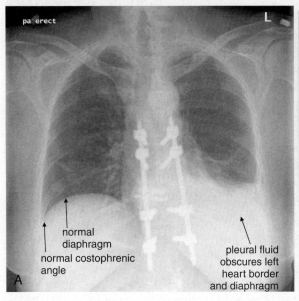
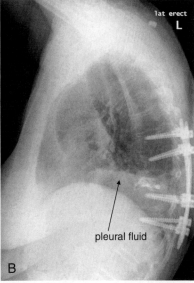

pa erect L

normal diaphragm
normal costophrenic angle

pleural fluid obscures left heart border and diaphragm

lat erect L

pleural fluid

Figure 6-139. Pleural effusions. Pleural fluid layers with gravity on upright chest x-ray. In the setting of trauma, fluid is assumed to represent blood. **A,** PA upright chest x-ray. **B,** Lateral upright chest x-ray. Compare these images with the thoracic ultrasound in Figure 6-140.

TABLE 6-6. Ultrasound Transducers (Probes) for Examination of the Thorax in Trauma[111]

Probe	Frequency	Depth of Penetration	Footprint	Mode	Application
Cardiac probe	1-5 MHz	35 cm	17-mm flat linear array	B	• Pericardial effusion • Hemothorax • Pneumothorax
Abdominal probe	2-5 MHz	30 cm	60-mm curved array	B M	• Pericardial effusion • Hemothorax • Pneumothorax
Linear high-frequency probe	6-13 MHz	6 cm	25-mm flat linear array	B M	• Hemothorax • Pneumothorax

From Sonosite. MicroMaxx: Transducers. (Accessed at http://www.sonosite.com/products/micromaxx/transducers/.)

injuries to these regions are suspected, CT is advocated, because it far surpasses the sensitivity of x-ray. Important questions today relate to the indications for CT in stable patients with normal chest x-rays and the correct clinical action for subtle injuries detected by CT but not by chest x-ray. We explore some of these questions here.

Do Patients with Normal Chest X-ray Require CT to Assess for Aortic Injury? Does a Normal Chest X-ray Sufficiently Exclude Aortic Injury?

Historically, patients with no evidence of traumatic aortic injury on chest x-ray did not routinely undergo aortography to exclude aortic injury definitively. A normal

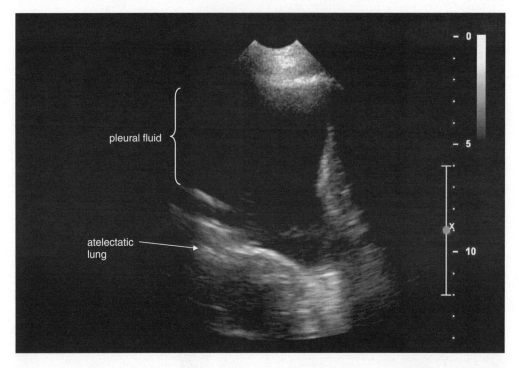

Figure 6-140. **Pleural fluid or hemothorax: Ultrasound.** Same patient as in Figure 6-139. An ultrasound of the chest was performed. The large black region is pleural fluid. Lung tissue is seen deep to this and has echo characteristics similar to abdominal solid organs, because it is atelectatic resulting from the pleural fluid. In this location, 10 cm of pleural fluid separates the chest wall and lung.

chest x-ray is reported in only about 7% of aortic injuries, for a sensitivity of around 93%.[20] Although this sensitivity is low for a life-threatening injury, aortic injury is relatively rare, occurring in only 274 patients in 2.5 years in a multicenter trial of 50 U.S. trauma centers—an average of only about 2 aortic injuries per trauma center per year.[20] Ungar et al.[16] reviewed 1096 consecutive blunt trauma patients at a major trauma center, all of whom had definitive imaging with CT, aortography, or both. The rate of traumatic aortic injury was only 2%. The authors derived a clinical decision rule for aortic injury based on chest x-ray and found that a chest x-ray without obscuration of the aortic knob, mediastinal widening, or displacement of the left paraspinous line had a sensitivity of 86% (95% CI = 65%-97%), a specificity of 77% (95% CI = 75%-80%), a positive predictive value of 7% (95% CI = 4%-11%), a negative predictive value of 99.6% (95% CI = 99.0%-99.9%), a positive likelihood ratio of 3.8 (95% CI = 1.1-12.9), and a negative likelihood ratio of 0.18 (95% CI = 0.05-0.61).[16] Despite relative low sensitivity, the negative predictive value of a normal chest x-ray is very high resulting from the rarity of the injury. An individual patient might deserve definitive aortic imaging despite normal radiography if other evidence of substantial trauma is present, such as hemodynamic instability without a clear cause. Although as many as 14% of aortic injuries might be missed by chest x-ray in the study by Ungar et al.,[16] the number needed to treat to detect 1 additional aortic injury using CT or aortography in patients with normal chest x-ray findings was high—nearly 300. Although the availability, speed, and ease of use of CT make it an attractive option to detect rare occult injuries, the cost and radiation exposure of CT may make the risk–benefit ratio of ubiquitous CT unfavorable.

Other Perspectives: Should Patients with a Normal Mediastinum on Chest X-ray but Other Evidence of Thoracic Trauma (e.g., Rib Fractures) Undergo CT? Should Patients with No Visible Evidence of Thoracic Injury Undergo Thoracic CT?

Other authors have argued that chest CT should be performed in every trauma patient regardless of the presence or absence of signs and symptoms of chest trauma. Exadaktylos et al.[74] reported on injuries detected by CT but missed on initial chest x-ray in 93 consecutive patients with blunt trauma. They reported that 73.1% showed at least one pathologic sign on chest x-ray and 26.9% had normal chest x-ray. Of those with normal chest x-rays, 52% had injuries detected at CT, including two aortic injuries (8% of those with normal chest x-rays), three pleural effusions, and one pericardial effusion. The authors conclude that the rate of serious injuries missed by x-ray justifies routine use of thoracic CT. However, their reported rates of injury exceeded those from other studies of blunt aortic injury, such as the Multicenter Trial of the American Association for the Surgery of Trauma,[20] strongly suggesting selection or spectrum bias. It is doubtful that the rate of injuries in trauma patients in community emergency departments would approach that in this study. Perhaps thoracic CT is routinely advisable in the high-risk patients seen in tertiary care trauma centers.

In a prospective study of 1000 patients, including 592 alert patients, Salim et al.[95] reported a rate of "significant" thoracic injuries of 19.6% in patients "without visible signs of thoracic trauma." Several criticisms of this study have been leveled, though it remains the

TABLE 6-7. Comet Tail Artifacts on Thoracic Ultrasound and Their Significance

B Lines
• Are a normal finding. Loss of B lines is a sign of pneumothorax. • Are vertical and bright lines arising from the pleural line and extending deep to the pleural line • Are well defined and narrow lines (sometimes described as "laser beam–like") • Spread to the deep edge of the screen (field of view) without fading • Erase A lines (horizontal repetition artifact lines that lie parallel and deep to the pleural lines) • Move with lung sliding
Z Lines
• Seen in both normal and pathologic states. Do not exclude or confirm pneumothorax. • Are ill-defined vertical lines arising from the pleural line and extending deep to it, in contrast to B lines, which are well defined • Fade after 2-5 cm of depth, in contrast to B lines, which continue without fading to the deep edge of the field of view • Do not erase A lines, in contrast to B lines, which do erase A lines • Are independent of lung sliding, in contrast to B lines, which move with lung sliding
E Lines
• Result from subcutaneous emphysema. May be a clue to pneumothorax but prevent assessment of motion at the pleural line. • Are bright lines arising superficial to the pleural line and preventing its visualization • Bat sign is not seen, as E lines obscure the pleural line • Extend deep to their origin and do not fade

From Lichtenstein DA, Meziere G, Lascols N, et al. Ultrasound diagnosis of occult pneumothorax. *Crit Care Med* 33(6):1231-1238, 2005.

TABLE 6-8. Diagnostic Accuracy of Ultrasound Findings of Pneumothorax[70,72,112]

Finding	Sensitivity	Specificity
Loss of sliding lung sign	95%-100%	78%-91%
Loss of sliding lung sign plus presence of A line sign	95%	94%
Lung point sign	66%-79%	100%

From Lichtenstein DA, Menu Y. A bedside ultrasound sign ruling out pneumothorax in the critically ill: Lung sliding. *Chest* 108(5):1345-1348, 1995; Lichtenstein D, Meziere G, Biderman P, et al. The "lung point": An ultrasound sign specific to pneumothorax. *Intensive Care Med* 26(10):1434-1440, 2000; Lichtenstein DA, Meziere G, Lascols N, et al. Ultrasound diagnosis of occult pneumothorax. *Crit Care Med* 33(6):1231-1238, 2005.

basis for many trauma protocols incorporating CT. First, the researchers focused on "visible signs of thoracic trauma" but did not evaluate for the presence or absence of other readily available evidence of injury, including complaints of chest or dyspnea or tenderness to chest palpation. Thus it is possible that most injuries detected by CT would have been suspected based on simple history or examination techniques. Perhaps a normal physical examination and the absence of chest symptoms (pain or dyspnea) in an alert patient might rule out significant injury, eliminating the need for CT. Evidence to this effect exists from studies of the indications for chest x-ray.[2-3]

Second, the authors included patients with significant alteration of mental status in their study. Patients who cannot be clinically assessed as a consequence of head injury, instability, intoxication, or intubation constitute a distinct population from those who are stable, alert, and awake. The former patients are likely also at greater risk for concurrent chest injuries than are alert patients. Although the authors stratified patient results by status ("evaluable" or "unevaluable"), these two groups should not be combined in clinical decision-making.

Third, the authors classified as "important thoracic injuries" virtually every finding identified on CT, including rib fractures, pulmonary contusions, and small pneumothoraces and hemothoraces. Only 7.9% of 809 patients with normal chest x-rays in this study had abnormal CT findings: 27 with occult pneumothorax or small hemothorax (3.3%), 2 with suspicion for aortic injury (0.2%), 27 with pulmonary contusion (3.3%), and 30 with rib fractures (3.7%) [percentages do not sum to 7.9%, because some patients had more than one of the above injury types]. It is not clear that detection of these injuries resulted in clinically beneficial changes in management of patients, justifying the cost and radiation exposure of CT. The authors demonstrated a very low rate of indisputably important injuries such as aortic trauma: 4 of 1000 total patients (0.4%) and only 1 of 592 "evaluable" patients (0.2%). Thus the number needed to treat to identify 1 aortic injury by their methods would be nearly 600 in alert patients without visible chest trauma and 1 in 400 with normal chest x-ray.[95]

In their publication in *Lancet*, Strohm, Hauschild, and Sudkamp[96] reported an association between use of pan-scan CT (CT of the head, spine, chest, abdomen, and pelvis) and reduced mortality, compared with patients undergoing more selective use of CT. This study (discussed in more detail in Chapter 10) is retrospective and can demonstrate only an association, not a causative relationship, between use of CT and survival. This study also lacks face validity in that many injuries detected by thoracic and abdominal CT (e.g., pulmonary contusions, rib fractures, and low-grade splenic and hepatic injuries) require only supportive management, so definitive diagnosis by CT would not necessarily be expected to alter management or outcome. Critics have pointed out numerous methodologic flaws in this study, including immortal time bias. This bias describes the fact that patients dying very early in their emergency department course would fail to undergo CT and would thus contribute to increased mortality in the selective CT group, whereas patients stable enough to survive through completion of a pan-scan would contribute to lower mortality in this group. A prospective, randomized, controlled trial is needed to examine the clinical value of pan-scan, and particularly thoracic CT, in more detail.[96]

When Injuries Are Detected by CT, What Interventions Are Appropriate? What Treatment Is Needed for Pneumothorax Detected Solely by CT?

CT is clearly more sensitive for multiple injury types than is chest x-ray, but less evident is the correct clinical action when subtle injuries are detected. Consider the case of small pneumothoraces detected by CT and not visible on chest x-ray. Is thoracostomy tube drainage necessary? Multiple small retrospective studies have examined this question, and collectively they suggest that thoracostomy tube drainage should not be routine. Even in the case of patients undergoing positive pressure ventilation, in whom a risk for tension pneumothorax might be assumed, routine thoracostomy drainage does not appear necessary. While a large prospective, randomized, controlled trial is needed to determine the value of thoracostomy tube for CT-only pneumothoraces, these studies call into question the benefit of CT detection of these injuries. It is possible that CT use simply results in the detection of more injuries requiring no specific management or that CT even results in patient harm by leading to unnecessary invasive procedures such as thoracostomy. We assess some of the studies on this topic here.

Ball et al.[97] retrospectively studied 761 trauma patients, documenting 103 pneumothoraces on CT scan. Of these, 55% were not evident on initial chest x-ray. The authors noted that pneumothoraces were more often occult on chest x-ray when located anteriorly or in basal or apical locations, all potentially identifiable using ultrasound (though the authors did not attempt to identify these pneumothoraces with ultrasound). In a separate report on the same patients, they noted that 4 of 17 (24%) patients with occult pneumothoraces underwent uneventful positive pressure ventilation without thoracostomy tube placement.[98]

Neff et al.[99] retrospectively reviewed the charts of 230 trauma patients with pneumothorax at admission and found that 126 (54.8%) were occult on chest x-ray, diagnosed instead by abdominal CT. The authors noted that 84 (66.7%) underwent thoracostomy tube placement and suggested that CT diagnosis of pneumothorax is beneficial. However, the necessity or benefit of this diagnosis is uncertain. It is possible that diagnoses of these occult pneumothoraces resulted in unnecessary thoracostomy with increased patient morbidity. Because of the retrospective methods of this study, it is not clear what percentage of patients with pneumothorax detected by CT alone had other signs or symptoms, such as hypoxia, which may have necessitated thoracostomy. Detection of occult pneumothorax may be beneficial in selected cases when patients require long intrahospital transportation or positive pressure ventilation that might result in progression to tension pneumothorax.

Brasel et al.[100] prospectively randomized 39 patients with occult pneumothorax (detected on CT but not chest x-ray) to thoracostomy or observation. In each group, 9 patients received positive pressure ventilation, and no patient developed respiratory distress attributed to the occult pneumothorax or required emergent thoracostomy. The authors concluded that occult pneumothoraces do not require routine thoracostomy, even in patients undergoing positive pressure ventilation. This small study does not rule out the possibility of infrequent significant worsening of an occult pneumothorax when not treated with thoracostomy.

Enderson et al.[101] performed a similar randomized controlled trial of 40 patients with occult pneumothorax. In this trial, 19 were randomized to tube thoracostomy, whereas 21 were observed without thoracostomy. While on positive pressure ventilation, 8 of 21 had progression of pneumothorax, with 3 developing tension pneumothorax. The authors concluded that patients with occult pneumothorax undergoing positive pressure ventilation should be treated routinely with thoracostomy.

Holmes et al.[102] prospectively studied 538 children who underwent both chest x-ray and abdominal CT. Pneumothorax occurred in 20 patients (3.7%). Of these, 9 (45%) had pneumothorax identified on initial chest x-ray, whereas 11 patients (55%) had pneumothoraces not seen on chest x-ray. Of these 11 patients, 10 (91%) were managed successfully without thoracostomy tube, including 2 undergoing positive pressure ventilation.

Renton, Kincaid, and Ehrlich[76] conducted a retrospective review and cost analysis to determine whether chest CT should replace chest x-ray as the initial imaging test in pediatric trauma. They noted that from 1996 to 2000, only 45 of 1638 pediatric trauma patients underwent CT at their institution, with 18 patients having injuries detected on CT that had not been recognized on x-ray. These included pulmonary contusions (12), hemothoraces (6), pneumothoraces (5), widened mediastinum (4), rib fractures (2), diaphragmatic injury (1), and aortic injury (1). They concluded that 8 patients (17.7% of the 45 undergoing CT) had clinical management changes as a result of CT findings: 5 with chest tube placement, 2 with aortography, and 1 with an operation performed. Based on an institutional cost of $200 per CT and a patient charge of $906 (compared with $96 for chest x-ray), they estimated that 200 thoracic CT scans would be required for each clinically significant change in management, at a patient cost of $180,000 and hospital cost of $40,000 per management change.

Which Patients Require CT to Evaluate Potential Thoracic Spine Trauma?

Imaging of thoracic spine injuries is discussed in detail in Chapter 3. Evaluation of thoracic spine injury is one of the major indications for chest CT today, because axial, sagittal, and coronal reconstructions of the spine can be performed from the data acquired from CT performed for evaluation of mediastinal and pulmonary injuries. CT has been shown to far surpass x-ray in sensitivity for these injuries. Indications for thoracic CT include spinal tenderness on exam; neurologic deficits potentially attributable to spinal trauma; obtundation, intoxication, or intubation preventing clinical assessment; thoracic spine abnormalities detected on imaging such as chest x-ray; and detection of cervical or lumbar fractures, because these injuries have been found to predict the presence of additional spinal injuries.

Can Imaging Detect Blunt Cardiac Injury?

Blunt cardiac injury (formerly called cardiac contusion) remains an area of controversy. Chest x-ray and CT scan offer no direct evidence of this diagnosis, although they may reveal associated pericardial hemorrhage or sternal fracture. Echocardiography provides the most clinically useful information regarding right and left ventricular ejection fracture, although formal echocardiography (rather than bedside echo as a part of the FAST examination) should not be routine in patients with blunt chest trauma. Indications for echocardiography are controversial but likely are restricted to patients with significant dysrhythmias or hemodynamic instability. Use of cardiac markers such as creatine kinase-MB isoenzyme and troponin I or T to detect blunt cardiac injury has fallen from favor resulting from a lack of supportive evidence.[60,103-104]

When Is Aortography Needed?

Aortography, the traditional gold standard for evaluation of blunt aortic injury, has been replaced almost entirely by chest CT for diagnosis. Modern CT provides sufficient anatomic detail to guide open surgical management and endovascular repair, which is used in some cases. Although some trauma surgeons have been vocal opponents of the use of CT, arguing for aortography, improvements in three-dimensional CT reconstructions have relegated aortography to a secondary role. It is most useful as a therapeutic modality allowing endovascular repair, or when CT is equivocal (see Chapter 16). Aortography has almost no role in primary diagnosis resulting from the availability of CT, which allows concurrent assessment of other important injuries, including intraabdominal and spinal trauma. In one retrospective study of 856 patients between 1997 and 2004, 24% of aortograms were preceded by CT; among 31 with confirmed aortic injury, 20 had preceding CT.[105] Rarely, a patient with a chest x-ray highly suggestive of aortic injury may be taken directly to the operating room with a plan for intraoperative aortography, depending on stability, suspicion for other injuries, local institutional protocols, and resources. Hunink and Bos[106] found CT before aortography to be more cost effective ($1468 per patient) than primary aortography ($2508 per patient) to pursue chest x-ray abnormalities suspicious for aortic injury in stable patients. For these reasons, in general, aortography is diminishing as an emergency department imaging study.

Can CT Guide Management of Penetrating Chest Trauma Such as Transmediastinal Gunshot Wounds and Stab Wounds to the Anterior Chest?

The speed of modern chest CT and its high spatial resolution have broadened its use for injury patterns that in the past were more commonly managed with surgery, angiography, bronchoscopy, esophagography, and esophagoscopy. Examples include transmediastinal gunshot wounds and stab wounds to the "cardiac box" (see Figs. 6-115, 6-116, and 6-118 through 6-120). Apparently stable patients with these injury mechanisms can have devastating injuries.[107] In some cases, CT can exclude or confirm cardiac, vascular, tracheobronchial, and esophageal injuries, eliminating the need for other diagnostic studies and determining the need for operative intervention. Hanpeter et al.[108] performed a prospective study of 24 stable patients with mediastinal gunshot wounds. One patient was taken for sternotomy and surgical removal of an embedded myocardial missile based on CT findings alone. Another 12 patients underwent additional imaging of the aorta or esophagus resulting from a missile track close to these structures; one had a bullet adjacent to the ascending aorta that was removed surgically. A further 11 patients had missile tracks not in proximity to the aorta, heart, or esophagus, and no further interventions were performed. Small studies such as this are just the starting point for more systematic research on the role of chest CT in penetrating thoracic trauma.

SUMMARY

Chest trauma is a common indication for diagnostic imaging. Clinical decision rules can identify patients requiring no imaging. In those who require imaging, chest x-ray is the initial test of choice resulting from low cost and low radiation exposure with substantial clinical information obtained. Ultrasound is a sensitive bedside tool for detection of hemo- and pneumothorax, as well as pericardial effusion. Chest CT and formal echocardiography play important roles in selected patients. The indications for chest CT remain in debate and require further study. Aortography has been largely replaced by CT for diagnosis but retains a therapeutic role for aortic injuries.

CHAPTER 7 Imaging of Pulmonary Embolism and Nontraumatic Aortic Pathology

Joshua Broder, MD, FACEP

In the two preceding chapters we discussed chest imaging in patients without a history of injury and in the setting of trauma. In this chapter, we focus on imaging of three particularly life-threatening conditions: pulmonary embolism (PE), spontaneous aortic dissection, and spontaneous thoracic aortic aneurysm rupture. These conditions share computed tomography (CT) as their primary diagnostic modality today. For each of these, we briefly review pathophysiology, pretest probability assessment, and the limited role of chest x-ray in diagnosis. We discuss the role of CT in detail, comparing CT to other imaging modalities, including the historical criterion standards, pulmonary angiography and aortography, which are more rarely performed today. We consider the role and diagnostic accuracy of alternative imaging modalities, including ventilation–perfusion (VQ) scan, magnetic resonance imaging (MRI), and echocardiography. We consider challenging clinical scenarios, such as the patient with contraindications to intravenous (IV) contrast, the unstable patient who may be at risk during imaging tests outside of the emergency department, the patient requiring exclusion of both PE and aortic pathology, and the pregnant patient with suspected PE. Along the way, we review critical imaging findings that may allow you to diagnose these important conditions before radiologist interpretation, allowing earlier initiation of therapy. In the chapter on interventional radiology (Chapter 16), interventions for PE and aortic disease are described, with a critical review of the evidence for these treatments.

BRIEF GUIDE TO FIGURES IN THIS CHAPTER

Figures in this chapter are grouped according to clinical case so that x-rays, CT scans, and other imaging studies from a single patient are clustered together for teaching purposes. This means that sometimes you are directed to a figure later in the chapter, illustrating a related imaging finding in a different patient. These cross-references to later figures are marked by the words *see also*. In addition, a summary of the figure content is listed in Table 7-1 for quick reference. We highly recommend looking at all figures corresponding to a given patient case. They are arranged to illustrate pearls and pitfalls of imaging.

We begin our discussion with PE. This discussion sets the stage for our review of aortic imaging, which has many features similar to those of PE.

PULMONARY EMBOLISM

PE occurs when thrombus, usually from lower extremity or pelvic veins, migrates to the pulmonary arteries, resulting in partial or complete obstruction of blood flow in the affected vessel. The lung segment supplied by this vessel may become infarcted, and atelectasis or pleural effusion may occur.[1] Pulmonary embolism is a life-threatening condition, although the range of reported mortality is very wide. In a large US emergency department sample of patients diagnosed with acute PE, 30-day mortality attributed to acute PE was only 1.1%, but all-cause mortality was 5.4%.[1a] Other studies suggest 30-day death rates of 15% in initially hemodynamically stable patients and almost 60% in patients presenting with hemodynamic instability, demonstrating the wide range of clinical severity.[1b]

Which Patients Require Imaging for Pulmonary Embolism? How Does Pretest Probability Influence Imaging Decisions?

Pretest probability assessment is a key part of planning for diagnostic imaging in emergency department patients with suspected PE. Pretest probability assessment first determines whether a patient requires imaging of any kind to assess for PE. Next, pretest probability strongly determines the reliability of the available diagnostic imaging modalities, influencing both the choice of modality and the clinical application of a negative or positive imaging test. As we discuss in detail later in the sections on VQ scan and CT, when imaging test results are at odds with clinical pretest probability, additional testing is warranted because of the possibility of false-positive and false-negative imaging results.

PE can be challenging to diagnosis clinically, as it can present with a variety of symptoms, including chest pain, dyspnea, and syncope. Let's consider how clinical risk assessment tools should be applied to patients with suspected PE. First, ask the binary question: Is

TABLE 7-1. Guide to Figures in This Chapter

Content	Figure Numbers
Pulmonary embolism figures	7-1 to 7-59
• Chest x-ray findings of pulmonary embolism	7-2, 7-3, 7-34, 7-38, 7-41, 7-51, 7-52
• Westermark sign	7-2
• Hampton's hump (visible pulmonary infarct)	7-3, 7-34, 7-38, 7-41, 7-51, 7-52
• CT findings of pulmonary embolism	7-8 to 7-33, 7-35 to 7-37, 7-39, 7-40, 7-42, 7-47, 7-55
• Contrast timing for CT pulmonary angiography	7-11, 7-12
• Saddle or central pulmonary emboli	7-13 to 7-27, 7-33, 7-39
• Cardiac thrombus and dilatation secondary to pulmonary emboli	7-16, 7-17
• Segmental and peripheral pulmonary emboli	7-28, 7-29, 7-36, 7-42
• Lung window findings of pulmonary infarction	7-30 to 7-32, 7-35, 7-37, 7-42
• Distinguishing pulmonary embolism from artifacts and adenopathy	7-39, 7-40, 7-47
• VQ findings of pulmonary embolism	7-43 to 7-46, 7-48 to 7-50, 7-53, 7-54
• Angiographic findings of pulmonary embolism	7-4, 7-5
• Tumor emboli	7-56 to 7-59
Aortic disease figures	7-60 to 7-102
• Chest x-ray findings of aortic disease	7-60, 7-65, 7-67, 7-69, 7-70, 7-73, 7-75, 7-78, 7-85, 7-88, 7-92, 7-95, 7-98, 7-99
• Classic chest x-rays of aortic aneurysm or dissection	7-60, 7-65, 7-67, 7-69, 7-70, 7-73, 7-75, 7-92, 7-95
• Normal x-ray despite aortic dissection	7-67, 7-78, 7-85, 7-88, 7-92
• Mediastinal abnormalities on chest x-ray unrelated to aortic dissection or aneurysm	7-98, 7-99
• CT scan findings of aortic disease	7-61 to 7-64, 7-66, 7-68, 7-69, 7-71, 7-74, 7-76, 7-77, 7-79 to 7-84, 7-86, 7-87, 7-89 to 7-91, 7-93, 7-94, 7-96 to 7-98, 7-100
• Contrast timing for CT aortography	7-80, 7-81
• Aortic branch vessel involvement	7-80, 7-82, 7-83 (brachiocephalic)
Iliac artery	7-64
Brachiocephalic artery	7-80, 7-82, 7-83
Renal artery	7-84, 7-91
Coronary artery	7-87
Mesenteric artery	7-90
• Imaging for concurrent PE and aortic pathology	7-96
• Aortic endovascular repair and endoleak	7-74, 7-93, 7-94
• Angiographic findings of aortic disease	7-72

PE a possible cause of the patient's presentation? If the answer is unequivocally "no," (for example, in a patient with pleuritic chest pain immediately after blunt chest trauma), further risk assessment is not needed and may trigger unnecessary testing. If the answer is "yes" (including "likely not," "possibly so," or "likely yes"), "further clinical risk stratification is needed. Several clinical assessment schemes exist, but they share the ability to sort patients into low-risk categories (not requiring imaging) and higher-risk categories (requiring imaging). Some risk stratification schemes incorporate lab testing

(D-dimer*), whereas others rely solely on clinical history and physical exam. We consider two risk stratification tools or clinical decision rules: Wells score and pulmonary embolism rule-out criteria (PERC).

Clinical decision rules are important guides to imaging decisions *once the diagnosis of PE has been considered*

---

*D-dimer is a fibrin degradation product present in blood after a clot is degraded by fibrinolysis. Its presence or absence can be used as a screening tool for the presence of clot.

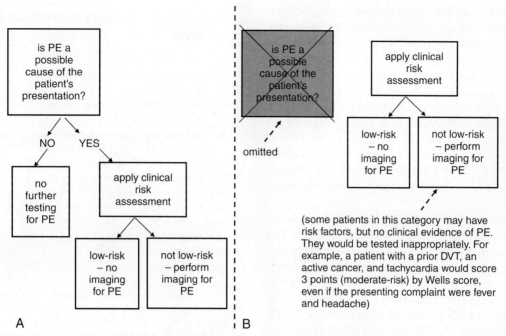

Figure 7-1. Two strategies for application of clinical risk stratification for pulmonary embolism (PE). Strategy **A** first asks the binary question: Could PE be the cause of the patient's presentation? Then it applies specific clinical risk scores. This avoids unnecessary testing of patients with presentations not compatible with PE. Strategy **B** applies a clinical scoring system first and may lead to inappropriate testing of patients who have no clinical signs or symptoms of PE but have risk factors. Indiscriminate use of D-dimer testing without clinical risk stratification leads to the same type of error.

based on clinical gestalt. This last statement is important, because the two clinical rules we discuss here could lead to unnecessary imaging if applied indiscriminately to patients with clinical presentations not suggestive of PE. For example, a 60-year-old patient presenting with fever, abdominal pain, heart rate of 120 beats per minute, and history of appendectomy 10 days prior may be an obvious clinical case of postoperative abscess but scores 3 points by Wells criteria (discussed later), falling into a moderate risk group for PE. Clearly, the patient should not be evaluated for PE solely based on these criteria, unless clinical signs and symptoms suggest PE. By the same concept, the patient would fail several of the PERC, but these should not be applied if the clinician does not suspect PE. Figure 7-1 demonstrates appropriate use of risk-stratification for PE, and also shows how inappropriate use of risk-stratification rules could lead to unnecessary imaging.

Wells criteria[2] (Table 7-2) are validated criteria to identify patients with a low clinical risk for PE. Wells and colleagues have investigated multiple cutoffs, including a low–moderate–high categorization, and a PE unlikely–likely categorization (see Table 7-2). In Wells' validation set, patients with a score less than 2 (low risk) had an overall PE rate of only 2.0%, regardless of D-dimer result. However, the confidence intervals were broad, with an upper limit of 7.1%, which would be unacceptably high for most clinicians. Ironically, low-risk patients with a negative D-dimer had a higher rate of PE (2.7%) than those with positive D-dimer testing (0%) in Wells' study, though no statistical difference between the groups existed. When the Wells Criteria are dichotomized into

TABLE 7-2. Wells Criteria for Pulmonary Embolism

Criterion	Score
Clinical signs and symptoms of DVT	3.0
PE is No. 1 diagnosis or equally likely	3.0
Heart rate > 100 bpm	1.5
Immobilization at least 3 days or surgery in past 4 weeks	1.5
Previous objectively diagnosed PE or DVT	1.5
Hemoptysis	1.0
Malignancy with treatment within 6 months, or palliative	1.0

Data from Douma RA, Gibson NS, Gerdes VE, et al. Validity and clinical utility of the simplified Wells rule for assessing clinical probability for the exclusion of pulmonary embolism. *Thromb Haemost* 101:197-200, 2009; Wells PS, Anderson DR, Rodger M, et al. Derivation of a simple clinical model to categorize patients' probability of pulmonary embolism: Increasing the models utility *with* the SimpliRED D-dimer. *Thromb Haemost* 83:416-420, 2000.

Total score: <2 gives low (1.3%) risk of PE, 2-6 gives moderate (16.2%) risk, >6 gives high (37.5%) risk. Score ≤ 4 plus negative D-dimer predicts a 2% risk for venous thromboembolic disease. When each criterion is assigned only 1 point, a score ≤ 1 plus a normal D-dimer gives a 0% rate of VTE at 3 months.

PE "unlikely" (score ≤ 4) and "likely" (score > 4) categories, an unlikely score plus a negative SimpliRed D-dimer predicts a PE risk for around 2% with an upper 95% CI of 6%.[2] Other studies suggest that the SimpliRed D-Dimer is not sufficiently sensitive and that ELISA D-dimer assays are superior.[2a-2c] More recently, a simplified dichotomized Wells Criteria has been described, although this rule requires additional prospective validation. Under this paradigm, each criterion is assigned only 1 point, and a score of no more than 1 combined with a normal D-dimer predicts a 3-month incidence of venous thromboembolism (VTE) of 0%, with a 95% confidence interval (CI) of 0% to 1.6%. Using this strategy, 26% of patients could avoid diagnostic imaging for PE.[3] The use of Wells criteria, in conjunction with D-dimer testing, to screen patients for possible PE is widely accepted and was endorsed by the American College of Emergency Physicians (ACEP) in its 2003 clinical policy on evaluation of adult patients with suspected PE, now retired.[4]

The PERC[5-6] are a prospectively derived and validated system to exclude PE without D-dimer testing. The advantage of such a system is the avoidance of unnecessary imaging prompted by false-positive D-dimer results, a problem often encountered with highly sensitive D-dimer tests. The criteria (Box 7-1) are meant to be applied only to patients judged to be at low risk for PE based on physician gestalt. Imaging decisions in patients not judged by gestalt to be at low risk of PE should not be based on PERC. In a prospective study of more than 8100 patients, the rate of 45-day VTE or death was less than 2% in PERC-negative patients. The rule can eliminate the need for diagnostic imaging in about 20% of patients with a low pretest probability (defined as <15%) based on physician gestalt. Multiple other clinical probability scores exist including the Charlotte Rule and Geneva Rule, with similar overall accuracy. These and experienced clinician gestalt can be used to determine pretest probability.[6a]

Formulating a pretest probability assessment of PE should be routine practice before the decision to perform a diagnostic imaging test for PE. In patients whose pretest probability assessment suggest a need for imaging to evaluate for PE, multiple imaging tests are available, but the usual first imaging step is chest x-ray.

How Is Chest X-ray Useful in the Evaluation of Pulmonary Embolism? What Is the Importance of Classic Abnormalities Such as Hampton's Hump and the Westermark Sign? Do Any Chest X-ray Findings Confirm or Exclude Pulmonary Embolism?

Chest x-ray plays a limited role in the diagnosis of PE, as an embolism is not directly visible on plain x-ray. The greatest importance of chest x-ray in assessment for PE is in evaluation of the differential diagnosis, which can include pneumonia, pneumothorax, malignancy, pleural effusion, pericardial disorders, and aortic or other mediastinal abnormalities. Chest x-ray is inexpensive, rapid to obtain, and exposes the patient to minimal radiation in comparison with CT and VQ scan. Consequently, it is an appropriate initial imaging test in virtually every patient with suspected PE, as it explores the differential diagnosis of complaints such as chest pain, dyspnea,

---

Box 7-1: Pulmonary Embolism Rule-Out Criteria

- **Age <50 years**
- **Pulse <100 beats per minute**
- **Sao2 >94%**
- **No unilateral leg swelling**
- **No hemoptysis**
- **No recent trauma or surgery (with general anesthesia) in past 4 weeks**
- **No prior PE or DVT**
- **No hormone use**

In a patient classified as "low risk" by clinician gestalt, PE is unlikely if all of the preceding criteria are fulfilled. Sensitivity is 97.4% (95% CI = 95.8%-98.5%), and specificity is 21.9% (95% CI = 21.0%-22.9%); likelihood ratio negative is 0.12 (95% CI = 0.07-0.19). The score is meant to be used without D-dimer testing.

From Kline JA, Courtney DM, Kabrhel C, et al. Prospective multicenter evaluation of the pulmonary embolism rule-out criteria. *J Thromb Haemost* 6:772-780, 2008; Kline JA, Mitchell AM, Kabrhel C, et al. Clinical criteria to prevent unnecessary diagnostic testing in emergency department patients with suspected pulmonary embolism. *J Thromb Haemost* 2:1247-1255, 2004.

---

and syncope. Chest x-ray also provides information that can predict the diagnostic utility of VQ scan or in some cases can even substitute for the ventilation portion of the VQ scan, reducing cost and radiation exposure. Prospective Investigation of Pulmonary Embolism Diagnosis (PIOPED) I, a multicenter trial from 1983 to 1989 that provided methodologically rigorous evaluation of diagnostic tests for PE, provides a rich source of information on the diagnostic value of chest x-rays in patients with and without PE. Normal chest x-rays occurred in only 12% of patients in this study published in 1990—although this was a high-risk patient population with a high incidence of PE. Normal chest x-rays may be more common in a lower-risk cohort, more typical of emergency department patients undergoing testing today. The most common chest x-ray findings in patients with PE were atelectasis, parenchymal areas of increased opacity, or both, but these findings occurred with similar frequency in patients without PE and therefore cannot be used to differentiate PE. Several classically described chest x-ray findings of PE were specifically investigated but found to have little diagnostic value (see Table 7-3). The Westermark sign (oligemia distal to a large vessel occluded by PE) (Figure 7-2) was found to be relatively specific but highly insensitive, found in only 8% to 14% of patients with PE. "Classic" findings that proved nonspecific and insensitive included the Fleischner sign (a prominent central artery caused by distension of a vessel by a large clot or by pulmonary hypertension from distal embolization) and Hampton's hump (a wedge-shaped pleural-based peripheral density with a convex medial border, representing parenchymal infarction)

TABLE 7-3. Chest X-ray Findings and Pulmonary Embolism Diagnosis

Chest X-ray Finding	Sensitivity	Specificity
Normal	12%	82%
Oligemia (Westermark sign)	8%-14%	92%-96%
Prominent central pulmonary artery (Fleischner sign)	20%	80%
Pleural-based area of increased opacity (Hampton's hump)	22%-24%	82%
Vascular redistribution	9%-10%	85%-87%
Pleural effusion	35%-36%	70%
Elevated diaphragm	14%-20%	85%-90%

From Worsley DF, Alavi A, Aronchick JM, et al. Chest radiographic findings in patients with acute pulmonary embolism: Observations from the PIOPED Study. *Radiology* 189:133-136, 1993.

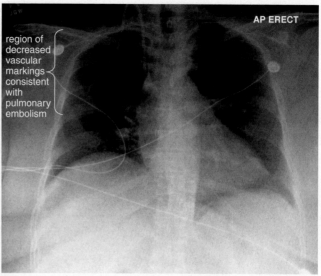

Figure 7-2. **Pulmonary embolism (PE), chest x-ray with the Westermark sign.** This 57-year-old female with ovarian cancer presented with worsening dyspnea and leg pain. She underwent ventilation–perfusion scan that was high probability for PE. Her chest x-ray shows an area in the right upper thorax with decreased pulmonary vascular markings compared with the left. This is consistent with the Westermark sign, an indication of a proximal PE blocking distal flow of blood to a lung segment. The Westermark sign is very insensitive but relatively specific, according to data from the Prospective Investigation of Pulmonary Embolism Diagnosis study. Occasionally, an abnormal region of lung parenchyma that is poorly ventilated because of bronchospasm or emphysema may have physiologic vasoconstriction, giving a similar appearance.

(Figure 7-3; see also chest x-rays in Figures 7-34, 7-38, 7-41, 7-51, and 7-52 and CT findings in Figures 7-30, 7-31, 7-32, 7-35, 7-37, 7-42, and 7-55).[7] Findings such as these should not be used to exclude or confirm PE, because they have excessively high false positive and false negative rates.

Several key points about chest x-ray bear emphasis:

- Chest x-ray abnormalities including pleural effusion, atelectasis, lung mass, and parenchymal densities can coexist with or be a consequence of PE. Chest x-ray findings must be considered carefully in the context of the patient's presentation and overall risk profile for PE. For example, a chest x-ray finding of parenchymal opacity can represent pneumonia or pulmonary infarction. In the context of fever and productive cough, the chest x-ray may provide sufficient information to diagnose pneumonia. However, in the setting of abrupt pleuritic pain and dyspnea, the same finding should be considered compatible with PE and should not prevent further testing for PE.
- No chest x-ray finding is sensitive enough to rule out PE.
- With the exception of the rare finding of oligemia (Westermark sign), no chest x-ray finding appears to be specific enough to rule in PE. If the diagnosis is seriously suspected, additional testing is warranted to confirm PE, regardless of suggestive chest x-ray findings such as Hampton's hump.
- A normal or near-normal chest x-ray is generally a prerequisite for VQ scan. As described in more detail later in this chapter, chest x-ray abnormalities often predict a nondiagnostic VQ scan, in which case CT may be a better choice.

A variety of chest x-rays from patients with pulmonary emboli are shown throughout the chapter, along with corresponding CT and VQ scans. The take-home point regarding chest x-ray is to avoid being misled by chest x-ray findings into inappropriately abandoning the hunt for pulmonary embolism in an at-risk patient.

What Modalities Can Be Used to Detect Pulmonary Embolism? How Does Pulmonary Angiography Diagnose Pulmonary Embolism?

As we discussed earlier, chest x-ray plays a limited role in the diagnosis of PE, as an embolism is not directly visible on plain x-ray. Instead, indirect or associated findings of PE may sometimes be visible, including pleural effusions and pulmonary parenchymal opacities associated with infarction. In general, these findings are neither sensitive nor specific for PE, so the major role of chest x-ray is in evaluation for other pathologic processes in the differential diagnosis. Common imaging tests for PE include VQ scan and CT pulmonary angiography, with niche roles for MRA and echocardiography in the evaluation of selected patients, as discussed later. The historical criterion standard diagnostic test was fluoroscopic pulmonary angiography (Figures 7-4 and 7-5). In this test, a catheter is inserted through a central vein and advanced through the right heart to the pulmonary artery. Contrast is injected through the catheter, filling the pulmonary arterial tree, which is then visible under fluoroscopy. A pulmonary embolus is visible as a filling defect within the stream of contrast. A fully

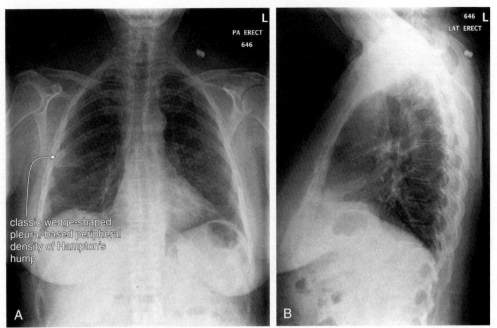

Figure 7-3. Pulmonary embolism (PE): Chest x-ray showing Hampton's hump. A, Posterior–anterior chest x-ray. **B,** Lateral chest x-ray. This 62-year-old female presented with sudden onset right pleuritic back pain awakening her at 2 AM. Her initial vital signs were pulse oximetry 96% on room air, blood pressure 153/70, heart rate 69 bpm, and temperature 38.0°C (100.4°F). This is an example of PE resulting in a peripheral wedge-shaped pleural-based infarction—Hampton's hump. Note how the density stops abruptly at the minor fissure (a pleural boundary) inferiorly. This was interpreted in the radiology report as "right axillary subsegment pneumonia, right upper lobe." Pneumonia and pulmonary infarction can appear identical on chest x-ray. Although neither sensitive nor specific for PE, Hampton's hump should be recognized as a possible finding of PE to avoid misdiagnosis of a patient with pneumonia. PE was strongly suspected in this patient because of sudden onset and recent hospitalization, and computed tomography confirmed the diagnosis (see Figure 7-32).

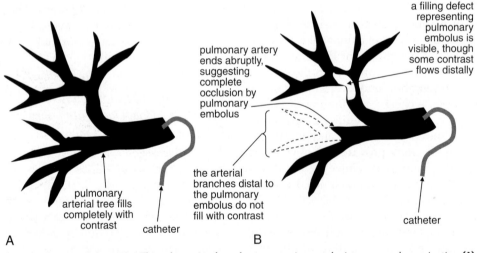

Figure 7-4. Pulmonary arteriogram: Schematic. This schematic of a pulmonary angiogram depicts a normal examination **(A)** and an examination consistent with pulmonary embolism (PE) **(B).** During pulmonary angiography, radiopaque contrast material is directly injected into the main pulmonary arteries, using a pulmonary arterial catheter. The pulmonary arterial tree is then visible under fluoroscopy. **A,** Contrast injected through a catheter in a main pulmonary artery completely fills the arterial tree, indicating that no obstructing pulmonary emboli are present. **B,** A branch of the tree does not fill (outlined here in dashed line). In addition, a filling defect in the stream of contrast is visible in another section of the arterial tree, although contrast does flow distal to the partially obstructing PE.

occlusive PE may completely block flow of contrast distally, whereas a partially occlusive thrombus or small peripheral thrombus may be subtler. As we discuss later, CT pulmonary angiography uses the same principles to detect thrombus and shares many of the advantages and pitfalls. Although pulmonary angiography is used as the "gold standard" diagnostic test in many studies

evaluating other imaging modalities, angiography is itself imperfect. Based on animal models, autopsy studies, and follow-up studies using subsequent diagnosis of PE to identify false-negative angiography results, pulmonary angiography is likely only about 87% sensitive (95% CI = 79%-93%), which as we discuss is comparable to CT sensitivity.[8-9] Pulmonary angiography is rarely

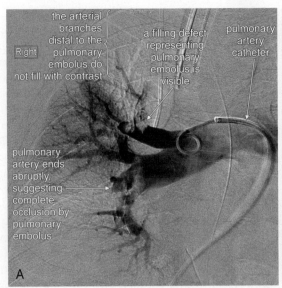
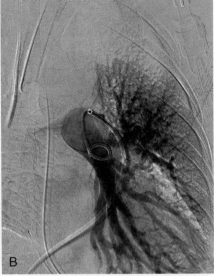

the arterial branches distal to the pulmonary embolus do not fill with contrast

a filling defect representing pulmonary embolus is visible

pulmonary artery catheter

Right

pulmonary artery ends abruptly, suggesting complete occlusion by pulmonary embolus

A

B

Figure 7-5. Pulmonary arteriogram. Pulmonary arteriography is the historical criterion standard diagnostic imaging test for pulmonary embolism—although recent studies suggest that computed tomography may be comparable in sensitivity and specificity. Today, the study is rarely performed unless other diagnostic imaging tests are inconclusive or an invasive therapy such as mechanical clot disruption or catheter thrombolysis is planned. In pulmonary angiography, a catheter is advanced through a central vein into the right heart and then into the right and left pulmonary arteries. Contrast is injected, and the pulmonary arterial tree becomes visible under fluoroscopy. Filling defects may be seen directly, or a branch of the tree may fail to fill, indicating a thrombus blocking flow of contrast to that region. **A,** The patient's right pulmonary arterial tree appears to be missing a major branch. Filling defects representing pulmonary emboli are also present. **B,** The left pulmonary arterial tree appears normal.

performed today as a primary diagnostic test for PE because of its invasive nature and morbidity.[10] Its role has largely been relegated to secondary investigation in cases in which other diagnostic modalities are inconclusive or when invasive therapy is needed for massive PE. The chapter on interventional radiologic techniques (Chapter 16) discusses pulmonary angiography in detail.

Next, we discuss the theory behind other common tests for PE, starting with CT.

CT Pulmonary Angiography

CT was independently invented in 1972 by British physicist Godfrey N. Hounsfield and American Allan M. Cormack, who in 1979 shared the Nobel Prize in medicine and physiology for their contributions.[11-15] CT was a breakthrough technology, because it allowed depiction of cross-sectional anatomy with soft-tissue detail unobtainable by conventional x-ray, discovered in 1895 by Wilhelm Roentgen.[16] The first CT scanner could accommodate only the human head and required more than 7 minutes to acquire a single image (slice). Early CT scanners used a single x-ray emitter and detector to acquire image data. Data was acquired one slice at a time, with the emitter and detector circling the patient once, and then the table moving a small distance between each image acquisition (Figure 7-6). The consequence was not only poor image resolution but also data gaps, because anatomic information between slices was unavailable. The ability of CT to diagnose subtle pathology, such as small pulmonary emboli, was limited by both resolution and data gaps. Initially CT was used to

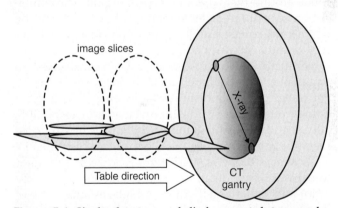

image slices

X-ray

Table direction

CT gantry

Figure 7-6. Single detector, nonhelical computed tomography. Individual slices were acquired by rotating a single, paired x-ray source and detector around the patient.

demonstrate not the PE but the infarcted lung segment, and it had a sensitivity of less than 50%.[17]

Computed Tomography Scan Characteristics
Two innovations known as "helical" and "multislice" technology improved CT image and data quality, enhancing diagnostic capability. Because of these improvements in CT technology, older studies on the diagnostic characteristics of single-slice CT do not apply to most CT scanners now in clinical use. CT scanners with helical or "spiral" capability acquire data continuously as the patient moves through the gantry (Figure 7-7). Although depending on the CT protocol some data gaps may remain, the amount of missing data is substantially reduced by this technology.[18-20] All modern scanners can acquire image data in this fashion. In the early years of

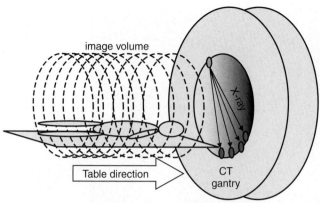

Figure 7-7. Multidetector, helical computed tomography (CT). An x-ray source and multiple x-ray detectors rotate helically around the patient to acquire a volume of image data. All modern scanners use this technology, so requesting a spiral CT for diagnosis of pulmonary embolism is not necessary. A 4-detector CT is shown, but CT scanners with 16, 32, 64, or 256 detectors are commonly available today.

CT, spiral CT for the diagnosis of PE was an important distinction, because nonhelical scanners were still in use at many institutions. Multislice CT introduces additional x-ray detectors. In scanners of this type, as the patient moves through the CT gantry, the emitter and detectors rotate around the patient in a circular path. The combination of continuous table motion and circular motion of the x-ray source and detectors results in a helical pattern of data acquisition.[21] Data is acquired as a three-dimensional volume. Slices may be reconstructed in any plane, or three-dimensional reconstructions can be generated using sophisticated software.[22-23] This technology offers substantial improvements in resolution, allowing structures less than a millimeter in size to be seen (the minimum slice thickness on most commercial CT scanners today is 0.625 mm). A tradeoff continues to exist between detail (resolution and signal-to-noise ratio) and radiation exposure. A high-resolution CT of the chest or abdomen exposes a patient to a radiation dose equivalent to approximately 400 chest x-rays.[24] A common misconception is that a higher "slice number" of a CT scanner indicates higher resolution. Instead, the slice number (4 slice, 16 slice, 64 slice, etc.) refers to the number of x-ray detectors, which determines the number of slices that can be acquired simultaneously. This is independent of the slice thickness, which determines resolution. A higher slice number does allow a body region such as the chest to be scanned more quickly, minimizing motion artifact and thus improving test performance. Chapter 8 discusses some technical aspects of CT in more detail in the context of cardiac CT.

On CT, the density of tissues is measured in Hounsfield units (HU). Air has a density of −1000 HU, water 0 HU, and bone +1000 HU. Fat, being less dense than water but denser than air, has a value of approximately −50 HU. Soft tissues such as muscle are somewhat denser than water and have an approximate value of +40 HU to +100 HU. A gray scale is then assigned spanning the range of densities, with the densest structures appearing white and the least dense appearing black. This gray scale can be shifted to accentuate tissues of interest. For example, if the user is interested in viewing details of bone, the computer reassigns the entire gray scale to values just below +1000 HU, allowing differentiation of subtle detail within bone. Detail of other structures is not visible on this setting, because all soft-tissue structures appear a fairly uniform gray whereas air remains black. If the user is interested in viewing lung detail, the gray scale is assigned to values near −1000 HU to accentuate details of low-density lung. Details of bone would be obscured on this setting, because all structures that are significantly denser than air would appear white. Most modern computerized picture archiving and communication systems (PACSs) allow the user to select from a list of useful preset variations in the gray scale, or windows. Typical window settings are lung, soft tissue (sometimes called vascular, chest–abdomen, or mediastinal), and bone. Most findings described in this chapter are seen best on soft tissue window settings, because these highlight detail of soft tissues and blood vessels. Some findings are seen best on lung windows, and these are specifically pointed out in the text and figure legends. Examples of window settings are shown in Figure 7-8.

How Does CT Pulmonary Angiography Detect Pulmonary Embolism?

As described earlier, traditional pulmonary angiography uses contrast material injected through a catheter in the main pulmonary artery to fill the pulmonary arterial tree. A filling "defect," or location where contrast fails to fill a vessel lumen, marks the presence of a PE (see Figures 7-4 and 7-5). CT pulmonary angiography relies on the same principle of filling defects in a stream of injected contrast (Figures 7-9 and 7-10). The technique can be augmented by acquiring additional CT images of the pelvis and lower extremities to assess for clot in these locations, a test called CT venography (discussed later in this chapter). Contrast material is injected, usually peripherally through a catheter in the antecubital fossa. For CT pulmonary angiography, the CT acquisition is timed in an attempt to coincide with the arrival of the contrast bolus in the pulmonary arteries, after it has first traversed veins of the upper extremity, the subclavian vein, the superior vena cava, and the right atrium and ventricle (Figure 7-11). An ideal scan is achieved with a rapid contrast bolus and perfect timing of the scan. A poor contrast bolus may fail to fill the pulmonary arteries, limiting diagnostic accuracy. A poor contrast bolus may cause either a false-negative or a false-positive result. In some cases, a vessel that is partially filled with contrast may simulate the filling defect of a PE, causing a false-positive result. More often, PEs may be missed because

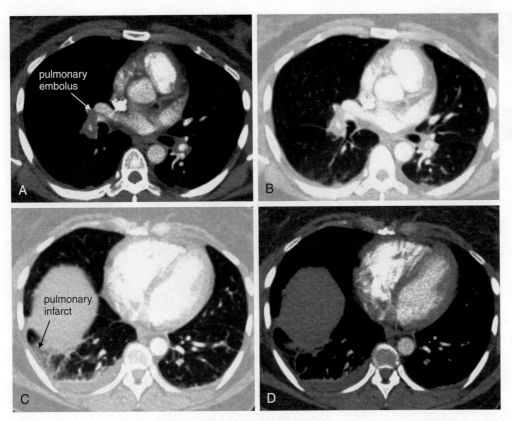

Figure 7-8. **Window settings highlight pathology: CT pulmonary angiography.** All images are from same patient with pulmonary embolism (PE) and pulmonary infarct. The PE is easily visible on soft tissue window **(A)** but not on lung window **(B)**. The parenchymal changes of the resulting infarcted lung are visible on lung window **(C)** but not on soft tissue window **(D)**. These findings are described further in later figures.

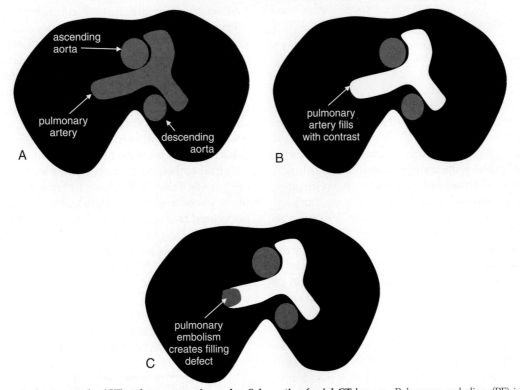

Figure 7-9. **Computed tomography (CT) pulmonary angiography: Schematic of axial CT images.** Pulmonary embolism (PE) is detected on CT scan by rapid injection of contrast. The dense contrast fills the pulmonary arteries, except where PE creates a "filling defect." Filling defects in the central pulmonary arteries are relatively easy to recognize, whereas distal branch vessels can be more difficult to evaluate because of their small size. Noncontrast CT is not useful for detection of PE, because liquid blood and thrombus share the same soft-tissue density. **A,** Noncontrast CT shows the aorta and main pulmonary artery filled with liquid blood, which has a dark gray appearance. **B,** Contrast has been injected, and the main pulmonary artery fills completely with contrast, eliminating the possibility of a thrombus in this location. **C,** A filling defect is present, where no contrast has filled the right pulmonary artery because of the presence of thrombus—a PE. Thrombi can have almost any shape, from irregular "blobs" to well-formed casts of the vessels from which they originate. It is common for some contrast to flow around thrombi, although in some cases they fully occlude the vessel in which they come to rest.

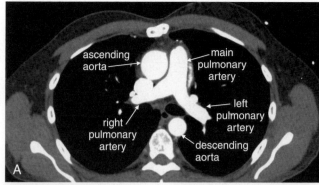

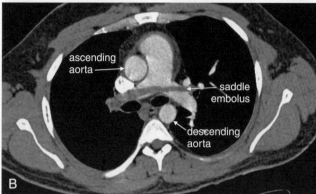

Figure 7-10. Computed tomography (CT) pulmonary angiography: Axial images. Compare these images with the schematic in Figure 7-9. **A,** A normal pulmonary artery fills completely with contrast. There are no filling defects to suggest pulmonary embolus. **B,** The stream of contrast is interrupted by a filling defect. This fully obstructs the right pulmonary artery and crosses through the left pulmonary artery—a "saddle" pulmonary embolus. An unenhanced CT cannot be used to identify pulmonary emboli, as the densities of thrombus and liquid blood are nearly identical without the use of injected contrast (see Figure 7-12).

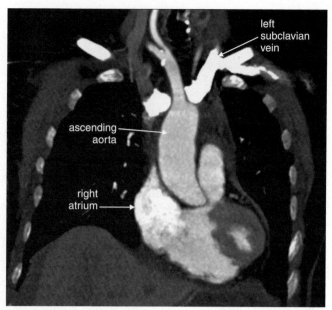

Figure 7-11. Contrast timing for computed tomography (CT) pulmonary angiography. Coronal CT image, demonstrating the effect of contrast timing on scan quality. In this patient, a contrast bolus (white) is present in the left subclavian vein and has reached the right atrium. The ascending aorta is not as well opacified with contrast. An optimal scan for aortic pathology or pulmonary embolism is timed so that the contrast bolus is in the vessel of interest at the time of the scan.

they are not visible unless surrounded by a bright bolus of contrast (Figure 7-12) (a noncontrast chest CT is therefore not useful to assess for PE). A poorly timed scan may result in an image in which the pulmonary arteries are poorly opacified with contrast, because the contrast bolus has not yet reached or has already passed through the pulmonary arteries. Today, automated bolus tracking software improves the timing of the bolus. A technician injects a small test bolus of contrast, and CT images at the level of the main pulmonary artery are acquired over a few seconds. Enhancement of the pulmonary artery is measured over this time interval, allowing selection of the optimal timing of the full contrast injection and complete CT scan (see Fig. 7-12).

Small-caliber catheters and distally placed catheters (in the hand, wrist, or forearm) may result in a suboptimal contrast bolus and a nondiagnostic scan. A discussion of flow rates through peripheral catheters is given in Chapter 4 in the context of cervical CT angiography. An optimal contrast bolus requires an automated pressure injector, with an injection rate of around 4 to 5 mL per second. Phantom studies show that peripheral catheters as small as 20 gauge allow adequate contrast injection

rates without exceeding safe pressure limits.[25] Many institutions bar the use of central venous catheters with power injectors because of theoretical concerns of embolization of catheter fragments. Embolization has also been described with peripheral venous catheters, but this appears to be a much rarer event.[26] Embolization occurs because of mechanical fragmentation of a catheter subjected to high pressures. Central venous catheters may be subject to fragmentation more than are peripheral catheters because of their length, which causes a linear increase in resistance to flow. In addition, a central catheter's tip usually lies in the superior vena cava, with little obstruction to embolization of a fragment. In contrast, a peripheral catheter fragment may be prevented from embolizing because of valves in peripheral veins. Despite these concerns, a number of studies suggest that pressure injection through central venous catheters is safe.[27-29] Some newer permanent and emergency devices are designed for high-pressure, rapid infusion. Examples include PowerPort and PowerLine, Bard Access Systems, which can tolerate 300 psi with a 5 mL per second maximum infusion rate (information from the manufacturer's website).

What Are the Diagnostic Findings of Pulmonary Embolism on CT Pulmonary Angiography?

Large pulmonary emboli may be recognized easily by familiarity with a few basic points. Box 7-2 outlines a simple approach to CT interpretation for PE. Figures 7-9 and 7-10 depict classic findings of PE on CT scan. On CT, a normal pulmonary artery fills with contrast and appears bright white when viewed with soft-tissue windows. A PE within the vessel displaces contrast, creating a filling defect, which appears as a dark gray region within the vessel. The majority of pulmonary emboli occur within a few bifurcations of the main pulmonary artery, so inspection of the central pulmonary arteries may allow detection of PE in many cases. In one study, 51% of pulmonary emboli were found in central or lobar vessels, and 27% were in segmental vessels. In only 22% were isolated subsegmental vessels involved.[30] More distal vessel branches may be more difficult to interpret because of their small size and the quality of the contrast bolus. Start your interpretation with inspection of the main pulmonary artery and its branches, because emboli in this location are both common and easily recognized (Figures 7-13 through 7-28). Inspect for saddle pulmonary emboli

(see Figures 7-10, 7-13, and 7-15) and right atrial and ventricular abnormalities (see Figures 7-16 and 7-17).

Several additional pieces of information may be helpful in the evaluation of the scan. First, pulmonary emboli are more common in vessels in lower lung segments (58% of cases), and these should be carefully inspected.[30]

Second, many pulmonary emboli do not completely obstruct the vessel, and a characteristic appearance of contrast leaking around the embolus is often seen (Figures 7-23 through 7-28).[30] A possible pulmonary embolus seen on one axial image should be tracked through multiple adjacent images to confirm or refute the finding (Figures 7-22 and 7-29; see also Figure 7-36). Coronal and sagittal plane images can also assist in this evaluation (see Figures 7-25 and 7-27).

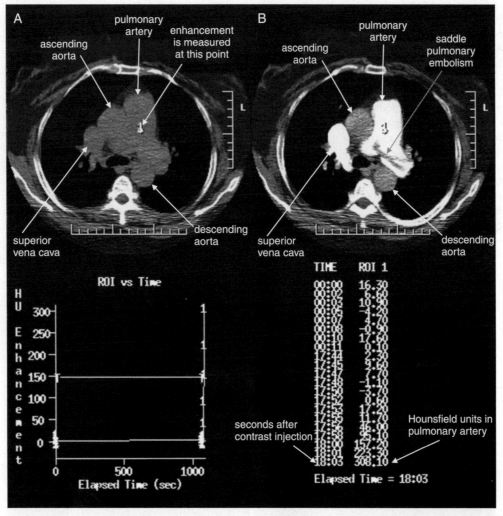

Figure 7-12. **Contrast timing for computed tomography (CT) pulmonary angiography.** This image dramatically displays why contrast is essential for the detection of pulmonary embolism (PE) and why timing of contrast is critical. **A,** No contrast has been given, and the pulmonary artery appears uniform. **B,** Contrast fills the pulmonary artery, and a huge saddle PE becomes visible. Automated contrast bolus tracking software is used to determine the optimal timing of the CT image acquisition, relative to the moment of contrast injection. A small test bolus of contrast is injected, and the intensity of enhancement in the pulmonary artery is measured over several seconds. In the bottom half of the figure, the software displays a graph and table of the Hounsfield unit enhancement versus time. The full CT scan is then performed using the time interval that produced the desired degree of enhancement. Studies in the radiology literature have clarified the degree of enhancement needed for a diagnostic scan.

Third, inspection of lung windows may aid in the detection of PE. As stated earlier, selecting lung windows simply refers to picking a default setting on a PACS that shifts the CT gray scale to accentuate the fine detail of low-density tissues such as lung. On lung

window settings, parenchymal abnormalities such as linear atelectasis and wedge-shaped peripheral opacities (representing infarcts) may be visible. Figures 7-30 through 7-42 demonstrate these CT lung window abnormalities, as well as the corresponding CT soft tissue window and chest x-ray findings. Once a parenchymal abnormality is noted on lung windows, the viewer should return to soft tissue window settings, where inspection of the vessels leading to the abnormal lung segment may reveal a PE. This step is necessary to differentiate pulmonary infarct, because a parenchymal density may also represent pneumonia or mass. Pleural effusions may be helpful in detection of a PE by pointing to a lung region of concern, but they are equally common in patients with and without PE, and their presence should not be interpreted as confirming PE.[30]

False-positive and false-negative CT pulmonary angiography results may occur due a number of factors. A poor contrast bolus may not opacify the pulmonary arteries sufficiently to allow the filling defect of a pulmonary embolus to be recognized. Ironically, a very dense contrast bolus can also lead to misdiagnosis because of streak artifact that can obscure thrombus (see Figures 7-21, 7-36, and 7-47). A slow scanner or an extremely tachypneic patient may result in a false-negative or nondiagnostic scan because of excessive motion artifact. Lymph nodes immediately adjacent to blood vessels appear dark gray and may be mistaken for pulmonary emboli by inexperienced readers. A blood vessel compressed by an adjacent structure such as a lymph node, airway, or mass may have an irregular contour that may be mistaken for the filling defect of a PE. Extremely obese patients may have poor-quality scans resulting from

---

Box 7-2: Algorithm for Interpreting CT for Pulmonary Embolism

1. **Choose soft tissue or vascular window setting. Some PACS systems have preset vascular windows. These alter the normal soft tissue window to decrease bloom artifact caused by the contrast bolus.**
2. **Assess contrast bolus quality.**
3. **Assess for motion artifact.**
4. **Locate the main pulmonary artery, and inspect for saddle embolism.**
5. **Moving cephalad or caudad, inspect each large-order vessel for emboli.**
   Pearls for Pulmonary Embolism
- **Look for more PEs in caudad vessels.**
- **Look for contrast leak around embolism.**
- **Use the patient's pain location as an aid.**
- **Check lung windows for evidence of pulmonary infarction.**
   Pitfalls for Pulmonary Embolism
- **Motion gives a false negative or positive.**
- **Tachypnea gives a false negative or positive.**
- **A slow scanner gives a false negative or positive.**
- **An obese patient gives a false negative or positive.**
- **Poor bolus gives a false negative or positive.**
- **Lymph nodes give a false positive.**
- **External compression gives a false positive.[30]**

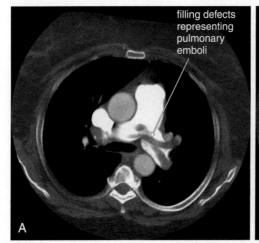 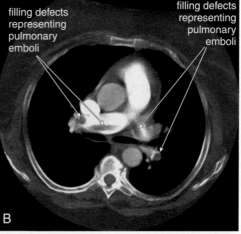

Figure 7-13. Pulmonary embolism (PE): Saddle embolus on CT pulmonary angiography. The main pulmonary arteries are a simple place to start when interpreting computed tomography (CT) for PE, as the anatomy is easily recognized and large clots are readily seen. **A, B,** Two axial CT images through the level of the main pulmonary artery. This 66-year-old female with a previous history of PE became short of breath while grocery shopping. Her vital signs were stable on emergency department arrival (blood pressure 143/75, heart rate 109 bpm, oxygen saturation 100% on 2 L). Her CT shows a remarkable saddle PE, with perfectly formed casts of the vessels from which the clots originated. Some of these are seen in long axis and have a tubular shape. Others are seen in cross section and appear circular.

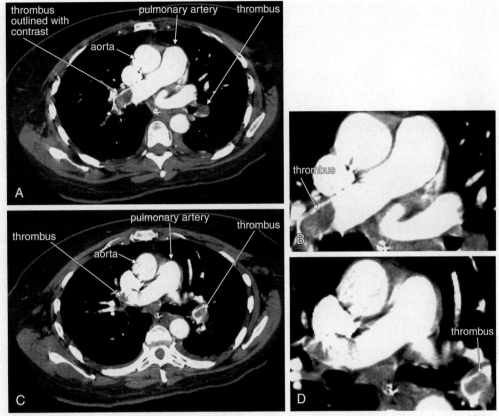

Figure 7-14. Pulmonary embolism: Multiple and bilateral emboli on CT pulmonary angiography. This 51-year-old female with metastatic ovarian cancer presented with dyspnea and pleuritic chest pain. A large filling defect is present in the right main pulmonary artery, surrounded by a thin stream of contrast. A large thrombus is also visible in a branch of the left pulmonary artery, again surrounded by contrast. **A, C,** Axial computed tomography images. **B,** Close-up from **A. D,** Close-up from **C.**

underpenetration of radiation.[30] Intentional inspiration and "breath hold" immediately before CT acquisition can introduce an artifact leading to false-positive interpretation by the following mechanism. With slower CT scanners, the patient is often instructed to take a deep breath and then to stop breathing during the scan to reduce motion artifact. Deep inspiration results in a sudden decrease in intrathoracic pressure, pulling noncontrasted blood into the right heart from the inferior vena cava. This can result in indeterminate or false-positive interpretation in a minority of cases, because the noncontrasted blood (which appears dark gray) may be mistaken for the filling defect of a PE.[31] Ironically, faster scanners might worsen this artifact if deep inspiration is encouraged, because the entire CT acquisition occurs rapidly during the peak of the effect of inspiration.

Do CT Findings Predict Acute Morbidity and Mortality from Pulmonary Embolism?

A number of scoring systems have been proposed for severity of PE by CT. Surprisingly, saddle PE does not predict high mortality.[32] CT can detect physiologic consequences of massive PE such as right ventricular dilatation, ventricular septal bowing, and decreased size of the left atrium and pulmonary veins from decreased pulmonary venous return.[33-35] To date, studies are equivocal, with some suggesting that CT evidence of right ventricular dysfunction may predict morbidity and mortality and thus might be a criterion for aggressive therapy using interventional radiologic techniques, which are described in detail in Chapter 16.[36-38]

CT Pulmonary Angiography Sensitivity: When Is a Negative Scan Enough?

Although many measures of CT sensitivity can be considered, let's start with two summary statements:

1. A normal CT predicts a very low risk for PE in patients with low to moderate pretest probability.
2. When very high clinical suspicion exists for PE, additional imaging is warranted following a negative CT pulmonary angiogram.

Later, we review the evidence for these statements.

CT as a diagnostic test for PE was attempted as early as 1978, but early attempts offered poor resolution, sensitivity, and specificity. This resulted from the use of single-slice, nonhelical technology. Because images were acquired at large distance intervals and with relatively

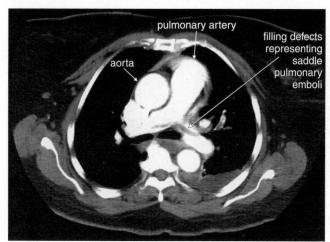

Figure 7-15. **Pulmonary embolism (PE): Saddle embolus with enlarged right ventricle on CT pulmonary angiography.** This 73-year-old female had recently undergone total knee arthroplasty when she experienced syncope and was found to have a systolic blood pressure of 80 mm Hg with tachycardia and hypoxia to 80% on room air. Her CT shows a large saddle PE. The patient underwent pulmonary angiography (see Figure 7-5) and thrombectomy. Her CT also showed right ventricular enlargement (See Figure 7-16).

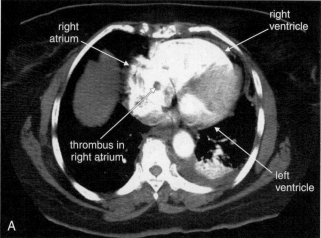

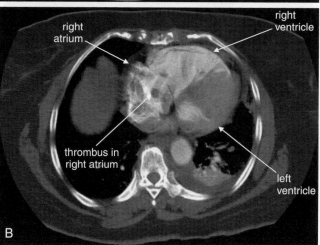

Figure 7-16. **Pulmonary embolism (PE): Saddle embolus with enlarged right ventricle on CT pulmonary angiography.** Same patient as Figure 7-15. Her CT showed a large saddle PE (prior figure). In addition, sections through the right atrium and ventricle showed enlargement of these chambers and filling defects suggesting thrombus in these chambers. Note the tubular and rounded cross sections, which could correspond to thrombus casts of lower extremity veins. **A, B,** Same slice with window settings adjusted to highlight clot and cardiac chamber anatomy.

thick slices, small pulmonary emboli were undetectable. Image acquisition speed was slow, resulting in motion artifact during respiration.[17,39] By the late 1990s, studies of CT using single-slice helical scanning began to report CT sensitivity of 87% to 91% with specificity of 78% to 98%, which compared favorably with the alternative diagnostic tests, VQ scan and pulmonary angiography.[40-41] By 2002 to 2005, reports emerged of modern helical multislice scans offering superior image resolution with visualization of subsegmental pulmonary arteries, limited gaps in data, and rapid scan acquisition, eliminating respiratory and cardiac motion artifact.[42-43] For these reasons, when evaluating studies on the sensitivity and other test characteristics of CT for PE, it is important to determine whether modern CT equipment was used in the study. Although CT remains a limited test, it uses the same basic principles as traditional pulmonary angiography as described earlier, and the test characteristics of the two modalities have converged as CT technology has continued to improve. The most current studies of CT show high sensitivity and specificity when compared with pulmonary angiography. Questions have begun to arise about the proper criterion diagnostic standard when comparing the two techniques, because pulmonary angiography itself is subject to false positives and false negatives.[8]

Before examining the evidence in detail, let's reexamine our goal in performing diagnostic imaging for detection of PE. CT accuracy can be evaluated using two general strategies. The first is a "disease-oriented outcome" standard, meaning the presence or absence of PE, as detected by some reference test and compared with CT. The second is a "patient-oriented outcome" standard, based on the clinical outcome (morbidity or mortality) for a patient with a normal CT scan who is not treated with anticoagulation. The second may be the more important standard, because our primary goal as emergency physicians is to prevent morbidity and mortality.

Literally hundreds of published articles exist on the topic of CT for PE; a PubMed search using the terms "CT," "pulmonary," and "angiography" found 1679 matches with more studies published each day. (The author performed that first search on March 8, 2010, but by March 21, 2011 the number of PubMed matches had grown to 2025). Here, we consider a few of the key studies underlying our understanding of CT sensitivity and specificity. Early studies of single-detector CT were haunted by questions of undetected subsegmental pulmonary emboli with possible significant patient morbidity and mortality resulting from undiagnosed and untreated

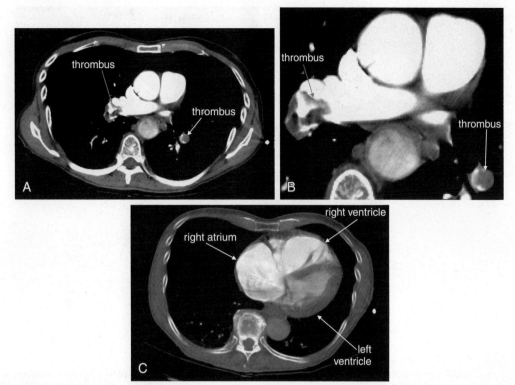

Figure 7-17. **Pulmonary embolism: Large bilateral PE with right ventricular enlargement on CT pulmonary angiography and echocardiogram.** This 79-year-old male with a history of pancreatic cancer experienced sudden dyspnea and presyncope while in the shower. Paramedics found the patient to be hypoxic to 80% oxygen saturation on room air with a systolic blood pressure of 80 mm Hg. The patient was noted to have bilateral large pulmonary emboli on CT (**A; B,** close-up). In addition, the right atrium and ventricle were noted to be dilated **(C),** concerning for right heart strain. This was confirmed on echocardiogram. **C,** The CT window has been adjusted to allow the internal structure of the heart to be better appreciated—the setting is closer to a normal bone window. Note the massive right atrium. The right ventricle is as large as the left.

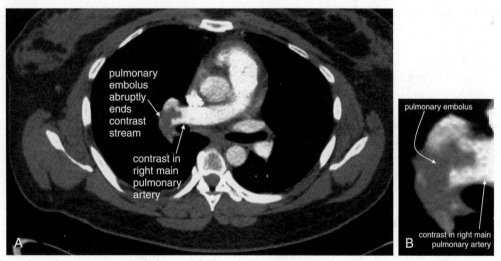

Figure 7-18. **Right main pulmonary artery embolus: Axial CT pulmonary angiography image. A,** A filling defect representing a pulmonary embolus obstructs contrast flow in the right main pulmonary artery. **B,** Close-up.

thrombus. However, new studies of multidetector CT demonstrate the ability to image subsegmental pulmonary arteries. Most importantly, patient outcomes after negative CT are similar to those after negative traditional pulmonary angiography. A 2005 review found that the incidence of PE 6 to 12 months after negative traditional pulmonary angiography was approximately 1.6%, whereas a negative CT pulmonary angiogram carried a

1.3% average incidence of VTE. Exceptions to this may include patients with symptoms of deep venous thrombosis (DVT), in whom further evaluation may be warranted if CT pulmonary angiography is negative.[8] To be fair, these outcome numbers are influenced not only by the sensitivity of the two tests, but also by the risk profile of the patient populations being tested. Patients subjected to formal pulmonary angiography are typically at

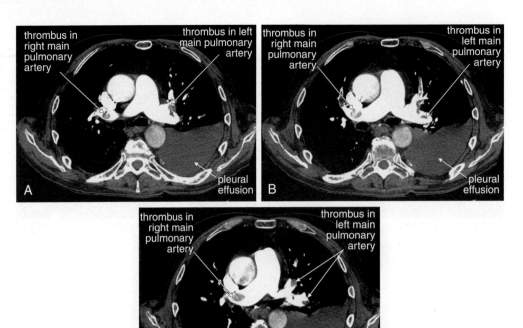

Figure 7-19. Pulmonary embolism: Emboli in main pulmonary arteries on CT pulmonary angiography. This 68-year-old male with esophageal cancer presented with an acute syncope episode and less acutely worsening dyspnea. **A** to **C,** Consecutive axial images through the level of the main pulmonary artery. These computed tomography slices show multiple filling defects characteristic of pulmonary emboli. Although these appear somehow suspended in the middle of the lumen of the pulmonary artery, remember that you are looking at individual slices through a larger three-dimensional structure. The thrombus may be caught on a vessel bifurcation and dangling like a streamer in the current. Learn the appearance of these large main pulmonary artery clots. These are easiest to recognize, but peripheral clots share the same features. These thrombi are dark filling voids within a contrast-filled vessel. They are not fully occlusive, more like pieces of Jell-O than like a cork in a wine bottle. It is common to see contrast outlining the margins of a thrombus. This will help you confirm that the filling defect is within the vessel, not outside of a vessel that is leaving the plane of the image.

high risk (high pretest probability) of PE, warranting the use of an invasive test for evaluation. Thus a low rate of PE following a negative angiogram in this population is impressive, reflecting high test sensitivity. In contrast, patients undergoing CT pulmonary angiography have a low overall risk of PE, so good outcomes following normal CT pulmonary angiography are as much a measure of the low pretest probability of disease as of the test's sensitivity. We will consider this issue in more detail in the discussion to come.

Outcome Studies Following Negative CT Pulmonary Angiography

A systematic review and meta-analysis (including both single and multidetector CT) published in *JAMA* in 2005[44] found that the likelihood ratio negative for PE following a negative chest CT was 0.07 (95% CI = 0.05-0.11). The likelihood ratio negative for mortality attributable to PE was 0.01 (95% CI = 0.01-0.02) at follow-up of 3 to 12 months. These values are similar to those reported for conventional pulmonary angiography. Other investigators have also reported good clinical outcomes (98% or greater survival without venous thromboembolic disease) in the 6 months after a negative chest CT, without additional DVT testing.[45] The Christopher Study, a prospective multicenter study of 3306 patients published in *JAMA* in 2006,[46] examined VTE outcomes in patients

with negative chest CT who were not anticoagulated. The 3-month rate of VTE was only 1.3% (95% CI = 0.7%-2.0%), with a mortality rate of 0.5% (95% CI = 0.2%-1.0%). A 2009 meta-analysis[47] found a similar 3-month incidence of VTE (1.2%, 95% CI = 0.8%-1.8%) following normal CT pulmonary angiography and conventional pulmonary angiography (1.7%, 95% CI = 1.0%-2.7%). Fatal pulmonary emboli were rare in the 3 months following a normal CT, occurring in 0.6%. The authors also evaluated the incremental safety provided by performing bilateral compression ultrasound to evaluate for DVT but found no statistically significant difference in 3-month risk for PE or fatal PE with this additional testing strategy.

In *JAMA* in 2007, Anderson et al.[48] reported a randomized, controlled, single-blinded noninferiority trial comparing CT and VQ scan to assess the safety of CT as an initial test for acute PE. The study examined a high-risk population of 1417 patients, all with a Wells score of 4.5 or greater or positive D-dimer results. Patients were randomized to assessment with either VQ scan or CT scan. Initial diagnosis with PE was made for 19.2% of patients in the CT group and 14.2% of patients in the VQ scan group. Patients with negative imaging results did not receive anticoagulation and were followed for 3 months to determine the interval development of either PE or proximal DVT. Only 0.4% of patients with negative

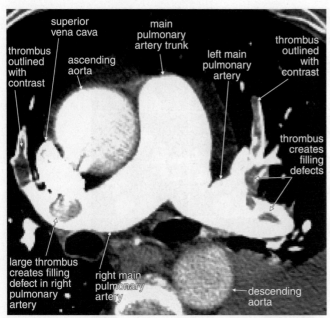

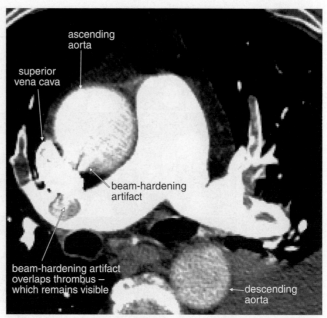

Figure 7-20. Pulmonary embolism in main pulmonary arteries on CT pulmonary angiography. Same patient as Figure 7-19. Look in closer detail at the main pulmonary artery, which is nicely seen with both major branches in this image. In the right main pulmonary artery, a large thrombus is visible. Just distal to this, the artery curves anteriorly and another thrombus is seen, outlined with a thin ribbon of contrast on each side. This is called "railroad tracking" and is a common feature of pulmonary emboli. In the left main pulmonary artery, a strand of thrombus is caught at a major bifurcation. The embolus winds in and out of the plane of the image and appears as several filling defects. Inspection of adjacent image slices would prove these to be part of the same long segment of clot. Again, railroad tracking surrounds the anterior portion of the clot.

Figure 7-21. Artifacts on CT pulmonary angiography. Same patient as Figure 7-20. Look in closer detail at the main pulmonary artery and its neighboring structures. The superior vena cava is visible as a bright kidney bean shape. It is so bright because of the continued injection of intravenous contrast that it is creating "beam-hardening artifact," which produces a sunburst pattern emanating from the superior vena cava. This sunburst is slightly overlapping the adjacent structures, interfering with their visualization. The pulmonary artery is well opacified with contrast, which has traveled through the superior vena cava, mixed with blood in the right atrium, and then been ejected by the right ventricle into the main pulmonary trunk and its branches. A moderate amount of contrast fills the ascending aorta, while less has reached the descending aorta. For the purposes of this imaging study, which seeks to evaluate filling defects in the pulmonary arteries, this is fine—but this would be a suboptimal study for evaluation of aortic dissection.

initial CT scan results and 1.0% of those with negative VQ scan results developed thromboembolism during the follow-up, with no statistical difference between the two groups. This study offers strong evidence that either CT scan or VQ scan is a safe initial approach to rule out PE in the emergency department, with a negative predictive value of 99%.

You may recall that negative predictive values are subject to variation depending on the rate of disease in the study population and are relatively discouraged as a reported measure of a test's accuracy for this reason. Consider the extreme example of a test that is always negative for PE and therefore has a sensitivity of 0%. If used in a study population consisting of 99 patients without PE and 1 patient with PE, the test would have a 99% negative predictive value, because only a single patient has the disease. Then, why should we accept a negative predictive value in Anderson et al.'s study? This study examined a high-risk population, with an overall rate of PE of 16.5%. This is likely a higher rate of thromboembolic disease than would occur in most emergency department cohorts being evaluated, so the test likely will perform with a similarly high negative predictive value in our patients. Consider how our hypothetical 0% sensitivity test would perform in this

population. It would fail to identify all patients with PE (16.5%), so the negative predictive value would be only 83.5%. Anderson et al.'s study[48] suggests that both VQ and CT perform well in sorting from a high-risk population those patients who can safely avoid anticoagulation. The authors point out that CT diagnosed more patients with PE than did VQ scan, yet those with negative CT or VQ fared equally well without anticoagulation. This implies that some of those diagnosed with PE by CT scan either did not really have the disease or did not require anticoagulation therapy for it. Overdiagnosis of PE remains a potential concern with CT scan, as this may subject patients to unnecessary anticoagulation.

CT, VQ scan, and Likelihood Ratios: Altering Pretest Odds With a Negative Diagnostic Imaging Test. Another measure of test diagnostic accuracy is likelihood ratio. Two likelihood ratios can be calculated for every test, based on the test's sensitivity and specificity. The likelihood ratio positive (LR+) is the probability of a person who has the disease in question testing positive divided by the probability of a person who does not have the disease testing positive. This is

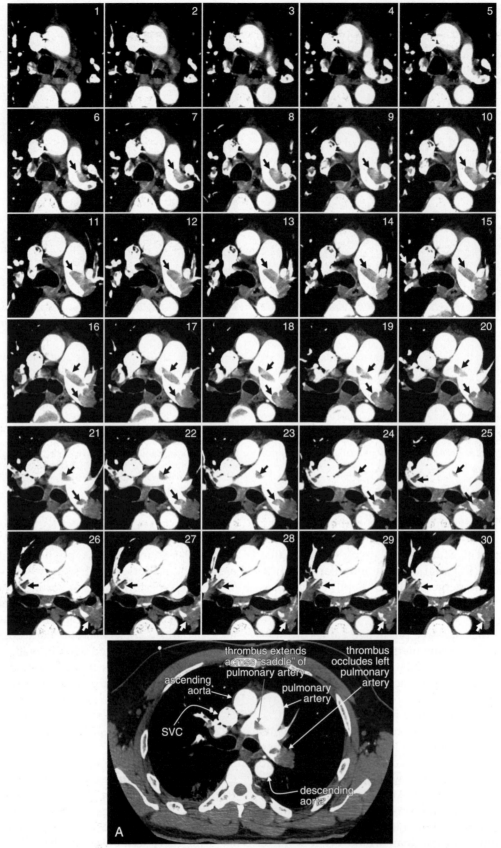

Figure 7-22. Pulmonary embolism (PE) in bilateral main pulmonary arteries on CT pulmonary angiography. This 50-year-old female developed acute dyspnea, pleuritic right chest pain, and syncope after a 3-day prodrome of left leg pain. A single image complete image **(A)** is shown for orientation, which is the same as usual for CT (patient's right is on left side of image). Coned-in views of the main pulmonary artery are also shown to allow you to follow the thrombus from slice to slice. The close-up corresponding to the complete computed tomography slice is number **21.** Although it cannot be seen in its entirety in a single slice, a saddle PE occludes much of the left pulmonary artery and extends across to the right. *Arrows* point out the thrombus in some images.

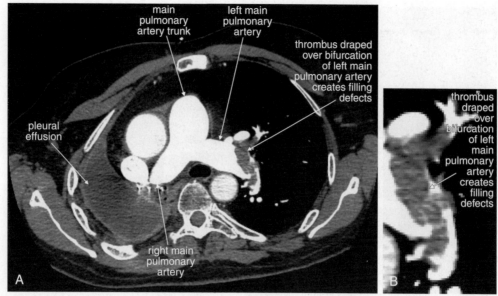

Figure 7-23. Pulmonary embolism in left main pulmonary artery on CT pulmonary angiography. This 58-year-old male with metastatic lung cancer presented with acute chest tightness and dyspnea. The patient described himself as "gasping for air." Again, a large central pulmonary embolus is seen as a filling defect, lodged at a bifurcation of the left main pulmonary artery. **B,** Close-up.

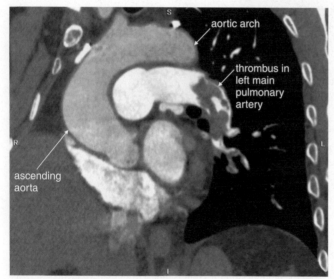

Figure 7-24. Pulmonary embolism (PE) in left main pulmonary artery on CT pulmonary angiography. Same patient as Figure 7-23. Some institutions routinely perform multiplanar reconstructions to further characterize PE. In equivocal cases, these may help to delineate true thrombus from various artifacts. In this patient, the diagnosis of PE is unequivocal, but additional reconstructions are shown to illustrate their capabilities. This oblique coronal view shows the left pulmonary artery, filled with an amorphous clot. As in other figures, the clot is seen to partially occlude the vessel with a thin rim of surrounding contrast.

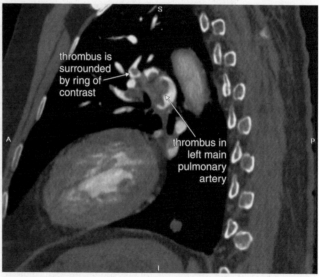

Figure 7-25. Pulmonary embolism (PE) in left main pulmonary artery on CT pulmonary angiography, sagittal view. Same patient as Figure 7-24. This sagittal view shows the left pulmonary artery, again with clot partially occluding the vessel. A circular rim of contrast surrounds the clot in some locations. This is a common appearance that should be recognized.

also mathematically represented as LR+ = sensitivity/(1-specificity). The likelihood ratio negative (LR-) is the probability of a person who has the disease in question testing negative divided by the probability of a person who does not have the disease testing negative. It is mathematically represented by LR− = (1-sensitivity)/specificity. The pretest odds of the diagnosis multiplied by the appropriate likelihood ratio determines the post-test odds. Odds and probability can be mathematically interconverted. Although the pretest odds cannot be specifically determined for an individual patient, it can be estimated by the physician based on factors such as the overall prevalence of disease in a given emergency department and the given patient's similarity to the overall population (e.g., more at risk or less at risk than an average patient). A likelihood ratio positive greater than 10 strongly increases disease probability, effectively ruling in disease for all but the lowest-risk patients. A likelihood ratio negative less than 0.1 strongly decreases disease probability, effectively ruling out disease in all

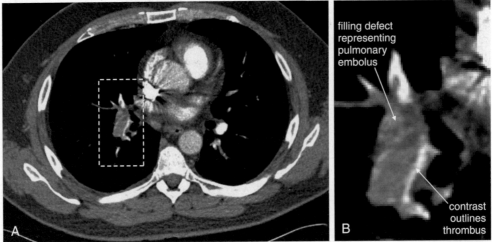

Figure 7-26. Railroad track sign of pulmonary embolism: Axial CT pulmonary angiography images. Pulmonary emboli often do not fully occlude a vessel. Contrast may be seen leaking around the periphery of a thrombus, helping to identify a true filling defect within a pulmonary artery. **A,** A filling defect representing a pulmonary embolus obstructs contrast flow in a segmental pulmonary artery. Contrast can be seen leaking around the thrombus, sometimes called the railroad track sign. **B,** Close-up.

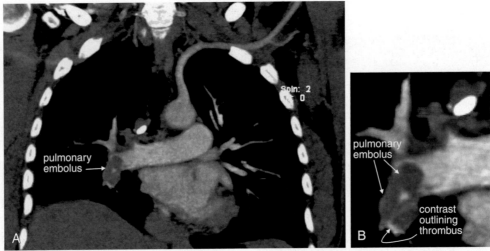

Figure 7-27. Right main pulmonary artery embolus: Coronal CT pulmonary angiography image. A, Coronal view of the same patient as in Figure 7-26. Multiplanar images can clarify the diagnosis when a filling defect is suspected on axial images. Sometimes the additional images will reveal the suspected thrombus to be a structure outside the blood vessel—for example, an adjacent lymph node. Here, a filling defect representing a pulmonary embolus obstructs contrast flow in the right main pulmonary artery. Contrast can be seen leaking around and through the thrombus, a variation of the railroad track sign. **B,** Close-up. The window setting has been adjusted to decrease the brightness of the contrast bolus from that seen with soft tissue windows. Excessively bright contrast can create "bloom artifact" that obscures adjacent tissues including thrombus. Bone windows minimize this effect while allowing evaluation of contrast-filled vascular structures. Some PACS interfaces have preset optimized "vascular window" settings. Others allow the user to adjust and then save window settings.

but the highest-risk patients. Given this background, what are the LR+ and LR− values for CT pulmonary angiography and VQ scan (a test for pulmonary embolism discussed later in this chapter)?

Roy et al.[49] performed a systematic review and meta-analysis of strategies for diagnosis of acute PE, published in *BMJ* in 2005. The authors provide likelihood ratios for CT and VQ scan, which are useful in our clinical decisions. Positive likelihood ratios were as follows: "high probability" VQ scan was 18.3 (95% CI = 10.3-32.5), CT was 24.1 (95% CI = 12.4-46.7), and lower extremity venous ultrasound was 16.2 (95% CI = 5.6-46.7). Because positive likelihood ratios greater than 10 are generally considered to be helpful in ruling in a disease process, all three diagnostic strategies could be considered confirmatory if positive in a patient with a moderate or high pretest probability of PE. Negative likelihood ratios were as follows: normal or near-normal VQ scan was 0.05 (95% CI = 0.03-0.10), and negative CT plus negative lower extremity ultrasound was 0.04 (95% CI = 0.03-0.06). Because a test with a likelihood ratio negative less than 0.1 is considered to provide strong evidence against a disease process, a normal VQ or CT plus ultrasound can be used to rule out PE in all but the highest-risk patients.[49] The authors

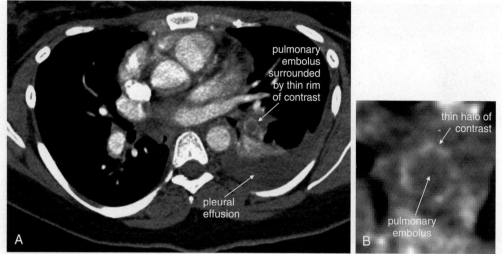

Figure 7-28. Segmental pulmonary embolism, CT pulmonary angiography. A, A filling defect representing a pulmonary embolus is visible in a segmental artery to the left lower lung segment. Contrast leaking around the thrombus is visible as a white halo around the thrombus, which appears as a dark circle in cross section. A pleural effusion is also present (dark gray "fluid density" on soft tissue windows). **B,** Close-up.

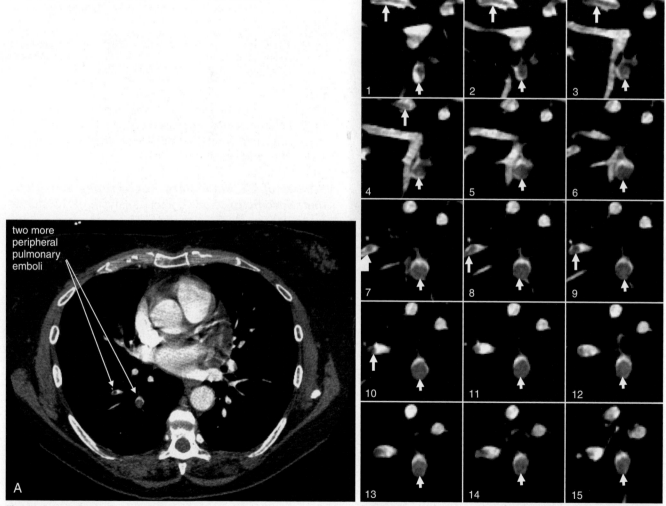

Figure 7-29. Pulmonary embolism, multilobar, seen with CT pulmonary angiography. This 54-year-old woman with recurrent ovarian cancer presented with progressive dyspnea over a 2-week period. The patient has pulmonary emboli involving more distal branches of the pulmonary arteries than those that we have considered previously. A single complete slice **(A)** is shown to illustrate one of the affected vessels in context. The series of coned-in images then tracks that vessel through the adjacent slices. The close-up corresponding to the full slice is number **9.** Some vessels are seen in short-axis cross section and have a circular appearance with circular clot. Other vessels are seen in long-axis cross section and contain clot that appears linear. *Arrows* have been placed to assist you in following a vessel and thrombus through multiple slices.

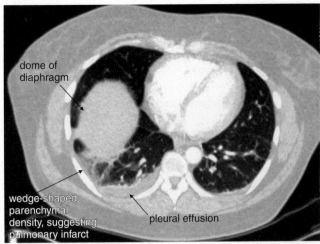

Figure 7-30. **Pulmonary infarction: Axial computed tomography (CT) image.** CT lung window in a patient with pulmonary embolism. A wedge-shaped, peripheral, pleural-based parenchymal density is visible in the right lung. This is the CT correlate of the classic x-ray finding, Hampton's hump. An adjacent pleural effusion is present. The dome of the liver is visible, because this is a slice through the lower thorax. Although the lung window can suggest pulmonary infarct, the appearance is also consistent with pneumonia, so the soft tissue window must be inspected to identify thrombus in a vessel supplying that lung region. The clot causing a parenchymal infarct may not be visible on the same slice, so inspect all slices.

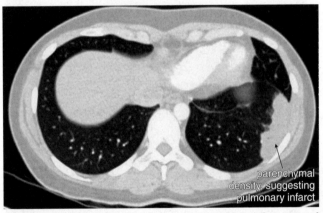

Figure 7-31. **Pulmonary infarction, subacute: Axial computed tomography (CT) image.** A CT lung window demonstrates a peripheral, pleural-based density in the left lung—the CT analogue of Hampton's hump. This patient presented nearly 1 month after an acute episode of pleuritic chest pain and dyspnea after an airplane trip. No filling defect was visible on any of the soft tissue window slices, presumably because of spontaneous lysis of a pulmonary embolus. In the right clinical context, this finding is compatible with pulmonary infarct from pulmonary embolus—but pneumonia or mass lesions can give a similar CT appearance, so inspection of the soft tissue window remains important.

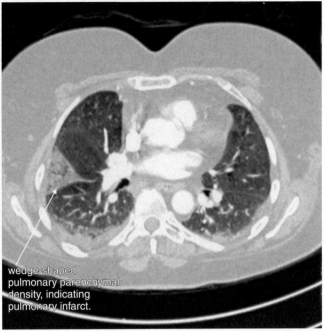

Figure 7-32. **Pulmonary embolism (PE): Hampton's hump.** Computed tomography scan from the patient in Figure 7-3. A lung window demonstrates the same wedge-shaped peripheral density seen on the patient's chest x-ray. This pulmonary infarct is in the watershed of the pulmonary artery obstructed by thrombus, a PE. Soft-tissue windows showing the PE are reviewed in Figure 7-33.

patients, a "low probability" VQ scan does not rule out PE. Likelihood ratios are based on sensitivity and specificity values, so what do published studies say about CT sensitivity and specificity?

Studies of CT Pulmonary Angiography Sensitivity and Specificity. A 2002 meta-analysis of 12 studies from 1990 to 2000 comparing CT to standard pulmonary angiography or high-probability VQ scan found an overall sensitivity of 74.1% and specificity of 89.5%, with broad reported ranges for both sensitivity (57% to 100%) and specificity (68% to 100%).[50] A systematic review and meta-analysis published in 2005 in *Radiology* (including single and multidetector CT) found the pooled sensitivity for CT to be 86% (95% CI = 80.2%-92.1%) with a specificity of 93.7% (95% CI = 91.1%-96.3%).[51] In other words, a positive CT is likely to rule in PE correctly, but a negative CT might miss as many as one in five patients with PE. A 2006 review reached similar conclusions, finding that CT pulmonary angiography alone was relatively insensitive but, when combined with lower extremity DVT diagnostic testing, had a false-negative rate of only 1.6%.[52]

In 2006, the results of the multicenter PIOPED II study were published in the *New England Journal of Medicine*. This National Institutes of Health–funded prospective study used a composite reference standard, including additional imaging results, to determine the accuracy of multidetector CT. The study included

noted that the likelihood ratio negative of a negative CT alone (without ultrasound) was only 0.11 (95% CI = 0.06-0.15) and therefore concluded that CT alone should only be used to rule out PE in low-risk patients. Adding ultrasound evaluation may be prudent in patients with higher clinical risk. A low-probability VQ scan had a negative likelihood ratio of 0.36 (95% CI = 0.25-0.50), meaning that it reduces the likelihood of PE but only moderately. In very-low-risk patients, this may equate to an acceptably low risk for PE, but in high-risk

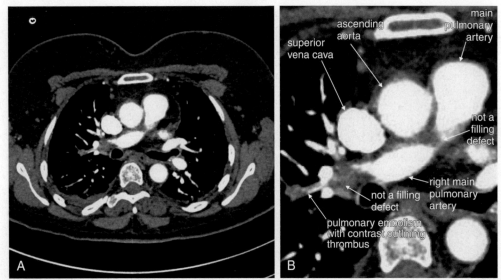

Figure 7-33. Pulmonary embolism (PE): Hampton's hump. Same CT pulmonary angiogram as Figure 7-32. **A,** Soft-tissue window. **B,** Close-up. A PE is present in a branch pulmonary artery, seen in long-axis cross section. This thrombus is outlined in contrast, a common finding sometimes called railroad tracking in the radiology literature. Interpreting chest CT for PE requires some getting used to. This figure has two other regions that appear to be occlusions on this single image, but review of adjacent images proves that these densities lie outside of the pulmonary artery. Novice readers might be deceived by the manner in which the pulmonary artery moves in and out of the plane of this image. We review many more examples that clarify this.

4-, 8-, and 16-detector CT scanners. Overall, the study found CT pulmonary angiography to be 83% sensitive (95% CI = 76%-92%) with a specificity of 96% (95% CI = 93%-97%). The likelihood ratio positive was 19.6 (95% CI = 13.3-29.0), indicating that a positive CT scan strongly predicts the presence of PE. The likelihood ratio negative was 0.18 (95% CI = 0.13-0.24), indicating that a negative CT substantially reduces but does not exclude the possibility of PE.[53] Remember that a test with a likelihood ratio positive greater than 10 is thought to suggest a disease process strongly, whereas a likelihood ratio negative less than 0.1 is necessary to exclude a diagnosis confidently. The investigators also reported the positive predictive values in patients with intermediate and high pretest probability and the negative predictive value of CT angiography in patients with low pretest probability. Positive predictive values of CT in intermediate- and high-risk patients were 92% and 96%, respectively. Negative predictive value was 97% in low-risk patients. As described earlier, positive and negative predictive values are influenced by the prevalence of disease in the subject groups and are generally discouraged as a means of describing test properties. However, in this case, reporting predictive values stratified by clinical pretest probability is appropriate, because validated tools (Wells score and others) are available to us as emergency physicians to allow us to identify patients with similar probability of disease. The authors concluded that a CT finding that is concordant with pretest probability is highly predictive, whereas discordant imaging and clinical risk assessment should be followed with additional testing. The relatively low sensitivity of CT pulmonary angiography in PIOPED II (83%) may come as a surprise, and deserves comment. The

reference standard for the diagnosis of PE in PIOPED II was designed to be extremely conservative, and included the diagnosis of DVT by venous ultrasound in a patient whose other diagnostic tests for PE were negative. Thus a DVT was assumed to be a surrogate for the diagnosis of PE, and a negative CT pulmonary angiogram in this setting was considered to be a false negative. While from a clinical perspective, patients with DVT require anticoagulation, it is not actually true that all patients with DVT also have PE. Thus, this reference standard exaggerates the false negative rate (and thus decreases the apparent sensitivity) of CT for PE. 13.5% of PE diagnoses in PIOPED II were based on such ultrasound findings. If these patients in truth had isolated DVT without PE, the negative CTs that occurred in some of these patients would be true negatives, not false negatives, and the sensitivity of CT would be higher than that reported by the PIOPED II investigators.[53a]

In another publication, the PIOPED II investigators recommended several diagnostic pathways based on clinical pretest probability.[54] They point out that a negative CT angiogram in a low-risk patient has an excellent negative predictive value (96%) and recommend against treatment in this group. They point out a slightly improved negative predictive value (97%) when CT venography (CTV) of the lower extremities is also performed, although controversy exists about this technique because the small additional diagnostic yield comes at the cost of considerable additional radiation exposure. Notably, they recommend additional diagnostic testing in low pretest probability patients with positive CT angiography results resulting from positive predictive values of only 68% for segmental PE and 25% for

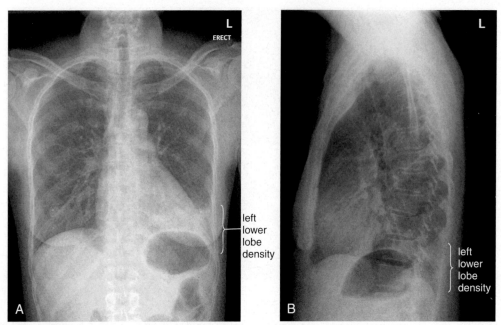

Figure 7-34. Pulmonary embolism (PE) with visible infarct on chest x-ray. This 48-year-old female presented with sudden onset of pleuritic pain along her left costal margin with dyspnea and hemoptysis. She had experienced some cough the prior 2 weeks. A left lower lobe opacity was noted on chest x-ray and is visible on both posterior–anterior (PA) **(A)** and lateral **(B)** views. The upper surface of the left diaphragm is obscured on the PA x-ray, and increased density overlies the heart on this view. On the lateral x-ray, the thoracic spine fails to become darker approaching the diaphragm (as is normal) because of the overlying lung density. This was interpreted as likely pneumonia by the radiologist. PE was suspected based on the sudden onset of symptoms, and CT pulmonary angiography was performed (Figure 7-35). Remember that pneumonia and pulmonary infarct are indistinguishable on chest x-ray.

Figure 7-35. Pulmonary embolism (PE) with visible infarct on chest x-ray. This computed tomography (CT) image (viewed on lung window settings) shows the same infiltrate as in the chest x-ray in Figure 7-34. Compare the normal right lung with the left lung, which shows a patchy, ground-glass appearance. This appearance can be caused by pulmonary infarction and hemorrhage (as in this case), atypical infection, or aspiration. The right lung has a central density, but this is the dome of the diaphragm or uppermost liver, because this slice is taken low in the chest near the upper abdomen. The critical teaching point is that chest x-ray findings suggesting pneumonia may represent pulmonary infarction. When PE is strongly suspected, chest CT should be performed to further evaluate the patient. Ventilation–perfusion (VQ) scan may be less helpful in this scenario, because an infiltrate on chest x-ray would likely result in a ventilation defect with a matched perfusion defect on a VQ scan—by definition, an intermediate probability scan for PE. VQ could be diagnostic if additional unmatched perfusion defects are found. The soft-tissue windows are shown in Figure 7-36 and confirm PE. Interestingly, the patient was found to be hyperthyroid and thrombocytopenic, perhaps contributing to pulmonary hemorrhage.

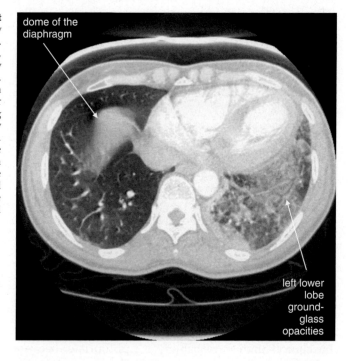

subsegmental PE. Segmental and subsegmental filling defects on CT are more prone to interobserver error and may result from poor contrast bolus or other artifacts, rather than PE. They are therefore less predictive of PE. If CT demonstrates main or lobar PE, for which positive predictive value is high (97%), the PIOPED investigators recommend treatment without further testing. Filling defects in main or lobar pulmonary arteries are usually readily recognized and easily distinguished from artifact; therefore, they are more predictive of PE.

For patients with moderate pretest probability assessment, the PIOPED II authors suggest treatment in accordance with CT results without further diagnostic testing because of good negative and positive predictive values in this group (89% and 92%, respectively).

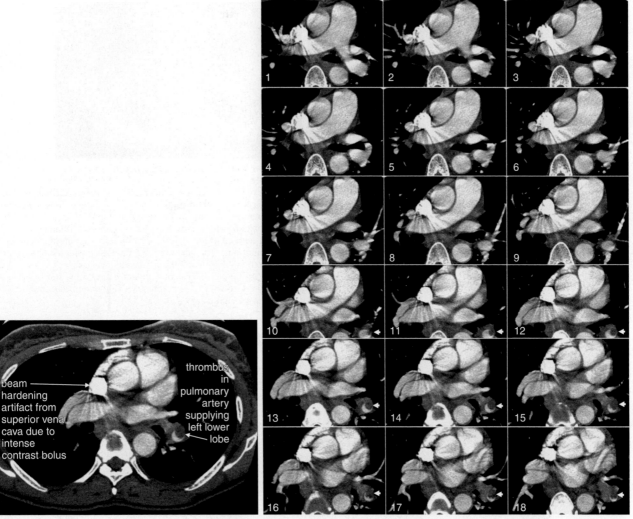

Figure 7-36. CT pulmonary angiogram from patient with visible pulmonary infarct on chest x-ray. Same patient as Figures 7-34 and 7-35, soft-tissue windows. A single complete slice is shown for orientation **(A)**, corresponding to image number **14.** Coned-in views of the main pulmonary arteries are shown to allow these vessels to be tracked through multiple slices. A large thrombus is seen in short-axis cross section, giving it a circular appearance. A crescent of contrast is seen partially outlining this thrombus, which does not completely fill the vessel at this level. The thrombus is a tubular cast of the vessel from which it originated and is visible on several adjacent slices because of its length. This thrombus lies in the pulmonary artery supplying the left lower lobe, explaining the infarct in that location. The superior vena cava is filled with very dense contrast, creating beam-hardening (streak) artifact with a sunburst appearance overlying adjacent structures.

In patients with high-probability clinical assessment, they recommend treatment for positive CT findings (positive predictive value = 96%) but further workup if CT is negative because of a negative predictive value of only 60% for CT angiography and 82% for CT angiography plus lower extremity CTV.

These recommendations from PIOPED II may be unnecessarily conservative, because they reflect a disease-oriented outcome based on CT sensitivity, not based on patient outcome. PIOPED II did follow patients to 3 and 6 months by phone interview, but the clinical outcomes of patients with negative CT were not reported. It is not clear from the study that PEs missed by CT scan resulted in patient deaths or significant morbidity. Other studies have shown a very low yield of routine lower extremity imaging for DVT in asymptomatic patients

with negative chest CT. Rates of additional DVT found using this technique are as low as 0.7% to 2.7%, with costs as high as $200,000 per additional isolated DVT diagnosed.[55-56] An overall algorithm incorporating pre-test probability and CT results in shown in Table 7-4.

What Is a Ventilation–Perfusion Scan? How Does It Detect or Exclude Pulmonary Embolism?

Ventilation-Perfusion (VQ) scan is a nuclear scintigraphy technique for detection of pulmonary embolism. VQ scanning is a two-phase test process (Figure 7-43). First, the patient inhales a radioactive isotope (usually xenon-133), and the distribution of this gas in the lung parenchyma is recorded by a gamma camera (also called scintillation camera) outside the patient's body. Next, a radioactive isotope (technetium-99m) is injected, and

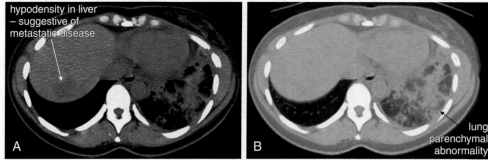

Figure 7-37. Pulmonary embolism (PE), massive: Visible infarct on noncontrast "renal protocol" computed tomography (CT). This 42-year-old female presented with left flank pain and cough. She had recently been diagnosed with likely lung cancer but had not undergone biopsy or other workup or treatment. The initial evaluation by the emergency physician suggested renal colic, and a noncontrast abdominal CT was performed. **A,** Soft-tissue window. **B,** Lung window for the same slice. The cephaladmost slices from abdominal CT routinely include the lower lung, and on the lung window a left lower lobe density was noted—interpreted appropriately by the radiologist as "heterogeneous opacities in the left lower lung, which may be the result of infection, aspiration, or spread of malignancy." However, another explanation for this appearance is pulmonary infarction from PE. The emergency physician obtained chest x-ray that also showed an appearance consistent with infiltrate (Figure 7-38). With this apparent diagnosis in hand based on imaging, the patient was admitted to an observation unit and treated for pneumonia. The next morning, PE was considered and confirmed by contrasted chest CT. The take-home point is that the appearance of pulmonary infarction and pneumonia can be identical on chest x-ray and CT lung window. In both cases, the density of lung tissue increases because of the presence of fluid, cellular debris, inflammatory cells, and possibly alveolar hemorrhage. When the clinical history suggests PE, the presence of an infiltrate on chest x-ray or CT is not diagnostic of pneumonia and does not rule out PE. Compare with the chest x-ray in Figure 7-38 and the CT pulmonary angiogram in Figure 7-39.

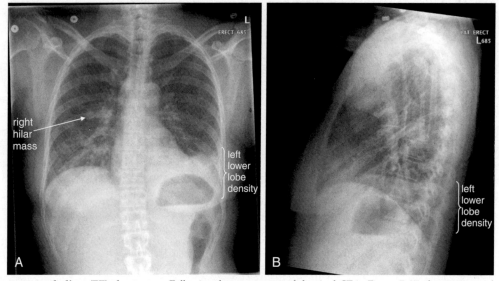

Figure 7-38. Pulmonary embolism (PE) chest x-ray. Following the noncontrast abdominal CT in Figure 7-37, the patient underwent chest x-ray, showing increased density in the left lower lobe. The diaphragm and left heart border are obscured on the posterior–anterior x-ray **(A),** and the retrocardiac space appears abnormally dense on the lateral view **(B)** (the "spine sign"—absence of the normal progressive lucency of the thoracic spine as it approaches the diaphragm). These abnormalities were interpreted as evidence of pneumonia by the emergency physician, though they were the result pulmonary infarction from PE (see Figure 7-39). The radiologist suggested infection, edema, or atelectasis but did not mention infarction. Pulmonary infarction and infectious infiltrate can have identical appearances on chest x-ray. The patient also has a known right hilar mass. Compare with the noncontrast CT in Figure 7-37 and the CT pulmonary angiogram in Figure 7-39.

the distribution of blood in the patient's pulmonary arteries is again recorded by an external camera. In a normal patient, the radioactive gas is well distributed through all lung segments, and blood flow is preserved to all lung segments. Several abnormal scenarios may occur, not all representing PE. For example, in a patient with pneumonia or atelectasis, a "defect" occurs in the ventilation image because little of the inhaled radioactive isotope is delivered to the abnormal alveoli of the affected lung segment. The normal physiologic response of the body is to decrease perfusion to poorly ventilated lung, so a corresponding decrease in signal is seen on the

perfusion portion of the scan, indicating low blood flow to the poorly ventilated lung zone. This is referred to as a "matched defect" and is considered abnormal but not clearly diagnostic of PE. This scenario of matched defect can occur with pneumonia, atelectasis, chronic obstructive pulmonary disease (COPD), asthma, or pleural effusion—or with a large PE resulting in parenchymal infarction. A matched defect may result in an "intermediate probability" interpretation of the VQ scan, which neither confirms nor excludes PE. In an uncomplicated PE without associated lung parenchymal infarction, gas exchange is normal, so no defect is expected on the

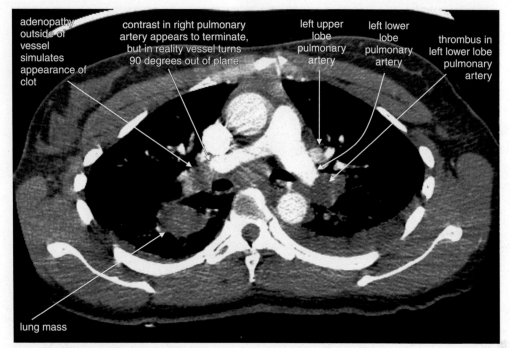

Figure 7-39. Pulmonary embolism with visible infarct. Same patient as in Figures 7-37 and 7-38. CT pulmonary angiography demonstrates a filling defect completely obstructing the left lower lobe pulmonary artery. On the right, a lung mass is seen, and hilar adenopathy adjacent to the right main pulmonary artery is seen. How can you distinguish a mass adjacent to the artery from a clot within? In some cases, they may be indistinguishable, but often inspection of several adjacent slices can allow the two to be discriminated. Thrombus and adenopathy or other soft-tissue masses share the same dark gray (soft-tissue density) on soft-tissue windows. Therefore it is not the color that should be relied upon. Instead, follow the vessel in question through several slices to determine whether the apparent cutoff is simply the result of the vessel turning and traveling outside of the plane of the single CT slice. If the contrast-filled vessel can be followed through several slices, the soft-tissue mass is likely extrinsic to the vessel. If the vessel does not appear to be filled with contrast in adjacent slices, the soft-tissue density is likely thrombus within the vessel—a pulmonary embolus. The next figure shows a series of coned-in views to allow you to see the distinction between thrombus and soft-tissue mass external to the vessel.

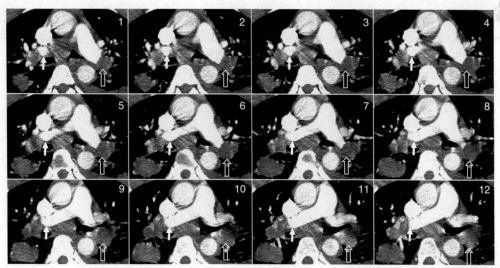

Figure 7-40. Pulmonary embolism (PE): Distinguishing adenopathy from thrombus. Image number **6** corresponds to the full computed tomography image in Figure 7-39—review that figure before proceeding with this one. Start with image **1** in the top left and track the normal right pulmonary artery (marked by a *white arrow*) as it turns and is visible as a contrast-filled circular cross section in several slices. It then is visible in long-axis section and merges into the pulmonary trunk. In none of the slices shown is it obstructed with thrombus. However, a lymph node outside of the vessel is easily mistaken for a PE. Now follow the left pulmonary artery (marked by an *open arrow*), and you will see that it remains obstructed in several adjacent slices. A branch to the right upper lobe diverges, but the branch to the left lower lobe *(open arrow)* remains obstructed in every slice and does not fill with contrast. Cases such as this are common and require careful attention by the radiologist to avoid misdiagnosis.

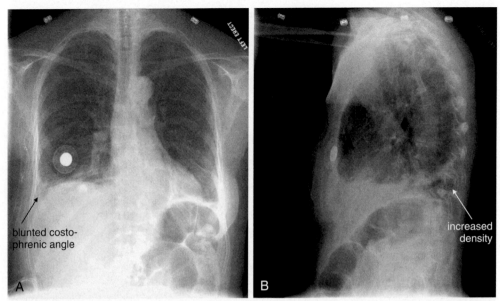

Figure 7-41. Pulmonary embolism (PE), massive. This 63-year-old female underwent mastectomy for breast cancer 5 days prior and awoke with pleuritic right chest pain and dyspnea. Her chest x-ray shows a blunted right costophrenic angle on the right on the posterior–anterior view **(A)** and increased density on the lateral view **(B)**. PE was suspected, and CT pulmonary angiography was performed (Figure 7-42).

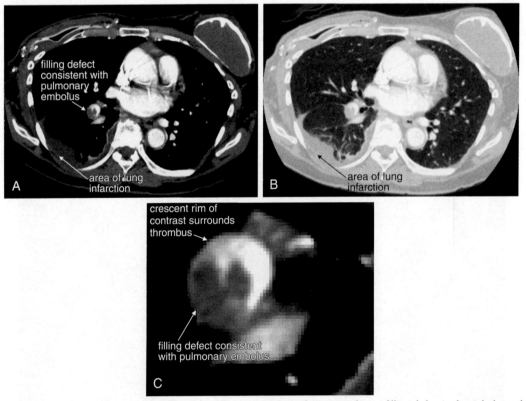

Figure 7-42. Pulmonary embolism (PE), massive. These CT pulmonary angiography images show a filling defect in the right lower lobe pulmonary artery, a PE. The watershed region of lung supplied by this vessel is infarcted, resulting in increased density on chest computed tomography and in the chest x-ray in Figure 7-41. **A,** Soft-tissue window. **B,** Lung window of the same slice. **C,** Close-up from **A** showing the thrombus in more detail.

ventilation phase of the VQ scan. The embolus blocks delivery of the injected radioactive isotope to a portion of the lung, resulting in a defect only on the perfusion images. The result is an "unmatched perfusion defect," which is considered high probability for PE. Although this finding is highly suggestive of PE, it is not pathognomonic, as we discuss later. When multiple unmatched perfusion defects are present, PE is by far the most likely cause. Figures 7-44 through 7-55 demonstrate high-probability VQ scans and the associated chest x-rays and

TABLE 7-4. Pretest Probability and CT Results*

| Pretest Probability of Pulmonary Embolism | CT SCAN RESULT | | |
| | | CT POSITIVE | |
	Normal CT	Segmental or Subsegmental Pulmonary Embolism	Main or Lobar Pulmonary Embolism
Low probability	Excludes PE	Does not completely confirm PE; consider additional imaging to confirm diagnosis (repeat CT, VQ, pulmonary angiogram, or lower extremity imaging for DVT)	Confirms PE
Moderate probability	PE unlikely, but consider lower extremity imaging for DVT	Confirms PE	Confirms PE
High probability	Does not completely exclude PE; consider additional imaging to confirm diagnosis (VQ, pulmonary angiography, or lower extremity imaging for DVT)	Confirms PE	Confirms PE

From Stein PD, Woodard PK, Weg JG, et al. Diagnostic pathways in acute pulmonary embolism: Recommendations of the PIOPED II investigators. *Radiology* 242:15-21, 2007; Stein PD, Woodard PK, Weg JG, et al. Diagnostic pathways in acute pulmonary embolism: Recommendations of the PIOPED II investigators. *Am J Med* 119:1048-1055, 2006.

*CT is most accurate when pretest probability and CT results are concordant. Discordant results or a CT scan showing peripheral pulmonary embolism should be considered nondiagnostic. The most reliable combinations of pretest probability and CT scan are highlighted.

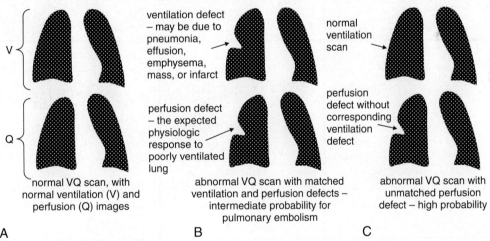

A — normal VQ scan, with normal ventilation (V) and perfusion (Q) images

B — abnormal VQ scan with matched ventilation and perfusion defects – intermediate probability for pulmonary embolism

C — abnormal VQ scan with unmatched perfusion defect – high probability

ventilation defect – may be due to pneumonia, effusion, emphysema, mass, or infarct

normal ventilation scan

perfusion defect – the expected physiologic response to poorly ventilated lung

perfusion defect without corresponding ventilation defect

Figure 7-43. Ventilation–perfusion (VQ) scan: Schematic. VQ scan is a nuclear medicine test used to evaluate for pulmonary embolism (PE). In the diagrams, the top images represent ventilation scans, each paired with a perfusion scan image below it. The blank space in the center of each image is the mediastinal silhouette, which results in a void space with little tracer. VQ scans are graded as normal or very low probability for PE (**A,** with normal ventilation and perfusion), low or intermediate probability for PE (**B,** with some areas of matched perfusion defects), or high probability for PE (**C,** with normal ventilation and single or multiple segmental and subsegmental perfusion defects). **A,** A normal lung should have uniform distribution of a gas through its parenchyma, which is demonstrated by administering an inhaled radioactive gas and acquiring a ventilation image (V). Normal pulmonary arteries should allow uniform blood flow throughout the lung, which can be demonstrated by injection of a radioactive isotope and acquisition of a perfusion image (Q). **B,** Abnormal lung parenchyma limits gas distribution, resulting in an abnormal ventilation scan. The normal physiologic response to a hypoxic lung region is vasoconstriction of the pulmonary arteries supplying that lung zone. This results in a "matched" perfusion defect, with decreased distribution of the injected radioactive tracer to the poorly ventilated lung zone seen on the perfusion scan. Any pathologic process that limits ventilation of a lung segment can result in a matched defect—including chronic obstructive pulmonary disease, pneumonia, pleural effusion, or lung mass. Sometimes PE results in a matched defect—if the embolism is large enough to result in pulmonary infarction with alveoli in the necrotic lung zone filling with fluid and cellular debris. **C,** More often, PE limits blood flow but not ventilation of the lung zone, resulting in a normal ventilation scan and an abnormal perfusion scan. This VQ mismatch is typical of PE but occasionally can result from other pathology. For example, a lung mass could result in extrinsic compression of a pulmonary artery, causing an abnormal perfusion scan but a normal ventilation scan. In a real VQ scan, multiple views from anterior, posterior, and oblique viewpoints are compared. A VQ scan is by nature low resolution—the scan is acquired over approximately 45 minutes, with a camera outside the patient registering emitted radiation. Respiratory motion and patient motion result in blurring of the image.

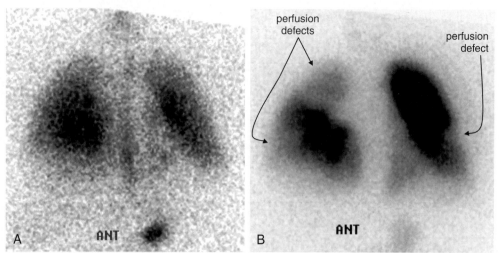

Figure 7-44. Pulmonary embolism (PE): Bilateral. A direct comparison of the ventilation–perfusion (VQ) scans in a 30-year-old female with bilateral PE. **A,** Ventilation scan image acquired with the detector anterior to the patient. Both lungs show distribution of inhaled radiopharmaceutical. **B,** Perfusion scan image acquired from the same anterior perspective. Multiple perfusion defects are seen; none matched on ventilation scan. This is a high-probability VQ scan, because no other process would be expected to cause multiple areas of poor perfusion with normal ventilation.

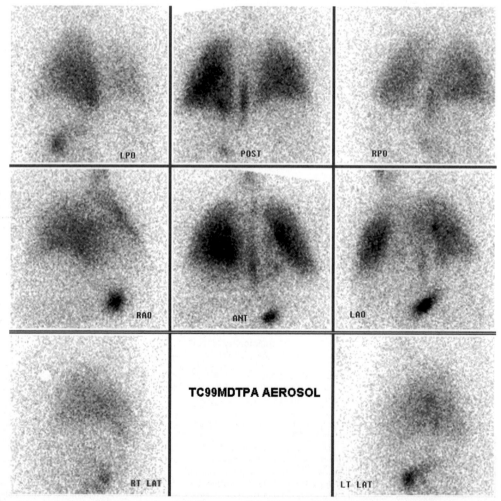

Figure 7-45. Pulmonary embolism (PE): Bilateral, ventilation scan. This 30-year-old female presented with flank pain and no identifiable risk factors for PE. Her initial vital signs were reassuring except for visible tachypnea, noted in the physician chart. Her ventilation–perfusion scan was read as high probability for PE. The inpatient team also performed chest computed tomography (Figure 7-47). We start by looking at the ventilation scan above; the perfusion scan is shown in Figure 7-46. This ventilation scan is essentially normal. Look at the central cell, showing an image captured with a detector anterior to the patient. Radioactive tracer is seen distributed through both lungs. The white region in the central chest, indicating absence of inhaled tracer, is the normal cardiac silhouette. The right diaphragm was felt to be slightly elevated. The other cells view the chest from varying angles (posterior, oblique, and lateral). Compare with the perfusion scan in Figure 7-46.

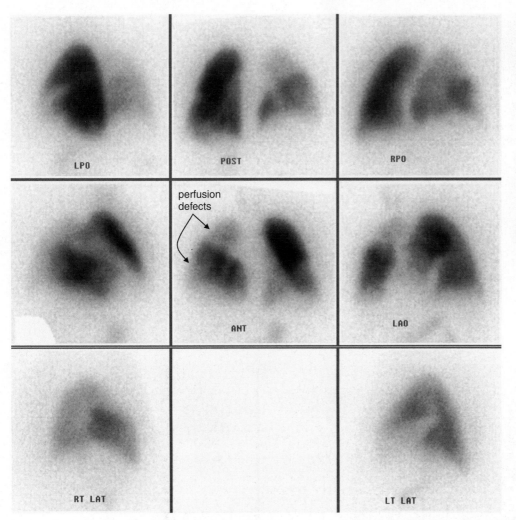

Figure 7-46. Pulmonary embolism (PE): Bilateral, perfusion scan. Same patient as Figure 7-45. Here we inspect the perfusion scan images. Look at the central cell, showing an image acquired with the detector anterior to the patient. Multiple perfusion defects are seen, none matched on ventilation scan (Figure 7-45). Together, Figures 7-45 and 7-46 constitute a high-probability ventilation–perfusion scan. The other images above view the chest from varying angles (posterior, oblique, and lateral). They confirm the same finding of multiple perfusion defects. Compare with the CT pulmonary angiogram from the same patient in Figure 7-47.

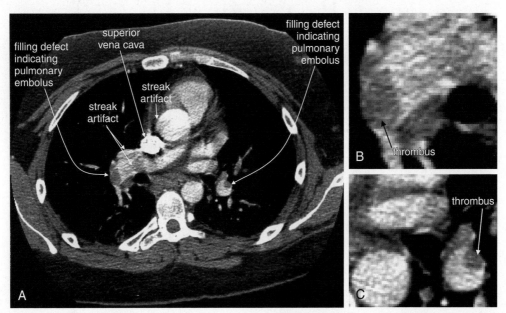

Figure 7-47. Pulmonary embolism (PE): bilateral with poor contrast bolus. Same patient as Figure 7-46. **A,** Axial computed tomography (CT) slice. **B, C,** Close-ups. Despite a relatively poor-quality scan with artifact and a suboptimal contrast bolus, bilateral pulmonary emboli are visible, indicated by filling defects in large pulmonary arteries. The superior vena cava is intensely enhanced with contrast, creating streak artifact that can confuse the diagnosis. Note the difference between these diffuse hypodense artifacts and the well-marginated real filling defects created by the pulmonary thrombus. In some cases, it may be impossible to differentiate artifacts from real emboli. Focus on identifying definite emboli to rule in the diagnosis.

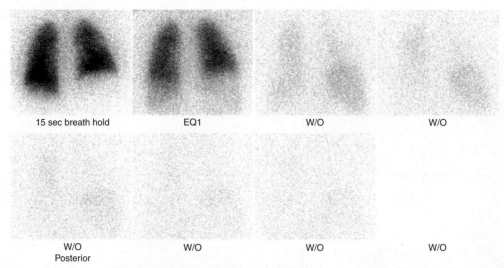

Figure 7-48. Pulmonary embolism ventilation–perfusion scan: High probability. This 48-year-old male with a history of recurrent deep venous thromboses presented with dyspnea and chest tightness. The previous week, he had visited his physician with left leg pain and was diagnosed with a muscle strain. This ventilation scan is normal. Compare with the perfusion scan from the same patient in Figure 7-49.

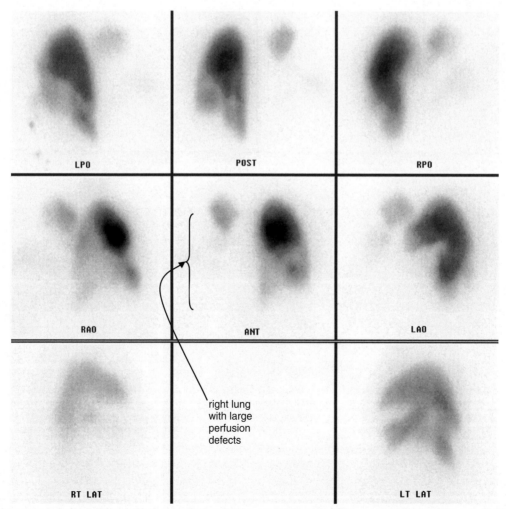

Figure 7-49. Pulmonary embolism (PE) ventilation–perfusion (VQ) scan: High probability. Same patient as Figure 7-48. This perfusion scan is markedly abnormal. There is virtually no perfusion of the right lung, and regions of the left lung also appear hypoperfused. Begin by looking at the central cell, which shows a perfusion image acquired with the detector anterior to the patient. Only the right lung apex shows perfusion. The left mid- and lower lung are also poorly perfused. The remaining cells confirm these perfusion defects, which are not matched on ventilation scan (Figure 7-48). This is a high-probability VQ scan for PE.

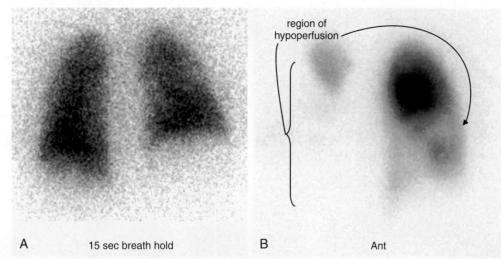

Figure 7-50. **Pulmonary embolism (PE) ventilation–perfusion (VQ) scan: High probability.** Same patient as Figures 7-48 and 7-49. These ventilation **(A)** and perfusion **(B)** images from the patient show multiple areas of VQ mismatch. Both were acquired with the detector anterior to the patient. The void in the center of the ventilation scan **(A)** is the normal mediastinal and cardiac silhouette. On the perfusion scan **(B),** nearly the entire right lung is not perfused, consistent with central PE. The left mid- and lower lung are also poorly perfused. This is a high-probability VQ scan for PE.

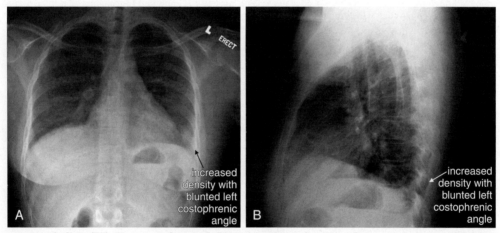

Figure 7-51. **Pulmonary embolism (PE): Hampton's hump. A,** Posterior–anterior chest x-ray. **B,** Lateral chest x-ray. Hampton's hump is a classic but insensitive and nonspecific finding of PE. It is described as a wedge-shaped peripheral density on chest x-ray, indicating pulmonary infarction. Its appearance is not distinguishable from an infiltrate from pneumonia. In a pulmonary infarction from PE, tissue necrosis leads to the accumulation of alveolar fluid and cellular debris, as well as reactive inflammatory cells and hemorrhage. This increases the tissue density from air density to water density, just as with bacterial pneumonia. Early in the course of PE, or with small nonocclusive PE, no infarction may occur, and Hampton's hump will not be visible. This 29-year-old female presented with acute onset of pleuritic left chest pain and dyspnea. Her chest was interpreted as normal, but look carefully at the left costophrenic angle. An increased density is present here. The finding is also seen on the lateral x-ray. Compare with the normal right side. Figure 7-52 shows her chest x-ray 2 days later. Her workup confirmed PE.

CT scans from the same patients. As you review the VQ scans, you may be surprised to see the grainy quality of the images. Current gamma cameras have a spatial resolution of only 1.8 cm at a distance of 5 cm from the camera face, meaning that two separate sources of gamma radiation must be at least 1.8 cm apart to be distinguished. Resolution rapidly diminishes with increasing distance of the radiation source from the camera.

Other pathology can disrupt blood flow without altering ventilation, resulting in a false-positive VQ scan. An example is a tumor embolism, classically a renal cell carcinoma, which can enter the inferior vena cava and then embolize to the lung. The VQ appearance would be identical to that for PE. CT could also misdiagnose this condition based solely on chest CT findings, but if a renal mass is suspected, additional CT of the abdomen could prove tumor involvement of the inferior vena cava (Figure 7-56). Another example of pathology that could create a false-positive VQ scan is a central lung mass that extrinsically compresses a pulmonary artery branch while preserving ventilation to the lung segment (Figures 7-57 through 7-59). Whereas one unmatched defect can suggest but not absolutely confirm PE, multiple bilateral defects strongly suggest PE because few other processes can lead to this pattern.

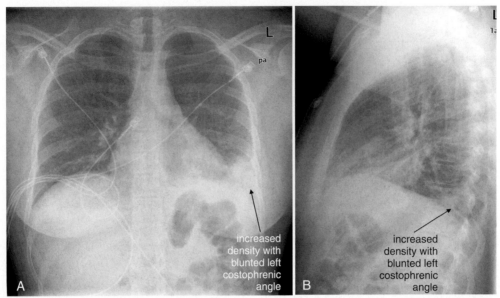

Figure 7-52. Pulmonary embolism (PE): Hampton's hump. A, Posterior–anterior chest x-ray. **B,** Lateral chest x-ray. Same patient as Figure 7-51, now 2 days later: 29-year-old female with sudden pleuritic left chest pain and dyspnea. Compare with the chest x-ray in the earlier figure. Now the increased density at the left costophrenic angle is more evident. This wedge-shaped pleural-based density is a pulmonary infarct—a finding sometimes called Hampton's hump. Although this finding is neither sensitive nor specific for PE, it is important to recognize that infarction and pneumonia can appear identical on chest x-ray. When the clinical history suggests PE, this appearance on chest x-ray should not lead to termination of the workup and diagnosis of pneumonia.

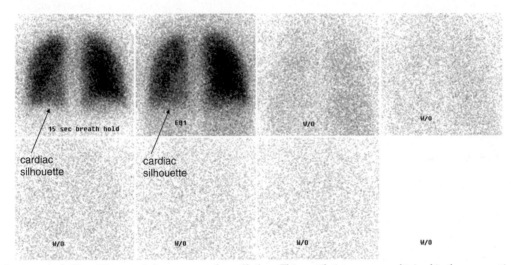

Figure 7-53. Pulmonary embolism: Hampton's hump, normal ventilation. This ventilation scan was obtained in the same patient as Figure 7-51. The perfusion scan is shown in Figure 7-54. The images in the upper left show even distribution of an inhaled radiopharmaceutical (11.3 mCi of xenon-133). A slight decrease in gas distribution is seen in the region overlying the cardiac silhouette, which appears on the left as these images are acquired with the detector behind the patient. The abnormal region near the left costophrenic angle (seen on the initial chest x-ray, Figure 7-51) is not visible on this ventilation scan—it is too small to be resolved. The remaining frames show the washout phase, which indicates that the inhaled gas is rapidly exhaled from the lung, with no air-trapping. Air-trapping would be evident as retained radiopharmaceutical and might be seen in chronic obstructive pulmonary disease or asthma.

Understanding of the technique behind VQ scanning allows identification of patients who would be poor candidates for this test. Patients with abnormal chest x-rays, for example, with pleural effusions or atelectasis, are likely to have matched defects on VQ scan. Consequently, VQ scan may be unreliable to rule out PE in these patients. Patients with COPD or asthma may also have matched defects on VQ because of poor gas exchange and a normal physiologic shunting of blood away from poorly ventilated lung. These patients may also have nondiagnostic VQ scans.[57-58]

What Are the Sensitivity and Specificity of Ventilation–Perfusion Scan?

VQ scans are rated on a structured scoring system with values of normal, very low probability, low probability, intermediate probability, and high probability.

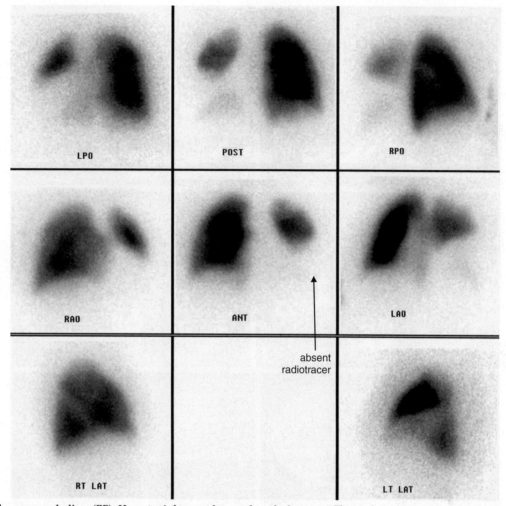

Figure 7-54. Pulmonary embolism (PE): Hampton's hump, abnormal perfusion scan. This perfusion scan was obtained in the same patient as Figures 7-51 through 7-53. The dark areas reflect distribution of an injected radiopharmaceutical (4.4 mCi of technetium-99m macroaggregate albumin). The abbreviations below the images indicate the relative position of the detector to the chest: LPO (left posterior oblique), POST (posterior), RPO (right posterior oblique), RAO (right anterior oblique), ANT (anterior), LAO (left anterior oblique), RT LAT (right lateral), and LT LAT (left lateral). Start by looking at the central image, which shows an anterior view. There is markedly decreased or absent tracer distribution in the left lower lobe and lingula. This is not accounted for by the cardiac silhouette, which does not project completely over this region. The other viewpoints confirm this finding. This, combined with the normal ventilation scan (Figure 7-53), constitutes a high-probability ventilation–perfusion (VQ) scan for PE. Another possible cause of this degree of VQ mismatch would be a large central mass compressing the pulmonary artery but not restricting airflow. Computed tomography was performed to exclude this alternative cause (Figure 7-55).

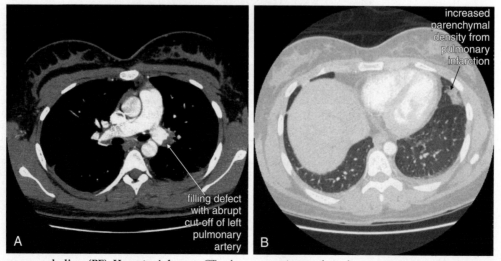

Figure 7-55. Pulmonary embolism (PE): Hampton's hump. CT pulmonary angiogram from the same patient as in Figure 7-54 showed a large left PE—accounting for the perfusion defect seen on ventilation–perfusion scan in that figure. On soft-tissue window **(A),** this is seen as a filling defect in the left main pulmonary artery. On lung window **(B),** an area of pulmonary infarction (corresponding to the abnormality on the patient's chest x-ray) is visible as increased parenchymal density. Compare with the patient's chest x-rays in Figures 7-51 and 7-52.

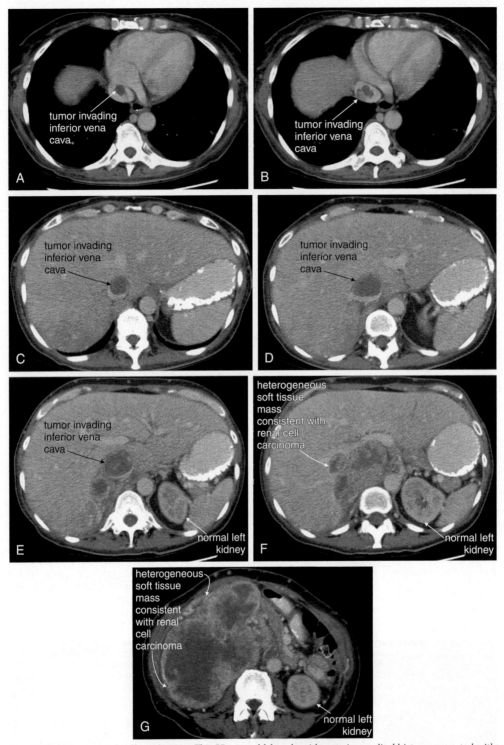

Figure 7-56. Tumor embolism from renal cell carcinoma. This 55-year-old female with no prior medical history presented with a 50-pound weight loss over the past 8 months, with a palpable abdominal mass and increasing dyspnea. Sadly, computed tomography (CT) of the chest **(A, B)** and abdomen **(C to G)** shows an enormous mass replacing her right kidney, invading the inferior vena cava, and extending to the right atrium. Other chest CT images (not shown) showed pulmonary emboli, which may have been tumor emboli rather than thrombus. Renal cell carcinomas classically invade the renal vein and inferior cava, resulting in tumor emboli. These create an intravascular filling defect on CT and would result in ventilation–perfusion (VQ) mismatch on VQ scan, exactly as with typical pulmonary embolism from thrombus. Emergency physicians must be aware of these alternative causes of abnormal VQ and CT pulmonary arteriograms.

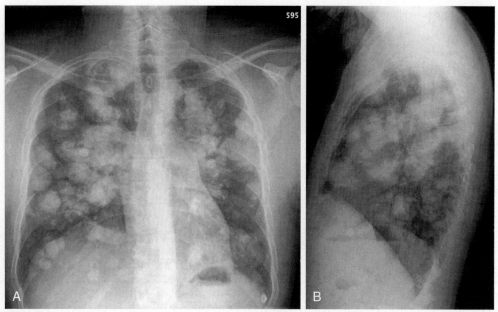

Figure 7-57. Metastatic disease with cannonball emboli. A, Posterior–anterior chest x-ray. **B,** Lateral chest x-ray. This patient with metastatic osteosarcoma has the classic appearance of pulmonary metastatic disease, with innumerable rounded bilateral nodules. These occur as tumor cells are carried hematogenously to the lungs, implant, and grow. Nodules of different sizes may have seeded at different times. Because of the markedly abnormal chest x-ray, ventilation–perfusion scan would be a poor choice for assessing this patient for pulmonary embolism. The CT in Figure 7-58 shows yet another reason that CT is a better choice in this patient.

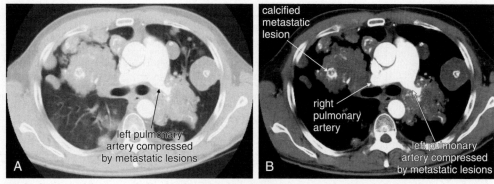

Figure 7-58. Metastatic disease with cannonball emboli and pulmonary artery compression. Same patient as Figure 7-57. **A,** Lung window. **B,** Soft-tissue window. Here, confluent metastatic lesions are creating a unique problem—the left pulmonary artery is surrounded and compressed. Compare the diameter of the right and left pulmonary arteries. Consider what would happen if this patient were to undergo ventilation–perfusion (VQ) scan for suspected pulmonary embolism (PE). Extrinsic compression of a pulmonary artery can create VQ mismatch, falsely suggesting PE. Even without the unusual compression of the left pulmonary artery, the multiple pulmonary masses would create matched VQ defects that would result in an indeterminate VQ scan. In these single images, the right pulmonary artery may appear to be obstructed by either tumor or thrombus, but remember that vessels can curve in and out of a single image plane. Look at the next figure to understand the true course of the vessel. Another feature of these osteosarcoma lesions is internal calcifications—although a noncontrast CT would demonstrate this more clearly. The white markings within the lesions are calcium deposits, not injected contrast material.

Based on an analysis of PIOPED II data, Sostman et al proposed a modified set of diagnostic criteria, simplifying the results of VQ to 3 categories: PE present, PE absent, or nondiagnostic (Table 7-5).[58a] When nondiagnostic categories are removed from analysis, and only the new categories of PE present and PE absent were considered, the sensitivity of VQ was 77.4% (95%CI 69.7% to 85.0%) and the specificity was 97.7% (95%CI 96.4% to 98.9%). If any VQ scan interpretation other than "normal" was considered positive for PE, the sensitivity was 99%, but the specificity was only 20%. This means that,

when only the extreme diagnostic categories are considered, the performance of VQ scan is similar to that of CT in PIOPED II.[59-60] Intermediate probability VQ scan results neither confirm nor exclude PE. Unfortunately, nondiagnostic results are common, with the majority of VQ scan results falling into neither the normal nor the high-probability categories. In PIOPED I, normal VQ results occurred in only 14% of subjects.[59] In PIOPED II, more than 25% of patients had nondiagnostic VQ scan results, compared with only 6% with nondiagnostic CT results.[60]

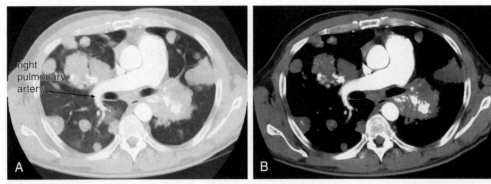

Figure 7-59. Metastatic disease with cannonball tumor emboli. Same patient as Figure 7-58. **A,** Lung window. **B,** Soft-tissue window. The right pulmonary artery remains patent despite encroaching metastatic lesions. Compare with the images in the prior figure.

TABLE 7-5. Modified PIOPED II Scintigraphic Criteria

Category	Finding
PE present (high probability)	Two or more segments of V/Q mismatch
PE absent (normal perfusion or very low probability)	Nonsegmental perfusion abnormalities; these were enlargement of the heart or hilum, elevated hemidiaphragm, costophrenic angle effusion, and linear atelectasis with no other perfusion defect in either lung
	Perfusion defect smaller than corresponding radiographic lesion
	Two or more matched V/Q defects with regionally normal chest radiograph and some areas of normal perfusion elsewhere in the lungs
	One to three small segmental perfusion defects (<25% of segment)
	Solitary triple-matched defect (defined as a matched V/Q defect with associated matching chest radiographic opacity) in the mid or upper lung zone confined to a single segment
	Stripe sign (a stripe of perfused lung tissue between a perfusion defect and the adjacent pleural surface; best seen on a tangential view)
	Pleural effusion of one-third or more of the pleural cavity with no other perfusion defect in either lung
Nondiagnostic (low or intermediate probability)	All other findings

From: Sostman HD, Stein PD, Gottschalk A, et al. Acute pulmonary embolism: sensitivity and specificity of ventilation-perfusion scintigraphy in PIOPED II study. *Radiology* 246(3):941-946, 2008.

Moreover, the pretest probability of PE affects the diagnostic accuracy of VQ, in much the same way that pretest probability affects the accuracy of CT, as reviewed earlier. A normal or very low probability VQ scan does not exclude PE in patients with a moderate or high pretest probability of PE; PIOPED I found PE rates in these patients to be as high as 16% to 40% with a negative VQ scan. Even with a low pre-test probability, the rate of PE was 7% in patients with very low probability VQ scan. In a retrospective analysis of data from PIOPED II, patients with very-low-probability VQ scan result and low pretest probability by Wells criteria had only a 3.1% rate of PE.[61] In a systematic review published in *Radiology* in 2005, VQ scan interpreted as "normal" was 98.3% sensitive to detect PE (95% CI = 97.2%-99.5%), meaning that a normal VQ scan effectively rules out PE in most patients. However, a "normal" VQ scan result was obtained in only 4.8% (95% CI = 4.7%-4.9%) of patients, meaning that most patients would have nonreassuring VQ results prompting further testing. A VQ scan interpretation of "high probability" was very specific for PE at 97.1% (95% CI = 96.0%-98.3%), effectively confirming the diagnosis in most patients. However, the sensitivity of a "high probability" VQ scan was only 39% (95% CI = 37.3%-40.8%) in this meta-analysis, meaning that 60% of patients with PE would have a false-negative or nondiagnostic VQ result. VQ results that are neither "normal" nor "high probability" fail to confirm or rule out the diagnosis, and additional testing should be performed.[51] The ACEP 2003 clinical policy on evaluation of adult patients presenting with suspected PE concluded that a normal VQ scan is adequate to exclude "clinically significant" PE in a patient with low to moderate pretest probability, but this policy predates the PIOPED II data.[4] Table 7-6 illustrates the relationship between pretest probability and VQ result in diagnosing PE. Note

TABLE 7-6. Pretest Probability and Ventilation–Perfusion Scan Results*

Pretest Probability of Pulmonary Embolism	VQ SCAN RESULT		
	Normal or Very Low Probability (PE absent)	Indeterminate (Low or Intermediate Probability)	High Probability (PE present)
Low probability	Excludes PE	Neither confirms nor excludes PE	Does not completely confirm PE
Moderate probability	PE unlikely	Neither confirms nor excludes PE	PE likely
High probability	Does not completely exclude PE	Neither confirms nor excludes PE	Confirms PE

From PIOPED Investigators. Value of the ventilation/perfusion scan in acute pulmonary embolism: Results of the prospective investigation of pulmonary embolism diagnosis (PIOPED). *JAMA* 1990;263:2753-9.

*VQ is most accurate when pretest probability and VQ results are concordant. Discordant results or an indeterminate VQ scan should be considered nondiagnostic.

the similarity in clinical application of VQ scan and CT results, incorporating clinical pretest probability. Concordant imaging test and clinical pretest probability results are generally correct, while discordant results requiring further testing.

Which Patients Are Candidates for Ventilation–Perfusion Scan? What Factors Favor the Use of Computed Tomography?

Table 7-7 illustrates factors favoring VQ or CT scan. Some patients may be candidates for VQ scan because of anticipated inability to undergo a diagnostic CT. Patients with poor IV access may not be able to undergo the rapid contrast bolus necessary for a high-quality CT. VQ may be necessary in patients with renal insufficiency or contrast allergy that are contraindications to CT. Obese patients may exceed the weight capacity of CT scanners (450 pounds for all major manufacturers, with some offering options up to 650 pounds). In addition, the gantry bore diameter of the CT scanner may limit CT in obese patients. The standard gantry diameter is 70 cm, with some manufacturers offering larger gantries up to 90 cm. A common myth is that large hospitals, zoos, and veterinary hospitals may have scanners with larger weight capacities and gantry size capable of scanning larger patients. However, tertiary care hospitals are limited to the same standard CT scanners found in most community hospitals. Veterinary hospitals and zoos are not licensed to care for human patients, and they are equipped with standard human CT scanners that have the same gantry diameter limits. Some have been modified with a specialized table to accommodate heavier animal bodies.[62-63]

Other considerations include patient stability—a chest CT requires minutes, whereas a VQ scan may take up to 1 hour to complete. The decision to use VQ scan as the initial diagnostic test for possible PE clearly should take into consideration the patient's pretest probability of PE. In addition, an understanding of the technique

TABLE 7-7. Factors Affecting Choice of Computed Tomography or Ventilation–Perfusion Scan

Patient Consideration	Favored Imaging Modality
Contrast allergy	VQ
Contrast nephropathy or poor renal function	VQ
Obese patient, exceeding CT table weight capacity or gantry diameter	VQ
Radiation exposure (young, pregnant, or female)	VQ or perfusion scan without ventilation scan
Poor or small-gauge IV access	VQ (does not require rapid contrast bolus)
Abnormal chest x-ray, chronic lung disease, or other factors predicting intermediate (nondiagnostic) VQ result	CT (provides alternative diagnoses)
Intermediate pretest probability	CT
Strong concern for alternative diagnosis (e.g., aortic pathology)	CT (provides alternative diagnosis)
Very high or very low pretest probability	Either CT or VQ as initial test; consider further investigation if imaging result is discordant with pretest probability

of VQ scanning (described earlier) can aid in patient selection for this test. Patients who are predicted to have matched VQ defects are poor candidates for this test, because the results will likely be nondiagnostic. Patients with moderate pretest probability of PE are also relatively poor candidates for VQ scan, the likelihood of a diagnostic VQ scan in this group is low. Patients who may be appropriate for VQ as the primary means of excluding PE may be those with normal chest x-ray, no history of COPD or asthma, and a low pretest probability of PE. A normal VQ scan in these patients likely excludes PE, perhaps to a greater degree than does a normal CT that has a small chance of missing subsegmental PE.[59] Older age, history of chronic lung disease such as emphysema, and chest x-ray findings of emphysema all predict nondiagnostic VQ scan, suggesting that CT may be a better choice in these patients unless contraindications to CT exist.[58] CT scan results in a higher radiation dose to breast tissue than does VQ scan, so VQ may be the favored test in young females, when all other considerations are equal. Phantom models suggest that a single chest CT may increase breast cancer risk by 0.4% to 4% relative to baseline, although shielding and other dose reduction techniques can be used.[64-66] Perfusion scanning without ventilation scanning is another option to reduce radiation exposure. In this technique, the chest x-ray is used as a surrogate for the ventilation scan, with chest x-ray abnormalities compared to defects on the perfusion image. A perfusion defect in the presence of a normal chest x-ray suggests PE. This technique has sensitivity and specificity similar to CT angiography and VQ scan, according to an analysis from PIOPED II data.[67] This technique may be preferable in pregnant women, in whom radiation dose to the fetus is a particular concern. Total effective whole-body radiation dose from this technique is approximately 0.8 mSv, compared with 1.6-8.3 mSv for CT pulmonary angiography.[67a] Radiation risks of CT and VQ scan in pregnancy are discussed later in this chapter.

Another factor in choosing between VQ scan and CT scan is the breadth of the differential diagnosis under consideration. VQ scan answers a binary question in the emergency department: Is a PE present? CT scan can provide alternative diagnoses and is the better test when a broad differential diagnosis is under serious consideration. A study of 1025 emergency department patients undergoing CT for suspected PE found that among the 921 patients without PE detected, 7% had a CT finding requiring "specific and immediate intervention." These findings included pneumonia (81%), aortic aneurysm or dissection (7%), and mass suggesting undiagnosed malignancy (7%).[68] Later in this chapter, we discuss diagnostic strategies when both PE and aortic dissection are serious concerns.

What Is the Position of the American College of Emergency Physicians on Diagnostic Testing for Pulmonary Embolism?

ACEP published a clinical policy on evaluation of adult patients presenting with suspected PE in 2003. In this evidence-based review, authors concluded that a normal VQ scan was adequate to exclude "clinically significant" PE in patient with low to moderate pretest probability.[4] In the same review, they cited as a level B recommendation the use of CT scan as an alternative to VQ scan for patients with suspected PE. Importantly, this clinical policy predates the publication of several of the meta-analyses described earlier on good clinical outcomes following negative CT scans. In addition, PIOPED II was completed and published after publication of this ACEP policy, which is now categorized by ACEP as "not current." ACEP clinical policies undergo review periodically to incorporate new clinical evidence, or are retired if such a review is not performed.

Magnetic Resonance Imaging in Diagnosis of Pulmonary Embolism

MRI is a more recently described modality in diagnosis of PE. Indications for MRI for PE include contraindication to CT because of dye allergy, radiation concerns, and nondiagnostic testing with CT or VQ scan. In a study of CT angiography (PIOPED II), 24% of patients had 1 or more relative contraindications to radiation or iodinated contrast, suggesting a need for MRI as an alternative.[53] MRI can be used to assess for both PE and lower extremity and pelvic DVT. Initial experience with MRI showed sensitivity and specificity comparable or superior to that of multidetector CT.[69] Several techniques, including real-time MRI, magnetic resonance angiography (MRA), magnetic resonance (MR) perfusion imaging, and MR venography, can be combined to take advantage of differential sensitivity and specificity of the techniques. When analyzed on a per-patient basis (as opposed to per-embolus basis), the sensitivity of real-time MRI, MRA, MR perfusion imaging, and a combined protocol was 85%, 77%, 100%, and 100%, respectively, compared with a reference standard of 16-detector CT in 62 patients. Specificity was 98%, 100%, 91%, and 93%, respectively. Real-time MRI is advantageous because it can be performed without use of contrast agents and is rapid, taking only 180 seconds. MR perfusion imaging requires gadolinium contrast and takes approximately 7 minutes. MRA also requires contrast and takes only a few minutes.[70-71] In another study comparing MRA to conventional pulmonary angiography, MRA had an overall sensitivity of 77% (95% CI = 61%-90%), with sensitivity of 40%, 84%, and 100% for isolated subsegmental, segmental, and central or lobar PE, respectively.[72-73] MRI may play a role in confirming or ruling out PE when other imaging studies are equivocal. PIOPED III, a prospective multicenter study of gadolinium-enhanced magnetic resonance pulmonary angiography and lower extremity venography, enrolled 371 patients at 7 hospitals from 2006 to 2008. MRA/MRV results were compared against a mixed reference standard consisting of CT, VQ, ultrasound, d-dimer, and clinical assessment. MRA was technically inadequate in 25% of patients. When only technically adequate images were considered, the sensitivity of MRA was 78% (95%CI

67%-86%) and specificity was 99% (95%CI 96%-100%). When technically inadequate MRA was included, sensitivity was only 57%. The combination of MRA and venography was 92% sensitive (95%CI 83%-97%) and 96% specific (95%CI 91%-99%) when only technically adequate images were considered, but 52% of patients had technically inadequate results. The high specificity of this test may make it particularly useful in patients with nondiagnostic or suspected false positive imaging results using other modalities. The limited sensitivity of MRA alone means that a negative MRA should not be considered to rule out PE. The large percentage of technically inadequate MRA and MRV exams should make this a second line imaging study in patients who qualify for other imaging strategies. The procedure is probably most useful at centers that frequently perform the exam and thus have a greater chance of obtaining technically adequate results.[74]

Echocardiography for Pulmonary Embolism Diagnosis

Both transthoracic echocardiography (TTE) and transesophageal echocardiography (TEE) can be used for assessment of PE. Echocardiography is not a first-line diagnostic test to exclude PE in most patients because of poor sensitivity. However, some echocardiographic findings are highly specific for PE and can be used to confirm the diagnosis. Other findings are suggestive of PE and in a critically ill patient can be used to plan confirmatory testing, empiric anticoagulation, or invasive therapy such as catheter-based thrombolysis or thrombectomy. If a patient is stable enough to undergo CT or VQ scan, these tests are generally preferred because of higher accuracy. Echocardiography is advantageous because it is portable and can be used at the bedside in the emergency department or intensive care unit. It does not require the administration of nephrotoxic contrast agents. It can provide information about serious alternative diagnoses such as pericardial effusion and tamponade or aortic dissection, potentially redirecting the diagnostic and therapeutic plan. Some echocardiographic findings have been correlated with mortality from PE and may suggest the need for intensive care unit admission or aggressive radiologic therapies, which are described in more detail in the chapter on interventional radiology (Chapter 16).

TTE has a reported sensitivity around 30% to 55%, with specificity between 85% and 95%.[75-76] In a single-center, prospective, single-blinded study, right ventricular dilatation by TTE had a sensitivity of only 31% (95% CI = 21%-41%) but was highly specific for PE (94%, 05% CI = 89%-99%). The maximum velocity of tricuspid regurgitation, a marker of high pulmonary artery pressures, was also assessed. Elevated values (>2.7 m per second) had a sensitivity of 51% (95% CI = 38%-64%) with relatively low specificity (88%, 95% CI = 81%-95%)

because any non-PE pathology causing pulmonary hypertension can result in this finding. If right ventricular hypertrophy (free right ventricular wall thickness > 6mm) was present, tricuspid regurgitation velocity should not be used in evaluation for PE, as right ventricular hypertrophy suggests a long-standing pulmonary hypertension rather than an acute cause such as PE. The presence of both RV dilatation and high tricuspid regurgitation velocity was poorly sensitive (29%, 95% CI = 19%-39%) but highly specific (96%, 95% CI = 92%-100%).[77] This study suggests that the combination of right ventricular dilatation, high tricuspid regurgitation velocity, and normal right ventricular free wall thickness has a specificity similar to that for CT scan and VQ scan and thus could be used for diagnosis of PE. The authors stressed that nonspecificity of individual echocardiographic criteria would mean that some patients would be erroneously diagnosed with and treated for PE if these were used in isolation. Still, in the sickest patients, TTE can increase the probability of the diagnosis of PE pending confirmatory testing. Other rare findings, such as free-floating right ventricular or inferior vena cava thrombus, may confirm the diagnosis of PE.[78-79]

TEE for definitive diagnosis of PE has been described in small studies. Pruszczyk et al.[80] reported 80% sensitivity and 100% specificity using this method to visualize pulmonary emboli in the main right and left pulmonary arteries directly—though in a series of only 32 consecutive patients. Other authors have suggested that direct visualization of PE may be difficult (sensitivity 26%), although suggestive right heart abnormalities may support the diagnosis of PE.[81] Other reports describe the value of TEE in detecting thrombus in the inferior and superior vena cava, right atrium, and right ventricle.[79]

The prognostic value of echocardiography for patients with PE confirmed by other modalities has also been studied. In a study of normotensive patients with acute PE, the predictive value of echocardiogram for in-hospital shock or intubation, death, recurrent PE, or severe cardiopulmonary disability at 6-month follow-up was assessed. Right ventricular dysfunction on initial echocardiogram was only 61% sensitive (95% CI = 46%-74%) and 57% specific (95% CI = 48%-66%) for an adverse outcome.[82] This gives LR+ of 1.4 and LR− of 0.7, values which do not substantially change pretest probability assessment. A systematic review found five studies of echocardiographic findings of right ventricular dysfunction, with a pooled risk ratio of 2.4 (95% CI = 1.3-4.4) for death among hemodynamically stable patients with acute PE.[36] Overall, these studies imply that right ventricular dysfunction is only a moderate predictor of inpatient morbidity, with larger studies needed to determine its role and accuracy in more detail.

ASSESSMENT FOR DEEP VENOUS THROMBOSIS

No discussion of PE assessment is complete without discussion of DVT. DVT is believed to be the source for most pulmonary emboli, and assessment for DVT can be a surrogate for assessment of PE. When a patient has signs or symptoms of PE (e.g., syncope, dyspnea, or chest pain) and DVT is confirmed, the diagnosis of PE is often assumed. When patients cannot undergo assessment for PE because of clinical instability or contraindications to CT or VQ scan, assessment for DVT is a reasonable alternative. Moreover, when tests for PE (CT or VQ) are negative but a high clinical pretest probability exists, additional exclusion of DVT provides a greater likelihood ratio negative for future risk for thromboembolic disease, bolstering the decision to withhold anticoagulation. PIOPED II demonstrated that lower extremity imaging for DVT detects about 7% more patients requiring anticoagulation than CT pulmonary angiography alone, increasing sensitivity from 83% to 90% when the techniques are combined.[83] Historically, DVT was assessed with venography—direct injection of contrast material into the lower extremity venous system. This technique was associated with a risk for inducing DVT and has been largely abandoned. The most common method for detection of DVT today is noninvasive serial compression ultrasonography, often referred to by emergency physicians as "Doppler." This is a bit of a misnomer, because DVT diagnosis by ultrasound does not require the use of Doppler capability. Normal veins of the lower extremities are readily compressible with an ultrasound probe, whereas thrombosed segments are incompressible (see Figure 14-132 illustrating this technique in the Chapter 14 on extremity imaging). An ultrasound technician or emergency physician can assess for DVT by incremental compression of lower extremity veins from the inguinal ligament to the level of the popliteal fossa. If all veins are compressible, no DVT is present. An incompressible segment is evidence of DVT. Depending on the age of the DVT, the ultrasound appearance may be hyper-, hypo-, or anechoic, so compressibility rather than echotexture is used to differentiate patent and thrombosed veins. Doppler can be used as a supplemental technique. Augmentation of Doppler flow with application of pressure to the calf can be used to prove patency of lower extremity veins, although Doppler has not been shown to improve accuracy over simple compression.[84] While many DVTs present with calf swelling or pain, the calf itself is not usually assessed, as superficial and deep calf vein thromboses are not usually treated with anticoagulation because of a low risk for subsequent PE or proximal extension. A meta-analysis of studies of ultrasound found the sensitivity of compression ultrasound for proximal DVT to be 93.8% (95% CI = 92.0%-95.3%) with specificity of 97.8%

(95% CI = 97.0%-98.4%).[85] Rare studies show a lower sensitivity of ultrasound, approximately 70%, with excellent specificity (100%).[86] Studies show the safety of withholding anticoagulation in patients with two negative ultrasound tests for DVT at 1-week intervals, with 3-month rates of thromboembolism of only around 0.6% (95% CI = 0.07%-2.14%). Guidelines call for repeat ultrasound in 1 week to confirm negative findings, partly because of the risk for progression of an undetected calf DVT.[87-88] However, repeat ultrasound appears to have a low additional diagnostic yield, around 1.3%.[85]

Ultrasound is advantageous because it is portable, is inexpensive, and does not require administration of contrast agents or radiation. It is therefore safe in pregnant patients and patients with contrast allergies or renal impairment that may limit use of CT and VQ scan for assessment of PE. Bedside ultrasound can be used in assessment of unstable patients, eliminating hazardous transportation.

CT venography (CTV) can be performed with CT pulmonary angiography (see Chapter 14, Figure 14-133). The chest CT contrast bolus is simply followed into the pelvis and lower extremities, eliminating or minimizing the need for additional contrast administration.[56] This is accompanied by a significant additional radiation exposure and cost, raising questions about the relative benefit of the technique. In a study of 427 emergency department patients evaluated with CT pulmonary angiography for PE, addition of CTV identified only a single additional case of isolated DVT without PE, at a cost of $206,400.[55] CTV adds between 2 and 6 mSv to the radiation exposure for the patient, including significant gonadal exposure.[56] PIOPED II suggests that lower extremity imaging increases sensitivity for thromboembolic disease from 83% (CT pulmonary angiography alone) to 90%.[83] The range of reported additional thromboembolic disease cases identified by addition of lower extremity imaging ranges from only 1%[89] to an astounding 27% in various studies.[90] A meta-analysis found the sensitivity of CTV to be 95.9% (95% CI = 93%-97.8%) with a specificity of 95.2% (95% CI = 93.6%-96.5%).[91] Some studies suggest lower sensitivity, closer to 70%.[86]

Pelvic thrombus appears to be rare, and a more radiation-sparing technique is CT solely of the lower extremities, skipping the pelvis (imaging from acetabulum down, rather than the iliac crest). This technique reduces radiation exposure by about 40% while missing only 4% of DVTs.[92] Another method for radiation reduction is use of discontinuous axial CT imaging, with 7.5-mm slices alternating with 15 mm of skipped anatomy. This technique approaches the sensitivity of continuous lower extremity CT imaging and would reduce pelvic irradiation by 75%.[93] Ultrasound of the extremities results in no radiation exposure and is a reasonable alternative.

When Is CT Venography a Preferred Approach Over Ultrasound?

CT and ultrasound assessment for DVT are diagnostically equivalent according to data from PIOPED II, so in an average patient, either test is reasonable when viewed purely from the perspective of diagnostic accuracy. The choice of test can be made based on safety, time, and expense in most patients.[83] Some patients cannot undergo lower extremity ultrasound because of the presence of overlying cast material or orthopedic external fixators. Obesity makes ultrasound a difficult test, with CT sometimes a better option. Open lower extremity wounds or infections may make compression with an ultrasound probe difficult or unacceptably painful for the patient, in which case CT is a reasonable alternative. When pelvic DVT is specifically suspected, CT or MR venography is preferred over ultrasound, which cannot detect thrombus within the bony pelvis.

Magnetic Resonance Venography for Assessment of Deep Venous Thrombosis

MRI can also be used as a diagnostic test for DVT. It shares many of the advantages of CT: it can be combined with MR pulmonary angiography and can assess for pelvic thrombus, as well as lower extremity clot. MR may be useful in many of the same clinical circumstances that make ultrasound difficult. Unlike CT, MR does not expose the patient to ionizing radiation, making it a reasonable choice in pregnant patients. Some MR sequences (e.g., time of flight and phase contrast venography) can identify clot without the use of contrast agents by using intrinsic properties of flowing blood or clot.[94] A meta-analysis showed diagnostic accuracy similar to that reported for both CT and ultrasound: sensitivity of 91.5% (95% CI = 87.5%-94.5% and specificity of 94.8% (95% CI = 93.9%-62.1%).[95] PIOPED III demonstrated an improvement in sensitivity for VTE to 92% when lower extremity MRV was combined with contrast-enhanced MR pulmonary angiography, compared with MRA alone (78% sensitivity). However, the combined technique was technically difficult, with 52% of patients having inadequate results.[95a] MRI is costly compared with other techniques and should not be used as a first-line examination.[96]

COST AND RADIATION EXPOSURE OF DIAGNOSTIC TESTS FOR THROMBOEMBOLIC DISEASE

Table 7-8 depicts approximate costs and radiation exposures for common tests used in evaluation of possible thromboembolic disease. Radiation risks of CT are described in more detail at the end of the chapter.

IMAGING OF NONTRAUMATIC AORTIC DISEASE: DISSECTION AND ANEURYSM

Let's move on to a discussion of aortic diseases. Physicians are often imprecise in their nomenclature, but when we discuss nontraumatic aortic pathology, we are dealing with two separate processes, aortic aneurysm (with risk for rupture and hemorrhagic shock) and aortic dissection (with risk for occlusion of branch vessels and retrograde extension to the pericardium and aortic valve). These may occur independently or may coexist in a given patient. While a complete discussion of the risk factors and pathology of the two processes is beyond the scope of this book, understanding the difference between the two categories of disease is essential to understanding diagnostic imaging for these. As you will see, aortic dissection may be extremely difficult to

TABLE 7-8. Approximate Costs and Radiation Exposures of Diagnostic Imaging Tests for Pulmonary Embolism and Deep Venous Thrombosis

Modality	Cost	Radiation Exposure
Pulmonary angiography	$6000	3.2-30.1 mSv
Contrast-enhanced CT pulmonary angiography	$1700	1.6-8.3 mSv
Contrast-enhanced CT lower extremity and pelvic venography	$500 surcharge in addition to CT pulmonary angiography	2.5-6 mSv
Ventilation–perfusion (VQ) scan	$900	1.2-2.0 mSv
Ultrasound of bilateral legs	$600	none
D-dimer (rapid ELISA)	$25	none
Chest x-ray (PA and lateral)	$50-$150	0.07 mSV
Echocardiogram	$250-$500	none
MRI pulmonary angiography or pelvic and lower extremity venography	$2000	none

From East Ohio Regional Hospital. Patient price information list. (Accessed at http://www.eastohioregionalhospital.com/pricelist.asp.); Harvard Pilgrim HealthCare. Massachusetts medical cost data. (Accessed at https://www.harvardpilgrim.org/portal/page?_pageid=253,192924&_dad=portal&_schema=PORTAL.); Hunsaker AR, Zou KH, Poh AC, et al. Routine pelvic and lower extremity CT venography in patients undergoing pulmonary CT angiography. *AJR Am J Roentgenol* 190:322-6, 2008; Johnson JC, Brown MD, McCullough N, Smith S. CT lower extremity venography in suspected pulmonary embolism in the ED. *Emerg Radiol* 12:160-3, 2006; Stein PD, Woodard PK, Weg JG, et al. Diagnostic pathways in acute pulmonary embolism: Recommendations of the PIOPED II investigators. *Radiology* 242: 15-21, 2007.

ELISA, enzyme-linked immunosorbent assay.

diagnose by x-ray when a concurrent aortic aneurysm is not present. The figures in this section are arranged to depict concepts about aortic disease, centered on clinical cases. Many cases show both x-ray and CT findings. Be sure to review all figures associated with a case to glean the most information.

Aortic aneurysm (Figures 7-60 and 7-61; see also Figures 7-67 through 7-74 and 7-92 through 7-94) is defined by an aortic diameter exceeding 3 cm (50% larger than the upper limit of normal, 2 cm). However, clinically significant thoracic aneurysms are substantially larger. The risk for rupture is proportional to diameter but must be weighed against the operative mortality risk. In general, ascending thoracic aortic aneurysms should be repaired at 5.5 cm diameter and descending thoracic aneurysms at 6.5 cm. Patients with Marfan's syndrome or familial aneurysms should undergo repair of the ascending aorta at 5 cm or the descending aorta at 6 cm.[97] Advancing age, cigarette smoking, and male gender are other significant risk factors for aortic aneurysm. Because aneurysm is a disease characterized by an enlarging aortic diameter, the chest x-ray silhouette is a better test for this disease than for aortic dissection—but from a clinical perspective, ruling out both diseases is usually necessary in a symptomatic patient, making chest x-ray a poor diagnostic exam.

Figures 7-62 through 7-98 demonstrate a series of cases of nontraumatic aortic dissection, with the chest x-ray, CT scan, and aortogram from the same patient grouped together when available. Figures 7-99 and 7-100 demonstrate a case of an abnormal mediastinum on chest x-ray

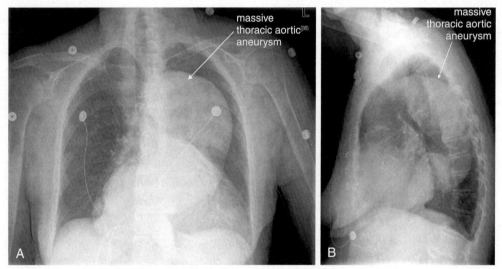

Figure 7-60. Thoracic aortic aneurysm. This 74-year-old female presented with myalgias and back pain. Her chest x-ray shows a massively dilated thoracic aortic aneurysm. A wide mediastinum may be an indication of aortic aneurysm. **A,** Posterior–anterior chest x-ray. **B,** Lateral chest x-ray.

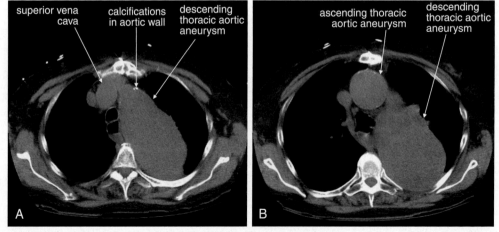

Figure 7-61. Thoracic aortic aneurysm. Same patient as Figure 7-60. The patient underwent noncontrast CT because of renal insufficiency. The ascending aorta measures 4.5 cm in diameter, whereas the descending aorta measures 7 by 10 cm. Without contrast, a superimposed dissection cannot be detected. **A, B,** Axial slices moving from cephalad to caudad.

that was not because of aortic dissection or aneurysm—a reminder of the limitations of chest x-ray.

Nontraumatic aortic dissection occurs as shear forces of blood flow initiate a tear in the intimal lining. This tear may extend proximally or distally, forming an intimal flap that divides the aorta into a true and a false lumen (see Figures 7-62 through 7-64). As the tear progresses, other layers of the aortic wall *may* be violated and blood *may* extravasate, in which case the classic chest x-ray findings of an indistinct aortic knob and widened mediastinum may be present (see Figure 7-65; see also Figures 7-70 and 7-75). However, the event begins as a purely intimal injury. As a consequence, the external aortic contour may not alter during aortic dissection.[98] Figures 7-78, 7-85, 7-88, and 7-95 demonstrate chest x-rays with a normal or near-normal mediastinum despite dramatic aortic dissections proven on CT. Review these chest x-rays and the accompanying CT scans (see Figures 7-79, 7-86, 7-89 through 7-91, and 7-96). Aortic dissections may extend into or occlude the origins of branch vessels, including coronary, carotid, extremity, renal, mesenteric, or spinal vessels (see Figures 7-64, 7-80, 7-82 through 7-84, 7-87, 7-90 and 7-91). Dissection may also lead to aortic valve regurgitation or pericardial tamponade. Risk factors for dissection include hypertension, connective tissue disorders such as Marfan syndrome (see Figures 7-67 and 7-68) and Ehlers-Danlos syndrome, bicuspid aortic valve, Turner syndrome, prior aortic valve replacement, and third-trimester pregnancy, when increased production of collagenase is thought to weaken the aortic wall.[99] Aortic dissection has been described in patients without evident preexisting aortic pathology. In these cases, a precipitating event, sometimes hypertension associated with drug use (cocaine)[100] or physical exertion (power weight lifting)[101] has been suggested as the cause.[102]

Who Needs Aortic Imaging? Can Clinical Risk Stratification Rule Out Aortic Dissection?

Unfortunately, no simple, accurate, and well-validated clinical scoring system exists to screen patients for aortic dissection. Shirakabe et al. described an emergency room acute aortic dissection score, using four clinical criteria: (1) presence of back pain, (2) mediastinal-thoracic ratio greater than 30%, (3) aortic regurgitation, and (4) aortic diameter greater than 30 mm on ultrasound. A score of at least three was 93% sensitive and 78% specific. However, the need for thoracic echocardiography limits the utility of this rule in screening chest pain patients for dissection and determining the need for CT. In many centers, CT may be more readily available than echocardiography. In addition, this scoring system has not been prospectively validated outside of the original study environment.[103] Acute aortic dissection is correctly suspected initially in only 15% to 43% of presentations, suggesting that the combination of risk factor analysis, history, and physical examination has poor sensitivity. A systematic review in *JAMA* in 2002[99] noted that a thorough chest pain history, including the quality, radiation, and intensity at onset, is associated with a higher initial diagnostic accuracy but still misses 10% of aortic dissections. This review notes that many classically described abnormalities of aortic dissection, including significant differences in interarm blood pressure measurements, have little evidence basis. The presence of upper extremity blood pressure differences greater than 20 mm Hg is sometimes recommended as a warning sign for aortic dissection, though studies show

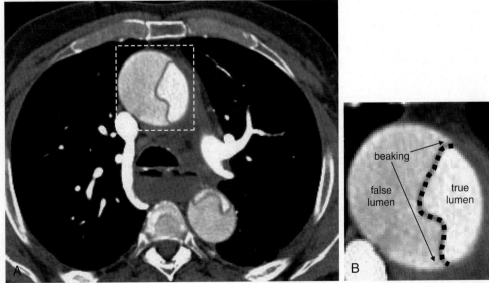

Figure 7-62. Anatomy of aortic dissection, CT angiogram. A, Axial CT image. **B,** Close-up. In aortic dissection, an intimal flap (*dotted black line in magnified view*) divides the aorta into a true and a false lumen. The characteristic sharp corners of the false lumen are known as "beaking."

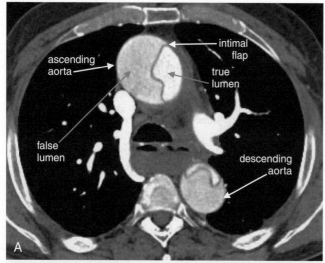

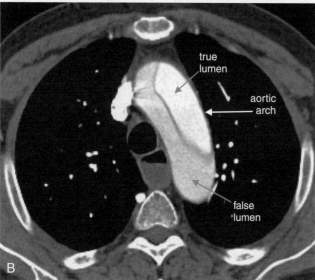

Figure 7-63. Aortic dissection, CT angiogram. Cross sections through the aorta, showing a large dissection. An intimal flap divides the aorta into a true and a false lumen. Here, the true lumen is brightly filled with contrast, whereas the false lumen appears darker because of a lower flow of contrast. The dissection involves the ascending aorta, arch, and descending aorta. There is no extravasation of contrast outside of the aortic lumen, and the patient's mediastinal silhouette on chest x-ray was normal. In this patient, the ascending aorta is somewhat dilated. The descending aorta is of normal size. **A,** Axial slice through the ascending and descending aorta. **B,** A more cephalad axial slice through the aortic arch.

that 18% of asymptomatic subjects with a history of hypertension and 15% of asymptomatic subjects with no such history have a blood pressure disparity exceeding 10 mm Hg between upper extremities.[103a,103b] A variety of classic signs and symptoms have poor discriminatory power when used alone. Table 7-9 reviews some history and physical examination findings that may increase or decrease the risk for aortic dissection. However, no single element of history or physical examination appears sensitive enough to rule out aortic dissection, meaning that definitive imaging should be performed when the diagnosis is seriously entertained.[99]

What Modalities Can Be Used to Diagnose Spontaneous Aortic Catastrophes?

Although chest x-ray is the initial imaging examination in most patients with chest pain, its sensitivity and specificity for aortic catastrophes is poor, as described in more detail later. Aortography (see Figure 7-72) is the historical gold standard for aortic dissection and thoracic aneurysm, but it has been replaced by CT with IV contrast as the predominant imaging modality in the emergency department. Today, aortography is restricted almost entirely to patients who have aortic disease detected with other imaging modalities and who require therapeutic interventions. As described in the chapter on interventional radiology (Chapter 16), aortography allows placement of stent grafts (see Figures 7-73, 7-74, 7-93, and 7-94) that can be used to repair some forms of dissections and aneurysms.

MRI without contrast, MRA with gadolinium contrast enhancement, TTE, and TEE can also be used to diagnosis aortic disease, but these are reserved primarily for patients with contraindications to CT. MRI and MRA are used predominately in patients with allergy to iodinated contrast agents used in CT. MRA was once used in patients with renal insufficiency because of concerns about contrast nephropathy related to iodinated contrast. However, the recent recognition of fatal nephrogenic systemic fibrosis in patients with renal disease who have received gadolinium has substantially eroded this indication for MRA. Gadolinium-associated nephrogenic systemic fibrosis is described in detail in Chapter 15. Gadolinium contrast-enhanced MRA has excellent test characteristics for aortic pathology but more limited availability in emergency departments. Multiplanar ECG-gated spin-echo MRI without use of gadolinium contrast also has excellent reported sensitivity and specificity for aortic dissection.[103c] Three-dimensional MRA without gadolinium contrast is a newer alternative, with preliminary experience suggesting similar diagnostic performance to gadolinium-enhanced MRA.[103d] Echocardiography and MRI or MRA share the ability to assess the aortic valve, pericardium, and left ventricular ejection fraction. CT can provide this information as well if retrospective electrocardiogram gating is performed (described in detail in Chapter 8) but at the cost of significant radiation exposure.

Echocardiography is a reasonable option in the patient who appears too unstable to undergo CT scan. The modality is portable and does not require administration of nephrotoxic contrast agents. TEE has excellent sensitivity and specificity (described later). It can be performed on an intubated patient in the emergency department or in the operating suite if a very high suspicion for aortic dissection exists.

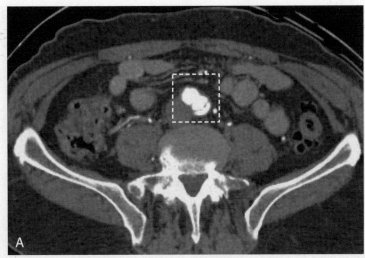
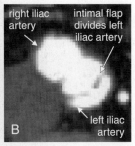

Figure 7-64. Aortic dissection with iliac artery dissection, CT angiogram. A, Axial image through iliac arteries at level of pelvis. **B,** Close-up. In this massive aortic dissection, the intimal flap extends into the left iliac artery. The right iliac artery is normal. Aortic dissection may involve any branch vessel. Consequently, the usual CT protocol for aortic dissection includes CT of the chest, abdomen, and pelvis to include the entire aorta and its major branches.

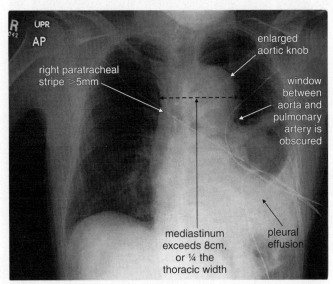

Figure 7-65. Aortic dissection with abnormal chest x-ray. This patient had experienced chest pain 1 week prior, which had spontaneously resolved, although dyspnea persisted. Chest x-ray demonstrates a wide mediastinum and aortic knob, confirmed on CT (Figure 7-66). The left pleural effusion was shown on CT to be a hemothorax from extravasating aortic blood. Other classic findings of aortic dissection are also seen here. Though none of these findings is reliable individually, in aggregate they are quite concerning for aortic pathology in this patient.

Interpreting the Chest X-ray for Aortic Pathology

Although a normal chest x-ray alone cannot exclude aortic pathology, some classic abnormalities may suggest aortic disease, and familiarity with these findings may assist with clinical risk stratification. Let's briefly describe the major chest x-ray abnormalities associated with aortic dissection and aortic aneurysm. These are also illustrated in figures throughout this section.

- *Widening of the mediastinum.* This finding implies either an aortic aneurysm or the presence of a mediastinal

hematoma associated with aortic dissection or aneurysm rupture. A width exceeding 8 cm at the level of the aortic knob or a ratio of mediastinal width to chest width exceeding 0.25 is considered abnormal. This finding is neither highly sensitive nor highly specific. Dissection can occur in an aorta of normal diameter, and no mediastinal hematoma may have accumulated. In addition, many other forms of mediastinal pathology, including adenopathy and masses, may widen the mediastinum. A **widened aortic knob** and **widening of the ascending and descending aorta** are also sometimes described for the same reasons.

- *Blurring of aortic knob or double density sign.* This finding implies dissection, with the double contour representing the intima and the muscularis layers. Blurring may also represent blood external to the normal aortic wall, trapped within the aortic adventitia or mediastinum—a mediastinal hematoma. For the same reasons described earlier, this finding may often be absent.

- *Pleural effusion.* Blood leaking from a ruptured thoracic aortic aneurysm or from an aortic dissection may accumulate in the pleural space. This finding is not specific for aortic disease, because pleural effusions may occur from many other causes. In addition, many dissections do involve not the loss of blood from the aorta but rather an isolated tear of the intimal lining, resulting in true and false lumens.

- *Widened right paraspinal shadow or paratracheal stripe.* Normally, a thin (1 to 4 mm) water-density stripe is visible between the air column of the trachea and the adjacent right lung. When this stripe is 5 mm or more in width, abnormal soft tissue or fluid such as blood is likely present. However, the finding may represent diseases of the trachea, mediastinum, or pleura and is not specific to aortic disease.[104]

Figure 7-66. Aortic dissection. **A,** Coronal image. **B,** Close-up from **A. C,** Axial image. **D,** Close-up from **C.** Same patient as in Figure 7-65. This aortic dissection occurred in an existing large thoracic aneurysm. Blood extravasated, causing hemothorax and collapsing the left lower lung. In the coronal images, note that the aorta immediately abuts the left main bronchus, explaining why displacement of this bronchus is seen on chest x-ray in some cases of aortic pathology.

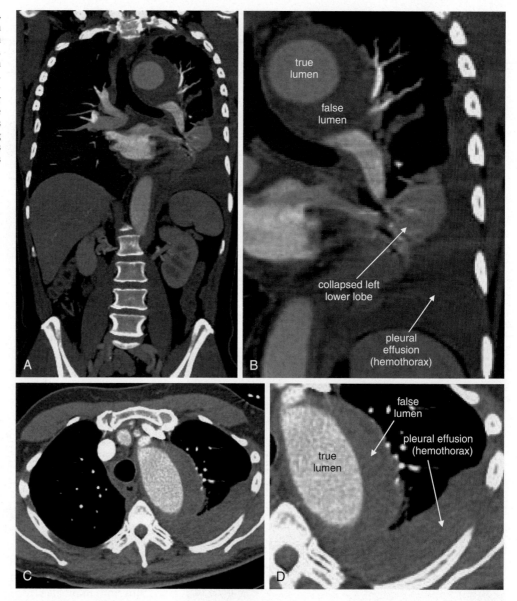

- *Tracheal shift* (usually to the right, with the center of the trachea to the right of the spinous process at the fourth and fifth thoracic vertebra). A mediastinal hematoma or aortic aneurysm may create mass effect within the mediastinum, displacing the trachea. A range of other pathology can result in tracheal shift, from other mediastinal pathology such as adenopathy or mass to pulmonary pathology such as atelectasis or lobar collapse. Even poor patient positioning can create the appearance of tracheal shift.
- *Distortion of the left main bronchus.* For similar reasons, mediastinal hematoma or aortic aneurysm can create mass effect, displacing the left main bronchus (see Figure 7-66). Again, this is not specific for aortic pathology but is an indication of mass effect.
- *Abnormal path of a nasogastric tube.* Mediastinal hematoma or aortic aneurysm can create mass effect upon the esophagus, resulting in displacement of a nasogastric tube. Again, this finding may not be present if dissection occurs without the development of a mediastinal hematoma. The finding is nonspecific, because other causes of esophageal displacement also result in this radiographic abnormality.
- *Displacement of soft tissues from aortic calcifications greater than 6 mm.* Calcifications are often found in the aortic wall in the absence of either aortic dissection or aneurysm. However, aortic dissection can lead to blood in a false lumen inside or outside of the calcified aortic rim. When soft-tissue density greater than 6 mm is seen outside of the calcifications in the aortic shadow, this finding suggests that aortic dissection, mediastinal hematoma, or aortic aneurysm is present. This is sometimes called the **eggshell sign.**[105]
- *Kinking or tortuosity of aorta.* This finding suggests aortic aneurysm or dissection but is quite nonspecific. The normal aorta should have a smooth arch and knob, with a fairly straight descending aortic

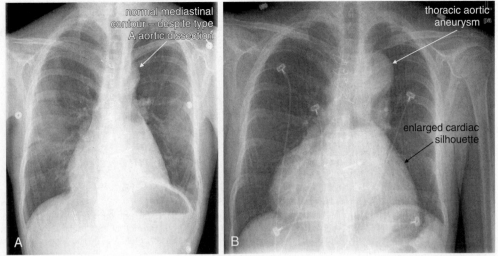

Figure 7-67. Aortic dissection versus aneurysm. Because aortic dissection may involve only the intima and may not violate the external contour of the aorta, the mediastinal silhouette may not change on chest x-ray. A normal chest x-ray occurs in approximately 12% of cases and cannot rule out aortic dissection when the condition is suspected clinically. Aortic aneurysm by definition involves a 50% or greater increase in aortic diameter, so the mediastinal silhouette is usually abnormal. This male patient with Marfan's syndrome had mitral valve replacement at age 13. At age 20, he developed chest pain and was found to have type A aortic dissection. He subsequently developed worsened aneurysmal dilatation of his aorta, chronic aortic dissection, and a dilated cardiomyopathy with an ejection fraction less than 15%. Compare his chest x-ray at age 20 on the date of his acute aortic dissection **(A)** with his chest x-ray a mere 4 years later **(B).** The widening of his mediastinum seen in **B** is a result of his thoracic aneurysm—he has type A aortic dissection at the time of both x-rays, but the aortic knob and mediastinum appear normal in **A.**

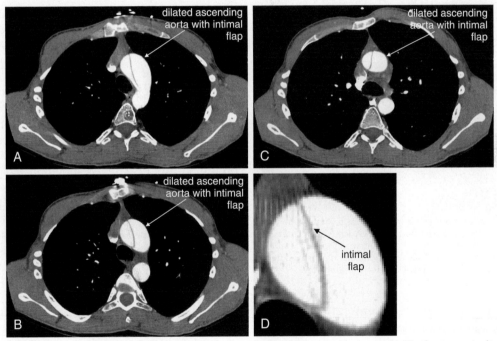

Figure 7-68. Aortic dissection. This 20-year-old male with Marfan's syndrome presented with chest pain. His chest x-ray is shown in Figure 7-67, **A,** and has a normal mediastinal silhouette. The CT images here demonstrate an intimal flap involving the ascending aorta and proximal arch, a type A dissection. The patient also has aneurysmal dilatation of the ascending aorta, which is nearly twice the diameter of the descending aorta. **A** through **C,** Axial images moving from cephalad to caudad. **D,** Close-up from **B.**

segment. Aneurysm may cause the descending aorta to be irregular in contour. In addition, mediastinal hematoma may displace the aorta or render its silhouette irregular or tortuous.

• *Opacification of the window between the aortic knob and the left pulmonary artery.* Normally, a lucent window (dark) is present between the aortic knob and the left pulmonary artery, which both have water density on chest x-ray (white) (see Chapter 5 for a discussion of tissue densities on chest x-ray). Mediastinal hematoma or aortic aneurysm can obscure this window.

• *Localized lump on the aortic arch distal to the great vessels.* This is another finding suggesting thoracic aneurysm or dissection with mural hematoma.

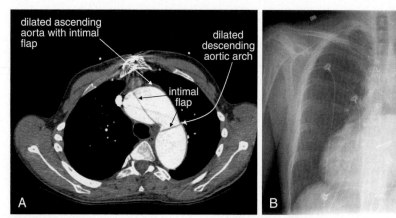

Figure 7-69. **Aortic dissection within an aneurysm.** Same patient as Figure 7-68, 4 years later. The patient now has a chronic type A dissection, with a markedly aneurysmal thoracic aorta. Compare this axial CT image **(A)** with that in Figure 7-68, noting that the descending aorta is now dilated as well. Compare the size of the aorta with that of the thoracic vertebral body. **B,** Chest x-ray at the time of the CT in **A.** The aortic aneurysm renders the aortic contour abnormal on chest x-ray. The intimal flap of dissection is not visible on chest x-ray.

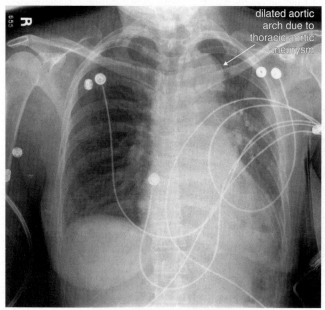

Figure 7-70. **Aortic dissection type B within thoracic aneurysm.** This patient with a known thoracic aneurysm developed acute chest and back pain. Her chest x-ray is abnormal—with a dramatically enlarged aortic knob and wide mediastinum—but these are old findings, unchanged from her prior chest x-rays. Her CT angiogram is shown in Figure 7-71.

See Figures 7-60, 7-65, 7-67, 7-69, 7-70, 7-73, 7-75, and 7-92, which demonstrate abnormal mediastinal findings on chest x-ray suggestive of aortic disease.

What Is the Role of Chest X-ray in Ruling Out Aortic Pathology? Does a Normal Chest X-ray Rule Out Aortic Pathology? If Not, When Is Computed Tomography Needed Following a Normal Chest X-ray?

Chest x-ray is insensitive for aortic pathology. In nontraumatic aortic dissection, chest x-ray is reported to have sensitivity as low as 81%, with specificity as low as 89%.[98-99,106-107] As described earlier, an intimal flap may occur in an aorta of normal caliber, and no extravasation of blood may occur, at least initially. In this scenario, the mediastinal silhouette seen on x-ray would not be expected to alter during dissection when compared with a chest x-ray taken before the dissection. Figures 7-78, 7-85, 7-88, and 7-95 show normal or unchanged chest x-rays in the setting of acute aortic dissection—review these and the associated CT images, which follow each x-ray. Chest x-ray may be abnormal in nontraumatic dissection if the dissection occurs in an aneurysmal aorta, if the dissection leads to formation of a large mural hematoma, or if extravasation of blood occurs into the mediastinum or pleural space. The likelihood ratio negative associated with a normal mediastinum and aortic contour is around 0.3—remember that a likelihood ratio negative less than 0.1 is needed to substantially decrease pretest odds of disease. As shown in Table 7-9, the combination of a normal chest x-ray, the absence of a classic aortic dissection clinical history, and the absence of pulse deficits or blood pressure disparities has a strong likelihood ratio negative. *However, it is essential to understand that a normal chest x-ray does not rule out aortic dissection when the disease is suspected clinically.* In addition, an abnormal mediastinum can result from nonaortic pathology, because the mediastinum contains numerous structures, including the heart, great vessels, trachea, esophagus, lymph nodes, and (sometimes) thyroid and thymus glands.

Chest x-ray findings suggestive of aortic dissection have been described, including a wide mediastinum, an abnormal aortic contour, displacement of soft tissues from aortic calcifications, tracheal deviation, and pleural effusions. A BestBETs review found four studies with mixed methodology—all of which found completely inadequate sensitivity of these findings to be useful clinically to rule out dissection. For example, displacement of soft tissues from aortic calcifications, which might be expected to occur as a dissection separates the intima from the aortic muscularis layer, has a sensitivity of only 5% to 9%. A widened mediastinum has a reported sensitivity of only about 47% to 65%. Even a normal chest x-ray may occur in the setting of dissection—reportedly in 12% to 40% of cases.[98] In a study of the interobserver agreement among radiologists for interpretation of these "classic" chest x-ray findings of aortic dissection, interobserver agreement was little better than that expected by chance. In a study of 75 patients with aortic dissection, only 25% had initial chest x-ray interpretations in which the radiologist prospectively stated that aortic dissection or aortic aneurysm was present or in which further aortic imaging was recommended.[108]

Jagannath et al. found that the classic chest x-ray features individually had poor interrater reliability, sensitivity, and specificity. When the radiologist's overall impression based on these findings was used, the sensitivity was 81%, with a specificity of 89%.[106] Hagan et al.[107] reviewed the International Registry of Acute Aortic Dissection database and found that no radiographic abnormalities were noted in 12% of aortic dissections. The mediastinum and aortic contour were normal in 21%. A widened mediastinum was noted in 62% and an abnormal aortic contour in 50%. An abnormal cardiac contour was present in 26% and pleural effusion in 19%. Displacement of aortic calcifications was noted in only 14%. Because the registry does not include patients without aortic dissection, specificity cannot be calculated.

Von Kodolitsch and colleagues[109] examined the likelihood ratios for individual chest x-ray findings in a high-risk cohort of patients with suspected aortic dissection. They reported likelihood ratios for individual findings, as well as sensitivity and specificity of the complete x-ray interpretation. Overall sensitivity was only 69%, and specificity was 86%. The negative likelihood ratios for classic findings such as widened mediastinum and displaced calcifications were between 0.4 and 1.1, which are not clinically useful to rule out disease.

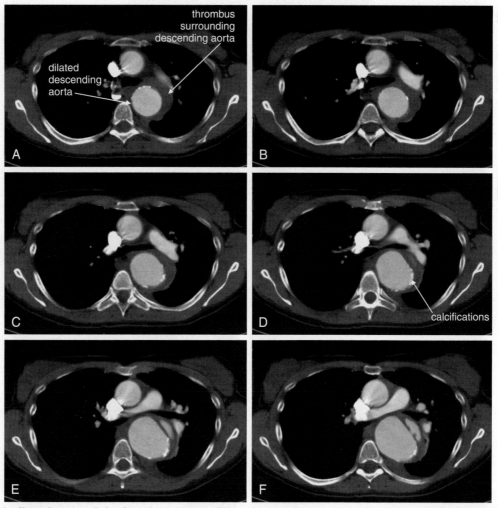

Figure 7-71. Aortic dissection type B in thoracic aneurysm, CT angiogram. Same patient as in Figure 7-70. **A** through **K,** Axial computed tomography (CT) images progressing from cephalad to caudad. This series of CT images shows an aneurysmal descending aorta, partially surrounded by a thombosed layer outside of vascular calcifications (bright white punctate lesions) within the aortic wall. This was described by the radiologist as a chronic type B aortic dissection (defined by its pviolvement of the descending aorta only). However, it may be a pseudoaneurysm of the descending aorta, arising from a true aneurysm. Regardless, contrast can be seen within a mushroom-shaped region on the left side of the patient's aorta.

Continued

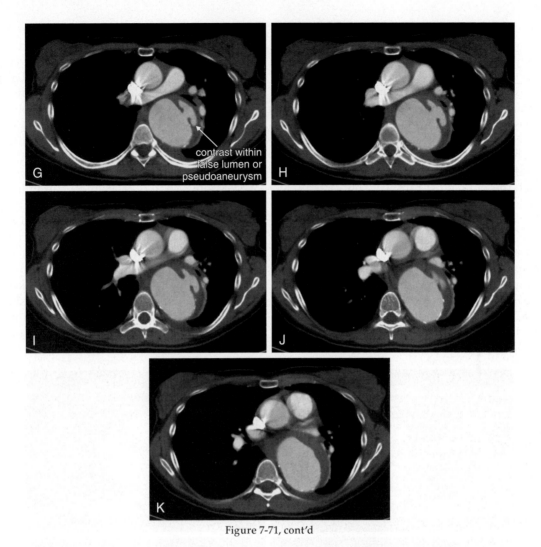

Figure 7-71, cont'd

Figure 7-72. **Aortic dissection type B in thoracic aneurysm.** Same patient as in Figures 7-70 and 7-71. This aortogram, performed during stent graft placement for repair of the chronic type B dissection and thoracic aneurysm, clearly shows the aneurysm but not the dissection. Because of its cross-sectional ability, computed tomography is particularly helpful at depicting the internal anatomy of the aorta.

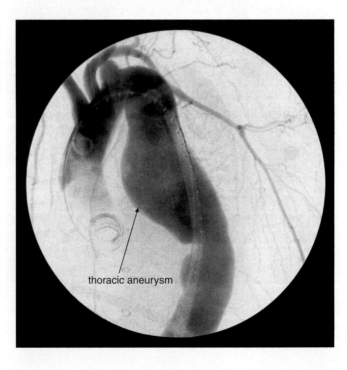

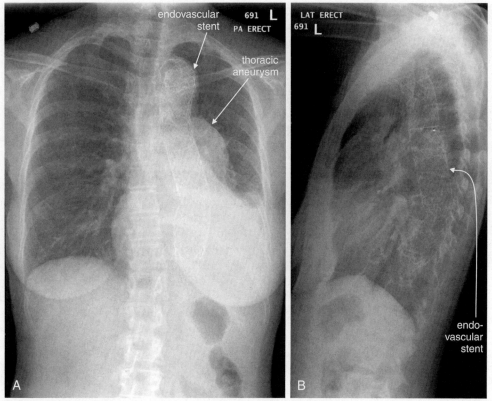

Figure 7-73. Thoracic aneurysm repair. A, Posterior–anterior chest x-ray. **B,** Lateral chest x-ray. The same patient as Figures 7-70 through 7-72, after endovascular stenting. The mediastinal silhouette remains wide, because the thoracic aneurysm sac has not been removed—the endovascular stent runs through it and protects against aneurysm rupture.

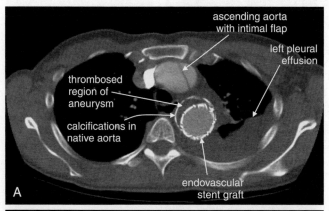

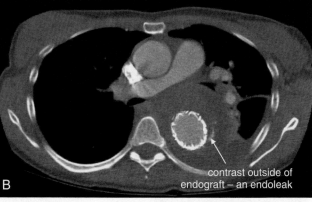

Figure 7-74. Complications of thoracic aneurysm repair: type A aortic dissection and endoleak. Same patient as Figure 7-73. This CT angiogram shows several findings. First, the endovascular graft is visible as a bright white ring (because of its metal composition). **A,** It is surrounded by the native calcifications of the patient's thoracic aneurysm. The lumen outside of the stent graft has thrombosed as expected and contains no contrast. The stent itself is patent and filled with contrast. The ascending aorta has an intimal flap—indicating a new type A aortic dissection. A pleural effusion is present. **B,** A more caudad slice shows a small amount of contrast outside of the stent graft but inside of the expected contour of the original aneurysm—an endoleak. Endoleaks are common after endovascular repair and are discussed in detail in Chapter 11. An endoleak is defined as the continued flow of blood into the aneurysm sac. Endoleaks are graded as one of four types. Type 1 endoleaks occur immediately at the time of placement of an endovascular graft, usually resulting from missizing of the graft, such that the proximal or distal ends of the graft are not sealed against the aorta. This requires placement of a larger graft, because type 1 endoleaks leave the aneurysm sac subject to systemic vascular pressures with continued risk for acute rupture. Type 2 endoleaks occur because of retrograde flow of blood through collateral vessels into the aneurysm sac. Common examples include filling of the aneurysm sac from spinal perforating arteries or intercostals arteries. Type 2 endoleaks are often observed without treatment, as they do not subject the aneurysm sac to full systemic vascular pressures and are at relatively low risk for rupture. Type 2 endoleaks that do not resolve spontaneously can be treated with angiographic embolization. Type 3 endoleaks occur when a tear in the fabric of the graft occurs, or if separation occurs between grafts consisting of multiple modules. This type of leak is relatively rare but leaves the aneurysm sac subject to systemic vascular pressures, requiring replacement of the graft because of continued risk for aneurysm rupture. Type 4 endoleaks occur from leaks through pores of the graft material and usually do not require repair. The type of endoleak can often be determined from CT. In this patient, the contrast was noted to arise from a single intercostal artery, making this a type 2 endoleak.

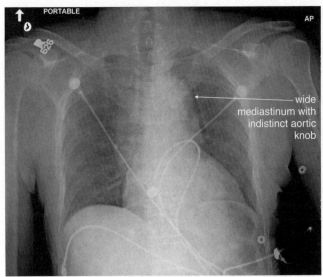

Figure 7-75. **Aortic dissection type A with abnormal chest x-ray.** This 50-year-old male presented with throat and abdominal pain, radiating to his legs. He was hypertensive (240 mm Hg systolic blood pressure), and aortic dissection was suspected, despite the absence of chest or back pain. His chest x-ray shows a wide mediastinum—but as the computed tomography (CT) in Figure 7-76 shows, this is due to a preexisting dilated ascending aorta. CT confirmed acute aortic dissection, but because the dissection was confined to the intima, it would not be expected to change the mediastinal contour on chest x-ray.

Does this mean that every patient with chest pain needs CT or other definitive imaging to evaluate the aorta, even with a normal chest x-ray? Not necessarily. Aortic dissection is a relatively rare disease, and the combination of a nonconcerning history, a normal chest x-ray, and the absence of blood pressure differentials or pulse deficits has a strong likelihood ratio negative (see Table 7-9). Consider the following scenario, depicted in Figures 7-101. A population of 1000 emergency department patients presents with chest pain. Imagine that 1% of that population has aortic dissection (10 patients), and that chest x-ray is 80% sensitive and 80% specific for detection of aortic dissection. This means that chest x-ray detects 8 of 10 patients with aortic dissection, leaving only 2 patients undetected. This gives a normal chest x-ray a negative predictive value of 99.7%. In 1000 patient encounters of this type, you would miss only 2 patients with aortic dissection by relying on chest x-ray as your imaging modality. If instead you chose to use CT as your diagnostic modality, you would need to perform CT in 794 patients with normal chest x-rays to identify 2 patients with dissection, giving a number needed to treat of almost 400. Consider a different scenario with a high-risk population, in

Figure 7-76. **CT angiogram in a patient with type A aortic dissection and abnormal chest x-ray.** This figure demonstrates several essential points. First, the intimal flap of aortic dissection cannot be seen without injection of vascular contrast material. Images **A** and **B** were acquired minutes apart. **A,** A section through the ascending and descending aorta without contrast. **B,** A section through the same level after contrast administration. The intimal flap is invisible in **A** but readily apparent in **B. C,** Close-up from **B.** The second essential point for this figure is the effect of aortic dissection on mediastinal contour. When nontraumatic dissection involves only the intima, the external contour of the aorta does not change. The mediastinum may or may not be widened—depending on the configuration of the aorta and other mediastinal structures before dissection occurred. This patient's mediastinum is wide, but not because of his dissection.

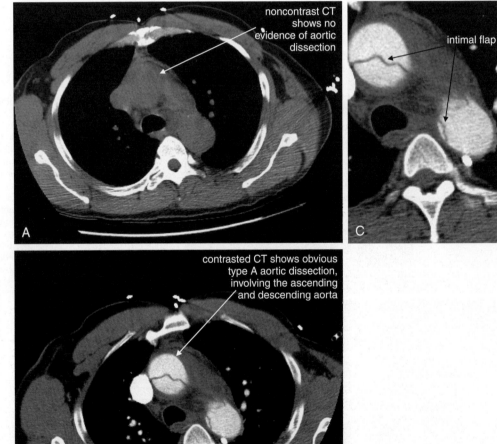

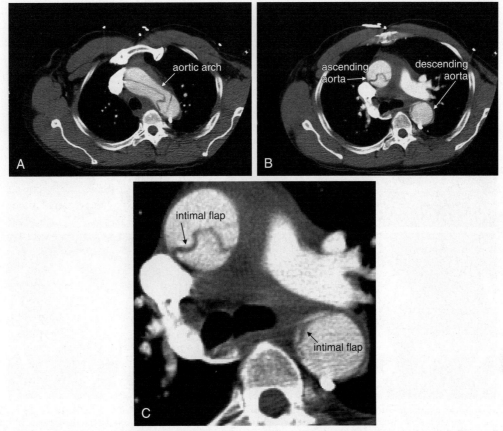

Figure 7-77. CT angiogram in a patient with type A aortic dissection and abnormal chest x-ray. Same patient as in Figures 7-75 and 7-76. **A,** An axial computed tomography (CT) slice through the aortic arch. **B,** A more caudad slice. **C,** Close-up from **B.** More images from the same patient depict the dissection flap in the ascending aorta, arch, and descending aorta. When the flap is located centrally within the lumen, it is readily apparent on contrasted CT. This is the case here in the ascending aorta and arch. However, in this patient, the true and false lumens are quite asymmetrical in the descending aorta and the intimal flap hugs the aortic wall, making it subtler. Inspect carefully for flaps along the aortic wall.

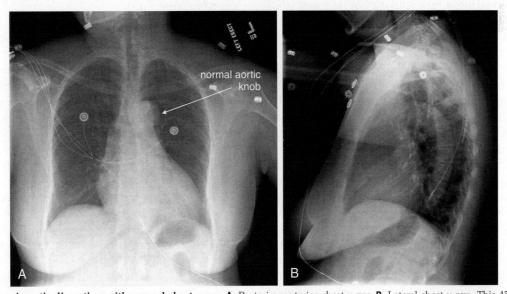

Figure 7-78. Type A aortic dissection with normal chest x-ray. A, Posterior–anterior chest x-ray. **B,** Lateral chest x-ray. This 45-year-old female with no past medical history presented with burning chest pain similar to her past indigestion. Her chest x-ray was interpreted as normal. Her aortic knob is well defined, and her mediastinum is not widened. She was admitted to an observation unit for assessment of possible cardiac ischemia. During an exercise stress echocardiogram, the patient developed leg pain and a dissection flap was noted on ultrasound. Her CT aortogram is reviewed in Figure 7-79. How can aortic dissection occur with a normal chest x-ray? Spontaneous aortic dissection affects the intima, so the external contour of the aorta may not acutely change. About one in eight dissections occurs with a normal chest x-ray.

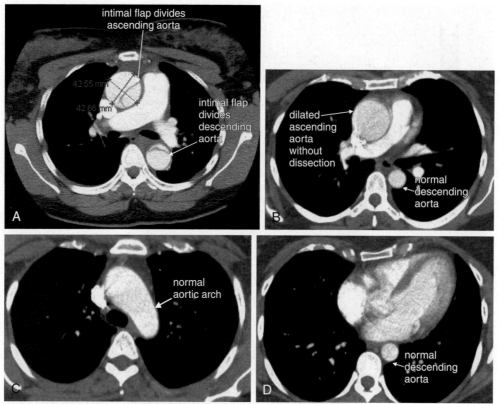

Figure 7-79. CT aortogram in a patient with type A aortic dissection and a normal chest x-ray. A, Same patient as in Figure 7-78, with Stanford type A aortic dissection. Compare with **B** through **D,** showing another patient with a dilated ascending aorta but no dissection. The normal aorta should be uniformly filled with contrast, without evidence of an intimal flap. The ascending and descending aorta should be circular in cross section. The arch is elliptic in cross section. Both of these patients have a dilated aortic root, a risk factor for aortic dissection. However, in neither patient did the ascending aorta result in a significantly enlarged mediastinum on chest x-ray.

which the 1000 patients encountered have a classic history of abrupt tearing interscapular pain (Figure 7-102). Let's allow that 30% of such patients (300 patients out of 1000) might have aortic dissection. If chest x-ray has 80% sensitivity and specificity, as in our first example, 80% of patients with aortic dissection (240 out of 300) would be identified by chest x-ray. As 60 patients with dissection would have normal chest x-rays, the negative predictive value of a normal chest x-ray would be only 90%, which is unacceptable given the morbidity of the disease in question. In this case, CT should be used to evaluate those patients with normal chest x-rays. Thus 620 patients would undergo CT to identify 60 aortic dissections, giving a number needed to treat of around 10. How does this hypothetical scenario help you understand when CT should be used to screen for dissection? Your clinical judgment, including factors from the history of present illness, past medical history, and physical exam, likely can select from all comers those patients who are at very low or high risk for aortic dissection. As demonstrated, if your pretest probability of aortic dissection is low (e.g., 1%), a normal chest x-ray has a good negative predictive value, and no further imaging for dissection should be performed. If your pretest probability is high (e.g., 30%), the negative predictive value of chest x-ray is relatively low, and further imaging for

dissection should be performed, even in a patient with a normal chest x-ray.

Notice that the relative rarity of aortic dissection means that even a fairly specific test results in a high false-positive rate—so most patients with abnormal chest x-ray findings do not have aortic dissection. As shown in Figure 7-101, in a population with a low incidence of aortic dissection (1%), false positives far outnumber true positives, and the positive predictive value of an abnormal chest x-ray is very low. An example would be a 20-year-old healthy patient with fever, noted to have a wide mediastinum on chest x-ray. This patient has a very low pretest probability of acute aortic dissection, and the mediastinal abnormality is likely not due to aortic pathology. Even in a high-risk population (30% rate of aortic dissection, see Figure 7-102), chest x-ray produces a large number of false-positive results, and the positive predictive value is less than 70%.

Overall, the pretest probability of aortic disease must be considered carefully when deciding how to proceed following a chest x-ray. A normal chest x-ray in a patient with a high pretest probability of disease demands further imaging. An abnormal chest x-ray in a patient

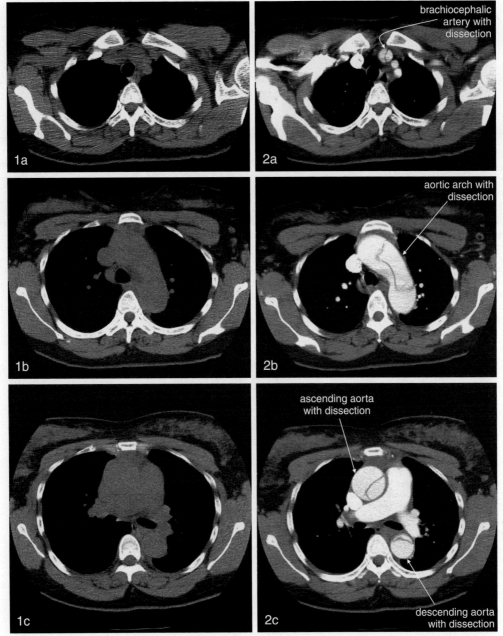

Figure 7-80. Contrast is essential to the CT diagnosis of aortic dissection. Same patient as Figure 7-78 and Figure 7-79, *A*. Series **1** (left column) shows noncontrast chest CT, moving from cephalad to caudad. Series **2** (right column) shows slices from the same positions, now with intravenous contrast. The importance of contrast for the diagnosis of aortic dissection cannot be overemphasized. The intimal flap is invisible without contrast.

with a low pretest probability of aortic disease does not strongly predict aortic pathology—although other causes of mediastinal widening (e.g., adenopathy or other mass) (see Figure 7-99 and 7-100) must be considered and may require imaging.

How Sensitive Are Advanced Imaging Modalities for Aortic Pathology?

Early CT studies for aortic dissection showed limited sensitivity, again because of the technologic limitations of single-slice, nonhelical CT.[110] Modern multislice helical CT offers high sensitivity and the advantage of three-dimensional reconstructions that depict branch vessel anatomy and may help with planning of surgical approach. By 1993, CT was described as nearing 100% sensitivity for detection of aortic dissection. A 1993 study by Nienaber and colleagues[111] in the *New England Journal of Medicine* compared CT, MRI without gadolinium contrast, TEE, and TTE in 110 patients with clinically suspected aortic dissection. The study had a strong gold standard, including operative findings in 62 patients, autopsy in 7, and contrast angiography in 64. The sensitivities were 98.3% for CT, 98.3% for MRI, 97.7% for TEE, and 59.3% for TTE. Specificities were 87.1% (CT), 97.8% (MR), 76.9% (TEE), and 83.0% (TTE). Further advances

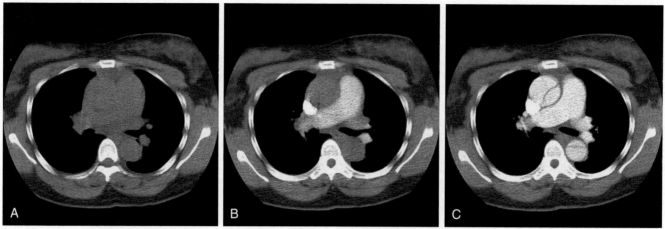

Figure 7-81. Contrast timing in the CT diagnosis of aortic dissection. Same patient as Figures 7-78, 7-79, *A*, and 7-80. For the diagnosis of aortic dissection, appropriate timing of the injected contrast bolus is essential. Fortunately, automated bolus tracking software allows a small test bolus to be performed, to gauge when the injected contrast will reach the vascular bed of interest. The images show the same patient during different phases of contrast injection. **A,** No contrast has been injected, and the aortic dissection is not visible. **B,** Contrast has reached the pulmonary artery—as would be the goal for a CT pulmonary arteriogram for the diagnosis of pulmonary embolism—and again, the aortic dissection is invisible. **C,** Contrast has reached the aorta and the dissection has finally become visible. The necessity for accurate contrast timing is an important concept for the emergency physician. It stresses the importance of informing your radiologist of your diagnostic priorities so that the CT protocol can be adjusted accordingly. In addition, the rapid contrast infusions necessary for high-quality CT angiograms require relatively large intravenous access.

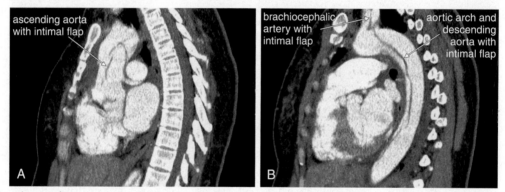

Figure 7-82. CT angiogram from a patient with type A aortic dissection and a normal chest x-ray. Same patient as Figures 7-78, 7-79, *A*, 7-80, and 7-81. **A, B,** Sagittal reconstructions from CT aortogram. These sagittal reconstructions reveal the aortic dissection to involve the aortic root and ascending aorta, the arch and descending aorta, and the brachiocephalic artery. Because the aorta does not lie in a single sagittal plane, the entire aorta is not visible in a single thin sagittal slice. Special curved reconstructions or thick slab reconstructions called maximum intensity projections can allow more of the aorta to be seen in a single image.

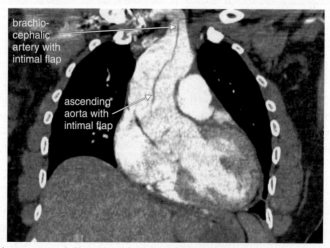

Figure 7-83. Multiplanar CT imaging can reveal dissection involving aortic branch vessels. Same patient as Figures 7-78, 7-79, *A,* and 7-80 through 7-82. This coronal reconstruction shows an intimal flap arising in the ascending aorta and extending into the brachiocephalic artery. Multiplanar reconstructions can help to define branch vessel involvement that can complicate aortic dissection.

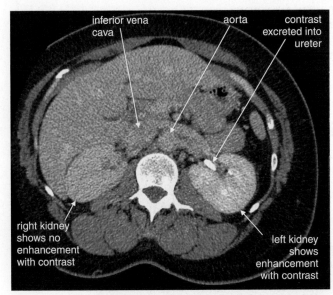

inferior vena cava

aorta

contrast excreted into ureter

right kidney shows no enhancement with contrast

left kidney shows enhancement with contrast

Figure 7-84. Delayed CT images can reveal organ hypoperfusion resulting from aortic dissection. Same patient as Figures 7-78, 7-79, A, and 7-80 through 7-83. Delayed images through the abdomen in the same patient reveal a lack of normal enhancement of the right kidney—an indication of ischemia from involvement of the right renal artery by the aortic dissection. The left kidney shows enhancement and is even beginning to excrete contrast into the ureter. The aorta and inferior vena cava do not contain contrast, since it has been several minutes since the contrast injection. As a consequence, the aortic dissection is again invisible.

in multidetector CT and three-dimensional postprocessing since that time have improved the diagnostic utility of CT. A 2003 study published in *Radiology* confirmed 100% sensitivity of CT for detection of type A aortic dissection compared with surgical findings. The study also examined the sensitivity and specificity of CT for important complications that can affect surgical planning, including detection of an entry tear (sensitivity = 82%, specificity = 100%), aortic arch branch vessel involvement (sensitivity = 95%, specificity = 100%), and pericardial effusion (sensitivity = 83%, specificity = 100%).[112]

CT Aortic Angiography Technique

CT for aortic pathology uses the same principles as for PE. In traditional aortic angiography, contrast injected through a catheter proximal to the aortic valve fills the aorta, revealing the aortic contour and size, as well as any intimal flaps. In CT aortic angiography, contrast is injected under pressure through a catheter in the antecubital fossa; traverses the upper extremity, subclavian vain, superior vena cava, right atrium and ventricle, and pulmonary vessels; and then returns to the left atrium and ventricle. The scan is timed to coincide with arrival of the contrast bolus in the aorta. As for CT pulmonary

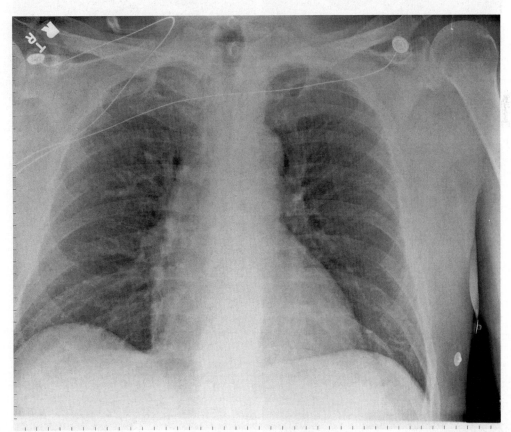

Figure 7-85. Aortic dissection type A with normal chest x-ray. A 72-year-old male with neck pain radiating into his chest. The patient was given aspirin and nitroglycerin by emergency medical services with improvement in his pain from 10 out of 10 to 2 out of 10. On electrocardiogram, the patient had ST segment depression in leads V3 through V5, and heparin was initiated. The chest x-ray appears normal, with a well-defined aortic knob and normal mediastinum. The emergency physician then suspected aortic dissection because of the migratory nature of the patient's pain, and chest CT was performed (Figure 7-86).

angiography (see discussion earlier in this chapter), a well-timed contrast bolus is essential to the diagnosis of aortic dissection. With rare exceptions in which calcifications in the aortic wall and high density thrombus in the false aortic lumen are visible, a noncontrast CT or poorly timed CT cannot detect aortic dissection (see Figures 7-80 and 7-81), although it may reveal aortic aneurysm (see Figure 7-61). Nondiagnostic scans result from poor contrast boluses, which may incompletely opacify the aorta. Poor scan timing limits sensitivity, because contrast may not yet have reached or may have already passed out of the aorta, preventing the intimal dissection flap from being recognized.[30,113] Typically, the entire aorta is imaged, from above the top of the aortic arch to below the aortic bifurcation, so CT spans the chest, abdomen, and pelvis.

Interpretation of Computed Tomography for Aortic Pathology

Normal Aorta. Interpretation of CT for aortic pathology is relatively simple compared with CT pulmonary angiography (Box 7-3 gives the recommended algorithm). The descending thoracic aorta is a tubular structure with a fixed location anterior and slightly to the left of the thoracic spine. Its normal size is defined as less than or equal to 2 cm. A normal aorta on a good-quality

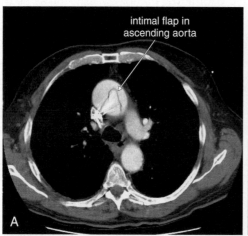
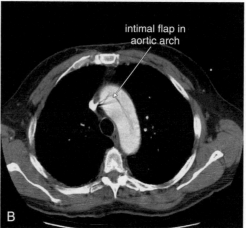

Figure 7-86. CT aortogram in a patient with type A aortic dissection and a normal chest x-ray. Same patient as Figure 7-85. This computed tomography with intravenous contrast shows an intimal flap within the ascending aorta **(A)** and aortic arch **(B)**. The ascending aorta is enlarged, measuring 5.4 cm in diameter. Because only the intima, not the muscularis layer, is affected, no blood has left the aorta. No mediastinal hematoma is present, and no increase in mediastinal diameter has occurred acutely. The result is the normal chest x-ray seen in this patient in Figure 7-85. Why did the ischemic electrocardiogram changes occur? The dissection flap may be intermittently occluding the coronary artery ostia.

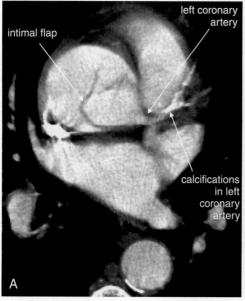
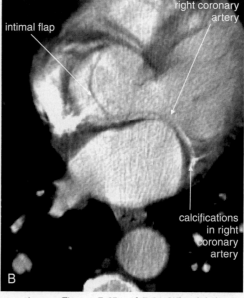

Figure 7-87. Aortic dissection with coronary artery involvement. Same patient as Figures 7-85 and 7-86. Why did the patient have ischemic electrocardiogram (ECG) changes? Again, the dissection flap may be intermittently occluding the coronary artery ostia. In these two panels, the intimal flap appears to lead into the ostia of the left **(A)** and right **(B)** main coronary arteries. The course of these arteries is marked by calcifications. This CT was not ECG-gated to reduce motion artifact, so the coronary arteries are not seen with optimal clarity. Chapter 8 discusses ECG-gating of CT in detail.

scan with an adequate contrast bolus should be completely opacified and should appear bright white on CT soft tissue windows. In cross section, the descending and ascending aorta appear as a smoothly outlined circle (see Figure 7-79). The aortic arch in cross section appears elliptic (see Figure 7-79). Calcifications in the aortic wall may be visible as bright white spots, even in the absence of contrast, and indicate atherosclerotic disease (see Figures 7-61, 7-71, and 7-74).[30]

Spontaneous Aortic Dissection or Aneurysm. Aortic aneurysm can be diagnosed on CT simply by measurement of the aortic diameter. Modern PACS software interfaces offer toolbar calipers for measurement. Diameters above 3 cm constitute aneurysm (see Figure 7-79). Aortic dissection may occur in aneurysmal aortas or aortas of normal caliber. Aortic dissection is diagnosed on CT by the presence of an intimal flap, visible as a line dividing the aorta into a true and a false lumen. There may be a differential enhancement or filling of the true and false lumens with contrast. This difference is not uniform; the true lumen may contain more or less contrast than the false lumen. In some cases, the false lumen may tear back into the true lumen, and the two channels may contain equal amounts of contrast. The false lumen (or more rarely, the true lumen) may be thrombosed and may contain no contrast, thus appearing dark on CT. Although it may be relatively unimportant for emergency medical management or diagnosis, the false channel often demonstrates "beaking" and cobwebbing (defined by the presence of thin strands of tissue connecting the dissected intimal flap to the aortic wall) (see Figures 7-62 and 7-63).[30] The extent of the dissection can be determined on CT, allowing classification by the Stanford or Debakey system (Box 7-4), which may determine medical or surgical therapy.[114] Blood products outside of the aorta may be seen, indicating leaking or rupture. Blood products that accumulated prior to the moment of CT appear dark on CT, with densities of approximately 40 to 70 HU. Extravasation of contrast material beyond the lumen of the aorta marks active bleeding at the time of CT—this appears bright white on CT soft-tissue windows, with densities between 130 and 200 HU, depending on the contrast bolus. Proximal

Figure 7-88. Aortic dissection Stanford type B with normal chest x-ray. This 63-year-old male experienced sudden, severe, sharp back chest pain radiating to the interscapular area and then to the upper abdomen. Aortic dissection was suspected resulting from the classic character of the patient's pain. Chest x-ray was normal, with a narrow mediastinum and well-defined aortic knob and course of the descending aorta. Computed tomography was ordered because of high pretest probability of aortic dissection (Figure 7-89). Remember that a normal chest x-ray does not rule out thoracic aortic dissection.

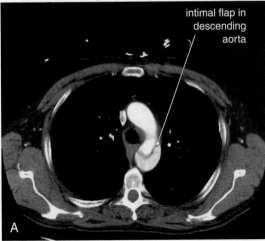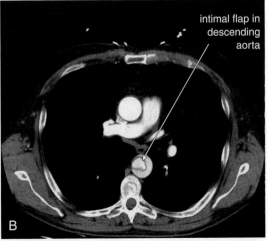

Figure 7-89. CT aortogram in a patient with Stanford type B aortic dissection and normal chest x-ray. Same patient as Figure 7-88. **A,** CT aortogram demonstrates an intimal flap involving only the descending aorta—a type B dissection. The aorta is of normal caliber. Because the intima is the only layer of the aortic wall involved, no blood has escaped the aorta, no periaortic hematoma is present, and no change in mediastinal contour is seen on chest x-ray (Figure 7-88). **B,** An interesting configuration of the intimal flap.

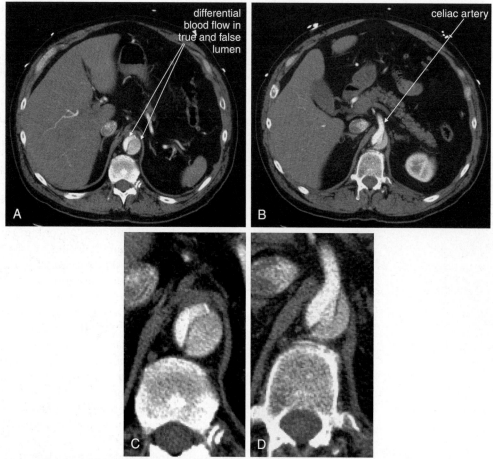

Figure 7-90. Branch vessel involvement from aortic dissection. Same patient as Figure 7-88 and 7-89. Imaging of the entire aorta is necessary when dissection is suspected. The dissection continues into the abdomen, involving the proximal celiac artery. Note the differential flow in the true and false lumens. Bright white contrast indicating brisk flow supplying the celiac artery. The darker lumen has a lesser amount of contrast within it, mixed with blood. **A,** Axial image just cephalad to the celiac artery. **B,** A few slices caudad to **A,** the celiac artery emerges from the aorta. **C,** Close-up from **A. D,** Close-up from **B.**

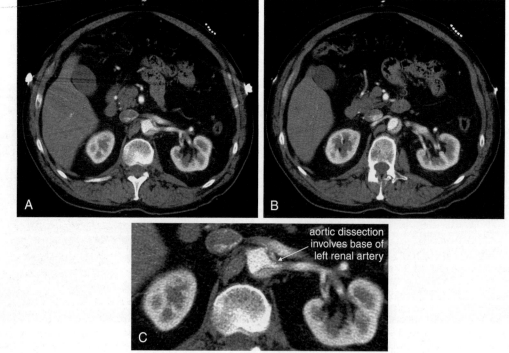

Figure 7-91. Branch vessel involvement from aortic dissection. A, B, Sequential images at the level of the renal artery. **C,** Close-up from **A.** Same patient as Figures 7-88 through 7-90. Here, the intimal flap and false lumen appear to involve the origin of the left renal artery, although the kidney does enhance with contrast.

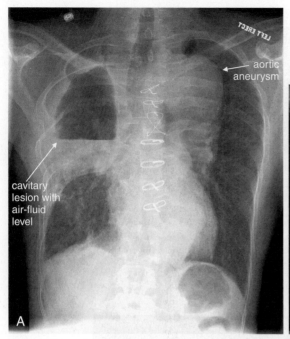

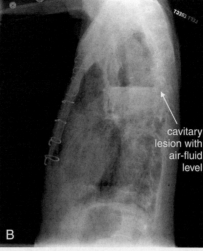

Figure 7-92. Aortic aneurysm and mycetoma. A, Posterior–anterior chest x-ray, **B,** Lateral chest x-ray. This 51-year-old male presented with fever, cough, and chest pain. The patient had a history of *Aspergillus fumigatus* mycetoma, accounting for the right upper lobe cavitary lesion. A superimposed lung abscess is also possible, and tuberculosis should be considered. Also notable is the wide mediastinum, consistent with a thoracic aortic aneurysm, which has previously undergone endovascular repair. Chest CT was performed to evaluate these abnormalities further (Figures 7-93 and 7-94).

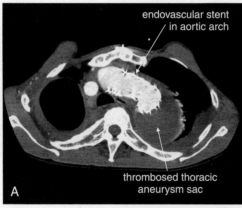

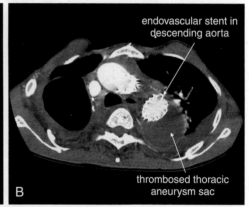

Figure 7-93. Aortic aneurysm with endovascular repair. A, B, Axial computed tomography images, moving from cephalad to caudad. Same patient as Figure 7-92. This 51-year-old male has had an endovascular repair of a large thoracic aortic aneurysm. The aneurysm sac persists but has thrombosed, resulting in a dark soft-tissue density when viewed on soft-tissue window—the expected result of the endovascular repair. The aortic stent is patent and fills with intravenous contrast, resulting in the bright white color within it. The contour of the aneurysm sac remains readily visible on the patient's chest x-ray (Figure 7-92).

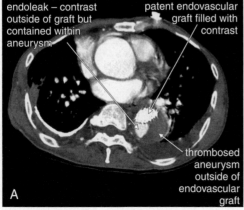

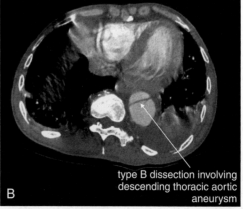

Figure 7-94. Endoleak and type B aortic dissection. Additional images from the same patient as Figures 7-92 and 7-93 reveal two complications. **A,** The descending aorta shows three compartments: an endovascular graft filled appropriately with contrast, a thrombosed segment of descending aortic aneurysm (the expected effect of excluding blood flow from the aneurysm with the endovascular stent), and a region of contrast that lies outside of the endovascular graft. This latter region is called an endoleak, meaning a region of blood leak outside of the endovascular graft but still contained within the aneurysm sac. This is a potentially serious failure of the endovascular stent, because blood leaking outside of the stent could leak from the aneurysm should it rupture. Small endoleaks are common and are often not treated, because they may thrombose spontaneously. Endoleaks are discussed in more detail in Chapter 11. **B,** An intimal flap of a type B dissection is seen, caudad to the termination of the endovascular graft.

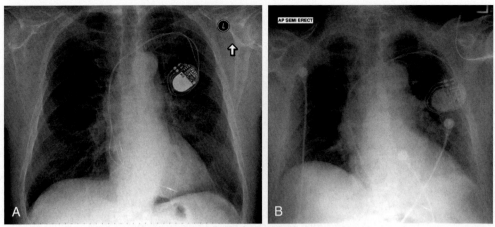

Figure 7-95. Aortic dissection type A, 1 year prior and on day of acute dissection. As described earlier, a spontaneous aortic dissection may not acutely change the aortic caliber or result in mediastinal hematoma—resulting in little or no change in the chest x-ray. The wide mediastinum often described may reflect a preexisting aortic aneurysm, which is a risk factor for aortic dissection. About 12% of aortic dissections occur with a normal chest x-ray. This patient had chest x-rays 1 year prior **(A)** and on the day of an acute type A aortic dissection **(B).** The radiology interpretation was, "Given differences in technique, cardiac and mediastinal contours are stable." Computed tomography images from the patient are shown in Figure 7-96.

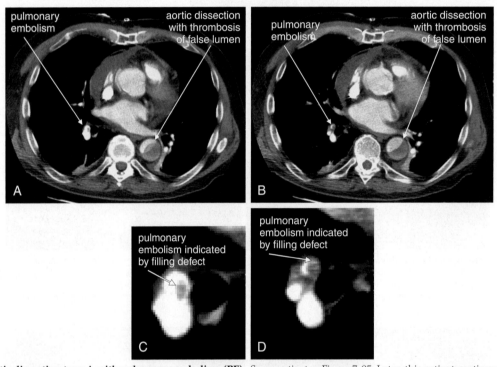

Figure 7-96. Aortic dissection type A with pulmonary embolism (PE). Same patient as Figure 7-95. Later, this patient continued to have a chronic type A aortic dissection, and has now developed an additional complication—a PE. The false lumen of the dissection is seen to be thrombosed—explaining the absence of contrast within it. PE is discussed in more detail earlier in the chapter. **A** and **B,** two adjacent slices through the chest, revealing the descending aorta and branches of the right pulmonary artery. **C** and **D,** close-ups from **A** and **B.**

extension of the dissection may be visible as pericardial blood, usually dark in appearance on CT unless active bleeding into the pericardium is ongoing. Branch vessels such as the coronary, carotid, subclavian, brachiocephalic, renal, mesenteric, and iliac arteries should be inspected for dissection as well (see Figures 7-64, 7-82 through 7-84, 7-87, 7-90, and 7-91).[30] Repeated CT of a body region after a brief delay is often performed, allowing contrast to be concentrated by end-organs. This can reveal normal and abnormal patterns of organ enhancement, in some cases disclosing poor perfusion

of organs resulting from aortic dissection. For example, failure of the kidneys to enhance on delayed images can indicate compromise of renal blood flow by the dissection (see Figure 7-84).

Computed Tomography Radiation and Cancer
Chest CT scan carries with it a radiation exposure of around 8 mSv, the equivalent of approximately 400 posterior–anterior chest x-rays.[115] The cancer risk associated with this exposure varies with age at exposure and with gender. For a 20 year old female undergoing

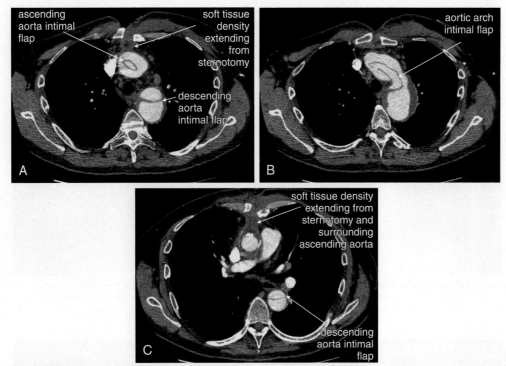

Figure 7-97. Aortic dissection type A with wound infection. This patient underwent open repair of a type A aortic dissection and returned with a poorly healing sternotomy wound. Computed tomography shows soft-tissue density extending from the wound and surrounding the ascending aorta—suspicious for invasive infection. In addition, intimal flaps remain. **A** through **C,** Axial slices at various aortic levels.

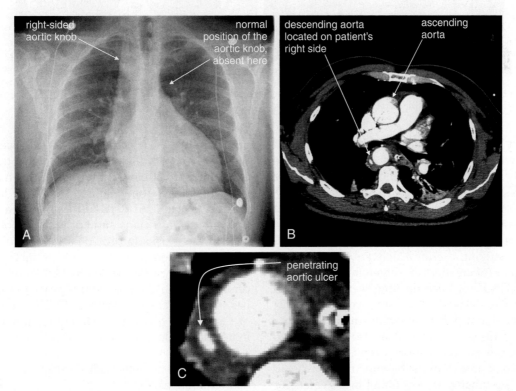

Figure 7-98. Right aortic arch. Variations in the appearance of the mediastinum on chest x-ray may occur because of congenital abnormalities. This 48-year-old male complained of chest pain and had a history of atrial fibrillation and stroke. **A,** His chest x-ray lacks the normal aortic knob—careful inspection reveals the aortic knob to be on the right. **B,** Chest computed tomography was performed and confirmed a right-sided aortic arch. A focal penetrating aortic ulcer or dissection was also noted (**C,** close-up). This connected to the main aortic lumen on an adjacent slice.

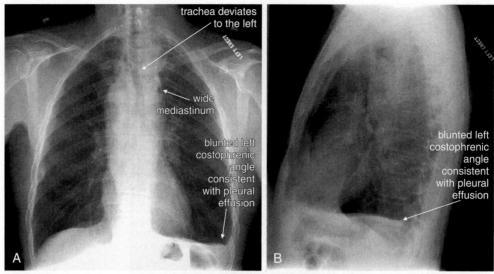

Figure 7-99. Right aortic arch and mediastinal mass. This 63-year-old male presented with 1 month of neck fullness and dysphagia. His chest x-ray shows a wide mediastinum, and the trachea deviates to the left just below the level of the clavicles. The clinical history was more concerning for mass than for aortic dissection. Computed tomography was performed and is reviewed in Figure 7-100. **A,** Posterior–anterior chest x-ray. **B,** Lateral chest x-ray.

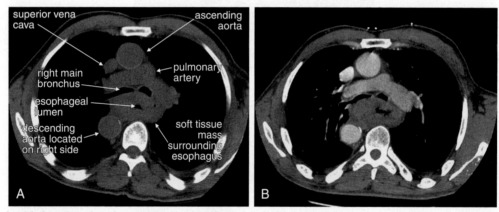

Figure 7-100. Right-sided aortic arch and mediastinal mass. Chest computed tomography from the same patient as in Figure 7-99. **A,** Noncontrast axial image. **B,** Image at the same level following IV contrast administration. Incidentally, the patient has a right-sided aortic arch. In addition, posterior to the main bronchi, a soft-tissue mass surrounds the esophagus. The esophageal lumen is filled with air and appears black. Workup revealed esophageal cancer. Not all mediastinal widening is the result of acute aortic pathology.

CT pulmonary angiography, the cancer risk is estimated at 1 in 330, while in a 60 year old female the risk is approximately 1 in 930. Males at these same ages have estimated risks of approximately 1 in 880 and 1 in 1770, respectively.[115a] This risk is cumulative and permanent (does not diminish with time since exposure), with no known safe exposure limit. A single x-ray photon of sufficient energy striking a critical deoxyribonucleic acid (DNA) base pair (or creating an oxygen free radical that interacts with DNA) can be the inciting event leading to a future cancer. This delayed risk must be weighed against the probability that a patient is today suffering from a life-threatening disease process. It is also important to recognize that this attributable risk from CT is still relatively small, compared with the baseline risk for cancer death, which is estimated at more than 1 in 5. Centers for Disease Control data indicate that cancer was the second leading cause of death in 2005, accounting for 22.8% of U.S. deaths.[24,116] In comparison, estimates of attributable

cancer induction (not death) from 64-slice cardiac CT (which carries a radiation exposure higher than that from CT pulmonary angiography, depending on the exact CT protocol) range from 1 in 143 (0.7%) for a 20-year-old woman to 1 in 3261 (0.03%) for an 80-year-old man.[117] Emergency physicians should be aware of the magnitude of these risks to provide a thoughtful risk–benefit analysis for their patients. In a 2004 survey, only 9% of emergency physicians stated that CT could increase cancer risk, though attention to this problem since that time has likely increased awareness.[118] The American Board of Emergency Medicine included reading on this topic in its 2009 Lifelong Learning and Self-Assessment Test.

Computed Tomography Radiation Exposure and Teratogenesis
As stated earlier, a single CT of the chest delivers a large radiation dose to the patient, approximately 8 mSv. However, risk for fetal malformation (teratogenesis)

TABLE 7-9. Clinical Factors and Likelihood of Thoracic Aortic Dissection

Clinical Factor	Positive or Negative Likelihood Ratio (LR) (95% CI)	Utility
Severe pain of abrupt onset	LR negative 0.3 (0.2-0.5) Positive LR 1.6 (1.0-2.4)	Decreases risk when negative
Migratory pain	LR positive 1.1-7.6 Negative LR 0.6 (0.5-0.7)	Increases risk when positive
Tearing or ripping pain	LR positive 1.2-10.8 LR negative 0.4-0.99	Increases risk when positive
Pulse deficits	LR positive 5.7 (1.4-23.0) LR negative 0.7 (0.6-0.9)	Increases risk when positive
Focal neurologic deficits	LR positive 6.6-33.0 LR negative 0.71-0.87	Increases risk when positive
Aortic regurgitation murmur (a diastolic murmur)	LR positive 1.4 (1.0-2.0) LR negative 0.9 (0.8-1.0)	Not useful
Combination of "aortic pain" (defined as severe, sudden-onset, tearing pain), blood pressure differential or pulse deficit in upper extremities, and wide mediastinum on chest x-ray	LR positive 66.0 (4.1-1062.0)	Increases risk substantially when all three factors are positive
Absence of *any* of these three classic findings: "aortic pain" (defined as severe, sudden-onset, tearing pain), blood pressure differential or pulse deficit in upper extremities, and wide mediastinum on chest x-ray	LR negative 0.07 (0.03-0.17)	Decreases risk substantially when all three factors are negative
Normal aorta and mediastinum on chest x-ray	LR negative 0.3 (0.2-0.4)	Decreases risk

From Klompas M. Does this patient have an acute thoracic aortic dissection? *JAMA* 287:2262-72, 2002.

Likelihood ratios are reviewed earlier in this chapter in the section on pulmonary embolism. LR+ ≥ 10 substantially increases odds of disease. LR− ≤ 0.1 substantially decreases odds of disease. LR + or − equal to 1 have no effect on odds of disease. Intermediate values have accordingly moderate effects on odds of disease.

	Disease + 10 patients	Disease − 990 patients	
Test + 206 patients	True Positive (TP) = 8	False Positive (FP) = 198	Positive Predictive Value (PPV) = TP/(TP+FP) = 4%
Test − 794 patients	False Negative (FN) = 2	True Negative (TN) = 792	Negative Predictive Value (NPV) = TN/(TN+FN) = 99.7%
	Sensitivity= TP/(TP+FN) = 80%	Specificity= TN/(FP+TN) = 80%	Number needed to treat (number of patients with normal chest x-rays who must be tested with CT to find one aortic dissection): 794/2 = 397

Figure 7-101. Examples of test performance of chest x-ray for detection of aortic dissection: low-risk population. Imagine 1000 emergency department patients with chest pain, of whom 1% (10 patients) have aortic dissection. Imagine that chest x-ray is 80% sensitive and 80% specific for aortic dissection. In this scenario, because aortic dissection is rare, even a sensitivity as low as 80% means that 99.8% of patients with normal chest x-rays do not have aortic dissection. Nearly 400 patients with normal chest x-rays would need to be imaged with computed tomography to find 1 patient with aortic dissection.

	Disease + 300 patients	Disease − 700 patients	
Test + 380 patients	True Positive (TP) = 240	False Positive (FP) = 140	Positive Predictive Value (PPV) = TP/(TP+FP) = 63%
Test − 620 patients	False Negative (FN) = 60	True Negative (TN) = 560	Negative Predictive Value (NPV) = TN/(TN+FN) = 90%
	Sensitivity= TP/(TP+FN) = 80%	Specificity= TN/(FP+TN) = 80%	Number needed to treat (number of patients with normal chest x-rays who must be tested with CT to find one aortic dissection): 620/60 = 10

Figure 7-102. **Examples of test performance of chest x-ray for detection of aortic dissection: high-risk population.** Imagine 1000 emergency department patients with chest pain, of whom 30% (300 patients) have aortic dissection. Imagine that chest x-ray is 80% sensitive and 80% specific for aortic dissection. In this scenario, because aortic dissection is common, a sensitivity as low as 80% means that up to 10% of patients with normal chest x-rays have aortic dissection. One dissection would be found for every 10 computed tomography scans performed in patients with normal chest x-ray.

Box 7-3: Algorithm for Evaluating Computed Tomography for Aortic Pathology

1. **Choose the soft tissue or vascular window setting.**
2. **Assess the contrast bolus quality.**
3. **Assess for motion artifact.**
4. **Measure the aortic diameter.**
5. **Inspect the ascending aorta, arch, descending aorta, and branch vessels for dissection of the intimal flap.**
6. **Look for a difference in contrast density in true and false lumens.**
7. **Inspect for extravasating contrast outside of the aorta.**
    Pitfalls in Aortic Imaging
- **Poor contrast bolus**
- **Aortic motion artifact**
- **Normal anatomic variants**

Box 7-4: Classification of Thoracic Aortic Dissection

- **Stanford**
  - A: Ascending aorta involved*
  - B: Ascending aorta not involved†
- **Debakey**
  - I: Ascending, arch, descending*
  - II: Ascending only*
  - III: Descending only, distal to left subclavian artery†

From Weisenfarth JD. Aortic Dissection in Emergency Medicine. (Accessed at http://emedicine.medscape.com/article/756835-diagnosis)
*Surgical therapy is usual.
†Medical therapy is usual.

resulting from diagnostic radiation exposure is not believed to be significant below a cumulative dose of 50 mSv. Radiation exposures should be avoided if possible in pregnancy, particularly in critical periods of organogenesis, from 2 to 8 weeks postconception. Despite this, American College of Obstetricians and Gynecologists guidelines state "Exposure to X-rays during pregnancy is not an indication for therapeutic abortion."[119,119a] The American College of Radiology, American College of Obstetrics and Gynecology, and National Council on Radiation Protection unanimously agree that no single diagnostic imaging procedure results in harmful fetal effects.[120] In contrast, physicians tend to overestimate the risk for fetal malformation resulting from exposure to diagnostic radiologic procedures.[121] In the pregnant patient, the usual considerations apply in selecting VQ or CT as a diagnostic test. With regard to fetal radiation exposure, a VQ scan exposes the fetus to approximately 0.32 to 0.36 mSv.[122] The dose can be further reduced by eliminating the ventilation scan, reducing ventilation imaging to a single breath-hold view, or reducing the amount of the perfusion agent.[122] Chest CT also is estimated to expose the fetus to less than 1 mSv.

Anthropomorphic phantom models suggest that fetal exposure from CT pulmonary angiography at 0 and 3 months are 0.24 to 0.47 mSv and 0.61 to 0.66 mSV, respectively, well below the recognized threshold for fetal effects.[122-123] Either modality may be reasonable, and other patient factors besides fetal radiation dose should likely drive the choice of imaging study.

Indications for Intravenous Contrast

IV contrast is indicated for the diagnosis of PE and aortic pathology. As described earlier, the presence of contrast material in pulmonary vessels allows recognition of filling defects caused by PE. In aortic dissection, intimal injuries and active bleeding are made visible by the presence of injected contrast. CT without contrast has quite limited sensitivity for these processes, although in extreme cases ruptured aneurysms or large pulmonary emboli may be visible without contrast.[30]

Intravenous Contrast and Allergy. Reaction to iodinated contrast agents is relatively rare, with an incidence of 3% to 15% for mild reactions but only 0.004% to 0.04% for very severe reactions. Fatal reactions occur in only 1 in 170,000.[124] Contrast reactions are termed "anaphylactoid" because they likely occur by slightly different mechanisms from those causing true allergic reactions, although the clinical presentation and treatment are the same.[126] Risk factors for contrast reaction include asthma (6- to 10-fold risk) and severe allergies to any other substance. Seafood allergies do not appear to constitute a specific additional risk factor, beyond the heightened risk seen in patients with a history of severe reaction to any allergen. Seafood allergies are thought to be mediated by proteins in seafood, not iodine. For a variety of reasons, new low-osmolality contrast agents have a lower potential for contrast reaction (5 times lower for mild reactions and 10 times lower for severe reactions) and should be considered for high-risk patients. These agents are somewhat more expensive than standard high-osmolality agents (approximately $40 per patient), which has prevented their universal use.[125] Most institutions have these agents readily available upon request.

Pretreatment to prevent contrast reaction can be performed, but most regimens require 12 to 24 hours of pretreatment and are impractical in the emergency department. In its *Manual on Contrast Media,* the American College of Radiology recommends a minimum of 6 hours between steroid and contrast administration, whether steroids are administered orally or intravenously, citing evidence that pretreatment 3 hours or fewer before contrast administration is not helpful.[126,128] A rapid pretreatment protocol beginning 1 hour before contrast has been described and is used in some institutions—though this is based on an uncontrolled case series of nine patients by Greenberger et al. (Box 7-5).[126-128] Breakthrough reactions may occur despite steroid premedication and may

> ## Box 7-5: Pretreatment to Prevent Anaphylactoid Reactions to Iodinated Contrast
>
> 1. **Avoid contrast if possible.**
>   - ❍ In the case of PE, consider an alternative imaging modality such as VQ scan.
>   - ❍ In the case of aortic disease, consider an alternative modality such as TEE or MR.
> 2. **If contrast must be used, *use a nonionic low-osmolality contrast agent.***
> 3. **Then, pretreat as follows:**
>
> In decreasing order of desirability, according to the ACR:
>
> 1. **Methylprednisolone sodium succinate (Solu-Medrol®) 40 mg or hydrocortisone sodium succinate (Solu-Cortef®) 200 mg IV every 4 hours until contrast study is required plus diphenhydramine 50 mg IV 1 hour prior to contrast injection**
>   **or**
> 2. **Dexamethasone sodium sulfate (Decadron®) 7.5 mg or betamethasone 6.0 mg IV every 4 hours until contrast study must be done in patient with known allergy to methylprednisolone, aspirin, or non-steroidal anti-inflammatory drugs, especially if asthmatic plus diphenhydramine 50 mg IV 1 hour prior to contrast injection**
>   **or**
> 3. **Omit steroids entirely and give diphenhydramine 50 mg IV. IV steroids have not been shown to be effective when administered less than 4 to 6 hours prior to contrast injection.**
>
> From American College of Radiology. Manual on Contrast Media. 7th ed: American College of Radiology; 2010.

be severe in 24% of cases,[129] so alternative methods of diagnosis should be considered in high-risk patients.

Intravenous Contrast and Nephrotoxicity. Nephrotoxicity from iodinated contrast is a major concern. Contrast nephropathy is defined as a rise of 25% or 0.5 mg/dL in measured creatinine from baseline. It occurs in an estimated 15% of contrast procedures, accounting for 150,000 cases per year in the United States. Contrast nephropathy is thought to be responsible for 10% of in-hospital renal failure. The contrast dose for chest CT approximates 150 mL and may place patients at risk for renal injury. A creatinine clearance below 60 mL per minute places a patient at risk. Estimated creatinine clearance can be calculated by a formula (Box 7-6) or by use of online or personal digital assistant calculators. Because creatinine clearance is a function of the patient's age, gender, weight, and measured creatinine, elderly patients with apparently normal measured creatinine values may have markedly abnormal creatinine clearance. For example,

Box 7-6: Creatinine Clearance Calculation*

$$\frac{[140 - age \ (yr) \times ideal \ body \ weight \ (kg)]}{Serum \ creatinine \ (mg/dL) \times 72}$$

Multiply by 0.85 for women.

---

*For automatic calculators, search online for "creatinine clearance calculator."

Box 7-7: Pretreatment to Prevent Contrast Nephropathy From Iodinated Contrast Agents

1. **Avoid contrast if possible.**
   - ○ In the case of PE, consider an alternative imaging modality such as VQ scan.
   - ○ In the case of aortic disease, consider an alternative modality such as TEE.
2. **If contrast must be used, *use a low-osmolality contrast agent.***
3. **In addition, use the following:**
   - ○ Normal saline
     1 mL/kg/hr 6-12 hours pre-contrast and 4-12 hours post-contrast
     or
   - ○ Sodium bicarbonate (not shown to be superior to normal saline)
     154 mEq/L (3 ampoules in 1 L D5W) administered at a rate of 3 mL/kg/hr IV for 1 hour before contrast and 1 mL/kg/hr IV for 6 hours after contrast
     plus
   - ○ N-acetylcysteine
     600 mg PO bid 1 day before and on day of contrast
     or
   - ○ N-acetylcysteine
     150 mg/kg in 500 mL normal saline over 30 minutes before contrast and then 50 mg/kg in 500 mL normal saline over 4 hours

---

From American College of Radiology. Manual on Contrast Media. 7th ed, American College of Radiology, 2010; Baker CS, Wragg A, Kumar S, et al. A rapid protocol for the prevention of contrast-induced renal dysfunction: the RAPPID study. *J Am Coll Cardiol* 41(12):2114-2118, 2003; Brar SS, Shen AY, Jorgensen MB, et al. Sodium bicarbonate vs sodium chloride for the prevention of contrast medium-induced nephropathy in patients undergoing coronary angiography: a randomized trial. *JAMA* 300(9):1038-1046, 2008; Trivedi HS, Moore H, Nasr S, et al. A randomized prospective trial to assess the role of saline hydration on the development of contrast nephrotoxicity. *Nephron Clin Pract* 93(1):C29-34, 2003.

an 80-year-old female weighing 72 kg with a measured creatinine of 0.95 mg/dL has a creatinine clearance less than 60 mL per minute and is at risk for nephrotoxicity. Congestive heart failure and diabetes are also risk factors. Fortunately, less than 1% of patients with contrast nephropathy require dialysis, but among those requiring dialysis, there is a 30% in-hospital mortality.[130-131]

Methods to decrease renal toxicity include use of low-osmolality contrast, prehydration with IV normal saline,[132-133] pretreatment with IV sodium bicarbonate,[134] and pretreatment with N-acetylcysteine (Box 7-7). Most N-acetylcysteine protocols require 24 hours of pretreatment, again making them of little utility in the emergency department, although an immediate N-acetylcysteine protocol has been described (see Box 7-7). Studies on pretreatment show only an effect on creatinine, not a patient-oriented outcome effect such as change in need for dialysis.[135-136] The latest randomized controlled trial comparing sodium chloride (normal saline) hydration to sodium bicarbonate showed no difference in rates of contrast nephropathy, contradicting an earlier promising trial with more limited methodology.[137] Overall, the best strategy is likely avoidance of contrast when possible through use of an alternative imaging modality. When contrast must be given emergently, the best strategy is normal saline hydration combined with low-osmolality contrast at the lowest possible volume to complete the CT.

In patients suspected of PE or aortic pathology who cannot undergo CT with IV contrast alternative diagnostic methods should be used, such as MRA (aortic pathology or PE), VQ (PE), or echocardiography (aortic pathology or PE). For patients with normal renal function who cannot receive iodinated contrast because of allergy, gadolinium can be used as a CT contrast agent, or MRA with gadolinium contrast can be used.[138-140] Gadolinium-enhanced MRA is no longer an alternative in patients with renal insufficiency who are at risk for contrast nephropathy from iodinated contrast. This is due to the recently recognized risk for gadolinium-induced nephrogenic systemic fibrosis, a rare but potentially fatal condition affecting patients with acute renal failure, those with chronic renal insufficiency with a poor glomerular filtration rate, and even patients already receiving dialysis. The risks of nephrogenic systemic fibrosis are described in detail in Chapter 15. In patients who can receive neither iodinated contrast nor gadolinium, some advanced MR techniques can assess for PE and aortic pathology without any contrast administration.

CRITICAL DIFFERENTIAL DIAGNOSIS: IMAGING WHEN BOTH PULMONARY EMBOLISM AND AORTIC DISSECTION ARE SUSPECTED

So far we have discussed imaging tailored for diagnosis of PE or aortic pathology. In reality, some patients present with histories, examination findings, vital signs, and risk factors compatible with both forms of pathology. What strategies are appropriate for diagnosis in this scenario? CT protocols for PE and aortic pathology differ, particularly in the timing of contrast relative to CT scan acquisition, as described in the earlier sections. An optimal scan for either form of pathology times the contrast to fill the vascular bed of interest, thus compromising assessment of alternative pathology (see Figures 7-11, 7-12, and 7-81). CT can be performed to assess for both PE and aortic dissection, as well as coronary artery disease (described in detail in Chapter 8). In brief, such "triple rule-out CT" requires a biphasic contrast injection (70 mL of contrast, followed by a 50:50 mixture of 25 mL of contrast and 25 mL of saline).[141] Occasionally, a CT performed for evaluation of one form of pathology may reveal the other—or even coexisting aortic dissection and PE (see Figure 7-96).

In any given patient, the importance of differentiating these diagnoses must be weighed against the additional risk for contrast nephropathy resulting from the increased contrast dose. In a patient with no renal disease, this risk may be minimal. Another strategy is to perform CT tailored to evaluate one form of pathology optimally, with the intention of performing a second diagnostic test or initiating empiric therapy for the second form of pathology if necessary. For example, CT can be performed to rule out aortic pathology as the first test. If negative, the patient can undergo VQ scan or can be treated empirically with anticoagulation. If PE is strongly suspected, imaging tailored for this diagnosis can be selected. In general, CT is often the best first diagnostic test in this scenario, because it may fortuitously reveal alternative diagnoses. VQ scan does not identify aortic pathology. MR can also be performed to evaluate aortic pathology or PE if initial CT is negative.

IMAGING IN THE UNSTABLE PATIENT WITH SUSPECTED PULMONARY EMBOLISM, AORTIC DISSECTION, OR BOTH

The unstable patient with suspected PE, aortic dissection, or both presents a particular dilemma. The two disease processes present competing treatment goals, limiting use of empiric medical therapy when both diseases are suspected. For example, use of heparin or thrombolytic agents for treatment of PE is contraindicated in the presence of aortic dissection. Similarly, the use of beta-blockers and vasodilators for empiric treatment of aortic dissection can decrease cardiac output and preload, causing hemodynamic collapse if large PE is present. Other competing diagnoses such as pericardial tamponade may present similarly and may be worsened by empiric therapy for PE or aortic dissection. Definitive diagnosis is important, and the risks and benefits of various diagnostic strategies must be weighed against the likelihood of mortality if no firm diagnosis is reached.

Bedside echocardiography including possible transesophageal approach can be of benefit, because it may reveal aortic dissection, evidence of PE, large pericardial effusion or tamponade, and cardiac wall motion abnormalities suggesting acute myocardial infarction. As a triage strategy, bedside transthoracic echocardiography is reasonable, because it does not require patient transport or administration of nephrotoxic contrast. It preserves the ability to continue resuscitation efforts in the emergency department.

As a rule, VQ scan is a poor choice in unstable patients, because it necessitates removing the patient from the emergency department for up to an hour. Although CT is often described as "a place where patients go to die," and the danger of an unstable patient in CT is undeniable, consider the alternatives if massive PE or aortic dissection is present. Neither of these diagnoses presents much opportunity for successful resuscitation in the emergency department if cardiac arrest occurs, and definitive diagnosis is essential to aggressive treatment. For example, massive PE can be treated by interventional techniques (described in Chapter 16), whereas type A aortic dissection requires emergency surgical treatment. The patient should be stabilized as much as possible with appropriate (and potentially prophylactic) airway management and vascular access. Empiric medical therapies should be considered, despite the risks described earlier. Once these measures have been taken, CT may be a reasonable option even in a patient who remains relatively unstable, because it may present the only path to diagnosis. Consider CT tailored for assessment of both PE and aortic pathology. Simultaneous consultation with thoracic surgeons, interventional radiologists, and cardiologists is also reasonable. The patient may benefit from transfer to an angiography suite or operating suite for procedures such as simultaneous right and left heart catheterization to evaluate the pulmonary arteries and aorta. The local resources strongly dictate the imaging approach, which must be closely tied to the therapeutic plan.

SUMMARY

A number of imaging modalities are available for emergency diagnosis of PE and aortic dissection or aneurysm. A normal chest x-ray cannot rule out these potentially fatal processes, so definitive imaging is needed when the diagnoses are strongly considered. CT of the chest has become the test of choice in the emergency department assessment of both conditions. VQ scan is a reasonable alternative to CT when the differential diagnosis is limited to PE. An understanding of pretest probability assessment is essential to selection and interpretation of an imaging test for PE and aortic dissection. When imaging results contradict clinical risk assessment, further imaging evaluation is warranted to exclude PE.

ONLINE CHAPTER 8 Cardiac Computed Tomography

Joshua Broder, MD, FACEP

For the complete chapter text, go to expertconsult.com. To access your account, look for your activation instructions on the inside front cover of this book.

In the previous three chapters, we discussed chest imaging for a variety of indications, ignoring one of the most obvious concerns—cardiac ischemia. Among chief complaints to the emergency department, chest pain is the second most common, according to the National Hospital Ambulatory Medical Care Survey,[1] and computed tomography (CT) has diagnostic value in ischemic chest pain evaluation and exclusion of pulmonary embolism and aortic dissection (discussed in detail in Chapter 7). CT scanners meeting the technical requirements for cardiac CT are widely available even in remote locations.[2]

In this chapter, we begin with some definitions of "cardiac CT" to provide a basis for understanding its diagnostic capabilities and limitations. We describe the major functions of cardiac CT, including calcium scoring, CT coronary angiography, CT assessment of left ventricular function, and assessment of noncardiac causes of chest pain. We explore controversial areas of relative risk and benefit, comparing CT to other diagnostic modalities and strategies for evaluating ischemia and cardiac function. We specifically consider issues of emergency department length of stay, crowding, and cost for which CT has putative benefits. We weigh these potential advantages against radiation exposure, potential for unnecessary testing (and increased costs), and risk for false-positive test results that may ensue from widespread use of cardiac CT.

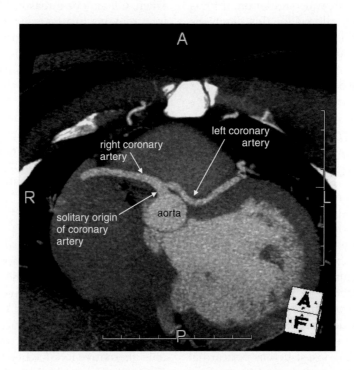

CHAPTER 9 Imaging of Nontraumatic Abdominal Conditions

Joshua Broder, MD, FACEP

Abdominal imaging is essential to clinical decision making in emergency medicine. According to the National Hospital Ambulatory Medical Care Survey,[1] about 8% of emergency department visits are for complaints potentially relating to the abdomen, including vomiting and abdominal pain. By 2005, 8% of adult patients visiting one tertiary care emergency department underwent abdominal computed tomography (CT).[2] Abdominal imaging must identify immediate life-threats such as leaking abdominal aortic aneurysm, conditions requiring urgent surgical intervention such as appendicitis, and conditions requiring antibiotic therapy such as diverticulitis without abscess. Ideally, imaging should also reliably identify patients who do not require any urgent or emergent therapy and can safely be managed as outpatients. In this chapter, we discuss the strengths, limitations, and indications for common emergency abdominal imaging modalities. We describe a systematic approach to interpretation of abdominal x-ray and CT and a focused approach to abdominal ultrasound interpretation. We conclude with a comprehensive survey of important abdominal pathology, describing the diagnostic accuracy and imaging findings for each of the commonly employed modalities for each condition.

Chapters 10, 11, and 12 review the imaging of abdominal trauma, abdominal vascular conditions, and genitourinary conditions, respectively. Chapter 16 delves into interventional radiologic procedures, including many for abdominal conditions. We refer to these chapters rather than repeating their content, recognizing that the clinical presentations of abdominal conditions can be quite nonspecific and that abdominal imaging sometimes must be selected to include an array of possible pathology, including traumatic, vascular, and genitourinary abnormalities.

Figures in this chapter are organized in general by type of pathology. In some cases, multiple modalities from the same patient are displayed together, because they depict a clinical story that can reveal strengths and weaknesses of various imaging modalities. For quick reference, Table 9-1 lists the content of figures in this chapter.

ABDOMINAL IMAGING MODALITIES

The most commonly used emergency department abdominal imaging modalities include plain x-ray, CT, and ultrasound. Nuclear scintigraphy and MRI are more rarely employed for selected conditions. Fluoroscopy for gastrointestinal (GI) studies and abdominal angiography have seen a decline in use with the increasing availability and diagnostic utility of CT scan for the same applications. We review each of these modalities here, pointing out some general principles about their diagnostic capabilities and limitations. These are elaborated upon in later sections on individual forms of abdominal pathology.

X-ray

Abdominal x-ray was the first abdominal imaging modality, used shortly after Roentgen's discovery of x-ray in 1895. Unfortunately, x-ray has limited utility in abdominal imaging. The abdomen contains four principal densities: air, fat, water (soft tissues and fluids such as blood), and calcified structures (e. g., bone, vascular calcifications, and ureteral calcifications). Although x-ray can distinguish among these according to principles discussed in more detail in Chapter 5, most pathologic processes are not well differentiated from normal findings by x-ray. Exceptions to this rule include radiopaque foreign bodies and gross bowel obstruction, as well as moderate to large amounts of pneumoperitoneum. Other inflammatory, infectious, vascular, and neoplastic abnormalities in the abdomen sometimes produce plain x-ray abnormalities, but these are inconsistently present and generally have poor sensitivity and specificity. Although early radiologists were ingenious at recognizing associations between pathology and subtle imaging abnormalities, today better imaging solutions are generally found through CT and ultrasound. Studies of abdominal x-ray generally find them to be diagnostically useful in a small minority of cases. Lack of sensitivity means that a normal x-ray does not exclude most disease processes, requiring either additional imaging or clinical observation to be performed. Similarly, lack of specificity means that many x-ray abnormalities require additional imaging confirmation before treatment can be initiated. The information required from imaging for clinical management of many abdominal conditions has grown over time, because more conditions are managed nonoperatively or with operative approaches that are tailored to specific disease features. As a consequence, abdominal x-rays should be ordered rarely. In unstable patients or patients with extremely high pretest probability of disease, portable x-rays can provide rapid information

TABLE 9-1. Guide to Figures in This Chapter

Content	Figure Number	Content	Figure Number
Abdominal x-ray, normal	9-1	Inflammatory bowel disease and colitis, CT	9-67 to 9-70
Hounsfield CT density scale	9-2	Necrotizing enterocolitis	9-71
Tissue densities on CT and fat as a contrast agent	9-3, 9-4	Cholelithiasis, x-ray	9-72
Fat stranding	9-5	Cholelithiasis, cholecystitis, and gallbladder polyps, ultrasound	9-73 to 9-87, 9-91, 9-111
Tissue enhancement with IV contrast, CT	9-6	HIDA nuclear scintigraphy	9-88 to 9-90, 9-101
Free air, x-ray	9-7, 9-8	Cholelithiasis, CT	9-92 to 9-94
Free air, CT	9-9, 9-10	Cholecystitis, CT	9-95 to 9-98
Bowel perforation, CT	9-11	Biliary ductal dilatation, ultrasound	9-99, 9-100
Pyloric stenosis, x-ray	9-12	Bile leak, CT	9-102
Pyloric stenosis, ultrasound	9-13	Cholangiography	9-103
Small-bowel obstruction, x-ray	9-14, 9-15, 9-18	Biliary tract obstruction and choledocholithiasis, CT	9-104 to 9-108
Small-bowel obstruction, CT	9-16, 9-17, 9-19	Pneumobilia, CT	9-109
Hernia, CT	9-20, 9-21, 9-34 to 9-36	Ascending cholangitis, CT	9-107, 9-110
Malrotation and midgut volvulus	9-22	Pancreatitis and complications including pseudocyst, CT	9-112 to 9-116, 9-119
Intussusception, CT	9-23, 9-24	Pancreatic mass, CT	9-117, 9-118
Intussusception, x-ray	9-25	Perirectal abscess, CT	9-120, 9-121
Intussusception, ultrasound	9-26, 9-28, 9-30	Liver abscess, CT	9-122 to 9-124
Intussusception, air-contrast enema	9-27, 9-29, 9-31	Postoperative abdominal abscess, CT	9-125, 9-126
Large-bowel obstruction, x-ray	9-32, 9-37, 9-38, 9-42, 9-44, 9-45, 9-46	Metastatic disease and splenomegaly, CT	9-127, 9-128
Large-bowel obstruction, CT	9-33; see also sigmoid and cecal volvulus CT	Ascites, x-ray	9-129
Sigmoid volvulus, x-ray	9-37, 9-38, 9-42	Ascites, ultrasound	9-130, 9-131
Sigmoid volvulus, CT	9-39 to 9-41	Ascites, CT	9-132
Sigmoid volvulus, barium enema	9-43	Hemoperitoneum, CT	9-133
Cecal volvulus, x-ray	9-44 to 9-46	Ingested foreign body, x-ray	9-134 to 9-137
Cecal volvulus, CT	9-47 to 9-49	Ingested foreign body, CT	9-138
Pseudo-obstruction of bowel, x-ray	9-50	Intestinal foreign body, macroparasite, CT	9-139
Appendicitis, CT	9-51 to 9-56	Adrenal imaging, CT	9-140 to 9-143
Appendicitis, ultrasound	9-57	Gastrointestinal bleeding, tagged red cell study	9-144, 9-145
Epiploic appendagitis	9-58	Mesenteric angiography for gastrointestinal bleeding	9-146
Mesenteric adenitis	9-59		
Diverticulosis, CT	9-60 to 9-62		
Diverticulitis, CT	9-62 to 9-66		

that may be adequate to determine treatment, such as laparotomy for perforated viscus. In patients with an extremely low pretest probability of disease, negative x-rays may provide adequate reassurance to allow discharge or observation without further imaging, although the emergency physician must always remember that negative x-rays do not rule out virtually any important disease process. As we discuss later, the frequently used terms *rule out free air* and *rule out obstruction* should be discarded, because they provide false reassurance based on the poor sensitivity of x-ray.

In the past, abdominal x-ray was considered a prerequisite for advanced imaging. However, for most

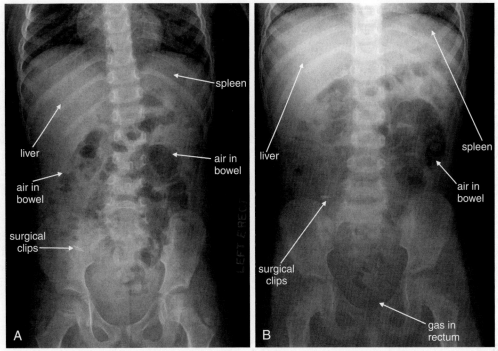

Figure 9-1. A normal abdominal x-ray series. A, Upright anterior–posterior (AP) x-ray. Scattered air and stool are seen in the bowel, with no distinct air–fluid levels or dilated loops of bowel. Surgical clips are visible in the right lower quadrant, because this patient has undergone prior appendectomy. No free air is seen under the diaphragm. **B,** Supine AP x-ray. A supine view would not be expected to demonstrate subdiaphragmatic free air or air–fluid levels, even in the presence of pneumoperitoneum or bowel obstruction, respectively. Gas is visible in the rectum, a normal finding.

conditions, the poor sensitivity and specificity of x-ray mean that x-rays should be avoided in patients with a moderate pretest probability of disease, because additional imaging is required in most cases, regardless of the x-ray findings. Advanced imaging should be performed without preceding x-ray in these cases.

Standard abdominal x-ray views include upright and supine anterior–posterior (AP) views (Figure 9-1). The upright view is sometimes called a KUB, for kidneys, ureters, and bladder—a misnomer because none of these structures are well seen on plain x-ray, though all are included in the field of view. A "three view of the abdomen" typically adds an upright chest x-ray to this series. A left lateral decubitus AP abdominal x-ray is sometimes used as well.[2a]

The **upright abdominal x-ray** (AP or PA) is performed to identify air–fluid levels, suggesting bowel obstruction. Air–fluid levels also rarely may be seen with intraabdominal abscesses, though the sensitivity of x-ray for this indication is likely so low that x-ray should not performed when abscess is suspected. The upright x-ray also may demonstrate dilated loops of bowel, again suggesting bowel obstruction. X-ray findings of bowel obstruction are discussed in more detail later in this chapter. Radiopaque foreign bodies (ingested, inserted rectally, or traumatically introduced into the abdomen) can be seen on this view as well. The upright abdominal x-ray is not generally useful for detection

of pneumoperitoneum, because the image is relatively overexposed and small to moderate amounts of subdiaphragmatic air are not usually visible.[2a]

The **supine AP abdominal x-ray** is generally less useful than the upright x-ray. On this view, dilated loops of bowel suggesting obstruction may be seen. However, air–fluid levels are not seen on the supine view, because air rises to the less dependent regions of the abdomen, layers in the plane of the x-ray film or detector, and does not form a visible interface with dependent fluids. Similarly, pneumoperitoneum rises to the anterior abdominal wall rather than the subdiaphragmatic region, layers in the plane of the x-ray detector, and is not generally visible. Radiopaque foreign bodies can be seen on this view.

The **upright chest x-ray** (AP or PA) is the most useful x-ray view for detection of free air (pneumoperitoneum). In the upright position, free air rises to the uppermost regions of the abdomen and collects beneath the diaphragm, forming a black silhouette between the denser liver on the right and sometimes the spleen or gastric wall on the left. The gastric air bubble on the left can be mistaken for pneumoperitoneum, a potential pitfall. Occasionally, colonic interposition (the presence of the air-filled transverse colon between the diaphragm and the liver) can also simulate free air. The sensitivity of upright chest x-ray is relatively low when the quantity of free air is small, as discussed later in this chapter. In addition, loculated free air, such as may be seen with an abscess or with a small perforation of bowel, may not rise to the subdiaphragmatic region and may therefore be invisible on x-ray.

The **left lateral decubitus abdominal x-ray** is occasionally used in patients who are unable to stand or to assume an upright position. The patient is placed on the left side, with the right side of the abdomen upright. An AP or PA x-ray image is then acquired. In this position, the lateral margin of the liver is the most superior abdominal organ, and free air may collect between the superior margin of the liver and the parietal peritoneal surface. The lateral decubitus x-ray can therefore substitute for an upright chest x-ray in particularly sick patients in a search for pneumoperitoneum. However, the same limitations to the sensitivity of upright chest x-ray described earlier apply to lateral decubitus x-ray. The lateral decubitus x-ray can also be used to visualize air–fluid levels, suggesting bowel obstruction. However,

in most cases today, if the patient is unable to undergo a standard three-view abdominal series, CT is a more sensible emergency department imaging test, for reasons outlined later.

Systematic Interpretation of Abdominal X-ray
Later in this chapter, we review x-ray findings of specific pathology. But as we stated previously, x-ray is both insensitive and nonspecific for many important conditions. For many conditions, our purpose in reviewing x-rays and comparing them with CT and ultrasound findings is to emphasize the poor diagnostic performance of x-ray, even when findings are quite overt with other imaging modalities. Nonetheless, abdominal x-rays remain important in some practice settings where CT and ultrasound may be unavailable. Here, we review a structured approach to abdominal x-ray interpretation, intended to glean as much information as possible from the image (Box 9-1).

Box 9-1: Structured Approach to Abdominal X-ray Interpretation

- **Free air**
  - Inspect subdiaphragmatic regions of upright x-ray for lucency
  - Avoid confusion with gastric air bubble on left
  - Free air is seen best on upright chest x-ray
- **Bowel obstruction**
  - Dilated loops of small bowel (>3 cm diameter)
  - Dilated loops of large bowel (>8 cm diameter)
  - Air–fluid levels
  - Sentinel loops
- **Other pathologic air**
  - Pneumobilia (consider ascending cholangitis)
  - Mural pneumatosis (mesenteric ischemia)
  - Gallbladder air (emphysematous cholecystitis)
  - Intrarenal air (emphysematous pyelonephritis)
  - Retroperitoneal air (abscess)
  - Peritoneal loculated air with air–fluid level (abscess)
- **Foreign bodies**
  - Surgical clips and stents (may provide clues to prior procedures in patients with unknown history)
  - Ingested foreign bodies
  - Shrapnel
- **Calcifications**
  - Gallbladder (calcified gallstones may be visible, though they do not confirm cholecystitis do not confirm cholecystitis; porcelain gallbladder of carcinoma has calcified rim)
  - Appendix (appendicolith suggesting appendicitis)
  - Vascular calcifications (abdominal aortic aneurysm and other advanced atherosclerotic disease)
  - Renal (nephro- or ureterolithiasis)
  - Pheloboliths (usually have a central lucency that differentiates them from ureteral stones; no pathologic significance)
  - Pancreatic calcifications (chronic pancreatitis)
  - Ovarian calcifications (dermoid cyst also known as teratoma may contain calcifications resembling teeth)
  - Hepatic (neoplasm or echinococcal infection)
  - Bladder (schistosomiasis infection)
- **Hepatosplenomegaly**
  - Enlarged silhouettes of liver and spleen
- **Ascites**
  - Diffuse ground-glass appearance, often with small bowel located centrally
- **Inflammation or hemorrhage in retroperitoneum**
  - Psoas fat stripe lost
  - Properitoneal line lost
- **Bones (pelvis, spine, or ribs)**
  - Lytic lesions
  - Fractures
- **Chest pathology causing abdominal symptoms**
  - Pneumonia
  - Pneumothorax
  - Pleural effusion
  - Pericardial effusion

As described earlier, a typical abdominal series consists of an upright chest x-ray (PA or AP), a single upright frontal projection (AP or PA) abdominal x-ray, and a supine AP abdominal x-ray.[2a] Review each of these in turn, seeking specific findings. X-rays of the chest and abdomen are typically displayed with the patient's right side on the left side of the viewing screen.

Begin by reviewing the upright chest x-ray for pneumoperitoneum (free air). This finding is reviewed in detail in Chapter 5. Pneumoperitoneum is visible as a black collection between the liver and the diaphragm on the right, the diaphragm and the inferior heart border medially, and the diaphragm and the stomach or spleen on the left. Air within the stomach may be mistaken for pneumoperitoneum on the left, although usually gastric air is distinguished by a thicker superior soft-tissue stripe, composed of the combination of the gastric wall and diaphragm. In contrast, when air is truly subdiaphragmatic, the diaphragm generally appears 2 to 4mm thick, depending on phase of respiration and diaphragm contraction. Free air can be minute in quantity, perhaps visible only as a thin black line, or massive, sometimes confusing novice x-ray readers by its sheer volume. Although CT is considered far more sensitive (as discussed later in this chapter), suspected free air is one of the primary remaining legitimate indications for abdominal x-rays (or more accurately, for upright chest x-ray) and thus deserves careful attention.

Next, examine the series for evidence of small- or large-bowel obstruction. Bowel obstruction is a second rational indication for abdominal x-ray, although the sensitivity of x-ray is believed to be significantly less than that of CT, as discussed later. Two key findings suggest small-bowel obstruction: dilated loops of bowel and air–fluid levels. Although normal bowel does contain both air and fluid, in the setting of obstruction, the small bowel becomes dilated to 3 cm or greater, and multiple stair-step air–fluid levels may be seen. Remember that air–fluid levels are expected only on the upright abdominal and chest x-rays; on the supine abdominal x-ray, air and fluid layer in the image plane and may not be seen. On both the upright and the supine images, small-bowel loops can be inspected for dilatation. Dilated loops of small bowel are usually recognizable by the plicae circularis (also called valvulae conniventes), which completely cross the diameter of the bowel lumen. In contrast, the haustra of the large intestine do not cross the complete width of the bowel. Large-bowel obstruction can be recognized by a dilated large bowel, measuring greater than 8 cm in diameter. Large-bowel air–fluid levels may also be seen on the upright x-ray. The distribution of gas in the bowel should also be noted. In a complete bowel obstruction, peristalsis distal to the point of obstruction may force air out of the bowel, leading to a gasless abdomen beyond the obstruction, including the rectum. If gas is present in the bowel through to the rectum, an obstruction is not ruled out, because it may be early in its course or may be incomplete. Bowel obstruction is discussed in more detail later in the chapter. Older texts describe multiple other bowel gas patterns that radiologists have attempted to correlate with other disease states, but unfortunately, these are quite nonspecific. Described gas patterns include adynamic ileus, "nonspecific bowel gas pattern," and incomplete obstruction—but these may be present in patients with normal abdomen, true mechanical bowel obstruction, or other pathologic processes, including surgical conditions such as appendicitis and mesenteric ischemia.

Next, a series of other findings should be sought, though each is individually relatively rare and may lack sensitivity and specificity for the acute cause of the patient's symptoms. Other **pathologic air** should be sought within the liver (pneumobilia), intestinal wall (mural pneumatosis intestinalis), gallbladder fossa (emphysematous cholecystitis), kidneys (emphysematous pyelonephritis), retroperitoneum, or loculated collections (abscess). Air in branching patterns particularly suggests air within abdominal ducts or vascular structures. Amorphous collections of gas can be impossible to localize, because they may represent bowel gas or extraluminal gas. Air which appears to outline both the internal and external surfaces of a loop of bowel suggests bowel perforation with extraluminal gas.

Calcifications can provide clues to disease, though again caution should be used, because calcified organs are not necessarily the acute cause of symptoms, and acutely diseased organs may lack calcifications. Calcifications may occur within the gallbladder (gallstones), kidneys or ureters (ureterolithiasis or nephrolithiasis), appendix (appendicoliths), pancreas (chronic pancreatitis), vascular structures (aortic aneurysm or other advanced atherosclerotic disease), pelvic structures (e.g., phleboliths or calcified partially formed teeth within a dermoid), liver (malignancy or echinococcal infection), and bladder (schistosomiasis). Pelvic vein calcifications (phleboliths) have no known pathologic significance but may be confused for appendicolith or ureteral calcifications. Phleboliths are usually recognizable by a tiny central lucency, not found in most other calcifications. Foreign bodies including surgical clips and stents, shrapnel, and ingested foreign bodies should be noted, because they can provide information not available from the patient history.

Sentinel bowel loops, isolated loops of bowel with localized ileus induced by adjacent inflammatory processes (e.g., pancreatitis) may hint at pathology but are neither sensitive nor specific. The silhouette of the liver and spleen may be visible and can suggest hepatomegaly or splenomegaly. Ascites may be recognized as a diffuse hazy or "ground glass" appearance, often associated with centralization of small bowel, resulting from bowel floating suspended in surrounding ascites. CT and ultrasound are extremely sensitive and specific for abdominal free fluid in comparison with x-ray, which has poor sensitivity and specificity. The psoas fat stripe can be obscured by inflammation or retroperitoneal hemorrhage, but x-ray should never be used to rule out these findings. The bones of the ribs, spine, and pelvis are visible within the field of view of an abdominal x-ray and should be assessed for lytic lesions or fractures. The chest x-ray should be scrutinized for chest pathology that may be the cause of abdominal pain, such as a lower lobe pneumonia, pneumothorax, or pleural or pericardial effusion. Interpretation of chest x-ray is reviewed in Chapter 5.

Computed Tomography

Abdominal CT scan is one of the most diagnostically useful abdominal imaging modalities. Despite its apparent high diagnostic accuracy for many conditions, questions remain about the clinical benefit to patient outcomes from increasing CT use. We explore some controversies surrounding CT throughout this chapter, including studies of outcomes in appendicitis diagnosed with CT and risks for radiation exposure from CT. Additional controversies include indications for oral, intravenous (IV), and rectal contrast, which we elaborate upon for specific indications. Here, we consider some general features of abdominal CT, which we refine as we review specific forms of pathology.

CT of the abdomen generally includes two separately ordered radiologic studies: CT of the abdomen and CT of the pelvis. For simplicity, we refer to these as abdominal CT. Abdominal–pelvic CT usually includes a cephalad–caudad range from the top of the diaphragm to the bottom of the bony pelvis so that it includes the entire peritoneal cavity and retroperitoneum. Occasionally, a more restricted or more extended CT is indicated; we specify this in the text.

Computed Tomography Technique

CT scan is a modality that uses ionizing radiation to expose detectors mounted on the opposite side of a circular gantry through which the patient passes. A complex computer algorithm constructs an image based on the relative attenuation of the x-ray beam by body tissues. We briefly compare early and modern CT technology, because this affects the diagnostic capabilities of modern scanners and means that older research on the diagnostic utility of CT is often outdated. Early CT scanners relied on single-detector, axial data acquisition. Modern scanners rely on multidetector, helical data acquisition.

The first CT scanners used a single x-ray emitter and detector, which rotated in a single circular path around the patient to construct each axial image slice. The table upon which the patient was positioned moved in steps through the gantry, with one axial image slice acquired following each step. The final CT image was composed of a "stack" of axial CT images, like slices of a loaf of bread. The thickness of the slices could be selected, with a typical slice thickness of 5 mm for abdominal CT. Early scanners were quite slow, so choosing a slice thickness represented a necessary trade-off between the resolution required for diagnosis and the amount of time required to perform the CT scan. If one slice were acquired per second, a 1-m (1000 mm) abdomen and pelvis divided into contiguous 5-mm slices would require 200 seconds to scan. Slice thickness is one determinant of image resolution. Consider the difference between a 1-mm and a 5-mm slice. For each pixel making up the image, a 5-mm slice gathers anatomic data from pixels in 5 mm of cephalad–caudad territory and then projects the average density values into a single pixel in the final image. This results in "volume averaging," meaning that if the 5-mm slice consists of multiple densities, the final image represents the average of those densities, rather than reflecting the true range of densities. In comparison, a 1-mm-thick slice averages the density values across only a 1-mm cephalad–caudad distance to generate the final image pixel. Thus relatively thick slices result in more volume averaging and can miss small pathology. For most abdominal pathology, a 3- to 5-mm slice thickness is adequate; very small abnormalities such as 1-mm renal stones might be missed by thick slices, although the clinical significance of such minute abnormalities is uncertain.

Because the patient table was stepped incrementally through the CT gantry with early CT technology, gaps existed between axial images using this technique, creating the possibility of missing small pathology lying between axial slices. Moreover, if an image in a plane other than the axial plane was desired, the gaps between the axial slices and the thickness of the axial data resulted in pixelated sagittal and coronal reconstructions marked by stair-step artifacts, with limited diagnostic utility.

Modern scanners rely on two major innovations to resolve these issues. First, modern scanners employ helical scanning, in which the patient table moves continuously through the CT scanner gantry. Although the gantry rotates in a simple circular pattern, the motion of the table through the gantry creates a helical (or spiral) pattern relative to the patient. As a consequence, a three-dimensional volume of image data is acquired across the entire cephalad–caudad extent of the abdomen, rather than the data consisting of a discontinuous stack of discrete axial slices. We explore the importance of this in a moment. The second innovation was an increase in the number of detectors; 16 and 64 detectors are common today, and even higher detector numbers are available (256 in some scanners). More detectors means that image data can be collected as thinner slices, while maintaining or improving the speed of the image acquisition. For example, if 64 detectors each collect 5 mm of cephalad–caudad anatomic data per gantry rotation, only three gantry rotations are required to cover 1 m of cephalad–caudad anatomy. Even if each detector is configured to acquire only 1 mm of anatomic data, because 64 detectors are at play, each gantry rotation can acquire 64 mm of anatomic data. Compare this with a single-detector CT scanner, which would acquire only 1 mm of cephalad–caudad anatomic data per rotation. Therefore modern multidetector, helical CT scanners can rapidly acquire "thin slice" three-dimensional volumes of anatomic data, free of data gaps and less subject to volume averaging. These three-dimensional volumes can be "resliced" in any plane, readily allowing axial, sagittal, and coronal planar reconstructions or true three-dimensional image reconstruction. Although axial images remain the primary images used diagnostically, some studies have examined the value of other imaging planes to detect pathology such as appendicitis.

One more feature of helical thin-slice CT technology bears mention. Although data can be acquired at very thin "slice thickness" (really, the width of anatomy projected onto each detector), it would be impractical to display all acquired data. For example, if each detector is set to capture 1 mm of anatomy thickness, and if the resulting data were displayed as 1-mm "thick" axial images, a single CT of a 1-m-long abdomen and pelvis would be composed of 1000 slices. Radiologists typically make compromises between the pragmatic need to have fewer images for review and the need to diagnose subtle pathology. Usually data is captured at a detector width compatible with the expected pathology and then displayed as thicker slices to reduce the number of resulting images. For example, if aortic dissection is suspected, data may be acquired at 1-mm detector width and then displayed as a series of 3- to 5-mm "thick" axial images. If more image detail is required at a particular anatomic area, the original 1-mm-thick data can be reconstructed selectively as thinner slices spanning that location.

Patient Positioning for Computed Tomography

During a CT scan, the patient is usually positioned supine on the scanner table. Some protocols use prone positioning—a common example is a "renal stone" protocol CT. The patient's position during the CT has important effects, for example, changing the expected locations of free air when compared with a conventional x-ray obtained with the patient in an upright position. These effects are discussed in more detail in sections that follow on specific pathologic conditions.

The Hounsfield Computed Tomography Density Scale and Tissues

In other chapters, we discussed the Hounsfield scale of CT densities, but it is particularly important in the abdomen. We review the general principles here, because they can assist you in problem-solving for both common and unusual pathology addressed later in this chapter.

The Hounsfield scale (named for one of the Nobel Prize–winning inventors of CT, the British physicist Godfrey N. Hounsfield) arbitrarily assigns water a density of 0 Hounsfield units (HU) and air a value of −1000 HU. Dense materials such as bone have density values approaching +1000 HU. The Hounsfield density of tissues reflects their attenuation of x-ray and is proportional to their physical density. To illustrate the relative density of common body tissues encountered in the abdomen and their CT appearance, imagine a glass of water into which various materials are placed. Air is less dense than water and remains suspended above the column of water. Oil (fat) floats on water, because it is less dense. A piece of meat (soft tissue) dropped into the water would sink to the bottom of the glass, because it is slightly denser than the water. Soft tissues are surprisingly similar in density to water—surprising until we consider that tissues are composed of cells, which are composed largely of water. A bone dropped into the water would sink readily to the bottom, because it is comparatively quite dense. Liquid blood has a density that is intermediate between simple water and soft tissues. This intermediate density makes perfect sense when we recall that blood is a "liquid tissue," composed of about 40% red blood cells (the hematocrit of the blood) and about 60% serous liquid (essentially water), with a small contribution from other cell types.

Windows and the Hounsfield Scale. The color scale assigned to tissues of various densities with CT can be varied to accentuate different tissues, a process called "windowing." The CT color scale is a gray-shade scale, from black to white. Less dense tissues appear blacker, denser tissues appear whiter, and tissues with intermediate densities occupy intermediate gray shades. Because the human eye and brain cannot perceive subtle variations in gray shades, it is usually not useful to distribute the available gray shades uniformly across the full range of densities when displaying the image. Instead, the distribution of the gray shades is varied depending on the tissue of greatest interest. In the case of abdominal structures, the most common window setting (a "soft-tissue" window) uses a fairly widely distributed gray scale, because the abdomen contains materials of highly variable density, from the normal air in the bowel (−1000 HU) to the subcutaneous, peritoneal, and retroperitoneal fat (-50 to -100 HU), to the liquid bile and blood (~+20 HU), to muscles and abdominal solid organs (~+40 to +100 HU), to the bones of the vertebral column, pelvis, and ribs (~+200 to +1000 HU) (Figures 9-2 and 9-3).

The lung window shifts the gray scale to accentuate the appearance of tissues of very low density—air and lung

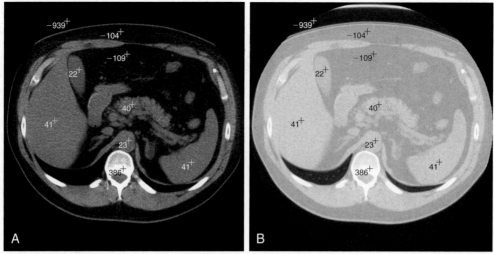

Figure 9-2. The Hounsfield CT density scale. On the Hounsfield scale, air is assigned a value of −1000 Hounsfield units (HU), water a value of 0 HU, and bone a value of several hundred to +1000 HU. Fat has a value of −50 HU, soft tissue a value of +40 HU. The grayscale color corresponding to these values varies, depending on the window setting selected. **A,** Body or soft-tissue window. The Hounsfield scale is centered on the tissues of interest, with white and black at the extreme ends of the spectrum. A cursor placed on various tissues displays the Hounsfield density. **B,** Lung window. By moving the gray scale toward low Hounsfield values, detail of low-density lung tissue is accentuated. Detail of high-density structures is lost. Although the tissue density numeric values are unchanged, the appearance is quite different.

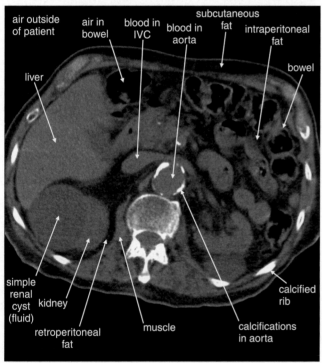

Figure 9-3. The Hounsfield CT density scale and fat as a contrast agent. Familiarity with the appearance of various tissue densities on CT is simple but essential. On a noncontrast CT viewed with a soft-tissue window, air appears black, fat appears nearly black, simple fluids are dark gray, and solid tissues are intermediate gray. Bone and calcifications are bright white. Fat can be a useful "contrast agent" on CT. To identify the appearance of fat, start with the patient's subcutaneous fat. Normal intraperitoneal and retroperitoneal fat have the same tissue density as subcutaneous fat. Notice how intraperitoneal fat separates loops of bowel and retroperitoneal fat separates the kidneys from paraspinal muscles. IVC, inferior vena cava.

tissue (see Figure 9-2). Although this window setting is designed to allow inspection of the lung parenchyma and to allow the differentiation of lung from surrounding pneumothorax, it is extremely useful in inspection of the abdomen, pelvis, and retroperitoneum for pathologic air or gas. On a typical soft-tissue window setting, small areas of abnormal air can be difficult to identify, because air (black on this setting) can appear similar to fat (a dark gray shade, depending on the exact window setting). On a lung window setting, all tissues except air or gas appear quite bright (white or nearly white) by comparison, drawing attention to air, which remains black. Even tiny quantities of free peritoneal air can be readily recognized using this setting. Air in other abnormal locations can also be more readily identified.

Throughout this chapter, unless otherwise specified, the appropriate window to evaluate for pathologic findings is the soft-tissue window. A window is defined by a center value and a width. The center value is the Hounsfield density to which the middle gray shade is assigned. The width is the number of Hounsfield units around the center value to which the brightest and darkest shades in the grayscale are assigned. The precise values used for soft-tissue and other window settings may vary from institution to institution, but common values are shown in Table 9-2.

Fat and Air as Contrast Agents. We soon discuss extrinsically administered contrast agents, but it is useful first to consider intrinsic contrast provided by normal differences in body tissue density. When we look at a CT image, we cannot distinguish two structures in physical contact with one another that share identical (or

TABLE 9-2. Common CT Window Settings

Window	Center	Width
Lung	−498 HU	+1465 HU
Bone	+570 HU	+3077 HU
Soft-tissue	+56 HU	+342 HU
Brain	+40 HU	+200 HU

HU, Hounsfield unit.
The center value is the Hounsfield density to which the central gray shade is assigned. The center value minus half the width is assigned black. The center value plus half of the width is assigned white. No standards have been established for CT window settings, so the exact values used by different institutions may vary.

even similar) densities. When a tissue of a different density intervenes, the transition from one tissue to another is clearly demarcated—tissue contrast. Because **air or gas** is dramatically less dense than other body tissues (−1000 HU, compared with the least dense competing tissue, fat, ~−50 HU), it provides outstanding tissue contrast. As a consequence, air can be recognized without the administration of any exogenous contrast agents. CT is therefore exquisitely sensitive for the detection of abnormal air or gas, as we discuss later in the section on pneumoperitoneum and other conditions in which pathologic gas assists in diagnosis.

A second key intrinsic contrast agent is **fat.** Again, fat is quite different in density from most other abdominal tissues and can separate other organs of similar density (see Figures 9-2 and 9-3). Fat is normally present in subcutaneous tissue, within the peritoneum, and in the retroperitoneum. In these locations, it separates normal organs from one another, allowing us to recognize individual loops of bowel in the abdomen or the demarcation of retroperitoneal organs such as the psoas muscles and kidneys, even without the addition of exogenous contrast agents. In the thinnest patients, a paucity of peritoneal and retroperitoneal fat is a diagnostic disadvantage, potentially increasing the necessity of exogenous contrast agents (Figure 9-4). In patients of average or somewhat above-average body mass index, fat actually provides helpful tissue contrast and may decrease the need for extrinsic contrast. Fat becomes a disadvantage in extremely obese patients, in whom it contributes to excessive image noise (Figure 9-5). Some very obese patients may actually exceed the CT scanner weight, size, and x-ray tube capacity, as described later.

Fat Stranding. Fat provides an additional diagnostic benefit, acting as the substrate for inflammatory fat stranding (see Figure 9-5). When inflammation occurs, microscopic lymphatic vessels within fat become relatively leaky, and the water content of adipose tissue increases. Because water is denser than normal fat, increasing the water content of adipose tissue increases its density. As you can anticipate from our earlier

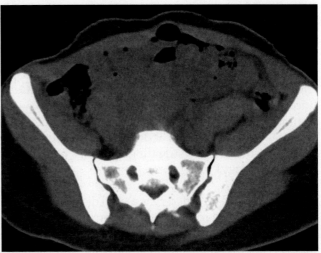

Figure 9-4. Fat, a useful "contrast agent" for CT. In very thin patients, the absence of intraperitoneal fat makes it extremely difficult to distinguish structures. Oral and intravenous contrast are particularly helpful in this setting. In this noncontrast CT of a very thin patient, anatomic structures are difficult to distinguish from one another, caused by the paucity of intraperitoneal fat.

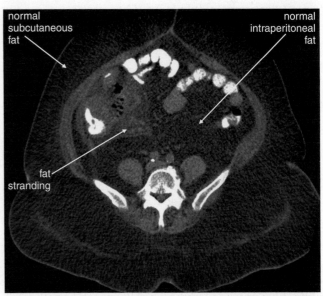

Figure 9-5. Fat stranding, CT without IV contrast. Fat stranding is an inflammatory change in fat, resulting from extravasation of fluid from tissue lymphatic vessels. When viewed with soft-tissue windows, stranding changes the appearance of fat from its usual near-black to a hazy gray. Compare the subcutaneous fat in this patient, which shows no stranding, to the intraperitoneal fat in the right abdomen, which shows stranding. Fat in the patient's left abdomen does not show stranding. The overall image quality of this scan is poor because of the patient's obesity, which results in a worsened signal-to-noise ratio.

discussion of density, increasing the density of a tissue increases the brightness or whiteness of the tissue on the CT image. Normal fat appears dark—nearly black on a standard soft-tissue window setting. Therefore inflamed fat appears whiter, assuming a smoky or hazy gray appearance called fat stranding. In the presence of an infectious or inflammatory process such as appendicitis, diverticulitis, cholecystitis, or colitis, the fat around the affected organ often demonstrates stranding, which can be a key diagnostic finding in these scenarios. In patients with little or no peritoneal fat, there is no substrate for stranding, and the diagnosis of these conditions can be difficult. For these reasons, "fat is our friend" in CT diagnosis. (The origin of this phrase is uncertain—the author's father is the only source known to him). Because inflammatory fat stranding accompanies many forms of acute abdominal pathology, where there is "smoke" (fat stranding) there is often "fire" (acute pathology).

Free Fluid. Free fluid deserves special discussion, partly because the familiarity of many emergency physicians with ultrasound might lead to confusion when interpreting CT scan. On ultrasound images, simple fluid appears black. On an abdominal CT image viewed on a typical soft-tissue window, simple fluid appears intermediate gray—a shade usually indicating a solid organ on ultrasound images. On this same CT window setting, air appears black and fat appears dark gray, or nearly black. If you are an emergency physician with extensive ultrasound experience, until you have become accustomed to viewing abdominal CT, you may mistakenly see fat as "fluid" on CT images and see fluid as "solid tissue."

Free fluid on CT can have several diagnostic meanings, depending on the scenario. Because CT differentiates tissues based on density and x-ray attenuation, CT cannot perfectly distinguish types of simple fluids (new advances in dual-energy CT, discussed later in this chapter, may help to alleviate this shortcoming). For example, blood, bile, purulent fluid, and ascites may differ in density by only a few Hounsfield units, depending on factors such as the hematocrit of the blood. As discussed in Chapters 10 and 12, in the setting of trauma, free fluid may be blood from solid-organ injury, fluid from bowel injury, or urine or bile resulting from injury to the relevant organ systems. In the setting of nontraumatic abdominal pain, fluid may be blood, ascites, purulent fluid, bile, or urine—clinical history, as well as other CT abnormalities, may help to narrow the differential diagnosis. Free fluid can be seen in infectious and inflammatory conditions, as well as mesenteric ischemia and bowel perforation. Although nonspecific, it is a potentially important sign of pathology and should be sought carefully. We discuss free fluid in more detail when we cover individual forms of pathology.

Computed Tomography Contrast Agents
As we discuss in more detail later in this chapter, considerable controversy exists about the need for contrast agents for some clinical indications, such as suspected appendicitis. In this section, we describe the core roles of contrast agents. Later we critically examine the need for contrast when evaluating for specific pathology. Contrast agents typically used for abdominal CT include IV

contrast, oral contrast, and more rarely, rectal contrast. In rare circumstances, contrast agents may be instilled retrograde into the bladder—this is discussed in detail in Chapter 12.

IV contrast agents are usually injected through a peripheral IV catheter. These contrast agents "go with the flow"; consequently, they highlight anatomic structures and pathologic processes with high blood flow. These include vascular structures; highly vascular end organs such as the kidneys, liver, and spleen; neoplastic processes; and inflammatory and infectious processes. Iodinated contrast agents are high in density, so organs receiving these agents experience an increase in their tissue density, called enhancement (Figure 9-6). The degree of enhancement depends on blood flow, so organs like the kidneys (receiving approximately 25% of the cardiac output) enhance intensely. Similarly, an infectious

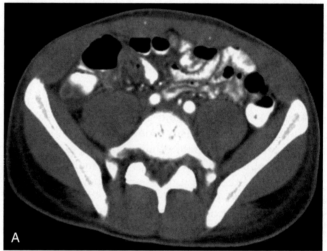

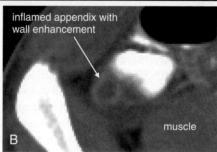

Figure 9-6. Enhancement, CT with IV contrast. Enhancement is an increase in density and brightness (Hounsfield units) after administration of IV contrast, seen in inflammatory, infectious, vascular, and neoplastic processes. The common feature of these conditions leading to enhancement is increased blood flow. In this case of appendicitis, the appendiceal wall shows enhancement. No specific Hounsfield unit value defines enhancement. If a noncontrast CT is performed first, comparison with the tissue density before IV contrast administration can be made. In most cases of emergency abdominal CT, a noncontrast CT is not performed before CT with contrast. In these cases enhancement is subjectively assessed by comparison of the tissue density with that expected of the normal tissue in question. In one study, enhancement of the appendix was considered present if the appendix was of higher Hounsfield units than were retroperitoneal muscles. **A,** Scan with IV and oral contrast. **B,** Close-up.

or inflammatory process typically receives increased blood flow and shows more enhancement than normal tissues. Sometimes a pathologic failure to enhance is diagnostic; for example, a renal infarction results in decreased blood flow and decreased tissue enhancement, which is readily evident when compared with areas of normal enhancement. IV contrast delineates the lumen of vascular structures, so stenoses or filling defects can be recognized. Without IV contrast, liquid blood within a blood vessel, thrombus adherent to the walls of the blood vessel or lodged within the vessel, and intimal defects such as the intimal flap of aortic dissection all share the same or similar densities and are indistinguishable on CT. When contrast is injected, the liquid-filled lumen of the vessel enhances, and "filling defects" within this channel become visible—including thrombus and dissection flaps. One more role of IV contrast is to identify areas of active hemorrhage or contrast extravasation. Contrast should not be seen outside of the blood vessels or the confines of vascular end organs. An amorphous "blush" of contrast outside of these locations indicates active bleeding at the moment that the CT scan was performed—usually an indication for some emergent intervention. Finally, IV contrast is concentrated and excreted by the kidneys and ultimately fills the ureters and bladder. Sometimes "delayed" CT images are obtained to visualize the excretion of injected contrast, as described in more detail in Chapter 12.

Intravenous Contrast Timing. Contrast injected into a peripheral vein should not allow immediate visualization of arterial structures or end organs. Depending on the vascular bed, organ, or pathology of interest, the timing of CT image acquisition relative to the moment of contrast injection is adjusted, allowing sufficient time for the injected contrast to traverse the right heart and lungs, enter the left heart and aorta, fill arteries, and reach target organs. For some disease processes, the timing of contrast is relatively unimportant. These include fixed structural abnormalities or inflammatory processes, for which the degree of enhancement may be less crucial. For other disease processes, contrast timing is critical. For example, for evaluation of mesenteric ischemia, contrast is desired first in the mesenteric arterial system and then in the portal venous system, because either may be affected. CT images are typically acquired first during the arterial phase, and then (after a delay of 60-90 seconds) additional images are acquired during a portal venous phase. Some neoplastic processes have characteristic enhancement properties when early, middle, and late phases of enhancement are compared on subsequent CT images, although these are generally not emergency department time-dependent diagnoses. Modern CT scanners use software to assist contrast timing, a process described in more detail in Chapter 7. As you can see, the timing of CT image acquisition relative to IV contrast administration can have diagnostic importance, so communication of the differential diagnosis to the radiologist is necessary to maximize diagnostic accuracy. A "generic" CT scan of the abdomen typically uses a delay of approximately 25 seconds, resulting in arterial-phase enhancement of organs. Some scanners use automated triggering software, which initiates the CT scan when the enhancement of the aorta or other target organs reaches a specific Hounsfield unit threshold, rather than using a fixed delay. This can provide better enhancement, because the rapidity of enhancement depends on factors such as the caliber and the location of the catheter used to infuse contrast, which vary from patient to patient.

Enteral Contrast (Oral and Rectal). Enteral contrast has several potential functions. Contrast can be administered into the intestine orally, by nasogastric or orogastric tube, or rectally (as described in more detail later). Enteral contrast agents can be "positive," "neutral," or "negative" contrast agents. The most common form of enteral contrast for emergency applications is positive contrast—meaning contrast that is radiographically dense and appears white on typical soft-tissue CT windows. Positive contrast agents include iodinated contrast agents such as Gastrografin (meglumine diatrizoate) and barium sulfate contrast agents, which can be used in patients with allergy to iodinated contrast agents. These have high density, positive on the Hounsfield scale. Neutral contrast agents are similar in density to water (~0 Hounsfield units) and include (not surprisingly) water, and Volumen, a low concentration barium suspension (0.1% barium). Although water is an excellent contrast agent, it is rapidly absorbed from the intestine and therefore is of little use in the jejunum and ileum.[3] Negative contrast agents are actually lower in density than water and include gases such as carbon dioxide,[4] used for applications such as CT colonography, that are not typically employed in the emergency department. We discuss the theoretical benefits of each type of contrast later.

All enteral contrast agents share two common properties: they distend the lumen of small and large bowel, and they distinguish bowel from "nonbowel" abdominal structures that may otherwise appear similar. The normal small bowel is a tubular structure, usually filled with some combination of fluid (near water density, 0 Hounsfield units, or moderately dark gray on soft-tissue CT window) and air (–1000 Hounsfield units or black on all window settings). Depending on the orientation of the bowel and the image plane, the small bowel may appear circular, elliptic, or tubular in cross section. Pathologic processes adjacent to the bowel can sometimes be difficult to distinguish from the normal bowel in the absence of positive enteral contrast, because they may have a similar appearance. For example, an abscess cavity adjacent to the bowel could have a similar appearance, with a circular cross section filled with dark gray fluid (pus) and air (black). Therefore one potentially important role of positive oral contrast agents is to identify the bowel, allowing structures that fail to fill with oral contrast to be identified as nonbowel structures.

A second potential role of positive enteral contrast is to identify a point of **obstruction** of the bowel. Conceptually, if the bowel is obstructed at a single point, orally administered contrast (or contrast given by nasogastric or orogastric tube) should fill the bowel to the point of obstruction but pass no farther; therefore oral contrast might be valuable in identifying not only the presence of an obstruction but also the exact location of the obstruction. In reality, oral contrast appears to be unnecessary in most cases of obstruction, as described in more detail later in this chapter in the section titled "Oral Contrast Agents and Computed Tomography of Suspected Small-Bowel Obstruction." The reason is simple: the bowel almost always contains some intrinsic neutral contrast composed of a slurry of swallowed saliva, partially digested food, and GI secretions. If the bowel is obstructed, it will appear distended, with this neutral contrast proximal to the point of obstruction. Distal to the point of obstruction, intestinal peristalsis will move this "contrast" farther along and the bowel will not appear distended.

A third potential role of positive enteral contrast is to reveal **intestinal perforation.** If enteral contrast is administered and then seen to collect in the peritoneal cavity, outside of the apparent lumen of the bowel, perforation can be diagnosed. As is the case for bowel obstruction, this theoretical advantage appears to be less useful in reality. Most intestinal perforations are likely fairly small, limiting the likelihood that enteral contrast would actually leak out of the bowel lumen. In addition, if a point of perforation is located not in a dependent loop of bowel but rather at a higher point (with the patient in the typical supine position for CT), enteral contrast may fail to leak out of bowel. Studies in the setting of blunt trauma show oral contrast to have limited or no utility in the diagnosis of bowel injury, as described in detail in Chapter 10.[5-6] Nonetheless, large perforations of bowel, or fistulas connecting the bowel lumen to other structures or cavities, might be revealed by positive enteral contrast.

Distension of bowel with enteral contrast can be important for determining the thickness of the bowel wall. **Bowel wall thickening** can suggest inflammation (as in infectious colitis or inflammatory bowel disease), ischemia (as in ischemic colitis or "shock bowel"), or a mass lesion (as in a sessile colonic polyp or small-bowel lymphoma). Without enteral contrast agents, the bowel may be relatively nondistended or even fully collapsed. In these cases, the thickness of the bowel wall can be difficult to estimate, because the wall may be folded upon itself or simply thickened because of lack of distension. Enteral contrast agents distend the bowel, helping to resolve this issue. Positive enteral contrast agents can obscure some details of the bowel wall, because

they are extremely dense relative to the bowel and can create image artifacts. Negative or neutral contrast agents may be more useful in depicting the bowel wall structure and the mucosal surface, but these agents are relatively rarely used today in emergency medicine.

Positive enteral contrast agents can obscure diagnostically important abnormalities of bowel wall enhancement with IV contrast. Bowel wall enhancement usually occurs to a limited extent in normally perfused bowel. Increased bowel wall enhancement indicates increased blood flow, which can be seen in infectious and inflammatory states, including appendicitis. Decreased enhancement can indicate hypoperfusion, for example, in a closed-loop bowel obstruction or embolic mesenteric ischemia. When positive enteral contrast is present immediately adjacent to the bowel wall, the degree of bowel wall enhancement with IV contrast can be obscured. As we discuss later in this chapter, positive enteral contrast can be relatively contraindicated for this reason when bowel wall enhancement is predicted to play an important role in the patient's diagnosis.[6a]

Positive enteral contrast agents also obscure extravasation of injected contrast agents into the bowel lumen, because both are quite dense and appear white on an soft-tissue CT window. Some new CT protocols for diagnosis of acute GI bleeding therefore do not use enteral contrast agents. We discuss these in more detail later in this chapter.

Finally, enteral contrast agents can assist in recognition of mass lesions within the bowel—though these are not usually emergency department diagnoses. When a contrast agent is used to distend the bowel and fill its lumen, mass lesions such as polyps are visible as "filling defects" within the bowel lumen. Accurate diagnosis of bowel mass lesions such as polyps requires a cleansing bowel prep to remove stool, which could otherwise have a similar appearance. Some protocols for CT colonography take an additional step, with the patient ingesting a contrast agent to "tag" stool with positive contrast, allowing any residual stool to be recognized. Usually such protocols use carbon dioxide gas as the negative enteral contrast agent to distend the bowel. Gases including atmospheric air and carbon dioxide appear black on CT, providing outstanding contrast against soft tissues. Carbon dioxide is often used, because it is rapidly reabsorbed from the gut lumen and exhaled, limiting discomfort from intestinal distension.

Rectally administered enteral contrast is rarely used for CT in the emergency department, but it has some putative benefits. The same potential advantages of enteral contrast agents described earlier apply to rectal contrast. Rectal administration of contrast can allow rapid opacification of the distal bowel without waiting for the transit of orally administered contrast, which can take hours, depending on factors such as the speed of intestinal peristalsis and the presence of ileus. Some protocols use rectal contrast for detection of appendicitis or diverticulitis for this reason. In cases of penetrating torso trauma, rectal contrast has been advocated by some radiologists to assist in detection of colonic perforation, because leaking contrast into the pelvis, peritoneum, or retroperitoneum might thus be seen. Rectal contrast could be useful in detection of perirectal or sigmoid abscesses by differentiating the bowel lumen from an adjacent fluid- and gas-filled abscess. Whether rectal contrast is necessary in these cases is discussed in more detail for individual conditions later in this chapter. Rectal contrast is usually administered as a retention enema of 400-800 mL of Gastrografin (3% meglumine diatrizoate–saline solution) through a rectal tube. The contrast is infused under gravity pressure only from a height of 3 feet over 2-4 minutes.[7]

Urinary Contrast Agents. Urinary contrast agents can be instilled into the bladder through a catheter for detection of bladder rupture or mass lesions, as discussed in Chapter 12.

Weight and Size Limits of CT Scanners

Obese patients may be unable to undergo CT scan because of physical constraints of equipment. Three factors can limit CT. First, the table upon which the patient is positioned typically has a weight limit of 450 to 650 pounds (200-295 kg). Second, the CT gantry (the circular opening through which the patient must pass for imaging) is typically 70 cm in diameter, though some manufacturers offer 90-cm models for obese patients. Patients with an abdominal or chest diameter extending this size cannot undergo torso CT.[8] Third, increasing patient size requires increased x-ray energy to penetrate the patient. Occasionally, problems with excessive heating of the x-ray tube may be encountered. Medical mythology suggests that obese patients can be transferred to the local veterinary hospital or zoo for CT imaging. This is not true for several reasons. CT scanners are not manufactured for animal imaging; most zoo and veterinary scanners are human CT scanners modified for veterinary use. Consequently, the gantry size remains a limiting factor, as described earlier. However, some veterinary scanners do have modified tables with higher weight capacities, allowing imaging of equine limbs.[9] Most animal facilities are not licensed for imaging of human patients.[9]

Contrast Injection Rate and Venous Catheter Size. The rate of contrast injection is important in vascular applications of abdominal CT. For CT angiography (CTA), rates of 4 to 5 mL per second are desirable to achieve sufficient opacification of vascular structures and thus allow recognition of filling defects, intimal flaps, and stenotic regions. Standard angiocatheters of a 14- to 20-gauge size are capable of achieving flow rates of 5 mL per second with power injectors using a pressure

limit of 325 psi. Catheters that are 22 gauge and smaller do not reach the desired flow rate before exceeding the safe pressure limit and are therefore not adequate for CTA.[10] Flow rates through catheters are inversely proportional to the catheter length and directly proportional to the radius raised to the fourth power, so a short, large-bore catheter is desirable for CTA. For nonangiographic applications, contrast flow rates are less important, and smaller catheters may be sufficient.

Contrast Controversies

We discussed in general terms the potential value of contrast agents in CT. Given the hypothetical advantages of IV and enteral contrast, why would we not administer these agents to all patients before abdominal CT? As we review here, vascular contrast agents have dangers of contrast reaction and nephrotoxicity. Enteral contrast agents are rarely associated with contrast reaction but result in diagnostic delays that can be significant to the individual patient and are problematic for efficient emergency department flow. Increasing evidence suggests that contrast agents may be unnecessary for many diagnoses, as we discuss in the sections on specific pathology.

Reactions to Iodinated Vascular Contrast. Contrast reactions are sometimes called contrast allergies, although the specific mechanism of these reactions is thought to be anaphylactoid, not mediated through true allergy. Nonetheless, from a practical clinical standpoint, they have effects much like those of true allergies and are treated similarly.

Incidence and Severity of Contrast Reactions. The incidence of contrast reactions with modern, low-osmolality, nonionic, contrast agents is very low, with mild reactions (e.g., urticaria or itching) occurring in about 3% to 15% of exposures. More severe reactions such as hypotension or respiratory distress occur in only about 0.04% to 0.004% of exposures. Fatalities are extremely rare (about 1 in 170,000 exposures). Older ionic and high-osmolality agents were more dangerous, with more frequent severe reactions, but are infrequently used today.[11-12]

Predicting Contrast Reactions: Risk Factors. Reactions to iodinated contrast agents are likely not caused by actual allergy to iodine. Elemental iodine is essential to human life, and allergy to iodine is unlikely. Similarly, seafood allergy is probably not related to iodine allergy and is instead thought to be mediated through protein allergens found in seafood. However, patients with severe prior allergic reactions to any allergen (including peanuts and hymenoptera sting) have an increased risk for contrast reaction. Patients with severe asthma also have an increased risk for contrast reaction. When possible, iodinated injected contrast should be avoided in these patients. Enteral contrast agents are minimally absorbed from the GI tract, and allergy to these agents is thought to be rare. Although enteral contrast agents can likely be used safely in patients with significant allergies to intravenous contrast, if concern exists about possible reaction to iodinated material, barium sulfate contrast agents can be used instead of iodinated contrast, eliminating the concern for a contrast reaction.[12]

Preventing Contrast Reactions: Choice of Contrast Agent and Premedication. When contrast reaction is a concern, because of either prior reaction to a contrast agent or severe allergy to another allergen, contrast should be avoided if possible. If the diagnosis requires injected contrast administration and cannot reasonably be made using noncontrast CT or another imaging modality, such as ultrasound or magnetic resonance imaging (MRI), an attempt at prophylaxis can be made using one of several published medication protocols (reviewed in Box 7-5).

The severity of a contrast reaction cannot be predicted based on prior reactions. Some patients with prior mild reactions progress to life-threatening reactions on reexposure.[12]

Treating Contrast Reactions. Contrast reactions should be treated like true allergic reactions. Administration of the contrast agent should be discontinued immediately. Treatment of allergic reactions is beyond the scope of this text, but epinephrine should be given for severe reactions, and IV fluid resuscitation, airway management, corticosteroids, and antihistamines should be used as for other allergic reactions.

Contrast Nephropathy. Contrast nephropathy is a serious potential consequence of exposure to iodinated vascular contrast. It is a leading cause of in-hospital renal failure, occurring in 150,000 cases per year in the United States. Contrast nephropathy is defined by a 25% increase in baseline creatinine or an absolute increase of 0.5 mg/dL within 48 hours after the administration of iodinated contrast. Less than 1% of patients experiencing contrast nephropathy require dialysis.[13] Contrast nephropathy is discussed in detail in Chapter 7.

Predicting Contrast Nephropathy. Patients with poor glomerular filtration rates (creatinine clearance) below 60 mL per minute are at increased risk for developing contrast nephropathy. The creatinine clearance, not the measured serum creatinine, is a better measure of risk for contrast nephropathy. Creatinine clearance is easily calculated with standard formulas or with online clinical calculators. Creatinine clearance depends on multiple factors, in addition to measured serum creatinine, including age, gender, race, and mass (particularly lean muscle mass, the source of creatinine).[12] In one study, use of the measured serum creatinine as a screen for risk for contrast nephropathy would have missed a significant proportion of at-risk patients: 55% with a creatinine cutoff

of 1.8 mg/dL, 40% with a creatinine cutoff of less than 1.5 mg/dL (the most commonly accepted cutoff for contrast administration), 19% with a threshold of 1.2 mg/dL, and 9% with a creatinine cutoff of 1.0 mg/dL.[14]

Other factors predicting risk for contrast nephropathy include diabetes, hypertension, congestive heart failure, diuretic use, and age older than 70 years. The American College of Radiology (ACR) recommends measuring serum creatinine before intravascular administration of iodinated contrast for the indications listed in Box 9-2.

Patients taking metformin are at risk for lactic acidosis following administration of vascular contrast, though this condition is extremely rare in patients with normal renal function. The risk is mediated through worsened renal clearance of metformin. Patients should be advised to discontinue metformin use for 48 hours after contrast administration. Patients with normal renal function can resume metformin use without having their creatinine rechecked. Patients with known renal dysfunction should be treated more cautiously, with creatinine being reassessed before resuming metformin use.[12]

Box 9-2: American College of Radiology Suggested Indications for Serum Creatinine Measurement Before Intravascular Administration of Iodinated Contrast Media[12]

- History of "kidney disease" as an adult, including tumor and transplant
- Family history of kidney failure
- Diabetes treated with insulin or other medications prescribed by a licensed physician
- Paraproteinemia syndromes or diseases (e.g., multiple myeloma
- Collagen vascular disease (e.g., scleroderma, systemic lupus erythematosa)
- Prior renal surgery
- Certain medications:
  ○ Metformin or metformin-containing drug combinations
  ○ Chronic or high dose use of non-steroidal anti-inflammatory drugs
  ○ Regular use of nephrotoxic medications, such as aminoglycosides
  ○ All inpatients

From American College of Radiology: ACR Manual on Contrast Media, version 7. 2010. Available at: http://www.acr.org/ SecondaryMainMenuCategories/quality_safety/contrast_ manual/FullManual.aspx.
Reprinted with permission of the American College of Radiology, Reston, VA. No other representation of this material is authorized without expressed, written permission from the American College of Radiology. Refer to the ACR website at www.acr. org/ac for the most current and complete version of the ACR Appropriateness Criteria®

Preventing Contrast Nephropathy. In patients with elevated risk for contrast nephropathy, iodinated vascular contrast should be avoided whenever possible. In some cases, the diagnosis can be made using CT without vascular contrast or other modalities, such as ultrasound or MRI. MRI with gadolinium contrast has its own risks in patients with poor renal function, as detailed in Chapter 15. When the severity and acuity of the suspected diagnosis demand IV contrast despite its risks, measures can be taken to mitigate the risk for contrast nephropathy. IV hydration with sodium chloride has been well studied and reduces the risk.[15-17] The ACR recommends administering normal saline at 100 mL per hour for 6 to 12 hours before and 4 to 12 hours after IV contrast administration.[12] Pretreatment and posttreatment of this duration are not feasible for most emergency department patients; however, efforts should be made to hydrate the patient before and after CT using saline boluses. Saline boluses have been shown to be equivalent to sustained overnight saline infusions when the outcome considered is change in creatinine at 24 and 48 hours, though a higher rate of transient creatinine increase is seen with boluses.[16] An initial study of sodium bicarbonate administration appeared promising,[18] but a methodologically strong randomized controlled trial showed no benefit of sodium bicarbonate compared with saline hydration.[19] Trials of *N*-acetylcysteine (NAC) have shown a small reduction in the degree of temporary creatinine elevation experienced by patients, although no trials have shown improvements in important patient outcomes such as permanent renal injury, progression to dialysis, or death. Most studies of NAC are in the setting of outpatient cardiac catheterization and allow 24 hours of oral pretreatment, which is not possible in the emergency department.[12,20] A single trial compared saline prehydration (12 hours pre contrast and postcontrast) with IV NAC (150 mg/kg in 500 mL of normal saline) 30 minutes before contrast administration and 50 mg/kg in 500 mL of normal saline for an additional 4 hours after contrast. This showed a reduction in serum creatinine but no difference in patient-oriented outcomes.[21] Prophylactic measures to prevent contrast nephropathy are summarized in Chapter 7, Box 7-7.

The risk for contrast nephropathy is related to the type of contrast agent used; low-osmolality, nonionic contrast poses a lower risk than high-osmolality, ionic contrast. The risk is also dose-related. Therefore discussion with the radiologist about measures to reduce the contrast dose should be considered. One such method, the saline-chaser method, reduces the contrast dose from 150 to around 75 or 100 mL while maintaining enhancement quality.[22-24]

Dialysis Patients and Iodinated Intravenous Contrast.
Iodinated IV contrast agents are safe in patients receiving long-term hemodialysis for renal failure.

Because these patients already have severe and irreversible renal dysfunction, contrast agents do not pose any additional risk for contrast nephropathy. In addition, the volume of contrast given is usually no more than 120-150 mL and does not generally pose a threat of vascular volume overload and pulmonary edema. Patients should be dialyzed as usual but do not require emergency dialysis following iodinated contrast administration.[12] This should not be confused with the situation for gadolinium contrast agents used for MRI. As discussed in Chapter 15 these agents pose a small but potentially life-threatening risk in patients with end-stage renal disease, including dialysis patients. Gadolinium should be avoided in these patients whenever possible, and dialysis should be performed as soon as possible after any administration of gadolinium.

Intravenous Contrast in Pregnancy. Intravascular iodinated and gadolinium contrast crosses the placenta, is excreted into the urine, enters the amniotic fluid, and is subsequently swallowed by the fetus. A small amount may then be reabsorbed from the fetal intestine and recycled throughout the duration of pregnancy. Animal studies have shown no mutagenic or teratogenic effects, but studies in pregnant women are lacking. The ACR recommends that these contrast agents be avoided when possible during pregnancy and that informed consent from the mother be obtained.[12] A small study found no effect on neonatal thyroid function of in utero exposure to nonionic iodinated vascular contrast for CT.[25]

Other Contraindications to Intravenous Iodinated Contrast. A number of other potential contraindications to intravascular iodinated contrast have been reported, though the evidence supporting these is limited. Intravascular iodinated contrast can exacerbate thyrotoxicosis and may decrease uptake of radioactive iodine used to ablate abnormal thyroid tissue (including carcinomas) by up to 50% 1 week after contrast administration. Increased serum catecholamine levels can occur in patients with pheochromocytoma receiving high-osmolality contrast but not after receiving nonionic contrast. Sickle cell anemia is believed to increase the risk for acute contrast reactions.[12] The ACR *Manual on Contrast Media* is freely available online and provides summarized guidelines, including contraindications to contrast administration.

Can Administration of Intravenous Contrast Disguise Pathology?

Administration of IV contrast can make recognition of high-density calcified structures more difficult or impossible, because calcium and iodinated contrast have identical CT appearances, with Hounsfield densities in the several hundreds. Some medical centers routinely perform noncontrast CT first, before CT with

IV contrast, to allow recognition of preexisting calcifications. Unfortunately, this doubles the radiation exposure for the patient, which may not be justified by the additional information gained in most cases. In the emergency department, a frequent concern on the differential diagnosis is urolithiasis, a diagnosis for which IV contrast is not required. If other concerns such as appendicitis or abscess exist and the decision is made to administer IV contrast for these indications, recognition of isolated ureteral calcifications may be impaired. Depending on the timing of the CT scan (as discussed earlier), IV contrast may be excreted into the ureters and hide small nonobstructing ureteral stones. However, diagnostic findings of hydroureter and hydronephrosis will remain visible. In the event of a large obstructing renal stone, typically contrast will not be excreted into the affected ureter, so the stone will remain visible. CT for urolithiasis is discussed in more detail in Chapter 12.

Dual-Energy Computed Tomography.

A new CT technique called dual-energy or spectral CT may eliminate some of these issues of obscuration of native tissues by exogenous contrast agents of similar density. In dual-energy CT, two x-ray tubes are used to scan the patient simultaneously, using two distinct x-ray voltages and x-ray tube currents. The combination of absorption spectra of a material at different energy levels of incident radiation gives the material a unique signature, allowing differentiation of two materials of similar density that may appear identical with conventional CT. This process could allow digital subtraction of iodinated contrast from an image, revealing calcifications having a different absorption spectrum. Bone structures can also be digitally removed, improving CTA. Although dual-energy scanners are commercially available, research into their applications is limited and they have not yet entered wide clinical use.[26]

Controversies Around Oral Contrast.

Oral contrast use for abdominal CT is a topic of significant controversy. Garra et al.[27] noted that the median interval required to consume 2 L of oral contrast was more than 100 minutes, with no significant difference between patients randomized to receive a prophylactic antiemetic and those receiving placebo. Consequently, oral contrast use can substantially increase the length of stay of an emergency department patient. For that individual, oral contrast use may lead to a delay in diagnosis, which could be clinically important for conditions such as appendicitis or, more critically, for vascular pathology such as abdominal aortic aneurysm or mesenteric ischemia. In addition to causing potential harm for the patient receiving contrast, the delay associated with oral contrast use may delay the care of other patients waiting to be seen, a critical issue in crowded modern U.S. emergency departments. The risks for these delays must be weighed against the potential benefit of increased

diagnostic accuracy that might result from oral contrast use. Numerous studies have attempted to determine the effect of oral contrast on diagnostic accuracy of CT for a range of conditions. We summarize these studies here, exploring them in more detail in individual sections on specific pathology.

Multiple studies suggest that CT without oral contrast is highly sensitive and specific for important emergency department diagnoses, including appendicitis, diverticulitis, pancreatitis, small-bowel obstruction, pneumoperitoneum, mesenteric ischemia, abdominal aortic aneurysm and dissection, and blunt abdominal injuries.[5-6,28-34]

What Other Risks Might Enteral Contrast Pose, and Do These Constitute Sufficient Grounds to Eliminate Enteral Contrast From Emergency Abdominal CT Protocols?

Some investigators have conjectured about the risk for **aspiration** of oral contrast in settings such as abdominal trauma. However, low-osmolality, water-soluble, iodinated contrast agents are completely absorbed from the lung and cause little morbidity.[12] Others have raised concerns about peritoneal irritation from enteral contrast in the event of bowel perforation. However, unlike barium sulfate solutions, low-osmolality, iodinated oral contrast agents such as Gastrografin induce little peritoneal reaction, and extraluminal leak of contrast appears rare, even when bowel perforation is present. Most likely, the greatest risk for enteral contrast agents is diagnostic delay resulting from the time required for contrast to be ingested or instilled and then allowed to migrate through the bowel before CT is performed. Although enteral contrast is likely unnecessary for many emergency diagnoses, it may increase sensitivity in some conditions. Approximately 35% of abdominal CT scans in the United States are performed with iodinated enteral contrast.[12]

In the end, the emergency physician must consider the risk and potential benefit of oral contrast case by case. Factors to be weighed include the specific differential diagnosis under consideration, the degree of illness of the individual patient, the time sensitivity of the suspected diagnoses, and the risk for repeated radiation exposure in the individual patient if CT without oral contrast is nondiagnostic and a repeated CT must be performed. If the differential diagnosis is solely conditions for which CT without oral contrast has been shown to be sensitive and specific, oral contrast likely should be omitted. In patients with concerning vital signs or clinical status, delay for oral contrast is most often not warranted. Even in patients with relatively reassuring vital signs and clinical appearance, if the suspected diagnosis is highly time-sensitive, such as mesenteric ischemia or leaking abdominal aortic aneurysm, delay for oral contrast should be avoided. Oral contrast may be reasonable in stable patients with relatively time-insensitive diagnostic concerns (e.g., diverticulitis, inflammatory bowel disease, or abscess) for which oral contrast is thought to have some diagnostic benefit. In young patients, repeated radiation exposures are a particular concern (as described elsewhere in this chapter and others), and it may be reasonable in a stable young patient to administer oral contrast to reduce the likelihood that the initial CT will be nondiagnostic. As discussed earlier in our overview of contrast agents, patients with little peritoneal fat can be difficult to diagnosis by CT because of the absence of fat stranding and intrinsic contrast provided by fat. If such a patient is stable and the differential diagnosis is less time-critical, administration of oral contrast may be wise.

Radiation Exposure From Abdominal and Pelvic Computed Tomography.

CT provides a relatively large ionizing radiation exposure, leading to growing controversy about its wide and repeated use, particularly in young patients. Radiation risks for CT are discussed later in this chapter in the sections titled *"Appendicitis Imaging in the Pediatric Patient"* and *"Imaging the Pregnant Patient With Possible Appendicitis."* Radiation risks are also discussed in Chapters 7 and 8.

Systematic Interpretation of Abdominal Computed Tomography

In the final section of this chapter, we discuss the CT findings of specific disease states in detail. Here, let's review two approaches to interpretation of abdominal CT scan. Many approaches are reasonable, as long as all key structures are reviewed. We first describe a systematic approach to interpretation, which we call the **focused abdominal computed tomography (FACT)** approach, and then discuss a more limited interpretation, in which the CT is only inspected for a few highly suspected diagnoses.

Focused Abdominal Computed Tomography Interpretation.

Although emergency medicine is already overflowing with abbreviations, we introduce one more here to emphasize a similarity to the **focused assessment with sonography in trauma (FAST)** ultrasound examination familiar to most emergency physicians. When performing a FAST examination (discussed in Chapter 10), the emergency physician looks at each of four anatomic regions in turn, answering a single yes-or-no question for each:

1. Right upper quadrant—Is free fluid present in the hepatorenal space?
2. Left upper quadrant—Is free fluid present in the splenorenal or subdiaphragmatic space?
3. Suprapubic region—Is free fluid present in the pelvis?
4. Subxiphoid region—Is fluid present in the pericardial sac?

The examination is thus brief, and the questions are clear and clinically-oriented. Although other structures may be seen in the field of view, the operator is trained to focus on a single question, avoiding distraction. The same approach can be used to interpret abdominal CT, which can otherwise baffle novices because of the number of structures and forms of pathology that can be seen. We call our focused interpretation FACT, because it follows the same principles as FAST.

Let's establish some simple rules for our discussion. First, we assume that you can only view axial images, because some centers do not yet routinely provide images in other planes. Second, we assume a familiarity with window settings and CT tissue appearances (discussed earlier), as well as with basic anatomy. Third, we assume that you are viewing the images on a digital computer workstation or picture archiving and communication system (PACS). The process is the same for reviewing printed images, although the window settings and other image characteristics cannot be modified. The axial images are conventionally displayed with the right side of the patient's body on the left side of the viewing monitor and the anterior abdomen facing the top of the screen. The viewpoint is that of an observer standing at the foot of the patient's bed, looking toward the head.

When interpreting abdominal CT using the FACT approach, you should focus your attention on one organ or structure at a time, with a single or limited number of questions for each organ. Although other structures may be visible in each axial image, you should intentionally ignore other structures to avoid distraction. Our approach requires you to make multiple passes through the stack of axial CT images, but you'll find that with practice you become extremely fast at this approach.

Our approach requires you to look through the abdominal CT images several times using three window settings: soft-tissue, lung, and bone. Most organs require inspection using the soft-tissue window, with a few exceptions deserving mention here. Free air (pneumoperitoneum) is often more readily recognized on lung window settings, because this setting leaves air or gas black while rendering all other tissues quite bright or white. On a standard soft-tissue window, fat is fairly black, and small quantities of free air may be difficult to recognize against this background. A lung window is also necessary when reviewing the cephalad axial slices for pneumothorax or pulmonary parenchymal opacity. A pneumothorax looks black on this setting, whereas the lung parenchyma is readily visible. On a soft-tissue window, both normal lung parenchyma and a pneumothorax appear black and can be indistinguishable. Perform your inspection of the chest and abdomen for free air and lung pathology using the lung window, and then switch to the soft-tissue window to complete your evaluation of other structures and pathology. A final window setting that may be more selectively used is the bone window. As the name suggests, a bone window allows detailed evaluation of bone for fracture or lytic lesions. The same images viewed with a soft-tissue window can obscure fine structural abnormalities of bone, because the bone appears bright white with "bloom artifact" obscuring cortical fractures or other abnormalities.[35] An unexpected use of a bone window includes evaluation for renal colic. Although ureteral calcifications are visible on a soft-tissue window, you may prefer to search for stones using bone window settings, which tend to render the abdomen in three primary shades: white for calcified structures, dark gray for soft tissues and fluids, and black for air. As a consequence, this window setting is also sometimes used to evaluate for free air.

To illustrate the FACT approach to interpretation, let's start with the example of evaluating the liver for traumatic injury, a topic examined in detail in Chapter 10. We won't belabor the findings of liver trauma here, because they are extensively reviewed in that chapter.

Begin your search by locating the liver, which is visible high in the abdomen, in a subdiaphragmatic position. The first several axial slices typically include chest structures above the diaphragm, but ignore these at the moment, because you are focused on a single question: Does the liver show signs of traumatic hemorrhage or contusion? The axial slices spanning the liver also show the spleen, aorta, stomach, pancreas, kidneys, and spine, but ignore these for now, concentrating on the liver. You will return to each of the other organs during your assessment. On each slice containing the liver, inspect the liver parenchyma and enhancement. Once you have passed through the caudadmost liver slice and are satisfied that you have answered your focused question, stop your evaluation and move to the next organ or disease process on your checklist. For example, in the case of nontraumatic abdominal pain, the aorta is a key organ to assess for abnormalities, particularly aortic aneurysm rupture or dissection. Because the aorta begins in the chest and continues through the pelvis after bifurcating into the iliac arteries, this inspection requires review of the entire stack of CT slices. However, the questions to be answered remain simple:
1. Is an aortic aneurysm (defined by an aortic diameter greater than 3 cm) present?
2. Is a dissection flap visible within the contrast-filled aorta?
3. Is blood or contrast visible outside of the confines of the aorta?

Again, intentionally ignore other chest, abdominal, and pelvic structures during your inspection of the aorta, which should take only seconds. The aorta normally appears as a rounded circular structure in cross section, with a fixed location, just anterior to the thoracic and lumbar spine and slightly left of the midline. Measure the aortic diameter on a single axial CT slice to develop a baseline understanding of its size, and then scroll through the digital stack of images from cephalad to caudad. Don't evaluate major aortic branches at this stage, though as you become more adept you may choose to incorporate their evaluation here.

This process is repeated for each of the major abdominal, pelvic, and retroperitoneal organs, as well as visible structures of the chest. A systematic approach requires that all structures be evaluated in this manner (Table 9-3). However, emergency physicians may elect to use a limited CT interpretation approach.

Limited Interpretation of Computed Tomography. Although a systematic approach minimizes the likelihood of missing pathology, in some cases the differential diagnosis is appropriately quite narrow and a more narrowly focused interpretation approach may be reasonable. A 23-year-old male with nontraumatic right lower quadrant tenderness likely has appendicitis, terminal ileitis, a ureteral stone, hernia, or testicular pathology. Abdominal aortic aneurysm and splenic rupture may be far from the differential, and it may be appropriate for the emergency physician to answer only a subset of the imaging questions for this patient, just as a focused history and physical examination may be appropriate. The radiologist bears a heavier burden, with responsibility for identifying even incidental findings of potential significance on the images. As an emergency physician, if you perform a limited initial interpretation of the CT, be sure that some system is in place for a more comprehensive interpretation by a radiologist and for any findings to be communicated to you and your patient.

Ultrasound

Ultrasound is a commonly-used and valuable diagnostic modality in emergency medicine. Advantages of ultrasound include portability and lack of ionizing radiation. The latter means that it can be safely used in pregnancy, can be used without concern in children, and can be repeated as necessary to assess for changes in the patient's condition. In this section, we briefly review some basic principles of ultrasound physics as they relate to the clinical utility of ultrasound. We then discuss common emergency department applications of ultrasound and review basic ultrasound terminology, which we use throughout the rest of the chapter. We review the ultrasound findings of specific abdominal pathology at the end of this chapter, along with diagnostic findings for these conditions using other imaging modalities. Applications of ultrasound in blunt abdominal trauma are discussed in Chapter 10. Vascular applications of ultrasound are discussed in more detail in

TABLE 9-3. Focused Abdominal Computed Tomography (FACT): An Approach to Computed Tomography Interpretation for the Emergency Physician*

Organ or Disease Process	Clinically Oriented Imaging Questions
Abdominal aortic aneurysm or dissection	• Is an aortic aneurysm present? • Is a dissection flap visible? • Is blood or contrast visible outside of the aorta? (See Chapter 11.)
Abscess	• Is fat stranding visible in the area of interest or tenderness? • Is a structure containing air and fluid visible that is not bowel? • Does the rim of the structure enhance with IV contrast?
Appendicitis	• Is fat stranding present in the right lower quadrant? • Is free fluid present in the right lower quadrant? • Is the appendix greater than 6 mm in diameter? • Is the appendiceal wall thickened? • Does the appendiceal wall enhance abnormally?
Ascending cholangitis	• Is evidence of biliary obstruction present? (See biliary obstruction in this table.) • Is evidence of cholecystitis present? (See cholecystitis in this table.) • Is air visible in a branching pattern within the liver?

Ascites	• Is free fluid present?
	  • If yes, how much?
	  • Is it diffuse or localized?
	  • What is the density in Hounsfield units?

Biliary obstruction	• Are the intra- and extrahepatic biliary ducts dilated? • Are gallstones present? • Is a pancreatic or hepatic mass present?
Blunt abdominal trauma	• Is blunt hepatic injury present? (See "Liver mass lesion or trauma" in this table.) • Is blunt splenic injury present? (See "Splenic mass lesion or trauma" in this table) • Is active hemorrhage present? • Is free fluid present (See Chapter 10.)
Bones	• Are fractures or lytic lesions present? (Review bone windows)
Chest findings	• Is a pneumothorax present? (lung windows) • Is a pulmonary parenchymal opacity present, suggesting pneumonia? (lung windows) • Are rib fractures present? (bone windows) • Is the aorta normal? (soft-tissue windows)
Cholecystitis	• Is the gallbladder wall thickened? • Is pericholecystic fluid present? • Is fat stranding present in the surrounding region? • Is abnormal enhancement of the gallbladder present? • Are gallstones present? • Are signs of biliary obstruction present? (See biliary obstruction in this table.)
Colitis	• Is the colon wall thickened? • Is fat stranding visible? • Is the region of abnormality diffuse or restricted to a segment of colon, suggesting a possible vascular etiology? • Are findings of diverticulitis present? (See diverticulitis in this table.)
Diverticulitis	• Is fat stranding visible along the course of the colon (ascending, transverse, descending, or sigmoid)? • Is the colon wall thickened? • Are diverticuli present? • Is an abscess present adjacent to the colon? (See abscess in this table.)
Inflammatory bowel disease	• Are segments of small, large, or both bowels thick-walled? • Is surrounding fat stranding present? • Is an adjacent abscess or fistula present? (See abscess in this table.) • Is a large vessel vascular occlusion present, suggesting an ischemic cause rather than inflammation?
Liver mass lesion or trauma	After administration of IV contrast: • Are areas of nonenhancing parenchyma seen, representing contusion or laceration? • Is active extravasation of contrast visible, indicating active hemorrhage (See Chapter 10.)

Continued

TABLE 9-3. Focused Abdominal Computed Tomography (FACT): An Approach to Computed Tomography Interpretation for the Emergency Physician*—cont'd

Organ or Disease Process	Clinically Oriented Imaging Questions
Mesenteric ischemia	• Are segments of small, large, or both bowels thick-walled? • Is surrounding fat stranding present? • Is an adjacent abscess or fistula present? (See abscess in this table.) • Is a large vessel vascular occlusion present, suggesting an ischemic cause rather than inflammation? • Is an aortic dissection present, possibly leading to bowel ischemia? • Are the celiac artery, SMA, inferior mesenteric artery, and portal vein patent? (see Chapter 11.)
Pancreatitis	• Is fat stranding or fluid visible around the pancreas? • Is a pseudocyst visible within the body of the pancreas? • If IV contrast was given, do areas of the pancreas fail to enhance, suggesting necrosis?
Penetrating abdominal trauma	• Is free fluid present? (See ascites in this table.) • Is free air present? (Review lung windows) • Is active vascular contrast extravasation present, indicating active hemorrhage? • Is enteral contrast extravasation present, indicating bowel perforation? • Is the projectile trajectory visible because of soft-tissue changes, and does it pass close to bowel? (See Chapter 10.)
Pneumoperitoneum (free air)	Use lung windows. • Is air visible outside of the apparent lumen of bowel? • Is air visible in the perihepatic subdiaphragmatic space, the left subdiaphragmatic space, or the anterior midline abdomen? • Are smaller, localized air collections visible that may be trapped by other abdominal structures?
Pyelonephritis	• Is perinephric fat stranding visible? • Is a perinephric fluid collection visible, suggesting abscess? • Does any fluid collection enhance peripherally, suggesting abscess? • Are signs of obstruction present, including hydronephrosis, hydroureter, or failure of contrast to be excreted into the ureter? (See Chapter 12.)
Renal colic	Use soft-tissue or bone windows. • Is a calcified stone visible within the apparent lumen of the ureter, anterior to the psoas muscle? • If a stone is present, what is its maximum diameter? • Proximal to any stone, is the ureter dilated relative to the contralateral side (7 mm is the upper limit of normal)? • Is hydronephrosis present? • Is free fluid present, suggesting urine leak? • Is perinephric stranding present? (See Chapter 12.)
Renal infarct	After administration of IV contrast: • Are wedge-shaped areas of nonenhancing parenchyma seen, representing infarct?
Small-bowel obstruction	• Is the small bowel dilated beyond 3 cm? • Is a transition point visible? • Is abnormal bowel enhancement or wall thickening present? • Is a closed-loop obstruction present?
Splenic mass lesion or trauma	After administration of IV contrast: • Are areas of nonenhancing parenchyma seen, representing contusion or laceration? • Is active extravasation of contrast visible, indicating active hemorrhage? (See Chapter 10.)
SMA thrombosis	See mesenteric ischemia in this table. Follow the SMA from its origin at the aorta distally. • Is there a filling defect, indicating occlusion? (See Chapter 11.)

*In FACT interpretation, the emergency physician concentrates on answering a single clinical question at a time, rather than attempting to interpret all structures in each image simultaneously. Several "passes" through the abdomen may be required to review all important structures and answer all important clinical questions. For each organ, disease, or injury focus your attention just on that organ while answering the clinical questions. Unless otherwise stated, soft-tissue is the appropriate window setting.

Chapter 11. Genitourinary applications of ultrasound are reviewed in Chapter 12. Many excellent dedicated books on bedside ultrasound techniques exist; we do not extensively review these in this text.

Ultrasound Physics

Ultrasound imaging relies on simple physics of sound transmission. An ultrasound probe (also called a transducer) contains **piezoelectric** crystals. These materials physically vibrate when subjected to an electric current, producing high-frequency sound waves. This supplies the ultrasound signal into the patient. These crystals also produce an electric current when subjected to the physical vibration from sound waves returning from body tissues, providing a signal that can be analyzed using complex computer algorithms to produce the ultrasound image. Various body tissues transmit, reflect, and absorb sound waves differently, allowing the returning sound waves and the electric current from the piezoelectric crystals to be interpreted. Ultrasound, like CT, is a **cross-sectional imaging technique.** The fan-like signal of ultrasound projecting from the ultrasound probe acts like a sonographic scalpel to provide image data in the plane in which the sound intersects the body.

Using ultrasound, a tissue that produces no echoes (reflected sound waves) produces no signal to the ultrasound probe, thus appears black, and is termed **anechoic.** A region that reflects sound waves extensively produces a strong returning signal to the ultrasound probe, appears white, and is termed **hyperechoic.** A region that reflects some sound while absorbing or transmitting a portion of the incident signal results in an intermediate signal returning to the ultrasound probe. These regions appear as an intermediate brightness or gray shade on the ultrasound image and are usually described as **hypoechoic**— although the terms *hyper-* and *hypo-* are relative terms used to compare one tissue to another in context.

Fluids are excellent transmitters of sound, because they propagate the physical sound wave with little attenuation or reflection. Solid abdominal organs also transmit sound relatively well because of their high water content, although significant internal reflection and attenuation of the sound wave occur. Dense materials such as bone reflect and absorb sound waves and prevent through transmission. Consequently, ultrasound cannot provide images deep to these structures. Air or gas is also a poor sound transmission medium, because sound waves are randomly scattered and reflected.

The ultrasound appearance of a tissue mirrors its physical properties. Simple fluids (urine, ascites, blood, and liquid bile) transmit sound without reflection or attenuation and therefore appear black (hypoechoic). Solid organs (the liver and spleen) transmit sound but also reflect and absorb a moderate amount of the signal,

appearing an intermediate gray. Dense bone reflects sound strongly and prevents through transmission. Therefore the cortex of bone appears as a bright white (hyperechoic) line or curve. Because no sound is transmitted beyond bone, the bone casts a dark acoustic shadow, just as a substance that is opaque to light casts a visual shadow. Acoustic shadows are seen with other physically dense materials that reflect sound and prevent its through transmission. These include gallstones and ureteral or kidney stones; thus acoustic shadowing has diagnostic importance, as discussed later in this chapter. Air scatters and reflects the sound wave, producing a bright returning signal and preventing visualization of deeper structures. This property can be used to diagnose abnormal gas, such as gas in subcutaneous tissues or the perihepatic space, where gas and its characteristic ultrasound appearance are not normally found. However, normal bowel gas also limits visualization of many deep abdominal organs. Ultrasound would be an even more powerful diagnostic tool if the abdomen contained no gas, because then excellent visualization of deep abdominal structures could be uniformly obtained.

The Doppler effect can also be used diagnostically in ultrasound. You may recall from physics that the Doppler effect describes the shifting frequency of sound waves as their source moves relative to an observer. Consider the example of a train whistle as a train first approaches you, passes, and then recedes into the distance. As the sound source approaches, the sound becomes higher in pitch (increases in frequency). As the train recedes into the distance, the pitch becomes lower (frequency decreases). The same effect is observed as ultrasound waves encounter flowing blood within a blood vessel. Blood flowing toward the ultrasound probe increases the frequency of the reflected sound, whereas blood flowing away decreases the frequency. This is represented visually on an ultrasound image as brighter and darker hues of red and blue. An important problem in diagnostic imaging is lack of standardization of the color scheme used to depict flow. Most ultrasound machines use color (blue or red) to denote the direction of flow relative to the ultrasound probe, not arterial or venous flow as would follow from a common and intuitive assumption, because many medical images depict arteries in red and veins in blue. In other fields of physics, such as astronomy, in which the Doppler effect is encountered, blue is usually assigned to shorter wavelengths, whereas red is assigned to longer wavelengths. However, in most medical applications of Doppler ultrasound, red denotes blood approaching the ultrasound probe and blue indicates blood flowing away from the probe—directly contradicting the wavelength and frequency properties of the Doppler signatures.

The speed of flow is depicted by the brightness of the hue; bright indicates faster flow, whereas dark hues by convention indicate slower flow. Many medical instruments actually measure the phase shift (time of arrival of the sound wave), rather than the frequency shift (Doppler shift), but with similar diagnostic effect. The term *Doppler* is widely applied to machines using this technique, though this is technically incorrect.

Based on these principles, common emergency department applications of ultrasound can be predicted. Ultrasound is excellent in depicting fluid-filled structures, solid organs, and vascular structures with directional blood flow. It cannot depict structures that lie deep to gas or bone. The bowel can sometimes be seen in great detail when it is pathologic and fluid-filled, as may be the case in bowel obstruction. However, air in normal or diseased bowel makes visualization of deeper structures impossible.

Common emergency department applications of ultrasound include the following:

- Blunt solid-organ trauma and hemoperitoneum (discussed in detail in Chapter 10)
- Gallbladder or biliary ductal pathology
- Renal disorders, hydronephrosis, or renal stones (discussed in detail in Chapter 12)
- Female pelvic pathology, including ectopic pregnancy, ovarian torsion, tuboovarian abscess, and ovarian cysts (Chapter 12)
- Bedside evaluation of abdominal aortic aneurysm (Chapter 11)
- Ascites
- Testicular torsion or epididymitis (Chapter 12)

Basic Ultrasound Modes and Image Interpretation

Two basic ultrasound modes are commonly used in emergency medicine today: brightness (B) mode and motion (M) mode. The commonly used two-dimensional planar grayscale images of ultrasound are B mode images—pixels in the image vary in brightness according to the reflectivity of the body tissue. M mode ultrasound images display a graph of the motion of tissues toward or away from the ultrasound probe along a line drawn through a point in a B mode image. The y-axis represents motion toward or away from the ultrasound probe, and the x-axis represents time. Pulsatile structures move cyclically toward and away from the ultrasound probe over time, generating a patterned sine wave on the M mode image. M mode is used in measurement of fetal heart rate, as described in detail in Chapter 12. B mode images are used to assess anatomic structures for nearly all other abdominal applications. Three-dimensional ultrasound is not routinely used in emergency medicine applications today, although it has become popular among patients for obstetric imaging.

Ultrasound Artifacts

Several image artifacts deserve mention here, because we encounter them later in the chapter. **Acoustic enhancement** is an artifact seen deep to fluid-filled structures, and it results in an artificially hyperechoic (bright) appearance of these structures, one that does not represent their true acoustic reflectivity. What is the source of this artifact? The computer algorithm that generates the ultrasound image "expects" idealized, uniform solid tissue (imagine a spherical hot dog or ball of dough). Such a tissue would result in a gradual linear decrease in the returning sound signal to the probe, caused by partial absorption of the sound beam proportional to increasing tissue depth. If the image were not corrected for this effect, the brightness of tissues would gradually decrease with increasing depth, even if their actual density and reflectivity were the same. The software algorithm is programmed to correct for this anticipated loss of signal by boosting the returning ultrasound signal proportionally with increasing depth of penetration. In the case of fluid-filled structures, the sound beam is attenuated to a lesser-than-expected degree, and the software correction therefore overcorrects relative to the actual degree of sound attenuation. Tissues immediately deep to fluid-filled structures such as the gallbladder or urinary bladder therefore normally appear bright because of this artifact.[36]

Ring-down artifact or reverberation artifact is seen when strong reflectors such as air bubbles or thin metallic structures are within the ultrasound beam. The reflector resonates and reflects the sound wave, creating a bright signal at the true location of the needle or gas interface. Additional reflections appear as a series of equally spaced, bright signals deep to the true location. This artifact is seen during ultrasound-guided procedures such as vascular access and can be seen during ultrasound-guided paracentesis and abdominal ultrasound when air is encountered.[36]

Mirror artifact is a mirror-image effect that is seen at the interface of two tissues of high reflectivity. Some sound waves may be reflected multiple times within this interface before returning to the ultrasound transducer, rather than being reflected immediately. Because of this longer path of reflection, the ultrasound software interprets these echoes as originating at a greater distance from the probe. As a consequence, the echoes are converted into an image of the object at an erroneously increased depth. Mirror artifact can occur at the inferior diaphragmatic surface, where high-density liver meets low-density lung on the opposite side. A reversed image of the liver is sometimes visible cephalad to the diaphragm and should be recognized as not representing real anatomy.[36]

Ultrasound Resolution, Depth of Penetration, and Probe Selection

Ultrasound imaging relies on physics of sound. Sound waves are sinusoidal waves. Assuming a fixed wave speed (v), the wavelength (λ) and frequency (f) of sound waves are inversely proportional, defined by the equation: $\lambda = v/f$. Long wavelength means low frequency, and short wavelength means high frequency. The depth of penetration of the ultrasound beam is determined by the wavelength, with long wavelengths allowing deep penetration of tissue for imaging of deep structures. The resolution of the ultrasound image is determined by the sound frequency, with high frequency yielding high image resolution for imaging of small structures. The simplest ultrasound probes emit a single frequency (really a narrow range of frequencies), so the frequency of the ultrasound probe determines both the resolution and the depth of penetration.

When selecting a probe for abdominal imaging, this trade-off must be considered, and the best probe for the suspected differential diagnosis must be chosen (Table 9-4). A typical abdominal ultrasound probe has a frequency of ~5 MHz, a 60-mm curved contact surface, and a depth of penetration of 20 to 30 cm. For deep structures, a low-frequency probe is necessary to provide sufficient imaging depth. For small structures, a high-frequency probe is needed to provide adequate resolution. If a structure is both deep and small, one solution is to place the probe closer to the object of interest; for example, an endocavitary ultrasound probe uses a high frequency (~8 MHz) to provide high resolution but is shaped to allow insertion into the vagina for imaging of deep structures. The curved surface is only about 11 mm in width and allows scan depth up to 10 cm.

Ultrasound probes also differ in their footprint (the surface contacting the patient and the shape and configuration of the ultrasound beam emanating from the probe). Typical abdominal ultrasound probes have a broad, curved, linear array (6 cm), creating a fan-shaped beam with a wide field of view.

Many parameters can be adjusted on modern ultrasound machines, and a full discussion is beyond the scope of this text. However, we address one common parameter and associated misconception here. The **gain** of an ultrasound machine can be adjusted, altering the brightness of the ultrasound image. Increasing the ultrasound gain increases the brightness of the image; decreasing gain decreases image brightness. Gain is the equivalent of the "listening intensity" of the ultrasound machine; although it boosts the returning signal strength, it proportionally increases the noise as well. Changing gain does not increase the intensity of the sound waves entering the patient. Improving the signal-to-noise ratio

would require increasing the energy of the sound waves interrogating the body tissues, which is not controlled by gain. Although higher-energy sound waves can be used, these can result in tissue heating and are not involved in most diagnostic ultrasound.

Interpretation of Ultrasound

Ultrasound differs somewhat from x-ray and CT in that often the examination is targeted to a single organ system or region of the abdomen and pelvis, such as the right upper quadrant. Consequently, entire organs or organ systems may be absent from the field of view. The ultrasound examination must be interpreted with specific clinical information in mind, depending on the specific diagnosis in question. We review key ultrasound findings of specific disease states in the last section of this chapter.

Fluoroscopy

Fluoroscopy is relatively rarely used today for abdominal imaging in the United States. Fluoroscopy uses an x-ray beam to expose a fluorescent receptor, generating either a moving video image or still x-ray images. Because the radiation exposure depends on the total duration of the x-ray beam exposure, prolonged fluoroscopic procedures can lead to significant radiation exposures, potentially even higher than those for CT. The technique does not reveal intraabdominal structures well, unless radiopaque contrast agents are used. Images acquired before contrast administration (called masks) can be digitally subtracted from postcontrast images, allowing static radiopaque structures such as bones and instruments to be removed from the image. When vascular contrast agents are used, the result is an angiogram, useful in diagnosis and treatment of conditions such as hemorrhage from solid organs, mesenteric ischemia, and intestinal hemorrhage. Some therapeutic applications of abdominal angiography are described in Chapter 16. Enteral contrast agents can be given, resulting in studies such as esophagography, contrast gastrography, small-bowel follow-through, and contrast colonography (e.g., barium or air-contrast enema). These studies have special utility in disorders affecting the bowel lumen, such as ulcer, volvulus, and intussusception. Contrast agents can also be instilled into the biliary system and urinary system. Overall, CT plays a broader diagnostic role today, with fluoroscopic procedures often assuming therapeutic roles once the diagnosis has been established. We discuss fluoroscopy in specific clinical settings later in this chapter.

TABLE 9-4. Ultrasound Probes for Abdominal and Pelvic Applications

Ultrasound Probe	Footprint	Frequency	Resolution	Depth of Imaging Penetration
Abdominal	~60 mm	Lower frequency (~5 MHz)	Lower resolution	Deeper penetration (20-30 cm)
Endovaginal	~11 mm	Higher frequency (~8 MHz)	Higher resolution	Shallower penetration (10 cm)

SYSTEMATIC GUIDE TO ABDOMINAL PATHOLOGY

In this final section, we review major forms of abdominal pathology. We describe which imaging modality is best when possible, and the evidence for that recommendation. We describe advantages and disadvantages of each modality for each diagnosis. We review the imaging findings for all major modalities that can be used to make the diagnosis. In some cases, we emphasize that a particular modality is insensitive or nonspecific and should not be relied upon. We often refer to the ACR appropriateness criteria, which provide succinct evidence-based guidelines for imaging in many common clinical scenarios (Table 9-5). Throughout other chapters

of this text, we emphasized well-validated clinical decision rules for imaging. Unfortunately, no single clinical decision rule governs imaging of the numerous, varied, and complex abdominal conditions. When possible, we highlight clinical guidelines that may alert the clinician to the need for imaging or provide reassurance that imaging may be deferred for the moment.

Pneumoperitoneum and Other Pathologic Gas

Figures 9-7 through 9-10 demonstrate imaging findings of pneumoperitoneum. Three modalities are commonly used to evaluate pneumoperitoneum: x-ray, CT scan, and ultrasound. X-ray has been the usual first choice and remains an appropriate first test in selected patients with a high probability of pneumoperitoneum based on

TABLE 9-5. Recommended Imaging Test, Based on American College of Radiology Appropriateness Criteria and Other Evidence-Based Guidelines

Leading Differential Diagnosis, Stable Patient*	"Best" Imaging Test†
Undifferentiated abdominal pain	• CT with oral and IV contrast
Abscess or postsurgical complication	• CT with oral and IV contrast
Aortic aneurysm	• CT with or without IV contrast; no oral contrast (ACR) • Bedside ultrasound in an unstable patient
Appendicitis	• CT with or without IV and oral contrast (ACR) • Ultrasound as a possible first-line test in young or pregnant patients • MRI possible
Blunt abdominal trauma	• CT with IV contrast • No oral contrast needed (ACR)
Cholecystitis	• Ultrasound; no radiation exposure • Cholescintigraphy (HIDA) • CT if adequate ultrasound views cannot be obtained
Diverticulitis	• CT with IV contrast, with or without oral or colonic contrast (ACR)
Free air	• Upright chest x-ray in an unstable patient • CT exquisitely sensitive without any form of contrast
Inflammatory bowel disease	• CT with oral and IV contrast (ACR) • Neutral rather than positive oral contrast (ACR)
Large-bowel obstruction	• CT with IV contrast • Enteral contrast possible
Mesenteric ischemia	• CT with IV contrast; no oral or rectal contrast, which may delay the diagnosis
Pancreatitis and complications (hemorrhage, abscess, pseudocyst)	• CT with or without IV contrast
Pelvic pathology (e.g., torsion or ectopic pregnancy)	• Ultrasound with Doppler capability • CT with IV contrast possible to evaluate for ovarian abscess, mass, or torsion; oral or rectal contrast may be useful
Penetrating abdominal trauma	• CT with oral, IV, and rectal contrast
Small-bowel obstruction	• CT with IV contrast; oral contrast unnecessary in most cases and may obscure pathology (ACR)
Ureterolithiasis	• CT without oral or IV contrast

*Unstable patients may require no imaging and may be best served by laparotomy. Patients with classic presentations of disease may require no imaging.
†Many factors may influence imaging decisions, including patient age, pregnancy status, clinical stability, allergies, and renal function. The ideal choice in a given patient may differ from that listed here.

history and examination findings or unstable vital signs. CT is more sensitive, as we discuss later, and is often the best, first, and only imaging study in stable patients with a broad differential diagnosis for their abdominal complaint. Ultrasound is not routinely used for detection of pneumoperitoneum in the United States, but a growing body of literature supports its use.

X-ray Technique and Findings of Pneumoperitoneum
Although emergency physicians often describe x-ray as "ruling out free air," this terminology is inaccurate, because studies suggest that x-ray is relatively insensitive for detection of pneumoperitoneum. If x-ray is used to assess for free air, it is upright chest x-ray, *not abdominal x-rays*, that are most sensitive. The upright position increases sensitivity by allowing air to collect under the diaphragm, where it provides a silhouette against the subjacent liver (right side) or stomach and spleen (left side; see Figure 9-7). In a patient positioned supine, air often collects in the midline abdomen in the highest position, near the anterior abdominal midline or anterior to the liver—and thus may not be visible under the diaphragm (see Figure 9-8). Studies with CT scan confirm that these are the common locations for intraperitoneal air to collect in the supine position, as described later. In this position, air does not form a silhouette against other abdominal organs and is not easily detected with

x-ray. Large amounts of pneumoperitoneum may sometimes be seen on supine abdominal x-ray. Gas may outline both the intraluminal and the extraluminal surface of the bowel wall, a finding called Rigler's sign. Gas can also collect along the falciform ligament (falciform ligament sign), around the perimeter of the peritoneal cavity ("football" sign), along the medial umbilical folds ("inverted V" sign), and over the liver (right-upper-quadrant gas sign). In one retrospective study, 59% of cases pneumoperitoneum exhibited one or more of these findings on supine x-ray, although this series was biased by the selection of cases of pneumoperitoneum and likely overstates the sensitivity of supine x-ray.[37]

The AP or PA upright chest x-ray can detect subdiaphragmatic gas, which appears black. Studies comparing the frontal and lateral views suggest that the lateral view may be more sensitive, particularly if air has not migrated to the most cephalad subdiaphragmatic position.[38-39] Woodring and Heiser[39] found that, in patients with known pneumoperitoneum, upright lateral chest x-ray detected 98% of cases, whereas upright PA chest x-ray detected only 80%. Maintaining the patient in an upright position for at least 5 minutes increases the sensitivity of chest x-ray. An upright abdominal x-ray is less sensitive than an upright chest x-ray because the abdominal x-ray exposure is greater

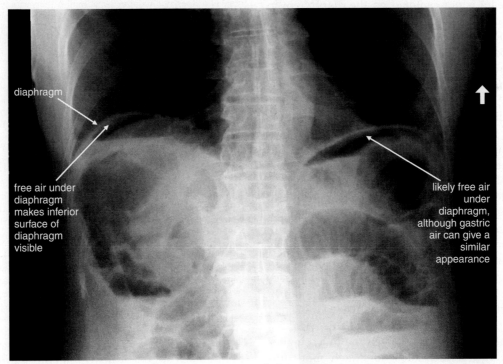

Figure 9-7. Free air (pneumoperitoneum). This upright chest x-ray reveals free air under both diaphragms. The upright chest x-ray is described as the most sensitive plain x-ray for detection of pneumoperitoneum. Positioning the patient upright for several minutes before obtaining the x-ray can improve sensitivity by allowing air to rise to the subdiaphragmatic region. Air can be most readily recognized beneath the right hemidiaphragm. Normally the inferior surface of the right hemidiaphragm is in contact with the liver, which shares the same density. Consequently, the inferior surface of the right hemidiaphragm is not normally seen. When air collects between the liver and right hemidiaphragm, the diaphragmatic surface is silhouetted against the adjacent extremely low-density air and becomes visible. Air under the left hemidiaphragm must be distinguished from air within the stomach, which is located beneath the left hemidiaphragm, normally contains air, and thus can simulate free air. Air in the colon under the right diaphragm can also simulate free air, as shown in Figure 9-46.

Labels on figure:
diaphragm

free air under diaphragm makes inferior surface of diaphragm visible

likely free air under diaphragm, although gastric air can give a similar appearance

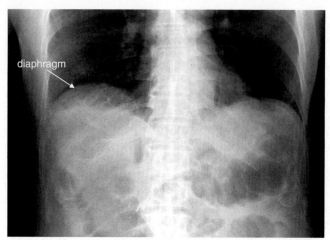

Figure 9-8. Free air (pneumoperitoneum) not visible on supine x-ray. Compare this supine abdominal x-ray obtained within minutes of the upright chest x-ray in Figure 9-7. No free air is visible, because the supine position allows truly free air to migrate to the anterior midline abdomen, rather than collecting under the diaphragm. Air in this location is dispersed in the horizontal plane of the image and does not silhouette solid organs. Loculated air might remain trapped under the diaphragm. Beware of supine x-rays that may not demonstrate free air. Also review the CT images in Figure 9-9 and 9-10.

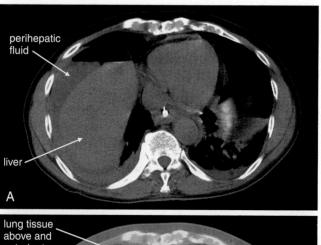

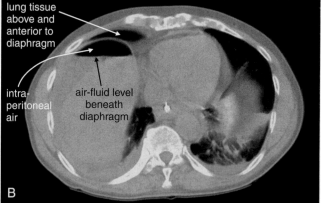

Figure 9-9. Free air (pneumoperitoneum), CT without IV contrast. Same patient as in Figures 9-7 and 9-8. Free air is readily visible on CT scan and does not require the administration of any contrast agents. By definition, air has a density of −1000 Hounsfield units, far less than the next least-dense tissue, fat, which has a density of -50HU. Air thus provides extreme intrinsic contrast. Air appears black on all window settings. These two images are the same axial CT slice, displayed on soft-tissue window settings **(A)** and lung window settings **(B).** This slice is taken from the upper abdomen—in the supine position, the liver and diaphragm are high enough in this patient that they are visible in the same slice with the lower portion of the heart. A soft-tissue window may seem the natural setting to use for inspecting for free air in the abdomen, but these images demonstrate that a lung window can clarify uncertain findings. With the soft-tissue window, the thin diaphragm is not readily visible, and air on each side of the diaphragm is difficult to discern. In addition, using a soft-tissue window, free air, aerated lung parenchyma, and fat all appear nearly black. The lung window demonstrates the diaphragm readily, and lung tissue is visible anterior to the diaphragm. The soft-tissue window is more valuable in discriminating the perihepatic fluid from liver parenchyma—these appear less distinct on the lung window. When free air is suspected, remember to review images using a lung window in addition to a soft-tissue window. Note this apparent conflict: On supine plain x-ray, air is not visible under the diaphragm, presumably because it has migrated to the anterior midline abdomen. Yet on CT in the supine position, a large amount of air remains visible under the diaphragm. This illustrates the relative insensitivity of plain x-ray for pneumoperitoneum, particularly in the supine position. Studies show that free air is more commonly found in the apex midline abdomen with CT as a result of the patient's supine position.

to allow penetration of abdominal organs, which are denser than lung tissue. This overexposes or "burns out" some regions of the abdomen, rendering even some soft tissues black on the x-ray image. Air may be hidden because of this effect. In addition, the central ray of the x-ray beam is not centered on the diaphragm in a typical abdominal x-ray, also reducing the sensitivity. Miller et al.[40] found that expiratory phase lateral decubitus and midinspiratory upright chest x-ray were most sensitive—using an interesting experiment in which two of the study authors were injected on separate occasions with 1 or 2 cm³ of intraperitoneal air. Another method to increase visibility of free air is perform an upright chest x-ray after the patient has been positioned in the right lateral decubitus position for 10 minutes, allowing air to collect under the left diaphragm.[41] In patients who cannot tolerate full upright positioning, a left lateral decubitus abdominal x-ray (left side down) can be performed. This allows pneumoperitoneum to collect between the right lateral margin of the liver and the abdominal wall, creating a silhouette. When peptic ulcer perforation is suspected, another method to improve visualization of free air is to insufflate the stomach with air using a nasogastric tube, a technique called a pneumogastrogram.[42] Lee et al.[43] found that this procedure increased the sensitivity of x-ray from 66% to 91% in 129 patients with suspected perforated gastric ulcer. Given the much higher sensitivity of CT (described later), it is likely more efficient to obtain CT in most cases than to perform multiple x-rays using these techniques.

Chest x-ray can be difficult to interpret for free air. The normal gastric air bubble can be mistaken for free air on the left side, although usually the superior wall of the stomach appears thicker than the diaphragm, allowing the two to be distinguished. On the right, the colon may become interposed between the liver and the diaphragm, in which case colonic air may simulate free subdiaphragmatic air (Chilaiditi syndrome).[44] Subphrenic fat is low in density and may be mistaken for air. Basilar atelectasis can create a linear density in the lower lung

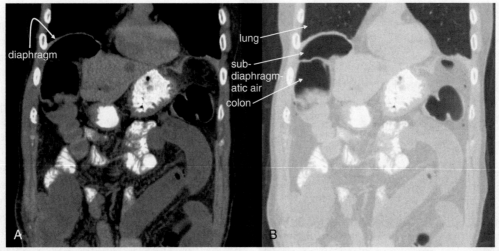

Figure 9-10. Free air (pneumoperitoneum), CT with oral contrast, no IV contrast. The same patient as in Figures 9-7 through 9-9, with coronal views set to soft-tissue **(A)** and lung **(B)** windows. Again, the lung window makes the subdiaphragmatic air clear-cut. Lung tissue above the diaphragm is visible on the lung window but not on the soft-tissue window. Air under the diaphragm is hard to discern from colonic air on the soft-tissue window, but the upper margin of the hepatic flexure of the colon is visible on the lung window, with subdiaphragmatic air visible outside the colon.

that can be mistaken for the diaphragm, in which case lung tissue above the actual diaphragm can be mistaken for intraperitoneal air. Loculated extraluminal air in the abdomen may fail to rise to a subdiaphragmatic location and may be missed.

Computed Tomography Technique and Findings of Pneumoperitoneum

CT scan is extremely sensitive for detection of gas in any location, including pneumoperitoneum (see Figures 9-9 and 9-10). Gas or air appears black on all CT window settings, because it is very low in density (−1000 Hounsfield units) compared with any other tissue. No contrast agents are needed to detect air because of the intrinsic extreme difference in density between air and other tissues. On a typical soft-tissue window setting, small amounts of air may be difficult to recognize, because fat within the peritoneum and retroperitoneum appears dark on these settings. The window level may be adjusted to make fat lighter in appearance. A simple solution is to select a lung or bone window, because either makes all other tissues lighter in hue, allowing black air to be readily detected. Because CT scan is usually performed with the patient in a supine position, intraperitoneal gas collects in a different location than is seen on upright chest x-ray. In one study, the most common locations for pneumoperitoneum were the anterior midline abdomen (pararectus and midrectus recesses) and the space anterior to the liver, although collections were also seen in the pelvis and mesentery.[45] Air may be trapped in other locations by normal organs, surgical adhesions, or the presence of a loculated abscess, so the entire abdomen should be inspected. The retroperitoneum should also be inspected, because some segments of bowel, including the duodenum and ascending and descending colon, are retroperitoneal. Another advantage of CT is that it may identify the source of

pneumoperitoneum, aiding surgical planning. Pinto et al.[46] found that the site of free air correlated with the site of perforation, particularly for gastroduodenal perforation. Free air did not occur with ruptured appendicitis in this study, which included only 40 patients.

Studies have compared the sensitivity of x-ray and CT for detection of pneumoperitoneum. Stapakis and Thickman[47] examined the performance of both modalities in patients who had undergone diagnostic peritoneal lavage for assessment of abdominal trauma—a procedure that introduced air into the peritoneum, providing an ideal setting to compare the two diagnostic tests. CT detected air in all patients, including collections as small as 1 mm. X-ray was far less sensitive, detecting no collections 1 mm or smaller, 33% of collections from more than 1 mm through 13 mm, and 100% of collections greater than 13 mm, for an overall sensitivity of 38% compared with CT. Earls et al.[45] found CT to be more sensitive than left lateral decubitus x-ray in detecting postoperative pneumoperitoneum, with x-ray detecting only 47% of gas collections detected by CT 3 or 6 days after surgery. CT detected gas collections with volumes as low as 0.3-5.8 mL.

If enteral contrast is given, contrast may leak out of bowel in some cases and be visible on CT—though studies in the setting of trauma show this to be a fairly rare event (Figure 9-11).

Ultrasound of Pneumoperitoneum

Ultrasound can be used to detect pneumoperitoneum. Gas is a poor acoustic transmitter and scatters the ultrasound beam, resulting in a highly echogenic signal, with dark acoustic shadowing occurring deep to any air collection. Air normally occurs within the abdomen,

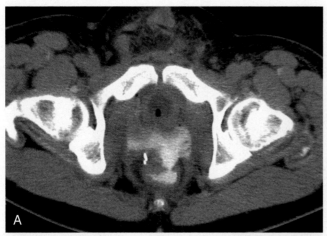

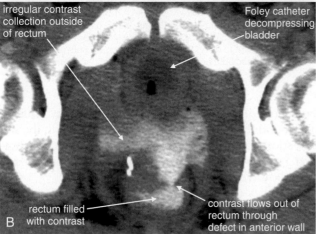

Figure 9-11. **Bowel perforation with enterial contrast leak, computed tomography.** Bowel perforation can result in free peritoneal air, as shown in earlier figures. In other cases, orally or rectally administered contrast may be seen in the peritoneal cavity. Less specific findings can occur—irritation from peritoneal soiling can result in ascites (free fluid) and fat stranding, which are also reviewed in other figures. This patient has orally administered contrast free in the abdomen. The patient had undergone prostatectomy and sustained a rectal injury. The rectal defect is visualized in this image, but do not expect to see defects in most perforations, because they may be quite small. More often, secondary findings such as pneumoperitoneum, free peritoneal fluid, fat stranding, or bowel thickening at the site of perforation may be seen. **A,** Scan viewed on soft-tissue window. **B,** Close-up.

contained within bowel, so the search for free air requires inspection of regions of the abdomen that are normally devoid of air. These include the right upper quadrant superficial to the liver. Subcutaneous air in this location has a similar appearance to free air but remains fixed in position, whereas true free air can be displaced by palpation with the ultrasound probe. Rib shadows can be mistaken for air, as both demonstrate bright acoustic signal and dark acoustic shadowing.

In some studies, ultrasound is comparable or superior in sensitivity to x-ray in the detection of pneumoperitoneum. Chen et al.[48] found ultrasound to have a sensitivity of 93% and specificity of 64%, compared with x-ray (sensitivity = 79%, specificity = 64%). In a second study, the same authors[49] found the sensitivity of ultrasound

to be 92%, compared with 78% for x-ray. Both modalities showed 53% specificity. Two problems occur in both of these studies. First, the populations in both studies are extremely spectrum biased, with most patients having hollow organ perforation. This compromises the external validity of the studies and their applicability to a general emergency department population with abdominal pain. Second, in both studies, the specificity of ultrasound is so low that it cannot be trusted to make the diagnosis of pneumoperitoneum accurately; some confirmatory study would be required, or a large number of patients would generally be expected to suffer an unnecessary operation. Braccini et al.[50] found ultrasound to be superior to x-ray in detection of pneumoperitoneum (ultrasound sensitivity 86%, specificity 83.5%; x-ray sensitivity 75.7%, specificity 89.2%). Moriwaki et al.[51] reported sensitivity of ultrasound for free air to be 85%, with higher specificity than in the prior studies (100%). Overall, the role of ultrasound in detecting free air is unclear. Although ultrasound may be superior to x-ray, it is less sensitive and specific than is CT. Ultrasound may be useful in patients in whom avoiding CT is particularly desired, but when a high degree of suspicion exists for pneumoperitoneum, CT should be performed.

Not all pneumoperitoneum detected by imaging is pathologic or is caused by abdominal pathology.[52-53] Rarely, pneumoperitoneum may occur because of pneumothorax or even entry of air through the female genital tract. Following surgery, gas may remain in the peritoneum and be visible on upright PA x-ray for up to 1 week.[45,54-55] However, the possibility of pathologic free air resulting from infection or iatrogenic bowel perforation should be considered if signs or symptoms are suggestive.

Bowel Obstruction

In the sections that follow, we discuss the radiographic diagnosis of bowel obstruction, beginning with proximal obstructions, continuing with small-bowel obstruction, and finishing with obstruction of large bowel. Figures 9-12 through 9-50 demonstrate imaging findings of bowel obstruction of various causes.

Gastric Outlet Obstruction

Gastric outlet obstruction is a variant of bowel obstruction. In adults, the diagnosis can be caused by neoplasm (including gastric lymphomas and carcinoma), ulcer, ingested foreign body, and rarely extrinsic compression. In infants, the process commonly occurs because of pyloric stenosis.

Although the principles of imaging for gastric outlet obstruction are the same as for small- and large-bowel obstruction, the proximal nature of the obstruction also offers the opportunity for direct visualization with

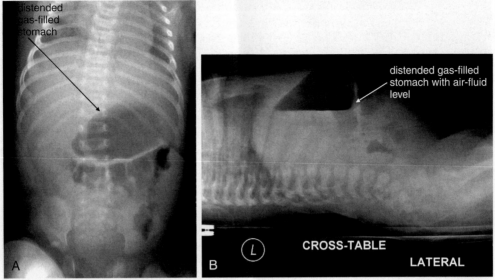

Figure 9-12. Pyloric stenosis (gastric outlet obstruction) x-ray, pediatric. Pyloric stenosis is usually diagnosed by ultrasound. This 3-week-old male patient with pyloric stenosis underwent abdominal plain x-rays first, which demonstrate a distended, gas-filled stomach. Although this is suspicious for pyloric stenosis, ultrasound is required to confirm the diagnosis. In adults, gastric outlet obstruction from causes such as tumor or ulcer can give a similar x-ray appearance. **A,** Supine anterior–posterior view. **B,** Cross-table lateral view. Compare with the ultrasound images from the same patient in Figure 9-13.

endoscopy. In addition, because the obstruction is so proximal, abnormalities on imaging are often limited to the stomach, though extrinsic compression of the stomach from adjacent pathologic processes is possible.

X-ray Findings of Gastric Outlet Obstruction. The x-ray findings of gastric outlet obstruction include a grossly distended stomach, with a paucity of gas in the remainder of the abdomen if sufficient time has elapsed for peristalsis to empty the bowel distal to the obstruction (see Figure 9-12). The stomach may displace the transverse colon inferiorly. If obstruction is caused by ulcer, free air may be seen.

Upper Gastrointestinal Series (Fluoroscopic Examination). A traditional means of assessing for gastric outlet obstruction is with contrast swallow study. In this case, contrast fails to move beyond the stomach. Irregularities in the mucosal surface, such as craters from ulcer, can be seen. The thickness of the stomach wall cannot be measured directly with this technique, because only the mucosal surface is visible.

Computed Tomography Findings of Gastric Outlet Obstruction. On CT, the stomach may appear grossly distended, and thickening of the pyloric region may be seen with gastric outlet obstruction. Gastric varices can be seen with IV contrast–enhanced CT. In rare cases of gastric volvulus, the stomach wall may fail to enhance normally and beaking at the point of volvulus may be seen, as described later for large- and small-bowel volvulus. If oral contrast is administered, it will not move beyond the stomach. Stomach anatomy can be difficult to visualize with CT, although thin collimation (slice

thickness) and coronal plane reformations can assist.[56] No large studies have examined CT for gastric outlet obstruction, so the description of the appearance is based on case reports.

Infantile Pyloric Stenosis. Pyloric stenosis causes gastric outlet obstruction in infants, with 95% of cases diagnosed between 3 and 12 weeks of age. A family history and male gender are risk factors, although sporadic nonfamilial cases and cases in female patients occur. The typical history is of projectile emesis immediately after feeding. In patients without the classic palpable olive on physical examination, the diagnosis was made historically using upper GI contrast studies, but today ultrasound is the predominant imaging modality. X-ray is nonspecific but usually shows gross gastric distension and often a paucity of distal bowel gas (see Figure 9-12). Ultrasound is highly sensitive and specific for pyloric stenosis and does not expose the patient to ionizing radiation, an important consideration in pediatric patients. Ultrasound findings of pyloric stenosis (see Figure 9-13) include a pylorus 14 mm or greater in length and 10 mm or greater in diameter. The use of a pyloric thickness 5.5 mm or greater does not improve diagnostic accuracy, although some authors suggested a thickness of 4 mm as a diagnostic criterion.[57]

Hernanz-Schulman et al.[58] studied 152 infants with suspected pyloric stenosis and found the sensitivity and specificity of ultrasound to be 100% for patients requiring surgery. Van der Schouw et al.[57] also found that ultrasound improved the diagnosis of pyloric stenosis in infants without a palpable abdominal olive suspected of pyloric stenosis. An ultrasound-measured

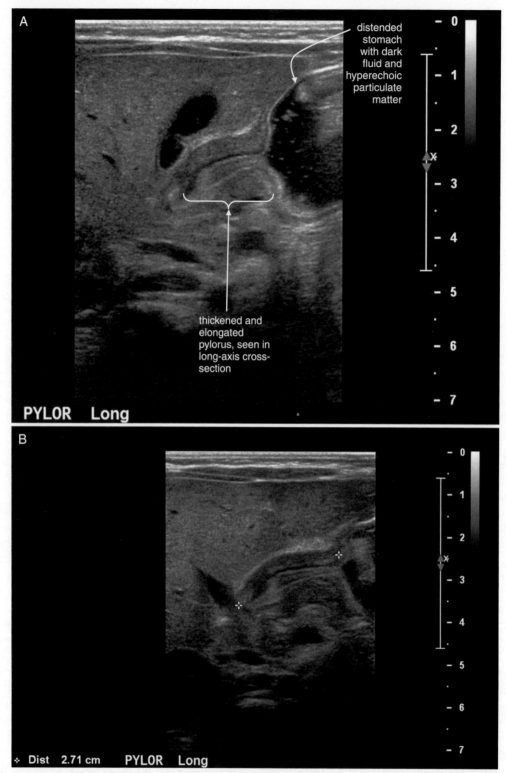

Figure 9-13. Pyloric stenosis, ultrasound. This 3-week-old male presented with 2 days of projectile, nonbilious emesis. His ultrasound shows typical findings of pyloric stenosis. In the long-axis views **(A** through **C),** a thickened and elongated pylorus is seen. The stomach proximal to the pylorus is distended with fluid and particulate matter. In the short-axis (transverse) view **(D),** a thickened pylorus is seen. The patient underwent pyloromyotomy and recovered uneventfully. Compare with the x-ray in Figure 9-12.

pyloric length of 14 mm or greater and a diameter of 10 mm or greater, along with the age at which vomiting began (<5 weeks), base excess, and a bicarbonate level of 28 mmol/L or greater, yielded high sensitivity and specificity.

Upper Gastrointestinal Series for Pyloric Stenosis. Because of the diagnostic utility of ultrasound, upper GI series is now rarely performed for evaluation of suspected pyloric stenosis.[57-58] Upper GI series requires radiation exposure, whereas ultrasound does not. When

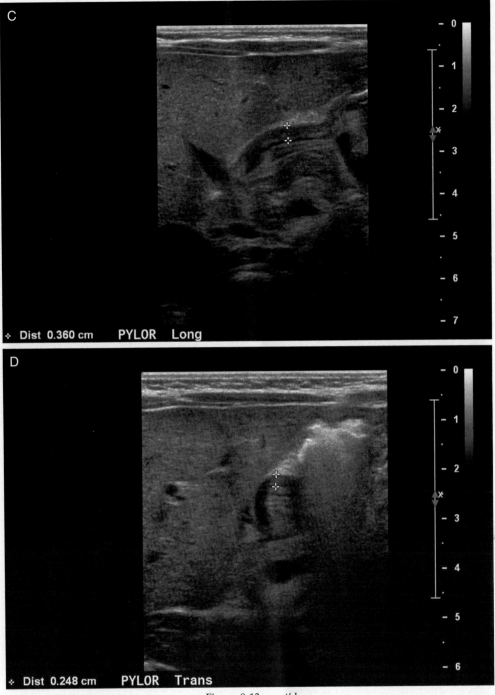

Figure 9-13, cont'd

ultrasound is equivocal, upper GI series can be performed. Enteral contrast introduced into the stomach by nasogastric tube is not seen beyond the pylorus.

Small-Bowel Obstruction

X-ray and CT are commonly used to evaluate small-bowel obstruction. Recent studies also support the use of ultrasound for this indication. X-ray has historically been used to "rule out" small-bowel obstruction, but this terminology is inaccurate, because x-ray has relatively poor sensitivity, as we discuss later. In the past,

contrast small-bowel series with fluoroscopy have been used to identify obstruction not evident on x-ray. This modality and contrast enteroclysis have little role today in the emergency department as a result of the diagnostic power of CT. MRI can also be used to evaluate small-bowel obstruction but is not routinely required in the emergency department, because CT provides the necessary information in most patients. MRI can be used instead of CT in the pregnant patient to eliminate radiation exposure.[59] Figures 9-14 through 9-19 show imaging findings of small-bowel obstruction.

X-ray of Small-Bowel Obstruction. X-ray diagnosis of small-bowel obstruction relies on two primary findings: dilated loops of small bowel and air–fluid levels (see Figures 9-14 and 9-15). Dilated loops of small bowel are visible on supine, upright, or lateral decubitus images. The small bowel is normally less than 3 cm in diameter, so a diameter exceeding this is considered pathologic. The small bowel is characterized by internal folds called plicae circularis (or valvulae conniventes), which completely traverse the diameter of the bowel. These distinguish the small bowel from the large bowel, which is marked by haustra, segmentations that do not completely traverse the bowel diameter. In a dilated loop of small bowel, the adjacent plicae circularis can give the tubular bowel the appearance of a "stack of coins."

Air–fluid levels are not visible on a supine x-ray, because air and fluid layer in the plane of the x-ray detector and do not form a silhouette against each other. Air–fluid levels are visible on upright or decubitus abdominal x-rays, because fluid settles into dependent loops of small bowel. Normal small bowel contains both air and fluid, so scattered air–fluid levels can be a normal finding or a finding in ileus. However, in the presence of a mechanical obstruction, multiple air–fluid levels occur. As loops proximal to the obstruction fill with fluid, displacing air, air–fluid levels may be replaced by tiny pockets of air, called the "string of beads" or "string of pearls" sign on the upright x-ray. On a supine x-ray, these air pockets may appear elongated and slitlike, caused by air trapped along plicae circularis—sometimes called the "stretch" sign.

Air is present in the small bowel primarily from swallowed air; gas within the large bowel is partly caused by gas production by anaerobic bacteria. Fluid is normally present in the small bowel because of swallowed fluids, including saliva and ingested materials, and gut secretions. In the presence of a mechanical obstruction, peristalsis distal to the point of obstruction may ultimately push air and fluid out of the distal bowel. Thus a classic appearance for small-bowel obstruction includes air–fluid levels, dilated loops of small bowel, and an absence of bowel gas in the distal bowel and rectum. However,

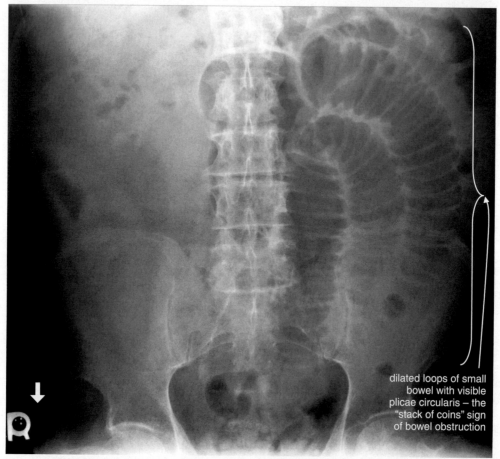

dilated loops of small bowel with visible plicae circularis – the "stack of coins" sign of bowel obstruction

Figure 9-14. Small-bowel obstruction, x-ray. A classic plain film finding of small-bowel obstruction is the presence of dilated loops of small bowel, characterized by markings of plicae circularis (valvulae conniventes), which span the entire lumen of small bowel. In contrast, the haustra of large bowel do not fully cross the luminal diameter. Dilated loops of small bowel can be seen on x-ray in upright, supine, or decubitus positions. In contrast, air–fluid levels, another common x-ray finding of small-bowel obstruction, are not. Why aren't air–fluid levels visible on supine x-ray? Imagine a glass of water, viewed from the side—the air–fluid level is visible, as on an upright x-ray. Now view the glass of water from above—the air–fluid level is not visible, as on the supine x-ray. Dilated loops of bowel with visible plicae circularis are sometimes said to have the appearance of a stack of coins.

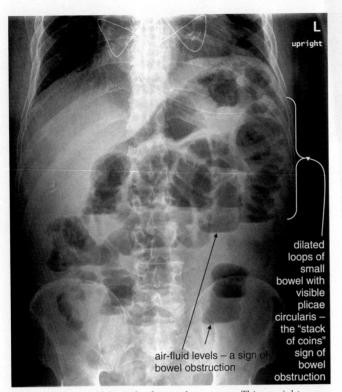

dilated loops of small bowel with visible plicae circularis – the "stack of coins" sign of bowel obstruction

air-fluid levels – a sign of bowel obstruction

mechanical bowel obstructions can occur along a spectrum, both in terms of severity (partial or complete) and in terms of duration of obstruction before x-rays are obtained, affecting the resulting images. Understandably, an x-ray obtained moments after the onset of even a complete obstruction may not yet show dilated bowel proximal to the obstruction or an absence of gas distal to the obstruction. A partial obstruction, which allows some bowel contents to traverse the point of obstruction, may never develop a classic x-ray appearance.

In the case of ileus, when small bowel is diffusely "stunned" or inactive, no focal point of obstruction is present. The bowel may appear dilated, and air–fluid levels may be seen, but air and gas are usually distributed throughout the bowel, including distally through the large bowel to the rectum. Classically, this appearance differs from that of a complete mechanical bowel obstruction, in which gas and fluid are evacuated from bowel distal to the point of obstruction by peristalsis. However, in reality, an ileus may appear identical to an early complete mechanical bowel obstruction or a partial bowel obstruction, so the presence of gas in the distal bowel cannot distinguish these or rule out complete obstruction. A number of other bowel gas patterns have been described, including a "nonspecific bowel gas pattern," but unfortunately, bowel obstruction may be present in patients with normal, nonspecific, ileus, or obstruction x-ray patterns. Air in the rectum should not be attributed to digital rectal examination, which does not introduce significant amounts of air.[60]

Figure 9-15. Small-bowel obstruction, x-ray. This upright x-ray from another patient shows the same finding of dilated loops of bowel seen in Figure 9-14—but the upright position also allows air–fluid levels to be seen. Air–fluid levels are a classic finding of small-bowel obstruction. Swallowed air becomes trapped in bowel, unable to move beyond the point of obstruction. Gas may also be produced by bacteria in obstructed bowel. Fluid is present from swallowed fluid and food and from bowel secretions. An ileus can have a similar appearance. Many air–fluid levels are visible here—a few are labeled, but look carefully and identify more.

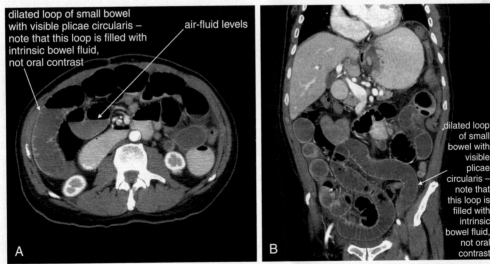

dilated loop of small bowel with visible plicae circularis – note that this loop is filled with intrinsic bowel fluid, not oral contrast

air-fluid levels

dilated loop of small bowel with visible plicae circularis – note that this loop is filled with intrinsic bowel fluid, not oral contrast

Figure 9-16. Small-bowel obstruction, CT with oral and intravenous contrast, soft-tissue window. This CT was performed in the same patient as the x-ray in Figure 9-15. The CT demonstrates air–fluid levels and dilated loops of bowel—similar in appearance to the plain x-ray. The normal diameter of small bowel is less than 3 cm, whereas this patient has loops nearly 4 cm in diameter. The patient also shows evidence of increased bowel wall enhancement and thickening, typical of ischemia complicating obstruction. A transition point—the location of the obstruction, where the dilated bowel gives way to bowel of normal caliber—was identified in the left lower quadrant. Air–fluid levels are visible on the axial views but not the coronal views, for the same reason that these cannot be seen on supine x-ray. The patient was treated with nasogastric tube drainage for 24 hours but failed to improve. At laparotomy, adhesions were identified binding the bowel to the anterior abdominal wall. **A,** Axial CT. **B,** Coronal CT reconstruction. Although this patient received oral and IV contrast, oral contrast is not necessary for diagnosis of high-grade small bowel obstruction. IV contrast is useful for identification of bowel ischemia resulting from obstruction.

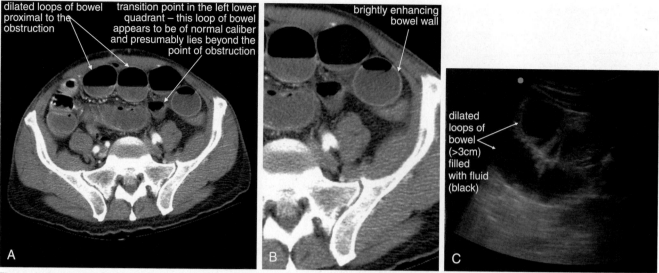

Figure 9-17. Small-bowel obstruction, CT and ultrasound. Same patient as in Figures 9-15 and 9-16. This figure demonstrates the concept of the transition point, the location where the dilated bowel proximal to the obstruction gives way to the normal-caliber bowel beyond the obstruction. Sometimes the specific cause of the obstruction is visible. Also note how brightly the small-bowel wall enhances with intravenous contrast, suggesting possible bowel ischemia. Bowel that fails to enhance with IV contrast is ischemic or infarcted--hence the failure to deliver IV contrast to that region. A bowel segment that enhances to a greater degree than adjacent segments may be ischemic, with increased deposition of contrast due to microvascular injury. **A,** Axial image, soft-tissue window. **B,** Close-up. **C,** Ultrasound image from the same patient demonstrates fluid-filled dilated loops of small bowel.

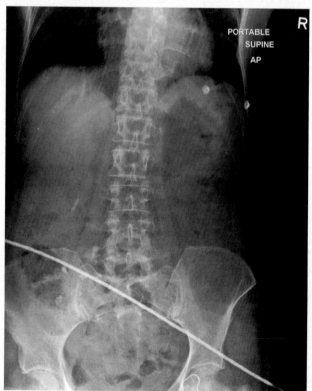

Figure 9-18. Small-bowel obstruction with closed loop on CT but normal x-ray. This 74-year-old female presented with acute abdominal pain beginning at 2 AM, 2 hours before emergency department arrival. This x-ray was interpreted as showing no signs of obstruction. This is a supine x-ray, so pneumoperitoneum and air–fluid levels would not be expected to be seen. Dilated loops of bowel might be seen if present but are not seen in this case. This image demonstrates the poor sensitivity of x-ray, which should not be relied upon to exclude serious abdominal pathology. CT was performed subsequently and is reviewed in Figure 9-19. Incidentally, the x-ray was mislabeled by the technician—with an "R" marker placed on the patient's left side.

X-ray is relatively poor for distinguishing ileus from mechanical obstruction. Air–fluid levels occurring at different heights within the same loop of bowel (called *differential* or *dynamic* air–fluid levels) have been described as more typical of mechanical obstruction than ileus, with an increasing likelihood of obstruction with increasing height differential. Harlow et al.[61] found that the presence of differential loops is only 52% sensitive and 71% specific for mechanical obstruction—inadequate for clinical utility. With height differentials greater than 20 mm, the specificity is 94%, with less than 25% sensitivity.[61]

This insensitivity of x-ray strongly limits its utility in the evaluation of small-bowel obstruction. Because a normal or nondiagnostic x-ray can occur in the presence of bowel obstruction (see Figure 9-18 and the related CT in Figure 9-19), CT (discussed later) is often performed following a normal x-ray. Moreover, because CT is commonly used to identify the point of obstruction, identify a cause such as hernia (see Figures 9-20 and 9-21), confirm the degree of obstruction, and identify ischemic bowel related to obstruction, an abnormal x-ray is commonly followed by CT today. Consequently, x-rays have little impact on patient management, other than introducing diagnostic delay and additional cost. Rarely, x-rays may be useful in the sickest patients (unsuitable for CT), when CT is unavailable, or in patients with such a low pretest probability of bowel obstruction that the physician is willing to accept an insensitive test result without further evaluation. X-rays can be performed portably, allowing other resuscitation measures to be continued in unstable or very ill patients. Early identification of

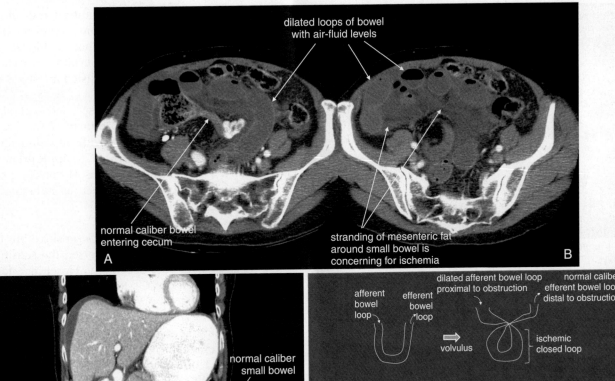

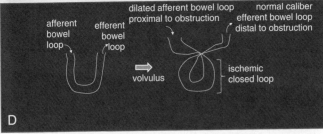

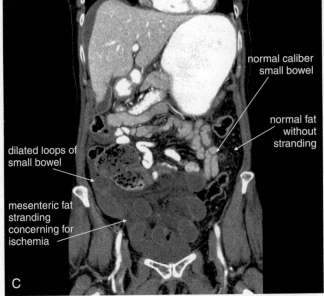

Figure 9-19. Small-bowel obstruction with closed loop, CT with oral and IV contrast. Despite a nondiagnostic abdominal x-ray (Figure 9-18), this CT shows strong evidence of small bowel obstruction. The small bowel is quite dilated, with air–fluid levels present. Normal-caliber small bowel is seen entering the cecum, suggesting a transition point just proximal to the ileocecal valve. Stranding of mesenteric fat and fluid in the pelvis suggest that the bowel is ischemic or inflamed. The patient was taken to the operating room, where a single adhesion was found obstructing both the proximal and the distal portions of a hemorrhagic bowel loop—a "closed loop" obstruction with ischemia of the strangulated section, which was resected. **A, B,** Axial CT images. **C,** Coronal CT image. **D,** Schematic demonstrating torsion of a loop of bowel, resulting in an ischemic closed loop obstruction.

free air or bowel obstruction with x-ray may facilitate care such as nasogastric tube placement or surgical consultation in these sickest patients.

What Are the CT Findings of Small-Bowel Obstruction?
The CT findings of small-bowel obstruction are similar to those found on x-ray: dilated loops of bowel and air–fluid levels (see Figures 9-16 and 9-17). Fukuya et al.[62] found that the optimal balance between sensitivity and specificity for obstruction was achieved using 2.5 cm as the definition for dilated small bowel. In this same study, a small-bowel diameter of 3 cm or greater was 100% specific for small-bowel obstruction.

Gazelle et al.[63] found obstruction was predicted by the presence of dilated loops of bowel greater than 2.5 cm in diameter from outer wall to outer wall proximal to a point of stenosis, giving way to undilated bowel distally. Air–fluid levels and the amount of intestinal fluid did not predict obstruction. Multiple planes of image reconstruction can be helpful in assessing for small-bowel obstruction; in some cases, curved or oblique planes may be useful in identifying the exact cause of obstruction.[64] Because CT scan is performed with the patient supine, rather than upright, air–fluid levels are seen on axial and sagittal planar images but not on images reconstructed in a coronal plane. Air appears black on

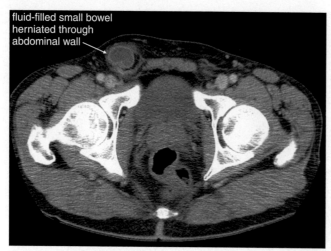

fluid-filled small bowel herniated through abdominal wall

Figure 9-20. Incarcerated inguinal hernia, CT with IV and oral contrast. This 46-year-old male presented with right inguinal pain and swelling. An attempt to reduce an apparent right inguinal hernia was unsuccessful. This axial slice shows a loop of small bowel entering a right inguinal hernia. Figure 9-21 shows a coned-in view focused on the region of the hernia. Whereas the radiologist identified this as an indirect inguinal hernia, the operative report noted a direct hernia through the inguinal ring.

a soft-tissue window, whereas native fluid within the bowel appears dark gray on this window setting.

Other CT findings of small-bowel obstruction have been described, including the string of pearls sign (similar to its x-ray counterpart), and the "small-bowel feces" sign.[65] The latter is defined by small gas bubbles mixed with particulate matter within dilated loops of small bowel proximal to a point of obstruction. Normally this mixture of gas and solid or liquid intestinal contents is seen only in the colon, but in the presence of bowel obstruction, bacterial action begins to produce gas in small-bowel contents, resulting in this sign, which has a reported specificity of 82% for small-bowel obstruction. The small-bowel feces sign has also been described as locating the transition zone.[66-68] Free fluid with bowel obstruction on CT has been associated with a higher rate of surgical intervention.[69]

Computed Tomography Findings of Complete Versus Incomplete Small-Bowel Obstruction. Using CT without oral contrast, high-grade obstruction is suggested by a 50% difference in the caliber of proximal dilated bowel and collapsed bowel distal to the transition point.[68] Using CT with oral contrast, complete obstruction is diagnosed if no enteral contrast passes the point of obstruction at delayed scans 3 to 24 hours after the initial CT.[68] Partial obstruction is diagnosed if some contrast material passes the point of obstruction.

Computed Tomography Findings of Bowel Ischemia Associated With Bowel Obstruction. On CT scan, a closed-loop obstruction can be seen, indicating a high risk for bowel ischemia (see Figure 9-19). In such an obstruction, characterized by a grossly distended

U-shaped loop of bowel with an abrupt transition to collapsed distal bowel loops, compression of the blood supply can lead to gangrene without rapid surgical intervention.[70] Other findings concerning for ischemia from strangulating obstruction are listed in Table 9-6.[71]

Although detection of ischemia associated with small-bowel obstruction is a prime indication for CT, the sensitivity and specificity have wide reported ranges in the medical literature. The ACR appropriateness criteria call CT an "excellent means of detecting complications of bowel obstruction such as ischemia and strangulation."[74]

Frager et al.[73] found CT to be 100% sensitive but only 61% specific. Balthazar et al.[75] reported the sensitivity of CT as 83%, with 93% specificity. Ha et al.[72] found the overall sensitivity of CT to be 85%, although individual findings such as poor bowel wall enhancement (sensitivity = 34%, specificity = 100%) or a serrated beak (sensitivity = 32%, specificity = 100%) were less sensitive but highly specific. Zalcman et al.[76] reported an overall sensitivity of CT of 96% and specificity of 93% for ischemia in the setting of small-bowel obstruction. Mallo et al.[77] conducted a systematic review from 1966 to 2004 and found 11 studies of CT for ischemia associated with small-bowel obstruction, with 743 patients. For ischemia, the aggregate sensitivity of CT was 83% (range = 63%-100%) and specificity was 92% (range = 61%-100%). Sheedy et al.[78] evaluated the prospective performance of CT for detection of small-bowel obstruction-associated ischemia in 60 patients and found poor sensitivity (14.8%) with high specificity (94.1%). Decreased segmental bowel wall enhancement with IV contrast was the most specific finding (100% specificity).

Jang et al.[79] compared simple visual assessment of bowel wall enhancement for evidence of ischemia with a quantitative measure (maximal attenuation of a region of interest) in which the Hounsfield unit enhancement of bowel wall was measured. Visual inspection had a sensitivity of 91.7% and specificity of 66.7%. In comparison, quantitative measurements provided better sensitivity and specificity. A maximum attenuation of less than 85 Hounsfield units was 100% sensitive but only 45% specific for ischemia. Adopting a lower threshold improved specificity at the expense of sensitivity. If the maximum bowel wall attenuation was less than 45 Hounsfield units, the sensitivity was only 25% but specificity was 100%. The authors also assessed a technique in which the Hounsfield density of the same region on a noncontrast CT (performed immediately before CT with IV contrast) was subtracted from the Hounsfield attenuation on IV-contrasted CT. This provided the best combination of sensitivity and specificity but would require that patients undergo two CT scans, increasing the radiation exposure.

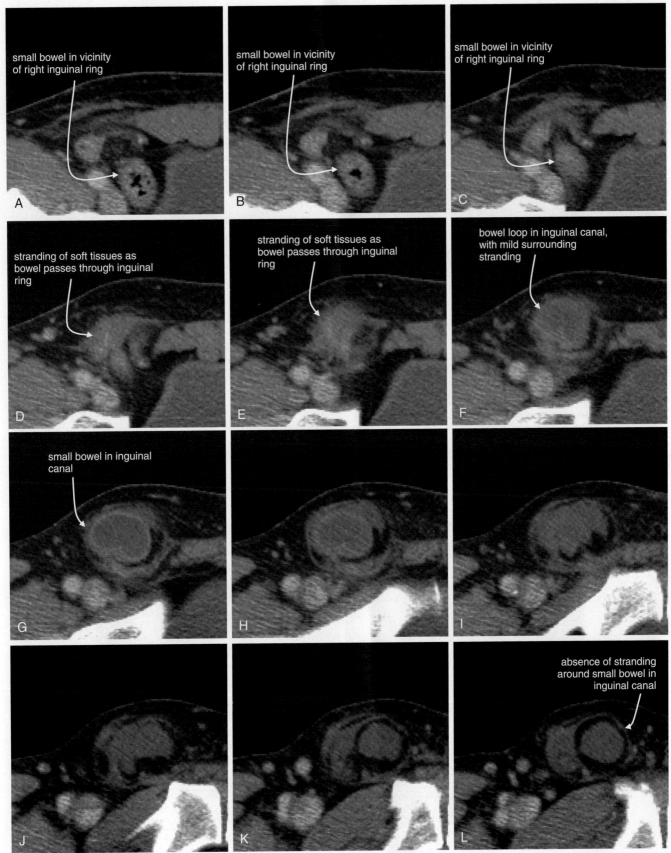

Figure 9-21. Incarcerated inguinal hernia, CT with IV and oral contrast, soft-tissue window. Same patient as Figure 9-20. This series of axial slices shows a loop of small bowel entering a right inguinal hernia. **A** through **L** progress from cephalad to caudad. The minimal stranding and absence of bowel wall thickening are reassuring, making frank bowel infarction less likely.

Oral Contrast Agents and Computed Tomography of Suspected Small-Bowel Obstruction. Just as small-bowel obstruction can be diagnosed with x-ray using no enteral contrast, CT without enteral contrast can demonstrate small-bowel obstruction.[34,74,79] In the case

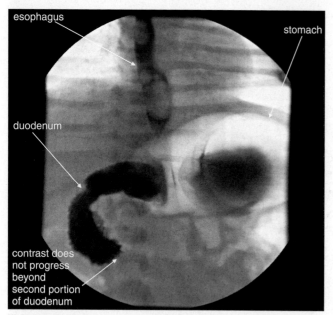

Figure 9-22. Pediatric midgut malrotation and suspected volvulus. This 10-day-old infant presented with bilious emesis. An upper gastrointestinal contrast study was performed and showed no contrast progressing beyond the second segment of the duodenum, suspicious for malrotation with midgut volvulus. Operatively, the patient was found to have malrotation without volvulus.

of obstruction, the small bowel is typically already distended with ingested saliva, partially digested food, and intestinal secretions—providing intrinsic enteral contrast. Unlike high-density enteral contrast agents (e.g., barium sulfate or Gastrografin, also called diatrizoate meglumine), which appear white on CT using soft-tissue window settings, native fluid within the bowel is relatively low in density, near water density. Low-density fluid appears dark gray on soft-tissue window settings and is readily differentiated from air and fat. High-density contrast agents are designated "positive" contrast agents, whereas low-density contrast such as native bowel contents are called "neutral" contrast agents. Multiple studies demonstrate that positive enteral contrast agents are not generally needed for the diagnosis of small-bowel obstruction. In its published appropriateness criteria, the ACR states that the use of positive enteral contrast may actually disguise bowel wall changes indicative of ischemia, which we discuss later.[74]

Intravenous Contrast Agents and Computed Tomography of Suspected Small-Bowel Obstruction. Small-bowel obstruction can be diagnosed without IV contrast, but the use of IV contrast can assist in diagnosis of bowel ischemia. Detection of ischemia is an important indication for abdominal CT in clinically suspected or x-ray-confirmed small-bowel obstruction, so IV contrast should be administered when possible. IV contrast may assist in other conditions with similar

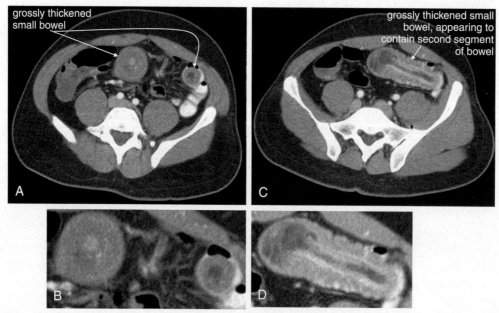

Figure 9-23. Adult intussusception, CT with IV and oral contrast, soft-tissue window. This 35-year-old male with multiple sclerosis presented with abdominal pain and vomiting for 4 days. CT scan shows an intussusception—pathology more commonly seen in children. The patient ultimately underwent laparotomy and resection of the intussusception. Pathology showed the intussusceptum to be a large, inverted diverticulum, likely a Meckel's diverticulum given the position in the terminal ileum, though no gastric mucosa was found. These axial CT images show a segment of small bowel with a thickened bowel wall. In some images, the bowel is seen in transverse (short-axis) cross-section, while in others it is oriented in long-axis section. The short-axis views **(A, B)** suggest that there is bowel within bowel, confirmed on the long-axis views **(C, D)**. **A, C,** Axial CT slices. **B, D,** Close-ups from **A** and **C,** respectively.

clinical presentations to small-bowel obstruction, as described in other sections of this chapter and chapters of this book.

Atri et al.[34] compared IV-enhanced CT with nonenhanced CT (no oral, IV, or rectal contrast). Unenhanced CT had a sensitivity of 88.1% and specificity of 77% for small bowel obstruction, not significantly different from the sensitivity and specificity of CT with IV contrast (87.6% and 75%, respectively).

What Is the Transition Point, and What Is Its Significance? With CT, the point of a mechanical obstruction can be identified and often the cause can be determined. Proximal to this point, the bowel appears dilated beyond 3 cm. Distal to the point of obstruction, bowel loops are decompressed (<3 cm).[62] The point of obstruction, at which dilated bowel loops give way to undilated bowel, is called the *transition point* or *transition zone*. Identification of a transition point helps to confirm a mechanical obstruction rather than ileus.[63]

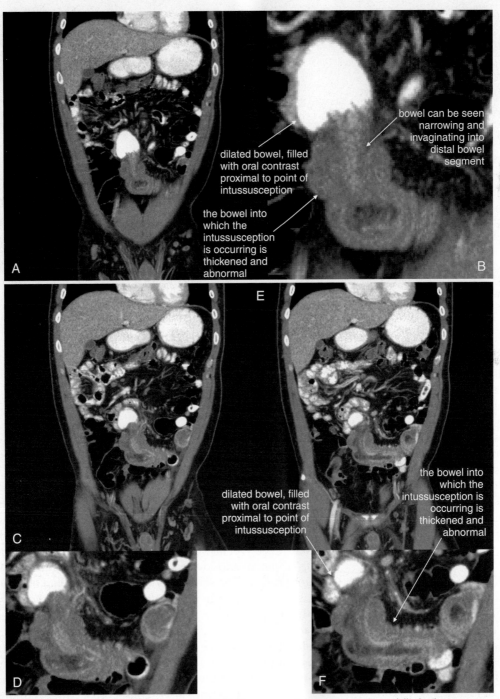

Figure 9-24. Adult intussusception, CT. Same patient as Figure 9-23. These coronal reconstructions beautifully display intussusception. The proximal bowel is filled with contrast, right up to the point when the bowel suddenly invaginates into the distal bowel segment. **A, C, E,** Coronal reconstructions. **B, D, F,** Close-ups from **A, C, E,** respectively.

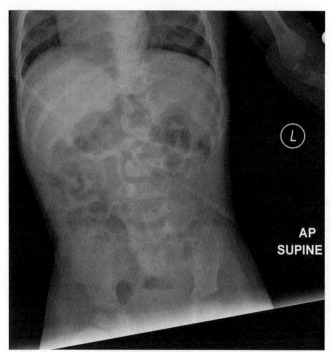

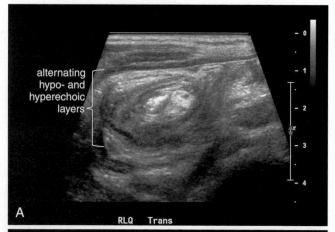

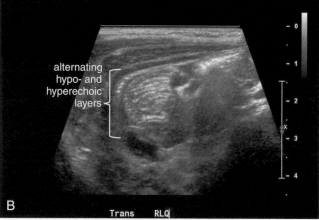

Figure 9-25. **Pediatric intussusception, x-ray.** Intussusception can be diagnosed by ultrasound in children, and this has become the primary screening modality in many institutions. X-ray is most often nondiagnostic, although findings consistent with obstruction may be seen. This 17-month-old male with proven intussusception had a nondiagnostic x-ray. Compare this with Figures 9-26 and 9-27, showing ultrasound and air-contrast enema in the same patient.

Figure 9-26. **Pediatric intussusception, ultrasound.** Same patient as the Figure 9-25. This 17-month-old male presented with 3 days of bilious emesis. A right lower quadrant tubular mass consistent with ileocolic intussusception is seen. The typical alternating hyperechoic and hypoechoic layers are seen. Intussusception can be diagnosed by ultrasound in children, and this has become the primary screening modality in many institutions. Ultrasound findings of intussusception include a concentric ring sign of bowel telescoped within bowel. Characteristically, there are alternating areas of increased and decreased echogenicity. **A, B,** Short-axis (transverse) views.

In addition, the cause of obstruction may be recognized as an abscess, mass, internal or external hernia (see Figures 9-20 and 9-21), volvulus, intussusception (see Figures 9-23 and 9-24), ingested foreign body, or inflamed bowel segment, aiding surgical planning.[80] Adhesions may be difficult to identify directly on CT but are a common cause of small-bowel obstruction in patients with CT evidence of small-bowel obstruction without a visualized cause.[62] Use of coronal plane images, in addition to axial images, may assist in detection of the transition point.[81] A recent study questions the clinical significance of the radiographic transition zone. Colon et al.[82] found no difference in the rate of immediate operative therapy or failure of nonoperative therapy in patients with and without transition zones. Transition zones correlated with operative findings in 63% of cases.

What Is the Sensitivity of Computed Tomography for Small-Bowel Obstruction? How Does This Compare With X-ray? X-ray and CT have been compared in sensitivity for detection of small-bowel obstruction. As with x-ray, the sensitivity of CT likely varies according to the severity of obstruction. The ACR[74] cites a range of sensitivities of x-ray (30%-90% in published series), as well as a high rate of misleading findings on plain x-ray (20%-40%).

In most studies, CT is considerably more sensitive than x-ray for the diagnosis of small-bowel obstruction,

although a small number of studies show comparable sensitivity and specificity.[83] In its appropriateness criteria, the ACR[74] cites the higher sensitivity and specificity of CT, as well as its ability to determine the degree and cause of obstruction and the presence of ischemia, as key reasons for the use of CT as the primary diagnostic modality for suspected small-bowel obstruction. Mallo et al.[77] conducted a systematic review from 1966 to 2004 and found 15 studies of CT for small bowel obstruction. The sensitivity of CT for complete obstruction was 92% (range = 81%-100%), and the specificity was 93% (range = 68%-100%).

Shrake et al.[84] retrospectively reviewed x-ray and enteroclysis (a rarely-used procedure in which the bowel is rapidly distended with fluid via an enteric tube prior to imaging) in 117 consecutive patients undergoing enteroclysis for suspected small-bowel obstruction. Among patients with normal or nonspecific x-rays, 22% had

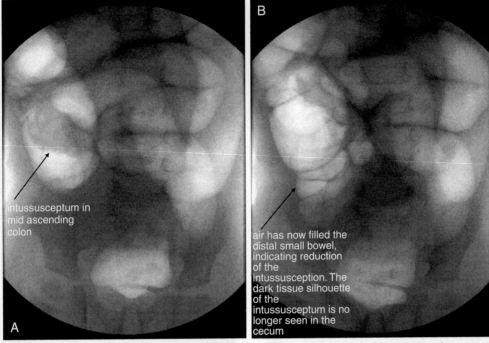

Figure 9-27. **Pediatric intussusception, air-contrast enema.** Same patient as Figures 9-25 and 9-26. The patient underwent air-contrast enema. To reduce the risk for bowel perforation, a manometer is used to monitor the pressure of insufflated air, and pressures are kept below 120 mm Hg. In an ileocolic intussusception, a successful reduction is marked by air refluxing through the entire colon and into small bowel. In this patient, the reduction was successful, as seen in **B. A, B,** Fluoroscopic air-contrast enema images.

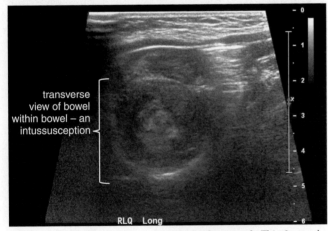

Figure 9-28. **Pediatric intussusception, ultrasound.** This 3-month-old presented with bilious vomiting and intermittent lethargy. Ultrasound shows intussusception, with the typical appearance of alternating hyperechoic and hypoechoic concentric layers. This mass extended into the right upper quadrant.

obstruction demonstrated by enteroclysis. Of patients with x-rays suggesting obstruction, 42% had normal enteroclysis or only minor adhesions. These results suggest that x-ray findings may imply the wrong diagnosis in 20%-40% of cases.

Megibow et al.[85] retrospectively viewed 84 CT scans from patients with suspected small-bowel obstruction and found a sensitivity of 94% and specificity of 96%. CT identified the cause of obstruction in 73% of cases.

Frager et al.[80] compared the accuracy of x-ray and CT in 85 patients, using a gold standard of surgical findings and clinical course. For complete obstruction, x-ray combined with clinical suspicion was 46% sensitive, whereas CT was 100% sensitive. For partial obstruction, x-ray with clinical suspicion was 30% sensitive, whereas CT was 100% sensitive. CT was false positive in three cases of ileus from causes including small-bowel infarction, pneumonia, and peritonitis from bladder rupture.

Maglinte et al.[83] retrospectively compared the sensitivity of x-ray and CT in 78 patients, using a gold standard of clinical outcome and enteroclysis. X-ray was 69% sensitive and 57% specific for small-bowel obstruction. CT was 64% sensitive and 79% specific. In subgroups classified as high-grade obstruction, x-ray was 86% sensitive and CT was 82% sensitive. In low-grade obstruction, x-ray was 56% sensitive and CT was 50% sensitive.

Suri et al.[86] reported that the sensitivity of CT was 93%, with 100% specificity. X-ray was 50% sensitive and 75% specific, and ultrasound was 83% sensitive and 100% specific. However, this prospective study included only 32 patients, 30 of whom had obstruction, suggesting significant selection and spectrum bias compared with a typical emergency department population.

Low-grade obstruction may be a relative CT blind spot, with fewer than 50% of patients diagnosed by CT in

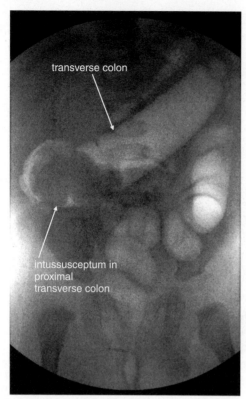

Figure 9-29. Pediatric intussusception, air-contrast enema. Same patient as Figure 9-28. After ultrasound showed intussusception, air-contrast enema was performed. The intussusceptum is seen as a soft-tissue density near the hepatic flexure, silhouetted by air. Although air did push the intussusceptum down to the level of the cecum, air did not reflux into the small bowel and the intussusceptum remained visible in the cecum. The patient underwent operative reduction of the intussusception.

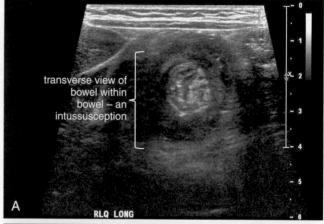

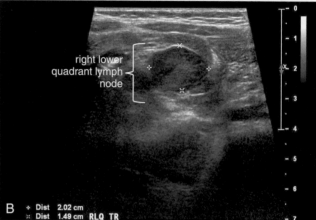

Figure 9-30. Pediatric intussusception, ultrasound. A, B, Transverse (short-axis) images. This 2-year-old presented with abdominal pain and vomiting. This ultrasound shows the typical mass of intussusception, with alternating hyperechoic and hypoechoic layers. The ultrasound also showed large lymph nodes **(B),** in keeping with the theory of an inflammatory leadpoint resulting in intussusception. After ultrasound confirmed intussusception, air-contrast enema was performed but was unsuccessful at reduction. The patient underwent laparotomy, and the intussusception was reduced. Large mesenteric lymph nodes were biopsied and subsequently grew adenovirus in culture.

two studies by Maglinte et al.[83,87] However, these studies included a nonconsecutive retrospective sample of patients referred for enteroclysis to confirm small-bowel obstruction, a group in whom presumably the diagnosis was relatively difficult (hence requiring enteroclysis). This may underestimate the sensitivity of CT in a typical population of emergency department patients.

Ultrasound for Small-Bowel Obstruction. Ultrasound is rarely used in the United States but often used internationally for the diagnosis of small-bowel obstruction. Advantages of ultrasound are portability, lack of any ionizing radiation exposure, and elimination of injected iodinated contrast, with its attendant risks.

Ultrasound findings of small-bowel obstruction are similar to those with other imaging modalities. Dilated loops of bowel greater than 3 cm diameter are seen proximal to a point of mechanical obstruction, with collapsed loops distally. Fluid-filled loops of bowel are readily seen with ultrasound, although air continues to pose a barrier to visualization, scattering the ultrasound beam. Associated ascites are readily recognized. The thickness of the bowel wall can also be assessed. Because ultrasound allows dynamic assessment of bowel motility, peristalsis

can be used as an additional criterion. In the presence of obstruction, increased bowel motility with a to-and-fro or whirling motion of intestinal contents may be seen. Conversely, in ileus, an absence of intestinal peristalsis is seen.[88] Hyperechoic ultrasound contrast agents can be administered intravenously to assess bowel wall perfusion. After administration of these agents, lesser echogenicity is seen in ischemic bowel wall compared with normally perfused bowel.

Ultrasound has been compared retrospectively and prospectively with x-ray for the diagnosis of small-bowel obstruction. Ko et al.[88] found ultrasound to be correct in 89% of 54 cases, compared with 71% of cases for x-ray. Sonography also more accurately predicted the degree and cause of obstruction. Ogata et al.[89] prospectively compared ultrasound and x-ray in 50 patients with suspected bowel obstruction, 22 ultimately diagnosed with small-bowel obstruction and 2 with large-bowel

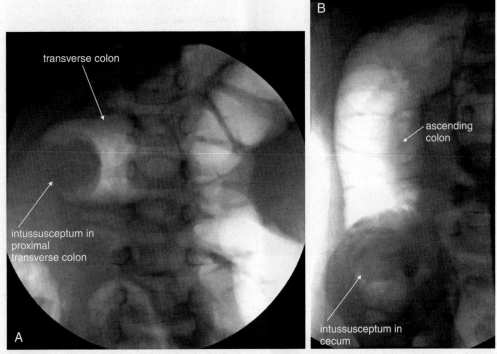

Figure 9-31. **Pediatric intussusception, air-contrast enema.** Same patient as Figure 9-30. **A, B,** Fluoroscopic air-contrast enema images show the intussusceptum (a dark soft-tissue mass, silhouetted by air) first at the level of the hepatic flexure and then in the cecum. But after repeated efforts, the intussusceptum could not be reduced further, necessitating laparotomy.

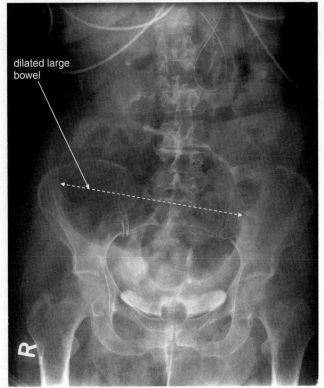

Figure 9-32. **Large-bowel obstruction from incarcerated inguinal hernia, x-ray.** This 90-year-old female presented with syncope and a right inguinal mass. X-ray shows a dilated large bowel. Review the CT in Figure 9-33.

obstruction. Ultrasound was 88% sensitive and 96% specific, whereas x-ray was 96% sensitive and 65% specific. This study is limited by selection biases and a small sample size with wide confidence intervals (CIs). Czechowski[90] compared x-ray and ultrasound in 96 patients and found ultrasound to be 91% sensitive in patients with strangulation, compared with 30% for x-ray. In cases of simple obstruction, ultrasound was 89% sensitive, compared with 78% for x-ray. However, the small number of cases (9 simple obstructions and 10 strangulation obstructions) results in wide CIs. As described earlier, Suri et al.[86] prospectively compared x-ray, CT, and ultrasound, finding ultrasound to be 83% sensitive and 100% specific, but with significant selection bias and a small patient population.

Hata et al.[91] studied contrast-enhanced ultrasound for assessment of small-bowel obstruction–associated intestinal ischemia in 51 patients with dilated bowel on x-ray. Ultimately, 15 patients were found to have bowel ischemia from strangulation, 5 from superior mesenteric artery (SMA) thromboembolism, and 31 patients had simple obstruction. Diminished or absent color signals from the bowel wall had a sensitivity of 85% for bowel ischemia (95% CI = 62%-97%) and specificity of 100% (95% CI = 91%-100%). Larger studies are needed to confirm these findings. The rate of SMA thrombosis in this series was extraordinarily high (10%) compared with the rate in the general population, suggesting selection bias in this study population.

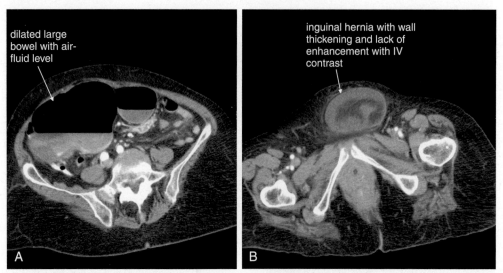

Figure 9-33. **Large bowel obstruction from incarcerated inguinal hernia, CT with oral and IV contrast, soft-tissue window.** Same patient as Figure 9-32. **A,** CT shows a dilated cecum (greater than 12 cm in this case). **B,** An inguinal hernia is present—the cause of the obstruction. Review the x-ray in Figure 9-32.

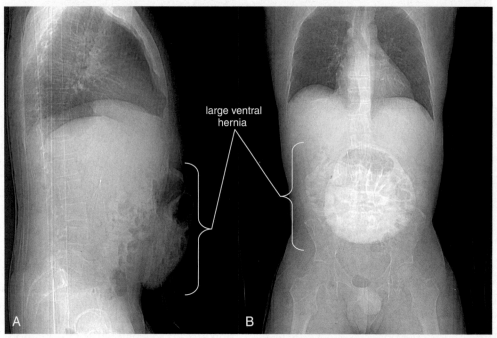

Figure 9-34. **Nonincarcerated ventral hernia, CT scout images.** Some hernias are so large that they are readily evident on examination and grossly obvious on CT. This patient has an enormous ventral hernia (10 cm in width) with bowel protruding into the subcutaneous space. This is an incisional hernia that developed after a snowmobile accident in which the patient sustained a grade V liver laceration and underwent exploratory laparotomy. These scout CT images demonstrate the extent of the hernia, which is explored in more detail in Figures 9-35 and 9-36. **A,** Lateral scout image. **B,** frontal scout image.

Midgut Volvulus With Resulting Bowel Obstruction and Ischemia in Adults.

Midgut volvulus can result in intestinal obstruction and acute bowel ischemia. The condition is not restricted to pediatric patients but represents a particular concern in preverbal infants who cannot communicate symptoms, sometimes leading to catastrophic diagnostic delay. In adults, midgut volvulus can occur as a result of undiagnosed midgut malrotation. It is a rare cause of mesenteric ischemia in young adults.[92] X-ray findings are nonspecific but can include

a "bird's beak" appearance because of rotation of the bowel around the point of volvulus. CT demonstrates this same appearance, with whirling of the mesentery.[93] Other CT findings of intestinal ischemia are often present, as described earlier.

Midgut Volvulus in Infants.

Midgut volvulus resulting from malrotation is a much feared pediatric emergency, occurring in an estimated 1 in 500 live births. Because 60% of cases present within the first month of

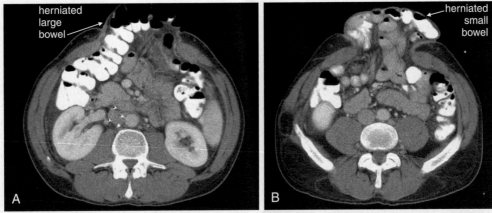

Figure 9-35. Nonincarcerated ventral hernia, axial CT with oral and IV contrast, soft-tissue window. Same patient as Figure 9-34. **A,** The contrast-filled colon is seen within the hernia sac. This demonstrates that no small-bowel obstruction exists, because the orally ingested contrast passed through the small bowel to reach the large intestine. **B,** The contrast-filled small bowel is seen in the hernia sac. The herniated bowel has normal wall thickness. Other signs of incarceration such as fat stranding do not appear to be present.

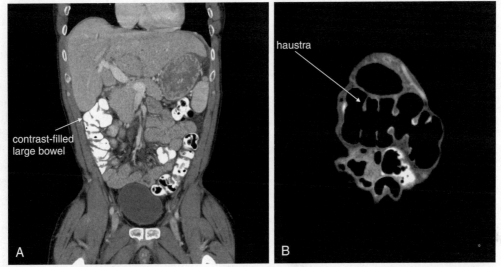

Figure 9-36. Nonincarcerated ventral hernia, CT. Same patient as Figures 9-34 and 9-35. **A,** A coronal reconstruction shows the large bowel to be filled normally with contrast, indicating that the hernia in this patient has not led to small bowel obstruction. **B,** The hernia sac protrudes well into the anterior abdominal wall so that it is seen alone in this anterior coronal plane. The haustra of the colon are visible.

life and another 20%-30% present before 12 months, diagnosis is difficult; the patients cannot communicate symptoms. Another 10% of cases present throughout life, including adults of any age. Mortality is around 15%, but short gut syndrome from extensive bowel infarction is a highly morbid consequence. The clinical presentation in neonates is bilious emesis.

X-rays for Midgut Volvulus. X-rays may demonstrate evidence of proximal intestinal obstruction, with a dilated stomach and proximal small bowel and an otherwise gasless abdomen. A "double-bubble" sign may also be seen. When x-rays suggest volvulus, the preferred radiographic technique for confirmation is upper GI series, although CT and ultrasound can also be used. Because x-rays are not sensitive for the diagnosis, a confirmatory study is needed whenever clinical suspicion exists.

Upper Gastrointestinal Series for Midgut Volvulus. Sizemore et al.[94] studied 166 patients and found upper GI series to be 96% sensitive for malrotation and 79% sensitive for midgut volvulus. Upper GI series demonstrates a classic beaking appearance of the small bowel at the point of volvulus, with no contrast passing this point. The configuration of the bowel is also abnormal, caused by malrotation, although the specific appearance is beyond the scope of this text. Figure 9-22 shows an upper GI series performed for suspected midgut volvulus.

Computed Tomography for Midgut Volvulus. CT scan can reveal midgut volvulus, as well as other serious causes of abdominal signs and symptoms, in infants. No large studies have examined its diagnostic performance, but multiple investigators have reported its use in pediatric patients.[95-98] The CT "perfusion cutoff" sign has been described in children and is seen as hyperenhancement

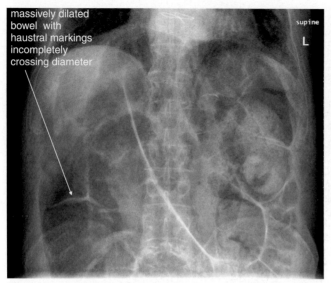

massively dilated
bowel with
haustral markings
incompletely
crossing diameter

supine
L

Figure 9-37. Sigmoid volvulus, x-ray. Sigmoid volvulus is a surgical emergency that can result in bowel perforation or bowel ischemia. The classic presentation is a bedbound nursing home patient who develops fecal impaction, followed by volvulus. Volvulus results in large-bowel obstruction and vomiting. The blood supply is compromised, and massive distension of bowel proximal to the point of obstruction occurs. This 84-year-old male presented with a history of 3 weeks of no bowel movements. He failed an attempt at treatment with colonoscopic decompression and underwent sigmoidectomy. An x-ray such as this, showing massively dilated bowel, should immediately raise the possibility of both volvulus and perforation. X-ray findings include massive dilatation of bowel with air. The dilated bowel is recognizable as the colon, because the markings of haustra do not cross the complete diameter of the bowel, in contrast to the plicae circularis of small bowel, which do. This x-ray simulates Rigler's sign, the visualization of both sides of a loop of bowel on x-ray. For bowel wall (soft-tissue density) to be seen in relief, it must be flanked on both the intraluminal and the extraluminal side by another density, in this case air density. Two scenarios allow this: (1) perforation with extraluminal air (Rigler's sign, also called the double wall sign) and (2) two adjacent bowel loops abutting each other so that the bowel walls appear as one and the intraluminal air in each loop is seen on either side of their abutting walls.

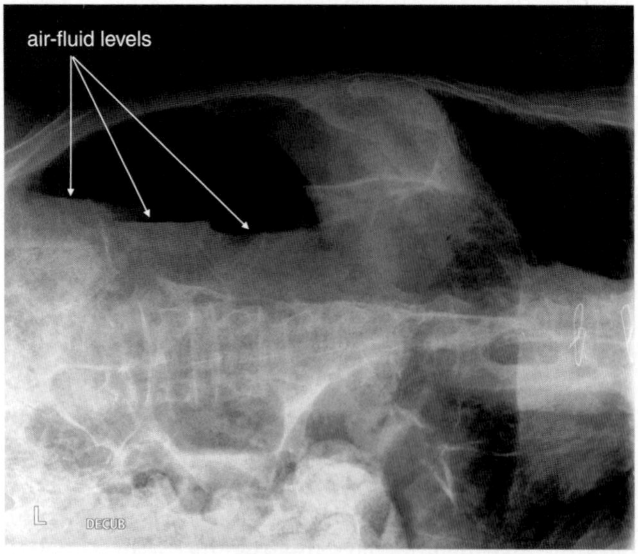

air-fluid levels

L   DECUB

Figure 9-38. Sigmoid volvulus, x-ray. This left lateral decubitus x-ray from the same patient as in Figure 9-37 shows stepladder air–fluid levels. No free air is seen.

of the bowel wall proximal to the point of volvulus, followed by an abrupt lack of enhancement of the bowel wall distal to the point of volvulus.[95] This finding is based on case reports, and the sensitivity is unknown.

Ultrasound for Midgut Volvulus. Ultrasound can assess for malrotation, the anatomic basis for midgut volvulus. Ultrasound can identify inversion of the normal positions of the superior mesenteric vein and artery and a "whirlpool" sign of twisted vessels, indicating midgut volvulus. The sensitivity for malrotation is reported to be 98%, whereas the specificity is only around 75%. Ultrasound thus may be useful to rule out malrotation but not to confirm malrotation or volvulus.[99]

Computed Tomography Findings of Intussusception With Resulting Bowel Ischemia.

Whereas intussusception in children (discussed in the next section) requires reduction with enema or surgery, in adults, intussusceptions are a rare and potentially incidental finding on CT scans. Sundaram et al.[100] reviewed 95,223 CT scans performed over 7 years and found 136 intussusceptions in 118 patients (0.13% of CT scans). In this study, 88.2% of intussusceptions were enteroenteric, 3.7% were enterocolic, and 4.4% were colocolic or other locations. The authors found 5.9% of patients required surgery, whereas 94.1% were nonsurgical. The discovery that 63% of surgical lesions involved the colon suggested that colonic intussusceptions is more likely surgical—though the small number of surgical cases in this series makes this finding uncertain. CT criteria were not specific for identifying enteroenteric lesions requiring surgery. Many nonsurgical enteroenteric intussusceptions were greater than 3.5 cm in length and thicker than 3 cm, suggesting that length and thickness had poor predictive value. A case of adult intussusception imaged with CT is shown in Figures 9-23 and 9-24.

Pediatric Intussusception. Intussusception is the leading cause of bowel obstruction and potential infarction in children 3 months to 6 years, with a peak incidence between 3 and 12 months. Most cases are ileocolic, with the terminal ileum carried through the ileocecal valve into the colon. Although a pathologic leadpoint is theorized to account for intussusception, 90%-95% of cases have no identifiable cause. The condition is fatal if not rapidly treated, although most patients recover if treated within 24 hours of onset. Intense colicky pain, vomiting, and currant jelly stools are classic but occur in only about one in five cases. Lethargy can occur. Rapid imaging is key to diagnosis and treatment (see Figures 9-25 through 9-31, which demonstrate imaging findings with multiple modalities).

X-rays can demonstrate a soft-tissue mass at the site of intussusception, a pattern of bowel obstruction, or perforation—but are often normal or nonspecific.

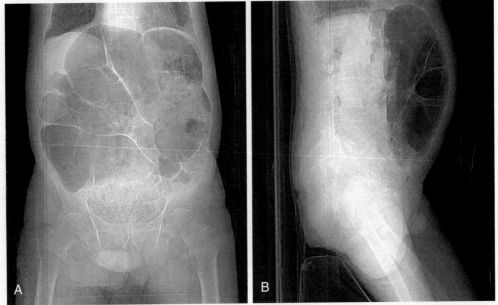

Figure 9-39. Sigmoid volvulus, CT scout images. Same patient as in Figurs 9-37 and 9-38. These scout imagesagain demonstrate massive large-bowel dilatation. **A,** frontal scout image. **B,** Lateral scout image.

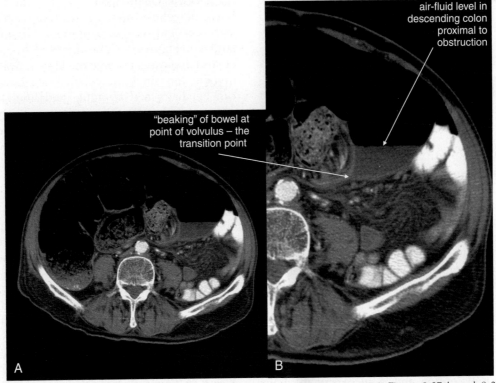

air-fluid level in descending colon proximal to obstruction

"beaking" of bowel at point of volvulus – the transition point

Figure 9-40. Sigmoid volvulus, CT with IV and oral contrast, soft-tissue window. Same patient as in Figures 9-37 through 9-39. Axial slice shows beaking of the colon at the point of volvulus in the sigmoid colon. This narrowed section results from twisting of the bowel, causing it to come to a point like a bird's beak. This finding was first described on x-ray and fluoroscopic views of the colon but is evident on CT scan as well. The point of "beaking" may also be called the transition point, marking the transition from proximal dilated bowel to nondilated bowel distal to the point of obstruction. **A,** Axial CT image. **B,** Close-up. Compare with the coronal images in Figure 9-41.

Sargent et al.[101] found that x-rays were equivocal in 53% of suspected cases of pediatric intussusception, positive in 21%, and negative in 26%. Smith et al.[102] reported a sensitivity of 80.5% and specificity of 58% for x-rays interpreted by full-time pediatric emergency physicians.

Morrison et al.[103] found that when interpreted by emergency physicians, x-ray had a sensitivity of 48% and specificity of 21%. Overall, x-ray appears too insensitive and nonspecific to confirm or exclude intussusception (see Figure 9-25).

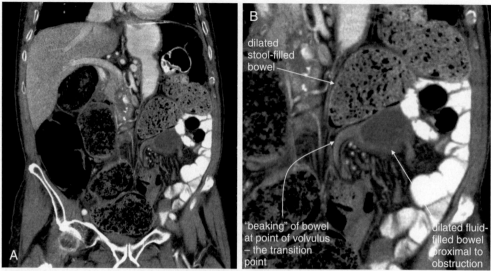

Figure 9-41. Sigmoid volvulus, CT with IV and oral contrast. Same patient as in Figures 9-37 through 9-40. Coronal reconstruction shows beaking of the colon at the point of volvulus in the sigmoid colon. Imagine a water-filled balloon, twisted near its central section. As the balloon twists, it narrows to a thin neck or "beak" on either side of the twisted section. This finding was first described on x-ray and fluoroscopic views of the colon but is evident on CT scan as well. **A,** Coronal CT image. **B,** Close-up.

Ultrasound has become the mainstay of diagnosis, because it is noninvasive and highly sensitive and specific. Hryhorczuk and Strouse[104] retrospectively reviewed 814 pediatric patients evaluated for intussusception with ultrasound and found ultrasound was 97.9% sensitive and 97.8% specific. Ultrasound is a desirability modality in children because of lack of radiation exposure. Findings include an appearance of alternating hyper echoic and hypoechoic layers (see Figures 9-26, 9-28, and 9-30).

CT is not usually required for the diagnosis of intussusception in children. However, CT may be obtained to assess for other conditions, such as appendicitis or mass, only to demonstrate intussusception.[105-106] CT demonstrates a "target" sign of alternating hyperattenuating and hypoattenuating bowel layers. Findings of bowel obstruction and ischemia (described earlier) may also be present, depending on the duration of the intussusception.

Air-contrast enema, once the mainstay of diagnosis, is usually used only therapeutically today after ultrasound diagnosis (see Figures 9-27, 9-29, and 9-31). Air is instilled into the rectum under controlled pressure to reduce the intussusception and is successful in about 85% of cases.[107-108] Water or barium contrast enema reduction is not commonly performed today because of the safety and efficacy of air-contrast enema. Unsuccessful reduction requires surgical therapy, as does perforation from the enema, which rarely occurs (in about 1.6% of cases).[108] When reduction with air-contrast enema is successful, recurrence takes place in about 7.5% of cases within 36 hours. However, recurrence is not associated with adverse outcomes, and routine admission after successful reduction may not be required.[109]

Large-Bowel Obstruction

Large-bowel obstructions including special cases, such as hernia and cecal and sigmoid volvulus, are demonstrated in Figures 9-32 through 9-50. About 25% of bowel obstruction cases involve the large bowel, whereas 75% involve the small bowel.[110] Large-bowel obstruction can be diagnosed by four modalities: x-ray, contrast enema, CT, and ultrasound. As previously discussed for small-bowel obstruction, x-ray is the historical standard but CT is more sensitive and specific, with the ability to provide information about the cause of obstruction and complications such as bowel ischemia. Contrast enema has become rare because of the diagnostic power of CT. Ultrasound is uncommonly used in the United States and thus is not discussed here, but it sees wider use internationally. Large-bowel obstruction can result from several processes, including intrinsic mass lesions, extrinsic compression by mass lesions or abscesses, adjacent inflammatory processes such as diverticulitis, surgical adhesions, hernias, and cecal and sigmoid volvulus. X-ray does not reveal the cause in most cases, although a characteristic appearance of cecal and sigmoid volvulus is sometimes seen, as described later.

X-ray in Large-Bowel Obstruction. The large bowel is located on the periphery of the abdomen and can usually be differentiated from the small bowel, which is normally located centrally within the abdomen.[111] The normal appearance of the large bowel on x-ray includes scattered irregular areas of gas, caused by the production of gas by anaerobic organisms in stool. Air–fluid levels are sometimes normally seen within the large bowel. Markings of haustra are sometimes seen; these soft-tissue ridges incompletely cross the diameter of the large bowel, in contrast to plicae circularis, which

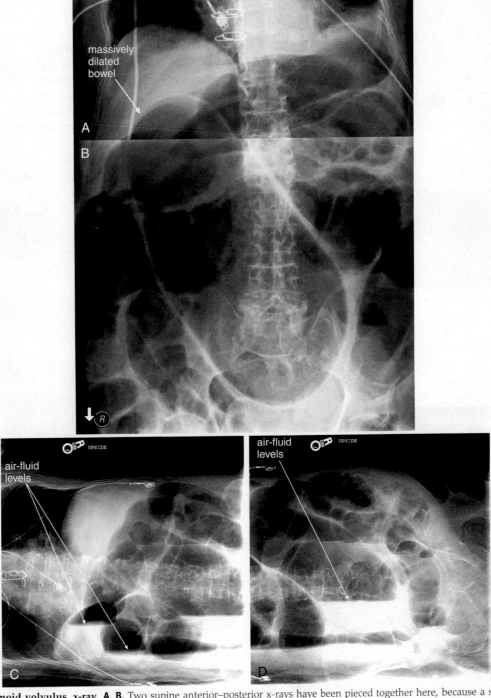

Figure 9-42. Sigmoid volvulus, x-ray. A, B, Two supine anterior–posterior x-rays have been pieced together here, because a single x-ray did not include the entire abdomen. **C, D,** Lateral decubitus x-ray images. Another example of sigmoid volvulus. This 88-year-old nursing home patient presented from a nursing home with increased abdominal distension. As expected, no air–fluid levels are seen on the supine views **(A, B).** Decubitus views **(C, D)** show air–fluid levels, as well as massively dilated bowel. Because of other medical conditions, the patient did not undergo surgery for this emergency condition. A barium enema was attempted for reduction (Figure 9-43) but was unsuccessful. The patient died the following day.

fully cross the diameter of the small bowel. The normal diameter of the large bowel on x-ray is less than 5 cm,[112] although dilatation beyond this degree can occur with ileus. A large bowel greater than 8 cm in diameter suggests mechanical obstruction, although diameters as great as 10 cm have been observed in ileus (see Figure 9-32).[111] If the ileocecal valve is not competent, large-bowel obstruction may lead to small-bowel dilatation, because large-bowel contents reflux through the ileocecal valve. When the ileocecal valve is competent, it can result in massive dilatation of the large bowel, because retrograde reflux of large-bowel contents is prevented. In this circumstance, the cecum may exceed 9 to 13 cm, with risk for perforation. Pseudoobstruction caused by fecal impaction can also occur and has a similar x-ray appearance with dilated large bowel (see Figure 9-50).

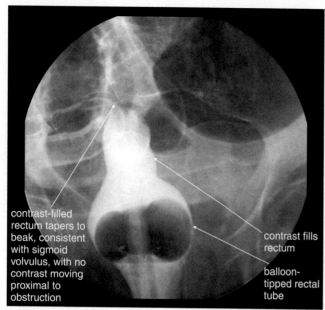

Figure 9-43. Sigmoid volvulus, barium enema. Barium enema from same patient as Figure 9-42. A rectal catheter and balloon have been inserted. Water-soluble contrast has been instilled, distending the rectum. However, contrast does not enter the sigmoid colon, ending instead in a narrow beak, consistent with sigmoid volvulus.

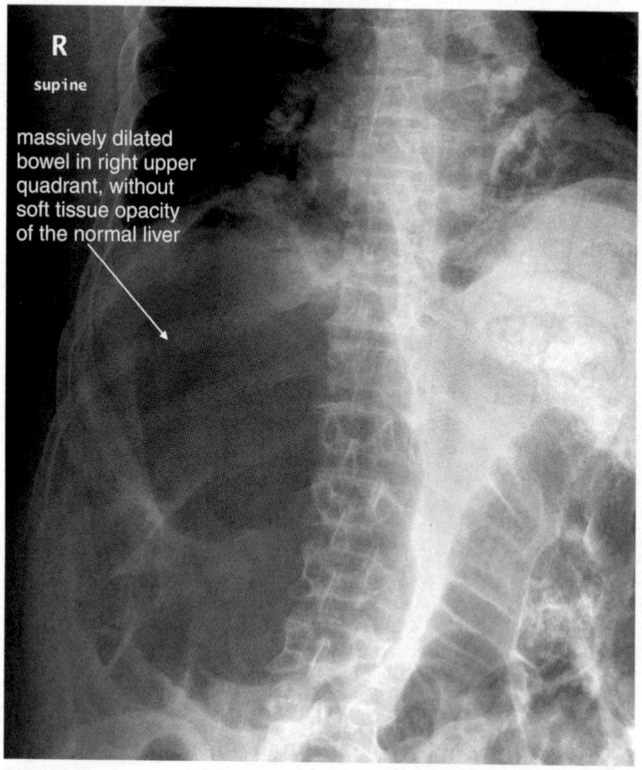

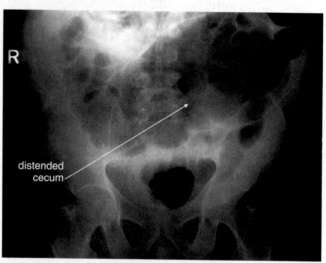

Figure 9-45. Cecal volvulus, x-ray. Same patient as Figure 9-44. Interestingly, the patient had been admitted on the trauma service the prior day following a fall, and plain x-rays of the abdomen had revealed a distended cecum at that time, located in the lower abdomen. Compare this initial image with the x-ray in Figure 9-44, taken at the time of the patient's return to the emergency department. Given the change in the position of the cecum, cecal volvulus appeared to be a strong possibility.

Prone and lateral decubitus x-rays are sometimes used to distinguish ileus from mechanical large-bowel obstruction. In ileus, air can fill the rectum with repositioning of the patient; in mechanical obstruction, air cannot pass the point of obstruction to reach the rectum. In most cases today, these additional x-ray maneuvers should be forgone in favor of CT, which provides more information about the nature and location of the obstruction, as well as complications such as perforation.

X-ray has a reported sensitivity of 84% and specificity of 72% for large-bowel obstruction, when clinical history

Figure 9-44. Cecal volvulus, x-ray. This 53-year-old male presented with severe abdominal pain and distension. The initial concern by the emergency physicians was a possible incarcerated hernia or perforation of bowel. X-rays showed a massively distended bowel segment in the right upper quadrant. This supine x-ray cannot assess for subdiaphragmatic air, but concerningly, the right upper quadrant is extremely lucent, without the usual soft-tissue opacity of the liver. Free air (pneumoperitoneum) was suspected. Abdominal computed tomography was performed (see Figures 9-47 through 9-49).

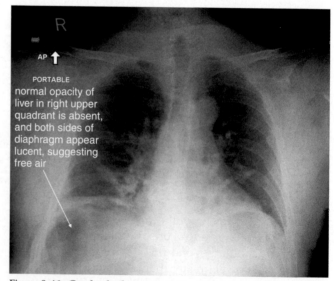

Figure 9-46. Cecal volvulus, x-ray. Same patient as Figures 9-44 and 9-45. This upright chest x-ray obtained on the day of the patient's return to the ED is concerning for free peritoneal air under the right diaphragm. The normal opacity of the liver is not present—both sides of the diaphragm appear lucent. Abdominal CT was performed (see Figures 9-47 through 9-49).

is provided to the radiologist.[113] However, large studies with appropriate blinding have not been performed.

Contrast Enema for Large-Bowel Obstruction.
Acute contrast enema is 96% sensitive and 98% specific[113]—but is rarely performed today in the emergency

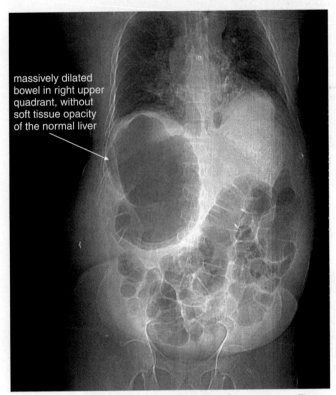

Figure 9-47. Cecal volvulus, CT scout image. Same patient as Figures 9-44 through 9-46. The scout image from the patient's CT again shows a massively dilated loop of bowel in the right upper quadrant.

department.[114] Contrast enema studies have lost favor as CT has improved the diagnosis of large-bowel obstruction and its complications, as well as that of alternative disease processes. Unlike contrast enema, CT can identify not only luminal narrowing and intrinsic masses but also extraluminal processes such as exophytic tumors and abscesses. Contrast enema can result in bowel perforation, again favoring CT for diagnosis when x-ray is nondiagnostic. Enema is contraindicated when ischemia, perforation, or peritonitis is suspected. Stewart et al.[115] performed a prospective study of 117 patients comparing x-ray and single contrast enema for the diagnosis of bowel obstruction. X-ray was only 52% specific, with enema showing free flow of contrast to the cecum in the remaining patients, consistent with pseudoobstruction.

Computed Tomography of Large-Bowel Obstruction.
Large-bowel obstruction diagnosis by CT relies on similar findings to those of small-bowel obstruction: the presence of dilated bowel proximal to a point of obstruction called the transition zone or point and collapsed bowel distal to this location (see Figures 9-33 through 9-36). Large bowel is considered dilated when the transverse diameter exceeds 8 cm by CT.[111] Without a transition zone to the collapsed distal colon, the degree of dilatation and the presence of air–fluid levels are not reliable for mechanical obstruction, because pseudoobstruction can result in diameters of 5 to 10 cm. Pseudoobstruction (also called Ogilvie's syndrome) is not a harmless condition, because massive dilatation of the colon caused by stool impaction can result in perforation. Cecal distension beyond 12 cm has been suggested as a threshold above which perforation is likely.[116-118] The point of obstruction of large bowel is

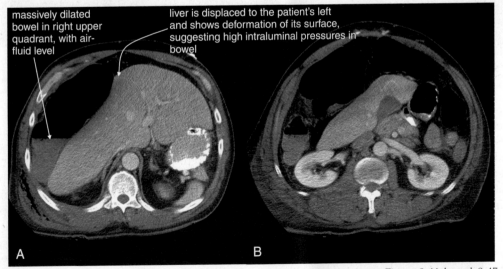

Figure 9-48. Cecal volvulus, large-bowel obstruction, CT with oral and IV contrast. Same patient as Figures 9-44 through 9-47. **A, B,** Axial images demonstrating massively dilated large bowel in the right upper quadrant. Air in this bowel segment is under such elevated pressure that it is exerting significant mass effect on the liver, deforming and displacing it to the patient's left. This is responsible for the plain x-ray appearance simulating free air on the x-rays in Figures 9-44 and 9-46. At laparotomy, the patient was found to have adhesions holding the cecum in the right upper quadrant, causing this obstruction. The patient underwent right hemicolectomy, appendectomy, and distal ileal resection because of poor viability of these structures.

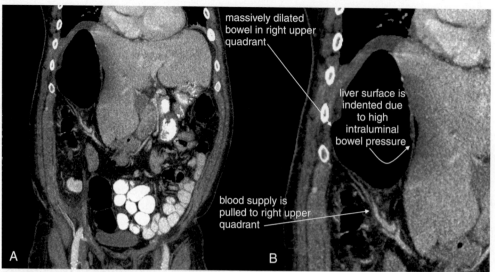

Figure 9-49. **Cecal volvulus, large-bowel obstruction, CT with oral and IV contrast, soft-tissue window.** Same patient as in Figures 9-44 through 9-48. On this coronal reconstruction, the dilated cecum is again seen in the right upper quadrant. Because it has changed its position, it has pulled its blood supply with it to the right upper quadrant. Again, mass effect on the liver is evident, suggesting very high intraluminal pressures in the cecum. **A,** Coronal image. **B,** Close-up.

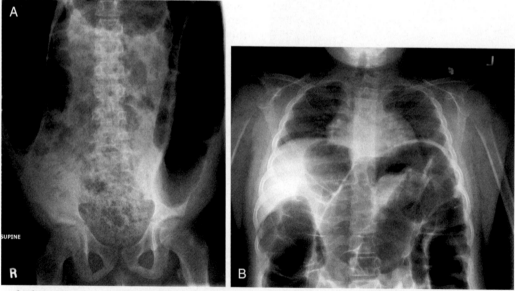

Figure 9-50. **Pseudoobstruction from fecal impaction, x-ray.** This 10-year-old boy presented with a history of chronic constipation and abdominal pain. His x-rays demonstrate massively dilated air-filled large bowel, and stool filling the most distal colon. He was suspected of Hirschsprung's disease and was taken to the operating room for disimpaction and biopsy, which was actually negative for Hirschsprung's. **A, B,** Supine x-ray images of the abdomen.

usually more easily recognized than the transition zone in a small-bowel obstruction, because the large bowel follows a predictable and readily traced course from the right lower quadrant to the hepatic flexure, across the posterior abdomen to the splenic flexure, and down the left lateral abdominal wall to the sigmoid colon and rectum.

False-positive CT results can occur when the distal colon appears collapsed in pseudoobstruction, with no colonic lesion seen at the transition zone. Stool within the colon may mimic an intrinsic mass (malignant polyp), appearing to narrow the lumen. Therefore, when

CT colonography is performed to evaluate the colon for polyps and cancers, cathartic bowel preparation is required to remove stool from the colon.[119-120] Some protocols also call for the patient to consume barium preparations with food before CT colonography to label any residual stool, preventing this diagnostic pitfall.[121] Stool typically contains air, whereas a malignant mass usually does not. A partially obstructing cancer can lead to an appearance with no or little proximal bowel dilatation, sometimes resulting in a false-negative CT. Gas production by bacteria distal to a point of obstruction can prevent the expected gasless appearance, again obscuring the diagnosis of obstruction. An ileus and a large-bowel

TABLE 9-6. CT Findings Suggesting Ischemia Complicating Small- or Large-Bowel Obstruction

CT Finding	Description
Triangular bowel loop	Suggestive of closed loop with strangulation
Abnormalities in the attached mesentery	Nonspecific, including increased or decreased enhancement
Beak sign[72]	Narrowing of the bowel lumen to a sharp point or beak at a point of tight obstruction or volvulus; insensitive but highly specific (sensitivity = 32%, specificity = 100%)
Bowel wall thickening >2 mm[73]	Suggestive of ischemia, inflammatory bowel disease, or infectious enteritis; Visible on CT without IV or oral contrast
Closed-loop obstruction	Grossly distended U-shaped loop of bowel with an abrupt transition to collapsed distal bowel loops, suggesting strangulating obstruction
Decreased bowel wall enhancement[72-73]	*After administration of IV contrast*, indicative of lack of blood flow to bowel and insensitive but highly specific (sensitivity = 34%, specificity = 100%)
Diffuse engorgement of mesenteric vasculature	Possibly suggestive of distal obstruction from volvulus or thrombosis
High attenuation in the bowel wall[75]	Bright appearance of the bowel wall, visible *without IV contrast*, indicative of hemorrhage into bowel wall and suggestive of bowel ischemia
Increased bowel wall enhancement[72-73]	*After administration of IV contrast*, suggestive of bowel ischemia but possible in reperfusion, infection, or inflammatory bowel
Large ascites	Nonspecific finding, because ascites can result from cirrhosis, heart failure, malignancy, or other causes other than ischemia; appears intermediate gray on soft-tissue CT windows, around 0-20 HU
Mesenteric fluid[73]	Intermediate gray with Hounsfield density around 0-20 HU, visible on CT with IV contrast, suggesting but not specific for bowel ischemia (normal mesenteric fat is darker due to fat content, around −50 to −100 HU)
Pneumatosis intestinali or pneumatosis coli	Gas (black) in bowel wall, suggesting infarction or presence of gas-forming organisms
Portal venous gas	Always abnormal and suggestive of bowel infarction
Target sign	Two concentric layers of enhancement of the thickened bowel wall
Two adjacent collapsed bowel loops at the site of obstruction[75a]	Represent the afferent and efferent bowel segments leading into a closed loop created by bowel volvulus.
Unusual course of mesenteric vasculature	Possibly suggestive of volvulus or malrotation
Whirl sign (also called the whirlpool sign)	A pinwheel appearance of blood vessels converging on a central point of volvulus

HU, Hounsfield unit.

obstruction can have a similar appearance, with dilated large and small bowel, sometimes leading to misdiagnosis of a more benign condition.

Causes of Large-Bowel Obstruction and Imaging Consequences. Large-bowel obstructions may result from intralumenal processes (e.g., fecal impaction or intussusceptions); intrinsic pathology, defined as processes affecting the colonic wall (e.g., carcinoma or inflammatory bowel disease); and extrinsic processes (e.g., adjacent diverticular abscess, volvulus, or hernias; see Figures 9-32 and 9-33). Carcinoma (60%), volvulus (10%-15%), and diverticulitis are the three main causes of large-bowel obstruction and are distinguished by CT.[111] Carcinoma complicated by perforation and diverticulitis (discussed in detail later in this chapter)

may be difficult to distinguish by CT. Both may demonstrate fat stranding adjacent to the colon and loculated or free extraluminal air. Adenopathy may be present in both conditions, although this should heighten concern for cancer. Regardless, initial emergency department therapy is similar, with antibiotics and possible surgery depending on severity of additional findings, such as evidence of perforation or ischemia.

Sigmoid volvulus (see Figures 9-37 through 9-43) accounts for about 70% of large-bowel volvulus and cecal volvulus (see Figures 9-44 through 9-49) makes up about 25%, with transverse colon accounting for the remainder. On x-ray, large-bowel volvulus leads to an enormously distended large bowel with fluid levels, usually in the left abdomen, and arising from the pelvis.

Sigmoid volvulus characteristically assumes a "coffee bean" shape on supine x-rays (see Figures 9-37, 9-38, and 9-42). Cecal volvulus (Figures 9-44 through 9-46) can result in displacement of the cecum to the left upper quadrant, although in almost half of cases it remains in the right lower quadrant. The volvulized cecum may also assume a coffee bean shape with haustral markings.[122] Historically, x-ray allowed prospective detection in only about 50% of cases of cecal volvulus—probably because of the associated appearance of dilated small bowel, suggesting ileus.[122] X-ray findings can be quite nonspecific for sigmoid volvulus, although in a study of 17 patients with sigmoid volvulus and 5 without, three signs appeared specific: the presence of the loop apex under the left hemidiaphragm, the convergence of the walls of the sigmoid colon in the inferior abdomen left of the midline, and the overlap of the walls of the volvulus with the descending colon.[123]

In the case of cecal or sigmoid volvulus, sometimes a bird's-beak appearance is seen on plain x-ray and on CT. This represents the point of volvulus, where twisting of the colon narrows the lumen, just as an air-filled balloon narrows when twisted at its midpoint.[111] In a variant called cecal bascule, the cecum folds anteriorly without twisting, also creating obstruction. Usually the cecum then appears as an enlarged bowel loop in the central abdomen.[124] If x-rays are not obtained, the CT topogram (also called the scout image) can reveal similar findings and can be helpful to review. CT findings of sigmoid or cecal volvulus include the "whirl" sign, composed of the collapsed colon, engorged mesenteric vessels, and twisted mesentery with a bird's beak appearance of the colon proximal and distal to the point of volvulus.[111,125-127] The bird's beak may not be oriented in the axial plane and may require additional imaging planes (e.g., sagittal, coronal, or oblique) for best demonstration. True three-dimensional rendering from the CT dataset can also clarify the form of volvulus.[124] Although axial CT images may suffice for diagnosis, Aufort et al.[64] and Filippone et al.[81] describe the use of multiplanar reformations, including coronal and curved sagittal reformations, to provide information such as the site and cause of bowel obstruction.

Identification of the form of volvulus is of therapeutic importance, because endoscopic detorsion of sigmoid volvulus is first-line therapy in the absence of signs of perforation. Cecal volvulus is usually treated surgically. Large-bowel obstruction from fecal impaction, foreign bodies, intussusception, diverticular disease, inflammatory bowel disease, or ischemic colitis may also occur.

Ischemic changes of large-bowel obstruction are similar to those found in small-bowel obstruction, including circumferential bowel wall thickening, stranding of adjacent fat, mural pneumatosis, and lack of large-bowel wall enhancement with administered IV contrast.[111] However, circumferential thickening can also be seen with infectious or ischemic colitis or with inflammatory bowel disease, any of which may lead to bowel obstruction.

How Sensitive and Specific Is Computed Tomography for Large-Bowel Obstruction? How accurately does CT detect large-bowel obstruction? Surprisingly, only two studies address this question explicitly. Frager et al.[128] prospectively compared CT with surgery, clinical course, contrast enema, or endoscopic findings in 75 patients with suspected large-bowel obstruction. CT was 96% sensitive for obstruction and 93% specific. The point of obstruction was identified correct in 94% of patients. Contrast enema was only 80% sensitive for obstruction. Beattie et al.[129] studied 44 patients with suspected large-bowel obstruction and found the sensitivity and specificity of CT to be 91%. In this study, most patients received IV but not enteral contrast. The authors supplemented typical supine position CT scanning with selective prone and decubitus position scans, so the reported sensitivity and specificity might not be achieved with routine scanning in the supine position. However, the positive and negative likelihood ratios (10.1 and 0.1, respectively) would make CT a valuable test to rule in or exclude large-bowel obstruction—if future studies confirm these findings.

Conditions Involving Inflammatory Changes of Bowel

In the sections that follow, we discuss three important diagnoses involving inflammatory changes of bowel: appendicitis, diverticulitis, and inflammatory bowel disease (including ulcerative colitis and Crohn's disease). X-ray is typically not helpful in the diagnosis of conditions involving bowel inflammation, because it does not directly visualize bowel inflammation and lacks sensitivity and specificity for these diseases. CT has become the most commonly applied emergency department modality for these conditions, although ultrasound plays an important role in the diagnosis of appendicitis in children and pregnant women.

Appendicitis

Figures 9-51 through 9-57 demonstrate imaging findings of appendicitis. Suspected appendicitis remains a key reason to obtain abdominal imaging. It also is a focus for many controversies in abdominal imaging, ranging from the need for or benefit from imaging of any form, to the value of contrast agents, to the optimal imaging modality. Appendicitis is one of the most intensively researched areas in emergency diagnostic imaging, yet questions remain. We divide our discussion into several sections. First, we present a simplified explanation about the potential use of a variety of common image modalities, avoiding areas of debate. Next, we ask a series of

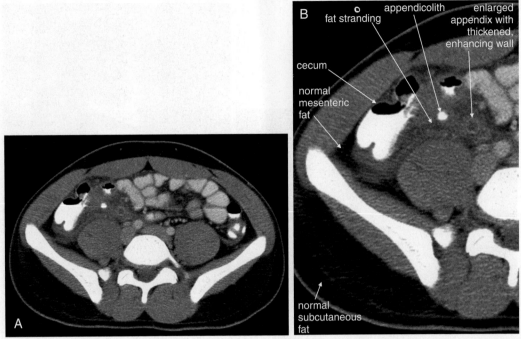

Figure 9-51. Appendicitis, CT with IV and oral contrast. This CT demonstrates classic findings of appendicitis in an 18-year-old male with right lower quadrant pain, as seen with CT with IV and oral contrast. Studies suggest that CT without contrast has similar sensitivity and specificity. An enlarged appendix is seen near the cecum as a right lower quadrant tubular structure in short-axis cross section, giving it a circular appearance. The surrounding fat shows stranding, a smoky appearance, indicating inflammation (compare with normal mesenteric and subcutaneous fat, which is nearly black). The appendiceal wall shows enhancement, a brightening after administration of IV contrast. This slice also shows an appendicolith, an occasional finding of appendicitis. It does not appear to be within the appendix in this slice, because the appendix bends in and out of the plane of this slice. An appendicolith usually appears as a calcified (white) rounded structure—visible without any contrast. **A,** Axial CT image. **B,** Close-up. Figure 9-52 demonstrates the appendix in long-axis cross section as it emerges from the cecum.

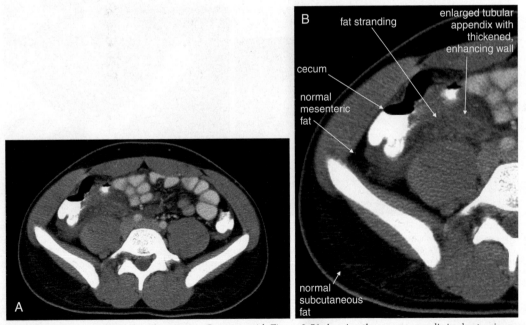

Figure 9-52. Appendicitis, CT with IV and oral contrast. Compare with Figure 9-51 showing the same appendix in short-axis cross section, with a circular appearance. When considering appendicitis, search carefully for either the circular cross section or the tubular profile, because the appearance depends on the orientation of the appendix relative to the slice. When perpendicular to the slice, the appendix appears circular. When oriented parallel to the plane of the slice, the appendix appears tubular. **A,** Axial CT image. **B,** Close-up.

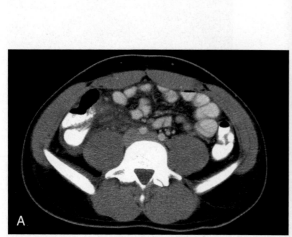
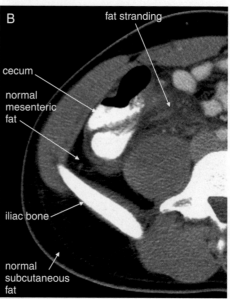

Figure 9-53. **Appendicitis, CT with IV and oral contrast.** Same patient as Figures 9-51 and 9-52. This CT slice is taken slightly cephalad to the prior two slices and shows fat stranding in the right lower quadrant. The appendix itself is not visible in this slice. Note the smoky gray appearance of mesenteric fat medial to the cecum, compared with the nearly black appearance of normal mesenteric and subcutaneous fat. Fat stranding should alert you to the possibility of appendicitis, even if the appendix itself is not visible. Orient yourself to your location: the iliac wings of the pelvis are visible, and the cecum is present in the right abdomen. Remember that fat stranding is a finding of inflammation, not of appendicitis specifically. Other diagnoses, such as cecal diverticulitis, colitis, and terminal ileitis, might cause right lower quadrant fat stranding. Occasionally, appendicitis can occur without significant fat stranding, so examine the CT carefully for the appendix. **A,** Axial CT image. **B,** Close-up.

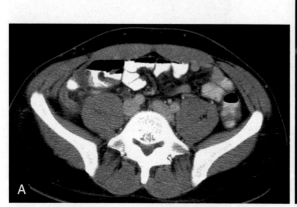
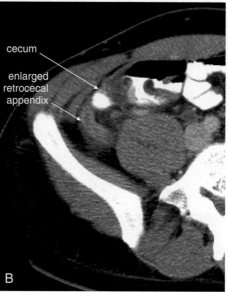

Figure 9-54. **Appendicitis, CT with IV and oral contrast.** This patient with appendicitis has a retrocecal appendix, located deep to the cecum and lateral to the psoas muscle. This slice captures the appendix in long-axis cross section, with its enlarged (>6 mm), tubular shape and thickened, enhancing wall. On this slice, less fat stranding is visible than in the previous figures, though stranding is visible on careful inspection. **A,** Axial image. **B,** Close-up. Remember that the appendix can have many orientations relative to the cecum, so the region anterior, posterior, medial, and lateral to the cecum must be inspected.

clinically oriented questions and examine the evidence available to answer these more controversial issues.

X-ray for Appendicitis. X-rays were a common historical starting point for evaluation of appendicitis, but they have little diagnostic value and should generally be avoided. The classic x-ray findings of appendicitis include a radiodensity in the right lower quadrant, called an appendicolith. Yet this is found on x-ray in fewer than 20% of cases of appendicitis.[130] Multiple studies have shown a low diagnostic yield for x-ray. Other findings sometimes seen on x-ray include obscuration of the normal right psoas muscle and properitoneal fat interface, presumably because of periappendiceal inflammation, but these are seen with equal frequency in patients with and without appendicitis

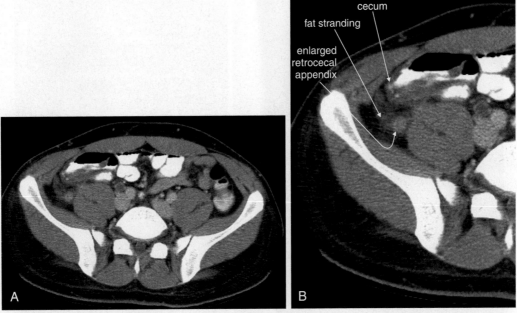

Figure 9-55. Appendicitis, CT with IV and oral contrast. Same patient as Figure 9-54. This slice captures the appendix in short-axis cross section, with an enlarged (>6 mm), circular shape and thickened, enhancing wall. Compare with the tubular appearance seen in Figure 9-54, seen two slices away in the same patient. On this slice, fat stranding is visible. **A,** Axial image. **B,** Close-up.

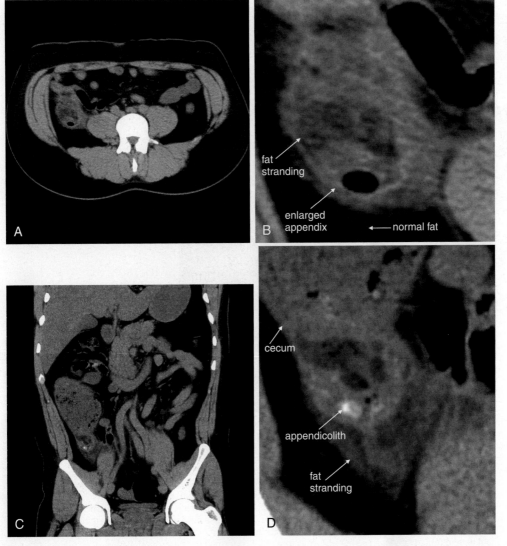

Figure 9-56. Appendicitis, noncontrast CT, soft-tissue window. This 34-year-old male complained of periumbilical pain and right flank pain. Noncontrast CT was performed following a typical protocol for renal stone diagnosis. **A,** An axial CT slice shows an enlarged appendix with surrounding fat stranding. **B,** Close-up. **C,** Coronal reconstruction shows similar findings. Dense material within the appendix may represent an appendicolith—one was identified by the pathologist after appendectomy. **D,** Close-up.

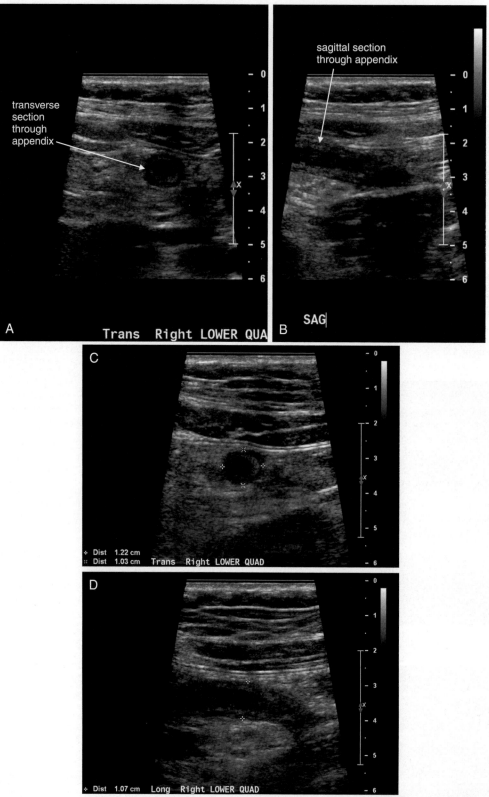

Figure 9-57. Appendicitis, ultrasound. Ultrasound is an alternative diagnostic imaging modality to CT for appendicitis. Unlike CT scan, ultrasound exposes the patient to no ionizing radiation, and it has been advocated as the first-line imaging modality in children, pregnant women, and thin adults. The appendix may be difficult to visualize in obese patients using ultrasound. Abnormal findings include a tubular structure exceeding 6 mm in diameter in the right lower quadrant, as well as right lower quadrant fluid collection that may indicate perforation and abscess formation. Hyperemia of the appendix may also be documented with Doppler technique. If the appendix is seen and tenderness is elicited by palpation with the ultrasound probe, this finding is the analogue of the sonographic Murphy's sign and may increase diagnostic specificity. Enlarged right lower quadrant lymph nodes may simulate appendicitis but should be distinguished on careful examination from the more tubular appendix. Ultrasound is reported to have lower sensitivity than CT but high specificity, so it can be used to rule in disease but not to rule out appendicitis. If the appendix is not clearly visualized, evaluation for appendicitis should continue with CT scan, clinical observation, or other strategies such as laparoscopy. This ultrasound shows a tubular right lower quadrant structure in transverse (short-axis, **A, C**) and sagittal (long-axis, **B, D**) cross sections. This structure is over 1 cm in diameter, concerning for appendicitis. The patient was 14 weeks pregnant at the time and underwent laparoscopic appendectomy that confirmed the ultrasound diagnosis.

and therefore have no discriminatory value.[131] Rao et al.[132] reviewed 821 consecutive patients hospitalized for suspected appendicitis, 78% of whom underwent x-ray. Radiographic abnormalities were seen in 51% of patients with appendicitis and 47% of those without appendicitis, with no radiographic finding being sensitive or specific. Even in the 10% of cases in which the x-ray suggested a specific condition, these failed to match the final diagnosis in 57%. Although the cost of x-ray was low ($67), the utility was so low that the cost per specific diagnosis was $1593, exceeding the cost for CT ($270).

One important reason for the lack of utility of x-ray is that treatment of appendicitis has evolved from open appendectomy to laparoscopic appendectomy for uncomplicated cases and frequent percutaneous drainage with antibiotic therapy in cases with complications such as loculated abscess. Even in the minority of cases in which x-ray findings of appendicolith support the diagnosis of appendicitis, x-ray does not provide additional information relevant to modern management strategies.

Barium Enema for Appendicitis. Before the advent of CT, barium enema was used periodically in assessment of appendicitis. Although a mass effect on the cecum and nonfilling of the appendix were described as diagnostic of appendicitis, these findings can be seen in nonsurgical disease processes such as small-bowel obstruction, enterocolitis, pelvic adhesions, and pelvic inflammatory disease.[133] Barium enema is generally no longer indicated for diagnosis of appendicitis. The ACR rates contrast enema as two or three (meaning "usually not appropriate") out of nine on its appropriateness scale, depending on the clinical scenario.[134]

Computed Tomography for Appendicitis. Despite intense research into CT for appendicitis, many controversies remain, which we address in the text that follows:
- What is the sensitivity of CT for appendicitis?
- What are the CT findings of appendicitis?
- Does abdominal CT reduce the rate of negative appendectomy and perforation? In which patient populations?
- Which patients benefit from abdominal CT for the diagnosis of appendicitis?
- Do clinical decision rules assist in selection of patients for imaging?
- Is oral, rectal, or intravenous contrast required for the diagnosis of appendicitis by CT? In which patients?
- When CT fails to visualize the appendix but is otherwise normal, is appendicitis excluded?
- When computed tomography findings are equivocal, what is the likelihood of appendicitis?
- What imaging approach is best in children?
- What imaging approach is best in pregnant women?

What Is the Sensitivity of Computed Tomography for Appendicitis? CT is given the highest rating by the ACR in its appropriateness criteria, for evaluation of adults with suspected appendicitis. CT is suggested as possibly appropriate by the ACR following negative or equivocal ultrasound in children and pregnant women.[134] There is little doubt that CT is a sensitive and specific imaging modality for appendicitis, capable of identifying alternative diagnoses and complications including perforation and abscess formation. A metaanalysis of prospective studies comparing CT and ultrasound found CT to be 94% sensitive and 95% specific.[135] Another systematic review of 23 studies found CT to be highly sensitive and specific, with or without oral contrast. The range of reported sensitivity is 83% to 97%, and for specificity the range is 93% to 98%.[32]

Computed Tomography Findings of Appendicitis. On CT scan, the normal appendix is a narrow tubular structure emerging from the cecum. It may occupy many different positions: descending into the pelvis, projecting medially or laterally from the cecum, or lying retrocecally. The upper limit of size of the normal appendix is 6 mm. The wall thickness is generally less than 1 mm.[136] The normal appendix may contain air or enteral contrast, but a calcified appendicolith is not normally present. The pericecal and periappendiceal fat normally show no inflammatory stranding or free fluid. These normal findings naturally give rise to criteria to identify an abnormal appendix.

An abnormal appendix is enlarged in cross-sectional diameter, is thick walled, and may contain an appendicolith. The surrounding fat often shows inflammatory stranding, a brightened appearance discussed earlier in this chapter. Free fluid may be present adjacent to the appendix or in dependent portions of the abdomen and pelvis. Air may be observed outside of the lumen of the appendix if perforation has occurred. An abscess or inflammatory phlegmon may be present in cases of perforation. The difference between true abscess and phlegmon is one of degree; an abscess typically has discrete borders and is fluid filled, whereas a phlegmon represents inflamed tissues without discrete abscess and may have less well-delineated margins.[137] All of these findings are potentially visible without the administration of any contrast agents. Enteral contrast (oral or rectal) theoretically might improve the diagnosis of appendicitis in several ways. First, by filling the cecum and terminal ileum with contrast, the bowel lumen is identified and can be discriminated from a fluid- and air-filled abscess. Second, a normal appendix might be expected to fill with enteral contrast, whereas an obstructed or edematous appendix might not. IV contrast might be expected to improve the diagnosis of appendicitis as well. In the presence of appendicitis, the appendix shows abnormally high enhancement with IV contrast, drawing attention to the appendix, which can be difficult to identify because of its small size and variable position. IV contrast may also cause rim enhancement of a periappendiceal abscess. The evidence for and against contrast is discussed later in this section. Table 9-7 lists CT findings of appendicitis with their reported sensitivity and specificity. Figures 9-51 through 9-56 demonstrate CT findings of appendicitis.

Because the appendix can be present in a variety of locations and with a variable course, images should be inspected for different cross-sectional appearances. In one study, the appendix was located more than 5 cm from McBurney's point in 36% of cases.[138] On axial slices, the cecum should be identified first, because the appendix arises from this structure. The cecum should be a large blind pouch filled with air (black) and stool

TABLE 9-7. Findings of Appendicitis Using Computed Tomography With Intravenous Contrast*

CT Sign	Sensitivity	Specificity
Abscess	9%	93%
Appendiceal intraluminal air	**21%**	**66%**
Appendiceal wall enhancement	75%	85%
Appendiceal wall thickening	66%	96%
Appendicolith	16%	100%
Enlarged appendix (>6 mm diameter)	93%	92%
Extraluminal air	8%	97%[137]
Extraluminal fluid	**17%**	**78%**
Focal cecal apical thickening	17%	100%
Intramural air	4%	100%
Lymphadenopathy	**41%**	**58%**
No identification of the appendix†	7%	98%
Periappendiceal fat stranding	87%	74%
Phlegmon	7%	99%
Segmental colonic wall thickening	**1%**	**87**
Segmental terminal ileal wall thickening	**6%**	**81**

Sensitivity and specificity are given for the most discriminatory CT findings.
Adapted from Choi D, Park H, Lee YR, et al: The most useful findings for diagnosing acute appendicitis on contrast-enhanced helical CT. Acta Radiol 44:574-582, 2003.
*Darkened rows indicate findings that are neither sensitive nor specific and therefore should not be used to rule-in or rule-out appendicitis.
†Subsequent publications suggest that failure to identify the appendix is not pathological when all other CT findings are normal.

(intermediate gray), located in the right lower quadrant. In most patients, the cecum lies near the level of the iliac crest. Another means of locating the cecum is to identify the ascending colon in the right upper quadrant medial to the liver and to follow the cecum through consecutive caudad slices until it terminates in the right lower quadrant. Three common appearances of the appendix occur on axial slices, depending on the orientation of the appendix relative to the axial plane. If the appendix is perpendicular to the axial plane, it will appear circular in cross section. If it is oriented parallel to the axial plane, it will appear tubular. And if the appendix is oriented obliquely to the axial plane, it will appear elliptic in cross section. Coronal imaging planes can assist in identification of an appendix not identified on axial planes.

Once the appendix is identified, it should be inspected for pathologic changes of appendicitis. The diameter should be measured; a diameter exceeding 6 mm is consistent with appendicitis. The wall thickness should be measured; a thickness greater than 1 mm suggests appendicitis.[136] If IV contrast has been administered, the appendiceal wall should be brighter than other normal bowel wall or the nearby psoas muscle. The presence of an intraappendiceal radiodensity (bright white on a soft-tissue CT window) is consistent with appendicolith, although its presence does not prove that the appendix is actively inflamed, in the absence of other findings. The fat surrounding the appendix should be inspected for stranding; comparison with fat in other locations, such as subcutaneous fat or remote intra peritoneal or retroperitoneal fat, may assist in recognition of subtle stranding. Normal fat should appear quite dark and homogeneous. Extremely thin patients with little intraperitoneal fat can present a diagnostic challenge, because they have no substrate for inflammatory fat stranding. Adjacent extraluminal air, free fluid, or abscess should be noted. We devised the mnemonic SCALPEL (Table 9-8) to guide assessment of the appendix for changes suggesting appendicitis.

Ultrasound for Appendicitis. Ultrasound is a common alternative diagnostic modality to CT scan for appendicitis. Advantages of ultrasound include portability, the absence of any exposure to ionizing radiation (a major concern with CT, especially in children, young adults, and pregnant women), and the absence of need for oral or injected contrast agents. Ultrasound disadvantages include operator dependence (a term used to describe the variable diagnostic performance of ultrasound in the hands of ultrasonographers of varying skill and experience) and limited ability to visualize the appendix in patients with significant fat stores or overlying bowel gas. Ultrasound is generally found to be quite specific (~93%-94% in multiple studies) but relatively insensitive (83%-88%) (Table 9-9).[135,139-141] In

TABLE 9-8. CT Findings of Appendicitis: SCALPEL Mnemonic

Term	Description
Stranding	Fat stranding suggests regional inflammation, possibly because of appendicitis.
Cecum	The appendix originates from the cecum, which should be identified first to help localize the appendix. The cecum may show wall thickening, suggesting appendicitis.
Air	Air outside of the lumen of the appendix is pathologic and suggests perforation. Air within the appendiceal wall is also abnormal.
Large	The normal appendix is <6 mm; an enlarged appendix >6 mm suggests appendicitis. Wall thickening >1 mm also suggests appendicitis.
Phlegmon	Inflammatory changes surrounding the appendix suggest a perforated appendix. A heterogeneous collection called a phlegmon may be seen. If the appendix has ruptured, a pericecal phlegmon may be the only remaining evidence, because the appendix itself may not be seen.
Enhancement	The wall of an abnormal appendix enhances with IV contrast and appears brighter than the normal bowel or the normal psoas muscle.
Lith	An appendicolith is a calcified stone sometimes found in the lumen of an inflamed appendix.

patients without appendicitis, the normal appendix can be difficult to identify, with as few as 2.4% of normal appendixes found in one study.[142]

Van Randen et al.[141] performed a metaanalysis of studies that compared CT and ultrasound in the same population and found that CT performed more accurately, though the performance of both tests was quite dependent on the prevalence of disease. In patients with low pretest probability and a positive ultrasound or CT, the possibility of a false-positive test should be considered. Overall, CT had a positive likelihood ratio of 9.29, indicating a high probability of appendicitis with a positive CT. Ultrasound had a positive likelihood ratio of only 4.5, which may not be adequate to rule in disease in cases of low pretest probability (recall that a positive likelihood ratio greater than 10 is generally felt to increase the probability of disease to a clinically actionable level). Negative likelihood ratios for CT and ultrasound were 0.1 and 0.27, respectively. Recall that a negative likelihood ratio less than 0.1 is felt to exclude disease with a high degree of certainty, except in cases of very high pretest probability. Thus a negative CT rules out appendicitis in most patients, whereas a negative ultrasound does not.

Multiple authors have proposed the following use of ultrasound. In patients in whom appendicitis is clinically suspected but additional confirmation is desired, ultrasound should be the first diagnostic imaging test performed. If ultrasound confirms appendicitis, no further imaging may be required because of high specificity. If ultrasound does not confirm appendicitis, CT may be required, as a result of the poor sensitivity of ultrasound. Target populations in whom ultrasound use as

TABLE 9-9. Sensitivity and Specificity of Ultrasound for Appendicitis, Compared With Computed Tomography

Study	Population	Ultrasound Sensitivity (95% CI)	Ultrasound Specificity (95% CI)	CT Sensitivity (95% CI)	CT Specificity (95% CI)
Doria et al.[135]	Pediatric metaanalysis, 26 studies, 9356 patients	88% (86%-90%)	94% (92%-95%)	94% (92%-97%)	95% (94%-97%)
Doria et al.[135]	Adult metaanalysis, 31 studies, 4341 patients	83% (78%-87%)	93% (90%-96%)	94% (92%-95%)	94% (94%-96%)
Terasawa et al.[140]	Adults and adolescents	86% (83%-88%)	81% (78%-84%)	94% (91%-95%)	95% (93%-96%)
Study	**Population**	**Ultrasound Positive Likelihood Ratio (95% CI)**	**Ultrasound Negative Likelihood Ratio (95% CI)**	**CT Positive Likelihood Ratio (95% CI)**	**CT Negative Likelihood Ratio (95% CI)**
Van Randen et al.[141]	Adults and adolescents, metaanalysis of 6 studies, 671 patients	4.5 (3.0-6.7)	0.27 (0.17-0.43)	9.29 (6.9-12.6)	0.1 (0.06-0.17)

the first diagnostic test should be encouraged are young patients and pregnant patients, arising from concerns about radiation exposures from CT. Thin patients of any age may be reasonable candidates for ultrasound. Conversely, ultrasound is likely to be nondiagnostic in obese patients, and CT may more reasonably be the first test. In older adults and the elderly, in whom radiation exposures from CT are of little concern and in whom multiple other serious abdominal conditions may be present, CT may be the more appropriate initial test.

Ultrasound for appendicitis is a focused examination. The examiner inspects the right lower quadrant, often starting with the location of tenderness identified by the patient. An abnormal appendix exceeds 6 mm in diameter and is incompressible. Sometimes a hypoechoic or heterogeneously echoic fluid collection representing abscess may also be identified. A normal appendix may be difficult to identify because of its small size. Figure 9-57 demonstrates ultrasound findings of appendicitis.

Magnetic Resonance Imaging for Appendicitis.
MRI represents a third option for imaging of suspected appendicitis. MRI is generally not a first-line test because of expense and limited availability but is useful in patients with equivocal results of other modalities or in patients in whom radiation exposures are a particular concern, such as children and pregnant females. The normal appendix on MRI is less than or equal to 6 mm in diameter and may be filled with air and oral contrast material. MRI findings of appendicitis include an appendiceal diameter greater than 7 mm and the presence of periappendiceal inflammatory changes.[143] MRI has high reported sensitivity and specificity. Pedrosa et al.[143] reported MRI to be 100% sensitive and 93% specific in a consecutive series of 51 pregnant patients—though only 4 patients in this series had appendicitis. In another study, Pedrosa et al.[144] reviewed 148 consecutive pregnant patients evaluated for acute appendicitis, 140 of whom had both ultrasound and MRI. MRI was 100% sensitive (14 of 14) and 93% specific, although the small number of patients in this study results in wide CIs.

Israel et al.[145] found MRI to be 100% sensitive and specific for appendicitis when the appendix was visualized, though only four patients with appendicitis were diagnosed by MRI. MRI was unable to identify the appendix in a fifth patient with appendicitis.

Cobben et al.[146] found MRI to be 100% sensitive and specific for appendicitis in pregnancy—but in a series of only 12 patients, 3 with appendicitis.

Chabanova et al.[147] examined a fast, unenhanced MRI technique in 48 patients and found sensitivity of 83% to 93% and specificity of 50%-83%. This study was not restricted to pregnant patients.

Basaran and Basaran[148] performed a systematic review and compared the pooled sensitivity and specificity of CT and MRI, following a nondiagnostic ultrasound in a pregnant patient. CT was 87.5% sensitive and 97.4% specific, whereas MRI was 80% sensitive and 99% specific. Although the studies on MRI in pregnancy are limited, the ACR[134] rates MRI as seven on its nine-point appropriateness scale, just below ultrasound (with a score of eight). In children, the ACR gives MRI a rating of five of nine, below both ultrasound (eight of nine) and CT (seven of nine).

Appendicitis Decision Rules.
Imaging in suspected appendicitis carries economic costs, radiation exposures (in the case of CT), and potential harms, including adverse effects of IV contrast administration for CT. In patients with acute appendicitis, therapeutic delays while awaiting diagnostic imaging could lead to perforation, with increased morbidity or even mortality. Therefore a clinical decision rule to stratify appendicitis risk could improve imaging utilization with cost, radiation, time, and morbidity benefits. Patients at low risk for appendicitis might require no imaging, only clinical observation for signs of worsening. Patients at high risk might require no imaging but, rather, empiric surgical management. Patients with intermediate risk might represent a group in whom imaging could provide benefit by preventing unnecessary appendectomy, reducing perforation rate, and identifying alternative diagnoses.

Several scoring systems have been proposed, though none are widely accepted at this time. The Alvarado score incorporates elements from the classic history, physical examination, and laboratory abnormalities associated with appendicitis (Table 9-10).[149] The mnemonic MANTRELS is sometimes used to indicate the criteria (see Table 9-10). In a retrospective validation study of 150 patients aged 7 or older, an Alvarado score of 7 or higher predicted appendicitis with 100% specificity, whereas a score of 3 or lower ruled out appendicitis without use of imaging (sensitivity = 96.2%). Patients with intermediate Alvarado scores (4-6) required further testing for appendicitis. Further study is required to narrow CIs.[150]

Other investigators have suggested that the Alvarado score is too nonspecific for clinical use without CT. Kim et al.[151] prospectively scored 157 patients using the Alvarado score and a separate clinical impression by an emergency physician, in which patients were judged to have "clinically evident appendicitis" or not. Of 71 patients with clinically evident appendicitis, 19 did not have appendicitis (specificity = 71.6%). Of 52 patients with Alvarado scores greater than or equal to 8 (predicted high likelihood of appendicitis), 14 did not have appendicitis (specificity = 79%). CT was 95.5% specific, leading the authors to suggest that CT should be used

TABLE 9-10. Alvarado Score for Appendicitis, Also Known by the MANTRELS Mnemonic[149-150]

Criterion	Points
Migration of abdominal pain to the right iliac fossa	1
Anorexia or acetone (ketones) in the urine	1
Nausea or vomiting	1
Tenderness to palpation of the right lower quadrant	2
Rebound tenderness	1
Elevated temperature (37.3°C)	1
Leukocytosis, or >10,000 white blood cells per microliter in the serum	2
Shift to the left (an increase in the percentage of neutrophils in the serum white blood cell count)	1

Alvarado Scores of 3 or lower rule out appendicitis (sensitivity = 96.2%). Scores of 7 or higher rule in appendicitis (specificity = 100%). Scores of 4 to 6 require imaging. This score requires further validation. Adapted from Alvarado A: A practical score for the early diagnosis of acute appendicitis. Ann Emerg Med 1986;15:557-64; and McKay R, Shepherd J. The use of the clinical scoring system by Alvarado in the decision to perform computed tomography for acute appendicitis in the ED. Am J Emerg Med 25:489-493, 2007.

TABLE 9-11. Pediatric Appendicitis Score[152]

Criterion	Point Value
Right lower quadrant tenderness	2
Hop tenderness (or tenderness with cough or percussion)	2
Anorexia	1
Fever >38°C	1
Emesis	1
Pain migration	1
Leukocytosis >10,000	1
Neutrophilia ≥75% neutrophils	1

A score of 4 or less excludes appendicitis (sensitivity = 97.6%, negative predictive value = 97.7%). A score of 8 or more confirms appendicitis (specificity = 95.1%, positive predictive value = 85.2%). Scores of 5-7 require imaging. This scoring system requires further validation.
Adapted from Bhatt M, Joseph L, Ducharme FM, et al: Prospective validation of the pediatric appendicitis score in a Canadian pediatric emergency department. Acad Emerg Med 16:591-596, 2009.

even in patients with apparently high pretest probability to prevent negative appendectomy.

The Pediatric Appendicitis Score similarly incorporates classic features of appendicitis to develop a risk assessment (Table 9-11).[152] In a validation study of 246 children with a 34% rate of appendicitis, the score performed well in reducing imaging, limiting the negative appendectomy rate, and avoiding missed appendicitis. A score of five or greater detected appendicitis with a sensitivity of 97.6%, meaning that children with scores of four or less need no imaging. A score greater than or equal to eight gave a specificity of 95.1%, indicating a need for appendectomy without imaging. Patients with scores of five to seven required imaging to exclude or confirm appendicitis. Using this rule would have eliminated 41% of imaging, achieved a negative appendectomy rate of 8.8%, and resulted in a missed appendicitis rate of 2.4%.[152] Larger studies are required to validate these findings.

Birkhahn et al.[153] prospectively derived an appendicitis likelihood model in 439 patients. Patients with a white blood cell count of less than 9500 x 10^9/L and either no right lower quadrant tenderness or a neutrophil count of less than 54% were classified as low likelihood. Patients were classified as high likelihood if they had a white blood cell count greater than 13,000 x 10^9/L and either rebound tenderness or voluntary guarding with a neutrophil count greater than 82%. The authors

suggest that patients with neither high nor low likelihood undergo imaging, whereas patients with high and low likelihood undergo laparotomy and observation, respectively. Compared with actual clinical practice in the study population, use of this model would have reduced the number of missed cases of appendicitis from 10% to 1% and negative laparotomy from 14% to 5.6% while reducing imaging from 71% to 62%. This study was underpowered to prove statistical significance of these findings.

Clinical scoring systems have not yet achieved wide acceptance, partly because of disparate results among studies and lack of broad external validation of studies with promising results.

Imaging Controversies: Does Abdominal CT Reduce the Rate of Negative Appendectomy and Perforation? In Which Patient Populations?

Before the advent of CT and other imaging tests for appendicitis, therapeutic decisions rested on history, physical examination, and laboratory assessment. Lewis et al.[154] reviewed 1000 appendectomies performed between 1963 and 1973. The overall negative appendectomy rate was 20%, whereas in women between the ages of 20 and 40 years, the rate was higher than 40%—with more than two thirds of surgeries performed for nonsurgical lesions such as mesenteric adenitis, gastroenteritis, abdominal pain of uncertain cause, and pelvic inflammatory disease. The appendiceal perforation rate in this series was 21%. The benefit of any imaging modality for appendicitis can be measured in terms of reductions in these two rates. Hypothetically, a diagnostic test that delayed surgery might have a negative effect by increasing rupture rates, even if achieving a lower rate of negative appendectomy.

Numerous studies have examined the association of imaging practices, particular CT use, on these two rates. Most studies of this type are retrospective observational studies, often comparing a historical control period without imaging to a later period with high CT utilization rates. In other cases, studies compare outcomes in contemporaneous patient groups, some undergoing imaging and some not, without randomization. Studies of this type measure associations, not causation, but authors often conclude that a causative relationship exists between imaging and patient outcomes. A cause–effect relationship cannot be determined from studies of this type for several reasons. Among the most important, without randomization, patients selected to undergo diagnostic imaging likely differ from patients who are managed without imaging. Patients undergoing imaging may represent more equivocal cases, with atypical histories, ambiguous physical examination findings, and uncertain laboratory results. Patients selected for surgical therapy without imaging, or observation without imaging, likely represent more classically abnormal or normal presentations. Comparing outcomes among these patient categories and attributing the outcomes to the use of imaging ignores these baseline differences. Some studies attempt to account for or even statistically correct for baseline differences, but in reality a randomized controlled trial is required to allow a fair comparison of two diagnostic and treatment strategies. We consider some examples of this type of study here.

Numerous studies have documented the historical rate of negative appendectomy and perforation, correlated these with rising rates of CT utilization, and attempted to draw conclusions about the effect of CT on these important outcomes. Overall, most of these reports suggest a correlation between CT use and reduced rates of negative appendectomy in women of childbearing age, with lesser or no benefit in men or older women. Some studies suggest benefits in older adults. In children, some studies suggest lower rates of negative appendectomy with CT, whereas others suggest no benefit from CT. A handful of studies suggest lower perforation rates with CT use, though others show no difference. Most of the studies we review here (Table 9-12) suffer from the same methodologic flaw: they are not randomized, so patients undergoing CT may differ in important ways from patients not undergoing CT. As a consequence, the differences in outcomes observed between the two groups may have more to do with those initial differences than with the choice of diagnostic strategy. Consider this example before we examine the study findings: Patients with a classic presentation of appendicitis may be relatively unlikely to be subjected to CT by the treating physician, whereas patients with

an atypical presentation may be more likely to be subjected to CT or other diagnostic tests. At the same time, classic-presentation patients may be more likely to have appendicitis (and therefore have a low rate of negative appendectomy) compared with patients with atypical presentations (who would therefore have a higher rate of negative appendectomy). If CT prevents unnecessary appendectomy in some patients with atypical presentations, the negative appendectomy rate in this group would decline but might remain equal to or higher than the rate in patients with classical presentations. Using a study design that compares the rates of negative appendectomy in patients with and without CT, it might appear that CT had no effect or benefit—when in truth it might have substantially decreased appendectomy in patients with equivocal presentations. With this in mind, consider some studies on CT and surgical outcomes.

Coursey et al.[155] retrospectively reviewed records from 925 patients undergoing appendectomy from 1998 to 2007 and found a dramatic increase in CT use from 18.5% to 93.2%. At the same time, the overall negative appendectomy rate remained unchanged, whereas the negative appendectomy rate fell in women 45 years and younger from 42.9% to 7.1%.

Balthazar et al.[156] retrospectively compared negative appendectomy and perforation rates in patients undergoing preoperative CT with historical rates from previous publications. The negative appendectomy rate was 4%, compared with historical rates of 15% to 20%. The perforation rate was 22%, similar to previous publications. In women ages 15 to 50 years, the negative appendectomy rate was 8.3%, with a 19% perforation rate.

Rao et al.[157] compared rates of negative appendectomy and perforation from 1992 to 1995 (before introduction of appendiceal CT) and from 1997, when 59% of patients underwent preoperative CT. Before appendiceal CT was introduced, the negative appendectomy rate was 20%, falling to 7% during a period of intensive use of preoperative CT. Perforation rates fell from 22% to 14% during the same period. Negative appendectomy rates fell from 11% to 5% in men, from 35% to 11% in women, from 10% to 5% in boys, and from 18% to 12% in girls. The authors advocated preoperative CT in most female and many male patients.

Karakas et al.[158] retrospectively reviewed the charts of 633 children and adolescents with suspected appendicitis, noted an increased risk for perforation in patients undergoing CT, and suggested a causal relationship. However, this retrospective study cannot prove causation, and it may be that patients with perforation are more difficult to diagnose and therefore are more likely to undergo CT than patients with unperforated appendicitis.

TABLE 9-12. Studies of the Association Between CT Scan Use and Clinical Outcomes in Appendicitis

Study	Design	Negative Appendectomy Rate With CT	Perforation Rate With CT	Special Populations or Outcomes
Coursey et al.[155]	Retrospective	Unchanged overall	Not reported	Negative appendectomy rates decreased in women younger than 46 years.
Balthazar et al.[156]	Retrospective	Decreased overall	Unchanged overall	Negative appendectomy rates decreased in women 15-50 years.
Rao et al.[157]	Retrospective	Decreased overall	Decreased overall	Negative appendectomy rates decreased in men, women, and children.
Applegate et al.[159]	Retrospective	Decreased overall	Unchanged overall	Study was exclusively of children.
McDonald et al.[160]	Retrospective	Unchanged overall	Unchanged overall	Patients older than 12 years
Bendeck et al.[161]	Retrospective	Unchanged overall	Not reported	Negative appendectomy rates decreased in adult women but not in other groups.
Fuchs et al.[162]	Retrospective	Decreased overall	Not reported	Negative appendectomy rates decreased in adult women.
Partrick et al.[163]	Retrospective	Unchanged overall	Not reported	Study exclusively of children
Torbati and Guss[164]	Prospective with historical control group	Not reported	Decreased	CT was associated with decrease in time to operative intervention in women.
Antevil et al.[165]	Retrospective	Decreased in all women and in all patients older than 30 years	Not reported	Negative appendectomy rates decreased in adult women and all patients older than 30 years.
Vadeboncoeur et al.[166]	Retrospective	Unchanged overall	Not reported	—
Chooi et al.[167]	Retrospective	Decreased overall	Decreased	Negative appendectomy rates were lower in males and females.
Riesenman et al.[168]	Retrospective	Not reported	Unchanged	Length of stay doubled without statistically significant change in perforation rate
Karakas et al.[158]	Retrospective	Unchanged overall	Increased	Study of children and adolescents

Applegate et al.[159] retrospectively examined rates of perforation and negative appendectomy in children. Perforation rates were similar with preoperative CT, preoperative ultrasound, and no preoperative imaging. Negative appendectomy rates were lower in patients undergoing CT alone (2%) than in patients with CT with or without prior ultrasound (7%), ultrasound alone (17%), and no imaging (14%).

McDonald et al.[160] observed no statistically significant change in negative appendectomy or perforation rates with increasing rates of CT utilization. In a retrospective study, Bendeck et al.[161] found the negative appendectomy rate to be significantly decreased, from 28% to 7%, in adult women undergoing CT compared with women undergoing no preoperative imaging, leading

the authors to suggest that women undergo preoperative CT when appendicitis is suspected. Negative appendectomy rates were not significantly different in men or male and female children, with or without CT imaging.

In a retrospective review, Fuchs et al.[162] noted a negative appendectomy rate of 11.9% in patients undergoing no CT versus 6.3% in patients undergoing preoperative CT. In women, the negative appendectomy rate was 23.5% without CT and 5.3% with preoperative CT.

In a retrospective study in 616 children, Partrick et al.[163] noted an increase in preoperative CT utilization from 1.3% in 1997 to 58% in 2001, with a nonsignificant decrease in negative appendectomy from 8% to 7%.

Torbati and Guss[164] prospectively observed 310 emergency department adult patients with suspected appendicitis. Patients with "clinically evident appendicitis" did not undergo CT, whereas those with equivocal presentations underwent CT. Comparison with historical controls was performed. In males, the perforation rate fell from 38% in historical controls to 25% with selective use of CT. In females, perforation rate fell from 23% historically to 6% with selective CT. This study also showed a decrease in time to operative intervention of nearly 5 hours in females with selective CT compared with historical controls.

Antevil et al.[165] retrospectively reviewed 633 adult patients undergoing appendectomy from 2000 to 2002, subdividing by age and gender. They found an association between CT use and lower rates of negative appendectomy in female patients of all ages and in patients of both genders older than 30 years (23% without CT vs. 8% with CT).

Vadeboncoeur et al.[166] compared the rate of negative appendectomy with selective CT use to a historical period before introduction of CT and found no significant difference (13.5% vs. 14.8%).

Chooi et al.[167] reviewed 380 patients undergoing appendectomy between 2000 and 2004 and found lower rates of negative appendectomy in both male and female patients undergoing (CT or ultrasound) imaging (11.4%) than in those without imaging (22.2%). The authors also reported a lower perforation rate in patients with preoperative imaging.

Riesenman et al.[168] compared emergency department length of stay and perforation rate in patients with and without CT for suspected appendicitis. Statistically, length of stay was significantly longer in patients with CT (606 vs. 321 minutes). Perforation rate was not significantly different between groups.

Randomized Controlled Trials on the Clinical Effect of Abdominal Computed Tomography for the Diagnosis of Appendicitis.
A better research methodology for determining the effect of diagnostic imaging on patient outcomes is a randomized controlled trial. In trials of this type, randomization attempts to create two equivalent patient populations before the study intervention, the use or not of diagnostic imaging for appendicitis. Several trials of this type have been conducted, using slightly different comparisons. All of these studies suffer from a lack of statistical power, so their results may not accurately depict the likely effect of imaging on negative appendectomy rates, rupture, or other patient outcomes. Although existing studies do not lay to rest questions about the clinical benefit of CT, we examine the evidence because it may shed light on future studies to resolve this debate.

Hong et al.[169] randomized 182 patients with suspected appendicitis to clinical assessment alone or clinical assessment with mandatory abdominal CT. The authors found clinical assessment to be more sensitive (100%) than CT (91%) but less specific (73% for clinical assessment vs. 93% for CT). Perforation rates were low in both groups and not statistically different (6% for clinical assessment vs. 9% for CT). Hospital length of stay and costs were equal in the two groups. Patients assessed without CT were operated upon more quickly. The authors concluded that CT was not routinely warranted.

Although this study begins to apply strong methodology to this important clinical question, it may fail to reveal a benefit of CT because of the inclusion of all patients with suspected appendicitis, regardless of pretest probability. It stands to reason that CT would be unlikely to benefit patients with classic clinical presentations of appendicitis, because these patients likely have the disease process. CT in these patients would be expected to delay operative care, raise costs, and potentially increase perforation rates by delaying operative care. Because most patients in this group would be expected to have appendicitis, CT would be unlikely to reduce the negative appendectomy rate, which would be near zero. CT would also be expected to have little benefit in patients with very low clinical probability of appendicitis. In these patients, appendicitis would be expected to be rare, and few would undergo appendectomy on clinical grounds if CT were not used. CT might identify patients in this group with unexpected appendicitis, but this would be expected to be a rare event. Consequently, CT use would be expected to raise costs while having little effect on important outcomes such as perforation and negative appendectomy rates. CT would be most likely to have clinical benefit in patients with intermediate pretest probability of appendicitis. In this group, a relatively high rate of negative appendectomy might be expected without CT; a relatively high rate of perforation might also be expected if appendectomy were delayed until clinical signs progressed. Hong et al.[169] might have found clinical benefit to CT if the patient population had been selected in this way based on pretest probability.

Lee et al.[170] randomized 152 adult patients with right lower quadrant pain to selective CT or mandatory CT use. CT was performed in 68% of patients in the selective group and 97% of patients in the mandatory group. Mandatory CT imaging showed a trend toward decreased negative appendectomy (11% reduction) and perforation rates (8% reduction), not reaching statistical significance. A larger study is required to determine whether the observed trends represent a true benefit of mandatory CT.

Lopez et al.[171] randomized 98 women of childbearing age with possible appendicitis to clinical observation alone or observation with CT scan. Charges and length of stay were similar in the two groups. Clinical observation alone was 100% sensitive and 87.5% specific, whereas CT was 89.5% sensitive and 95.6% specific. The study was underpowered to determine superiority of one method over the other. While acknowledging this limitation, the authors concluded that CT reliably identified patients requiring operation and appeared equivalent to observation. In addition to limitations because of poor statistical power, this study again suffers from inclusion of patients with very low and very high pretest probability of appendicitis, extremes at which CT would be predicted to have little benefit. The authors included patients with Alvarado scores of 2 to 8 (see Table 9-10). Alvarado scores of 7 or greater strongly predict appendicitis, whereas scores of 3 or less strongly exclude the diagnosis.[150] Inclusion of patients with these scores dilutes the possible benefit of CT in patients in whom true clinical uncertainty exists.

Contrast Controversies: Is Oral, Rectal, or Intravenous Contrast Required for the Diagnosis of Appendicitis by CT? In Which Patients? What Forms of Contrast?

A major controversy in appendicitis imaging today is the benefit or requirement for oral and IV contrast for CT. In its appropriateness criteria, the ACR acknowledges the mixed evidence for and against enteral and IV contrast. The ACR[134] states that oral or rectal contrast use should be determined by institutional preference. For nonpregnant adults, the ACR rates CT with IV contrast 8 of 9 on its appropriateness scale and CT without IV contrast 7 of 9. Oral contrast represents a potentially serious barrier to CT use, because it adds a median of more than 100 minutes to the emergency department stay, even when antiemetics are administered prophylactically.[27] IV contrast represents a risk for contrast allergy and contrast nephropathy. In addition, in some settings, up to an hour delay may occur for creatinine measurement before administration of IV contrast is allowed. Delays such as these could increase the risk for appendiceal rupture and could be critical in other time-dependent abdominal conditions, such as aortic aneurysm or mesenteric ischemia. Therefore the question of the need for contrast agents is an important one to emergency physicians.

An ideal study to determine the incremental value of oral, IV, and rectal contrast agents would randomize patients to receive unenhanced CT, CT with each contrast agent individually, or CT with each possible combination of contrast agents. Such studies are rare; instead comparisons are often made among separate studies that determine the sensitivity and specificity of a single CT protocol. Critics of this approach point out that comparisons of this type can be confounded by differences in the study populations so that differences in the performance qualities of various CT protocols may not be valid. While acknowledging this limitation, let's examine the available evidence. We summarize the findings using available metaanalyses and systematic reviews where possible, because the number of studies of CT for appendicitis is large, with more than 800 publications in PubMed.

A number of studies suggest that oral contrast is not needed for the diagnosis of appendicitis. Anderson et al.[32] performed a systematic review to compare the performance of CT with and without oral contrast. The authors identified 23 studies, and the sensitivity of CT without oral contrast was not statistically different from that of CT with oral contrast (95% vs. 92%). The specificity of CT without oral contrast was 97%, whereas the specificity of CT with oral contrast was 94% ($p < 0.0001$). The authors suggest that a prospective head-to-head comparison of the two protocols be performed to confirm the findings. This study, although suggesting that oral contrast is unnecessary, pools results from a variety of different CT protocols. Some studies used no oral contrast but applied rectal or IV contrast. Interestingly, in the subgroup of 1510 patients receiving no contrast, sensitivity was 93% and specificity was 98%. In the 750 patients receiving only rectal contrast, sensitivity and specificity were 97%. For the 914 patients receiving oral and IV contrast, sensitivity and specificity were 93%. None of the included studies used IV contrast alone.

Studies have also examined the performance of CT with IV contrast alone. Iwahashi et al.[172] found CT with IV contrast only to be 92% sensitive and 88% specific in a population of 78 patients. Mun et al.[173] retrospectively reviewed 173 patients undergoing CT with IV contrast only for appendicitis and found sensitivity of 100% and specificity of 97%. Anderson et al.[174] prospectively randomized 303 patients to CT with IV contrast alone or CT with oral and IV contrast and found similar performance for the diagnosis of appendicitis: sensitivity of 100% and specificity of 97% for both protocols. Keyzer et al.[175] prospectively randomized 131 patients with suspected appendicitis to CT with or without oral contrast. All patients underwent two CT scans, before and after administration of IV contrast. Performance of unenhanced, IV only, oral only, and oral and IV contrast CT were similar, with variation in accuracy depending more on the radiologist interpreting the images than on the contrast protocol. Seo et al.[176] performed CT with IV contrast (and no oral or rectal contrast) in 207 adults with suspected appendicitis, using both standard and low-radiation dose CT techniques. Sensitivity was 98% to 100% for low-radiation dose and 100% for standard radiation dose. Specificity was 95% to 97% for low dose and 93% to 97% for standard radiation dose.

Other studies suggest that noncontrast CT (with no oral, IV, or rectal contrast) is adequate for the emergency department diagnosis of appendicitis in adults (see Figure 9-56). Hlibczuk et al.[177] performed a systematic review, identifying seven methodologically rigorous studies from more than 1258 publications. The included studies used a representative emergency department patient spectrum and strong reference standards for diagnosis and provided a pooled sample of 1060 patients. The pooled sensitivity of noncontrast CT for appendicitis was 92.7% (95% CI = 89.5%-95.0%) and specificity was 96.1% (95% CI = 94.2%-97.5%). The positive likelihood ratio was 24, and the negative likelihood ratio was 0.08. Positive likelihood ratios greater than 10 are generally considered to confirm disease confidently, whereas negative likelihood ratios less than 0.1 are generally considered to exclude disease. Although this review does not specifically compare the performance of noncontrast CT to CT with various contrast agents, it suggests that unenhanced CT is accurate for the diagnosis of appendicitis. This review does not address the question of alternative diagnoses in patients without appendicitis, so the results should be treated with caution when applied to patients with a broad differential diagnosis. For example, unenhanced CT does not exclude subtle vascular pathology such as iliac artery dissection.

Other authors have suggested that unenhanced CT be performed as the initial test, with contrast being administered for inconclusive cases. Tamburrini et al. (2007) found that unenhanced CT was conclusive in 75% of patients, with a sensitive of 90% and specificity of 96%. In the 25% of patients with inconclusive initial noncontrast CT, a repeat CT scan with IV and oral or rectal contrast yielded a sensitivity of 96% and specificity of 92%. The authors conclude that a noncontrast CT is an appropriate first test, with contrast reserved for equivocal cases. However, this approach would also result in two radiation exposures in 25% of patients. Such exposure might be acceptable in older patients but quite undesirable in young patients, so the choice of unenhanced CT or enhanced CT should include consideration of factors such as patient age and differential diagnosis.

Other factors may influence the sensitivity of CT and the benefit of contrast agents. Thin patients including many children have little intraperitoneal fat, providing little substrate for inflammatory fat stranding that can be important to the diagnosis of appendicitis. Some authors have suggested that thin patients and children should receive oral and IV contrast because of this limitation. Kaiser et al.[178] found that unenhanced CT (no IV, oral, or rectal contrast) limited to the lower abdomen was only 66% sensitive but 96% specific for appendicitis in 306 children. Addition of IV contrast and widening of the region of the CT to the entire abdomen increased sensitivity to 90%, with a 94% specificity.

Grayson et al.[179] demonstrated that decreased peritoneal fat reduces visualization of the normal appendix in pediatric patients. Benjaminov et al.[180] observed that the normal appendix was more difficult to identify in patients with lesser degrees of intraperitoneal fat, using unenhanced CT.

When CT Fails to Visualize the Appendix but Is Otherwise Normal, Is Appendicitis Excluded?

In approximately 13% to 15% of CT scans performed for evaluation of appendicitis, the appendix is not visualized, preventing direct commentary on the findings of appendicitis described earlier.[181-182] With modalities such as ultrasound, lack of visualization results in a nondiagnostic test—additional assessment is required by some other means (e.g., CT, observation, or laparoscopy) to determine whether appendicitis is present. When the appendix is not visualized on CT, are additional imaging studies required? Multiple studies have investigated the rate of appendicitis in patients with a nonvisualized appendix on CT, with more than 750 adults and 1100 pediatric patients included (Table 9-13). A nonvisualized appendix *in the absence of additional signs of inflammation, such as fat stranding or free fluid,* yields a negative predictive value of 98%—the equivalent of a CT that visualizes a normal appendix. Consequently, a normal CT with or without visualization of the appendix effectively rules out appendicitis in most patients.[181-183]

When CT Findings Are Equivocal, What Is the Likelihood of Appendicitis?

In some instances, CT findings are equivocal for appendicitis, because the appendix may appear enlarged without surrounding inflammatory change or inflammatory changes may be present in the right lower quadrant

TABLE 9-13. Rate of Appendicitis When CT Is Normal but the Appendix Is Not Visualized

Study	Population	Rate of Appendicitis
Nikolaidis et al.[182]	366 consecutive adults	2% rate of appendicitis when appendix not seen and no secondary signs of appendicitis (one female patient with paucity of right lower quadrant fat)
Ganguli et al.[181]	400 consecutive patients, 20% with appendicitis	2%
Garcia et al.[183]	1139 children	Negative predictive value of 98.7% for nonvisualized appendix, 100% for partially visualized, 99.6% for fully visualized—not statistically different

without evident abnormalities of the appendix. In other cases, the appendix is not seen but inflammatory changes of the right lower quadrant are present.

Daly et al.[184] reviewed 1344 consecutive patients undergoing CT for suspected appendicitis between 1998 and 2002. They found that 172 patients (12.8%) had equivocal CT results. Of these, approximately 30% were ultimately diagnosed with appendicitis. Consequently, when CT findings include some abnormalities but appendicitis is not diagnosed specifically, the diagnosis is not ruled out.

Appendicitis Imaging in the Pediatric Patient.
Imaging for appendicitis in the pediatric patient warrants several special considerations. First, the differential diagnosis for acute abdominal pain is usually far more restricted than in adults. Often a binary question can be asked: Is the cause of the patient's pain appendicitis? No further diagnostic testing is required when the answer is no. In contrast, a multitude of important causes in adults may simulate appendicitis, including ovarian pathology, obstructing renal stones, and vascular pathology. Although a broad differential diagnosis should be considered in pediatric patients, the requirement for an imaging test to fully evaluate all possible causes of abdominal pain is diminished. As a consequence, ultrasound, with its more limited ability to assess right lower quadrant abdominal pain, becomes a reasonable alternative to CT (see Figure 9-57).

Second, radiation exposures are a growing concern in pediatric patients, with risks varying depending on age at exposure. Brenner and Hall[185] estimate lifetime attributable mortality from a single abdominal CT to be approximately 1 in 700 if performed at birth, 1 in 1000 if performed at 5 years, and 1 in 2000 if performed at age 25. In contrast, the attributable risk is thought to be less than 1 in 5000 if CT is performed at 35 years, with a continued decrease with advancing age. Whereas these risks are small for the individual patient compared with baseline risks for cancer death in the United States (~22%, according to Centers for Disease Control and Prevention data from 2005),[186] on a population level these risks are estimated to translate into as many as 500 additional pediatric deaths annually in the United States.[187] Again, a diagnostic imaging test with no ionizing radiation exposure becomes more desirable; ultrasound and MRI meet this criterion.

Third, the CT diagnosis of appendicitis depends partly on the presence of intraperitoneal fat, the substrate for inflammatory fat stranding. Although CT has been shown to be relatively sensitive (84%) and highly specific (99%) for appendicitis in children,[158] some thin pediatric patients have little intraperitoneal fat, which may make diagnosis more difficult.[179] At the same time, a low body mass index typically improves the diagnostic performance of ultrasound.

Therefore a growing trend has emerged toward ultrasound as the first diagnostic imaging test for pediatric patients. As we discussed earlier, ultrasound is quite specific but relatively insensitive. Consequently, the ACR recommends that ultrasound be used as the first diagnostic test in children younger than 14 years, followed by CT for equivocal ultrasound results (e.g., nonvisualization of the appendix by ultrasound).[134] MRI is another option, although its expense and limited emergency availability make it a less viable strategy in many centers.[134]

Imaging the Pregnant Patient With Possible Appendicitis.
Pregnant patients with possible appendicitis pose another clinical diagnostic dilemma. Appendicitis is one of the most common surgical emergencies in pregnancy. Changes in the location of the appendix have been posited as causing atypical presentations in pregnant patients, although there is little supporting evidence in the medical literature. Leukocytosis is a normal finding in pregnancy, also complicating the diagnosis. Missed appendicitis can lead to fetal loss, so accurate diagnosis through the use of imaging is particularly desirable. As with the pediatric patient, minimizing radiation exposure in the pregnant patient is a priority. Consequently, alternatives to CT imaging using ultrasound or MRI are often sought.

Ultrasound is the first-line imaging modality in pregnant patients with suspected appendicitis. In pregnant patients, ultrasound has limited sensitivity (~50%) but is highly specific (100%) for appendicitis when the appendix is seen.[145] Ultrasound may fail to visualize the appendix in a large minority of pregnant patients, resulting in a nondiagnostic study. Shetty et al.[188] found that CT was 100% sensitive for appendicitis in pregnancy, compared with only 46% for ultrasound. Given the low sensitivity of ultrasound for appendicitis, further imaging is prudent in patients with negative or equivocal ultrasound.

Ironically, physicians generally overestimate the radiation risk from CT in pregnancy. The radiation dose from a single CT of the abdomen and pelvis is approximately 8 mSv, below the cumulative radiation exposure generally held to result in a measurable increase in risk for fetal anomaly or loss.[189-190] Despite this, physician knowledge lags behind, perhaps resulting in unnecessary fear of CT by physicians and patients. Ratnapalan et al.[190] surveyed family physicians and obstetricians on the risk for fetal anomaly following a single CT scan in pregnancy. In the survey, 61% of family physicians and 34% of obstetricians rated the likelihood of anomaly as greater than 5%—although the consensus among experts in this field is that no appreciable risk results from these exposures. This is not to say that CT should be used with abandon in pregnancy. Some evidence suggests that in utero radiation exposures might result in an increased risk for childhood leukemias, so if other imaging or diagnostic options are available, they should be considered. Ultrasound and MRI are reasonable options, with CT used when these are unavailable. Currently the ACR recommends right lower quadrant ultrasound, followed by MRI and CT when ultrasound is nondiagnostic for suspected appendicitis in pregnancy (Table 9-14).[134,191] Neither ultrasound nor MRI exposes the patient to radiation. Both ultrasound and MRI can evaluate for appendicitis and other causes of right lower quadrant or pelvic pain. Gadolinium safety in pregnancy is unknown; avoid gadolinium use when possible.

Complications and Treatment of Appendicitis: Abscess and Percutaneous Drainage

A frequent complication of appendicitis is perforation with abscess formation. Today, when CT detects periappendiceal abscess, surgery is often delayed or avoided in favor of antibiotic therapy with percutaneous drainage (discussed in detail in Chapter 16). Randomized controlled trials show a high rate of resolution with this approach. In long-term follow-up, the risk for recurrent appendicitis appears low, suggesting that routine appendectomy following percutaneous drainage may be unnecessary.

Limited Computed Tomography Versus Computed Tomography of Entire Abdomen for Suspected Appendicitis

In the pediatric patient and in adults with localized right lower quadrant pain and tenderness, appendicitis may be the leading diagnosis, and complete imaging of the abdomen may be unnecessary. When the differential diagnosis is constrained, a more restrictive CT imaging approach could be sufficient, reducing radiation exposure. Rao et al.[192] explored the sensitivity of z-axis restricted CT for the diagnosis of appendicitis, using a CT confined to the lower abdomen, and reported a sensitivity of 100% and specificity of 95%. The same group reported a cost savings of more than $45,000 per 100 patients using this technique, compared with clinical assessment alone.[193] Fefferman et al.[194] retrospectively reviewed 93 CT scans performed in children for assessment of appendicitis and determined that a CT limited to the region below the lower pole of the right kidney would be 97% sensitive and 93% specific while limiting radiation exposure. Mullins et al.[195] found focused CT to be 97% sensitive and 99% specific in 199 children.

Broder et al.[196] used a CT strategy guided by the location of abdominal tenderness, rather than guided by anatomic landmarks. Although the study was designed to assess for multiple forms of abdominal pathology, in the subset of patients with appendicitis, the technique was 93% sensitive. They found 38% to 69% of radiation exposure could be avoided by this technique, though additional study is required.

TABLE 9-14. American College of Radiology Appropriateness Criteria: Right Lower Quadrant Pain —Suspected Appendicitis, Fever, Leukocytosis, Pregnant Woman

Radiologic Procedure	Rating	Comments
Ultrasound abdomen right lower quadrant	8	With graded compression. Better in first and early second trimesters
MRI abdomen and pelvis without contrast	7	May be useful following negative or equivocal ultrasound
Ultrasound pelvis	6	
CT abdomen and pelvis with IV contrast	6	Use of oral or rectal contrast depends on institutional preference.
CT abdomen and pelvis without IV contrast	5	Use of oral or rectal contrast depends on institutional preference.

From American College of Radiology: ACR appropriateness criteria: Right Lower Quadrant Pain — Suspected Appendicitis. 2010. Available at: http://www.acr.org/SecondaryMainMenuCategories/quality_safety/app_criteria/pdf/ExpertPanelonGastrointestinalImaging/RightLowerQuadrantPainDoc12.aspx.
Rating Scale: 1,2,3: usually not appropriate; 4,5,6: may be appropriate; 7,8,9: usually appropriate.
This table is abbreviated from the complete ACR appropriateness criteria. Only the primary imaging recommendations (i.e., procedures rated as "usually appropriate") and alternatives (i.e., procedure rated as "may be appropriate") are included in this truncated list.
Reprinted with permission of the American College of Radiology, Reston, VA. No other representation of this material is authorized without expressed, written permission from the American College of Radiology. Refer to the ACR website at www.acr.org/ac for the most current and complete version of the ACR Appropriateness Criteria®."

Appendicitis Mimics

Multiple disease processes can mimic appendicitis and may be detected with imaging performed for evaluation of appendicitis. CT can visualize obstructing renal stones, ovarian pathology (including tuboovarian abscess, ovarian torsion, ovarian mass, and ectopic pregnancy), hernias, vascular abnormalities, right-sided diverticulitis, and inflammatory bowel disease such as colitis or terminal ileitis.[197] Two common appendicitis mimics deserve special attention because they may be unfamiliar to emergency physicians and are frequently visualized with CT: epiploic appendagitis and mesenteric adenitis.

Epiploic appendagitis (Figure 9-58) occurs when fat appendages attached to the taeniae coli, called epiploic appendages, become inflamed. This may occur primarily, caused by torsion of the appendage with ischemic infarction, or secondarily, caused by adjacent inflammatory processes such as diverticulitis. The diagnosis is made on CT when a round or oval pericolonic structure is identified with rim enhancement and adjacent fat

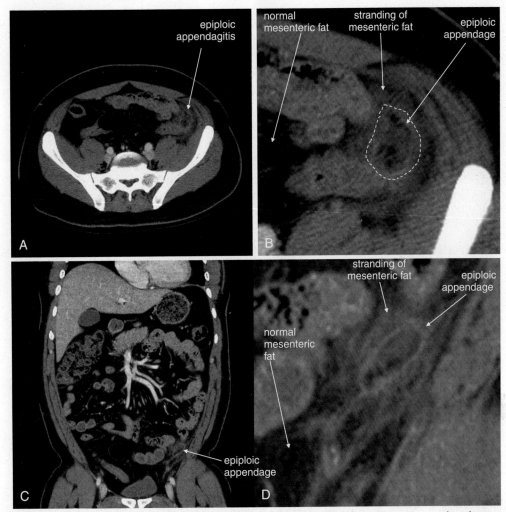

Figure 9-58. Epiploic appendagitis, CT with IV contrast, soft-tissue window. Epiploic appendagitis occurs when fat-containing appendages from the colon undergo torsion and ischemic infarction. The epiploic appendage appears as a dark and well-circumscribed structure of fat density. Surrounding the epiploic appendage is inflammatory change with stranding in the surrounding mesenteric fat. **A,** Axial view. **B,** Close-up from **A. C,** Coronal view. **D,** Close-up from **C.**

stranding.[198] Fever and leukocytosis, as well as abdominal pain, may occur with epiploic appendagitis. Primary epiploic appendagitis does not require surgery in many cases, although historically the condition was often discovered at surgery for suspected appendicitis and the torsed epiploic appendage was often removed.[199] Some authors advocate antibiotics,[200] although no systematic evidence exists for their use because the condition is believed to be caused by vascular insufficiency of the appendage, not infection. Conservative management with nonsteroidal antiinflammatory drugs and analgesics may be sufficient in most cases.[201]

Mesenteric adenitis (Figure 9-59) is enlargement of mesenteric lymph nodes and may occur with viral or bacterial enteritis (including pathogens such as *Clostridium difficile, Yersinia enterocolitica, Salmonella typhi, Mycobacterium tuberculosis,* and *Mycobacterium avium* complex), inflammatory bowel disease, lupus, appendicitis, diverticulitis, human immunodeficiency virus, and malignancy.[202-203] When enlarged nodes are found

without another cause of inflammation, primary mesenteric adenitis is diagnosed. When another cause is found, secondary mesenteric adenitis is diagnosed. The enlarged nodes may cause right lower abdominal pain and tenderness, whereas the underlying infection or inflammatory process can cause diarrhea and fever, simulating appendicitis. Adenovirus is a classically described cause of mesenteric adenitis.[204] Treatment of primary mesenteric adenitis is supportive care, whereas a search for an underlying cause such as bacterial enteritis may be warranted. Surgery is not required for primary mesenteric adenitis. Antibiotics are required only if indicated for the underlying infection. In one study, 8.3% of patients undergoing CT for acute abdominal symptoms had mesenteric adenitis, with 3.3% having primary adenitis.[205] Rao et al.[206] found that mesenteric adenitis was the final diagnosis in 7.7% of 651 consecutive patients admitted with suspected appendicitis. In this same group of patients, it constituted about 20% of the final diagnoses in patients without appendicitis, indicating that it is a frequent appendicitis mimic.

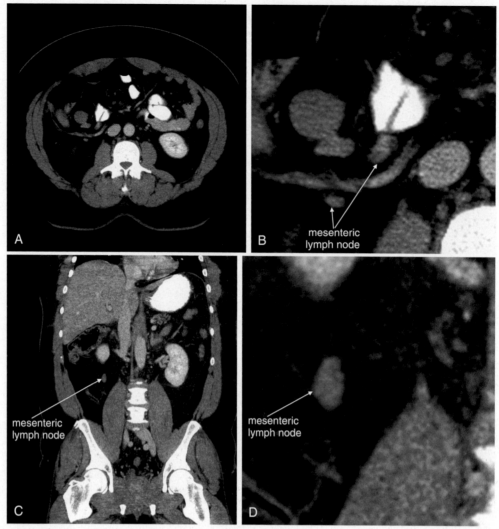

Figure 9-59. **Mesenteric adenitis, CT with IV and oral contrast, soft-tissue window.** Mesenteric adenitis can mimic appendicitis in its clinical presentation. Enlarged lymph nodes are visible on CT. Lymph nodes have soft-tissue density and appear as discrete, rounded structures. On a single image they may appear similar to blood vessels or to the appendix, but on inspection of adjacent images it becomes clear that lymph nodes are rounded, not tubular like a blood vessel or the appendix. **A,** Axial image. **B,** Close-up from **A. C,** Coronal reconstruction. **D,** Close-up from **C.**

CT criteria for the diagnosis of mesenteric adenitis include a cluster of three or more mesenteric lymph nodes, each measuring 5 mm or more. With CT, lymph nodes appear as rounded structures with soft-tissue density, usually surrounded by mesenteric fat. They usually enhance homogenously with IV contrast. Necrotic lymph nodes associated with malignancy may be hypoattenuating with an enhancing rim. Because mesenteric lymph nodes can enlarge from serious processes, including appendicitis and malignancy, the CT must be reviewed carefully for other findings.

Diverticular Disease
Figures 9-60 through 9-66 demonstrate imaging findings of diverticulosis and diverticulitis.

Diverticulosis. Diverticulosis (see Figures 9-60 through 9-62) is the presence of diverticuli, small outpouchings of the bowel, most common in the colon. Risk

factors include low-fiber diets, common in the United States and rare in the developing world. Diverticuli occur with increasing frequency in older patients but are present in patients in the United States as early as age 30. Diverticulosis occurs in 10% of U.S. adults younger than 40 and 50%-70% of adults 80 years or older.[207] Thus diverticulosis is not a condition restricted to the elderly in the United States. Colonic diverticuli more commonly occur in the distal colon, where stool is more solid in consistency; the sigmoid and descending colon are the most frequent sites, though ascending and transverse colon diverticuli occur.[207] Pseudodiverticuli, composed only of mucosa and submucosa with no muscular layer, can occur at entry sites of perforating arteries, which represent weak areas in the muscle wall.

Diverticuli are not seen on x-ray. Historically, contrast barium enema was used to diagnosis diverticuli, but today the diagnosis is more commonly made using CT

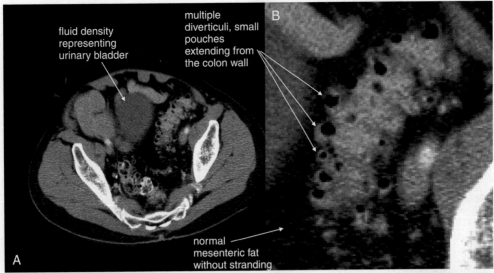

Figure 9-60. Diverticulosis, CT with oral and IV contrast, soft-tissue window. This patient had known diverticulosis from prior colonoscopy. His scan shows diverticuli without evidence of inflammation such as fat stranding, abscess, or free air. This slice is through the pelvis and visualizes a section of the sigmoid colon, a common location for both diverticulosis and diverticulitis. Note the normal, dark appearance of the fat surrounding the sigmoid colon. **A,** Axial image. **B,** Close-up. Future figures examine cases of diverticulitis, which are revealed by the smoky appearance of inflammatory fat stranding. This patient did receive intravenous (IV) and oral contrast. Diverticulitis can be recognized without contrast, using findings such as fat stranding and abscess, but IV contrast assists by providing bowel wall enhancement, and oral contrast may assist by revealing the margins of bowel versus an adjacent abscess.

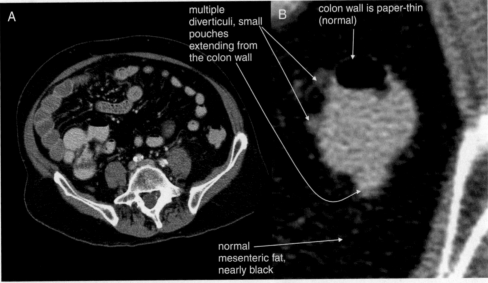

Figure 9-61. Diverticulosis, CT with oral and IV contrast, soft-tissue window. The descending colon in the same patient as in Figure 9-60 also shows scattered diverticuli. Again, note the normal surrounding fat and extremely thin (normal) colon wall. **A,** Axial image. **B,** Close-up.

in U.S. emergency departments. On contrast enema, the appearance is of small outpouchings, often with a narrow neck. A similar appearance is seen with CT scan, although no enteral contrast is needed to identify diverticuli. Imaging of diverticular bleeding is discussed in the later section on GI hemorrhage.

Diverticulitis. When food particles become entrapped within diverticuli, infection and inflammation of diverticuli may occur, termed diverticulitis (see Figures 9-62 through 9-66). Mirroring the locations of diverticuli,

diverticulitis occurs in the descending and sigmoid colon in 90% of cases. CT is the preferred imaging modality for diagnosis of diverticulitis, because it can display inflammatory change, complications of diverticulitis such as perforation or abscess formation, and alternative diagnoses including ischemic or infectious colitis, cancers, ureteral stones, and aortic aneurysm. Ultrasound and MRI are alternatives, though studies are limited. X-ray plays little role in the diagnosis. The ACR appropriateness criteria for imaging of suspected diverticulitis are shown in Table 9-15.[208]

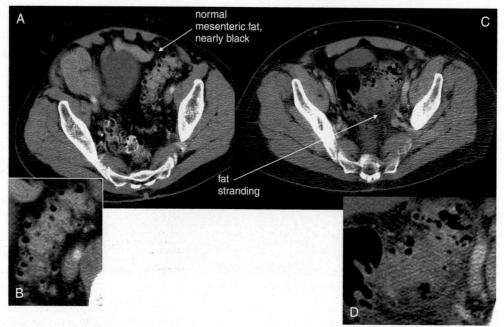

Figure 9-62. Diverticulosis compared with diverticulitis, CT. Compare the axial image in **A,** showing uninflamed sigmoid diverticuli, with that in **C,** showing sigmoid diverticulitis. The normal fat surrounding the sigmoid colon appears nearly black with a soft-tissue window in **A,** whereas the inflamed fat in **C** shows stranding, giving it a gray or smoky appearance. Whereas the borders of the uninflamed sigmoid colon are quite distinct in **A,** the margins of the sigmoid are blurred in **C,** reflecting inflammation of the bowel wall and surrounding fat. **B, D,** Close-ups from **A** and **C,** respectively.

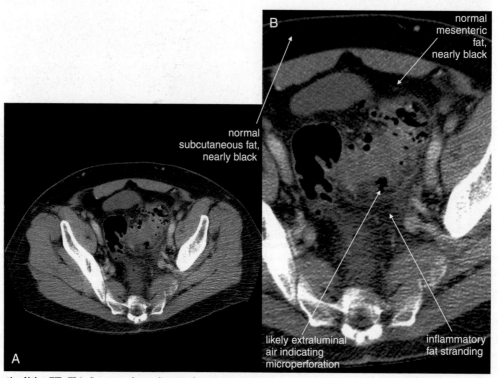

Figure 9-63. Diverticulitis, CT. This figure explores diverticulitis in more detail. Again, note the appearance of fat stranding. Several foci of air along the margins of the sigmoid colon may be in extraluminal fat, rather than within diverticuli. Although it may appear intuitive that this would indicate perforation or abscess formation requiring surgical drainage, this is a common feature of diverticulitis and may resolve with medical therapy. This 69-year-old male was treated with intravenous ciprofloxacin and metronidazole with resolution of his symptoms and did not require surgery. **A,** Axial image. **B,** Close-up.

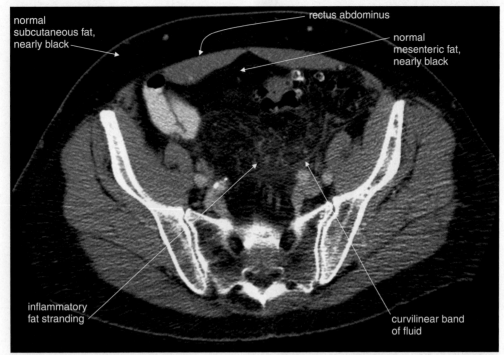

Figure 9-64. Diverticulitis, CT with IV and oral contrast, soft-tissue window, showing sentinel fat stranding. Even before an inflamed area of diverticulitis is seen, fat stranding gives away an inflammatory process in the region. Look at this pelvic section, taken a few slices cephalad to the image from Figure 9-63. A smoky region of stranding is seen. Compare this with the normal subcutaneous fat—a convenient standard present in nearly every patient. A curvilinear band may be a thin line of fluid tracking in a tissue plane, rather than true fat stranding, which usually has a less organized appearance. The fat becomes more normal in appearance just deep to the rectus muscles. When seeking any inflammatory process, look for the smoke (fat stranding) that gives away the presence of the fire (inflammatory process).

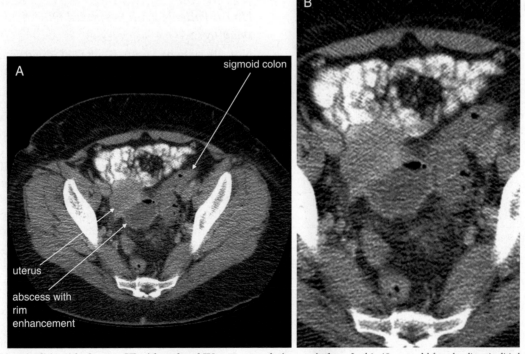

Figure 9-65. Diverticulitis with abscess, CT with oral and IV contrast, soft-tissue window. In this 48-year-old female, diverticulitis has progressed to abscess formation. The abscess is seen as a rounded, fluid-filled structure with an air–fluid level and an enhancing rim in this CT with intravenous and oral contrast. The sigmoid colon is seen to the patient's left; no definite diverticuli are seen on this scan, although the patient has known diverticuli from prior studies. **A,** Axial image. **B,** Close-up. When viewing CT scans of the pelvis, it is important to identify normal landmarks to ensure that normal structures are not mistaken for pathology, and vice versa. Theoretically, a loop of fluid-filled bowel could have a similar appearance to an abscess on a single slice, but inspection of slices above and below this one in the complete CT proved that this abscess was cystic, not tubular like bowel. The uterus lies slightly anterior and right of the abscess, and the bladder lies deeper in the pelvis, not visible on this slice. Figure 9-66 shows a coronal reconstruction that illustrates this relationship. Large discrete fluid collections such as this one usually require drainage, rather than medical therapy alone. This patient underwent ultrasound-guided drainage, with a percutaneous drain left in place. Cultures from the abscess grew beta-hemolytic *Streptococcus* group F, *Candida albicans,* and *Bacteroides fragilis.*

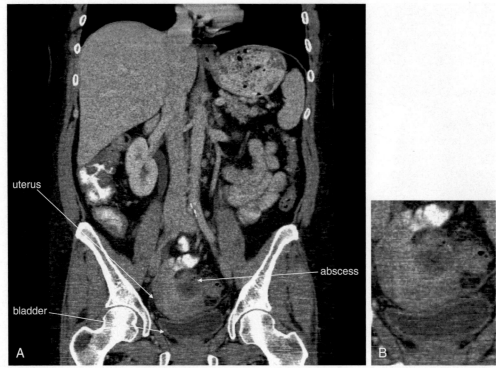

Figure 9-66. Diverticulitis with abscess, CT with oral and IV contrast, soft-tissue window. A coronal section (**A; B,** close-up) from the same patient as Figure 9-65 shows an abscess arising from a sigmoid diverticulum. The uterus and bladder lie close together. When looking for abscesses in the pelvis, be sure to identify normal anatomic structures; these may otherwise be taken for pathology, and vice versa. Distinguish between bowel and abscess by examining adjacent slices to determine whether a structure is tubular or cystic.

TABLE 9-15. American College of Radiology Appropriateness Criteria: Left Lower Quadrant Pain, Older Patient With Typical Clinical Presentation for Diverticulitis

Radiologic Procedure	Rating
CT abdomen and pelvis with IV contrast—Oral and/or colonic contrast may be helpful for bowel luminal visualization	8
CT abdomen and pelvis without IV contrast	6
X-ray contrast enema	5
Ultrasound abdomen transabdominal with graded compression	4
Ultrasound abdomen, transrectal or transvaginal	4
X-ray abdomen and pelvis	4
MRI abdomen and pelvis with or without contrast	4

From American College of Radiology: ACR appropriateness criteria: Left lower quadrant pain, 2008. (Accessed at http://www.acr.org/SecondaryMainMenuCategories/quality_safety/app_criteria/pdf/ExpertPanelonGastrointestinalImaging/LeftLowerQuadrantPainDoc8.aspx Rating Scale: 1,2,3: usually not appropriate; 4,5,6: may be appropriate; 7,8,9: usually appropriate.
The full ACR Appropriateness Criteria document includes other clinical variations with additional imaging recommendations.
Reprinted with permission of the American College of Radiology, Reston, VA. No other representation of this material is authorized without expressed, written permission from the American College of Radiology. Refer to the ACR website at www.acr.org/ac for the most current and complete version of the ACR Appropriateness Criteria®.

Do All Patients With Suspected Diverticulitis Require Imaging?

Not all patients with suspected diverticulitis require emergency imaging. Some practitioners may empirically treat suspected diverticulitis with antibiotics, reserving imaging for patients with history or examination findings concerning for complications or in whom an alternative diagnosis is seriously considered. Some preliminary work has been performed to derive clinical decision rules for imaging of diverticulitis, though no rule has received wide acceptance. Lameris et al.[209] found that direct tenderness only in the left lower quadrant, the absence of vomiting, and a C-reactive protein of more than 50 mg/L was 98% specific for diverticulitis but only 36% sensitive. In this same study, sensitivity based on clinical judgment before CT was 71%. Toorenvliet et al.[210] found that clinical diagnosis of diverticulitis had a positive predictive value of 65% and a negative predictive value of 98%. Imaging improved accuracy but changed management in only 7% of cases. Other authors have suggested broad application of CT in most patients to define the severity of disease, complications of diverticulitis, and alternative diagnoses.[211,213]

Diagnostic Accuracy of CT for Diverticulitis. Lameris et al.[212] performed a metaanalysis of studies on diagnostic accuracy of CT and ultrasound for diverticulitis. CT was 94% sensitive (95% CI = 87%-97%) and 99%

specific (95% CI = 90%-100%). Ultrasound was 92% sensitive (95% CI = 80%-97%) and 90% specific (95% CI = 92%-95%). Although there was no statistically significant difference between ultrasound and CT in sensitivity or specificity, CT was more likely to identify alternative diagnoses. Other authors have found similar sensitivity and specificity for CT. [207] Although CT is likely highly sensitive and specific for diverticulitis, Liljegren et al.[214] performed a systematic review of the literature on diagnostic imaging of diverticulitis and found relatively poor methodologic quality as a result of poor reference standards and selection bias in most studies.

What Are the CT Findings of Diverticulitis?

We review the CT findings of diverticulitis here and consider the potential value of contrast agents (Box 9-3). Figures 9-60 through 9-66 demonstrate CT findings of diverticulosis, diverticulitis, and diverticular abscess.

Essential to the CT diagnosis of diverticulitis is the presence of diverticuli, plus the presence of inflammatory changes. On CT, diverticuli are visible without the administration of any contrast agents. They appear as small outpouchings from the colon, particularly in the descending and sigmoid colon. Usually they contain some air (black on soft-tissue windows).

Inflammatory changes associated with diverticulitis include stranding of the adjacent fat, giving it a "smoky" appearance, which is brighter than uninflamed fat elsewhere in the abdomen, in the retroperitoneum, or in subcutaneous fat stores. When doubt exists about the presence of fat stranding, compare the fat region in question with an unaffected region to assess for differences in brightness. As described earlier in this chapter in the general discussion of CT, fat stranding results from increased water content of fat and is visible without the administration of any contrast agents. The bowel wall may appear thickened in the region of the affected diverticulum. If IV contrast is administered, the bowel wall may show increased enhancement in this region. CT grading systems for diverticulitis divide the condition into mild, moderate, and severe disease. Table 9-16 defines each grade by CT findings.[215] The Hinchey classification for diverticulitis is based on surgical findings and predicts mortality (Table 9-17).[207] CT accurately correlates with Hinchey classification in most cases (93% in one study).[216]

Perforation of a diverticulum can occur, so the peritoneum or retroperitoneum surrounding the diverticulum should be carefully inspected for extraluminal air. Because air is black and fat surrounding the colon is quite dark in appearance on a soft-tissue window, the window setting should be modified to accentuate the

---

Box 9-3: CT Findings of Diverticulitis

- **Diverticuli**—Appear as small pockets emerging from the colonic wall, most often in the transverse, descending, and sigmoid colon. Their presence is necessary but not sufficient for the diagnosis of diverticulitis.
- **Abscess**—May occur in perforated diverticulitis. Fluid or air-fluid-containing structure adjacent to colon.
- **Colon wall thickening**—May indicate colitis or mass if diverticuli not seen.
- **Free fluid**—Nonspecific finding, suggesting microperforation.
- **Mural air**—Can be seen within the bowel wall with diverticulitis but also with colonic ischemia.
- **Perforation**—May appear as localized or diffuse extraluminal air.
- **Stranding**—Nonspecific finding of inflammation.

TABLE 9-16. CT Grading of Diverticulitis

Grade of Disease	CT Findings
Mild	Diverticula with bowel wall thickening ≤3 mm and pericolic fat stranding
Moderate	Bowel wall thickening >3 mm with small abscess or phlegmon formation
Severe	Bowel wall thickening >5 mm, perforation with localized or subdiaphragmatic free air, and abscess >5 cm

Adapted from Buckley O, Geoghegan T, O'Riordain DS, et al: Computed tomography in the imaging of colonic diverticulitis. *Clin Radiol* 59:977-983, 2004.

TABLE 9-17. Hinchey Classification of Diverticulitis Severity

Grade	Findings	Mortality
1	Small, confined pericolic or mesenteric abscesses	5%
2	Larger abscesses, confined to pelvis	5%
3	Ruptured peridiverticular abscess with purulent peritonitis	13%
4	Rupture of an uninflamed and unobstructed diverticulum into the peritoneal cavity with fecal contamination	43%

Adapted from Jacobs DO. Clinical practice. Diverticulitis. *N Engl J Med* 357:2057-2066, 2007.

difference between fat and air. A lung or bone window makes air more visible and may be useful. Extraluminal air is also visible with no contrast agents. Perforation can also lead to free fluid in the abdomen, which appears an intermediate gray on a soft-tissue window. No contrast is needed to identify free fluid, which typically pools in dependent regions of the abdomen and pelvis, between bowel loops, solid abdominal organs, and pelvic organs. When enteral contrast is given, it may be found in the peritoneal cavity in up to 35% of cases of perforation.[216]

Abscess formation adjacent to an area of diverticulitis may occur. An abscess typically is an irregular, sometimes rounded collection with a mixture of fluid and air densities. Fluid appears an intermediate gray on an a soft-tissue window; air appears black. An abscess may be visible without the administration of any contrast agents. Fat stranding surrounding an abscess is common and can be seen without IV contrast administration. Contrast agents can be useful in some circumstances in differentiating an abscess from adjacent bowel. The colon normally contains air, liquid, and solid stool; this can have a similar appearance to an abscess, filled with air and heterogeneous purulent contents. Addition of enteral contrast (orally or rectally administered) identifies the bowel lumen; an abscess would not be expected to fill with enteral contrast. IV contrast typically causes rim enhancement of an abscess, which is not expected in normal colon. However, in some cases, an abscess may be readily distinguishable from adjacent bowel based on the other characteristics described, without use of contrast agents.

Colonic obstruction can occur in about 6% to 10% of cases of diverticulitis.[215,217] Findings of large-bowel obstruction were discussed earlier in this chapter. Ureteral obstruction can also occur; findings of ureteral obstruction are discussed in Chapter 12. Fistula formation may complicate diverticulitis. Colovesical fistula is the most common form and is characterized by thickening of the colon adjacent to the bladder and air within the bladder.[215]

Are Contrast Agents Required for the CT Diagnosis of Diverticulitis?

When CT is performed, controversy exists about the preferred technique. The ACR appropriateness criteria for left lower quadrant pain recommend CT with IV contrast and acknowledge conflicting evidence for the need for enteral contrast.[208] Some institutions use oral contrast, whereas others use rectally administered contrast. CT without any contrast agents has been shown to have high sensitivity and specificity, though no single study has compared unenhanced CT, CT with IV contrast, and CT with enteral contrast to determine the incremental benefits of each contrast type.

Tack et al.[29] compared sensitivity and specificity of CT for diverticulitis, using low-radiation-dose unenhanced CT (no oral, rectal, or IV contrast) and standard-radiation-dose CT with IV contrast in the same patient. No significant difference in sensitivity was found between the two protocols, with four readers achieving sensitivities between 85% and 100% with both protocols. Specificity was also equivalent for the two protocols, between 92% and 100%.

Werner et al. (2003) performed CT with IV and rectal contrast only in 120 patients and reported a sensitivity of 97% with 98% specificity. Perforation was detected with a sensitivity of 100% and a specificity of 91%; abscess was detected with a sensitivity of 100% and a specificity of 97%. As with many studies, the reference standard in this study was mixed, with some patients having surgery, others undergoing additional diagnostic imaging, and some having clinical follow-up only. This is a common problem in studies of diagnostic imaging modalities and calls into question the accuracy of the reported sensitivity and specificity, because the true diagnosis in all patients is not confirmed using the same technique.

Cho et al.[218] compared CT and barium enema in 56 patients with suspected diverticulitis based on left lower quadrant pain and tenderness, fever, and leukocytosis. CT was 93% sensitive and 100% specific. Barium enema was 80% sensitive and 100% specific. CT demonstrated alternative diagnoses in 69% of patients without diverticulitis, whereas barium enema found alternative diagnoses in only 10%. This study is compromised by a poor gold standard, in that more than half of the patients were diagnosed with diverticulitis based on improvement with antibiotic therapy—calling into question the validity of the reported CT and barium enema performance.

Rao et al.[7] reported the performance of CT using only rectal contrast (no IV or oral contrast) and found sensitivity of 97% with specificity of 100%. Alternative diagnoses were found in 58% of patients who did not have diverticulitis.

Computed Tomography and Complications of Diverticulitis. Ambrosetti et al.[219] reported that 16% of cases of diverticulitis diagnosed by CT had an associated abscess. They found that 40%—mostly mesocolonic abscesses—were treated with antibiotics without surgery and resolved.

Ambrosetti et al.[220] also reported that poor outcomes in diverticulitis could be predicted from CT findings. When CT demonstrated only mild changes, including localized thickening of the colon wall and pericolic fat inflammation, only 16% of patients experienced complications such as persistent or recurrent diverticulitis, abscess, or fistula formation. In contrast, 48% of patients with severe CT findings, such as abscess, extraluminal air, or extraluminal enteric contrast, experienced bad outcomes requiring surgery.

Ambrosetti et al.[221] later found CT to be 97% sensitive for diverticulitis and to predict complications requiring surgery. Abscess formation and extracolonic gas and enteral contrast predicted failure of medical management in this series.

Image-Guided Drainage of Diverticular Abscesses. Image-guided drainage of diverticular abscesses using CT or ultrasound can be performed, with several potential advantages. In some cases, surgery may be avoided altogether. In other cases, resolution of the acute abscess with percutaneous drainage allows time for colon cathartic cleansing before resection of diseased colon. This allows a single procedure partial colectomy with primary anastomosis, rather than colostomy followed by takedown, which would typically be required for unprepped emergency partial colectomy. Particularly in the elderly or in patients who are poor operative candidates because of comorbidities, percutaneous drainage may be the primary or only therapy. The evidence for this approach comes primarily from small retrospective nonrandomized case series, not large prospective randomized studies.

Bernini et al.[222] examined outcomes in abscesses associated with intestinal disease, drained percutaneously under CT guidance. They found 23% were diverticular abscesses and 100% of unilocular abscesses resolved without surgery. Even with complicated abscesses, drainage was successful in more than half of cases.

Siewert et al.[223] retrospectively reviewed 181 patients with a CT diagnosis of diverticulitis and found 17% with associated abscess. Abscesses less than 3 cm in diameter resolved with antibiotics alone, without CT-guided drainage or surgery. In addition, 50% of abscesses between 3.4 and 4.1 cm in diameter resolved with antibiotics alone. Abscesses larger than 4 cm were successfully treated with CT-guided percutaneous drainage, without acute surgery.

Singh et al.[224] retrospectively reviewed 16 patients undergoing percutaneous diverticular abscess drainage under CT or ultrasound guidance. Even large abscesses were successfully managed initially with percutaneous drainage, although fistula formation complicated 38% and half of patients in this series had surgical resection ultimately.

Sparks et al.[225] reported two cases of percutaneous image-guided diverticular abscess drainage and noted that by treating abscess initially by this approach, an emergent colonic resection and colostomy were avoided.

Stabile et al.[226] reviewed 19 patients with large diverticular abscesses (mean = 8.9 cm) treated with percutaneous drainage. No complications occurred as a result of catheter placement, and resolution of sepsis was seen within 3 days in 89%. Fistula formation occurred in 47%. In addition, 74% of patients were successfully treated with single-stage partial colectomy and primary anastomosis.

Mimics of Diverticulitis on Computed Tomography. Several mimics of diverticulitis should be considered. An inflammatory mass resulting from a colonic neoplasm can have a similar appearance, and it is often recommended that a repeated CT be performed following antibiotic treatment to assess for resolution of CT findings. Follow-up colonoscopy may be performed (in addition to, or sometimes instead of, repeated CT imaging) to help identify neoplasms simulating diverticulitis. CT morphologic criteria, including length of involved bowel, presence of a mass, pericolonic inflammation, and pericolonic lymph nodes, have relatively poor ability to discriminate colon cancer from diverticulitis, because characteristics overlap between the two conditions. Early work using CT perfusion scanning to identify cancers suggests better sensitivity and specificity but these are too low for clinical application.[227] If diverticuli are not identified but regional inflammatory changes such as stranding, bowel wall thickening, and altered bowel wall enhancement are seen, colitis should be considered (ischemic, infectious, or resulting from inflammatory bowel disease). These conditions are discussed in more detail in this and other chapters.

Ultrasound of Diverticulitis. Transabdominal ultrasound has been investigated for detection of diverticulitis and has a reported sensitivity of 77% to 98% and specificity of 80% to 99%.[228-231] Overall, ultrasound is likely less sensitive and specific than CT. In women, transvaginal ultrasound can be used and can differentiate left lower quadrant abnormalities such as ectopic pregnancy, tuboovarian abscess, and ovarian torsion. Ultrasound carries no radiation exposure, unlike CT. The ACR recommends ultrasound as the initial test in women of childbearing age with left lower quadrant abdominal pain for this reason.[208]

Ultrasound findings of diverticulitis include bowel wall thickening greater than 4 mm and a relatively hypoechoic colonic wall. Dilated and fluid-filled colon may be seen. In some cases, air-containing diverticuli or abscesses may be identified.[230] A target-like appearance of the bowel in transverse view can be seen. Tenderness of the abdomen during graded compression over a segment of colon has also been described.[229]

Magnetic Resonance Imaging of Diverticulitis. MRI is rarely used in diagnosis of diverticulitis, and studies are limited. The indications for MRI are relatively few, because patients with allergies to IV contrast can undergo unenhanced CT or CT with enteral contrast only. Patients in whom radiation exposures must be limited, such as pregnant patients, can undergo ultrasound as an initial test. More studies are required to validate the sensitivity and specificity of MRI. If MRI becomes more widely available, inexpensive, and rapid, it may become a more widely accepted alternative to CT, given the advantage of no ionizing radiation exposure.

Ajaj et al.[232] compared T1-weighted dark-lumen MRI using an aqueous enema with IV gadolinium contrast to conventional colonoscopy for the diagnosis of sigmoid diverticulitis in 40 patients. MRI findings of diverticulitis included increased wall thickness and pericolic mesenteric fat infiltration. MRI was 83% sensitive and 81% specific. MRI missed cases of mild inflammation detected by colonography and misclassified as diverticulitis some cases of colon cancer identified by colonography.

Heverhagen et al.[233] performed MRI in 20 patients with established acute diverticulitis, using diagnostic criteria including presence of at least one diverticulum, pericolonic inflammatory change, and colon wall edema. MRI detected 95% of cases, although this performance might not be replicated in an unselected patient sample. In addition, because only positive cases were included, the specificity of MRI cannot be determined from this study.

Schreyer et al. (2004) performed MRI in 14 consecutive patients with suspected diverticulitis and found the performance was identical to CT.

Bleeding from Diverticuli. Bleeding from diverticuli can be identified using one of three imaging modalities: tagged red blood cell study (a nuclear medicine procedure), mesenteric angiography, or CTA. These procedures are discussed in more detail in the section on GI bleeding.

Bowel Abnormalities: Inflammatory Bowel Disease, Infectious Colitis, and Enteritis

Inflammatory bowel disease and infectious colitides and enteritides have similar imaging findings, which must be correlated with clinical history to determine the likely cause (Figures 9-67 through 9-71). X-ray is of little utility. CT scan can demonstrate typical inflammatory findings, can identify complications of inflammatory bowel disease such as abscess or fistula formation, and can demonstrate alternative diagnoses such as bowel ischemia, diverticulitis, appendicitis, or neoplasm. Ultrasound, MRI, and nuclear scintigraphy are alternatives, though these are rarely used in the emergency department for this indication. In the emergency department, CT is the most commonly used modality in the United States because of its wide availability and ability

to diagnose complications and alternative disease processes. CT is likely the most appropriate initial test in the patient without known inflammatory bowel disease as well, as a result of its ability to evaluate for multiple disease processes.

A dedicated CT technique called CT enteroclysis can be used to evaluate the small bowel. In this technique, a nasoenteric tube is passed into the small bowel at the duodenal–jejunal junction under fluoroscopic guidance and low-density contrast material (usually water) is rapidly instilled in large volumes to distend the small bowel. This allows identification of abnormal bowel wall thickness and morphology. The technique is not commonly used in the emergency department, partly because of poor patient tolerance of nasoenteric intubation.[234]

Sensitivity of Diagnostic Modalities for Inflammatory Bowel Disease. The sensitivity and specificity of CT, MRI, ultrasound, and nuclear scintigraphy have been compared in a metaanalysis of prospective studies. Horsthuis et al.[235] evaluated 33 studies and found similar diagnostic performance among the modalities on a per-patient basis, as opposed to a per-bowel-segment diagnostic basis (Table 9-18). The authors suggest that MRI and ultrasound be considered for disease monitoring, because these modalities do not result in ionizing radiation exposure.

Other authors have found better sensitivity of dedicated CT techniques such as CT enteroclysis, though the number of included patients is small. Boudiaf et al.[236] reported CT enteroclysis to have a sensitivity of 100% and specificity of 95% for small-bowel diseases including small-bowel masses, Crohn's disease, small-bowel tuberculosis, small-bowel lymphoma, and low-grade small-bowel obstruction. However, the total number of patients in this study was only 107 and represented a range of disease processes, so the sensitivity and specificity of CT for each disease process have wide CIs. In small studies, CT enterography has been shown to correlate with disease progression, may reveal clinically unsuspected bowel strictures, and may rule out clinically suspected strictures.[237-238]

Computed Tomography Findings of Inflammatory Bowel Disease. Figures 9-67 through 9-70 demonstrate CT changes of inflammatory bowel disease. On CT scan, hallmarks of bowel inflammation include bowel wall thickening (often visible with no contrast agents) and surrounding fat stranding (also visible without contrast agents). Bodily et al.[239] found that increased wall thickness and increased mural attenuation correlated with disease activity measured by endoscopy and histology. Lymphadenopathy may be seen. Findings such as free abdominal fluid may be present and should raise concerns about perforation. Inspection for extraluminal air should also be performed. If IV contrast is administered,

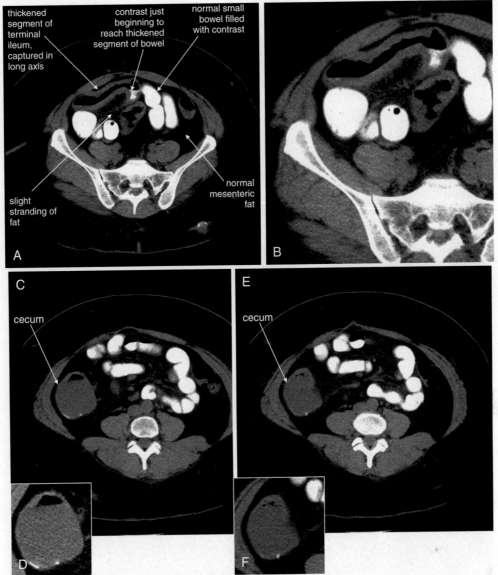

Figure 9-67. Inflammatory bowel disease: Crohn's disease, CT with oral contrast, soft-tissue window. This patient with confirmed Crohn's disease presented with abdominal pain and has thickening of the terminal ileum typical of Crohn's disease, although the CT appearance is not pathognomonic and could be mimicked by infectious causes. **A, C, E, G, I, K, M,** Axial images. **B, D, F, H, J, L, N,** Close-ups from **A, C, E, G, I, K, M,** respectively. Note the abnormal bowel wall thickness—compare with the normal small bowel in the same slice. The patient received oral contrast, which has just started to reach the terminal ileum but did not fill the affected segment. Theoretically, oral contrast might help to distinguish the bowel lumen from the bowel wall, but in this case air in the thickened bowel segment performs this function. The diagnosis could have been made in this patient without oral contrast. The patient did not receive intravenous contrast for unclear reasons. The normal bowel to the patient's left has an extremely thin wall. The oral contrast in the normal bowel lumen is discretely contained, but the wall itself is hardly visible—oral contrast marking the lumen gives way to the mesenteric fat surrounding the bowel. The abnormal bowel segment is also surrounded by fat that appears to show slight stranding (*gray* in comparison to the dark fat surrounding normal bowel). These images also prove that the inflamed segment is the terminal ileum. Following retrograde from **C** to **N,** the thickened ileum emerges from the cecum. Wall thickening of the ileum is present, and fat stranding can be seen. The thickened small bowel has a "doughnut" appearance in short-axis cross section.

the bowel wall should be inspected for increased enhancement, consistent with inflammation, infection, or ischemia, and decreased enhancement—which suggests bowel ischemia. Mural pneumatosis suggests regional bowel gangrene, which can occur from ischemia or infection. Occasionally, fistula formation may be visible without enteral contrast, but enteral contrast can assist in the diagnosis by demonstrating extraluminal contrast leak via the fistula. Abscess formation can occur with inflammatory bowel disease and appears the

same as described in the earlier section on diverticulitis or in the later section on abscesses.

The "fat halo" sign is a finding of submucosal fat deposition in the bowel wall, associated with Crohn's disease. A density of less than −10 Hounsfield units is diagnostic. The ileum and ascending colon are the most common locations. It is not a marker of acute inflammation but is thought to occur with increasing duration of disease. In one study, the fat halo sign was seen in

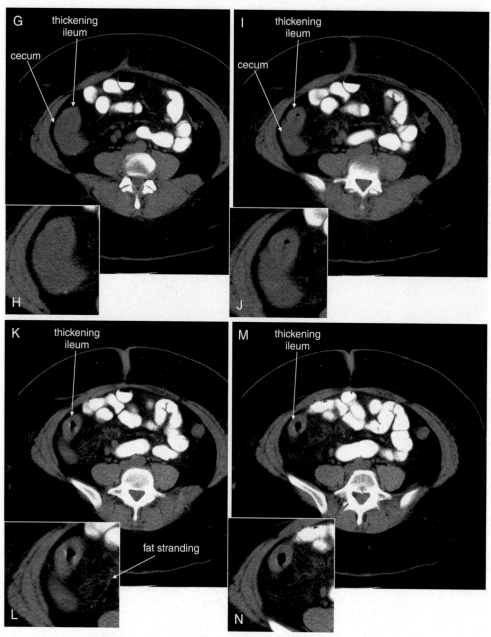

Figure 9-67, cont'd

only 3.8% of patients with disease duration of less than 1 year and in 21.9% of patients with longer duration of disease.[240] Unfortunately, the fat halo sign may also be seen in obese patients with no apparent inflammatory bowel disease and is thus nonspecific.[241]

Differentiating the cause of bowel abnormalities by CT criteria may be difficult or impossible, and clinical history or other testing such as microbiologic or endoscopic findings may be required. Some clues from CT can narrow the differential diagnosis (Table 9-19). First, diverticuli should be sought; their absence generally rules out diverticulitis. However, sometimes severe inflammation around diverticuli may mask their presence. If previous CT or other imaging from the patient is available, it

may be useful to review that imaging for the presence of diverticuli. The bowel should be followed sequentially from the rectum proximally, including both the small and the large bowel, for signs of inflammation. Ulcerative colitis should demonstrate only contiguous regions of inflammation starting at the rectum and moving proximally. In contrast, Crohn's disease is well known for discontiguous regions of inflammation (sometimes called "skip lesions"), which can involve any part of the intestine from mouth to anus. Vascular disease causing ischemic bowel can appear identical to other inflammatory or infectious abnormalities of bowel; it is discussed in detail in Chapter 11. However, clues to a vascular cause include a region of inflammation or bowel abnormality matching a common vascular distribution. Inspection of

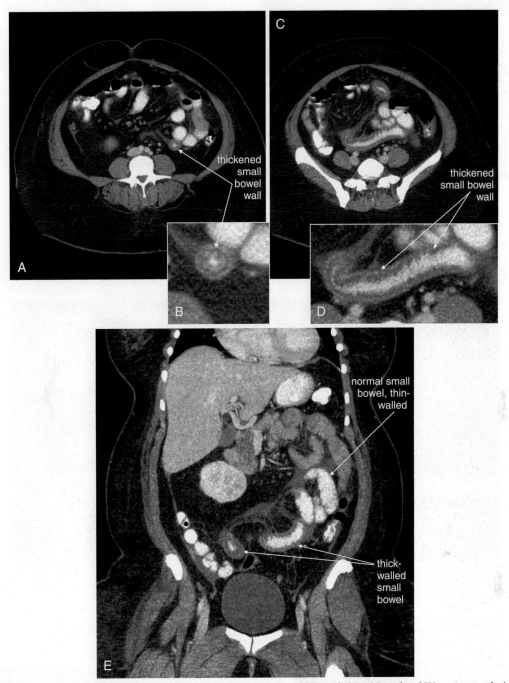

Figure 9-68. Inflammatory bowel disease, Crohn's disease, positive oral contrast in bowel, CT with oral and IV contrast, soft-tissue window. In another patient with Crohn's disease, oral contrast has reached a thickened segment of small bowel. Note the remarkable degree of thickening of the small-bowel wall, remembering that the normal wall is nearly invisible. **A, C,** Axial images. **B, D,** Close-ups from **A** and **C,** respectively. **E,** Coronal view. **A** shows a thickened section in short-axis cross section, with a typical doughnut appearance, whereas **B** shows a thickened segment in long-axis cross section. The lumen of the bowel in **A** is nearly obliterated, with just a narrow column of oral contrast remaining (the "doughnut hole"). **E** shows a coronal reconstruction. Compare the normal and abnormal small-bowel segments in **E.** Technically, CT cannot determine whether there is a fixed point of stricture from bowel wall thickening, because CT is a static study capturing a moment in time. Perhaps the bowel segment was undergoing peristaltic contraction at the moment of CT. Note also the relative lack of fat stranding—this CT shows a relative remission for this patient, who has had chronic bowel wall thickening and at times has had more inflammatory stranding. Remember also that a differential diagnosis exists for these findings. Bowel wall tumors such as lymphomas can present with bowel wall thickening. Infection and ischemia, as well as inflammatory bowel disease, may cause bowel wall thickening.

blood vessels for filling defects can allow direct detection of stenosis or thrombosis; this requires IV contrast administration. Beware the possibility of bowel ischemia; a noncontrast CT cannot fully discriminate bowel ischemia and inflammatory or infectious bowel disease.

Neoplastic disease can result in bowel wall abnormalities and inflammation, sometimes mimicking infection or benign inflammatory bowel disease. Inspection of solid organs may reveal lesions consistent with metastatic disease, suggesting a malignant cause of the bowel

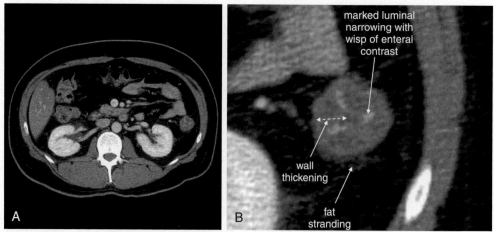

Figure 9-69. Colitis, likely infectious, CT with oral and IV contrast, soft-tissue window. This 41-year-old male with no past medical history presented with abdominal pain and bright red blood per rectum. The wall of the descending colon is quite thickened, leaving only a ribbon of lumen with enteral contrast. Some surrounding fat stranding is present. These findings are consistent with colitis, though the cause is not determined by CT. Infectious colitis, inflammatory bowel disease, or ischemia colitis could have similar appearances. **A,** Axial image. **B,** Close-up.

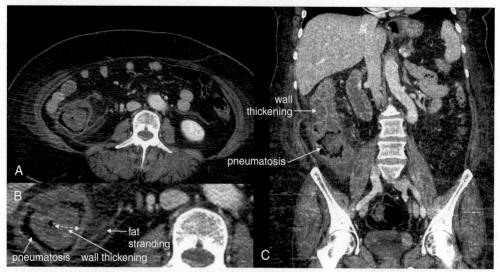

Figure 9-70. Colitis, CT with oral and IV contrast, soft-tissue window. CT findings of colitis include large-bowel wall thickening and stranding of surrounding fat. CT often cannot distinguish the cause, though subtle findings may suggest infectious, inflammatory, or ischemic causes. Ischemic colitis may be recognized by explicit identification of a vascular occlusion or may be suspected when the affected portions of bowel follow a specific vascular distribution. This patient had concerning findings for ischemia and underwent laparotomy—but no resection was performed because the bowel appeared viable. The patient recovered uneventfully with antibiotics and fluids. **A,** The axial CT slice (**B,** close-up) shows significant bowel wall thickening and pneumatosis coli of the cecum and ascending colon. Fat stranding is also present. **C,** A coronal reconstruction shows similar findings. Bowel ischemia is discussed in detail in Chapter 11.

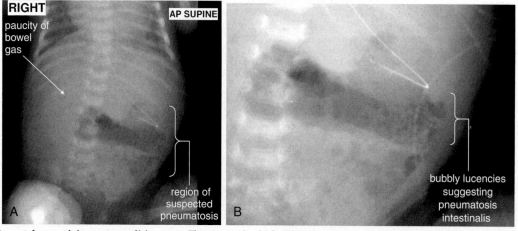

Figure 9-71. Neonatal necrotizing enterocolitis, x-ray. This 1-month-old female infant was in the intensive care unit for treatment of a complex congenital heart defect when she developed bloody stools. Her x-ray is concerning for necrotizing enterocolitis, with small bubbles consistent with pneumatosis intestinalis and a paucity of luminal bowel gas. **A,** Supine x-ray. **B,** Close-up.

TABLE 9-18. Diagnostic Performance of Modalities for Inflammatory Bowel Disease

Modality	Sensitivity	Specificity
CT	84.3%	95.1%
MRI	93%	92.8%
Nuclear scintigraphy	87.8%	84.5%
Ultrasound	89.7%	95.6%

Adapted from Horsthuis K, Bipat S, Bennink RJ, Stoker J. Inflammatory bowel disease diagnosed with US, MR, scintigraphy, and CT: meta-analysis of prospective studies. *Radiology* 247:64-79, 2008.

abnormalities. Lymphadenopathy can occur with infectious, inflammatory, or malignant disease. Radiation colitis typically causes circumferential bowel wall thickening and adjacent fat stranding, but the appearance is nonspecific. Graft-versus-host disease in patients with a history of bone marrow transplant can result in a similar appearance.[242]

Infectious enteritis or colitis, including *C. difficile* colitis, can appear similar to other forms of inflammatory or ischemic disease and should be considered.[242] Fishman et al.[243] described the CT findings of *C. difficile* pseudomembranous colitis, including significant bowel wall thickening with a mean thickness of 14.7 mm, and enteric contrast trapped between broad transverse tissue bands. The entire colon or localized segments can be involved. An accordion appearance can be seen, in which the colon wall is so thickened that only a thin string of contrast is seen within the lumen between abutting walls. The appearance is not specific and must be correlated with the clinical presentation. Toxic megacolon from *C. difficile* or other causes can be evaluated with CT. Perforation and septic thrombosis of the portal system complicating toxic megacolon can be identified with CT.[244]

Bowel disease can be further evaluated with a variety of modalities when CT does not adequately differentiate disease. Angiography can further explore bowel ischemia. Upper GI or lower GI contrast studies, including enteroclysis and contrast enema, can assist in identifying changes of inflammatory bowel disease. Direct endoscopic visualization can also assist when imaging is nondiagnostic. MRI, ultrasound, and nuclear scintigraphy provide other options but are rarely indicated in the emergency department.

Typhlitis

Typhlitis is cecal inflammation and necrosis first described in leukemia patients but subsequently observed in patients with AIDS, lymphoma, aplastic anemia, immunosuppression for organ transplant, and chemotherapy-induced neutropenia. It can involve the appendix and terminal ileum and, in severe cases, potentially the entire colon. The condition is seen in

TABLE 9-19. CT Findings Suggesting Inflammatory, Infectious, or Ischemic Colitis, or Colonic Neoplasm

CT Finding	Implication
Bowel wall thickening	Nonspecific
Differential bowel wall enhancement	Decreased enhancement suggests ischemia; increased enhancement is nonspecific
Diverticuli	Nonspecific—may coexist with other pathology
Fat halo sign	Nonspecific—correlates with duration of Crohn's disease, not acute inflammation
Free air	Nonspecific—can occur with ischemia, inflammation, infection, or neoplasm
Free fluid	Nonspecific
Lymphadenopathy	Lymphadenopathy greater than 1 cm concerning for malignancy rather than infection or inflammation
Metastatic disease in solid organs	Suggestive of bowel malignancy, although other acute bowel pathology (e.g., ischemia) and other primary malignancy may be present
Skip lesions	Intermittent areas of abnormal bowel, with intervening normal regions, suggestive of Crohn's disease
Vascular lesions	Occlusive mesenteric disease is specific for mesenteric ischemia
Vascular territories	Abnormal bowel corresponding to a single vascular territory suggests ischemia

patients with absolute neutrophil counts less than 1000 per microliter. The exact cause is unknown, although GI mucosal cytotoxicity from chemotherapy agents is thought to play a role in iatrogenic cases. Cytomegalovirus infection has also been implicated. Mucosal ischemia may allow transmural penetration of bacteria, leading to perforation. Intramural hemorrhage may also be seen. Although rare, the condition has a mortality of 40% to 50%, related to sepsis from bowel perforation.

Computed Tomography Findings of Typhlitis

The normal cecum thickness on CT is 3 mm or less, and when the cecum is distended with stool, it normally appears paper thin. The pericecal fat does not normally show inflammatory stranding. With typhlitis, the cecal wall thickens; a symmetrical pattern is common, but eccentric thickening can occur. Pericecal fat stranding is typical. Hemorrhage in the colonic wall may appear higher in attenuation than the normal wall. Complications such as pneumatosis coli, pneumoperitoneum, and abscess may be seen and have the CT characteristics described elsewhere in this chapter. Overall, the CT appearance is nonspecific, resembling other forms of colitis, but is diagnostic in the setting of severe immunocompromise and neutropenia.[245-246]

Ultrasound of Typhlitis

Ultrasound can be used to diagnose typhlitis and demonstrates decreased or absent peristalsis, a thickened and hypoechoic bowel wall, and a thickened and echogenic mucosa. Ultrasound findings should be augmented with CT to evaluate for complications such as abscess or perforation.

X-ray of Typhlitis

As with most other conditions described in this chapter, x-ray is nonspecific for typhlitis. Thumbprinting of the cecal wall, pneumatosis, and free air may be seen.

Bowel Ischemia

Mesenteric ischemia encompasses a family of disorders, including acute thrombosis of the SMA, chronic mesenteric artery thrombosis, ischemic colitis, portal vein thrombosis, and ischemia caused by mechanical effects such as bowel obstruction or volvulus (described earlier). These conditions are not accurately diagnosed by x-ray, which only rarely shows findings of advanced disease such as pneumatosis intestinalis from bowel infarction. Historically, catheter angiography was used to identify vascular occlusions and stenoses, but modern CTA has largely replaced this. CT with IV contrast has the advantage of identifying other causes of acute abdominal pain, as well as secondary bowel injury related to vascular occlusion. MRI is rarely used in the emergency department to identify bowel ischemia but is comparable in performance to CT and can be used when contraindications to CT exist. Imaging of bowel ischemia is discussed in detail in Chapter 11.

Hepatobiliary Imaging

In the sections that follow, we discuss the imaging of hepatobiliary disorders, including cholelithiasis, cholecystitis, choledocholithiasis, biliary ductal obstruction, and biliary ductal leaks. Figures 9-72 through 9-110 demonstrate hepatobiliary imaging with a variety of modalities.

Cholelithiasis and Cholecystitis

Cholelithiasis and its complications can be imaged with multiple modalities, including ultrasound, nuclear scintigraphy, CT and MRI. Although x-rays occasional demonstrate calcified gallstones (see Figure 9-72), they lack sensitivity or specificity for cholecystitis and should not be used for this diagnosis.[247] Clinical signs and symptoms and laboratory testing are relatively nonspecific and insensitive, meaning that imaging is often necessary to exclude or confirm disease.[248] Gruber et al.[249] found that 71% of patients with nongangrenous cholecystitis were afebrile and 32% lacked leukocytosis. In gangrenous cholecystitis, 59% of patients were afebrile and 27% lacked leukocytosis.

Ultrasound of Cholelithiasis and Cholecystitis. Ultrasound is commonly used for the diagnosis of cholelithiasis and cholecystitis and is increasingly performed by emergency physicians. The test is portable, requires no radiation exposure, and can rapidly provide diagnostic

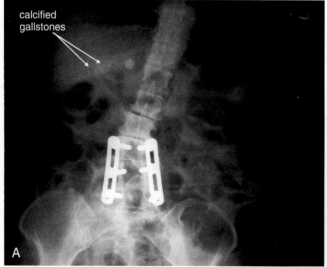
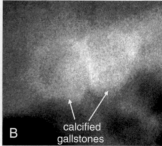

Figure 9-72. X-ray demonstrating calcified gallstones. X-ray is a poor modality for diagnosis of biliary disease, although gallstones are sometimes incidentally noted. X-ray typically does not provide the necessary additional information to differentiate asymptomatic gallstones, symptomatic gallstones, or acute cholecystitis. Additional imaging with ultrasound, nuclear medicine studies, or computed tomography is usually required. **A,** X-ray. **B,** Close-up. The contrast in **B** has been adjusted to improve the visibility of the gallstones.

information. Ultrasound findings of cholecystitis must be differentiated from those of cholelithiasis—because the presence of gallstones is not sufficient for the diagnosis of cholecystitis. Although gallstones are present in most cases of cholecystitis, acalculous cholecystitis can occur in critically ill patients, particularly following burns or trauma, during sepsis, and while receiving total parenteral nutrition.[250] Currently ultrasound is recommended by the ACR as the most appropriate imaging test in patients with right upper quadrant pain.[251]

Ultrasound Findings of Cholelithiasis. With ultrasound, gallstones are visible as hyperechoic (bright white) structures within the gallbladder, casting dark acoustic shadows (see Figures 9-73 through 9-87). Gallstones are typically mobile (see Figure 9-80) unless lodged in the gallbladder neck (see Figure 9-83), cystic duct, or common bile duct—distinguishing them from gallbladder polyps, which are immobile and do not cast acoustic shadows (see Figure 9-84). Gallstone mobility can be assessed by rolling the patient during the ultrasound examination to observe any resulting motion of gallbladder contents. Smaller gallstones may be as small as a grain of sand or even finer particles—leading to terms such as "gallbladder sand" and "sludge." Even at these small sizes, gallstones remain hyperechoic and are mobile. Gallbladder sludge forms a dependent layer within the gallbladder but may not be so dense as to cast an acoustic shadow. When the gallbladder is completely filled with stones, an appearance called the wall–echo–shadow sign may be seen. In this case, the ultrasound beam reflects off of stones immediately deep

to the superficial gallbladder wall. Deeper structures are not seen. This appearance can be similar to that seen with a heavily calcified gallbladder (porcelain gallbladder; Figure 9-111), which is associated with gallbladder carcinoma. In one recent study, this association has been found to be less strong than previously described.[252] In addition, in gangrenous cholecystitis, air within the gallbladder wall creates a bright echo and posterior shadowing.[253]

Findings of cholecystitis include gallbladder wall thickening (>3-4 mm), pericholecystic fluid, and sonographic Murphy's sign.[253-254] The normal gallbladder wall is a pencil-lead-thin (2-3 mm) hyperechoic line (see Figures 9-73 and 9-85). With inflammatory change, the wall thickens and may take on a striated appearance (see Figure 9-86). Thickening may occur in other disease states besides cholecystitis, including cirrhosis, viral hepatitis, heart failure, hypoalbuminemia, and chronic renal failure.[255] Pericholecystic fluid appears hypoechoic (black) on ultrasound (see Figure 9-87). The finding is nonspecific in isolation, because fluid may be present in the gallbladder fossa from other processes including diffuse ascites. A sonographic Murphy's sign is the presence of tenderness to direct palpation over the gallbladder with the ultrasound probe. The sensitivity of this finding in isolation for acute cholecystitis is only around 86%, with 35% specificity.[256] Some radiologists decline to comment on the sonographic Murphy's sign in a patient who has received analgesics. An enlarged gallbladder is another nonspecific sign of possible cholecystitis. The normal size of the gallbladder is 7-10 cm in length and 2-3 cm in

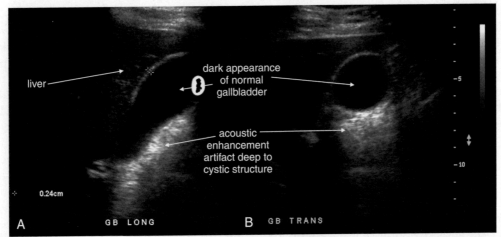

Figure 9-73. Normal gallbladder, ultrasound. The normal gallbladder is thin-walled, hypoechoic (*black*, with no internal echoes), and has no pericholecystic fluid (which would appear black with ultrasound). Although the exact size and position of the gallbladder varies from patient to patient, in general it is a pear-shaped structure, elliptic in the long-axis view **(A),** and circular in short axis **(B).** It narrows to a neck (infundibulum) at one end, leading to the cystic duct. At this end, it may have one of more folds that are normal anatomic variants. Normal liquid bile is an excellent medium for sound transmission without reflection, resulting in the black appearance of the normal gallbladder. This in turn leads to an image artifact, called acoustic enhancement. This is an artificial brightening of the image deep to any cystic structure. This is not caused by the tissues deep to the gallbladder being more echogenic. Rather, more sound is transmitted through the gallbladder than through solid tissues at a similar depth. Put another way, the gallbladder and other cystic structures attenuate ultrasound transmission to a lesser extent than do solid tissues. As a consequence, more ultrasound signal remains to be reflected back by deep tissues. Ultrasound software is typically written to brighten the tissue appearance to account for an expected uniform loss of signal with increasing depth. When less signal is lost than is expected, the software over-corrects, resulting in acoustic enhancement artifact.

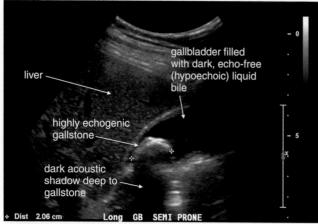

Figure 9-74. Cholelithiasis, ultrasound. The standard modality for assessment of gallbladder pathology is ultrasound. Cholelithiasis, the presence of gallstones, is demonstrated readily on ultrasound. Liquid bile is black on ultrasound because liquid is an excellent medium for sound transmission, with little internal reflection (echoes). Gallstones cause significant reflection of sound waves, making them quite bright or echogenic. In addition, because sound waves are mostly reflected and not transmitted well beyond the location of the stone, the stone typically casts a black acoustic shadow on ultrasound. Gallstones may be single or multiple. Normally cholelithiasis without cholecystitis shows gallstones without accompanying gallbladder wall thickening, pericholecystic fluid, or sonographic Murphy's sign. Here, a classic example of a gallstone is shown. This large gallstone (2 cm) has a highly echogenic surface, with acoustic shadowing occurring deep to the gallstone.

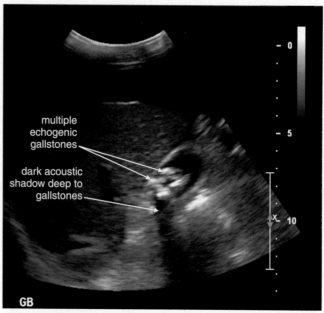

Figure 9-75. Cholelithiasis, multiple stones, ultrasound. Stones may vary in size from sandlike (sometimes called "sludge"), to pea-sized ("gravel"), to quite large "stones." This patient has multiple smaller stones, piled upon one another, compared with the previous patient, in Figure 9-74. These stones share the same highly echogenic appearance and posterior acoustic shadowing on ultrasound.

width. A transverse diameter greater than 5 cm suggests cholecystitis.[254]

Sensitivity and Specificity of Ultrasound and Nuclear Scintigraphy for Acute Cholecystitis. Numerous studies have evaluated the sensitivity and specificity of ultrasound and nuclear scintigraphy (described shortly) for cholelithiasis and acute cholecystitis. Most studies suggest that ultrasound is highly sensitive and specific for gallstones. It is sensitive but less specific for cholecystitis. Nuclear scintigraphy is considered more sensitive and specific than ultrasonography for acute cholecystitis—but is more costly and time-consuming and exposes the patient to ionizing radiation.[251] Shea et al.[257] performed a metaanalysis of studies of ultrasound and nuclear scintigraphy and corrected the calculated sensitivity and specificity for a common methodologic bias: verification bias. This error occurs when a gold standard test is not performed in all patients to confirm the findings of the test whose performance is being evaluated. This can result in inaccurate calculation of sensitivity and specificity, because the true presence or absence of disease is not confirmed. The authors found that the sensitivity of ultrasound and nuclear scintigraphy were likely lower than previously reported, when corrected for verification bias (Table 9-20). They recommended that a sensitivity midway between corrected and uncorrected values be assumed.

False-positive ultrasound findings can occur in a number of settings. Gallbladder wall thickening can occur

postprandially because of normal gallbladder contraction.[254] Consequently, some centers require that the patient fast at least 4 hours before gallbladder ultrasound. As previously mentioned, pericholecystic fluid may represent fluid within the abdomen from another source such as ascites, rather than inflammatory fluid related to gallbladder pathology.

Nuclear Scintigraphy (Hepatobiliary Iminodiacetic Acid Scan) of Cholecystitis and Biliary Obstruction. Hepatobiliary iminodiacetic acid (HIDA) nuclear scintigraphy (also called cholescintigraphy, hepatobiliary scintigraphy, or a hepatobiliary scan) represents another means of assessing the gallbladder and biliary tree for pathology. In this test, HIDA labeled with a radioactive tracer (usually technetium-99m) is injected intravenously, is taken up by the liver, and is excreted into the bile. It then travels in bile from the liver through the biliary ducts to the gallbladder and on to the small intestine. A series of images is captured over time with a gamma camera, recording the sequence of passage of bile. In a normal HIDA scan, the liver becomes visible first, followed by the hepatic duct. The gallbladder then becomes visible, because it fills retrograde through the cystic duct. Filling of the common bile duct also occurs, followed by transit of bile through the Sphincter of Oddi into the small bowel. Patients are usually required to fast for 2 hours before cholescintigraphy.

In cases of obstruction of biliary ducts, portions of the biliary system distal to the obstruction are not

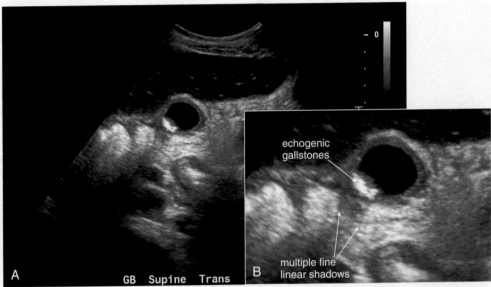

Figure 9-76. Cholelithiasis, multiple stones, ultrasound. A, Short-axis (transverse) view of the gallbladder. Fine, sandlike gallstones are echogenic but cast relatively small shadows. A close-up **(B)** shows the thin linear shadows cast by these stones. This gallbladder also shows abnormal wall thickness, which is discussed in a future figure.

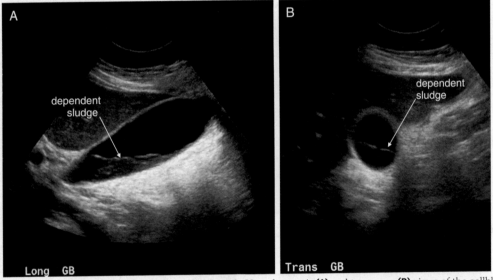

Figure 9-77. Cholelithiasis, multiple stones and sludge, ultrasound. Here, long-axis **(A)** and transverse **(B)** views of the gallbladder show sludge in the gallbladder. This material is denser than liquid bile but does not have discrete stones. Sludge may be asymptomatic or could be present in a case of acalculous cholecystitis. Sludge typically does not cast an acoustic shadow. This patient underwent a CT scan, which showed additional findings suggesting acute cholecystitis, including fat stranding in the region of the gallbladder.

visualized, because HIDA-labeled bile does not pass the point of obstruction. If the cystic duct or gallbladder neck becomes obstructed by a stone, as is common in cases of cholecystitis, the gallbladder is not visualized. In cases of choledocholithiasis, distal portions of the common bile duct and small bowel do not receive HIDA-labeled bile and are not visualized. An abnormal HIDA scan is not specific for biliary obstruction by a stone, because obstruction by a mass or stricture would have a similar appearance.

In some cases of cholecystitis or gallbladder dysfunction leading to chronic abdominal pain, the gallbladder fills normally but does not contract normally. When the gallbladder is visualized on cholescintigraphy but doubt remains about the function of the gallbladder, cholecystokinin can be administered intravenously and the response observed. Usually brisk emptying of the gallbladder is observed, with subsequent nuclear scintigraphy images showing an absence of the gallbladder in the image after HIDA-laden bile is expelled. In the case of an abnormal gallbladder, the gallbladder image remains on images acquired after administration of cholecystokinin, because HIDA-labeled bile remains within the gallbladder. Quantitative measurement of the gallbladder ejection fraction can be performed; an ejection

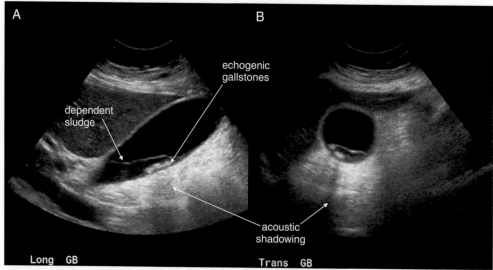

Figure 9-78. Cholelithiasis, multiple stones and sludge, ultrasound. Same patient as Figure 9-77. Sludge and stones can coexist. Dependent sludge is present, and small stones have settled to the bottom of the sludge layer. Long-axis **(A)** and transverse **(B)** views both show these findings. Posterior acoustic shadowing is seen in both views.

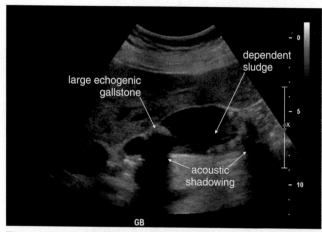

Figure 9-79. Cholelithiasis, multiple stones and sludge, ultrasound. Sludge and stones can coexist. In this patient, not currently complaining of any abdominal pain, large and small stones are present, along with sludge. But no pericholecystic fluid or wall thickening is present, and the patient does not have a sonographic Murphy's sign. The patient does not have acute cholecystitis.

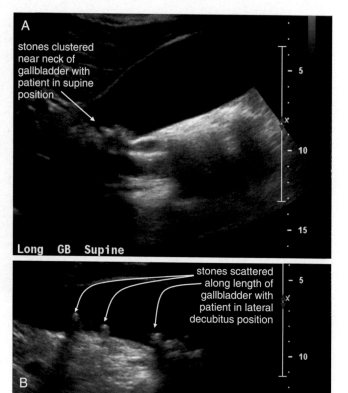

Figure 9-80. Cholelithiasis, mobile stones, ultrasound. Stones are typically mobile, shifting in the gallbladder if the patient changes position, such as rolling from a supine to a decubitus position. In contrast, gallbladder polyps are not mobile, because they are fixed to the gallbladder wall with a stalk. A gallstone may also be immobile if it is lodged in the neck (infundibulum) of the gallbladder—a setup for cholecystitis even if other sonographic findings are not yet present. **A, B,** Long-axis views of the gallbladder. In this patient, gallstones are clustered near the neck of the gallbladder when the patient is supine **(A)**. In the next image **(B)**, the patient has rolled to a left lateral decubitus position, scattering the stones along the length of the gallbladder. These stones are not impacted.

fraction less than 50% after cholecystokinin is abnormal.[258] Figures 9-88 through 9-90 demonstrate normal and abnormal HIDA studies.

HIDA–nuclear scintigraphy can be used to assess for conditions other than cholecystitis, biliary obstruction, and gallbladder dysfunction. Because the test traces the route of bile excreted from the liver, it can be used to assess for bile leaks, as may occur as a complication of hepatobiliary surgery. If radiotracer accumulates in an unexpected location, a leak can be diagnosed (see Figure 9-101). If tracer accumulates locally, a biloma may be diagnosed. If tracer is distributed diffusely in the abdomen, a bile leak into the peritoneal cavity is present. HIDA scintigraphy can also diagnose iatrogenic

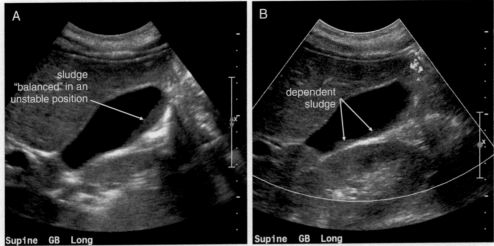

Figure 9-81. Cholelithiasis, mobile sludge, ultrasound. Sludge is also freely mobile, settling to a dependent position as the patient is repositioned. **A, B,** Long-axis views of the gallbladder. In this patient, sludge is seen sloped in an unstable position along the wall of the gallbladder. A moment later, a "landslide" occurs, and the sludge is seen settled in a more dependent position.

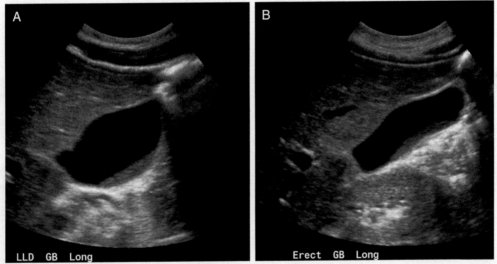

Figure 9-82. Cholelithiasis, mobile sludge, ultrasound. A, B, Long-axis views of the gallbladder. In this patient, sludge is seen in a dependent position with the patient positioned in left lateral decubitus **(A)** and erect **(B)** positions.

obstruction, such as inadvertent clipping of the common bile duct during surgery. Because the method records scintigraphic emission from bile, it provides no specific information about the cause of the obstruction (tumor, stone, stricture, or surgical clip), because the body tissues themselves are not imaged.

The high sensitivity and specificity of HIDA cholescintigraphy is achieved with imaging up to 4 hours after radiotracer administration, an important limitation to use in the emergency department. Sensitivity and specificity are decreased to only 80% to 88% when imaging is continued for only 1 hour. Administration of morphine can be performed if the gallbladder is not seen by 40 to 60 minutes after administration of radiotracer and if tracer is seen in the small bowel. Morphine is thought to cause some constriction of the sphincter of Oddi,

enhancing retrograde filling of the gallbladder when the cystic duct is patent. Cholescintigraphy with morphine augmentation in this manner has been shown to achieve high sensitivity (94.6%) and specificity (99.1%) with only 1.5 hours of imaging.[259]

The sensitivity and specificity of HIDA cholescintigraphy has been studied extensively (see Table 9-20).[251,257] It remains a second-line test to ultrasound in most circumstances, because it may take 2 to 4 hours to complete, exposes the patient to ionizing radiation, and is more expensive than ultrasound. In addition, it does not directly visualize organs, unlike ultrasound and CT, and so may be less useful in evaluating for alternative pathology. Although metaanalysis data suggests high specificity, some studies have suggested very low specificity of HIDA scans, as low as 38%.[260]

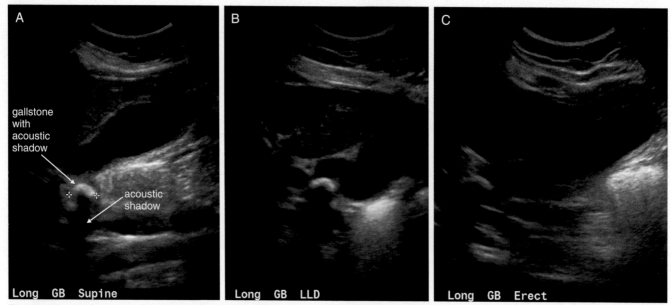

Figure 9-83. **Cholelithiasis, immobile stones, ultrasound. A,** Long-axis view of the gallbladder with the patient supine. **B,** Long-axis view of the gallbladder with the patient in a left lateral decubitus position. **C,** Long-axis view of the gallbladder with the patient erect. In this 38-year-old presenting with abdominal pain and vomiting, a single large gallstone is seen in the neck of the gallbladder. It remains in the same location as the patient is taken from supine **(A),** to a left lateral decubitus position **(B),** and even to an erect position **(C).** This suggests impaction of the gallstone in the gallbladder neck, which will lead to acute cholecystitis. Cholecystectomy was performed, confirming the ultrasound findings.

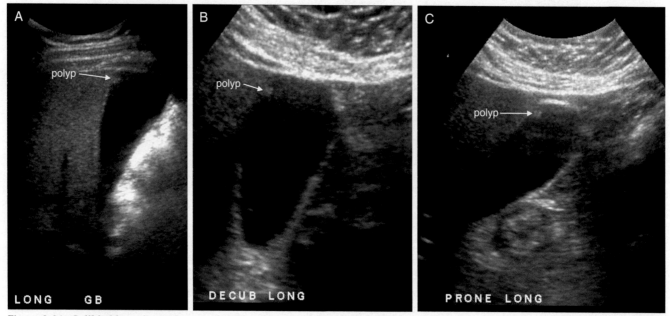

Figure 9-84. **Gallbladder polyps, ultrasound.** When echogenic foci are seen within the gallbladder, gallbladder polyps should also be considered. These can strongly resemble gallstones, but several features may distinguish them. First, because they are comparatively lucent to sound waves, polyps usually do not cast a posterior acoustic shadow, in contrast to gallstones that most often do. Second, polyps are immobile, because they are attached to the gallbladder mucosa. Gallstones may be immobile as well, but usually only when they are lodged in the neck of the gallbladder. In contrast, polyps remain immobile as the patient is moved from supine through decubitus and upright positions, even when the polyps are located in the fundus of the gallbladder. In these long-axis views of this patient, an echogenic focus is seen in the fundus of the gallbladder. It does not move as the patient transitions from supine **(A),** to a left lateral decubitus position **(B),** and finally to a prone position **(C).** This is a gallbladder polyp. This image has been adjusted to accentuate the low-density polyp with its faint echo, resulting in a noisy appearance with other internal echoes seen in the gallbladder.

Computed Tomography for Cholelithiasis and Acute Cholecystitis. CT is generally not considered the first-line test for cholecystitis and related biliary disorders, because ultrasound is well-studied and offers an imaging option free from radiation or the use of potentially nephrotoxic contrast agents. However, CT is frequently used for the imaging of nonspecific abdominal pain and sometimes reveals biliary pathology as the source of pain. CT can disclose the presence of gallstones, although many gallstones are isodense with bile by CT and are not seen. Normal bile has a density somewhat greater than water (~20 Hounsfield units),

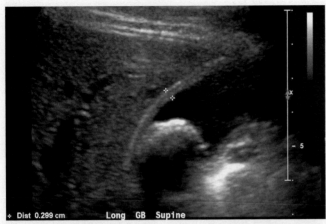

Figure 9-85. Cholelithiasis—assessing wall thickness, ultrasound. The normal gallbladder wall thickness is less than 3 mm, a pencil-thin hyperechoic appearance to the eye without measurement. Thickening greater than 4 mm is suggestive of acute cholecystitis—although a rule of thumb is that a normal gallbladder wall is hardly visible. Thickening of the gallbladder wall normally occurs after eating, as a consequence of gallbladder contraction. This can lead to a false-positive ultrasound, suggesting cholecystitis when inflammation is not present. Ultrasound technicians typically ask that the patient not take anything by mouth for 4-6 hours before ultrasound to avoid this problem. However, an early ultrasound with a normal wall can exclude cholecystitis, and a markedly thickened wall with other features of cholecystitis can rule in the disease even if the patient has not been kept from oral ingestion.

and appears dark gray on a CT soft-tissue window. Bile does not normally enhance with IV (or oral) contrast. The gallbladder wall is normally a pencil-thin line and isodense or slightly denser than bile, thus appearing as a slightly brighter line around the gallbladder. The normal gallbladder fossa does not contain fluid. Gallstones may be visible as hyperdense (brighter) rounded or irregular structures in a dependent position within the gallbladder. Figures 9-92 through 9-94 demonstrate gallstones seen with CT.

Fidler et al.[261] reported the CT findings of acute cholecystitis in 29 patients with proven disease (Table 9-21). Gallbladder wall thickening may be seen as thickness greater than 4 mm. The gallbladder may appear distended. An abnormal gallbladder wall may enhance with IV contrast, appearing bright. A gangrenous gallbladder may fail to enhance. Pericholecystic fluid may be visible within the gallbladder fossa and appears an intermediate gray, around 0 to 20 Hounsfield units. CT cannot assess for the presence of a Murphy's sign. Complications of gangrenous cholecystitis, including gas in the gallbladder, gallbladder wall, or gallbladder

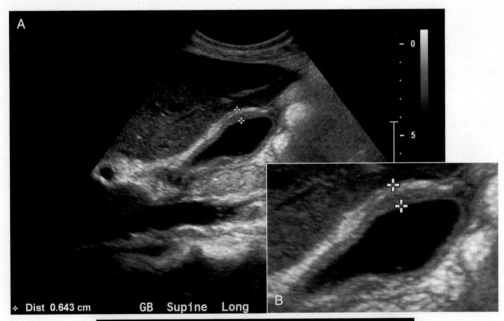

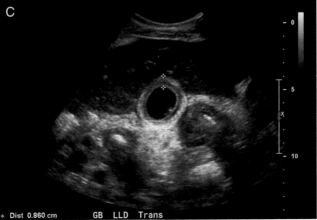

Figure 9-86. Acute cholecystitis with gallbladder wall thickening, ultrasound. A, Long-axis view of the gallbladder. **B,** Close-up from **A. C,** Transverse view. Edema and inflammation of the gallbladder wall thickens it, resulting in an abnormal ultrasound. This patient has significant thickening of the gallbladder wall, more than twice that of normal. The wall has a banded appearance, illustrated in **B.** As discussed in Figure 9-85, normal contraction of the gallbladder after a meal thickens the gallbladder wall and can cause a false-positive ultrasound.

Figure 9-87. **Acute cholecystitis with gallbladder wall thickening and pericholecystic fluid, ultrasound.** Pericholecystic fluid, or fluid in the gallbladder fossa, is a sign of acute cholecystitis. Alone, it is neither specific nor sensitive. In combination with other findings, it gains significance—this patient has gallbladder sludge, as described in earlier figures. As we saw in an earlier figure, cholecystitis may be present without pericholecystic fluid. In addition, disease states with diffuse ascites (cirrhosis, congestive heart failure, malignancy, and hypoalbuminemia) may result in pericholecystic fluid without cholecystitis. **A,** Long-axis view of the gallbladder. **B,** Short-axis view.

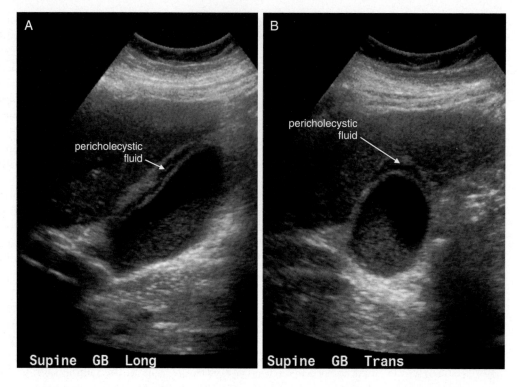

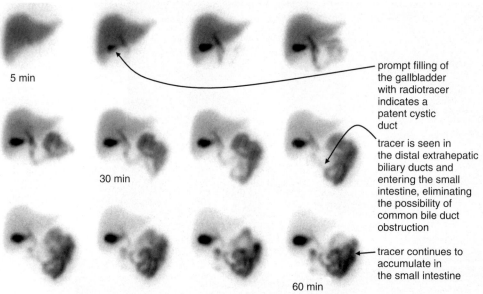

Figure 9-88. **Hepatobiliary iminodiacetic acid (HIDA) scan.** When ultrasound or CT is nondiagnostic, hepatobiliary nuclear scintigraphy can be useful to detect acute cholecystitis and obstruction of the biliary ducts. In this imaging test, a radiopharmaceutical (usually technetium-99-labeled HIDA) is administered intravenously. A gamma camera is positioned over the patient to detect emitted radiation, and a series of images are generated at 5-minute intervals over 1 hour or longer. The radiopharmaceutical is rapidly taken up by the liver and excreted in bile. In a normal study, this radiolabeled bile becomes visible in all bile-containing structures: the liver, gallbladder, the intrahepatic and extrahepatic biliary ducts, and ultimately the small intestine as bile enters the bowel through the sphincter of Oddi. In acute cholecystitis, the obstructed gallbladder does not fill with radiolabeled bile and thus does not appear. In chronic cholecystitis, the gallbladder may fill but not empty. In a case of distal biliary ductal obstruction, radiolabeled bile does not move beyond the point of obstruction, so structures beyond the obstruction do not appear on the images. Cholecystokinin can be administered to stimulate gallbladder contraction. A gallbladder that contracts and empties normally shows progressive loss of radiotracer.

fossa, may be seen. Inflammatory fat stranding may be seen surrounding the gallbladder. In some cases, an abscess in the gallbladder fossa may be seen, with rim enhancement, air, and fluid.[262] Figures 9-95 through 9-98 demonstrate CT findings of cholecystitis.

Additional complications such as ascending cholangitis are discussed later.

X-ray for Gallstones and Biliary Disease. Some gallstones are visible on x-ray (see Figure 9-72), but many

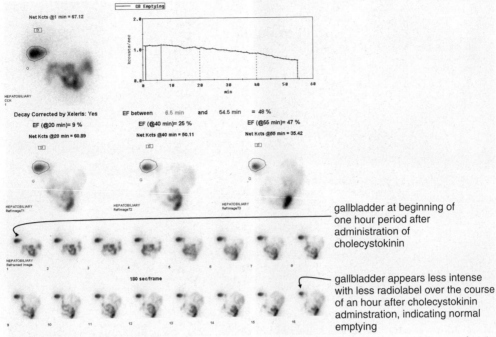

Figure 9-89. Hepatobiliary iminodiacetic acid (HIDA) scan. In the same patient as Figure 9-88, cholecystokinin was administered at 1 hour, and additional images were acquired over the next hour. There is progressive loss of radiotracer from the gallbladder, indicating emptying of the gallbladder. A quantitative measurement can be made, giving the gallbladder "ejection fraction."

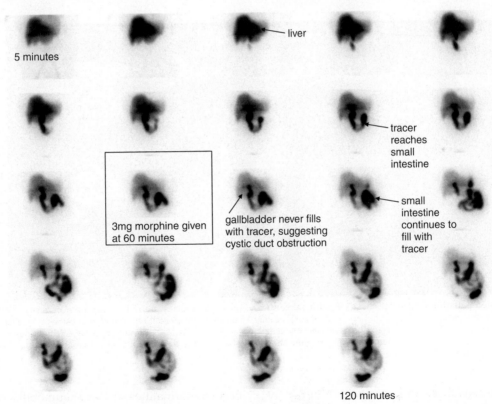

Figure 9-90. Abnormal hepatobiliary iminodiacetic acid (HIDA) scan consistent with acute cholecystitis (images taken at 5-minute intervals). In acute cholecystitis, the obstructed gallbladder does not fill with radiolabeled bile and thus does not appear. In this patient, the liver intensifies with radiolabel and labeled bile enters the extrahepatic bile ducts and progresses to the small intestine. However, the gallbladder does not appear, suggesting obstruction of the cystic duct and cholecystitis. Compare with the normal images in Figures 9-88 and 9-89. Interestingly, ultrasound in this patient was read as negative for cholelithiasis or cholecystitis. CT performed after ultrasound showed a distended gallbladder with slight thickening of the wall and trace pericholecystic fluid. In addition, the liver parenchyma was noted to be enhancing around the gallbladder, sometimes seen in acute cholecystitis. This prompted a HIDA scan. Morphine was administered in an attempt to constrict the sphincter of Oddi to increase back-filling of the gallbladder through the cystic duct, with no apparent effect. Cholecystectomy was performed, and pathology showed chronic cholecystitis and a single gallstone.

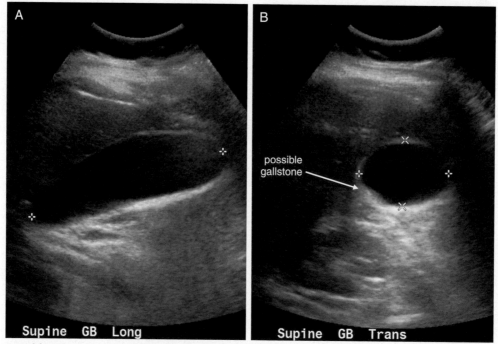

Figure 9-91. Ultrasound from patient with abnormal hepatobiliary iminodiacetic acid (HIDA) scan consistent with acute cholecystitis. Same patient as in Figure 9-90. This ultrasound was performed before a HIDA scan and was interpreted as normal—although in retrospect a possible stone is seen in the gallbladder. No definite posterior acoustic shadowing is seen. The gallbladder wall appears of normal thickness, and no pericholecystic fluid is present. **A,** Long-axis view of the gallbladder. **B,** Short-axis view.

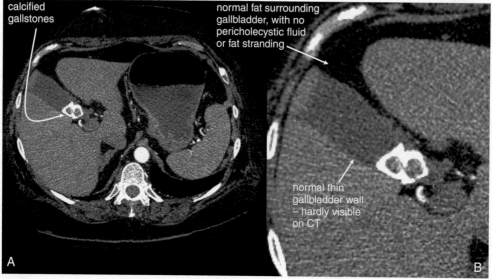

Figure 9-92. Calcified gallstones, seen on chest CT with IV contrast. These gallstones were noted on the lower slices of a chest CT with IV contrast performed to assess for possible pulmonary embolism. They had been observed as well on an earlier chest x-ray. Gallstones may be seen on CT scan, depending on the degree on calcification and density relative to liquid bile. These gallstones are more calcified than most, making them readily visible. This patient has no other findings to suggest acute cholecystitis by CT. The gallbladder wall is extremely thin, and no fluid surrounds the gallbladder. **A,** Axial image. **B,** Close-up.

are not, and the sensitivity and specificity of x-ray for clinically important conditions such as cholecystitis are too low for clinical utility. In some complicated cases such as ascending cholangitis, air may be seen on x-ray overlying the gallbladder fossa, or branching over the liver, suggesting biliary duct or portal venous gas. Generally, x-rays should not be obtained for assessment of suspected biliary pathology. Rothrock et al.[247] found that major abnormalities such as pneumobilia were extremely rare in patients with biliary disease—and did not occur in their series of patients. Minor findings possibly suggesting biliary disease (e.g., right upper quadrant calcifications, ileus, and right basilar atelectasis) occurred with equal frequency in patients with and without acute biliary disease—making them useless to differentiate biliary and nonbiliary sources of symptoms.

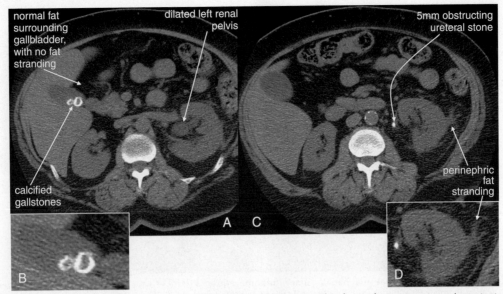

Figure 9-93. Noncontrast CT ("renal colic protocol CT") showing cholelithiasis. This figure demonstrates two important points. First, some gallstones are visible on noncontrast CT—CT with no oral, intravenous, or rectal contrast. The reason is simple: Gallstones can be detected by the difference in density between liquid bile and solid stones or sludge. The density of these is not affected by contrast, because typical CT contrast agents do not enhance bile or stones (although special contrast agents for bile are available). Second, gallstones detected on CT are not necessarily the acute cause of the patient's pain or other symptoms. Other pathology must be considered and sought. In this patient, left flank pain was the chief complaint. Although two calcified gallstones are readily seen, the adjacent fat shows no inflammatory stranding. The left kidney shows enlargement of the renal pelvis (pelviectasis) and perinephric stranding, and an obstructing 5-mm ureteral stone is seen a few slices caudad—the cause of this patient's pain. A, C, Axial images. B, D, Close-ups from A and C, respectively.

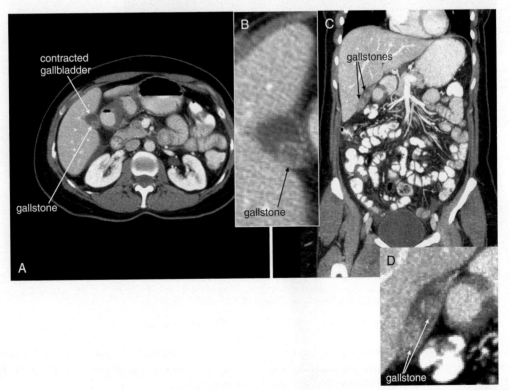

Figure 9-94. Cholelithiasis, CT with oral and IV contrast, soft-tissue window. A, Axial image demonstrating incidental cholelithiasis. B, Close-up from A. The gallbladder is not dilated, and no free fluid is present in the gallbladder fossa. No inflammatory stranding is seen. C, Coronal view from the same patient. D, Close-up from C.

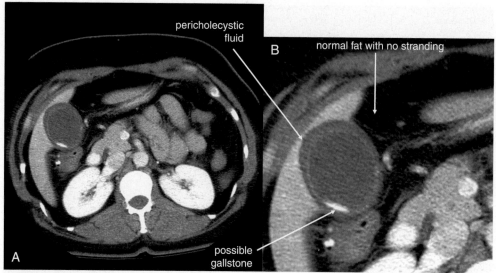

Figure 9-95. CT from a patient with an abnormal hepatobiliary iminodiacetic acid (HIDA) scan consistent with acute cholecystitis. See also this patient's HIDA scan in Figure 9-90 and ultrasound in Figure 9-91. This CT was performed following ultrasound and before a HIDA scan and was interpreted as abnormal, with pericholecystic fluid and a likely gallstone. However, the gallbladder wall itself appears thin, and the adjacent fat shows no stranding. The take-home point is that no diagnostic imaging test is perfect. When clinical examination and history suggest pathology, care must be taken not to rely excessively on apparently normal or nondiagnostic imaging. The HIDA scan suggested acute cholecystitis, and surgery confirmed chronic cholecystitis. **A,** Axial image. **B,** Close-up.

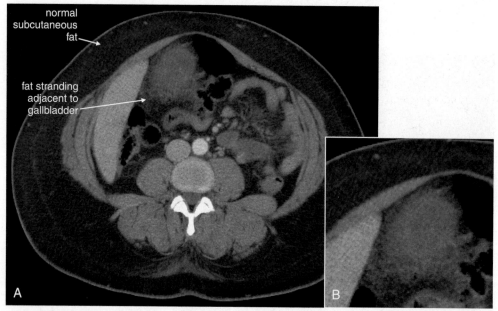

Figure 9-96. CT showing cholecystitis. In this 37-year-old woman with choledocholithiasis, stranding is present in mesenteric fat adjacent to the gallbladder. This supports a diagnosis of cholecystitis, despite the absent of gallbladder wall thickening on her ultrasound. Operative and pathology findings confirmed the diagnosis. **A,** Axial image, with intravenous contrast. **B,** Close-up.

Contrast-Biliary Imaging for Gallstones. Contrast biliary studies using fluoroscopy and contrast agents injected directly into the biliary tract represented the first imaging method to visualize the biliary system—before the advent of ultrasound, CT, or MRI. Today the modality is primarily used for interventions such as placement of percutaneous biliary drains or stents under image guidance (see Figure 9-103). The ACR does not generally recommend these studies, except in hospitalized

patients in whom invasive cholangiography with percutaneous cholecystostomy can be both diagnostic and therapeutic.[251]

Magnetic Resonance Cholangiopancreatography for Biliary Obstruction and Cholecystitis. Magnetic resonance cholangiopancreatography (MRCP) allows visualization of the gallbladder, biliary ducts, and pancreas. The method can detect obstruction and can often reveal

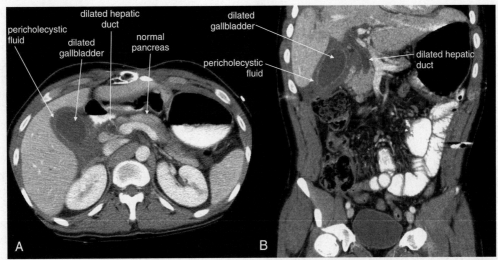

Figure 9-97. Cholecystitis and choledocholithiasis, CT with IV and oral contrast, soft-tissue window. This scan demonstrates cholecystitis. Findings include a dilated gallbladder and pericholecystic fluid. No stones are seen within the gallbladder—a finding that may be caused by gallstones that are isodense with liquid bile, by acalculous cholecystitis, or by choledocholithiasis with an obstructing gallstone outside of the gallbladder in the cystic duct or common bile duct. In both the axial **(A)** and the coronal **(B)** images, dilated extrahepatic bile ducts are visible, consistent with distal obstruction. This patient underwent endoscopic retrograde cholangiopancreatography that confirmed an 8-mm obstructing stone in the common bile duct.

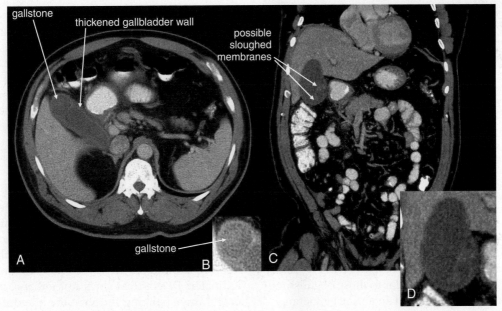

Figure 9-98. Acute cholecystitis, CT with IV and oral contrast, soft-tissue window. CT demonstrating acute cholecystitis with visible gallstones. As in our prior examples, the gallbladder wall is thickened, and the gallbladder is dilated. Gallstones are visible as hyperdensities within the gallbladder. The density of gallstones on CT may vary from isodense with liquid bile to hyperdense. When calcified, gallstones are quite hyperdense on CT. **A,** Axial image. **B,** Close-up from **A. C,** Coronal image. **D,** Close-up from **C.** The more linear appearance in **D** may indicate sloughed membranes within the gallbladder, a finding of acute cholecystitis.

the cause, including gallstone, extrinsic compression from mass, and intrinsic obstruction from neoplasm. This technique is used more often in the diagnosis of painless jaundice from presumed pancreatic mass than in the diagnosis of cholecystitis, because less expensive and more available alternatives exist.[264]

MRI has been compared with ultrasound for the diagnosis of acute cholecystitis. Hakansson et al.[265] studied 35 patients with both MRI and ultrasound and found

that MRI was more sensitive. Loud et al.[266] also reported that MRI was useful in the preoperative evaluation of 14 patients with suspected acute cholecystitis, though no comparison with other modalities was made.

Acalculous Cholecystitis. Acalculous cholecystitis can be a difficult diagnosis, with nonspecific imaging findings. Large prospective studies do not exist because of the rarity of the condition. Mirvis et al.[260] retrospectively reported findings in 56 patients during a 6-year

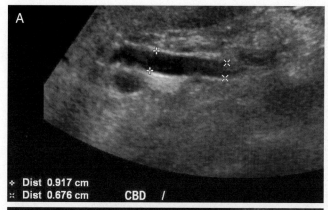

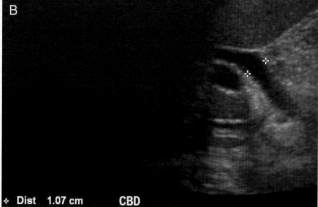

Figure 9-99. Biliary ductal dilatation, ultrasound. A normal common bile duct (CBD) measures 5 mm or less, although some increase in size with age can be normal. Dilatation of the CBD is concerning for distal obstruction, with possible causes including CBD stone, stricture, extrinsic compression (e.g., from a pancreatic head mass), or intrinsic narrowing from a neoplasm such as cholangiocarcinoma. The CBD can be measured by ultrasound, computed tomography, or magnetic resonance imaging. A cholangiogram can also be performed, using endoscopic instillation of contrast material through the sphincter of Oddi by intraoperative cholangiography, or by percutaneous injection into the biliary ducts. **A, B,** Long-axis views of the CBD.

period. Ultrasound and CT were sensitive (92% and 100%, respectively) and specific (96% and 100%, respectively), whereas cholescintigraphy with HIDA was only 38% specific. Findings were similar to those of gallstone-associated cholecystitis, but with an absence of stones.

Choledocholithiasis and Biliary Ductal Obstruction. Choledocholithiasis is the presence of bile stones within the biliary ducts. It can be assessed with several modalities, including ultrasound, magnetic resonance, CT, cholescintigraphy, and contrast fluoroscopy.

Ultrasound of Choledocholithiasis and Biliary Ductal Obstruction. Ultrasound readily measures the caliber of the major biliary ducts, although distal segments may be hidden by overlying bowel gas. A stone obstructing the common bile duct may be directly visualized and has the same characteristics as a stone within the gallbladder—hyperechoic with acoustic shadowing—but is immobile once trapped within the duct (see Figures 9-99 and 9-100). Sometimes the source of obstruction (stone, mass, or extrinsic compression) is not directly seen with

ultrasound, but biliary ductal dilatation proximal to the obstruction is seen. The normal diameter of the common bile duct is around 5 mm but increases with age.[267] The extrahepatic bile duct (including the common bile duct) increases in diameter by about 0.4 mm per year in patients older than 50 years. In elderly patients, a diameter of 8.5 mm has been suggested as the upper limit of normal.[267]

Magnetic Resonance Cholangiography of Choledocholithiasis and Biliary Ductal Obstruction. Magnetic resonance similarly can demonstrate biliary ductal obstruction and is considered the current optimal noninvasive imaging test for stones and tumor.[268-271] Soto et al.[272] reported sensitivity for detection of bile duct stones of 96% for MR, with 100% specificity. In the case of malignancy, magnetic resonance can demonstrate ductal infiltration and lymph node metastases.[264] Magnetic resonance is also useful in assessment of patients with postoperative complications of biliary surgery and can demonstrate anastomoses.[273]

Computed Tomography of Choledocholithiasis and Biliary Ductal Obstruction. CT can reveal both intrahepatic and extrahepatic biliary ductal dilatation (see Figures 9-104 through 9-108). In some cases, the source of obstruction may be evident with CT, including obstructing stone or extrinsic compression such as from pancreatic mass. A stone within a duct can sometimes be seen as a bright filling defect, with a surrounding rim of darker bile called the target or crescent sign.[274] In other cases, the stone may be isodense with bile and thus invisible. The stone's location may then be inferred by the transition from dilated to nondilated biliary duct. Bile does not enhance with standard IV or oral contrast agents, and the normal density of bile is approximately 20 Hounsfield units, making it a dark gray on a soft-tissue window. Hemobilia (blood in bile) gives blood a higher density, around 40 to 60 Hounsfield units. Although iodinated IV contrast does not enhance bile, it can be useful in visualizing intrahepatic bile ducts by enhancing the surrounding liver parenchyma and adjacent portal triad. This triad is composed of hepatic vein, portal vein, and biliary duct. Without IV contrast, the density of bile, blood in vessels of the portal triad, and surrounding liver parenchyma are similar—around 20 to 40 Hounsfield units. Consequently, without IV contrast, the intrahepatic biliary ducts may be difficult to identify, and dilatation may be difficult to recognize. Enhancement of liver parenchyma with IV contrast leaves unenhancing dilated biliary ducts in relief. IV contrast can thus be important in assessment of ductal patency. However, some bile duct stones are calcified and are better seen on unenhanced CT. Some noncalcified stones are visible on unenhanced CT because they have higher density than surrounding liquid bile. Very small stones, 6 mm or smaller, can be difficult to detect.[274] Specialized oral contrast agents that are concentrated in bile are also

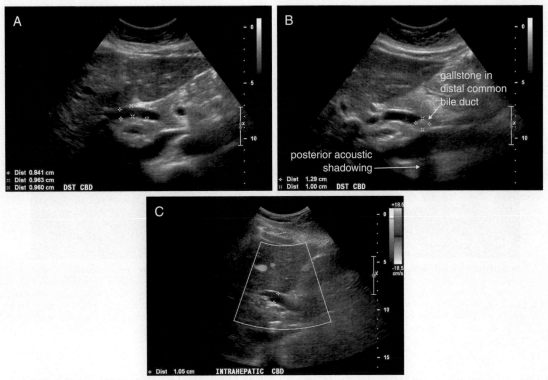

Figure 9-100. Common bile duct dilatation with choledocholithiasis, ultrasound. As described earlier, common bile duct dilatation may be a normal age-related phenomenon or may be caused by intrinsic or extrinsic obstruction of the duct. In this 37-year-old female with known cholelithiasis, extrahepatic biliary ductal dilatation was noted on ultrasound. Her common bile duct measures nearly 1 cm, clearly abnormal given her age. Careful inspection of the duct showed a 1-cm echogenic structure with posterior shadowing—a gallstone in the common bile duct, or choledocholithiasis. This is an important finding that requires either endoscopic retrograde cholangiopancreatography or surgery for stone removal. The intrahepatic biliary ducts were also noted to be enlarged on this patient's ultrasound. **A, B,** Long-axis views of the common bile duct. **C,** Long-axis view with Doppler ultrasound. Doppler helps to identify vascular structures with flow. The bile duct does not appear to have flow, because bile flow is normally quite slow and is not present in this obstructed duct. The intrahepatic common bile duct is dilated here.

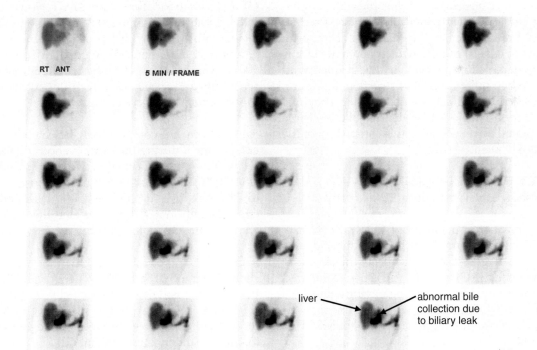

Figure 9-101. Abnormal hepatobiliary iminodiacetic acid (HIDA) scan consistent with bile leak. A HIDA scan is not just a test for cholecystitis and biliary obstruction. In a postoperative patient, HIDA can assess for a bile leak. In this patient, radiotracer accumulates in an abnormal position overlying the liver and never appears to fill the bowel. This is concerning for a bile leak. Why use HIDA for this purpose? Why wouldn't CT be a better test? This is a complex patient who has undergone a liver and kidney transplant. He did undergo CT, which showed massive ascites (Figure 9-102). Bile leaking into ascites cannot be recognized on CT, because bile and ascites are of similar fluid density. Moreover, as they mix, they become identical in density. In addition, as a result of the patient's recent renal transplant, intravenous contrast was not given, though it is doubtful this would have changed the diagnostic ability of the CT. Here, HIDA played a key role in diagnosis.

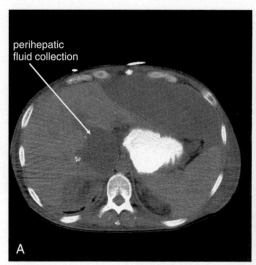
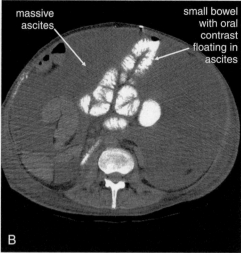

Figure 9-102. CT in patient with bile leak shown on hepatobiliary iminodiacetic acid (HIDA) scan. The patient in Figure 9-101 had a bile leak demonstrated by HIDA scan. CT was performed before the HIDA scan but was nondiagnostic. A fluid collection is seen adjacent to the transplanted liver, but the cause is unclear. The patient has massive ascites, so the perihepatic fluid could be ascites, bile, blood, or an abscess—all essentially indistinguishable by CT. **A, B,** Axial images with oral contrast but no intravenous (IV) contrast. IV contrast might help to identify an abscess, but the patient had undergone recent renal transplant and IV contrast was withheld because of a creatinine of 1.4 mg/dL. HIDA scan was key to the diagnosis by confirming bile leak. Because the injected radiotracer accumulates only in bile, the collection was confirmed to be biliary. Paracentesis had been nondiagnostic because the ascites diluted the bile substantially.

available (e.g., iopodic acid) and are sometimes used for dedicated CT cholangiography.[272] Accurate delineation of the cause of biliary ductal obstruction with CT requires thin-section image acquisition and reconstruction, because biliary ducts have normal diameters in the range of a few millimeters.

When biliary duct obstruction is not present, intrahepatic biliary ducts are nearly invisible, because they are decompressed and quite small in diameter. The portal triad appears to consist of only two components in this instance, the hepatic and portal veins, both filled with IV contrast. When biliary ductal obstruction is present, the intrahepatic biliary ducts become dilated proximal to the point of obstruction. Low-density bile is visible within the dilated ducts, allowing this component of the portal triad to be seen.

Studies of CT with protocols dedicated to biliary duct assessment show high sensitivity and specificity.

Soto et al.[272] compared unenhanced CT, oral contrast–enhanced CT cholangiography using iopodic acid, and MRCP for the diagnosis of choledocholithiasis in 51 patients. Unenhanced CT was 65% sensitive, compared with 92% sensitivity for CT cholangiography and 96% sensitivity for MRCP. Specificity was 84% for unenhanced CT, 92% for CT cholangiography, and 100% for MRCP.

Ahmetoglu et al.[275] performed CT using only IV contrast without an oral cholangiographic contrast agent. The sensitivity and specificity were 93% and 89%, respectively, for biliary stone. For malignant obstruction, the sensitivity and specificity were 94%.

Anderson et al.[274] compared unenhanced and IV contrast–enhanced CT without the use of a bile-specific oral contrast agent. For study purposes, two observers interpreted the CT scans specifically with choledocholithiasis in mind. For the two observers, the sensitivity ranged between 69% and 87% for unenhanced CT and was 87% for enhanced CT. Specificity was 92% for unenhanced CT and 83% to 88% for enhanced CT. However, the original CT interpretation, performed at the time of patient evaluation, was only 46% sensitive (unenhanced) and 33% sensitive (enhanced), with high specificity (98%-100%). This serves as a strong reminder that real-world sensitivity and specificity may differ substantially from those found in a study setting.

Anderson et al.[276] compared 64-slice CT with IV contrast enhancement during the portal venous phase to MRCP. CT was moderately sensitive (70%-78%) and very specific (100%) for detection of biliary stenosis. CT was 72% to 78% sensitive for choledocholithiasis and 96% specific—though in a setting in which the CT interpreters were specifically looking for biliary duct abnormalities.

Kim et al.[277] reported sensitivity and specificity of CT cholangiography for stones to be 97% and 96%, respectively. The sensitivity and specificity for bile duct stricture were 86% and 100%, respectively. Multiplanar reconstruction was used in this and the previous studies to improve diagnostic performance.

Fluoroscopic Contrast Biliary Studies for Biliary Ductal Obstruction. Fluoroscopic assessment of biliary ductal patency can be performed but usually is reserved for interventions to treat obstruction, following diagnosis

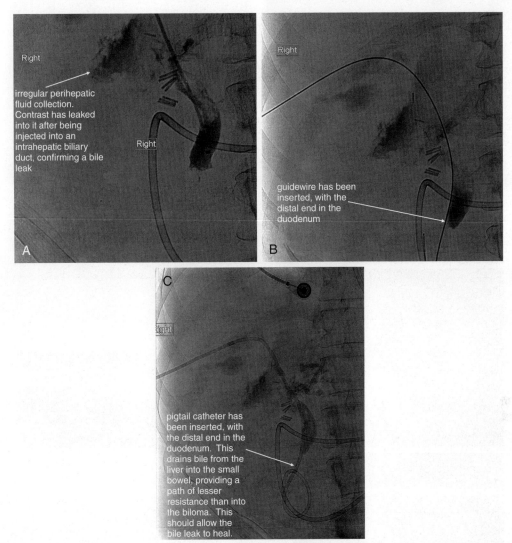

Figure 9-103. Cholangiogram for bile leak. A, B, C, Fluoroscopic cholangiogram images. Same patient as in Figures 9-101 and 9-102. Cholangiography is not a common emergency department diagnostic imaging procedure, but this case concludes with the patient undergoing diagnostic and therapeutic cholangiography. This procedure is included to illustrate the importance of making the correct diagnosis to treat the patient appropriately. Wise use of diagnostic imaging led to the correct diagnosis. Although cholangiography could have been used instead of a hepatobiliary iminodiacetic acid (HIDA) scan to make the diagnosis, the HIDA scan is noninvasive, whereas cholangiography is an invasive procedure performed by an interventional radiologist. In this procedure, an intercostal location in the right midaxillary line was sterilely prepped and a needle was introduced through the liver into a bile duct under fluoroscopic guidance. Contrast injection confirmed intrabiliary puncture, and a guidewire was advanced into the biliary system, common bile duct, and duodenum. A pigtail catheter was then placed over the guidewire to drain the collection. **A,** The image shows irregular extravasation of injected contrast into the biloma. **B,** A guidewire has been placed. **C,** The pigtail catheter is present.

with another imaging modality. In these procedures, an intrahepatic biliary duct is cannulated, often using ultrasound guidance. A radiopaque contrast agent is then injected, allowing visualization of the biliary ducts using fluoroscopy. An obstructing lesion prevents contrast from progressing distally. A stent or catheter can sometimes be placed across the point of obstruction using this technique. In other cases, percutaneous external drainage is performed.

Cholescintigraphy of Choledocholithiasis and Biliary Ductal Obstruction. Cholescintigraphy is discussed in the earlier section on cholecystitis. Biliary ductal obstruction can be recognized by failure of HIDA-labeled bile to progress distal to a point of obstruction.

Ascending Cholangitis. Ascending cholangitis is a life-threatening infection of the biliary ducts, usually in the context of biliary ductal obstruction. Imaging plays both direct and indirect roles in the diagnosis. The primary role of imaging is to rule out other causes of symptoms such as abdominal pain, tenderness, jaundice, and fever. In addition, imaging may reveal biliary ductal obstruction from an intrinsic process, such as gallstone, or extrinsic obstruction from a compressing mass or abscess. In some cases, imaging may reveal more direct evidence of ascending cholangitis such as gas within the biliary ducts or portal venous system, caused by the presence of gas-forming anaerobic organisms. Direct evidence of ascending cholangitis may not be present; the emergency physician may need to infer the presence

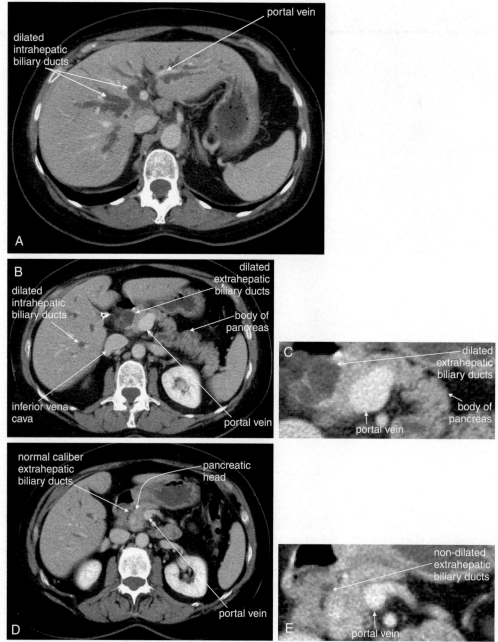

Figure 9-104. Biliary tract obstruction, CT with IV and oral contrast, soft-tissue window. Intra and extrahepatic biliary ductal dilatation from cholangiocarcinoma. The patient presented with painless jaundice and had a remote history of cholecystectomy. The scan suggests that the obstruction is in the distal bile duct, because the proximal extrahepatic biliary ducts and intrahepatic biliary ducts are markedly dilated. The patient was found to have a cholangiocarcinoma resulting in a biliary stricture. **A, B, D,** Axial slices. **C, E,** Close-ups from **B** and **D,** respectively. **B** and **C** show a more caudad slice relative to **A.** Biliary ducts are dilated throughout the liver. These can be distinguished from vascular structures such as portal veins on this scan with intravenous contrast. The vascular structures are strongly enhancing *(white)* because of the injected contrast. The biliary ducts have a *dark gray* appearance on this soft-tissue window because they contain low-density fluid—bile. In cross section, some of these ducts have a circular appearance similar to hepatic cysts, but they can be followed through multiple slices, revealing their tubular shape. The pancreas is seen draped anterior to the portal vein. **D** and **E,** more caudad slice compared with **B,** show extrahepatic ducts that have assumed a normal nondilated size. The pancreatic head lies just right of the portal vein. The transition zone where the biliary ducts lose their dilatation and assume a normal size marks the location of the obstruction, stricture, or external compression.

of ascending cholangitis from imaging findings of biliary obstruction, in the presence of other clinical findings such as fever, jaundice, altered mental status, or hypotension. Treatment requires decompression of obstruction, which can be performed surgically, endoscopically by endoscopic retrograde cholangiopancreatography, or by percutaneous biliary drainage under ultrasound or fluoroscopic guidance. Thus imaging plays a role in both diagnosis and treatment. Treatment need not relieve the actual site of pathologic obstruction; instead, as a temporizing measure, percutaneous drainage of the biliary system can suffice.

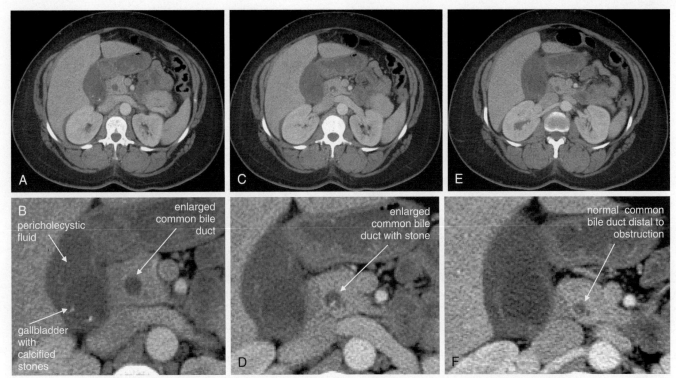

Figure 9-105. CT with IV contrast of choledocholithiasis and biliary ductal dilatation. In this 37-year-old female, a gallstone has obstructed the distal common bile duct—a condition called choledocholithiasis. In this series of slices, moving from cephalad **(A)** to caudad **(E)**, the common bile duct is seen to be enlarged at and above the level of the obstructing stone and smaller in caliber below the obstruction. Interestingly, this patient has evidence of cholecystitis by CT (pericholecystic fluid), which was not recognized by ultrasound the same day. Operative findings and pathology results confirmed cholecystitis. **A, C, E,** Progressively more caudad axial CT slices. **B, D, F,** Close-ups from **A, C, E,** respectively.

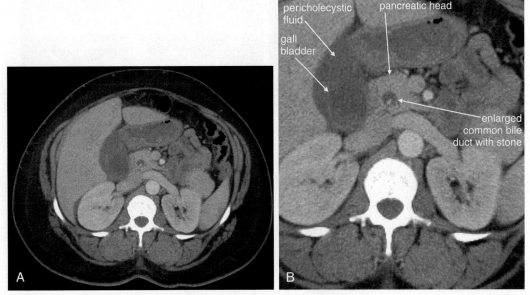

Figure 9-106. CT with IV contrast of choledocholithiasis and biliary ductal dilatation. Same patient as Figure 9-105. The gallbladder with dependent sludge or gallstones is visible, and pericholecystic fluid is present. To the patient's left, the common bile duct is seen in cross section in its normal position within the pancreatic head. A bright stone is visible in the duct. Notice how the common bile duct is filled with bile, which has the same fluid density as bile in the gallbladder. The stone in this case is denser than liquid bile, likely partially calcified. **A,** Axial image. **B,** Close-up.

X-ray for Ascending Cholangitis. X-ray is insensitive for ascending cholangitis and should not be relied upon to confirm or exclude the diagnosis However, gas in a branching pattern overlying the liver can suggest pneumobilia from gas-forming organisms in the biliary system.

Computed Tomography for Ascending Cholangitis. In ascending cholangitis, CT findings may include signs of biliary obstruction as described earlier (see Figures 9-107 and 9-108), as well as gas within the intrahepatic biliary ducts (see Figures 9-109 and 9-110). Gas in this location

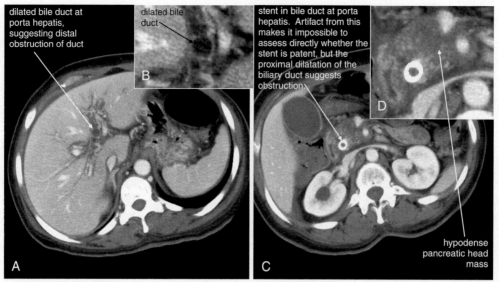

Figure 9-107. Ascending cholangitis, dilated bile ducts, CT with IV contrast. Obstruction of the biliary ducts can lead to devastating ascending infection—cholangitis. This is largely a clinical diagnosis, because classic imaging findings such as pneumobilia can lag behind clinical deterioration. Fever, jaundice, abdominal pain, and altered mental status should prompt immediate antibiotic therapy and surgical consultation, regardless of imaging findings. **A, C,** Axial images. **B, D,** Close-ups from **A** and **C,** respectively. This patient with a known pancreatic mass and a previously placed biliary stent presented with right upper quadrant abdominal pain. She became febrile during her emergency department stay. Her scan shows biliary ductal dilatation, suggesting obstruction of her stent. In addition to antibiotic therapy, a procedure to relieve obstruction is needed. Her blood cultures subsequently grew *Escherichia coli,* consistent with ascending cholangitis.

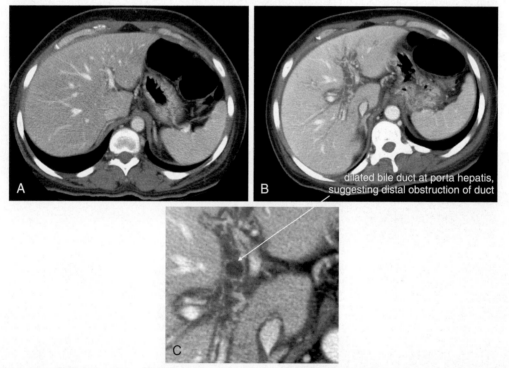

Figure 9-108. Comparison of dilated and nondilated intrahepatic biliary ducts, CT with IV contrast. Same patient as in Figure 9-107. Patient with stent in the common bile duct for treatment of malignant biliary stricture. **A,** The stent (not seen in this axial slice because it lies in the extrahepatic biliary ducts) is patent and the intrahepatic biliary ducts are not dilated. They are essentially invisible on this scan because they are draining normally and are empty of bile. **B,** The stent has become obstructed, and the intrahepatic biliary ducts are becoming dilated. **C,** Close-up from **B.** The patient became febrile, and blood cultures grew *Escherichia coli,* consistent with ascending cholangitis. Biliary evidence of biliary ductal dilatation suggests obstruction, and ascending cholangitis should be suspected if clinical features are present, even if imaging does not show dramatic findings such as pneumobilia.

appears black on a soft-tissue window and may have a branching pattern. Gas in biliary ducts may be difficult or impossible to differentiate from gas in portal venous branches. Balthazar et al.[278] reported that CT identified biliary dilatation suggesting obstruction in 78% of patients with ascending cholangitis, detected the level of obstruction in 65%, and identified the cause in 61%. Five patients (22%) had air within the biliary tree, and three patients (13%) had hepatic abscesses. Lee et al.[279] similarly reported biliary obstruction to be a common

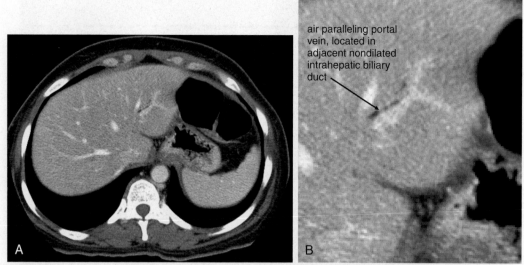

Figure 9-109. Pneumobilia, CT with IV contrast. This patient's CT demonstrates pneumobilia (air in the biliary tree), which is worrisome for ascending cholangitis if abdominal pain, fever, jaundice, leukocytosis, altered mental status, or signs of biliary obstruction are present. Air is black on CT. **A,** Axial image. **B,** Close-up. In this patient, this pneumobilia is iatrogenic, caused by placement of a biliary stent 15 days prior. The patient has adenocarcinoma of the pancreatic head that had resulted in a stricture of the common bile duct. There is no biliary ductal dilatation (see Figures 9-104 through 9-108 demonstrating this), implying that the biliary stent is not obstructed.

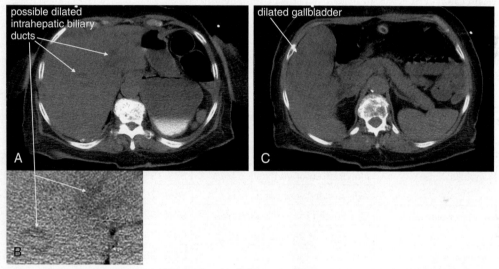

Figure 9-110. Ascending cholangitis, CT without IV contrast, no biliary air. This patient presented with altered mental status, hypotension, fever, and a history of abdominal pain. CT without IV contrast was performed because the patient was in acute renal failure. CT showed a markedly dilated gallbladder. Ascending cholangitis was suspected—a percutaneous cholecystostomy tube was placed by interventional radiology. Fluid from that drain, as well as blood cultures, grew *Enterococcus faecalis*. CT findings in this patient are more difficult to recognize in the absence of IV contrast. Without IV contrast, the liver parenchyma, vessels, and biliary tree are nearly isodense (fluid and tissue densities). If IV contrast had been given, the liver parenchyma would have enhanced, making the nonenhancing biliary tree more evident. **A, C,** Axial images. **B,** Close-up from **A. A,** The biliary tree is slightly hypodense relative to the liver parenchyma and appears to be dilated. **B,** The gallbladder is hypodense relative to the liver and appears markedly enlarged. Again the patient had ascending cholangitis without classic features such as biliary air, which would have been visible (*black*) on this CT without IV contrast. The patient did receive oral contrast through her gastrostomy tube, which does not contribute to the diagnosis because it is pooled in the stomach.

finding. Papillitis and inhomogeneous liver enhancement were also associated with cholangitis in this study.

Ultrasound for Ascending Cholangitis. Ultrasound in ascending cholangitis also provides supporting but not direct evidence of the diagnosis. Ultrasound findings may include those of acute cholecystitis and biliary ductal dilatation (intra hepatic and extrahepatic). An obstructing stone in the common bile duct may

be seen (see Figures 9-99 and 9-100). Ultrasound can demonstrate air within bile ducts; air scatters the ultrasound beam, resulting in "static" in the ultrasound image. Normally this artifact is not seen within the liver parenchyma, allowing intrahepatic air to be recognized or suspected.

Magnetic Resonance Cholangiography for Ascending Cholangitis. Magnetic resonance can demonstrate biliary

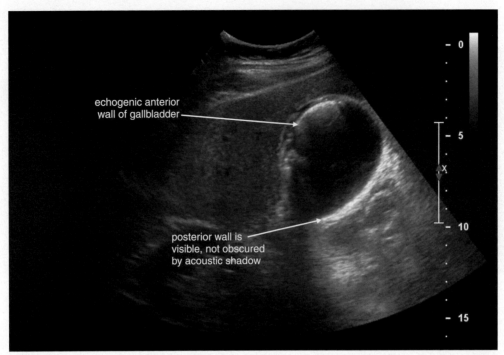

echogenic anterior
wall of gallbladder

posterior wall is
visible, not obscured
by acoustic shadow

Figure 9-111. Porcelain gallbladder versus air in gallbladder wall, ultrasound. Porcelain gallbladder, a finding concerning for carcinoma of the gallbladder, can be recognized on ultrasound by a highly echogenic anterior wall of the gallbladder with posterior acoustic shadowing. This patient has findings that do not quite meet this definition. The anterior wall is highly echogenic, but the posterior wall is visible. With a true porcelain gallbladder, the densely echogenic anterior gallbladder wall would create a dense shadow, preventing visualization of the posterior wall. Other possible causes of this finding in this patient are air within the gallbladder wall (which scatters and reflects the ultrasound signal) or confluence of "comet tail artifact" from multiple adjacent cholesterol crystals. In this case, the patient had severe pulmonary disease and was not an operative candidate, so no pathology report is available. His CT suggested acute cholecystitis, and he was treated successfully with percutaneous drainage and antibiotics.

TABLE 9-20. Sensitivity and Specificity of Ultrasound and Nuclear Scintigraphy for Cholelithiasis and Cholecystitis

Modality	Condition	Assumptions	Sensitivity (95% CI)	Specificity (95% CI)
Ultrasound	Cholelithiasis	Unadjusted for verification bias	97% (95%-99%)	95% (88%-100%)
		Adjusted for verification bias	84% (76%-92%)	99% (97%-100%)
	Acute cholecystitis	Unadjusted for verification bias	94% (92%-96%)	78% (61%-96%)
		Adjusted for verification bias	88% (74%-100%)	80% (62%-98%)
Nuclear Scintigraphy	Acute cholecystitis	—	97% (96%-98%)	90% (86%-95%)

Adapted from Shea JA, Berlin JA, Escarce JJ, et al. Revised estimates of diagnostic test sensitivity and specificity in suspected biliary tract disease. *Arch Intern Med* 154:2573-2581, 1994.

ductal dilatation and in some cases can determine the cause. Like CT, magnetic resonance does not prove the diagnosis of ascending cholangitis but rather confirms biliary obstruction, a risk factor for cholangitis. Bile-specific contrast agents such as gadolinium ethoxyben-zyl diethylenetriamine pentaacetic acid can assist in the diagnosis.[280-281]

Pancreatitis and Pancreatic Masses

Figures 9-112 through 9-119 demonstrate imaging findings of the normal pancreas, pancreatitis, and pancreatic masses. Imaging in pancreatitis can serve several purposes, the most clear-cut being to identify cases of pancreatitis resulting from an obstructing gallstone in the

common bile duct. Gallstone obstruction of outflow of pancreatic secretions is a leading cause of pancreatitis and is treated by stone removal with endoscopic retrograde cholangiopancreatography. Obstruction of biliary ducts can be identified using ultrasound, CT, or MRI as described earlier.[282]

The role of diagnostic imaging for the diagnosis of pancreatitis itself is less clear. Laboratory assessment of pancreatitis can be insensitive, particularly in chronic pancreatitis, where elevations of amylase and lipase may not occur. Isolated amylase elevations can occur without pancreatic inflammation, from sources including bowel and salivary gland, making laboratory assessment

TABLE 9-21. CT Findings of Acute Cholecystitis

Finding	Description	Frequency
Gallbladder distension	>5 cm short axis or 8 cm long axis	41%
Gallbladder wall thickening	≥4 mm at a midpoint of the wall, not near the fundus	58%
Gas in gallbladder wall and lumen	Gas from anaerobic gas-forming organisms appears black on all CT windows	0% in this study; has been described in other studies as a finding of gangrenous cholecystitis[263]
High attenuation bile	Increased attenuation relative to water density	24%
Pericholecystic fat stranding	Fat stranding isolated to the pericholecystic region	52%
Pericholecystic fluid	Fluid in the gallbladder fossa without diffuse ascites	31%
Sloughed membranes	Irregular linear soft-tissue densities within the gall bladder	3%
Subserosal edema	Defined by a central region of low attenuation within the gallbladder wall, also called a halo	31%

Adapted from Fidler J, Paulson EK, Layfield L. CT evaluation of acute cholecystitis: findings and usefulness in diagnosis. *AJR Am J Roentgenol* 166:1085-1088, 1996.

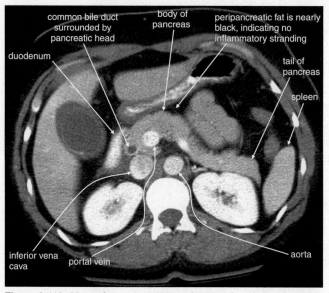

Figure 9-112. **Normal pancreas, CT with IV and oral contrast, soft-tissue window.** This scan shows a normal pancreas. In many patients, the pancreas is not so horizontally oriented and is therefore difficult to see in a single slice. Here, the common course of the pancreas is seen. The pancreatic head is draped over the portal vein. The tail of the pancreas crosses the midline and then moves posteriorly. It crosses the left kidney and ends medial to the spleen. The duodenum is to the right of the pancreatic head, filled with oral contrast. The common bile duct is seen as a hypodense area within the pancreatic head, because it is filled with bile. The contrast between the dark bile and the bright pancreatic tissue is increased by the administration of IV contrast, because the pancreas enhances as a result of high blood flow. The fat surrounding the pancreas is dark, which is normal and indicates the absence of inflammatory stranding—almost the entire pancreas is outlined in fat and has distinct border. Incidentally, the patient has an abnormal dilated gallbladder with pericholecystic fluid. Given this finding, the prominent common bile duct should be inspected further for an obstructing stone.

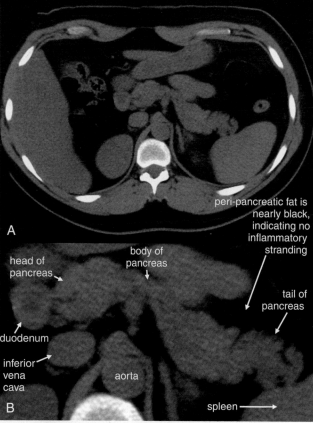

Figure 9-113. **Normal pancreas, CT without IV or oral contrast, soft-tissue window.** Without oral and IV contrast, the pancreas can be a bit harder to identify. Here, another common course of the pancreas is seen. The pancreatic head is anterior to the inferior vena cava and medial to duodenum. The body of the pancreas crosses the midline and then moves posteriorly. The pancreatic tail ends anterior to the spleen. **A,** Axial image. **B,** Close-up.

nonspecific as well. Still, in most cases, pancreatitis is diagnosed by a combination of clinical features and laboratory abnormalities. No well-validated decision rule for the use of diagnostic imaging in pancreatitis has been developed, either for patients with normal lab

assessment or for patients with apparent pancreatitis based on laboratory abnormalities. Diagnostic imaging can identify complications of pancreatitis such as abscess, pseudocyst, and hemorrhagic or necrotizing pancreatitis. Which patients require imaging to assess

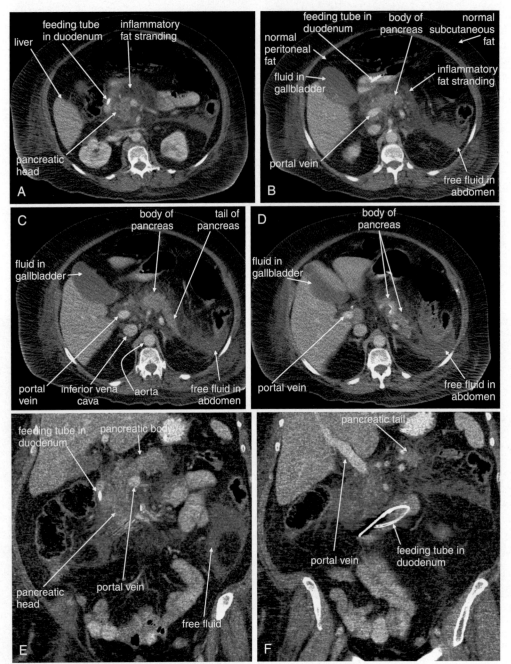

Figure 9-114. Pancreatitis, CT with IV contrast, soft-tissue window. For novice readers, pancreatitis can be one of the most difficult diagnoses to recognize on this CT, perhaps because the normal pancreas attracts so little attention. **A** through **D,** Axial images. **E, F,** Coronal images. This series of four axial slices shows an inflamed pancreas, starting at the pancreatic head **(A)** and moving progressively cephalad to its tail **(C, D).** The entire pancreas here is surrounded by inflamed peripancreatic fat that shows marked stranding. Near the tail, free fluid is evident. Find the pancreas by recognizing the company it keeps. The pancreatic head normally lies medial to the gallbladder, in the vicinity of the portal vein. If necessary, trace the portal vein backward from the liver to the center of the abdomen. In addition, the pancreas typically lies at the level of the celiac artery as it emerges from the aorta. The body and tail of the pancreas then continue to the patient's left, typically terminating near the left kidney and spleen. The splenic artery feeds branches to the pancreas and is usually parallel to the pancreas, so one method of finding the pancreas is to follow the splenic artery backward from the spleen to the aorta. **A,** The pancreatitic head is visible, just left of the duodenum that is marked by a bright feeding tube. Compare the inflamed fat around the pancreas with normal subcutaneous and peritoneal fat (labeled in **B**). **C,** The body and tail of the pancreas are visible, starting at the midline anterior to the aorta and progressing left and posteriorly. A fluid collection is visible in the left abdomen—its density is similar to that of fluid in the gallbladder. Normal structures such as the aorta are labeled to assist you in getting your bearings. Frustrated? This process is easier using a digital picture archiving and communication system (PACS), because you can find familiar landmarks before looking for a less familiar structure such as the pancreas. **E, F,** Coronal reconstructions from the same patient may help you to understand the orientation.

for these complications is debated, though a cogent case can be made for imaging in critically ill patients, patients with a history of these complications, patients with pancreatitis and fever, or patients with metabolic derangements such as multiple Ranson's criteria. The grading of

severity of pancreatitis with imaging has some prognostic value, although no studies have shown clinical benefits to patients based on management changes resulting from imaging. Imaging today provides much information with little apparent effect on patient treatment or

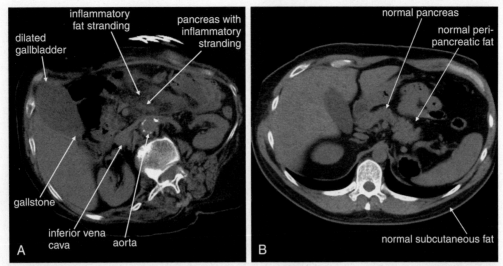

Figure 9-115. **Gallstone pancreatitis and normal pancreas for comparison, axial CT without contrast. A,** Gallstone pancreatitis CT. A dilated gallbladder is visible with a hyperdense dependent lesion consistent with a gallstone. The region of the pancreas shows significant inflammatory stranding In this patient, the pancreas lies just anterior to the left renal vein, which can be seen crossing anterior to the aorta and entering the inferior vena cava. **B,** A normal pancreas is visible. This pancreas is surrounded by uninflamed fat, which is dark (nearly black). Compare this normal fat with normal subcutaneous fat.

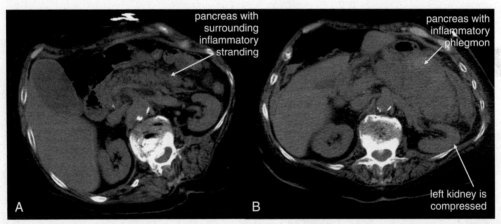

Figure 9-116. **Gallstone pancreatitis, progressing to hemorrhagic pancreatitis over a 13-day period, CT without contrast, soft-tissue window. A,** The inflamed pancreas is visible on the initial scan. **B,** An expanding region of pancreatic inflammation and hematoma is visible 13 days later. Notice how the left kidney is compressed by the inflamed pancreas in **B,** compared with **A.**

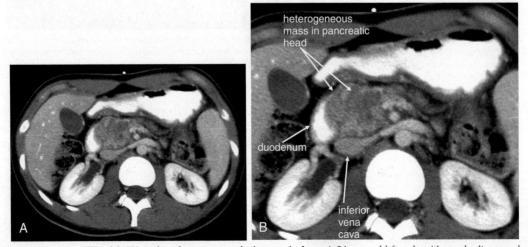

Figure 9-117. **Pancreatic mass, CT with IV and oral contrast, soft-tissue window.** A 24-year-old female with newly diagnosed pancreatic head mass, ultimately diagnosed as a solid pseudopapillary tumor. This was an aggressive malignancy that rapidly metastasized. On this scan with intravenous and oral contrast performed around the time of initial diagnosis, the mass is seen in abutting the inferior vena cava and duodenum. From our earlier discussion of pancreatitis, you'll recognize that much of the pancreas is not seen in this slice. **A,** Axial image. **B,** Close-up.

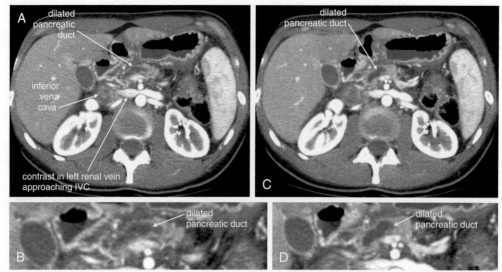

Figure 9-118. Pancreatic mass. Same patient as Figure 9-117. This CT with IV contrast shows dilatation of the pancreatic duct up to 8 mm. Normally the pancreatic duct is quite subtle on CT, but obstruction of the duct in the pancreatic head by the mass has resulted in its prominence here. The mass itself is not visible in these images. The dilated pancreatic duct is a dark gray—fluid density, because we have reviewed previously. The mottled appearance of the spleen is caused by the early arterial phase of injected contrast; this can mimic splenic infarction or injury. You can recognize that this is an early-phase CT, rapidly performed after contrast injection, as the inferior vena cava has not yet filled with contrast. Contrast is seen in the left renal vein about to enter the inferior vena cava. Images obtained slightly later would result in a more homogeneous appearance of the spleen as venous structures fill with contrast. **A, C,** Axial CT images. **B, D,** Close-ups from **A** and **C,** respectively.

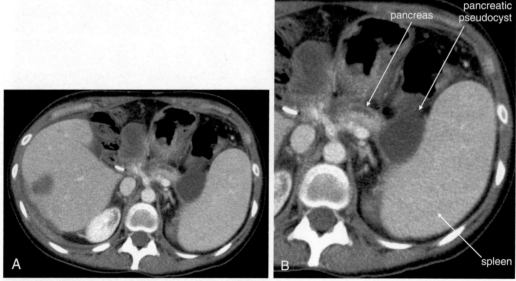

Figure 9-119. Pancreatic pseudocyst, CT with IV contrast. This patient has a known pancreatic head mass (adenocarcinoma). After an episode of pancreatitis caused by malignant obstruction of the pancreatic duct, a cystic lesion developed in the tail of the pancreas abutting the spleen. This lesion was followed by CT over the course of months and slowly decreased in size, consistent with a pancreatic pseudocyst. Notice the large spleen as well. **A,** Axial CT image. **B,** Close-up.

outcomes. Perhaps future advances in therapy will use imaging findings to guide patient treatment decisions. We review diagnostic imaging findings of pancreatitis here and discuss grading of severity.

X-ray in Pancreatitis

X-ray findings of pancreatitis are insensitive and nonspecific; x-ray should not generally be used to assess the condition. Nonspecific findings such as ileus may occur, and in chronic pancreatitis calcifications of the pancreas may be present. Pancreatic calcifications may

be present during quiescent periods between acute flares and thus have little clinical value. Calcified gallstones may occasionally be visible, but x-ray can neither confirm nor exclude the diagnosis of pancreatitis, nor does it provide prognostically or therapeutically useful information in most cases. Davis et al.[283] reviewed abdominal x-rays in 100 patients with pancreatitis and found pancreatic calcification in only one case. Biliary abnormalities including a visible gallbladder, gallstones, or biliary gas were seen in only 10%. Nonspecific so-called sentinel bowel loops representing dilated duodenum or jejunum were seen in around 30% of patients. In its appropriateness guidelines for acute pancreatitis, the ACR[282] does not provide any rating or discussion of x-ray—because x-rays are not typically indicated.

Ultrasound of Pancreatitis

The primary role of ultrasound in evaluation of pancreatitis is to assess for biliary ductal obstruction by a gallstone or mass, as described earlier. Ultrasound also can identify secondary signs of pancreatitis such as free abdominal fluid and complications such as pseudocyst or abscess. Fluid collections in the pancreatic bed appear hypoechoic (black); an abscess may have a more complex architecture with internal echoes. The ACR[282] recommends ultrasound as the most indicated imaging test in a first episode of pancreatitis, as a result of its ability to assess for gallstone pancreatitis. Even when alcoholic pancreatitis is suspected, the ACR recommends assessment for biliary obstruction using ultrasound. Visualization of pancreatic abnormalities such as intraparenchymal and retroperitoneal fluid collections with ultrasound is difficult in acute pancreatitis because of the frequent presence of overlying bowel gas.

Computed Tomography of Pancreatitis

The ACR[282] recommends CT, with or without contrast, for the evaluation of acute pancreatitis. The ACR rates CT as indicated for first episodes of pancreatitis of unknown cause, though ultrasound is recommended as the first-line imaging test in this circumstance. In other pancreatitis scenarios, including severe abdominal pain, elevated lipase and amylase, fever and leukocytosis, hemoconcentration, oliguria, or tachycardia, the ACR recommends CT be performed. The ACR credits CT as useful for differentiating pancreatitis from other disease processes, as well as for identifying complications of pancreatitis such as necrosis, severe inflammation, and fluid collections. The ACR states that CT is insensitive for detection of biliary calculi, although as we have reviewed in the earlier section on choledocholithiasis and biliary obstruction, some studies show CT to have sensitivity comparable to MRI.

Computed Tomography Findings of the Normal Pancreas and Pancreatitis. The normal pancreas is an intermediate gray band of soft-tissue density (~+40 Hounsfield units) in the upper abdomen (see Figures 9-112 and 9-113). The pancreatic head is located just right of the midline, with the pancreatic body crossing to the patient's left anterior to the abdominal aorta. The pancreatic tail terminates in the left abdomen medial to the spleen and anterior to the left kidney. The surface of the normal pancreas has a frondlike or crenellated appearance. The surrounding fat is quite black, with no inflammatory change. No free fluid is seen around the normal pancreas. When IV contrast is administered, the

normal pancreas enhances uniformly. Oral contrast is not needed to assess the pancreas.

CT findings of pancreatitis include peripancreatic free fluid, peripancreatic fat stranding, and edema of the pancreas, with loss of the normal crenellated appearance (see Figures 9-114 through 9-116).[284] The adjacent fat appears smoky or hazy, and the borders of the pancreas become indistinct. A pancreatic mass or pseudocyst may also be seen (see Figures 9-117 through 9-119). Pancreatitis can be recognized by CT without oral or IV contrast. However, if IV contrast is given, areas of necrosis will fail to enhance and remain dark, whereas less-affected areas will enhance and appear brighter.[285] The demarcation between areas of normal enhancement and necrotic unenhancing regions is often sharp.[284] The pancreatic head is often spared because of a redundant vascular supply.[284] Several investigators have shown a correlation between lack of pancreatic parenchymal enhancement on CT with IV contrast and surgically proven pancreatic necrosis.[285-286] Areas of necrosis identified by CT do not recover enhancement but rather eventually resorb in survivors.[287] Mesenteric edema surrounding blood vessels creates a low-attenuation cuff around the contrast-enhanced blood vessel. A pancreatic pseudocyst may be seen as a well-circumscribed area of hypodensity (typically close to 0 Hounsfield units, or dark gray by CT with a soft-tissue window) within or immediately adjacent to the pancreas, often with an enhancing rim. This may be difficult to differentiate from abscess, although abscesses may be more heterogeneous, sometimes containing air, as well as fluid and semi-solid debris. Patients with extrapancreatitic phlegmon and pancreatic necrosis are at high risk for complications and poor clinical outcomes.[288] CT severity of pancreatitis has been shown to be more predictive of clinical outcomes than are clinical scoring systems such as Ranson's criteria in some studies, although this remains an area of research (described in detail later).[289-290]

Is Intravenous Contrast Detrimental in Pancreatitis? Is it Necessary to Diagnosis or Prognosis?

As described earlier, use of IV contrast allows identification of nonenhancing regions of the pancreas, reflecting pancreatitic necrosis. Some authors have cautioned against the use of IV contrast, because its administration in some animal models is associated with worsened pancreatitis.[291] McMenamin and Gates[292] retrospectively studied 95 patients with acute pancreatitis and found that IV contrast–enhanced CT was associated with longer hospitalization, suggesting the possibility that IV contrast might worsen pancreatitis. The authors found no difference in initial Acute Physiology and Chronic Health Evaluation (APACHE) II scores in patients who underwent IV contrast–enhanced CT and those who did not. Consequently, they concluded that IV-contrasted CT was likely the cause of worsened outcome, not simply a marker of patient disease severity. However, a prospective randomized trial would be required to determine a causal relationship. The ACR[282] currently states that no prospective human data supports an adverse effect of IV contrast in pancreatitis and that benefits outweigh risks. On the other hand, no prospective trial has demonstrated improved outcomes in patients undergoing IV contrast–enhanced CT, so it is difficult to determine the benefit of CT.

Spitzer et al.[33] determined the association of CT without any contrast agents performed within 48 hours with patient mortality in acute pancreatitis and found a strong correlation. Consequently, if patients are unable to receive IV contrast because of contraindications, unenhanced CT may provide similar prognostic information.

Clinical and Computed Tomography Grading Systems for Pancreatitis. Ranson's criteria for pancreatitis are a clinical grading scale that correlates with mortality—though validation of these criteria in subsequent trials shows less impressive predictive power than some proposed CT systems. Nonetheless, it is interesting to observe a qualitative relationship among Ranson's criteria, CT findings, and the pathophysiology of pancreatitis (Table 9-22). Ranson's criteria include several clinical parameters that may have visible CT analogues.[293]

A number of grading systems for the severity of pancreatitis have been developed, based on CT criteria. Increasing severity by CT predicts increasing mortality. A direct relationship between CT findings and therapeutic interventions has not been developed, so although CT may have prognostic significance, the clinical benefit to patients is not proved. Presumably, additional information about the severity of pancreatitis would improve clinical care by allowing treatment of complications such as abscess. We examine some of the studies on CT severity scores here.

TABLE 9-22. Ranson's Criteria for Pancreatitis and Related CT Findings

	Pathophysiology	CT Correlate
At Admission		
Age >55 years	—	None
White blood cell count >16,000 cells/mm^3	—	None
Blood glucose >10 mmol/L (>200 mg/dL)	Pancreatic injury reducing insulin production	Pancreatic necrosis with lack of enhancement on CT
Serum aspartate aminotransferase >250 IU/L	—	None
Serum lactate dehydrogenase >350 IU/L	—	None
At 48 Hours		
Serum calcium <2.0 mmol/L (<8.0 mg/dL)	Fat saponification because of digestion of retroperitoneal fat and sequestration of calcium in the resulting soap	Inflammatory change (stranding) in retroperitoneal fat
Hematocrit fall >10%	Hemorrhagic pancreatitis	Hemorrhagic pancreatitis with fluid in retroperitoneal space
Oxygen (hypoxemia PO$_2$ < 60 mm Hg)	Systemic inflammatory response syndrome with development of acute respiratory distress syndrome	Possible diffuse infiltrates on lung window
Blood urea nitrogen increased by ≥1.8 mmol/L (≥5 mg/dL) after IV fluid hydration	Inflammatory change with increased vascular permeability	Possible anasarca and ascites on CT
Base deficit (negative base excess) >4 mEq/L	Third spacing of fluid results in intravascular hypovolemia and poor end-organ perfusion	Possible anasarca and ascites on CT
Sequestration of fluids >6 L	Inflammatory change with increased vascular permeability	Possible anasarca and ascites on CT
Ranson's Score	**Predicted Mortality**	
0-2	2%	
3-4	15%	
5-6	40%	
7-8	100%	

Adapted from Ranson JH, Rifkind KM, Roses DF, et al. Prognostic signs and the role of operative management in acute pancreatitis. *Surg Gynecol Obstet* 139:69-81, 1974.

Balthazar et al.[294] graded 83 patients with acute pancreatitis based on CT findings and correlated CT severity with clinical outcome (Table 9-23). Length of hospitalization correlated positively with CT severity. Abscesses occurred in 21.6% of all patients, no patients with grades A and B, and 60.0% of patients with severe pancreatitis (grade E). Pleural effusions were more common in grade E patients. No patients with CT grade A or B died. The authors concluded that early CT had prognostic value for morbidity and mortality. Whether early CT results in improved care has not been studied and would require a prospective study randomizing patients to CT or no CT to determine the effect on outcome.

Subsequently, Balthazar et al.[295] correlated the degree of pancreatitic necrosis identified with CT in 88 acute pancreatitis patients with morbidity and mortality. Based on these findings, they developed a CT severity index to predict morbidity and mortality (see Table 9-23).

Clavien et al.[296] compared early CT findings (within 36 hours) and clinical scores to clinical course in 202 patients with acute pancreatitis. The authors classified CT findings in three categories and clinical scores as three groups, which correlated with mortality (Table 9-24). In patients with CT grade III and clinical score 2 or 3, mortality was particularly high: 32% or 58%, respectively. Complications developed in all survivors in these two groups, and all but two pancreatic abscesses developed in patients with CT grade III. The authors suggested that early CT be performed in all patients with a clinical score of 2 or 3, given the high mortality in these groups. This study did not explicitly examine any therapeutic inventions performed in response to CT findings, so it is unproven that the additional information provided by CT would alter management or improve mortality.

London et al.[297] studied 126 patients with acute pancreatitis undergoing contrast-enhanced abdominal CT within 72 hours of presentation. Several CT criteria including pancreatic enhancement, loss of peripancreatic tissue planes, and a pancreatic size index (calculated by multiplying the maximum AP diameter of the pancreatic head and body) correlated with severity of pancreatitis. A pancreatic size index of at least 10 cm^2 was 71% sensitive and 77% specific for a severe attack—but was less predictive than the modified Glasgow criteria (similar to Ranson's Criteria), which were 85% sensitive and 79% specific.

Basterra et al.[298] compared Ranson's criteria with Balthazar's CT criteria in 100 consecutive patients admitted with pancreatitis and found CT criteria to have superior sensitivity and specificity in predicting outcomes. Pancreatic necrosis was most predictive of outcome.

Ju et al.[300] compared clinical scores (Ranson's criteria) with three CT scoring systems: the Balthazar ABCD score, the Balthazar CT severity index (see Table 9-23),

TABLE 9-23. CT Pancreatitis Severity Index, Which Combines the Balthazar Grading System With Additional Points for Degree of Pancreatic Necrosis

Balthazar CT Grade	CT Findings	Points Assigned
A	Normal pancreas	0
B	Pancreatic enlargement	1
C	Pancreatic inflammation, peripancreatic fat stranding, or both	2
D	Single peripancreatic fluid collection	3
E	Two or more fluid collections, retroperitoneal air, or both	4
Pancreatic Necrosis	Points Assigned	
0%	0	
<30%	2	
30%-50%	4	
>50%	6	
Pancreatitis severity index (0-10)	Sum of points from Balthazar CT grade and percentage necrosis	

Adapted from Balthazar EJ. Acute pancreatitis: assessment of severity with clinical and CT evaluation. *Radiology* 223:603-613, 2002.

TABLE 9-24. CT Findings and Clinical Scores in Pancreatitis, Compared With Mortality

CT Grade	Description	Mortality
I	No phlegmonous extrapancreatic spread	0%
II	Phlegmonous extrapancreatic spread in one or two areas	4%
III	Phlegmonous extrapancreatic spread in three or more areas	42%
Clinical Score	**Description**	**Mortality**
1	0-1 positive Ranson sign	0%
2	2-4 positive Ranson signs	13%
3	≥5 positive Ranson signs	35%

Adapted from Clavien PA, Hauser H, Meyer P, Rohner A. Value of contrast-enhanced computerized tomography in the early diagnosis and prognosis of acute pancreatitis. A prospective study of 202 patients. *Am J Surg* 155:457-466, 1988.

and London's pancreatic size index. Ranson's criteria and the pancreatic size index performed best, with the pancreatic size index being more predictive of local complications. Earlier investigators had found little additional prognostic benefit to CT compared with clinical scores.[301]

Rickes et al.[302] reported the sensitivity and specificity of contrast-enhanced ultrasound (using an IV sonography contrast agent) for detection of severe pancreatitis, defined by a Balthazar score of D or E or CT evidence of pancreatic necrosis. Compared with CT, ultrasound was 82% sensitive and 89% specific.

Magnetic Resonance Imaging of Pancreatitis
Lecesne et al.[303] compared contrast-enhanced CT to MRI in predicting morbidity. Unenhanced MRI and MRCP both correlated well with patient outcome and with CT. Ward et al.[304] found MRI and contrast-enhanced CT to be comparable in identifying areas of pancreatic necrosis. MRI was better at characterizing fluid collections and identifying gallstones, whereas CT was superior in detection of gas and pancreatic calcification. MRI is thus an option in patients with nondiagnostic CT or contraindications to CT.

Urologic Emergencies

Imaging of conditions of the urinary tract including renal and ureteral stones, pyelonephritis, and perinephric abscess is discussed in detail in Chapter 12. Noncontrast CT is the most versatile emergency department study for these conditions because of its ability to evaluate nonurinary conditions that may have overlapping clinical presentations. Other imaging modalities, including IV urography and ultrasound, are discussed in Chapter 12.

Abdominal Aortic Aneurysm and Dissection

Abdominal aortic aneurysm and dissection are life-threatening and time-dependent conditions. In unstable patients, no imaging may be possible, and immediate laparotomy may be required. Ultrasound provides a portable imaging solution for patients with concerning vital signs, whereas CT provides more definitive imaging in patients who appear temporarily stable. X-ray plays virtually no role in evaluation of patients with suspected abdominal vascular emergencies. Imaging of nontraumatic abdominal aortic pathology is discussed in detail in Chapter 11.

Obstetric and Gynecologic Emergencies

Obstetric and gynecologic emergencies may overlap substantially with other abdominal and urinary conditions in their clinical presentation, and the emergency physician must prioritize the imaging evaluation based on the most dangerous, time-dependent, or likely diagnosis. Ultrasound is the preferred initial imaging test for most obstetric and gynecologic conditions, because it causes no radiation exposure (and is thus safe in pregnancy and in young female patients), can be performed portably, provides dynamic blood flow information for conditions such as ectopic pregnancy and ovarian torsion, and has good sensitivity and specificity for many gynecologic conditions. Often imaging with CT must be considered as well, because competing diagnoses such as appendicitis may sometimes be impossible to rule out with ultrasound. Imaging of conditions including ectopic pregnancy, ovarian torsion, ovarian masses, and tuboovarian abscess is discussed in detail in Chapter 12.

Abscesses, Cysts, and Masses

Abscesses, cystic masses, and solid masses may be detected with a number of modalities. CT, ultrasound, and MRI are generally accurate for masses, with sensitivity and specificity greater than 95%.[305] Figures 9-120 through 9-128 demonstrate findings of abscess and mass.

X-ray of Abscesses, Cysts, and Masses
X-ray findings of abscess, cyst, and solid mass are insensitive and nonspecific. Any of these may lead to obstruction of bowel, with findings described elsewhere in this chapter. Abscesses may occasionally demonstrate air–fluid levels, though these may be difficult to distinguish from air–fluid levels within bowel. Solid masses can increase x-ray attenuation. Some solid masses such as ovarian dermoid tumors (teratomas) may have internal calcifications, visible on x-ray. Other modalities are more sensitive and specific. The ACR rates CT with or without contrast as most definitive but continues to suggest

---

Box 9-4: Modified Glasgow Criteria for Pancreatitis

Clinical scores and CT grading systems have been compared in the research setting to determine their prognostic accuracy. In many studies, CT is more predictive than clinical criteria.

On Admission
- **Age >55 years**
- **White blood cell count >15 × 10⁹ per liter**
- **Blood glucose >200 mg/dL (no diabetic history)**
- **Serum urea >16 mmol/L (no response to IV fluids)**
- **Arterial oxygen saturation <60 mm Hg**

Within 48 Hours
- **Serum calcium <2 mmol/L**
- **Serum albumin <32 g/L**
- **Lactate dehydrogenase >219 IU/L**
- **Aspartate aminotransferase or alanine aminotransferase >96 IU/L (removed from modified criteria)**

Adapted from Corfield AP, Cooper MJ, Williamson RC, et al. Prediction of severity in acute pancreatitis: Prospective comparison of three prognostic indices. *Lancet* 2:403-407, 1985.

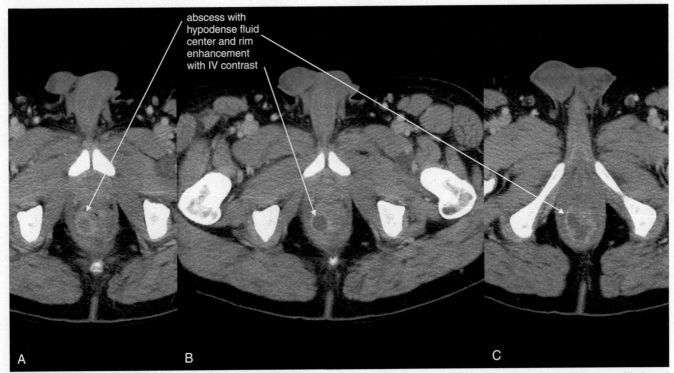

Figure 9-120. Perirectal abscess, CT with IV and oral contrast, soft-tissue window. This patient presented with rectal pain but was afebrile and had only a mild leukocytosis (10.6×10⁹/L, with the upper limit of normal being 9.8×10⁹/L). Rectal examination did not reveal an obvious mass. **A, B, C,** Axial images, cephalad to caudad. An abscess abuts the rectum on the right. The abscess reveals typical findings: a hypoattenuating (fluid-density) center and an enhancing rim, which results from the administration of IV contrast. The orally administered contrast had not transited to the rectum at the time of this CT and was of no diagnostic benefit.

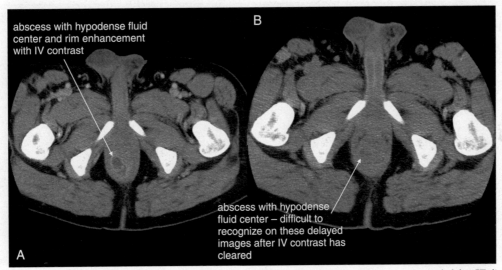

Figure 9-121. Perirectal abscess, CT with IV and oral contrast, role of contrast agents. Are contrast agents needed for CT diagnosis of abscess? Contrast agents can be helpful, although many abscesses can be detected without any contrast. **A,** The appearance of a perirectal abscess after administration of IV contrast. The abscess shows rim enhancement, which makes the rim brighter than the surrounding soft tissues. The center of the abscess is quite hypodense relative to the enhancing rim. **B,** Delayed images taken after the bolus of IV contrast had dissipated. The rim of the abscess is not as conspicuous, and the center, although hypodense, is not as obvious because of the lesser degree of tissue contrast. An experienced reader would likely make the correct diagnosis, although the extent of the abscess might be less certain. The orally administered contrast had reached several slices higher but did not play a role in the diagnosis. Occasionally, rectal (or orally administered) contrast might help to differentiate the bowel lumen from an adjacent abscess.

x-ray as a reasonable initial study for a possible mass and to exclude bowel obstruction as a possible cause of an apparent mass. Interestingly, a mass is found in only about 16%-38% of patients referred for imaging of a possible mass.³⁰⁵

Ultrasound of Abscesses, Cysts, and Masses
Ultrasound can be used to assess for abscesses, cysts, and solid masses.³⁰⁵ Abscess cavities typically display heterogeneous contents, with both anechoic or hypoechoic (black) fluid contents and hyperechoic (white) semi-solid

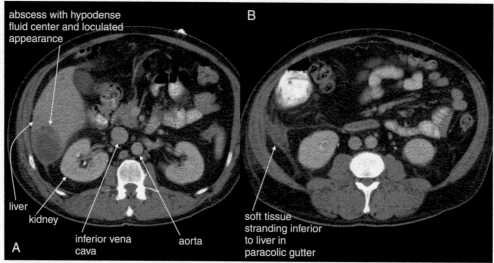

Figure 9-122. Liver abscess, CT with oral and IV contrast. This 50-year-old male presented with high fever and rigors. He had undergone a laparoscopic appendectomy several weeks prior, complicated by a right lower quadrant abscess that had been percutaneously drained. CT scan of the abdomen was performed to assess for abscess. **A,** Axial CT shows a hypodense lesion in the liver, with a loculated appearance—consistent with abscess. **B,** Inflammatory soft-tissue stranding inferior to the liver also suggests that this is an infectious abscess. No abscess was seen in the right lower quadrant. The patient grew *Clostridium ramosum* from blood cultures, and a mixture of anaerobes was cultured from the abscess after CT-guided percutaneous drainage. Compare these images to Figure 9-121. Why is rim enhancement not present here? IV contrast was administered, but these images were taken after a delay (the patient underwent a chest CT with IV contrast first to evaluate for pulmonary embolism resulting from recent surgery). Look at the aorta, inferior vena cava, kidneys, and liver. They all show a small degree of enhancement compared with the psoas muscle but not the intense blush seen when CT is performed immediately upon IV contrast administration. A CT performed slightly earlier after IV contrast administration would have demonstrated rim enhancement of the abscess. This abscess likely would have been diagnosed without any contrast administration, because it is rather large and hypodense. To be fair, the difference in density between the liver and the abscess here is accentuated because the liver is moderately enhanced by the IV contrast. Oral contrast was also given, because of concern for appendiceal abscess, but played no role in the diagnosis of this hepatic abscess. In general, solid organ lesions do not require oral contrast for diagnosis.

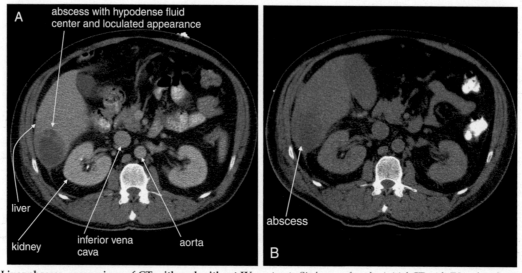

Figure 9-123. Liver abscess, comparison of CT with and without IV contrast. Six hours after the initial CT with IV and oral contrast, the patient underwent CT-guided needle aspiration. No additional contrast agents were given at that time. **A,** The initial CT, performed shortly after IV and oral contrast administration. **B,** A slice through the same level, 6 hours later. The IV contrast has been cleared by the kidneys at this point, so this scan is a CT without IV contrast. Oral contrast remains in the descending colon. The abscess is visible without IV contrast, although the difference in contrast between liver parenchyma and fluid in the abscess is less pronounced.

components. Air within an abscess may be evident as scattering of the ultrasound beam with acoustic shadows occurring deep to the air, a consequence of lack of through-transmission of sound. Simple cystic structures are often visible as spheroid structures with homogeneous anechoic or hypoechoic (black) fluid contents. Some cysts are more complex and display internal echoic septations, although the contents remain primarily anechoic. Solid masses are typically hyperechoic (bright), though the tissue density may vary between hypoechoic and hyperechoic relative to the adjacent organs. Calcifications within a solid mass are highly echoic (bright white) and cast acoustic shadows, much like gallstones. Ultrasound can also display the presence of blood flow

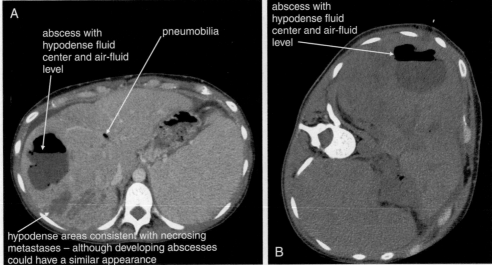

Figure 9-124. Liver abscess with air–fluid levels, comparison of CT with and without IV contrast. This 28-year-old patient has a large hepatic abscess, in this case with a dramatic air–fluid level. The patient has metastatic pancreatic cancer (low-density lesions spread throughout liver) and had undergone a radiofrequency ablation and other invasive procedures, including biliary stent placement. Her CT also shows pneumobilia, which had been noted on prior CT scans following her biliary stent. She likely became bacteremic or seeded her biliary system with gastrointestinal flora, with areas of necrotic liver metastases then acting as a perfect culture medium for circulating bacteria. This abscess was percutaneously drained under CT guidance. The patient grew ampicillin- and vancomycin-resistant enterococci from blood and from the abscess aspirate. Cultures from the abscess also grew *Klebsiella pneumoniae.* This patient received oral and IV contrast for her CT, because the cause of her symptoms was not clear initially and a broad differential diagnosis was considered. The patient presented with intermittent fevers for 3 weeks, as well as chronic right upper quadrant pain, and was receiving chemotherapy. She also had a history of pancreatic pseudocyst, so a long list of abdominal disorders was considered. In retrospect, no contrast was needed to make this diagnosis. Air in the abscess does not require contrast for diagnosis, because it appears black without any contrast agents. The fluid in this abscess is extensive and quite hypodense relative to the liver parenchyma, although the difference in density is accentuated by the IV contrast enhancement of the liver. Oral contrast was a reasonable choice given the broad differential diagnosis being entertained, though it did not assist with the diagnosis of hepatic abscess. A, An axial slice from the patient's CT with IV and oral contrast, obtained with the patient in the usual supine position. Air in the abscess has risen to the top of the cavity, while fluid remains dependent. B, For comparison, a slice through the same region is shown from the patient's CT-guided drainage procedure the following day, during which no contrast agents were given. The patient is in a lateral decubitus position for the procedure, and the air–fluid level has shifted accordingly.

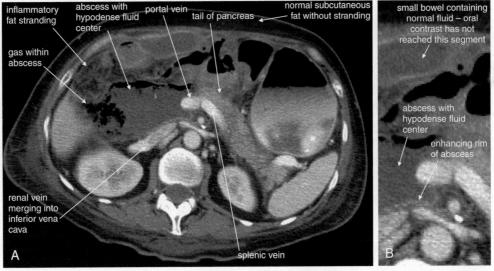

Figure 9-125. Abdominal abscess, developing in postoperative patient following Whipple procedure. CT with oral and IV contrast, soft-tissue window. An abscess is visible in the region of the resected pancreatic head (the pancreatic tail was not removed). For orientation, several other structures are labeled. The abnormalities typical of an abscess include a fluid collection, rim enhancement with IV contrast, gas or air within the fluid collection, and stranding of adjacent fat. Compare this abnormal fat with normal subcutaneous fat that does not show stranding. **A,** Axial CT image. **B,** Close-up. Could this abscess have been detected without contrast? The hypodense abscess fluid, the fat stranding, and the gas within the abscess would all have been visible. The overall appearance might have been more confusing, because the pancreas, liver, blood vessels, and bowel in the region would have been more isodense with the abscess without the administered contrast agents. The boundaries of the abscess are likely better recognized with contrast, especially in this busy region of the central abdomen.

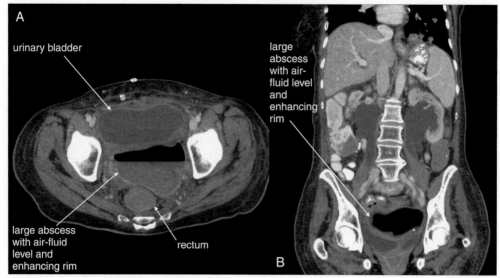

Figure 9-126. Pelvic abscess, developing following pelvic exenteration for mass, CT with IV and oral contrast. This 63-year-old female with metastatic ovarian cancer presented with chills following resection of a pelvic mass. **A,** Axial image. **B,** Coronal image. An abscess is visible in the pelvis, deep to the urinary bladder. This abscess demonstrates classic findings of an air–fluid level and rim enhancement with IV contrast. The rectum is visible deep to the abscess **(A).**

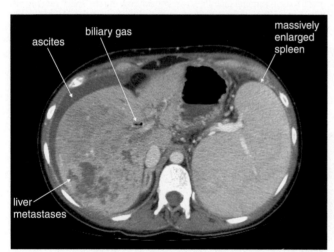

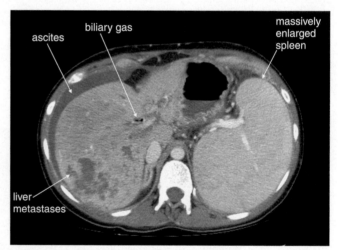

Figure 9-127. Metastatic disease, CT. This patient has metastatic pancreatic cancer and related splenomegaly. Other findings in this CT (splenomegaly, biliary gas, and ascites) are discussed in detail elsewhere in this text. The liver is a common site of metastatic disease from many sources, including pancreatic and colon cancers. On IV contrast–enhanced CT, liver metastases frequently show rim enhancement with central hypodensity, reflecting central necrosis as these lesions outgrow their blood supply. Remember that a differential diagnosis exists for this appearance, including liver injury (contusion or hematoma) in the setting of trauma and abscess in the setting of suspected fever. On noncontrast CT, these lesions remain hypodense compared with the surrounding liver parenchyma, though less so than on IV contrast–enhanced CT, because normal liver enhances brightly with IV contrast. Hepatic cysts are typically more rounded than metastatic disease, although they too can be multiple. Other lesions that appear hypodense on noncontrast CT, such as hemangiomas, can be distinguished from metastases by their pattern of enhancement on IV-contrasted CT, including their contrast appearance on delayed images (taken periodically as time elapses from the time of contrast administration). Primary hepatic neoplasms such as hepatomas may have a similar appearance to these for the nonspecialist. Differentiating the multitude of hepatic lesions by their CT appearance is beyond the scope of this text, although it is important for the emergency physician to recognize the existence of a differential diagnosis to avoid misdiagnosis.

Figure 9-128. Splenomegaly, CT with IV contrast. Splenomegaly can occur from many causes. A normal spleen can be difficult to measure with ultrasound, because it lies sheltered by the left costal margin in many cases. An enlarged spleen can usually be seen with ultrasound. CT readily reveals splenomegaly, as does magnetic resonance imaging (MRI). This patient has metastatic pancreatic cancer and related splenomegaly. The spleen is nearly as large as the liver in this cross section. This may be partly caused by thrombosis of the portal vein (not seen in this image, but noted in other CT images and confirmed with MRI in this patient). Remember that the splenic vein drains ultimately to the portal vein, so thrombosis of the portal vein may lead to splenomegaly. Other findings in this CT (biliary gas, metastatic disease, and ascites) are discussed in detail elsewhere in this text.

within vascular lesions, including hypervascular solid masses and primary vascular anomalies such as hemangiomas and hemangioblastomas. The use of ultrasound for assessment of solid and cystic gynecologic conditions is discussed in more detail in Chapter 12. In general, ultrasound is useful for detection of abscesses, masses, and cystic structures within or adjacent to solid organs, which provide excellent acoustic windows for the ultrasound beam. Abscesses and masses associated with bowel may be more difficult to assess as a result of poor transmission of the ultrasound beam through bowel gas. Nonetheless, ultrasound diagnosis of appendiceal and diverticular abscesses can be performed, and percutaneous drainage of these lesions under ultrasound guidance is possible. The ACR[306] recommends ultrasound as the most appropriate imaging modality for suspected abdominal abscess in the pregnant patient.

Computed Tomography of Abscesses, Cysts, and Masses

Abscess, cysts, and solid lesions are well-characterized by CT.[305-306] With CT, a simple cyst is seen as a spherical structure with homogeneous contents, with a typical fluid density near or just above water density (0 HU) (see Figure 9-3). Simple cysts are visible without any contrast agents. Usually these structures do not enhance with IV contrast administration—in contrast to abscesses and vascular lesions such as hemangiomas. For example, a variety of cystic-appearing liver lesions can occur, sometimes differentiated on CT only by their temporal pattern of IV contrast enhancement. Differentiation of these lesions is beyond the scope of this text but may require CT with additional delayed image acquisition.

An abscess can be recognized on CT by several common features (see Figures 9-120 through 9-126). These include the presence of heterogeneous contents, including fluid contents 0 to +40 Hounsfield units in density (dark gray on a soft-tissue window), denser solid and semi-solid debris, and occasionally gas caused by bacterial metabolism (black or −1000 HU). Because of high blood flow, the rim of an abscess usually enhances with administration of IV contrast, giving it a bright appearance. IV contrast can make abscesses within solid organs more prominent by demonstrating abnormalities of enhancement. Fat surrounding an abscess may demonstrate inflammatory stranding. Enteral contrast may assist in differentiating adjacent loops of bowel (containing fluid and air) from an abscess. Enteral contrast delineates the bowel lumen, whereas an abscess would not be expected to fill with enteral contrast. Abscesses within solid organs such as the liver do not require enteral contrast for diagnosis—though often the emergency physician cannot suspect the specific site of abscess based on history or examination. Consequently, enteral and IV contrast should generally be administered when abscess is suspected, particularly if the abscess is believed to lie adjacent to bowel. Exceptions may include soft-tissue abscesses not thought to involve the peritoneal cavity, some suspected retroperitoneal abscesses such as perinephric abscesses, and solid-organ abscesses such as hepatic abscesses when their presence has already been disclosed by another modality such as ultrasound.[306] CT with IV contrast can differentiate perirectal abscess from cellulitis. Usually enteral contrast (most often rectal) is also given to identify bowel and potential fistula.[307] CT can be used to guide percutaneous drainage of abscesses. Studies show good outcomes in percutaneous drainage of periappendiceal abscess, with approximately 80% resolving without surgery (see Chapter 16 for a more detailed discussion).[308]

Mass lesions including metastatic disease can be recognized by CT (see Figures 9-127 and 9-128). IV contrast enhancement patterns can be important to the diagnosis, because certain lesions have a typical spatial and temporal pattern of enhancement (e.g., filling from the periphery or filling selectively during arterial or portal venous phases of enhancement). Characterizing mass lesions based on these criteria is beyond the scope of this text.[309]

Magnetic Resonance Imaging of Abscesses, Cysts, and Masses

MRI can be used to identify abdominal abscesses and masses—though usually it is not required for this purpose in the emergency department, as a result of the excellent sensitivity and specificity of CT.[305-306,309]

Ascites, Hemoperitoneum, and Other Peritoneal Fluids

Free fluid in the abdomen can be diagnosed by a number of imaging modalities. Imaging cannot accurately determine the exact composition of intraabdominal fluid, though the cause is sometimes evident from history, examination, other clinical findings, or other imaging findings. For example, fluid within the abdomen may be suspected to be blood when solid abdominal organ injury is discovered or when an abdominal aortic aneurysm is diagnosed. However, a differential diagnosis for abdominal fluid, including simple ascites, infectious ascites, malignant ascites, blood, and urine, should be considered. Often, direct sampling of the fluid is necessary for specific diagnosis. Imaging of peritoneal fluids is demonstrated in Figures 9-129 through 9-133.

X-ray of Peritoneal Fluid

X-ray is insensitive and nonspecific for the detection of abdominal fluid. Large amounts of fluid may give the entire abdomen a ground-glass appearance. In the case of large ascites or other fluid, the small bowel may be suspended within the fluid and assume a central location in the abdomen (see Figure 9-129). Overall, ultrasound and CT provide such superior diagnostic capabilities that x-ray should not be ordered for this indication.

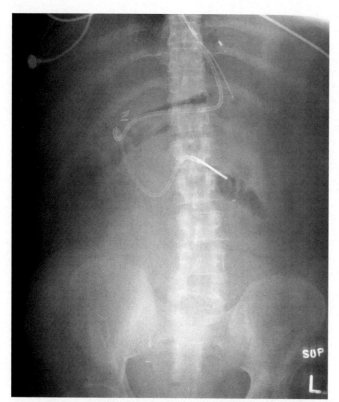

Figure 9-129. Ascites, x-ray. X-ray is a poor modality for diagnosis of ascites. However, ascites can produce x-ray findings suggesting diffuse abdominal fluid. Typical findings include a diffuse hazy appearance, centralization of bowel gas (caused by bowel floating in the peritoneal fluid), and a paucity of bowel gas. These findings are nonspecific and relatively insensitive. Other diagnoses are not excluded by these x-ray findings, and the presence of ascites is not confirmed. Note the paucity of bowel gas and hazy appearance in this x-ray. Bowel obstruction can give a similar appearance as gas is expelled distal to the point of obstruction. This is a supine x-ray, so air–fluid levels would not be expected to be seen. The patient has a feeding tube terminating in the distal duodenum. Compare this x-ray with the ultrasound and CT from the same patient in Figure 9-130 through 9-132.

Ultrasound of Peritoneal Fluid

With ultrasound, abdominal fluid appears black (anechoic) and usually homogeneous (see Figures 9-130 and 9-131). Blood may be suspected based on a more heterogeneous appearance, with anechoic and echoic components (representing liquid and coagulated blood, respectively). Sometimes fibrinous strands can be seen with ultrasound, adhered to other structures such as bowel. The use of ultrasound to detect traumatic hemoperitoneum is discussed in Chapter 10. Simple ascites, infected ascites as in spontaneous bacterial peritonitis, and fluids such as bile or urine leaking from their respective ductal systems have a similar anechoic appearance. Consequently, when the cause of the fluid is important to diagnosis and treatment, sampling of the fluid should be performed, rather than relying upon imaging criteria. Some recent studies have examined the use of injected vascular contrast agents to allow detection of hemoperitoneum with active bleeding (discussed in more detail in Chapter 11, and briefly in Chapter 10).[310]

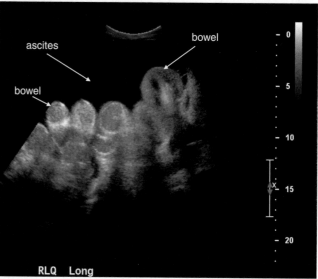

Figure 9-130. Ascites, ultrasound. Ultrasound is useful for detection of ascites. Simple fluids such as ascites are excellent sound transmission media, reflecting almost no sound waves. As a consequence, they appear quite hypoechoic (*black*) on ultrasound. This view of the right lower quadrant in the same patient as Figure 9-129 shows loops of bowel surrounded by fluid. During the ultrasound, the bowel loops would be seen to undergo peristalsis and drift back and forth in the ascitic fluid with patient movement. Ultrasound cannot distinguish the composition of the fluid—ascites, liquid blood, liquid bile, urine, and infectious fluids have a similar appearance, with a few exceptions. Blood may coagulate and form septations within the fluid collection. Infectious fluids also frequently form loculated fluid collections that may be recognized on ultrasound, although the exact composition cannot be determined.

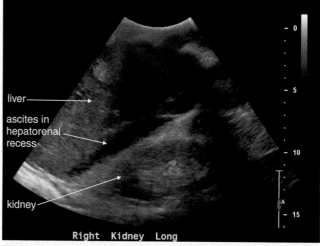

Figure 9-131. Ascites, ultrasound. Ultrasound is excellent for detection of ascites. In this view of the right upper quadrant from the same patient as Figures 9-129 and 9-130, fluid is visible in Morison's pouch (hepatorenal recess), separating the liver and right kidney. Ascites has settled in this location because it is the most dependent portion of the abdomen in a supine patient. Were this a trauma patient, this fluid could represent blood and this view would constitute a positive Focused Assessment with Sonography for Trauma (FAST). Ultrasound cannot determine the composition of the fluid directly, because simple fluids such as ascites, urine, and liquid blood look alike.

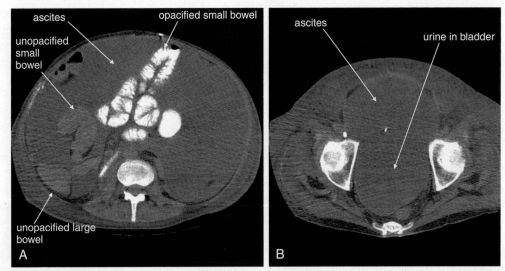

Figure 9-132. Ascites, CT with oral contrast, soft-tissue window. Free fluid in the abdomen can be recognized on CT without the administration of contrast. Depending on its composition (ascites, blood, bile, intestinal contents, urine, or pus), its density may vary somewhat. Simple ascites and urine have densities similar to water, zero Hounsfield units (HU). Blood varies in density (see Table 9-25).The density of fluid can be measured to estimate the likely composition; however, this can be unreliable. For example, mixing of two types of fluid (e.g., blood and ascites) can occur, or blood of varying hematocrits may have varying densities. In this patient, massive ascites were present after a liver and kidney transplant. No intravenous contrast was given. Oral contrast was given but did not fill all of the small bowel **(A).** The ascites are a low-density *(dark gray)* fluid, slightly less dense than unopacified small bowel, which is also fluid-filled. Urine in the bladder is slightly less dense than the ascitic fluid and appears slightly darker as a consequence **(B).** **A, B,** Axial images.

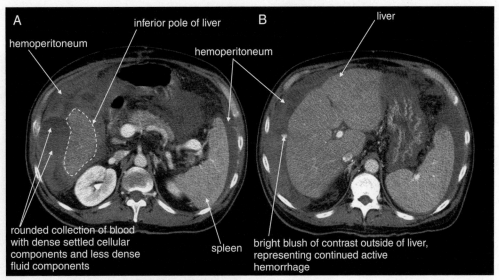

Figure 9-133. Hemoperitoneum, CT with IV contrast, soft-tissue window. This 55-year-old liver transplant patient presented with hypotension developing during a liver biopsy. Bedside ultrasound showed free fluid, which could have represented existing ascites or hemoperitoneum. Peritoneal aspiration showed frank blood, and the patient was treated with emergency angiographic embolization of a bleeding vessel. **A, B,** The axial CT images were obtained after that procedure to determine whether hemostasis had been achieved. The images show complex fluid of multiple densities surrounding the liver and spleen, representing blood in various stages of coagulation. A rounded area with a fluid–fluid level is visible, representing blood with a hematocrit level resulting from settling of cellular components. **B,** Injected contrast material is seen next to the liver, representing continued hemorrhage at the moment of CT.

Large quantities of free abdominal fluid may be immediately visible from any location using ultrasound. More subtle free fluid can be difficult to detect. The hepatorenal space is a dependent region that can trap small amounts of fluid and should be inspected, as in the FAST examination (discussed in more detail in Chapter 10). Fluid appears as a dark stripe between the liver and the kidney. The rectovaginal space can be inspected as well, using a midline sagittal position of the ultrasound probe.

Fluid appears as a dark stripe separating the posterior wall of the vagina and the anterior wall of the rectum (discussed in more detail in Chapter 12).

Computed Tomography of Peritoneal Fluids
CT provides additional information about the density of peritoneal fluid, as well as offering a panoramic view of other abdominal organs with possibly related pathology. On a soft-tissue window, ascites appears intermediate

gray, with a density usually between 0 and +30 Hounsfield units (see Figure 9-132).[311] Water has a density of 0 Hounsfield units, so it comes as little surprise that fluids such as urine and simple ascites may be indistinguishable with routine CT. CT techniques to assess for urine leak are discussed in Chapter 12. Dense fluid (~+40 Hounsfield units) detected by CT is more likely to be pathologic, including blood.[311-312] Hemoperitoneum has a widely variable CT appearance (Table 9-25; see Figure 9-133).[311]

Free abdominal fluid requires no contrast agents for diagnosis with CT. However, contrast agents can sometimes reveal the source of fluid. For example, injected contrast agents may leak into the peritoneal cavity from blood vessels, revealing existing abdominal fluid to be blood. On delayed CT images, injected contrast agents may be concentrated and excreted by the kidneys and can then leak into the peritoneal cavity or retroperitoneum—suggesting existing fluid in these locations to be urine.[311] Oral contrast agents may leak through bowel perforations, although in reality this occurs rarely and oral contrast agents have been shown to have rare value in diagnosis of conditions such as traumatic bowel injury. Infectious fluids may have variable densities, from near zero HU (e.g., spontaneous bacterial peritonitis) to near solid-organ density in the case of thick purulent material. Enhancement of ascites on delayed images after administration of IV contrast has been described but is nonspecific, occurring in both malignancies and benign conditions.[311] Like ultrasound, CT cannot always discriminate among fluids as different as ascites, blood, bile, and urine, so sampling of fluid may be necessary to determine its composition.

Large amounts of abdominal fluid are usually readily visible using CT, because they are distributed throughout the abdomen. Bowel may float within abdominal fluid and assume a centralized location. Smaller amounts of free fluid are more subtle. Dependent portions of the abdomen and pelvis should be examined for free fluid. Morison's pouch (the hepatorenal space) and the pouch of Douglas (rectovaginal space) should be inspected. Fluid between loops of bowel in the abdomen and pelvis may have an irregular contour, because it occupies any potential space. The paracolic gutters may also contain free fluid.

Magnetic Resonance Imaging of Peritoneal Fluid

MRI can be used to assess abdominal fluid, although it is rarely indicated in the emergency department because of the diagnostic accuracy of ultrasound and CT. MRI can reveal peritoneal or ascites enhancement, suggesting infectious peritonitis or malignant ascites.[313] Nonetheless, sampling of fluid is usually required to determine the exact cause, so the advantage of MRI is limited.

Foreign Body Ingestion or Insertion

Orally ingested, rectally inserted, or living enteric (parasitic) foreign bodies can be detected by a variety of imaging modalities, as shown in Figures 9-134 through 9-139. Foreign bodies from penetrating trauma and medical devices can also be identified.

X-ray of Abdominal Foreign Bodies

Metal, stone, and glass are usually visible on plain x-ray—in contrast to a common misconception that only leaded glass is visible on x-ray (see Figures 9-134 through 9-137).[314]

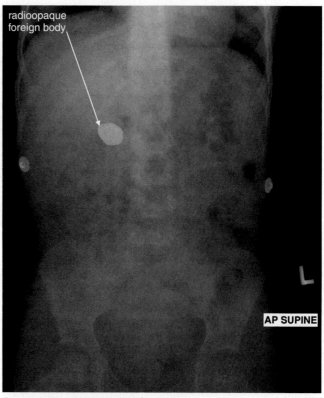

radioopaque foreign body

L

AP SUPINE

Figure 9-134. Ingested foreign body, x-ray. This 3-year-old patient swallowed a single magnetic stone measuring 2.5 × 1.5 cm. It was allowed to pass spontaneously and did so without complication. X-rays of the abdomen have little utility in most scenarios. Ingested foreign body is one exception, where x-ray may confirm ingestion, allow characterization of size and shape, and allow tracking of the progress of the foreign body through the gastrointestinal track.

TABLE 9-25. CT Appearance of Hemoperitoneum

Blood Product	Hounsfield Density
Fresh unclotted blood	30-45 Hounsfield units
Clotted blood	60-100 Hounsfield units
Serum (after clotting)	0-20 Hounsfield units
Fresh blood with "hematocrit effect"	Settling of cellular component can create a fluid–fluid level, with the more dependent and higher-density layer being cells

Adapted from Gayer G, Hertz M, Manor H, et al: Dense ascites: CT manifestations and clinical implications. *Emerg Radiol* 10:262-267, 2004.

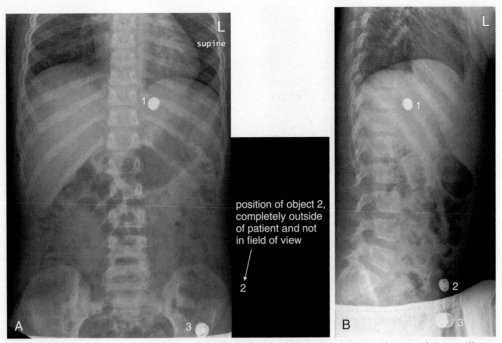

position of object 2, completely outside of patient and not in field of view

Figure 9-135. Ingested foreign body, x-ray. This 7-year-old child was "washing" a button battery in her mouth in an effort to fix her electric toy when she reported accidentally swallowing the battery. Parents were uncertain whether any ingestion had occurred. The anterior–posterior (AP) supine view **(A)** reveals two radiopaque objects; the lateral view **(B)** reveals three. Did the patient ingest multiple batteries? Only object 1 is projected in a consistent location overlying the abdomen on both views and is intraabdominal. The other two objects are external to the patient. Object 3 on the lateral corresponds to the caudad object on the AP view. Object 2 on the lateral view is so far lateral that it is not visible on the AP view. The patient underwent upper endoscopy but the battery had moved beyond the pylorus and could not be retrieved. Plain x-rays obtained 24 hours later confirmed passage of the battery.

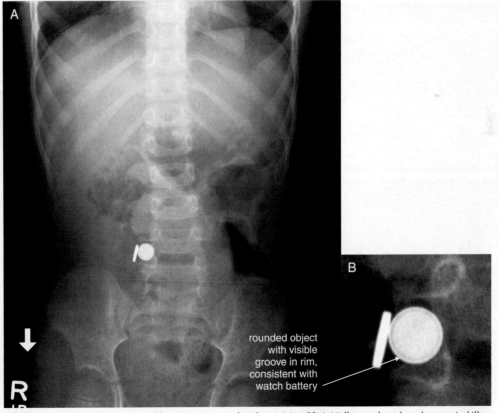

rounded object with visible groove in rim, consistent with watch battery

Figure 9-136. Ingested battery, x-ray. This 3-year-old patient presented with vomiting. He initially was thought to have a viral illness, but he continued to be symptomatic over 23 hours of emergency department observation and developed substantial leukocytosis. This abdominal x-ray revealed the surprise finding of two foreign bodies, one corresponding in size and shape to a lithium watch battery (note the slightly lucent band around the rim). **A,** Anterior–posterior upright x-ray. **B,** Close-up from **A.**

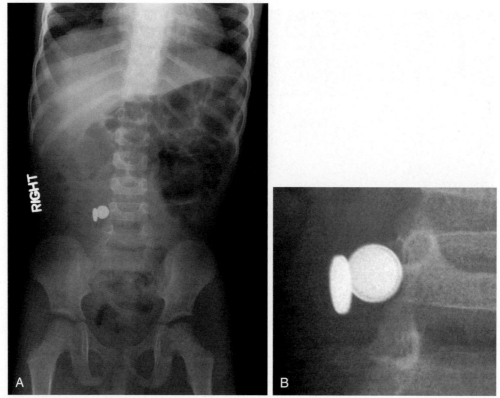

Figure 9-137. Ingested battery, x-ray (obtained 3 days after the x-ray in Figure 9-136**).** This 3-year-old patient was found to have ingested two objects, one suspected to be a watch battery. X-rays over the course of 3 days showed no significant change in the location of the ingested foreign bodies—and peculiarly, they remained touching each other. **A,** Anterior–posterior supine x-ray. **B,** Close-up from **A.**

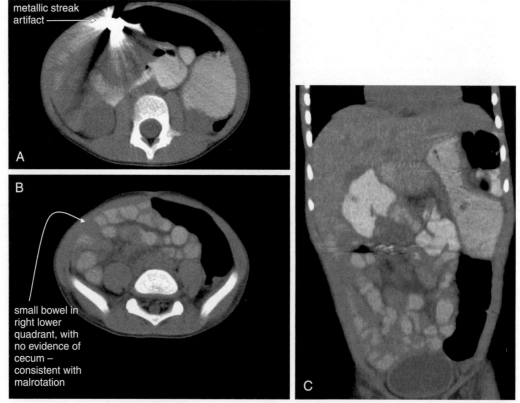

Figure 9-138. Ingested battery, CT with oral contrast. Same patient as Figures 9-136 and 9-137. CT was performed to further evaluate the location of the ingested foreign bodies but provided little additional detail because of metallic streak artifact. Unexpectedly, it revealed malrotation, with the small bowel in the right abdomen. **A, B,** Axial images. **C,** Coronal CT reconstruction clarifying the malrotation. The small bowel is seen occupying predominantly the right abdomen, whereas the large bowel occupies the left. Laparotomy was performed to repair the malrotation and retrieve the foreign bodies, which were found to be a battery and a magnet, magnetically attracted to one another in two adjacent loops of small bowel.

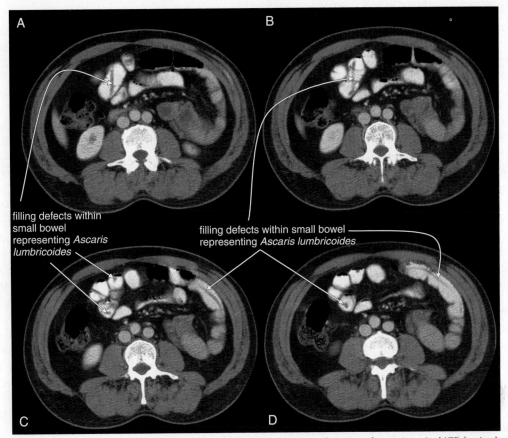

Figure 9-139. Intestinal foreign body—*Ascaris lumbricoides.* Oral contrast can assist in detection of gastrointestinal (GI) foreign bodies. Traditionally, an upper gastrointestinal series would be performed to identify an intraluminal foreign body, which appears as a filling defect in the column of enteral contrast. In this case, the patient underwent abdominal CT for suspected appendicitis. The diagnosis was instead infection with the GI macroparasite *A. lumbricoides,* a giant roundworm. These worms appear as tubular filling defects within the small bowel when seen in long section and as circular filling defects when seen in short-axis cross section. Without oral contrast, these worms would have a similar density to surrounding intestinal contents and would not be identified. *A. lumbricoides* infection is the one of the most common parasitic infections worldwide, with an estimated prevalence of 1.25 billion cases. In the United States, the infection is rarer but may have a prevalence as high as 4 million cases, concentrated in the southern states. The parasite is endemic in tropical regions worldwide and should be considered as a cause of abdominal pain in immigrants and returning travelers. *Ascaris* infections can be complicated by small-bowel obstruction, appendicitis, and biliary ductal obstruction. **A** through **D,** Axial CT slices.

Ingested bone may be visible on x-ray, depending on the density. Small or poorly calcified bones such as fish bones are often not visible on x-ray.[315] X-ray can also reveal complications such as perforation or obstruction, with the caveat that the sensitivity of x-ray is limited (as discussed earlier in this chapter). Lower-density materials including plastic, meat, and wood are often invisible on x-ray. One small study found that ingested cocaine packages were invisible on x-ray in 40% of cases.[316]

Two orthogonal x-ray views are required for localization of a foreign body. An object located posterior to the patient, for example, in a skin fold or trapped in clothing, can appear to be within the patient on a single frontal projection. A lateral view can confirm the location within or outside of the patient (see Figure 9-135).

Contrast Studies of Gastrointestinal Foreign Bodies
Fluoroscopic GI studies using enteral contrast agents (e.g., Gastrografin swallow esophagography, small-bowel series, or barium enema) can detect low-density

intraluminal foreign bodies not seen with standard x-ray. The contrast agent surrounds the foreign body, creating a recognizable void or filling defect.

Computed Tomography of Abdominal Foreign Bodies
When an ingested or intraabdominal foreign body is not visible on x-ray, CT offers an alternative that can localize the object three-dimensionally. CT can reveal foreign bodies with a range of densities, including plastics and organic food material. However, low-density material may be impossible to distinguish from normally occurring food materials in the digestive tract. Enteral contrast agents can outline a foreign body, making it more evident. Macroscopic intestinal parasites can be detected by this same mechanism (see Figure 9-139).[317] Although CT easily detects dense materials such as metal, stone, and glass, these may create metallic streak artifact that can make precise identification of the object and exact determination of its location impossible (see Figure 9-138). Therefore x-ray can actually be superior to CT for identification and localization of dense objects.

Ultrasound of Abdominal Foreign Bodies

Ultrasound can detect some ingested objects in the small bowel; in one study, 60% of ingested cocaine packages were identified with ultrasound.[316] However, ultrasound is often nondiagnostic because of the presence of bowel gas that interrupts and scatters the ultrasound beam.

Adrenal Gland Pathology

Adrenal gland pathology is rarely the indication for abdominal CT in the emergency department, but CT can provide information about pathologic processes affecting these glands. The normal adrenal glands are thin, lambda-shaped structures located in the retroperitoneum at the cephalad pole of each kidney. Adrenal masses or hemorrhage can distort or obscure these structures. Figures 9-140 through 9-143 demonstrate normal adrenal glands and adrenal pathology.

Esophageal Abnormalities

Esophageal abnormalities are often assessed by direct visualization with upper endoscopy. However, in some cases, diagnostic imaging can provide information not readily available from endoscopy or when endoscopy is contraindicated.

X-ray of Esophageal Abnormalities

Plain x-ray provides limited information about the esophagus. Radiodense esophageal foreign bodies may be seen, as described earlier. Frank perforation of the esophagus may be evident from air within the mediastinum (pneumomediastinum), discussed in more detail in Chapter 5.[318] Low-density esophageal foreign bodies such as impacted bread or meat are not usually visible on x-ray, though an air–fluid level in the esophagus may be seen in some cases.[319]

Barium Versus Gastrografin Swallow Studies for Esophageal Abnormalities

When esophageal injury is suspected, as in the case of recurrent vomiting or hematemesis, swallowed foreign body (see Chapter 4, Figures 4-35 and 4-36), or penetrating chest trauma, an esophagram can demonstrate partial- or full-thickness injury. A radiodense contrast material is ingested, and residual contrast retained within mucosal tears or extravasating into the mediastinum can be seen. Gastrografin is recommended as the initial contrast agent, because it is relatively nontoxic to the mediastinum when a full-thickness esophageal injury is present. However, Gastrografin is low in viscosity, resulting in less material being retained in small esophageal defects. If Gastrografin study is normal but injury is still suspected, higher-viscosity barium sulfate can be used to achieve higher sensitivity. Barium is more toxic than Gastrografin when full-thickness tears are present, so it is not the suggested first-line contrast agent.[320-321] Ingested contrast agents can make subsequent endoscopy more difficult.[322]

Computed Tomography of Esophageal Abnormalities

CT is not commonly used for assessment of esophageal injury in the emergency department. However, CT can demonstrate abnormalities including thickening of the

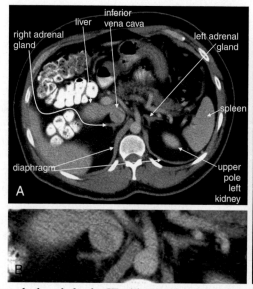
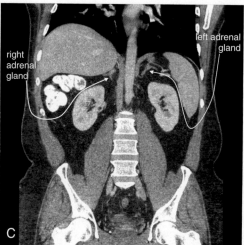

Figure 9-140. Normal adrenal glands, CT with IV and oral contrast. The normal adrenal glands are located superior to the kidneys, tucked into the recess below the diaphragm on each side of the midline. They commonly have a thin lambda (λ) shape in both axial and coronal cross section. Depending on the amount of retroperitoneal fat, they may be separated from the adjacent kidney by several centimeters in both an anteroposterior and a cephalad–caudad direction. In thin patients, they may be immediately adjacent to the kidney, liver *(right),* spleen *(left),* and other retroperitoneal structures, such as the inferior vena cava. We look at several examples of normal adrenal glands to demonstrate the range of their normal size, shape, and location. **A (B,** close-up), In this patient, the adrenal glands are separated from adjacent solid organs by a moderate amount of retroperitoneal fat. The right adrenal gland abuts the inferior vena cava. **C,** In a coronal view from the same patient, the right adrenal gland lies close to the liver.

esophagus at sites of injury, mediastinal air and fluid in cases of esophageal perforation, and foreign body.[322-323] Oral contrast agents usually are not retained well within the esophagus in the supine position used for CT, unless complete esophageal obstruction is present—but they may leak from the esophagus in cases of perforation. In a small prospective study comparing swallow fluoroscopy, CT with oral contrast, and endoscopy, CT and swallow fluoroscopy were comparable, detecting 88% of leaks.[324]

Gastrointestinal Hemorrhage

Imaging plays little role in the diagnosis of upper GI hemorrhage, because lesions within the stomach and proximal small bowel lie within reach of an endoscope for both diagnosis and treatment. Bleeding from the middle and lower intestine presents a greater endoscopic challenge, particularly in emergency situations without preceding bowel cleansing. Three imaging modalities present diagnostic solutions: nuclear scintigraphy, mesenteric angiography, and CT mesenteric angiography.

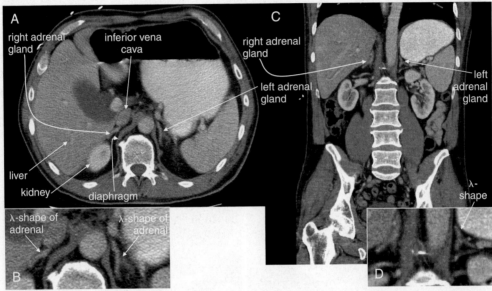

Figure 9-141. Normal adrenal glands, CT with IV and oral contrast. This patient is thinner than the previous patient and has less retroperitoneal fat. The adrenal glands are even more closely abutting adjacent structures, though a thin layer of fat separates them from the surrounding organs. Without this layer of fat, they would be virtually indistinguishable because they share the tissue density of liver, contrasted inferior vena cava, and spleen. Note the lambda (λ) shape of the adrenals. Realize that this cross-sectional shape may vary from patient to patient and slice to slice. Some cross sections may appear more V shaped. Look for enlargement beyond this thin wispy shape, which may signal adrenal mass or hemorrhage. **A,** Axial view. **B,** Close-up from **A. C,** Coronal image. **D,** Close-up from **C.**

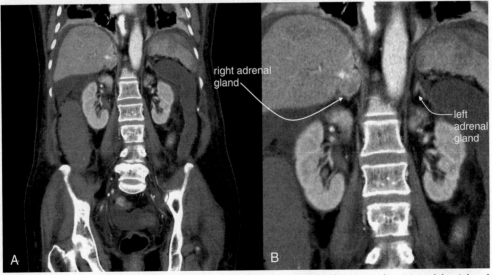

Figure 9-142. Adrenal adenoma, CT with IV contrast. This CT shows a rounded mass in the expected position of the right adrenal gland. At first glance, it may look like a portion of the liver, but note the normal thin lambda-shaped (λ) left adrenal. Scrolling through the entire CT, you would readily note the absence of a normal right adrenal gland. Technically, this adrenal mass cannot be classified as an adenoma based on the CT, although this is the most likely diagnosis. **A,** Coronal image. **B,** Close-up.

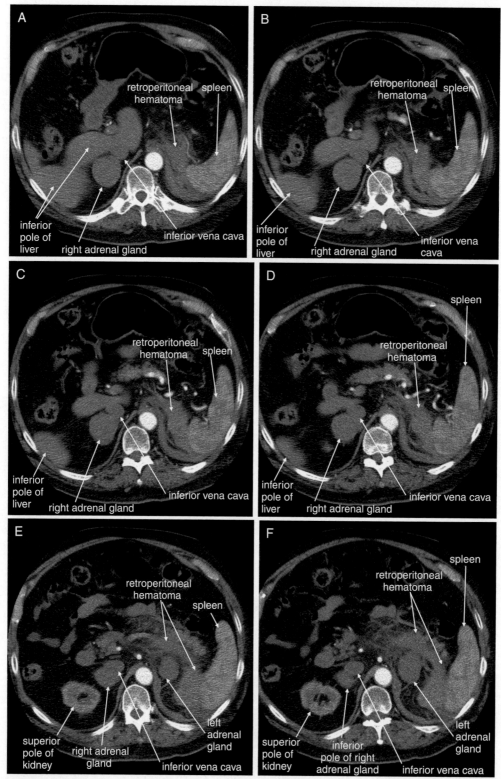

Figure 9-143. Adrenal hemorrhage, CT with IV contrast. This 72-year-old male presented with acute flank pain, diaphoresis, and hypotension. He was being treated with coumadin for deep venous thrombosis. The leading diagnosis was catastrophic aortic pathology—rupture or dissection. CT without contrast, followed by IV-contrasted CT, was performed. **A** through **H,** Sequential axial images from CT with IV contrast. Noncontrast CT showed a normal-caliber aorta with significant retroperitoneal hemorrhage present, extending from the level of the spleen to the iliac bifurcation. The apparent source was the left adrenal gland. CT with IV contrast confirms no aortic dissection and no active extravasation of IV contrast. The patient was noted to have bilaterally enlarged adrenal glands on CT, and his cortisol level was subsequently found to be low. He remained hypotensive disproportionate to his apparent blood loss, even after transfusion. His blood pressure improved with steroid therapy for apparent Addison's disease (adrenal insufficiency) resulting from adrenal hemorrhage. This case raises several interesting points. First, given the concern for aortic catastrophe, clinical management, including volume resuscitation and surgical consultation, takes precedence over imaging.

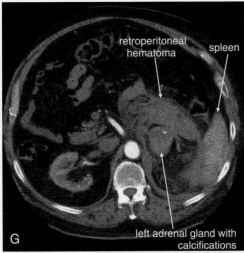

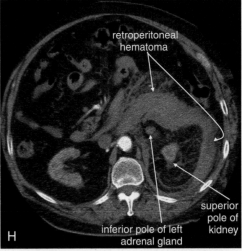

Figure 9-143, cont'd Bedside imaging with ultrasound to evaluate for aortic aneurysm or free peritoneal fluid is a wise initial option. Oral contrast plays no role in the diagnosis of aortic pathology and would result in unacceptable delay in this case. Aortic rupture can be diagnosed without IV contrast; thus noncontrast CT should be performed immediately if a question exists about the patient's renal function or allergies to contrast. IV contrast should be administered to evaluate for aortic dissection or active extravasation of contrast if the noncontrast CT does not provide all desired diagnostic information. In this patient, noncontrast CT demonstrated a large retroperitoneal hematoma, ruled out aortic aneurysm, and appeared to identify the source of hemorrhage as the left adrenal gland. IV contrast confirmed the absence of aortic dissection and demonstrated no active bleeding, an important finding for management, because active retroperitoneal bleeding might require angiographic embolization for hemostasis. How can the adrenal glands be recognized on CT? Emergency physicians may pay little attention to the adrenal glands on CT—they are a rare source of emergency pathology, and the normal glands are inconspicuous. In this case, knowledge of normal anatomy and process of elimination guides the diagnosis. The normal location of the adrenal glands is just cephalad and anterior to the kidneys on each side. The adrenals are often separated slightly from the kidneys by retroperitoneal fat. Look closely at the series of images. **A,** Cephalad and anterior to the right kidney, a rounded structure is seen, right of the spine and abutting the inferior vena cava. Because the CT was obtained during an arterial phase of injection, to maximize contrast enhancement of the aorta, the vena cava does not contain contrast, and the adjacent adrenal gland is easily mistaken for the inferior vena cava. The right adrenal gland might also initially be mistaken for the superior pole of the right kidney, but the kidney comes into view as a separate structure several slices caudad **(C).** Reviewing these images, you'll realize that the normal lambda (λ)-shaped adrenal glands cannot be found—instead, rounded structures have replaced them, suggesting adrenal mass or internal hemorrhage within the adrenal glands.

Nuclear Scintigraphy for Gastrointestinal Hemorrhage

Nuclear scintigraphy allows detection of relatively slow GI bleeding. The technique can identify bleeding anywhere within the GI tract, although its primary use is for suspected lower GI bleeding. In this test, red blood cells are harvested from the patient, tagged with a radionuclide (technetium-99m), and reinfused. Alternatively, a technetium-99m sulfur colloid may be injected.[325] A gamma camera positioned outside of the patient detects scintigraphic emission. A series of images are taken over time, demonstrating accumulation of the radionuclide. A normal image shows counts concentrated over the aorta and iliac arteries, with a low background resulting from blood flow in other organs. When blood carrying the radionuclide tracer leaks into the intestinal lumen because of GI hemorrhage, the gamma camera records abnormally high signal outside of normal blood vessels and organs. The intensity of the counts increases over subsequent images if bleeding is ongoing. The location of the signal may appear to migrate distally over the time course of the images, caused by continued peristalsis (Figures 9-144 and 9-145).

Nuclear scintigraphy is performed over approximately 1 hour, with advantages and disadvantages. An advantage of the technique is relatively high sensitivity for even slow rates of bleeding, as low as 0.1 to 0.4 mL per minute.[326] Intermittent bleeding may also be detected by this technique. Paradoxically, this high sensitivity can also be a disadvantage, because slow bleeding detected by nuclear scintigraphy may have ceased spontaneously by the time an intervention is undertaken to stop bleeding. In one study, almost half of patients with positive scintigraphy had no bleeding detected by angiography.[327] Nontherapeutic invasive procedures may result, although the rate of positive angiography is more than twice as high in patients who have been screened for active bleeding first using scintigraphy.[327] Another disadvantage of scintigraphy is the need to remove a potentially unstable patient from the emergency department for a relatively extended period. However, positive scintigraphy can accurately predict the site of bleeding, which is advantageous in patients with continued bleeding requiring surgical resection.[328]

Mesenteric Angiography for Gastrointestinal Hemorrhage

Mesenteric angiography can be performed to assess the source of GI bleeding and to treat ongoing hemorrhage. In this technique, the major mesenteric arteries are sequentially cannulated using a catheter introduced through the femoral artery. Contrast is injected into each mesenteric branch, and extravasation of contrast is observed if active bleeding is present (Figure 9-146). Small branches of mesenteric arteries can be cannulated and embolized to terminate bleeding (discussed in more

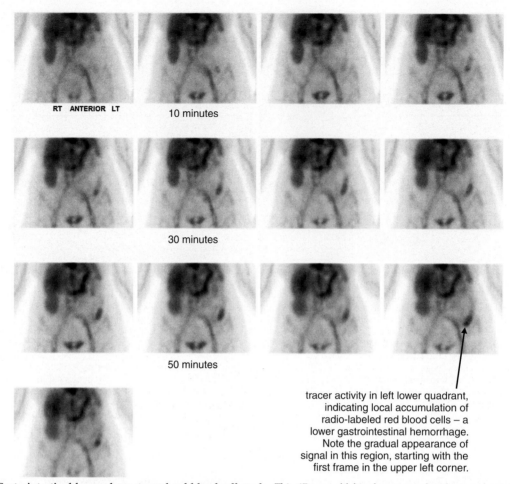

RT   ANTERIOR   LT   10 minutes

30 minutes

50 minutes

tracer activity in left lower quadrant,
indicating local accumulation of
radio-labeled red blood cells – a
lower gastrointestinal hemorrhage.
Note the gradual appearance of
signal in this region, starting with the
first frame in the upper left corner.

Figure 9-144. Gastrointestinal hemorrhage, tagged red blood cell study. This 67-year-old female presented with several episodes of bright red blood per rectum at home. In the emergency department, she had another significant episode of rectal bleeding. In addition, over 10 hours of observation, her hematocrit fell from 37 to 26. Tagged red blood cell study was performed, with images generated at 5-minute intervals. Tracer activity is visible in the left lower quadrant within 10 minutes and becomes progressively more evident in the region of the descending colon. The patient subsequently underwent mesenteric angiography that was negative for active bleeding. Why the disparate test results? The patient undoubtedly was actively bleeding during the tagged red blood cell study. However, by the time of the angiogram, bleeding had spontaneously stopped. Mesenteric angiography is performed over a briefer period—extravasation of injected contrast (indicating active bleeding) is only witnessed if bleeding is occurring during the moment after contrast injection, when the fluoroscope is turned on. If bleeding is intermittent, angiography can fail to detect even moderate bleeding.

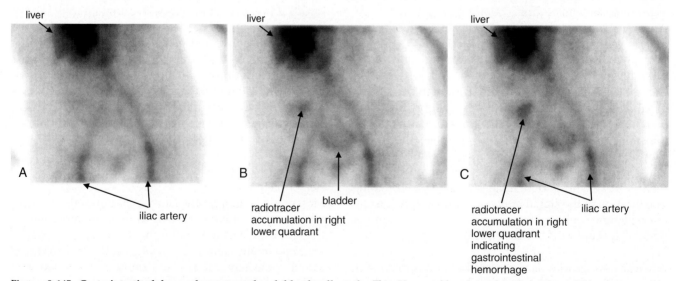

liver

liver

liver

A   iliac artery

B   radiotracer accumulation in right lower quadrant   bladder

C   radiotracer accumulation in right lower quadrant indicating gastrointestinal hemorrhage   iliac artery

Figure 9-145. Gastrointestinal hemorrhage, tagged red blood cell study. This 58-year-old presented with bright red blood per rectum. A technetium-99m tagged red blood cell study was performed. **A,** Acquired 10 minutes after injection of the labeled red cells. **B,** Acquired 45 minutes after injection. **C,** Acquired 55 minutes after injection. A focus of radiotracer activity is seen gradually accumulating in the right lower quadrant, consistent with hemorrhage within the cecum. Normal tracer is also seen in the region of the liver (because this is a vascular organ), in the iliac arteries, and in the urinary bladder. Compare this with the angiogram in Figure 9-146.

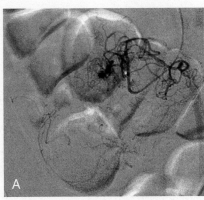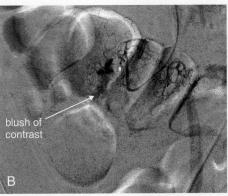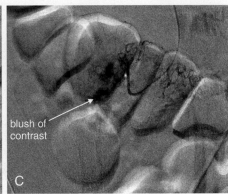

Figure 9-146. Gastrointestinal (GI) hemorrhage imaged with mesenteric angiography. A, B, C, Close-up fluoroscopic images of the cecum during angiography, separated in time by a few seconds. This patient presented with rectal bleeding and underwent a tagged red blood cell study showing radiotracer accumulation in the right lower quadrant (Figure 9-145). Mesenteric angiography was performed and shows active extravasation of contrast in the region of the cecum arising from a branch of the ileocolic artery. This was selectively embolized with a combination of particles and coils. Selective arteriography following embolization showed no further active extravasation of contrast. These images show sequential frames from a digital subtraction angiogram, cropped to show just the region of the cecum. A faint blush of contrast is seen developing over a few seconds, representing active GI hemorrhage.

detail in Chapter 16). Advantages of this technique include a therapeutic ability, which is not seen with nuclear scintigraphy. This is an invasive procedure with risks including arterial injury and contrast nephropathy or allergy. The technique requires the services of an interventional radiologist, not routinely available at all hours even in large medical centers. Mesenteric angiography is less sensitive than nuclear scintigraphy, because bleeding must be ongoing at the time of contrast injection and imaging to be detected. Overall, the sensitivity of digital subtraction angiography for active bleeding is approximately 60%, with 100% specificity.[329] The disparity between the relatively high sensitivity of nuclear scintigraphy and the lower sensitivity of mesenteric angiography means that many positive nuclear scintigraphy studies (showing bleeding) are followed by negative and nontherapeutic mesenteric angiograms, because bleeding may have stopped spontaneously by the time angiography is performed.

Computed Tomography Angiography for Gastrointestinal Hemorrhage

CTA for detection of GI bleeding is a relatively newly described technique.[330-339] CTA relies on similar principles to those of standard catheter angiography. If bleeding is actively occurring at the time of CT, injected contrast will be seen in the intestinal lumen. No oral contrast is needed for this technique; in fact, it should not be administered, because positive enteral contrast disguises extravasating injected contrast. Advantages of the technique include speed and availability, because it uses standard CT equipment widely available in many hospitals. In some cases, not only the location but also the cause of the hemorrhage can be determined.[336] A potentially unstable patient must be removed only briefly from the emergency department for the procedure. A disadvantage of the technique is that intermittent or slow bleeding may not be detected, because bleeding must be ongoing during the brief duration of the CT (seconds) to be detected.

However, intermittent bleeding not detected by CT may not require angiographic embolization. Another disadvantage is that the patient is exposed to iodinated contrast with its attendant risks. Because the technique has no therapeutic option, a positive CT must be followed by a standard mesenteric angiogram for treatment, requiring a second exposure to iodinated contrast. Despite this, some authors have proposed that patients be screened with CT before undergoing invasive angiography to increase the therapeutic yield of angiography.

Abdominal Trauma

X-rays play relatively little role in evaluation of abdominal and retroperitoneal blunt mechanism injuries, although chest and pelvic x-rays are routinely obtained for evaluation of associated thoracic and pelvic injuries, discussed in detail in Chapters 6 and 13, respectively. Abdominal and chest x-rays are often used in the evaluation of penetrating abdominal trauma. Ultrasound plays a useful bedside role in blunt trauma to identify hemoperitoneum or hemopericardium in unstable patients. CT scan is today the key imaging modality for patients with blunt abdominal trauma not requiring immediate operative therapy. It plays a growing role in patients with penetrating abdominal and flank injuries, allowing some to be managed nonoperatively. Abdominal trauma imaging is discussed in detail in Chapter 10.

SUMMARY

Abdominal imaging remains an area of intense utilization and research. X-ray is of little value for most emergency abdominal conditions. Ultrasound provides important clinical information about many disorders, particularly right upper quadrant and pelvic pathology, without radiation exposure. CT provides detailed information about a multitude of disorders, but controversy remains about the necessity for contrast agents and the clinical benefit to patients from the information obtained.

Abdominal trauma presents challenges in diagnostic imaging. Patients with abdominal trauma may have multiple, concomitant life-threatening injuries to the head, spine, chest, and extremities. For the unstable patient, the greatest challenge may be prioritizing injuries for diagnostic and therapeutic interventions. Often, emergency department imaging of these patients must be kept to a minimum before operative intervention. For the stable patient, the challenge is often to avoid unnecessary imaging, which may lead to undesirable radiation exposure and costs of care.

In this chapter, we discuss imaging modalities useful in blunt and penetrating abdominal trauma and imaging of the unstable and the stable patient. For computed tomography (CT) in trauma, we discuss the evidence and indications for contrast agents. We review the interpretation of ultrasound, plain radiographs, and CT images, with a focus on common and serious injury patterns. We also discuss clinical decision rules for blunt abdominal trauma, which may identify patients at low risk for injury who may safely forgo imaging. We consider the safety of discharge from the emergency department following a negative imaging evaluation in blunt and penetrating trauma. Finally, we review trauma imaging in the pregnant patient and radiation exposure in trauma imaging.

IMAGING MODALITIES IN TRAUMA

Plain Radiographs

Plain x-ray plays a limited role in the evaluation of blunt abdominal trauma. X-rays of the chest and pelvis are often obtained to evaluate for concurrent thoracic or pelvic injuries (discussed in dedicated chapters), but normal x-rays do not rule out injuries to solid or hollow abdominal organs. Abnormal chest x-ray findings of pneumothorax and rib fractures are associated with intraabdominal injuries and are indications for abdominal imaging if a mechanism for multisystem trauma is present.[1] Chest x-ray may reveal free air, suggesting hollow organ injury, although this finding is both rare and nonspecific in blunt trauma. Pneumoperitoneum can also result from thoracic injuries, with air tracking into the abdomen, and is thus not an absolute indication for laparotomy.[2-4] Diaphragmatic rupture may also be seen, although Smithers et al.[5] reported a sensitivity of chest x-ray of around 60% for

diaphragm rupture within 48 hours after injury. X-rays of the abdomen are *not* useful in blunt trauma because they do not assess for solid organ injuries, which are the most commonly injured organs with blunt mechanisms.

In high-velocity, penetrating abdominal trauma such as gunshot wounds, plain radiographs are commonly obtained, including anterior–posterior (AP) and lateral x-rays of the abdomen, upright AP chest radiograph, and pelvis x-ray. In the case of gunshot wounds, x-rays identify the location and number of retained projectiles. Chest and pelvis x-rays are obtained because of the erratic path of tumbling missiles, which can lead to extra-abdominal injuries. Common findings include free abdominal air (pneumoperitoneum), pneumothorax, and hemothorax. The upright chest radiograph is most sensitive for free air. In penetrating trauma, pneumoperitoneum is generally considered an indication for laparotomy, because of the likelihood of bowel perforation as the source. Plain radiographs may also reveal important bony injuries. Plain radiographic findings of hemoperitoneum and solid organ injury are unreliable, and other imaging modalities are usually relied upon to assess for these.

In abdominal stab wounds, plain radiographs of the chest and abdomen are usually obtained, again to assess for pneumoperitoneum, pneumothorax, or hemothorax, any of which can occur from high abdominal or flank stab wounds.

Ultrasound

Ultrasound has become a common part of the initial assessment of blunt abdominal trauma. Ultrasound serves a screening function because it assesses for the presence of free fluid in the abdomen or pericardium but does not explicitly identify the source. The focused assessment with sonography in trauma (FAST) (also sometimes called focused abdominal sonography in trauma or focused abdominal sonography for trauma) examination has been a standard part of the diagnostic algorithm since the 1990s in most U.S. trauma centers. In the FAST exam, the right upper quadrant (Morison's pouch, or hepatorenal recess), the left upper quadrant (splenorenal recess), the suprapubic space (pelvis), and the pericardium (usually via a subxiphoid approach) are inspected for anechoic material representing fluid— which in the setting of trauma is assumed to be blood.

Advantages of ultrasound include portability (allowing it to be used in the trauma bay during resuscitation), lack of ionizing radiation exposure, repeatability (allowing evaluation of changes in patient condition), and rapidity of the exam. Disadvantages include significant operator dependence, meaning that equal results are not achieved with ultrasonographers of varying experience and ability. Ultrasound is considered most useful in detection of solid organ injuries with associated hemoperitoneum. It is considered insensitive for the detection of bowel or retroperitoneal injuries. More recent studies have focused on the ability of ultrasound to detect pneumoperitoneum[6] and hemopneumothorax (discussed in Chapter 6 on chest trauma). Moriwaki et al.[6] found ultrasound was 85% sensitive and 100% specific for detection of free air in a prospective study of 484 patients. Some small studies have also investigated the utility of ultrasound contrast agents to detect active bleeding.[7-8]

Ultrasound is relatively sensitive for free abdominal fluid. In one study, in which fluid was instilled into the abdomen in 100-mL aliquots during diagnostic peritoneal lavage (DPL), the median amount of fluid required for identification of an anechoic stripe in Morison's pouch was 700 mL with the patient in a supine position. Positioning the patient in Tredelenburg (head down) position reduced the detection limit to 400 mL.[9] In a second study, continuous scanning of Morison's pouch during infusion of DPL fluid revealed a mean detection limit of 619 mL. Only 10% of ultrasonographers (attending physicians and residents in emergency medicine, radiology, and surgery) detected volumes less than 400 mL. The sensitivity at 1 L was 97%.[10]

Ultrasound has been extensively studied in the hands of both emergency physicians and surgeons. In one prospective study of 55 patients, the sensitivity and specificity of ultrasound were 91.7% and 94.7%, respectively, for detection of intraabdominal injury.[11] Another prospective study of 200 blunt trauma patients found ultrasound to be 83% sensitive and 100% specific—although the authors concluded that only a single missed injury was significant.[12] Ma et al.[13] reported sensitivity of 90% and specificity of 99%. A review in 1996 found a paucity of prospective trials of ultrasound and numerous methodologic flaws in those studies.[14] A systematic review and meta-analysis found 123 trials, of which 30 trials met methodologic criteria for inclusion. These trials included 9047 patients and gave a composite negative likelihood ratio of 0.23. Recall that a negative likelihood ratio of 0.1 is generally considered to provide strong evidence of the absence of pathology. In a patient with a pretest probability of abdominal injury of 50%, a negative ultrasound reduces the probability of injury only to around 25%. Ultrasound is not sufficiently sensitive to exclude intraabdominal injury, limiting its utility as a definitive test for abdominal trauma.[15]

What is the role of ultrasound in blunt trauma evaluation? When first introduced, ultrasound was viewed as a potential replacement for DPL.[12] DPL was extremely sensitive for abdominal injuries (100% in many series), but its lack of specificity led to many nontherapeutic laparotomies. Because ultrasound requires the accumulation of greater amounts of peritoneal fluid for detection, it may fail to detect subtle injuries—leading to fewer laparotomies for minor solid organ injuries but also risking missed bowel injuries. With the growth of CT use in evaluation of blunt abdominal injury from the mid-1980s, nonoperative management of most blunt solid organ injuries became the norm, and the information provided by ultrasound became less useful in this setting. Given that a negative ultrasound does not exclude abdominal injury, CT is usually performed in stable patients with possible injury, even following negative ultrasound. CT is also usually performed in stable patients with positive ultrasound findings because further characterization of the source and degree of bleeding can allow nonoperative management, sometimes with angiographic embolization (see Chapter 16).

Ultrasound remains useful in the unstable patient. Following blunt trauma, hemodynamic instability is most often because of hemorrhage, with six potential sources: chest, abdomen, pelvis, retroperitoneum, large extremity compartments, and external bleeding sources (Table 10-1). Ultrasound can be used to exclude or confirm substantial abdominal and pelvic free fluid. A negative FAST suggests other sources of hemorrhage. A positive FAST suggests that abdominal bleeding is a significant contributor, potentially leading to immediate laparotomy. In a retrospective study, Farahmand et al.[16] evaluated the performance of ultrasound in hypotensive blunt abdominal trauma patients. Whereas ultrasound was only 85% sensitive for detection of any injury, it was 97% sensitive for surgical injuries with 82% specificity in these patients, suggesting utility in patients too unstable for CT. The treatment priorities for the patient depend on the overall scenario, including the results of chest and pelvis radiographs and the presence of head injury. Patients with significant pelvic bleeding may require angiographic embolization, either before or after laparotomy. Patients with concurrent chest injuries may require thoracotomy or endovascular repair.

The role of ultrasound in patients with penetrating abdominal trauma is limited. As described later, CT is increasingly used to evaluate stable patients with penetrating abdominal injury, avoiding laparotomy in some. Because ultrasound does not distinguish between free fluid from penetrating solid organ injury (often managed nonoperatively) and that from hollow viscus injury (managed operatively), it is of little use in stable patients. Unstable patients with penetrating abdominal injury typically are taken rapidly to the operating suite, regardless of ultrasound findings.

TABLE 10-1. Sources of Hemorrhage in Blunt Trauma, With Imaging Modality Used to Evaluate

Bleeding Source	Diagnostic Modality	Comments
Chest	Chest x-ray	A negative chest x-ray (normal mediastinum and no hemo- or pneumothorax) substantially reduces the risk of thoracic hemorrhage as the cause for hemorrhagic shock.
Abdomen	Ultrasound (FAST examination)	A negative FAST (ultrasound) examination excludes abdominal bleeding as a likely source of shock, though it does not rule out abdominal injuries. A positive FAST examination identifies significant abdominal bleeding sources.
Pelvis	Pelvis x-ray	A normal pelvis x-ray excludes significant pelvic bleeding in most patients. Fractures that destabilize the pelvic ring may be associated with substantial pelvic bleeding (see Chapter 13).
Retroperitoneum	CT	Retroperitoneal injury is not readily evident from examination, though ecchymosis of the flanks or abdominal wall may be present. X-ray and ultrasound do not screen for this injury well, although by excluding hemorrhage sources in the chest, abdomen, and pelvis, they may identify retroperitoneal injury as a likely source of hemorrhage by process of elimination. CT scan is usually necessary to confirm or exclude retroperitoneal injury.
Extremities	Physical examination, x-ray	Examination may reveal significant limb swelling and possible unstable fractures. X-rays confirm fracture.
External sources	Physical examination	External bleeding is usually readily visible on examination.

Ultrasound can be useful in penetrating abdominal trauma in assessing for hemopericardium. Penetrating abdominal wounds can enter the chest, causing this injury pattern.

Does ultrasound improve clinical outcomes in patients with blunt abdominal trauma? Melniker et al.[17] conducted a prospective randomized controlled trial of ultrasound in the initial evaluation of blunt abdominal trauma. The measured outcomes were time from emergency department arrival to transfer for operative care, CT use, hospital length of stay, complications, and charges. They enrolled 262 patients, and all measured outcomes favored patients undergoing ultrasound and reached statistical significance. Time to operative care was 64% less for ultrasound patients compared to control patients, and ultrasound patients underwent fewer CTs (odds ratio = 0.16), spent 27% fewer days in the hospital, and had fewer complications (odds ratio = 0.16). Charges were 35% less compared to control patients.[17] Although this study appears at first glance to demonstrate a resounding advantage, the study was conducted in centers in which operative management of blunt solid organ injuries was common—not the case in most U.S. medical centers today. As a consequence, the reductions in time to operating room entry, CT use, and cost are unlikely to be reproduced. The study included penetrating and blunt trauma patients, two populations treated with different diagnostic and treatment algorithms in most centers. Other methodologic flaws limit the study, including lack of blinding, failure to enroll consecutive patients, and significant dropout rate (17%) after enrollment. The study did not control for the availability of operative care, which may have

been the largest factor in the measured difference in time to operating room entry.

Computed Tomography

CT is discussed in detail later, including sensitivity for solid and hollow organ injuries in the setting of both blunt and penetrating trauma. For most stable trauma patients, CT has become the definitive imaging modality of choice when intraabdominal injury is suspected. CT is rapid and highly sensitive and specific for many important injury types. The information provided by CT allows prognosis of injury and selective nonoperative management in both blunt and penetrating trauma. CT is less sensitive for some important injuries, including bowel and diaphragmatic trauma, a limitation that must be recognized to prevent clinical errors following a negative CT.

IMAGING ALGORITHMS IN THE UNSTABLE AND STABLE ABDOMINAL TRAUMA PATIENT

Patients with hemodynamic instability should be assumed to have hemorrhagic shock as the most likely source, with obstructive shock (tension pneumothorax or pericardial tamponade) or distributive shock (spinal cord injuries) being exceedingly rare by comparison. Imaging in the emergency department should be performed quickly, with the goal of triage to the operating room or angiography suite if necessary. Sources of hemorrhage fall into six categories (see Table 10-1), which can be evaluated in the trauma bay using ultrasound and portable plain radiographs. Pericardial tamponade can be evaluated with bedside ultrasound as described in Chapter 6. Although tension pneumothorax is often described as a clinical diagnosis never to be made radiographically, rapid chest x-ray or bedside ultrasound can be used to evaluate for this condition (see Chapter 6).

No further emergency department imaging may be needed in a hemodynamically unstable patient with a single identified source of hemorrhagic shock. Patients with shock and abdominal or chest injuries typically are taken to the operating suite for surgical intervention. Patients with pelvic injuries resulting in shock usually receive external pelvic fixation and pelvic angiographic embolization of actively bleeding vessels. Preperitoneal packing is also sometimes used to tamponade bleeding. Patients with extremity hemorrhage or active external bleeding are usually treated with limb splinting and local compression to limit bleeding. If these interventions plus fluid resuscitation succeed in stabilizing the patient, then additional imaging with CT can be performed to evaluate more comprehensively for injuries.

Hemodynamically stable patients can be evaluated with plain radiographs followed by CT in patients with suspicion of injury, based on clinical judgment or published clinical decision rules (described later). Some patients with minimal trauma mechanism and no signs or symptoms of injury require no imaging. Stable blunt trauma patients with suspected abdominal injury usually undergo CT. In some centers, stable penetrating trauma patients without pneumoperitoneum on x-ray also are evaluated with CT, allowing nonoperative management for those without CT evidence of peritoneal violation and in those with isolated solid organ injury. In other centers, laparotomy or laparoscopy is performed rather than diagnostic imaging with CT.

COMPUTED TOMOGRAPHY IN TRAUMA: INDICATIONS FOR CONTRAST AGENTS

Blunt Trauma: Indications for CT Contrast Agents

For the evaluation of blunt abdominal or flank trauma, intravenous (IV) contrast should be routinely used, but oral contrast should not. The American College of Radiology recommends the use of 150 mL of intravenous contrast, infused at 2-4 mL per second, with CT being performed after a 60 second delay.[17a] Without any contrast agents, CT can reveal several important imaging findings. Free air, while rare following blunt trauma, is readily seen without any contrast agents.[2-4] Air appears black on all window settings and is even more readily visible on lung or bone windows than on soft-tissue (abdominal) window settings (see Chapter 9). Free abdominal fluid representing hemoperitoneum is also readily seen on noncontrast CT. Simple fluid such as simple ascites or urine has a Hounsfield density on CT of 0 Hounsfield units (HU), whereas blood has a density of

around 45 HU (though the exact value likely varies with time since hemorrhage and hematocrit).[18] Using a digital radiology display called a picture archiving and communication system (PACS), the density of organs and fluid collections can be measured. On a noncontrast CT, blood appears slightly darker gray on soft-tissue windows than do solid organs such as the liver and spleen because these organs are slightly denser (around 100 HU).

The liver, spleen, kidneys, vascular structures, bones, bladder, and peritoneal fat are also visible on noncontrast CT. Use of bone windows and reconstructions to evaluate the spine and bony pelvis is discussed in Chapters 3 and 13. With the addition of IV contrast, several additional important features can be seen. First, solid organs such as the liver, spleen, and kidneys are highly vascular and intensely enhance with injected contrast on arterial phase imaging (CT images acquired at a moment coinciding with the injected contrast bolus reaching arterial beds). Enhancement is visible as a brightening or whitening of the organ because of the distribution of high-density injected contrast throughout the organ parenchyma. A normal solid organ enhances relatively uniformly. Injured areas of these solid organs fail to enhance with IV contrast because they no longer receive a normal blood supply. These regions appear darker than ("hypodense" relative to) the surrounding normally perfused organ. Areas of injury are variously described as *contusions, lacerations,* and *contained hematomas*—but these terms are essentially synonyms for regions of solid organs that do not enhance with IV contrast, indicating poor perfusion of that organ segment. Without the addition of IV contrast, these regions may be less conspicuous because the density of normal solid organs is similar to that of an injured region without IV contrast. A large area of injury may be visible on noncontrast CT if the density is sufficiently decreased by accumulated blood.

IV contrast serves a second important function: revealing active hemorrhage from injuries. With the injection of contrast, a blush of contrast on arterial phase imaging within a hypodense injured solid organ indicates active bleeding. This must be distinguished from normal enhancement of vessels within solid organs, such as portal and hepatic vessels within the liver. These normal vessels are surrounded by enhanced normal tissue on CT images. On the other hand, active bleeding within an area of injured organ appears as a bright white spot of contrast, surrounded by the hypoattenuated (darker gray) region of injury. Active bleeding into the peritoneal cavity can also be seen with injection of IV contrast. In this case, blood that had escaped into the peritoneal cavity before the moment of contrast injection and CT acquisition appears dark (around 45 HU) on soft-tissue windows. Active bleeding at the moment of CT acquisition appears as a bright white spot or amorphous patch within this hypoattenuated region of injury.

If noncontrast CT can reveal hemoperitoneum and even large areas of solid organ injury, why is IV contrast of value? In a stable patient, hemoperitoneum and even large regions of solid organ injury are often managed nonoperatively. On the other hand, active bleeding revealed by injected IV contrast predicts the need for either operative management or, more commonly today, angiographic embolization to stop hemorrhage. Angiographic embolization is discussed in more detail in Chapter 16.

IV contrast can also reveal hypoperfused organs resulting from vascular pedicle injuries. In this case, the organ appears hypodense (dark gray), failing to enhance normally following IV contrast administration. This is an indication for laparotomy, either for vascular repair to salvage the organ or for organ removal to prevent hemorrhage. Active bleeding from an injured vessel may be visible but may be limited acutely by vasospasm. Bowel injuries are sometimes recognized with the addition of IV contrast. A regional bowel injury may result in hypoattenuation of the bowel wall because IV contrast does not perfuse the injured segment.

Other injuries can be revealed by injected IV contrast. Although contrast is injected intravenously, not intraarterially, for CT, the CT image acquisition is usually timed to coincide with arterial perfusion, so arterial bleeding may be seen directly. The timing of the CT may be intentionally selected to represent an intermediate phase of perfusion, when both arterial and venous structures are filled with contrast. Sometimes, additional "delayed" CT images are acquired following the initial CT. These additional images are obtained seconds to minutes after the injected contrast bolus to allow visualization of venous structures, venous phases of solid organ perfusion, and even renal perfusion and excretion of contrast. The use of delayed images to evaluate renal and ureteral injuries is discussed in detail in Chapter 12.

Oral contrast is not indicated for the evaluation of blunt trauma patients. Intuitively, it seems logical that addition of oral contrast might assist in recognition of bowel injuries. A bowel injury might result in bowel perforation, characterized by leak of contrast from the bowel lumen into the peritoneal cavity. Alternative, a contused and thickened bowel wall might be more visible if the bowel lumen were opacified with contrast. These theoretical benefits have not been demonstrated in clinical trials. In multiple large studies, CT without oral contrast performed comparably to CT with oral contrast. In its appropriateness criteria for blunt abdominal trauma, the American College of Radiology states "CT evaluation of the abdomen and pelvis for blunt trauma does not require the use of oral contrast."[17a]

Clancy et al.[19] reviewed 492 abdominal CTs for blunt trauma and compared CT interpretation with operative findings and clinical follow-up. Oral contrast was used in only 8 patients. Only 1 of 372 patients with a negative non–oral contrast CT required surgery. Five bowel injuries were found in 42 patients who underwent operation, and the authors claimed that oral contrast would not have ensured preoperative diagnosis, although their retrospective methods cannot prove this assertion.

Stafford et al.[20] randomized 594 adult blunt trauma patients to receive oral contrast or no oral contrast before CT with IV contrast. Six bowel injuries were identified at laparotomy in the oral contrast group, and three were identified in the non–oral contrast group. One small-bowel injury was missed by CT in the 199 patients receiving oral contrast. No small-bowel injuries were missed by CT in the 195 patients receiving no oral contrast.

Allen et al.[21] prospectively enrolled 500 consecutive adult blunt trauma patients and performed CT with IV contrast only to determine the sensitivity for blunt bowel and mesenteric injury. They compared the initial clinical CT interpretation to a composite criterion standard of laparotomy results, autopsy results, a research study–only CT reading, and clinical follow-up to determine the presence or absence of injury. CT without oral contrast was 95% sensitive and 99.6% specific, comparing favorably with the reported sensitivity of oral contrast–enhanced CT. In a separate report from the same study, the authors reported the sensitivity and specificity of CT without oral contrast for blunt diaphragmatic injury (66.7% and 100%, respectively).[22]

Stuhlfaut et al.[23] retrospectively reviewed records of 1082 patients undergoing multidetector CT without oral contrast to determine the sensitivity of CT for bowel and mesenteric injury requiring surgical repair. The criterion standard was a composite of laparotomy report and hospital course. CT was considered positive for bowel or mesenteric injury if findings included pneumoperitoneum with other secondary findings ($n = 4$), mesenteric hematoma and bowel wall abnormality ($n = 2$), mesenteric hematoma only ($n = 4$), or bowel wall thickening only ($n = 4$). CT was considered negative for bowel or mesenteric injury if findings included no intraabdominal injury, solid organ injury only, or free fluid only. Sensitivity was 82%, with a 95% confidence interval (CI) of 52% to 95%, and specificity was 99% (95% CI = 98%-99%), similar to prior studies of CT with oral contrast.

Holmes et al.[24] retrospectively reviewed records of 6052 consecutive blunt trauma patients undergoing CT with IV but without oral contrast to determine the sensitivity of CT for gastrointestinal injury. Injuries were confirmed by laparotomy, autopsy, or additional (non-CT) imaging studies. Out of 106 patients with confirmed gastrointestinal injuries, CT was abnormal in 91 patients

(86%, 95% CI = 78%-92%). CT specifically suggested gastrointestinal injury in 81 patients (76%, 95% CI = 67%-84%). CT specifically suggested gastrointestinal injury in 58 of 64 patients (91%, 95% CI = 81%-96%) with major gastrointestinal injuries, defined as gastrointestinal perforation, active mesenteric hemorrhage, or mesenteric devascularization.

Why did these trials fail to demonstrate an anticipated benefit of oral contrast? Several factors may contribute. First, some bowel injuries are seen on CT without oral contrast. Bowel injuries may be suggested from free air, hypoperfusion of a segment of bowel following IV contrast administration, thickening of the bowel wall, infiltration of the mesenteric fat surrounding the bowel, or free peritoneal fluid without an evident solid organ injury. None of these findings requires oral contrast for detection. Although these findings are nonspecific, they may be sufficient to prompt appropriate management (observation or surgical exploration). Second, many bowel injuries do not result in frank perforation, at least initially. Instead, the bowel wall may be contused but not violated. As a result, oral contrast may not leak into the peritoneal cavity. Other injuries may be microperforations that seal spontaneously or do not lie in dependent loops of bowel where contrast could escape. Third, if CT is performed rapidly following oral contrast administration, or if injuries or drugs slow gastrointestinal transit of contrast, orally administered contrast may not reach an injured segment of bowel to aid in diagnosis.

Finally, bowel injuries are quite rare, occurring in only about 1% of blunt abdominal trauma. Consequently, even large studies may fail to demonstrate a moderate benefit of oral contrast. For example, in a population of 1000 blunt trauma patients, only about 10 bowel injuries would be expected. If oral contrast enabled detection of 8 of 10 injuries, whereas 5 of 10 were detected without oral contrast, a real difference might exist, but the difference would be too small to be statistically significant. A very large study of thousands of patients would be required to confirm a difference of this magnitude. From a practical standpoint, however, the number needed to treat (by administering oral contrast) to detect a single additional bowel injury would be several hundred. While bowel injuries are important and might seem to justify the treatment of many patients to prevent a single missed injury, oral contrast has potential harms. Oral contrast takes time to ingest and transit through bowel before CT, potentially wasting precious time in a patient with other life-threatening injuries. In addition, many blunt abdominal trauma patients are intoxicated, have head injuries, or are immobilized supine because of suspected spine trauma—making ingestion of oral contrast a potential aspiration hazard, though likely a rare event. In one retrospective review of 506 consecutive trauma patients undergoing CT with

oral and IV contrast, one patient was noted to have instillation of enteral contrast through a nasogastric tube inadvertently placed into the right main bronchus rather than the stomach.[25]

Penetrating Trauma: Can "Triple-Contrast CT" Guide Nonoperative Management?

Historically, penetrating trauma of the abdomen or flank was evaluated with surgical exploration (laparotomy), laparoscopy to inspect for peritoneal violation, or local wound exploration. More recently, selected stable patients have been evaluated with so-called triple-contrast CT (CT with oral, IV, and rectal contrast). IV contrast in this setting serves the same functions as in blunt trauma, discussed in detail earlier. Oral and rectal contrast agents are used for the theoretical benefit of demonstrating leak of contrast from the bowel lumen into the peritoneum or retroperitoneum.

As we discussed earlier, oral contrast has not been shown to be diagnostically beneficial in blunt abdominal trauma. Theoretically, oral and rectal contrast might be more useful in penetrating injuries, in which bowel penetration is a more common injury, and in which larger defects in the bowel wall might be expected. However, multiple studies have failed to show contrast leak from the bowel lumen to be a sensitive indicator of hollow viscus injury. In one prospective study of 200 patients, only 19% of patients with proven bowel injury had contrast leak from bowel observed on CT. In comparison, a wound track near the bowel was 77% sensitive.[26] Given this, are oral and rectal contrast agents truly essential in the setting of penetrating trauma? A single study has evaluated the sensitivity and specificity of "single-contrast CT" (CT with IV contrast and no oral or rectal contrast) for penetrating abdominal or flank injuries.[27] Ramirez et al.[27] retrospectively reviewed 10 years experience with IV contrast–only CT for evaluation of penetrating torso trauma in 306 hemodynamically stable patients. CT predicted "need for laparotomy" with 98% sensitivity and 90% specificity, a positive predictive value of 84%, and a negative predictive value of 99%. In 222 patients with gunshot wounds, the authors reported 100% sensitivity and a 100% negative predictive value, whereas they found 92% sensitivity and a 97% negative predictive value in patients with stab wounds. Although the authors did not compare the sensitivity and specificity of CT with IV contrast to triple-contrast CT, their results are comparable to those reported in studies of triple-contrast CT, described later. Like many retrospective studies, this study suffers from a mixed criterion standard that includes laparotomy and clinical course. The authors did not report the duration of clinical follow-up and losses to follow-up, raising the possibility that some injuries might have been missed by CT. Unlike some other studies, this study focused on prediction of "need for laparotomy" rather than sensitivity for peritoneal violation. Unfortunately, the authors did not categorize the laparotomy results (therapeutic, nontherapeutic, and negative). Because the surgeons in this study were not blinded to the CT results, they assuredly were influenced by the CT findings in their decision to operate. As a consequence, the reported performance of the CT is affected by incorporation bias. Nevertheless, the authors pointed to significant time savings by avoiding oral and rectal contrast agents.

Demetriades et al.[37] prospectively studied alert hemodynamically stable patients without findings of peritonitis on examination following penetrating abdominal injury. Unstable patients, patients with peritonitis, and those who could not be evaluated clinically underwent immediate laparotomy. Of 152 patients, 61 (40.1%) met criteria for CT evaluation with IV but without oral or rectal contrast. Patients without CT findings of hollow viscus injury were observed with serial exams and laboratory evaluation for falling hematocrit or developing leukocytosis. The authors found that 43 patients with 47 solid organ injuries (liver, spleen, and kidney) had no CT evidence of hollow viscus injury by CT. Because of CT evidence of active bleeding, 4 patients underwent angiographic embolization of the liver. Whereas 41 patients (27% of total) were managed nonoperatively, 3 patients failed nonoperative management but recovered without complications after laparotomy, and 2 patients underwent laparoscopy to evaluate for possible diaphragm injury, given the relatively low reported sensitivity of CT for this injury pattern.

Inaba and Demetriades[38] reviewed the indications for laparotomy in penetrating abdominal injury. Hemodynamically stable patients without examination findings of peritonitis can be managed nonoperatively with careful observation. Gunshot wounds to the abdomen can be imaged with CT to determine projectile trajectory and likely injuries. Peritoneal violation on CT without evidence of organ injury can be managed nonoperatively with careful serial examinations. Solid organ injuries can be managed with endovascular therapies, primarily embolization for control of hemorrhage. Evidence of hollow viscus injury on CT warrants surgical exploration.

Mitra et al.[39] retrospectively reviewed all patients with penetrating abdominal injury over a 5-year period and found 36 hemodynamically stable patients undergoing CT for evaluation. The authors did not identify the CT protocol used, although they specified that triple contrast was not used. They reported a 77.8% combined sensitivity of CT and ultrasound in these patients.

Beekley et al.[40] retrospectively reported on 145 stable patients in a military combat support hospital without peritonitis following penetrating abdominal shrapnel wounds. Patients were routinely evaluated with CT with IV contrast; oral contrast was used "rarely" and rectal contrast was used in 2 cases. Patients with no CT findings of intraperitoneal or retroperitoneal penetration were managed nonoperatively. Based on CT, 85 (59%) of patients were managed nonoperatively, and 60 (41%) underwent laparotomy. The authors reported that 75% of laparotomies were therapeutic. Negative CT missed 1 patient with an intraabdominal injury requiring laparotomy (sensitivity = 97.8%, specificity = 84.8%, negative predictive value = 99%).

A number of studies have evaluated the safety and sensitivity of the triple-contrast CT approach. Multiple large series and a metaanalysis report good outcomes with conservative nonoperative management following a CT showing no evidence of bowel injury. We discuss these shortly, but first consider some limitations. First, publication bias may skew the reported literature on this topic, with authors not reporting failures of this technique. Second, many of the published studies suffer from limited clinical follow-up, raising the possibility of missed injuries not recognized by the researchers. Third, the indications for conservative management with CT include a reassuring physical exam. Because different physicians may interpret the physical examination differently, it is unclear how safe the practice would be outside of the major trauma centers that are the source of much of the data.

Hauser et al.[28] retrospectively reviewed 40 cases of posterior abdominal penetrating injuries evaluated with CT using IV, oral, and rectal contrast. They found 6 of the 40 cases to have abdominal injury by CT, confirmed by laparotomy. Although 34 patients without CT evidence of peritoneal or retroperitoneal organ injury were observed for 72 hours and discharged without laparotomy, lack of long-term follow-up prevents certainty that no injuries were missed.

Himmelman et al.[29] prospectively enrolled 88 hemodynamically stable patients with penetrating back or flank wounds. In 9 patients, CT suggested surgical injuries; 5 of these underwent laparotomy, with 2 having significant injuries. The other 79 patients had no CT findings suggesting need for surgery, and 77 of them were observed for 48 hours without complications. Because of positive DPL, the remaining 2 patients underwent laparotomy, negative in both cases. The authors concluded that a reassuring CT had a 100% negative predictive value for injuries requiring surgical repair.

McAllister et al.[30] reported on 53 hemodynamically stable patients with stab wounds to the back, evaluated with triple-contrast CT if local wound exploration showed muscle fascia penetration. Of the 53 patients, 51 had negative CT or injuries not requiring surgery and did well with nonoperative management. Two CTs demonstrated injuries requiring therapeutic celiotomy. The authors concluded that CT was accurate in detection of occult injury but was costly and did not contribute to clinical management decisions—a peculiar conclusion given that the authors did not assess the planned management from clinicians blinded to the CT results.

Soto et al. reported on 32 stable patients examined with triple-contrast CT and serial ultrasound following penetrating abdominal stab wounds. One patient had CT findings of extensive hepatic laceration and massive hemoperitoneum and was managed operatively. The other 31 patients were managed nonoperatively based on CT and ultrasound findings and were asymptomatic at 28-day follow-up. Of these patients, 21 had some form of intraperitoneal injury but without evidence of bowel injury.[31] The small number of patients in this series, and the limited number of significant injuries, limit the external validity of this study.

Chiu et al.[32] retrospectively reviewed 75 hemodynamically stable patients undergoing triple-contrast CT following penetrating torso trauma. Patients with negative CT or isolated solid organ injury were observed, whereas those with any other evidence of peritoneal violation (free air or fluid, contrast leak, or nonsolid visceral injury) underwent laparotomy. In patients with negative CT, 47 of 49 (96%) had successful nonoperative management, 1 had negative laparotomy, and 1 had a left diaphragmatic injury. In patients with positive CT, 15 of 18 had therapeutic laparotomy. Whereas 5 patients had isolated hepatic injuries, 2 had hepatic and diaphragmatic injuries, managed with angiographic embolization and thorascopic diaphragmatic repair. The authors concluded that CT is useful in selecting patients for nonoperative management, although solid organ injuries and diaphragmatic injuries may require invasive therapies.

Shanmuganathan et al.[33] prospectively studied triple-contrast helical CT in predicting peritoneal violation and need for laparotomy following penetrating torso trauma in 104 hemodynamically stable patients (54 gunshot wounds and 50 stab wounds). A positive CT was defined as evidence of peritoneal violation or injury to the retroperitoneal colon, a major vessel, or the urinary tract. Laparotomy was performed in patients with a positive CT except in those patients with isolated liver injury or free fluid. Patients with negative CT were initially observed. Among those with positive CT, 19 (86%) had therapeutic laparotomy. Whereas 9 patients with isolated hepatic injury on CT were successfully managed nonoperatively, 67 of 69 patients (97%) with negative CT had successful nonoperative management. The authors reported 100% sensitivity and 96% specificity of CT, although they failed to account for the operative management in 2 patients with negative CT.

In a separate report, Shanmuganathan et al.[26] reported on 200 hemodynamically stable penetrating trauma patients without peritoneal signs or radiographic (x-ray) findings of pneumoperitoneum. The group included 86 patients with gunshot wounds, 111 with stab wounds, and 3 sharp impalements. Triple-contrast CT was prospectively evaluated by three radiologists for peritoneal violation and injury to intra or retroperitoneal solid organs, bowel, mesentery, vascular structures, diaphragm, and urinary tract. CT was 97% sensitive for peritoneal violation requiring laparotomy and diagnosed 28 hepatic, 34 bowel or mesenteric, 7 splenic, and 6 renal injuries. Laparotomy based on CT findings was therapeutic in 87% of patients. Two patients with negative CT required therapeutic laparotomy.

Conrad et al.[34] retrospectively reviewed the charts of 81 patients who had emergency department workup for penetrating truncal trauma using triple-contrast CT. Following negative CT, 62 patients were discharged from the emergency department. Two missed injuries were identified but had no complications according to the authors. The authors concluded that emergency department discharge is a safe disposition; unfortunately, nearly one third of those discharged had no follow-up, rendering uncertain the outcomes of this strategy. If a significant percentage of the patients lost to follow-up had missed injuries, emergency department discharge following a negative CT would be unacceptable.

Loberant and Goldfeld[35] provided a case report of a patient undergoing a negative laparotomy because of a bony fragment mistakenly identified as contrast extravasation on triple-contrast CT.

Dissanaike et al.[36] reported a series of 9 patients evaluated with triple-contrast CT, with no missed injuries following nonoperative management of patients with negative CT. Clearly, the small numbers of patients in this series limit the value of the study.

Goodman et al.[41] performed a metaanalysis to determine the predictive value of CT for laparotomy in hemodynamically stable patients with penetrating abdominal trauma. They identified 180 studies but included only 5 because of methodologic concerns. The pooled sensitivity, specificity, negative predictive value, positive predictive value, and accuracy were 94.90%, 95.38%, 98.62%, 84.51%, and 94.70%, respectively. This metaanalysis included studies using both single-contrast and triple-contrast techniques and thus does not clarify the necessity for contrast agents.

Overall, triple-contrast CT appears to be a safe management strategy in highly selected stable patients without peritonitis on examination. Losses to follow-up, variable inclusion criteria, and the likelihood of publication bias favoring positive outcomes in the published studies all contribute to a need for caution with a negative CT. Multiple studies have demonstrated the possibility of missed diaphragmatic injuries and, rarely, missed operative bowel injuries. Following a negative triple-contrast CT, observation or close follow-up should be ensured. Further study is needed to determine the true diagnostic value of oral and rectal contrast in this setting.

INTERPRETATION OF IMAGES

Interpretation of X-Ray

Interpretation of chest and pelvis x-rays for trauma is described in detail in Chapters 6 and 13, respectively. In blunt abdominal trauma, abdominal radiographs are not useful and should not be obtained. The chest x-ray should be evaluated for signs of free air (see Figures 6-11 and 9-7), although the trauma chest x-ray is usually obtained in a supine position and is insensitive for pneumoperitoneum. The chest x-ray can reveal **diaphragmatic rupture** (see Figures 10-30 and 10-33 later in the chapter), more commonly on the left than on the right. Signs of diaphragm rupture include an elevated hemidiaphragm and herniation of abdominal contents into the thorax. If a nasogastric tube has been placed, it may be seen curling in the thorax. The gastric air bubble may be seen in an abnormally elevated position.

In penetrating abdominal trauma, an upright chest x-ray should be obtained to increase the sensitivity for free air. The subdiaphragmatic region should be inspected for lucencies suggesting *pneumoperitoneum* (see Figures 6-11 and 9-7). The abdominal, chest, and pelvis x-rays should be inspected for **retained missile fragments** (see Figure 10-9) in the case of gunshot wounds. Bony injuries, particularly spine and pelvic fractures, should be sought. Hemothorax (see Figures 10-9 and 10-35) and pneumothorax are other common findings in this setting.

Interpretation of Ultrasound

The key radiographic finding in ultrasound of blunt and penetrating abdominal trauma is free fluid, which is assumed to be **hemoperitoneum** in the setting of trauma. Patients with medical conditions causing preexisting ascites can have false-positive ultrasound exams in this setting. Fluid is anechoic (black) on ultrasound. In the case of small amounts of hemoperitoneum, fluid may be visible only as an anechoic stripe separating the liver and the kidney on the right (Figure 10-1), or the spleen and the kidney on the left (Figure 10-2). Fluid may also accumulate between the spleen and diaphragm. Free fluid pooled in the pelvis is visible as anechoic collections lateral to the bladder on a transverse view (Figure 10-3). Free fluid may also be visible in the rectouterine recess (pouch of Douglas) in females using a sagittal view (see Figure 10-3). In cases of gross

hemoperitoneum, loops of bowel may be seen floating in blood (Figure 10-4). In some cases, coagulated blood may take on a more echogenic appearance or fibrinous strands may be seen suspended in anechoic collections. Abdominal trauma can also cause hemopericardium, visible as an anechoic layer surrounding the heart on a subxiphoid view (Figure 10-5).

Pneumoperitoneum is also sometimes visible on ultrasound. Air is hyperechoic and disrupts the ultrasound beam, preventing visualization of deeper structures. Because bowel gas is normally present in the anterior midline abdomen, free air should be sought overlying the liver, where air is not normally present.[6]

Interpretation of Computed Tomography

Approach to Abdominal CT

For the emergency physician, a systematic and targeted approach allows rapid and accurate identification of important injuries on abdominal CT. Because multiple injuries are common following abdominal trauma, it is extremely important to inspect all major abdominal structures. A common pitfall is to end the search after detection of a single injury. Three window settings are useful in evaluating abdominal structures: soft-tissue (sometimes called abdominal or vascular) windows, lung windows, and bone windows. Soft-tissue windows are used to assess solid organs and hollow organs, to detect free fluid, and to detect free air. Lung windows are used to assess for pneumothorax (recall that the lower lungs and pleural spaces are visible on the cephalad-most abdominal CT slices) and pneumoperitoneum, as described later. Bone windows are used to assess for fractures but can also reveal pneumoperitoneum. We recommend evaluating soft-tissue windows first, followed by lung windows, followed by bone windows. Window settings are discussed in more detail in Chapter 9. In the descriptions of traumatic injuries that follow, soft-tissue windows are the appropriate setting for evaluation unless stated otherwise.

On soft-tissue windows, evaluate each organ in turn, rather than attempting to evaluate multiple structures on each slice. For example, follow the spleen through all CT slices in which it appears, evaluating for splenic injury. Do not attempt to evaluate the liver, kidneys, or pancreas during this process, even though they are visible, because this may distract you from a splenic injury. After completing evaluation of the spleen, repeat this process with other organs.

Common and Serious Injury Patterns on Computed Tomography

Imaging Findings of Shock: Inferior Vena Cava and Bowel. In cases of severe volume depletion (generally from hemorrhagic shock following trauma), the infrahepatic **inferior vena cava (IVC)** appears flattened

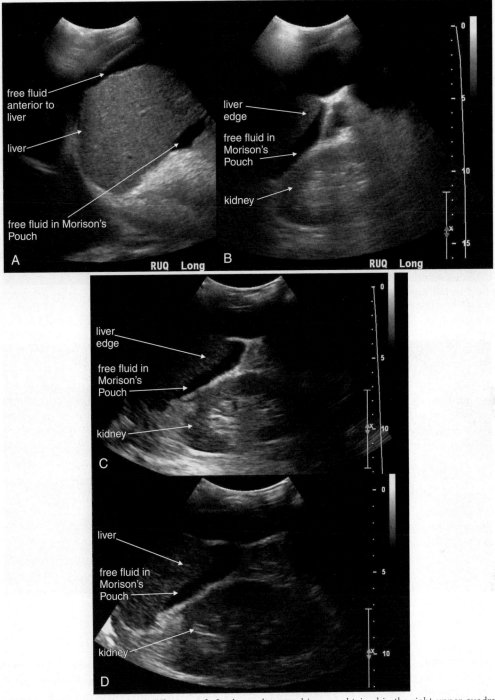

Figure 10-1. Free fluid in right upper quadrant: Ultrasound. In these ultrasound images obtained in the right upper quadrant, free fluid in the abdomen is visible as a black (anechoic) collection separating the liver and the right kidney in Morison's pouch **(A-D).** Fluid is also seen anterior to the liver **(A).** It is important to realize that the location of free fluid may not correlate with its source because fluid pools in dependent regions of the abdomen when the patient lies supine. Around 700 mL of fluid is required for detection with the patient supine. Fluid should be assumed to be hemoperitoneum in the setting of trauma, although preexisting ascites may have a similar appearance. Solid organ injury with hemoperitoneum is the most common cause of free fluid on ultrasound following trauma. Other causes of abdominal free fluid include bowel, mesenteric, and urinary tract injuries.

(Figure 10-6; see also Figure 10-20).[42] This appearance can occur in patients before the development of clinical hypotension or hemodynamic collapse and demands immediate volume resuscitation. Rarely, it may be a normal variant. In a series of 100 trauma patients, a flattened IVC occurred in 7, 6 of whom had other evidence of severe blood loss. In 100 patients without trauma, a flattened IVC was not seen.[42]

Shock bowel is a term for secondary bowel injury resulting from sustained systemic hypotension. The CT appearance includes *diffuse* bowel wall thickening,

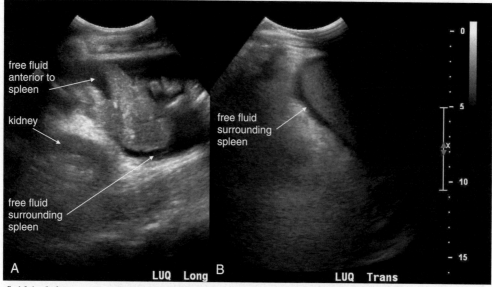

Figure 10-2. Free fluid in left upper quadrant: Ultrasound. In these ultrasound images obtained in the left upper quadrant, free fluid in the abdomen is visible as a black (anechoic) collection separating the spleen and the left kidney **(A, B).**

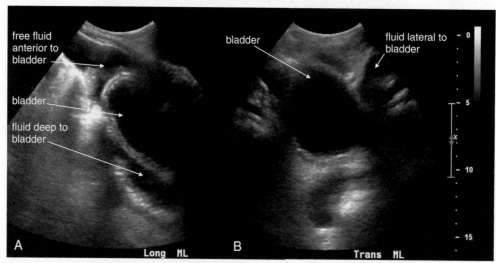

Figure 10-3. Free fluid in pelvis: Ultrasound. The suprapubic view of the FAST examination assesses for free fluid in the pelvis. A full bladder appears as a round, well-circumscribed, midline anechoic structure. **A,** A midsagittal (long-axis midline) view. Fluid is visible anterior and deep to the bladder. **B,** A transverse view. Fluid is visible lateral to the bladder.

visible on CT without oral contrast (Figures 10-7 and 10-8). This is in contrast to primary small-bowel traumatic injuries, which usually show *focal* regions of bowel wall thickening. Shock bowel is variably associated with IVC and aortic flattening, abnormal pancreatic enhancement and peripancreatic fluid, and poor enhancement of the spleen and liver because of hypotension. This constellation of findings is sometimes called the **CT hypotension complex** and has been reported in other conditions, including head and spine injury, post–cardiac arrest, septic shock, and diabetic ketoacidosis.[43]

Pneumoperitoneum. Pneumoperitoneum is rare following blunt abdominal injury but can indicate bowel perforation. When detected on CT, it is not specific for bowel injury because air tracking from thoracic injuries can collect in the abdomen.[2-3] Following penetrating abdominal injury, pneumoperitoneum detected on CT is likely to indicate bowel perforation and prompts laparotomy in most cases.

On soft-tissue windows, air including pneumoperitoneum appears black (Figures 10-9 and 10-10; see also Figure 10-24). Large amounts of pneumoperitoneum are usually visible on this window setting, but smaller collections are more difficult to recognize because intraperitoneal and retroperitoneal fat appears quite dark on soft-tissue windows. On lung windows, all soft tissues and bones appear white, leaving only air black—thus emphasizing both pneumoperitoneum and bowel gas (see Figures 10-10 and 10-24, **B**). On bone windows, bone appears white or light gray, and all soft tissues

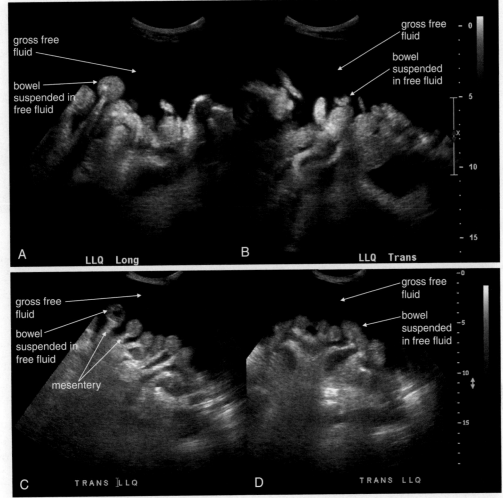

Figure 10-4. Gross free peritoneal fluid: Ultrasound. Free fluid in the abdomen is common following blunt or penetrating abdominal trauma. After trauma, fluid in the abdomen should be considered to be a sign of hemorrhage until proven otherwise—although preexisting fluid such as ascites would have a similar appearance. A rarer source of fluid following trauma is bowel injury. Free fluid is anechoic (black) on ultrasound. When gross free fluid is present, loops of bowel may be seen suspended within it **(A-D).** The mesentery is also visible as "stalks" tethering the bowel **(C, D).**

are an intermediate gray, making black air readily visible. During trauma CT, the patient is generally supine, so pneumoperitoneum collects in the anterior midline and perihepatic spaces preferentially (60% in one study) rather than in a subdiaphragmatic location, as occurs on upright chest x-ray.[44] Air can collect in other locations, including the pelvis and mesentery. CT can detect air collections as small as 1 mm.[45]

Hemoperitoneum and Free Abdominal Fluid. CT is believed to be highly sensitive for abdominal hemorrhage and free fluid. Hemoperitoneum is approximately 30 to 45 Hounsfield units (HU) in density and appears dark gray on CT soft-tissue windows (Figures 10-11 to 10-19 and 10-21 to 10-24).[18] The density of fluid can be measured using the PACS cursor. Simple fluids such as urine or ascites have densities around 0 HU. Free fluid may also accumulate because of bowel injury and may have an intermediate density between the density of water and that of blood. Free fluid or hemoperitoneum generally collects by gravity in dependent regions of

the abdomen and pelvis, so the location does not necessarily correspond to the source of bleeding. Inspect the perihepatic and perisplenic regions, including the hepatorenal recess (Morison's pouch) and splenorenal recess. In addition, inspect the pelvic, paracolic gutters, and central abdomen because these regions may contain free fluid. Free fluid may be seen outlining bowel loops (see Figures 10-21 and 10-22).

When free fluid is seen, a careful search for accompanying solid organ, bowel, and mesenteric injury must be performed. Although solid organ injury is the most common source of free fluid following trauma, the presence of a solid organ injury does not rule out concomitant hollow viscus or mesenteric injury. When free fluid is observed in the absence of solid organ injury, bowel or mesenteric injury must be strongly suspected. Unfortunately, the finding is nonspecific. In a study of 259 pediatric blunt trauma patients, 24 patients (9%) had free fluid as the only abnormal finding. Among the 16 patients with a small amount of free fluid, only 2 (12%)

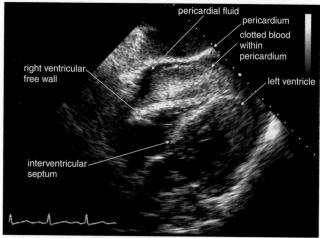

Figure 10-5. **Hemopericardium: Ultrasound.** The FAST examination for blunt trauma includes inspection of the pericardium for blood. Usually a subxiphoid approach is used (as in this case), although in some patients long-axis parasternal or four-chamber apical views may be necessary. In this 57-year-old male who struck a telephone pole while riding a bicycle, a large pericardial effusion is visible (black, or anechoic). The pericardium appears bright, or hyperechoic. Clotted blood within the pericardium but outside the right ventricle is evident. The right ventricular free wall is bowed into the ventricular chamber. In the context of the hypotensive patient, these findings indicate pericardial tamponade.

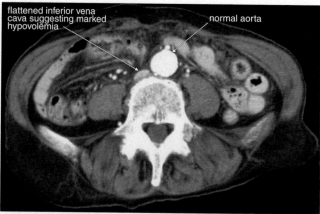

Figure 10-6. **Inferior vena cava (IVC) flattening, a sign of hypovolemia and shock.** CT with IV contrast, soft-tissue window. The size of the IVC has been suggested as a surrogate for intravascular volume status. A flattened IVC can indicate impending hemodynamic collapse and should prompt immediate volume resuscitation. In this 77-year-old trauma patient, who had been traveling in a car struck by a train, the IVC is extremely flat, suggested marked hypovolemia. Compare with the aorta, which has a normal caliber (2 cm). The patient had multiple injuries noted on CT, including pulmonary contusions, a periaortic hematoma, free fluid around the liver, and pelvic superior rami fractures. She also suffered a closed head injury with subarachnoid and subdural hemorrhage. Her initial lactate was elevated. Three hours after CT, the patient suffered a pulseless electrical activity arrest and could not be resuscitated. Autopsy found more than 500 ml of hemoperitoneum, as well as mediastinal hemorrhage.

required laparotomy. Among the 8 patients with a moderate amount of free fluid, including free fluid in multiple areas on CT, 50% required operation.[46] In a study of 2299 adult blunt trauma patients, 90 patients had free abdominal fluid without solid organ injury, but only 7 (8%) had documented intestinal injuries.[47]

Active Bleeding. As described earlier in the section on indications for contrast agents, **active bleeding** is revealed by IV contrast (see Figures 10-12, 10-15, 10-19, and 10-21 through 10-24). On soft-tissue windows, parenteral contrast leaking into regions of solid organ injury or into existing hemoperitoneum is readily visible as a bright white "blush" or amorphous collection (see Figures 10-12, 10-15, 10-19, and 10-21 through 10-24). The surrounding area of hypoperfused solid organ, contained hematoma, or hemoperitoneum appears darker gray, corresponding to around 45 Hounsfield units. Normally perfused, uninjured solid organs appear brighter than hematoma but less bright than the area of active hemorrhage. Depending on the timing of CT image acquisition relative to contrast injection, normal vascular structures within solid organs may be visible as bright white linear or circular markings. These should not be confused with areas of active hemorrhage. Normal vascular structures are surrounded by moderately enhancing normal solid organ parenchyma (intermediate or bright gray) (see examples of normal livers in Figures 10-11 and 10-12;). Areas of active hemorrhage usually are surrounded by hypoattenuating or nonenhancing areas of hematoma or injured solid organ parenchyma, which appear dark

gray on soft-tissue windows (see Figure 10-12). Pooling of extravasated parenteral contrast is an indication for angiographic embolization (described in more detail in Chapter 16) or laparotomy.[48]

Spleen Injuries. CT with IV contrast is highly sensitive for spleen injuries. **Spleen injuries** are evaluated using soft-tissue windows (see Figures 10-11 through 10-16). On this window setting, a normal spleen enhances with IV contrast and appears bright gray (see Figure 10-11). As described earlier in the section on indications for IV contrast, areas of splenic parenchymal injury or contained hematoma fail to enhance and appear dark gray, with a density around 45 HU (see Figure 10-11). Areas of hemoperitoneum (see Figures 10-11 and 10-12) may surround the spleen, or may settle in dependent regions of the abdomen or pelvis, remote from the bleeding source, as described earlier. **Active hemorrhage** is visible as a bright blush, as described earlier. If an area of blush increases in size on delayed phase images acquired 60 to 70 seconds and again 5 minutes after contrast injection, this likely represents active bleeding rather than contained vascular injury.[49]

Spleen injuries are graded in severity based on CT appearance using a five-point scale (Table 10-2) (see Figure 10-11).[50-51] Grading schemes can be used to select patients for nonoperative therapy including angiographic embolization, described in Chapter 16. Even high-grade injuries can sometimes be managed nonoperatively with embolization.[52] For the emergency physician

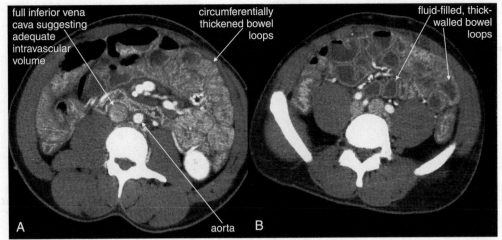

Figure 10-7. Shock bowel, a sign of severe sustained hypotension. A and **B,** CT with IV contrast viewed on soft-tissue windows, demonstrating shock bowel in a trauma patient. Shock bowel refers to the appearance of bowel that has been hypoperfused for an extended period. Under these conditions, the bowel ceases peristalsis and assumes an appearance similar in some respects to small-bowel obstruction. In other respects, the bowel appears similar to a case of mesenteric ischemic—but the process is diffuse, rather than being restricted to a single vascular territory. As bowel becomes ischemic, it develops edema of the bowel wall, and the bowel wall develops a hyperenhancing pattern following administration of intravenous contrast, resulting from microvascular leak of the injected contrast. The bowel wall thus looks thick and bright, unlike its normal inconspicuously thin appearance. Loops of fluid-filled bowel are common, and the internal structure of the bowel becomes exaggerated. Sometimes plicae circularis become visible; at other times, the degree of bowel edema is so great that the lumen becomes effaced. This patient developed hemorrhagic shock from a traumatic amputation of his right arm, leading to shock bowel. By the time of the CT, the patient had been volume resuscitated, as indicated by the prominent inferior vena cava (compare with Figure 10-6).

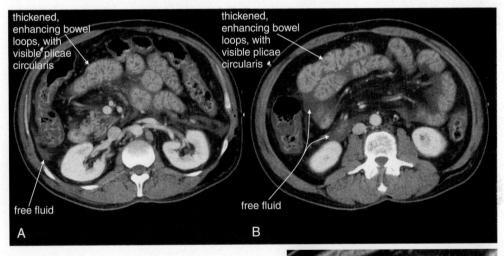

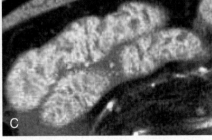

Figure 10-8. Shock bowel. CT with IV contrast, soft-tissue window. No oral contrast has been given. **A-C,** Another example of shock bowel. This patient underwent exploratory laparotomy to assess for traumatic bowel injury because some free fluid was noted in the abdomen on CT. No abdominal injuries were found at laparotomy. **C,** Close-up from **B.**

interpreting CT, recognition of normal mild, moderate, and severe splenic injuries is probably sufficient in most cases, with formal grading being unnecessary.

Liver Injuries. CT with IV contrast is highly sensitive for liver injuries. **Liver injuries** follow a similar pattern to spleen injuries. The liver is a highly vascular solid organ and enhances with IV contrast, giving its normal parenchyma a bright appearance on soft-tissue windows (see Figure 10-17). Areas of injury are typically hypoperfused and do not enhance with IV contrast, making them darker gray (hypoattenuated) (see Figures 10-17 through 10-19 and 10-36). Areas of active hemorrhage may be visible as a blush of contrast (see the earlier

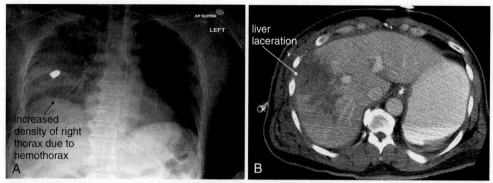

Figure 10-9. Penetrating abdominal injury with hemothorax. This patient sustained a right upper quadrant gunshot wound. The trajectory of the bullet crossed the liver and diaphragm, entering the thorax. **A,** Chest x-ray shows a retained bullet and increased density of the right thorax, consistent with hemothorax. No meniscus is seen because this is a supine chest x-ray. **B,** CT with IV and oral contrast (soft-tissue window) shows a large hypodense area indicating hepatic laceration. Always consider chest injury with abdominal or flank gunshot wounds because the trajectory of the missile is unpredictable.

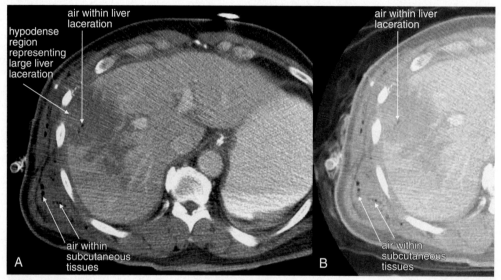

Figure 10-10. Intraperitoneal gas. Same patient as the prior figure. Penetrating abdominal injuries can introduce exogenous air into the peritoneum and retroperitoneum. In addition, if perforation of a viscus occurs from a penetrating injury, air may escape into the peritoneum as a result. This patient sustained a gunshot wound to the right upper quadrant. CT shows air in the subcutaneous tissues, as well as air within the large hepatic laceration that resulted from the injury. Air appears black on all CT window settings, regardless of the administration of contrast. However, sometimes small collections of air may be difficult to identify on soft-tissue windows **(A)** because peritoneal fat is dark, nearly black, on this setting. Two other settings are useful to highlight air: bone and lung windows. On bone windows, bone is white, air is black, and all other tissues are intermediate gray. **B,** The same slice as **A** viewed on a lung window. Air is nearly black, whereas all other tissues appear white.

section on active bleeding). Liver injuries are graded on a six-point scale that guides nonoperative management (Table 10-3).[51] As with spleen injuries, specific grading of liver injuries may be unnecessary for the emergency physician interpreting CT. Differentiating normal, mild, moderate, and severe injuries is essential to management decisions. Mild injuries rarely require intervention, whereas severe injuries often require angiographic embolization or laparotomy.

Renal Injuries. **Renal injuries** are discussed in detail in Chapter 12. They follow a pattern similar to that of other solid organs. The normal kidneys are well perfused and enhance brightly with IV contrast. Areas of hypoperfusion resulting from injury appear dark gray. Perinephric fluid collections appear dark gray and may represent blood or

urine. Chapter 12 discusses the use of delayed CT images to differentiate urine leaks from hemorrhage. In general, images acquired during an arterial phase of contrast enhancement may show active extravasation of contrast, indicating bleeding. If contrast extravasation is seen on delayed images obtained minutes later during renal excretion of contrast, a urine leak is present (see Chapter 12).

Biliary Tract Injuries. **Biliary tract injuries** are rare following blunt trauma, occurring in only around 2% to 3% of patients undergoing laparotomy, a select group in today's era of nonoperative management of many injuries.[56] Gallbladder injuries are difficult to recognize because of the common occurrence of adjacent organ injury. A collapsed gallbladder or thickening or disruption of the gallbladder wall suggests injury (see Figure 10-19).

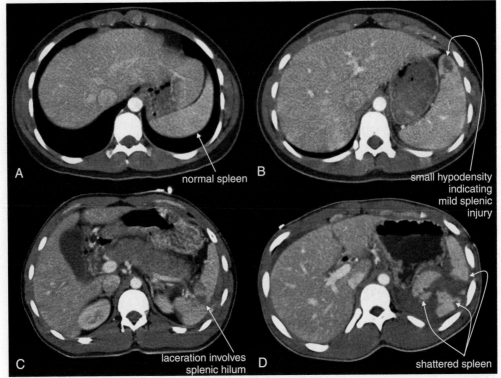

Figure 10-11. Spectrum of splenic injuries. Injuries to the spleen are generally easy to recognize as hypoattenuated (*dark*) regions on CT with IV contrast. With the administration of intravenous (IV) contrast, the normal spleen enhances quite homogeneously to a fairly bright gray. Injured areas within the spleen (variously referred to as lacerations, contained hematomas, or contusions) fail to enhance with IV contrast, because they are avascular. Depending on the timing of the CT relative to the injection of contrast, normal vessels within the spleen may appear brighter than surrounding parenchyma and should not be confused with active bleeding. Active bleeding (demonstrated in Figure 10-12) appears as a blush of bright contrast but is typically surrounded by hypodense areas of injury. **A,** Uninjured spleen. **B,** Minimally injured spleen (grade I). This injury is unlikely to cause hemodynamic compromise acutely because it is small, contained within the spleen, shows no active hemorrhage, and does not involve the hilum. **C,** Moderately injured spleen (grade III or IV). This injury, though relative small, involves the splenic hilum and may become life-threatening. This injury type is often treated with angiographic embolization to prevent further bleeding. **D,** Severely injured spleen (grade V). This spleen is shattered and may require embolization or splenectomy.

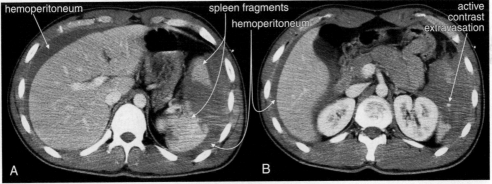

Figure 10-12. Grade IV spleen injury with hemoperitoneum and active extravasation of contrast material. A, B, This 20-year-old male was ejected 15 feet from a vehicle and was found to have a high-grade splenic injury on CT with IV contrast. This injury was called "large" by the radiologist, "grade IV" by the surgeons. In this text, we focus on identifying injuries and accurately estimating severity, but specific scores are given less importance. CT findings include marked fragmentation of the spleen, gross hemoperitoneum, and active extravasation of injected contrast. Several points bear emphasis. First, note the quantity of fluid (blood) surrounding the liver even though the spleen is the injured organ. The location of free fluid is determined by gravity and tissue planes, not necessarily by the location of the injured organ. Free fluid appears dark gray compared with the brighter solid organs after administration of IV contrast. This is because of enhancement of the solid organ, which is receiving blood flow carrying contrast material. The free fluid accumulated before the administration of IV contrast and thus does not enhance. An exception is a region of active bleeding, which shows a bright blush of injected contrast at the moment of CT acquisition. This patient has such as blush, indicating active bleeding, in the bed of the spleen. How can active extravasation be discriminated from the normal appearance of vessels within the liver and spleen? These are, after all, extremely vascular organs. Depending on the timing of the CT scan relative to the injection of contrast material, the liver may show enhancement of hepatic arteries or veins, as well as portal veins. The liver parenchyma may remain somewhat enhancing, even after the major vessels have cleared of contrast. However, in each case, normal contrast enhancement of vessels can be recognized and discriminated from active extravasation. Active extravasation occurs in a location with an injury, which is hypodense (darker than surrounding tissue). In general, this means that the blush of active extravasation is surrounded by a darker tissue density of unenhancing fluid (blood) or poorly perfused injured tissue. Look for the bright spot with a dark background. The patient underwent exploratory laparotomy that confirmed a splenic injury with bleeding from the short gastric arteries. No other injuries were detected, and the patient underwent splenectomy. Grade IV and V splenic injuries are occasionally treated with embolization rather than splenectomy, even in the presence of active contrast extravasation, although the evidence for this approach is limited (see Chapter 16). Figures 10-13 to 10-15 explore this patient's injury in more detail.

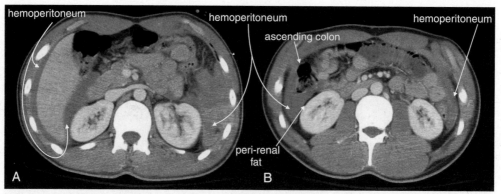

Figure 10-13. Hemoperitoneum in the setting of a grade IV spleen injury. CT with IV contrast. These images are more caudad than those in Figure 10-12 for the same patient. **A,** Hemoperitoneum is present in a perihepatic location, including Morison's pouch between the liver and the right kidney. This patient would have a positive FAST examination with fluid detected in the right upper quadrant. The liver itself was uninjured in this patient; the location of hemoperitoneum does not indicate its source. On the patient's left, this slice is now below the level of the spleen, but a large amount of hemoperitoneum is present in this location as well. **B,** Still farther caudad, free fluid (hemoperitoneum) is seen in both paracolic gutters. Again, this would be seen on a FAST examination. A thin strip of fat separates the free fluid from the abdominal wall and from the kidneys, which are retroperitoneal. A common point of confusion is the appearance of fluid on CT, perhaps because emergency physicians use ultrasound so frequently. Whereas fluid appears black on ultrasound, on CT fluid appears an intermediate to dark gray (using soft-tissue windows). Fat appears nearly black on this window setting.

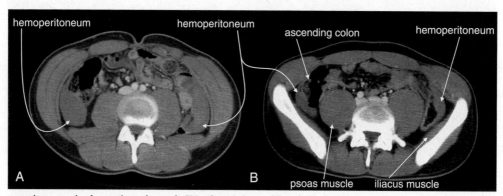

Figure 10-14. Hemoperitoneum in the setting of a grade IV spleen injury. CT with IV contrast, soft-tissue window. These images are more caudad than those in Figure 10-13 for the same patient. Free fluid (hemoperitoneum) is seen in both paracolic gutters **(A, B),** extending into the pelvis **(B).** Again, this would be seen on a FAST examination. A thin strip of fat separates the free fluid from the iliacus muscle, which hugs the internal surface of the iliac bone of the pelvis, and the psoas muscle, which is paravertebral. Fat plays an important role as a contrast medium here, because without the interposed fat it would be difficult or impossible to identify the limits of the hemoperitoneum.

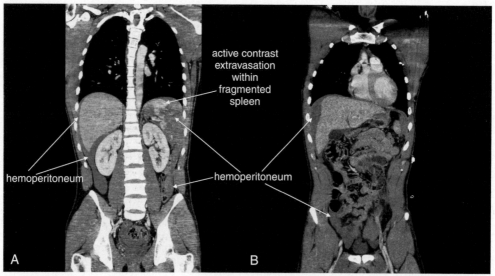

Figure 10-15. Grade IV spleen injury with hemoperitoneum and active extravasation of contrast material. CT with IV contrast, soft-tissue window. Same patient as Figures 10-12 through 10-14. **A, B,** Coronal CT reconstructions are shown. Although these were not needed to make the diagnosis, they help illustrate the degree of hemoperitoneum, the fragmentation of the spleen, and the active extravasation of contrast indicating ongoing bleeding.

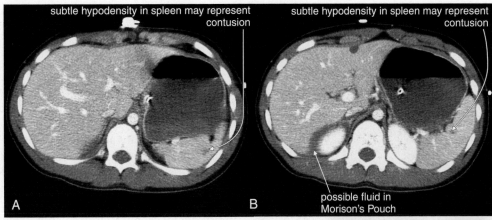

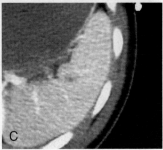

Figure 10-16. Grade I spleen injury. CT with IV contrast, soft-tissue window. **A-C,** This 14-year-old male fell 15 feet from a tree. CT showed a subtle spleen injury. This injury would be characterized as grade I. Is free fluid present in Morison's pouch? The patient did have pelvis fractures that could be a source. The patient was observed and did well without intervention. **C,** Close-up from **B.**

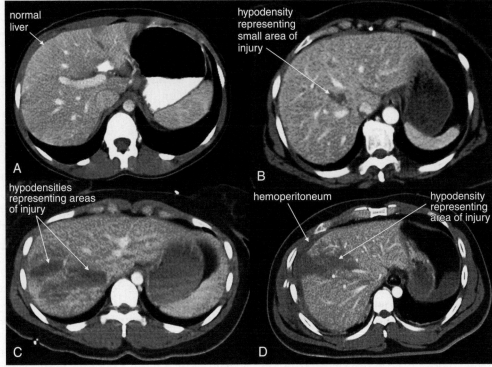

Figure 10-17. Spectrum of liver injuries. CT with IV contrast, soft-tissue windows. In **A,** oral contrast is also present in the stomach. The normal liver enhances relatively uniformly with administration of intravenous contrast. Depending on the timing of the CT acquisition relative to the injection of contrast, portal and hepatic vessels are visible as bright linear markings. Injuries to the liver are generally easy to recognize as hypoattenuated (dark) regions because these regions have lost their blood supply and do not enhance. Areas of injury may be referred to by terms including hematoma, contusion, and laceration, which are essentially synonymous when describing CT findings. Hepatic injuries are graded from I to VI (see Table 10-3), but for the emergency physician, the key discriminatory categories are normal, low-grade injuries not requiring invasive therapy, and moderate- to high-grade injuries likely to require intervention (angiographic embolization or laparotomy). **A,** Uninjured liver. Dark areas here represent the normal anatomic divisions of the liver. **B,** Minimally injured liver (grade I). This injury is unlikely to cause hemodynamic compromise acutely because it is small, contained within the liver, shows no active hemorrhage, and does not involve the major vascular structures. **C, D,** Moderately to severely injured liver (grade III). **C,** The hematoma appears contained. **D,** The liver surface appears torn, and there is associated hemoperitoneum (dark gray crescent surrounding the liver). These injuries may progress, requiring embolization or laparotomy.

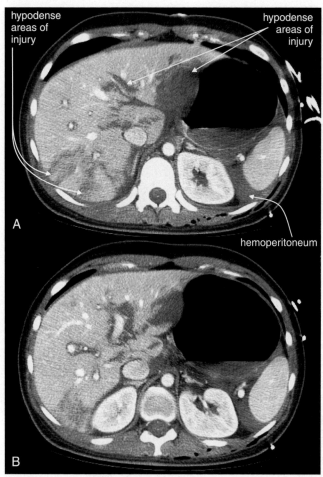

Figure 10-18. Hilar liver laceration. CT with IV contrast, soft-tissue window. This patient sustained multiple life-threatening injuries in a motor vehicle collision, including a multifocal liver laceration extending to the liver hilum **(A, B).** Hemoperitoneum is present, particularly around the spleen. The patient was treated with angiographic embolization. Patients with higher grades of liver injury are sometimes too hemodynamically unstable even to undergo CT. The FAST examination may be positive, and the liver injury may be diagnosed during laparotomy or angiography.

Pericholecystic fluid is nonspecific because it may accumulate from other sources. Layering of dense fluid within the gallbladder can suggest hemorrhage in the gallbladder. Bile duct injury can result in free fluid.

Small Bowel, Mesentery, Stomach, or Colon Injuries. **Injuries to the bowel** (including stomach, small bowel, and large bowel) and **mesentery** are difficult to detect with CT. The reported sensitivity of CT varies from around 60% to as high as 95% in some series.[20,21,24,53] Findings suggesting bowel or mesenteric injury include free peritoneal fluid without evidence of solid organ injury, mesenteric infiltration (an increased density, brightening, or smoky appearance of the normally nearly black mesenteric fat), thick-walled bowel, and free air (see Figures 10-20 through 10-24).[54] As discussed earlier in the section on indications for contrast agents, oral contrast is not recommended for blunt trauma but is commonly used for penetrating trauma. Even when enteral contrast is used, leak of enteral contrast is not routinely seen with bowel injuries; however, when present, it is proof of bowel perforation.[55] Other abdominal injuries are commonly present when bowel injuries occur.

Pancreatic Injuries. **Pancreatic injuries** are rare, occurring in around 2% of blunt trauma patients, and can be difficult to recognize on CT.[56] Single-detector CT was reportedly only about 80% sensitive for pancreatic injuries, and reports of the sensitivity of multidetector CT with narrow slice thickness are lacking.[56] A common mechanism for pancreatic injury is a direct blow to the epigastrium as in a handlebar injury or crush injury against the underlying spine. Pancreatic injuries are rarely isolated (<10%) and can accompany bowel injury. CT findings include abdominal free fluid with or without other solid organ injury, peripancreatic stranding or fluid, and direct evidence of pancreatic parenchymal injury (Figure 10-25). Like other solid organs, the normal pancreas is well perfused and enhances with IV contrast. Injured regions are hypoperfused and appear hypoattenuated or dark gray on soft-tissue windows. The body of the pancreas may appear completely transected or comminuted. Active hemorrhage is sometimes seen. Fluid between the splenic vein and the pancreas also suggests pancreatic injury. Injury to the pancreatic duct, which requires repair, can be difficult to recognize but is strongly suggested by deep lacerations of the pancreas (>50% of the pancreatic thickness).[56-57]

Adrenal Injuries. **Injury to the adrenal glands** can occur in blunt trauma. In addition, adrenal hemorrhage is thought to occur spontaneously in some patients with shock and may subsequently lead to adrenal insufficiency. The normal adrenal glands are thin, lambda-shaped structures capping the kidneys bilaterally (Figure 10-26). Adrenal hemorrhage usually results in an enlarged, rounded appearance (see Figure 10-26). The normal adrenal glands enhance with IV contrast, whereas contained adrenal hematoma is usually hypoattenuating. Stranding around the adrenal glands may also occur.[58-60]

Retroperitoneal Injuries. **Retroperitoneal injuries** such as **psoas muscle hemorrhage** are readily seen on CT. The presence of retroperitoneal fat assists in recognition of these injuries, acting as a natural contrast agent. Fat appears nearly black on soft-tissue windows, whereas the normal psoas muscle appears an intermediate gray. Blood in the retroperitoneum has a similar density to psoas muscle and can obscure fat planes (Figure 10-27).

Abdominal Wall or Flank Injuries. Muscles of the anterior abdominal wall or flank can be damaged, resulting in herniation of abdominal contents. On CT, abdominal contents may be seen in subcutaneous fat (Figures 10-28 and 10-29).

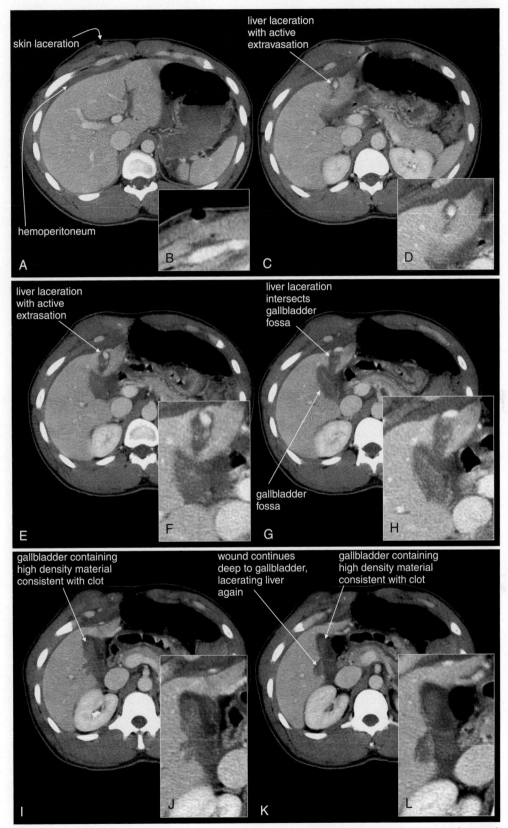

Figure 10-19. Gallbladder and biliary injuries. A-L, Series of computed tomography (CT) slices, with close-ups from each slice. This patient sustained a single stab wound to the right upper quadrant. CT with intravenous contrast demonstrates a wound track through the liver into the gallbladder. The gallbladder has high-density material within it consistent with clot—higher in density than normal bile. The liver laceration, though small, shows evidence of active contrast extravasation. The patient underwent laparotomy, confirming a through-and-through gallbladder laceration that was treated with cholecystectomy.

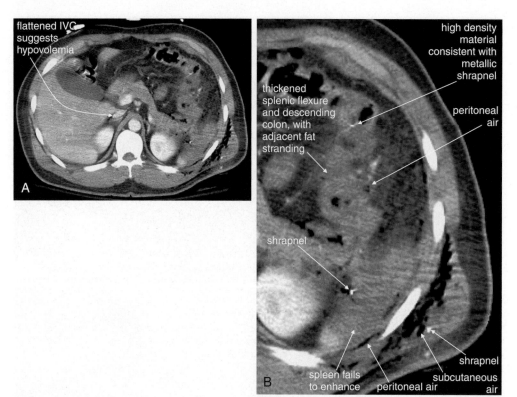

Figure 10-20. Bowel injuries or perforation from penetrating trauma. A, This patient sustained a gunshot wound to the left chest, which entered the left upper abdomen, injuring the splenic flexure and descending colon. **B,** The area of injury has been enlarged to allow inspection for small foci of air and metal shrapnel. On soft-tissue windows, metallic material is bright white (remember, calcium in bone is technically a metal). Air is black. Air is visible in the subcutaneous tissues, in the abdomen around the region of the spleen, and scattered outside the colon. The splenic flexure and descending colon appear ill-defined, with a hazy appearance of the surrounding fat—inflammatory stranding. Without a history of trauma, a case of colitis or diverticulitis could have a similar appearance. One of the metal fragments appears to lie within the colon. Laparotomy confirmed perforation of the distal transverse colon, which was resected. The spleen also shows a lack of enhancement (compare with the liver and kidneys)—suggesting a splenic arterial injury resulting in hypoperfusion. The inferior vena cava (IVC) is flattened, suggesting hypovolemia.

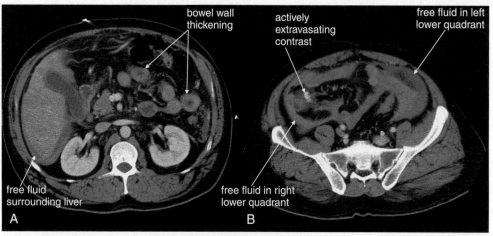

Figure 10-21. Penetrating bowel and mesentery injuries. A, B, This male sustained a gunshot wound to the right hip. CT with intravenous contrast reveals free fluid throughout the abdomen, as well as extravasation of intravenously injected contrast in the right lower quadrant in the region of the small-bowel mesentery. Several areas of bowel wall thickening are visible. These findings indicated the need for laparotomy, which confirmed both mesentery and distal ileal injuries. The CT findings are explored in more detail in Figures 10-22 and 10-23.

Diaphragm Injuries. Overt **diaphragm injuries** with herniation of abdominal contents into the thorax are readily detected by CT (Figures 10-30 through 10-34). However, when the chest x-ray is normal and the diaphragmatic injury is subtler, CT is less sensitive. Improvements in CT technology, particularly the use of helical CT and coronal and sagittal reconstructions, appear to have improved sensitivity. Nonetheless, studies of diaphragm rupture are limited by the rarity of this injury, with wide confidence intervals because of small studies (described later). Overall, CT likely has a sensitivity of around 60% to 80%, with a specificity of 80% to 100%.

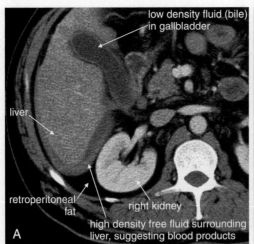
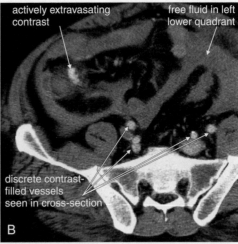

Figure 10-22. Penetrating bowel and mesentery injuries with active bleeding. Same patient as in Figures 10-21 and 10-23. Several clues on this CT with IV contrast suggest active bleeding. **A,** Fluid surrounding the liver and bowel is high density, more suggestive of blood than of serous fluid such as ascites. Compare the appearance of the fluid surrounding the liver to the appearance of lower-density fluid (bile) in the gallbladder. On CT scan, regardless of window setting, denser substances are brighter (whiter) and less dense substances are darker. Fluid is identifiable around the liver because it is less dense than the solid liver but denser than retroperitoneal fat, which is nearly black on this soft-tissue window setting. Dark retroperitoneal fat surrounds the right kidney. **B,** Injected contrast is seen extravasating in the right lower quadrant. How can this be identified as active bleeding? This patient received no oral contrast, so high-density material in this region must be injected contrast. The contrast does not have the typical well-circumscribed, rounded shape of contrast within vessels (compare with other vessels on this image). On the digital PACS, the blush of contrast does not communicate with a well-defined vessel as we search cephalad and caudad through the stack of images.

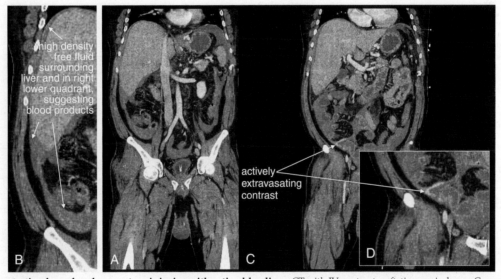

Figure 10-23. Penetrating bowel and mesentery injuries with active bleeding. CT with IV contrast, soft-tissue windows. Coronal reconstructions from the same patient as in Figures 10-21 and 10-22. help illustrate the extent of intraabdominal hemorrhage and the location of the active bleeding. **B,** Close-up from **A. D,** Close-up from **C.**

CT findings of subtle diaphragmatic injury include a discontinuous diaphragm and waistlike constriction of abdominal viscera (sometimes called the "collar sign"), the most common finding in one study.[61] An additional finding, the "dependent viscera sign," may also be sensitive for diaphragm injury and is described here. Normally, an intact diaphragm prevents the upper one third of the liver from contacting the posterior ribs on the right and the stomach and bowel from contacting the posterior ribs on the left. When the diaphragm is ruptured, these organs become dependent (hence the term *dependent viscera sign*) and contact posterior ribs in a patient

positioned supine during CT.[61] The diaphragm itself may be obscured by hemothorax or hemoperitoneum.[62] In some cases, the presence of a diaphragm injury can be inferred from injuries on both sides of the diaphragm, though the diaphragmatic defect itself may not be seen (Figures 10-35 and 10-36).

The sensitivity of CT for diaphragmatic injury has improved over the past 20 years due to technological improvements, while chest x-ray sensitivity has remained static. Gelman et al.[63] reported the sensitivity of chest x-ray as 46% for left-sided diaphragmatic

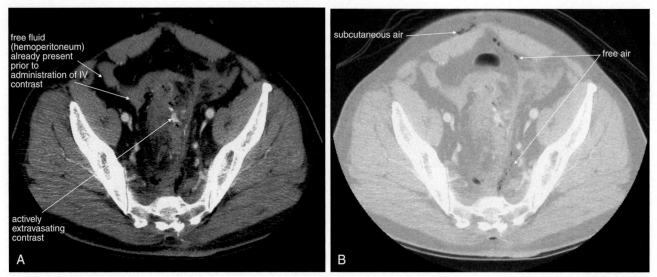

Figure 10-24. Penetrating mesenteric injuries. CT with IV contrast. This patient sustained a gunshot wound below the umbilicus. On a soft-tissue window **(A),** intravenous contrast extravasation is seen just left of the midline, indicating active bleeding. Free air is seen well on the same slice using a lung window **(B).** Air is present just deep to the rectus muscles in the peritoneal cavity, as well as just anterior to the sacrum. This air does not appear to be contained in bowel.

TABLE 10-2. American Association for the Surgery of Trauma Splenic Injury Scale

Grade[*]	Type	Description of Injury
I	Hematoma	• Subcapsular, <10% surface area
	Laceration	• Capsular tear, <1 cm parenchymal depth
II	Hematoma	• Subcapsular, 10%-50% surface area • Intraparenchymal, <5 cm in diameter
	Laceration	• 1-3 cm parenchymal depth • Does not involve a trabecular vessel
III	Hematoma	• Subcapsular, >50% surface area or expanding • Ruptured subcapsular or parenchymal hematoma
	Laceration	• >3 cm parenchymal depth or involves trabecular vessels
IV	Laceration	• Involves segmental or hilar vessels and produces major devascularization (>25% of spleen)
V	Laceration	• Completely shattered spleen
	Vascular	• Hilar injury that devascularizes the spleen

*Advance one grade for multiple injuries up to grade III.
From Tinkoff G, Esposito TJ, Reed J, et al. American Association for the Surgery of Trauma Organ Injury Scale I: Spleen, liver, and kidney, validation based on the National Trauma Data Bank. *J Am Coll Surg* 207:646-655, 2008.

rupture but only 17% for right-sided rupture. An additional 18% of left-sided ruptures had abnormalities not diagnostic of diaphragm rupture but prompting additional imaging. At that time (1991), CT was only 14% sensitive.

Smithers et al.[5] (1991) reported a sensitivity of chest x-ray around 60% for diaphragm rupture within 48 hours after injury.

Murray et al.[62] (1996) reported the performance of three radiologists for detection of diaphragm rupture on CT in a case-control study (11 cases, 21 controls). Sensitivity for detecting diaphragmatic rupture was 54% to 73%, and specificity was 86% to 90%. Average sensitivity for

the three observers was 61% (95% CI = 41%-81%), and average specificity was 87% (95% CI = 76%-99%).

Killeen et al.[61] (1999) reported on helical CT with sagittal and coronal reconstructions in 41 patients, 23 with proven diaphragm injury. Sensitivity for detecting left-sided diaphragmatic rupture was 78%, and specificity was 100%. Sensitivity for the detection of right-sided diaphragmatic rupture was 50%, and specificity was 100%.

Bergin et al.[64] (2001) described the dependent viscera sign (discussed earlier). In their sample of 28 patients, 10 with diaphragm injury, the finding was 100% sensitive for left-sided rupture and 83% sensitive for right-sided

TABLE 10-3. American Association for the Surgery of Trauma Liver Injury Scale

Grade	Type	Description of Injury
I	Hematoma	• Subcapsular, <10% surface area
	Laceration	• Capsular tear, <1 cm parenchymal depth
II	Hematoma	• Subcapsular, 10%-50% surface area • Intraparenchymal, <10 cm in diameter
	Laceration	• Capsular tear, 1-3 cm parenchymal depth, <10 cm long
III	Hematoma	• Subcapsular, >50% surface area of ruptured subcapsular or parenchymal hematoma • Intraparenchymal, >10 cm or expanding
	Laceration	• >3 cm parenchymal depth
IV	Laceration	• Parenchymal disruption involving 25%-75% hepatic lobe or 1-3 Couinaud segments[*]
V	Vascular	• Parenchymal disruption involving >75% of hepatic lobe or >3 Couinaud segments[*] within a single lobe • Juxtahepatic venous injuries, i.e., retrohepatic vena cava or central major hepatic veins
VI	Vascular	• Hepatic avulsion

*The liver is divided into eight Couinaud segments. Each is functionally independent, with its own vascular inflow, outflow, and biliary drainage. The center of each segment contains a branch of the portal vein, hepatic artery, and bile duct. The periphery of each segment contains vascular outflow through hepatic veins.

From Tinkoff G, Esposito TJ, Reed J, et al. American Association for the Surgery of Trauma Organ Injury Scale I: Spleen, liver, and kidney, validation based on the National Trauma Data Bank. *J Am Coll Surg* 207:646-655, 2008.

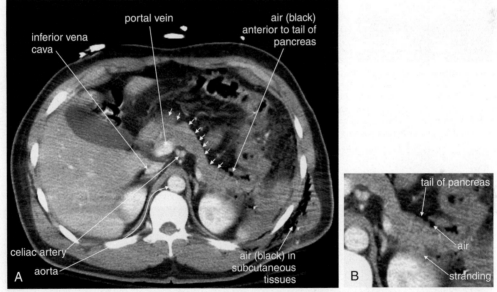

Figure 10-25. Pancreatic injuries. A, This patient sustained multiple gunshot wounds to the left thorax, resulting in injuries to the diaphragm, transverse colon, and pancreas that were confirmed at laparotomy. CT with intravenous contrast (soft-tissue window) shows air in the subcutaneous tissues of the left chest wall. The pancreas (*small arrows*) can be seen in its usual position, draped over the portal vein and celiac artery and then crossing just anterior to the left kidney. Air is present along the anterior border of the pancreatic tail, perhaps having been introduced by the gunshot wound or having escaped from the injured colon. The fat plane that normally separates the pancreas and kidney is obscured by stranding. The inferior vena cava also is flattened, consistent with blood loss. **B,** Close-up from **A.**

rupture. The authors claimed a consecutive sample of patients undergoing CT and laparotomy was studied, but the high incidence of diaphragm injury in this series (36%) far exceeds other reports and strongly suggests selection bias.

Allen et al.[22] (2005) reported CT without oral contrast to have a sensitivity and specificity for diaphragm injury of 66.7% (95% CI = 29.9%-92.5%) and 100% (95%

CI = 99.2%-100%), respectively, although their study included only nine injuries.

Vascular (Aorta and Inferior Vena Cava) Injuries.
The abdominal aorta is relatively rarely injured with blunt mechanisms of trauma. However, severe trauma (e.g., falls from great height or extremely high-speed collisions) can disrupt the abdominal aorta. The normal aorta is circular in cross section, does not exceed 3 cm in

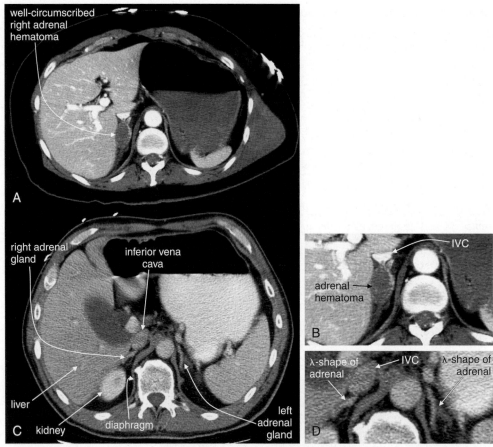

Figure 10-26. Adrenal injuries. A, CT with IV contrast, soft-tissue window. This patient sustained an adrenal hematoma in the setting of severe blunt trauma that also resulted in multiple rib fractures, thoracic spine fractures, and a pneumothorax. Adrenal hematomas may result from the stress of severe injury, rather than from direct trauma to the gland. No injury to the surrounding liver, kidney, or adjacent ribs or vertebrae occurred. The inferior vena cava is anterior to the adrenal hematoma and filled with contrast. **B,** Close-up from **A. C,** CT with IV and oral contrast in a different patient. Normal adrenal glands for comparison. The adrenal glands are normally inconspicuous and may be difficult to locate. They usually lie just cephalad of the kidneys and have a lambda (λ) shape. **D,** Close-up from **C.**

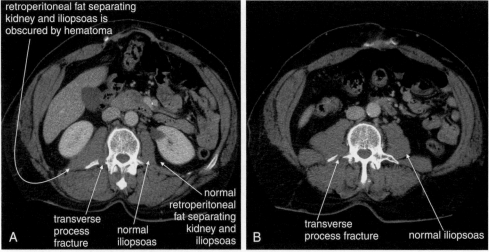

Figure 10-27. Retroperitoneal hemorrhage (iliopsoas hematoma). This patient fell 12 feet from a ladder, sustaining transverse process spinal fractures and a pneumothorax. In addition, this CT with IV contrast (soft-tissue window) demonstrates a right iliopsoas muscle hematoma. The source of the hemorrhage is evident—a transverse process fracture of the adjacent L2-5 lumbar vertebrae. Hemorrhage can be subtle because fresh blood and muscle have similar density on CT—both appear medium gray on soft-tissue window settings. In this case, comparison with the normal left side reveals asymmetry of the right iliopsoas resulting from an adjacent hematoma. The retroperitoneal fat separating the right kidney from the right iliopsoas is also obscured. **A,** A slice through the level of the kidneys. **B,** Two lumbar levels lower.

diameter, and has a smooth contour. It has a uniform location anterior to the spine, making it easy to inspect. With IV contrast, the aorta should fill uniformly with contrast, with no filling defects or intimal flaps visible. In older patients, aortic aneurysms and mural thrombus may be incidentally detected, unrelated to trauma (see Chapter 11). In cases of trauma, the aortic contour may be irregular, and active extravasation of contrast may be seen as a bright blush (Figure 10-37). Any periaortic hematoma that accumulated before the administration of IV contrast appears dark gray, approximately 45 Hounsfield units. Aortic injuries from penetrating trauma have a similar appearance to those seen with blunt trauma, if the patient is stable enough to undergo CT.

Injuries to the IVC are more common in penetrating trauma than in blunt trauma. The IVC has a uniform location to the right of the patient's aorta. Its size is generally smaller than that of the aorta but varies with the patient's intravascular volume status. The IVC may be circular or elliptical in cross section. In hemorrhagic shock, the IVC appears flattened (see Figures 10-6 and 10-20).[42] Active extravasation of contrast can be seen with IVC injuries.

Spine and Pelvis Injuries. Body CT performed for the evaluation of blunt or penetrating abdominal trauma also yields detailed information about bony structures. Axial, sagittal, and coronal reformations help characterize injuries in three dimensions (see Figure 10-37). Although injuries can be evaluated directly from the abdominal images by switching to bone windows, finer detail can be seen using special bone reconstruction algorithms on the original image dataset. Evaluation of these injuries on CT is discussed in Chapters 3 and 13.

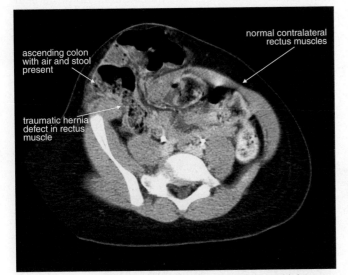

Figure 10-28. Abdominal wall injuries. This 6-year-old boy was injured falling off a bicycle while riding down a hill and presented with right lower abdominal pain and a protuberant abdomen. CT shows a large hernia defect in the rectus muscle of the right abdominal wall, through which the bowel has herniated into the subcutaneous tissues. Laparotomy was performed, and the hernia was found to contain both the small and the large bowel, with a contusion of the terminal ileum and a serosal tear of the cecum, which was repaired primarily. Compare the injured side with the normal muscles of the left abdominal wall. The patient is tilted slightly in the CT scanner, accounting for the apparent asymmetry of the pelvis.

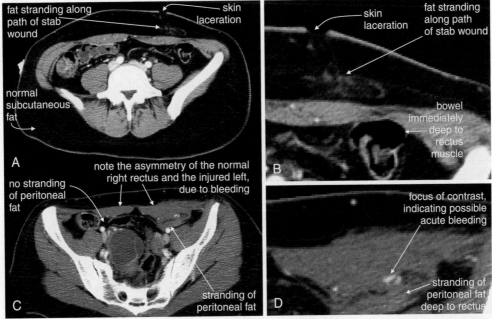

Figure 10-29. Penetrating abdominal trauma with abdominal wall injury. This patient presented with a self-inflicted stab wound to the lower abdomen. **A, C,** CT with oral and intravenous contrast was performed. **A, B,** axial CT slices through the pelvis, viewed on soft-tissue windows. **B,** Close-up from **A. D,** Close-up from **C.** The CT shows fat stranding consistent with blood in the subcutaneous tissues deep to the stab wound. Compare with the normal appearance of uninjured subcutaneous fat (dark gray). Of greater concern, the bowel lies just deep to the rectus muscle. Though no definite bowel injury is seen, a second slice at a more caudad level **(B)** shows stranding of intraperitoneal fat just deep to the rectus muscle. This suggests the stab has penetrated the peritoneum, possibly injuring the bowel. In addition, a tiny focus of contrast may represent active bleeding. The patient was observed without laparotomy despite these findings and did well.

CLINICAL DECISION RULES: WHICH STABLE BLUNT TRAUMA PATIENTS REQUIRE ABDOMINAL CT?

Adult Blunt Trauma Decision Rules

Following blunt trauma, stable adult patients can be evaluated safely using CT, which has been shown to have an excellent negative predictive value for serious injuries requiring treatment (see the section on safety of discharge following a negative CT). However, CT imaging of all stable blunt trauma patients would be costly, would be time consuming, and would result in large radiation exposures (see the later section on radiation) with little clinical benefit. Studies show that around 80% of adults

and 84% of pediatric patients undergoing CT for blunt abdominal injury have completely normal CT.[47,65] A clinical decision rule to identify patients at low risk for serious injury could spare many stable patients unnecessary CT.

Some studies have suggested that adults with no clinical findings of blunt torso trauma may have intraabdominal injuries, a result that (if true) would suggest that CT is required in apparently uninjured patients, based on trauma mechanism. However, methodologic problems cast doubt on the findings. Salim et al.[66] studied 1000 patients without obvious signs of torso trauma and reported that 8.3% (83 patients) had an abnormal abdominal CT suggesting or confirming injury. However,

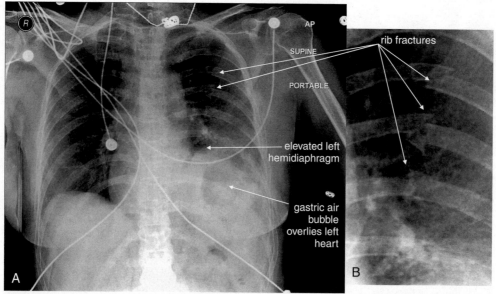

Figure 10-30. Left-sided diaphragmatic rupture from blunt trauma. A, supine portable AP chest x-ray. Several features of this x-ray strongly suggest traumatic diaphragm rupture. First, the left hemidiaphragm is elevated relative to the right. Normally, the right hemidiaphragm is slightly higher than the left because the liver is larger than the spleen. Second, the apparent gastric air bubble overlies the heart in the left chest. Third, the costovertebral angle is not clear on the left, though this is a nonspecific finding. The patient has multiple left posterior rib fractures, suggesting a high-energy trauma mechanism that might also produce diaphragm rupture. The patient's CT is explored in Figures 10-31 and 10-32. **B,** Close-up from **A.**

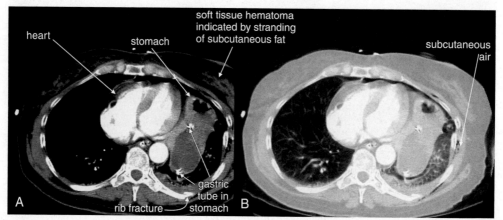

Figure 10-31. Left-sided diaphragmatic rupture from blunt trauma. Same patient as in Figures 10-30 and 10-32. CT with IV contrast, axial images. **A,** Soft-tissue window of a slice through the T6 level. The stomach is seen in the left chest abutting the heart. A gastric tube is seen passing through the stomach. These findings confirm diaphragm rupture, even without direct visualization of the diaphragm injury. These findings could be recognized without the use of any contrast agents. This patient received intravenous but not oral contrast. A soft-tissue contusion is seen in the left chest wall. A posterior fracture of the sixth rib is visible—this could be inspected in more detail on a bone window. **B,** Lung window showing subcutaneous air but no large pneumothorax.

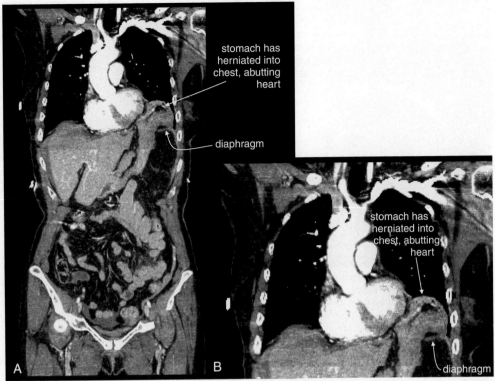

Figure 10-32. Left-sided diaphragmatic rupture from blunt trauma. Same patient as in Figures 10-30 and 10-31. **A,** In this coronal reconstruction, the stomach abuts the heart, having herniated through a diaphragmatic injury. **B,** Close-up from **A.**

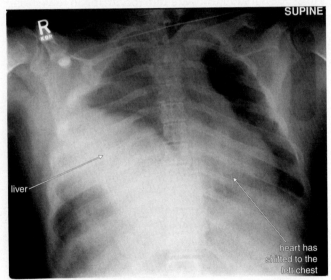

Figure 10-33. Right-sided diaphragmatic rupture from blunt trauma. AP supine chest x-ray. Though rarer than left-sided ruptures, right diaphragm ruptures can occur and must be recognized. This 17-year-old male presented in respiratory distress after a motor vehicle collision. He has herniated the entire liver and segments of colon into the right chest, resulting in mediastinal shift to the left. His respiratory distress is likely because of complete compressive atelectasis of the right lung, as well as compression of the left lung by the shifted mediastinum. The patient's CT is explored in Figure 10-34.

nearly half of patients with injuries detected by CT had abnormally depressed mental status, preventing reliable abdominal examination. The authors admitted to not examining the patients with normal mental status for signs of injury such as costal tenderness.[66] It is possible

that simple physical examination and history could exclude abdominal injuries in awake and alert patients.

Other studies have suggested that physical examination and complaints correlate poorly with injury. In a prospective study of more than 2000 adult blunt trauma patients, 19% of patients with CT demonstrating abdominal injury had no abdominal tenderness—although the rate of intoxication and altered mental status in this group was not documented. Among those with abdominal tenderness or bruising, only 22% had a positive CT.[47] Abdominal tenderness and bruising alone appear insufficient to select patients for CT.

Another clinical scenario for which abdominal CT is often obtained is "clearance" of the abdomen in patients requiring urgent extraabdominal surgery. Often, patients with no abdominal signs or symptoms undergo CT, with the rationale for CT in this instance being the inability to observe for worsening signs or symptoms in a patient under general anesthesia for operative treatment of other injuries. Do patients of this type require abdominal CT? In a prospective observational study, Schauer et al.[67] enrolled 201 patients scheduled to undergo extraabdominal surgery for orthopedic (91%), facial (8%), soft-tissue (3%), vascular (2%), neurosurgical (1%), urologic (1%), and ophthalmologic (0.4%) injuries. Patients were excluded if they had isolated extremity injuries (with no mechanism for blunt abdominal injury), signs or symptoms of abdominal injury (including systolic blood

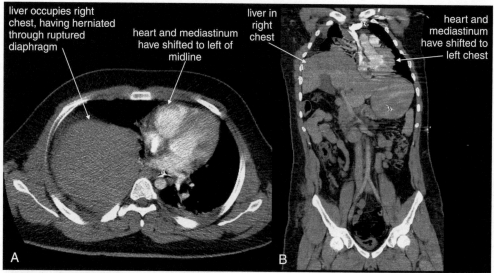

Figure 10-34. Right-sided diaphragmatic rupture from blunt trauma. Same patient as in Figure 10-33. CT with IV contrast, soft-tissue windows. A right diaphragm rupture has occurred. **A,** Axial image. At the level of the scapula, the liver is seen in the right thorax adjacent to the heart, which has been displaced into the left chest. Kinking of the superior mediastinum results, similar to the case in a tension pneumothorax. **B,** A coronal reconstruction highlights the mediastinal shift.

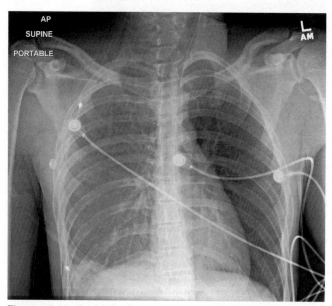

Figure 10-35. Transhepatic gunshot wound with hemothorax and diaphragm injury. This patient sustained a gunshot wound to the abdomen but was hemodynamically stable on arrival. Chest x-ray shows veiling of the right thorax, suggesting a hemothorax. This appearance is typical on a supine chest x-ray, whereas an upright chest x-ray usually would show a meniscus because of dependent thoracic fluid. The patient underwent abdominal CT, shown in Figure 10-36. Always consider chest injury with any penetrating abdominal or flank wound because the course of a penetrating injury may cross the diaphragm.

pressure <90 mm Hg; abdominal, flank, or costal margin tenderness; abdominal wall contusion or abrasion; pelvic fracture; and gross hematuria), or unreliable findings on abdominal examination as a consequence of a Glasgow Coma Scale (GCS) score below 14, paralysis, or mental retardation. Three patients had abdominal injuries detected at CT (1.2%; 95% CI = 0.2%-3.4%), including two splenic injuries managed with simple observation.

One patient (0.4%; 95% CI = 0%-2.2%) underwent splenectomy; this patient had multiple abdominal injuries, including kidney and pancreatic injuries sustained in a motorcycle collision.[67] The authors concluded that intraabdominal injuries are rare (occurring in fewer than 2%) in patients with normal mental status and no examination evidence of abdominal injury.

A large prospective study to further characterize the criteria for abdominal CT in blunt trauma patients was needed. Holmes et al.[1] prospectively derived and then internally validated two clinical decision rules for stable adult patients with blunt abdominal trauma in a cohort of more than 5000 patients (Box 10-1). The first rule, intended to identify injuries requiring intervention (laparotomy or angiographic embolization) consisted of hypotension, a GCS score less than 14, costal margin tenderness, abdominal tenderness, a hematuria level greater than or equal to 25 red blood cells per high-power field, and a hematocrit level less than 30%. This rule was 100% sensitive (95% CI = 93.4%-100%).[1]

The second (more conservative) rule, intended to identify all intraabdominal injuries, consisted of a GCS score less than 14, costal margin tenderness, abdominal tenderness, femur fracture, a hematuria level greater than or equal to 25 red blood cells per high-power field, a hematocrit level less than 30%, and an abnormal chest radiograph result (pneumothorax or rib fracture) (Box 10-2). This rule was 95.8% sensitive (95% CI = 91.1%-98.4%), was 29.9% specific (95% CI = 27.5%-32.3%), and had a negative predictive value of 98.6% (95% CI = 97.1%-99.5%) in a high-risk population (1595 patients, in whom 9% had abdominal injury).[1] The authors advocated use of the combined set of criteria to

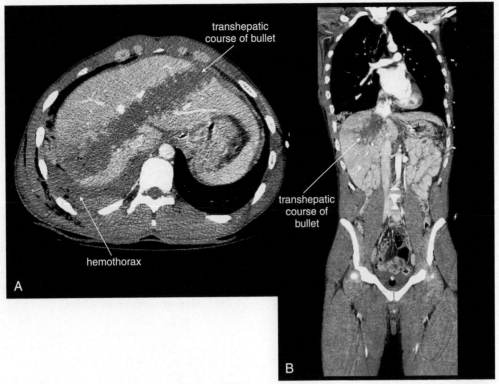

Figure 10-36. Transhepatic gunshot wound with diaphragm injury. Same patient as in Figure 10-35. **A,** Axial view. **B,** Coronal view. CT with IV contrast (soft-tissue windows) shows a transhepatic gunshot wound with an associated hemothorax. The presence of simultaneous chest and abdominal injuries suggests a diaphragmatic perforation, which was confirmed at surgery.

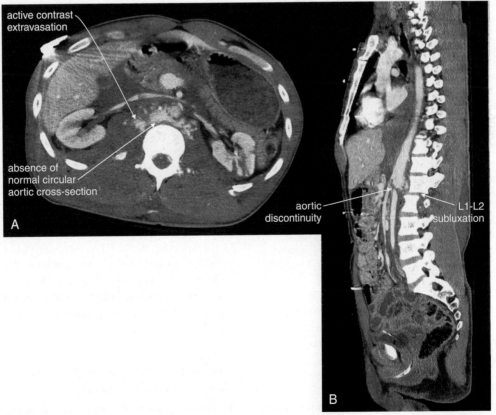

Figure 10-37. Abdominal aortic injury from blunt trauma. This patient sustained a traumatic L1-2 spinal subluxation resulting from a fall from great height. The abdominal aorta was torn at the site of spinal trauma, an unusual injury following a blunt mechanism. CT with IV contrast, soft-tissue windows. **A,** Axial view shows an absence of the normal circular cross section of the aorta, as well as the presence of abnormal contrast extravasation. **B,** Sagittal view shows the aortic discontinuity at the level of spinal injury. Following an emergent aortic repair, the patient survived with relatively normal neurologic and vascular function.

Box 10-1: Clinical Decision Rule for Abdominal/Pelvic CT in Adults Following Blunt Trauma, detects injuries requiring intervention

This clinical decision rule identifies adult patients who require laparotomy or angiographic embolization following blunt abdominal trauma. Patients meeting any single criterion are at risk. Patients meeting none of the criteria are at low risk and are unlikely to benefit from abdominal CT.

- **Hypotension**
- **GCS score <14**
- **Costal margin tenderness**
- **Abdominal tenderness**
- **Hematuria level ≥25 red blood cells per high-powered field**
- **Hematocrit level <30%**

Adapted from Holmes JF, Wisner DH, McGahan JP, et al. Clinical prediction rules for identifying adults at very low risk for intraabdominal injuries after blunt trauma. *Ann Emerg Med* 54:575-584, 2009.

Box 10-2: Clinical Decision Rule for Abdominal/Pelvic CT in Adults Following Blunt Trauma, detects any injury

This clinical decision rule identifies adult patients with any intraabdominal injury following blunt abdominal trauma. Patients meeting any single criterion are at risk. Patients meeting none of the criteria are at low risk and are unlikely to benefit from abdominal CT.

- **GCS score <14**
- **Costal margin tenderness**
- **Abdominal tenderness**
- **Femur fracture**
- **Hematuria level ≥25 red blood cells per high-powered field**
- **Hematocrit level <30%**
- **Abnormal chest radiograph result (pneumothorax or rib fracture)**

Adapted from Holmes JF, Wisner DH, McGahan JP, et al. Clinical prediction rules for identifying adults at very low risk for intraabdominal injuries after blunt trauma. *Ann Emerg Med* 54:575-584, 2009.

Box 10-3: Clinical Decision Rule for Abdominal/Pelvic CT in Pediatric Patients Following Blunt Trauma, detects any injury

This clinical decision rule identifies pediatric patients with any intraabdominal injury following blunt abdominal trauma. Patients meeting any single criterion are at risk. Patients meeting none of the criteria are at low risk and are unlikely to benefit from abdominal CT.

- **Low age-adjusted systolic blood pressure**
- **Abdominal tenderness**
- **Femur fracture**
- **Increased liver enzyme levels (serum aspartate aminotransferase concentration >200 U/L or serum alanine aminotransferase concentration >125 U/L)**
- **Microscopic hematuria (urinalysis >5 red blood cells per high-power field)**
- **Hematocrit level <30%**

Adapted from Holmes JF, Mao A, Awasthi S, et al. Validation of a prediction rule for the identification of children with intraabdominal injuries after blunt torso trauma. *Ann Emerg Med* 54(4):528-533, 2009.

identify patients at low risk for injury, not requiring CT. Use of these rules would have safely eliminated CT in around 30% of study patients. These rules have not been externally validated.

Pediatric Blunt Trauma Decision Rules

The same imperatives for a clinical decision rule for blunt trauma take on even greater significance in pediatrics (Box 10-3). Here, concerns about radiation exposure are heightened, with models suggesting a higher risk for radiation-induced cancers from CT exposures in younger patients.[68-70] The estimated attributable mortality risk from a single abdominal CT in a 1-year-old is 0.18%.[68] Moreover, young patients may require sedation to undergo CT, with attendant procedural risks. Holmes et al.[71-73] derived and validated a clinical decision rule to identify pediatric patients with any abdominal injury after blunt abdominal trauma. The rule consisted of six variables: low age-adjusted systolic blood pressure, abdominal tenderness, femur fracture, increased liver enzyme levels (serum aspartate aminotransferase concentration >200 U/L or serum alanine aminotransferase concentration >125 U/L), microscopic hematuria (urinalysis >5 red blood cells per high-power field), or an initial hematocrit level less than 30%. Patients meeting none of these criteria were at very low risk of injury. In a validation cohort of 1119 patients, the rule was 94.9% sensitive (95% CI = 90.2%-97.7%) and 37.1% specific (95% CI = 34%-40.3%). Use of the rule would have reduced CT use by 33%. The rule missed 8 patients, only 1 of whom underwent laparotomy, which was nontherapeutic (identifying a serosal tear and mesenteric hematoma not requiring intervention). This rule requires external validation.

Is There a Role for Pan-Scan CT in Patients With Blunt Abdominal Trauma?

In contrast to the admonition for limited CT based on clinical decision rules, other authors have cautioned that significant injuries are often present in patients with no signs of symptoms of abdominal trauma. Several studies have concluded that so-called pan-scan CT (CT of the head, neck, chest, abdomen, and pelvis) is required following all blunt trauma—though these studies have serious methodologic flaws and have been widely criticized. We discuss some of these flawed studies here. Many of these studies suffer from both selection and spectrum bias. The studies are typically conducted in large, high-acuity, high-volume centers, and application of techniques developed in these settings is unlikely to yield similar results when used in centers with lower patient acuity and volume. In addition, studies of this type frequently suffer from poor collection of history and examination data. In one case, the authors titled their study "Whole Body Imaging in Blunt Multisystem Trauma Patients Without Obvious Signs of Injury," but in questions following their oral presentation, the investigators admitted failing to assess for obvious physical findings such as chest and spine tenderness.[66] Some studies also included both patients with abnormal mental status and those with normal mental status—two populations whose examination findings may be different in their reliability.[66]

Sampson et al.[74] reported a retrospective series of 296 patients undergoing comprehensive CT, including noncontrast CT of the head and cervical spine with contrast-enhanced CT of the chest, abdomen, and pelvis. The authors reported the detection of "unsuspected injuries," including 19 cervical spine injuries, 97 pneumothoraces, and 19 splenic injuries. Whether these injuries were truly unsuspected based on history and examination is not clear from the study design and manuscript. Moreover, the clinical importance of some injuries, including small pneumothoraces detected by CT, is unknown and not measured in this study. It is possible that detection of subtle injuries resulted in worsened patient outcomes by prompting unnecessary interventions such as thoracostomy. Despite this, the authors advocated comprehensive CT in blunt trauma patients, with little evidence to guide their selection of patients. The authors stated that all hemodynamically stable blunt trauma patients with more than two body systems involved were imaged. However, this study is highly selection biased because only 296 patients in a 7-year period were imaged in this manner, with an annual emergency department census of 85,000 visits. It is likely that only relatively sick patients were selected to undergo comprehensive CT. Application of this imaging strategy to all blunt trauma patients in other practice settings would likely result in imaging of less injured patients, with less potential benefit from intensive imaging. The cost and radiation exposure of this strategy would likely not be warranted.

Huber-Wagner et al.[75] retrospectively reported survival in 1494 patients undergoing whole-body CT for evaluation of blunt trauma, compared with 3127 not undergoing whole-body CT. They reported a 25% reduction in mortality risk in patients undergoing whole-body CT, compared with the predicted mortality using previously published trauma scores. The authors concluded "whole-body CT… significantly increased the probability of survival in patients with polytrauma." Unfortunately, retrospective studies such as this can demonstrate only association, not causation, as the authors suggested. Many confounding factors may cause studies such as this to reach precisely the wrong conclusions. Although the authors attempted to control for factors such as trauma-center type and year, this is not a randomized controlled trial and bias likely played an important part in outcomes in the two groups. Patients not undergoing whole-body CT may have differed in important but unmeasured ways from patients undergoing whole-body CT. For example, more stable patients may have been recognized by the treating physicians and selected for CT imaging, giving the false appearance that CT caused improved survival.[75] The type of physicians caring for the patients may have been the biggest determinant of outcome, with the use of CT as simply a marker of physician training. The local infrastructure at hospitals practicing whole-body CT may have differed from those not performing whole-body CT. The authors skipped an important step in demonstrating any cause–effect relationship when they failed to demonstrate injuries found on CT that plausibly could have been treated to reduce mortality. In commentaries upon this study, other authors pointed out that early deaths, before the completion of whole-body CT, could contribute to the worsened outcomes in the group not receiving whole-body CT.[76-79] In the first hour, 58 patients died in the non–whole-body CT group, compared with only 8 in the whole-body CT group. Although the authors of this study proposed a prospective randomized controlled trial, others have criticized them for aggressively suggesting whole-body CT based on their study.

Can Patients Be Safely Discharged Following a Normal CT for Blunt Abdominal Trauma? What Injuries Can Be Missed?

Historically, patients with blunt abdominal trauma were typically observed to allow repeat clinical examination and detection of evolving abdominal injuries. The introduction of CT allowed earlier detection of injury, but the safety of discharge following a normal abdominal CT was unknown. Reports of missed injuries such as bowel, mesenteric, and diaphragmatic injury prompted frequent admission even following a normal abdominal–pelvic CT.

Livingston et al.[47] (1998) prospectively studied 2299 adult blunt abdominal trauma patients using a standardized protocol with abdominal CT, followed by admission and observation. CT was negative in 1809 patients. Among these patients, 9 underwent celiotomy, including 6 therapeutic laparotomies for 3 bowel, 1 bladder, 1 kidney, and 1 diaphragmatic injury. Another 2 patients had nontherapeutic laparotomy, and 1 had a negative laparotomy. The negative predictive value of abdominal CT for celiotomy was 99.63% (lower 95% CI = 99.31%, lower 99% CI = 99.16%). The authors concluded that admission and observation are not required in patients following negative abdominal CT. This study benefits from its prospective design, protocol-driven follow-up, and high rate of injury (17% with abnormal CT). However, several important limits should be emphasized. Bowel injuries are rare following blunt abdominal injury, occurring in only 25 patients in this study (1% of patients). As a result, even a poor test will have an excellent negative predictive value for this injury. A fixed guess of "no bowel injury" will be correct in 99% of cases. However, in patients with a high pretest probability of bowel injury, a negative CT should be treated with caution. For example, a patient with increasing abdominal pain and tenderness and abdominal bruising should likely be observed despite normal CT. In this study, CT was only 88% sensitive for bowel injury, meaning that 1 in 8 patients with a bowel injury could be missed. The same principle applies to diaphragm injuries, which are also rare and difficult to detect with CT, with sensitivity as low as 66% in some studies.[22]

In pediatric patients, the safety of discharge following a negative abdominal CT has also been investigated. Awasthi et al.[65] prospectively enrolled 1295 patients younger than 18 years undergoing CT with IV contrast for evaluation of blunt abdominal trauma. Of these patients, 210 had injuries detected on CT. The authors then followed the 1085 patients with normal abdominal CT. Only two intraabdominal injuries were noted in patients with normal CT: a mesenteric hematoma and serosal tear discovered during nontherapeutic laparotomy and a perinephric hematoma on repeat CT not requiring therapy. The negative predictive value of a normal abdominal CT was 99.8% (95% CI = 99.3%-100%). This study is strengthened by excellent follow-up, large numbers, and a high-risk population, with 16% of the initial cohort having an abnormal CT indicating injury. The authors concluded that the probability of an injury requiring intervention is low in pediatric patients with normal abdominal CT and that routine admission is not necessary. As with the adult population, observation should be considered for patients with a high suspicion for injury based on examination and history because of the limited sensitivity of CT for bowel, mesentery, and diaphragm injuries.

Can Patients Be Safely Discharged Following a Normal CT for Penetrating Abdominal Trauma? What Injuries Can Be Missed?

The sensitivity of CT for penetrating torso injuries was described in detail earlier in this chapter. Based on a meta-analysis, the sensitivity, specificity, negative predictive value, positive predictive value, and accuracy were 94.90%, 95.38%, 98.62%, 84.51%, and 94.70%, respectively.[41] However, multiple studies document missed bowel and diaphragm injuries, suggesting that observation should be strongly considered following a negative CT. Studies that claim good outcomes with emergency department discharge following a negative CT suffer from significant losses to follow-up that may invalidate their results.[34]

Radiation Exposure in Trauma Imaging

Radiation exposures in trauma patients have received increasing attention in recent years. Winslow et al.[80] reported substantial radiation exposures during the first 24 hours of trauma care. In a sample of 86 patients meeting "less acute major trauma criteria," they noted a median effective dose of 40.2 mSv, equivalent to approximately 1005 chest radiographs. Hubert-Wagner et al.[75] also noted significant radiation exposures in patients undergoing whole-body CT but defended the exposure based on a calculated mortality risk reduction from CT of nearly 25%, compared with a cancer mortality risk in the range of 1 in 1250. This mortality benefit of CT has been strongly questioned (see the earlier discussion on pan-scan CT). Even the most vocal hawks regarding radiation risk for abdominal CT concede that "the risk–benefit balance is still strongly tilted toward benefit."[68] However, as the threshold to image patients with relatively minor mechanisms of trauma becomes lower, the risk–benefit ratio becomes less favorable. Because the cancer risk from CT-radiation exposure in an individual is small, this ratio always appears to favor use of CT, but on a population basis increased cancer rates result from unnecessary imaging. Radiation exposures can be reduced in low risk patients by use of clinical decision rules, clinical observation without CT, and imaging with ultrasound, which does not expose patients to ionizing radiation.

Can CT Be Performed in Pregnant Patients With Abdominal Trauma? What Is the Radiation Risk?

In the pregnant female, radiation to the abdomen and pelvis should be minimized because of concerns for fetal effects. However, unrecognized abdominal or pelvic injuries pose a threat to both the mother and the fetus. Contrary to common physician belief, a single abdominal or pelvic CT delivers a radiation dose below the threshold known to cause teratogenic or neurologic effects.[81-82] If significant concern exists for maternal injury, CT should be performed. An increase in pediatric cancers, particularly leukemias, is a theoretical risk for in utero irradiation.[82-83] If possible, a well-considered imaging plan should be develop to avoid redundant radiation exposures. For example, if CT is required, plain radiographs of the pelvis and lumbar–sacral spine should be avoided because these deliver fairly high radiation doses and provide no information that could not be gleaned from CT. When the suspicion for maternal injury is lower, alternative strategies such as observation with serial physical examination, serial ultrasound, and trending of laboratory data can take the place of immediate CT.

What Is the Risk From Intravenous Contrast?

IV contrast crosses the placenta in small quantities. Animal studies do not show fetal teratogenic or mutagenic effects or effects on fertility.[83a]

Are Special Findings Seen on CT During Pregnancy?

Pregnancy results in special findings on CT.[84] Hydronephrosis (resulting from compression of the ureters by the enlarged uterus) and enlarged ovarian veins are normal findings in later pregnancy. Diastasis of rectus abdominus muscles and widening of sacroiliac joints and pubic symphysis are normal in the third trimester. Nonenhancing regions of the placenta on IV contrast–enhanced CT (dark gray or hypoattenuating in appearance) can indicate placental infarction or abruption. These should not be confused with normal placental cotyledons that have central areas of low attenuation with surrounding high-attenuation rings. CT can demonstrate uterine rupture, characterized by extrauterine fetal parts or by oligohydramnios with free maternal abdominal and pelvic fluid. Fetal parts are not usually seen until late first trimester on CT, and direct detection of fetal injuries is rare. Hemorrhage in the amniotic cavity may be seen. Fetal loss is most often because of placental abruption or maternal hypotension.

Although MRI can be used to evaluate traumatic injuries, in most centers it is not rapidly available, making it impractical for patients with potentially serious and time-sensitive injuries.[84]

Can Imaging Rule Out Placental Abruption?

Placental abruption can occur with even minor trauma and should be considered in every patient with blunt abdominal trauma beyond 22 to 24 weeks.[85] Ultrasound is considered insensitive for detection of placental abruption, with sensitivity, specificity, and positive and negative predictive values of 24%, 96%, 88%, and 53%, respectively.[86] Retroplacental hematomas can be isoechoic with the placenta and uterus and may not be recognized.[87] Consequently, even if ultrasound appears reassuring, patients should undergo fetal heart rate monitoring for several hours for signs of fetal distress, such as bradycardia or tachycardia, that may the earliest signs of abruption.[88]

SUMMARY

Modern imaging techniques allow sensitive detection of many important traumatic abdominal injuries. Bowel and diaphragm injuries remain difficult to detect with CT. Ultrasound and plain radiography play important roles in patients who are too unstable to undergo CT. Clinical decision rules are being developed to identify patients at low risk for injury who can forgo CT.

CHAPTER 11 Imaging Abdominal Vascular Catastrophes

Joshua Broder, MD, FACEP

Abdominal vascular conditions demand special attention in diagnosis. First, despite highly variable presentations, they must be suspected by the clinician so that appropriate imaging can be performed. Routine abdominal imaging without vascular contrast agents can be normal in the presence of these life-threatening processes. Second, diagnostic imaging must be performed without delay, because these conditions are time sensitive and often fatal. Unfortunately, in many cases, the optimal test cannot be performed because of the patient's hemodynamic condition, renal insufficiency, or contrast allergy. Even when the best available tests are performed, the sensitivity of diagnostic imaging for some key conditions is not perfect, so the emergency physician must remain vigilant for the possibility of a false-negative test result. We begin by defining the disease conditions and then briefly discuss their epidemiology and presentation. Although no formal clinical decision rules exist for these conditions, some risk stratification strategies can improve patient selection for diagnostic imaging. We also discuss the sensitivity and specificity of available imaging tests and interpretation of imaging findings.

ABDOMINAL VASCULAR CATASTROPHES

Abdominal vascular catastrophes constitute a family of disorders sharing some key features but differing in details. Overall, these conditions primarily affect older patients, although rarely young patients with no apparent medical problems may be afflicted. Therefore vascular causes should always be considered in patients presenting with acute abdominal pain. According to Centers for Disease Control data, abdominal vascular diseases become an important cause of death by around age 50, with aortic aneurysm and dissection accounting for more than 13,000 U.S. deaths in 2006.[1] Mesenteric ischemia may be more common than epidemiologic data suggest, because it may be misdiagnosed and may be a cause of death in elderly patients not undergoing premortem definitive diagnostic testing or autopsy. Here, we define each of these disease states, pointing out risk factors as well as some common misconceptions about the presentation that may prevent timely recognition.

GENERAL APPROACH TO THE PATIENT WITH POTENTIAL ABDOMINAL VASCULAR CATASTROPHE

The clinical presentations of abdominal aortic aneurysm (AAA) rupture, abdominal aortic dissection, and mesenteric ischemia can overlap substantially, and a unified imaging approach to evaluate for all is best when any of the three is suspected. General resuscitation measures, preoperative preparation, and surgical consultation should occur simultaneously with imaging. Because perforation of a viscus with pneumoperitoneum can present with sudden abdominal pain simulating vascular catastrophes, an upright portable chest x-ray is a reasonable bedside screening examination (Figure 11-1, and CT for comparison Figure 11-2), although it provides no specific information about abdominal vascular disorders. Other plain radiographs should be minimized, because these provide little diagnostic information and can waste precious time. Rarely, frank pneumatosis intestinalis may be seen on plain radiographs (Figure 11-3), but more often x-rays may provide false reassurance or misdiagnosis of a more benign abdominal condition. Bedside imaging with ultrasound by the emergency physician to assess for AAA should occur at the time of initial physical examination (Figures 11-4 to 11-11). If AAA is not recognized by ultrasound, rapid computed tomography (CT) without oral contrast should be obtained in the stable patient. Intravenous (IV) contrast should be used when possible, as explained later. The presentation of vascular catastrophes can also overlap considerably with other important abdominal conditions, which are discussed in Chapter 9. Fortunately, CT without oral contrast provides substantial information about many other abdominal conditions.

Abdominal Aortic Aneurysm

AAA is defined as dilatation of the aorta to a size greater than 3 cm in the abdomen. Risk factors for AAA include advancing age, male gender, cigarette smoking, atherosclerotic disease, and family history of AAA.[4] Diabetes, female gender, and black race are negatively associated with AAA.[4] However, advancing age is the greatest risk factor, and no patient can be considered at no risk unless aortic imaging has been performed. Risk of acute aneurysm rupture increases with increasing aneurysm size,

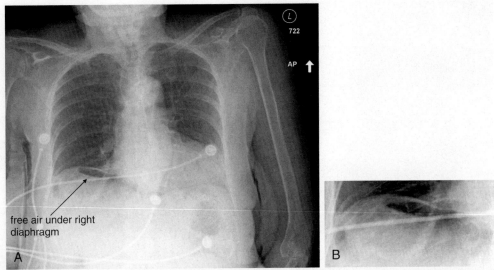

Figure 11-1. Pneumoperitoneum: X-ray. A, AP upright chest x-ray. **B,** Close-up from **A.** This 88-year-old female presented with sudden onset of severe abdominal pain, diaphoresis, and nausea. A wide differential diagnosis, including cardiac ischemia and abdominal catastrophes such as mesenteric ischemia, was considered. Ironically, the chest x-ray shows free air, but the patient had already been transported for computed tomography (CT) before the chest image was visible on the picture archiving and communication system. When abdominal vascular catastrophes are considered, an upright chest x-ray is a reasonable bedside examination for the competing diagnosis of intestinal perforation, particularly in an unstable patient. Unless the patient is too unstable for CT, other plain films should generally be avoided, because they are insensitive and nonspecific and can waste precious time. Plain x-ray can be avoided entirely, because CT has the advantage of simultaneously assessing for vascular catastrophes and a multitude of other causes of abdominal pain, including free air. Compare the above x-ray with CT in Figure 11-2.

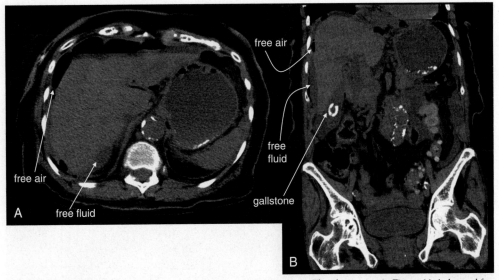

Figure 11-2. Pneumoperitoneum: CT without contrast. Same patient as Figure 11-1. The chest x-ray in Figure 11-1 showed free air, but the patient had already been transported for CT before the chest image was visible on the picture archiving and communication system (PACS). In the operating room, the patient was found to have a perforated duodenal ulcer. **A,** Axial image on soft-tissue window shows free air *(black)* outlining the liver. Free fluid *(gray)* is also visible. **B,** A coronal view shows similar findings. An incidental gallstone is also seen. Many forms of pathology can be detected without oral contrast, as described in Chapter 9.

which correlates with increasing wall tension. Above a diameter of 5 cm in women and 6 cm in men, the risk of rupture dramatically increases.[2-3] Lederle et al.[3] reported the 1-year incidence of rupture was 9.4% for AAAs of 5.5 to 5.9 cm, 10.2% for AAAs of 6.0 to 6.9 cm, and 32.5% for AAAs 7 cm or greater. Brown et al.[2] reported the rupture rate for aneurysms of 5.0 to 5.9 cm to be 1% per year in men and 3.9% per year in women. The rupture rate increased dramatically for both men and women with aneurysms of 6 cm or greater, reaching 14.1% and 22.3%, respectively. A rapid increase in the rate of aneurysm expansion also may predict rupture, although the mean difference in expansion rates between AAAs destined to rupture and those that do not rupture is small—an increase of less than 0.5 cm per year.[2]

The presentation of AAA rupture can be extremely variable. The classic presentation includes sudden abdominal and back pain, associated with hemodynamic collapse. This may be the most common presentation

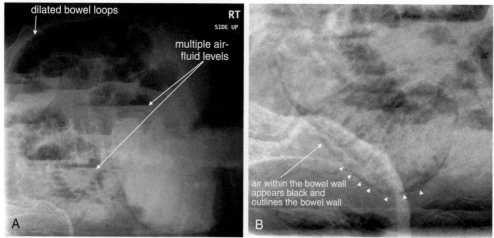

Figure 11-3. Mesenteric ischemia with pneumatosis: X-ray. This 77-year-old male presented with abdominal distension and vomiting, along with aching abdominal pain, for 2 days. He was suspected of having bowel obstruction, and plain films were obtained. His initial white blood cell count was 8.6, with normal bicarbonate and no anion gap. Minutes after this x-ray, he arrested in the emergency department and could not be resuscitated. **A,** Left lateral decubitus abdominal x-ray shows multiple air–fluid levels and dilated bowel loops, suggesting small-bowel obstruction. **B,** A closer look reveals mural pneumatosis. This patient may have had a closed loop obstruction leading to bowel ischemia or diffuse ischemia leading to ileus. Unfortunately, x-ray findings such as these occur after frank bowel necrosis, making them insensitive for early ischemia when intervention may be most beneficial. X-rays should generally not be obtained when bowel ischemia is suspected, because x-rays can be falsely reassuring and can waste precious time. Computed tomography with intravenous contrast is usually more definitive and should be performed as soon as possible. Delay for oral contrast is unnecessary and should be avoided when ischemic bowel is suspected.

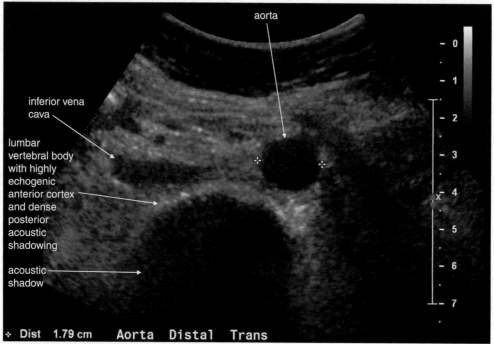

Figure 11-4. Normal aorta: Ultrasound. Bedside ultrasound in the hands of emergency physicians has been shown to be sensitive for the presence of abdominal aortic aneurysm. Ultrasound is considered poorly sensitive for rupture. In the presence of symptoms suggestive of aortic rupture, identification of an aneurysm by bedside ultrasound should be acted upon as if diagnostic of rupture. This ultrasound demonstrates a normal aorta, viewed in short-axis (transverse) cross section. The aorta should be examined in cross section from the xiphoid process to the umbilicus, the usual location of the aortic bifurcation to form the iliac arteries. The majority of aortic aneurysms are infrarenal, and this area should be examined in detail. If measurements are made only at the subxiphoid and umbilical levels, an aneurysm might be missed, because the aortic diameter may be quite normal proximal and distal to a sacular aneurysm. Several features of the normal aorta should be recognized. First, the normal abdominal aorta lies just anterior and to the left side of the lumbar vertebral bodies. These are identified by their highly echogenic anterior surface (the bony cortex), which reflects sound waves and casts a dense posterior acoustic shadow. This should not be confused for an aortic aneurysm and is a reliable landmark for orientation. The normal aorta should be less than 3 cm in diameter and have a circular cross-sectional contour. The inferior vena cava (IVC) should lie just anterior to the lumbar vertebral bodies, on the right side. The IVC should be the same size or smaller than the aorta. Depending on the patient's intravascular volume status, the IVC may be round or may have a flattened, elliptical shape. The IVC often varies in size and shape with respiration, but this should not be mistaken for the pulsatile aorta.

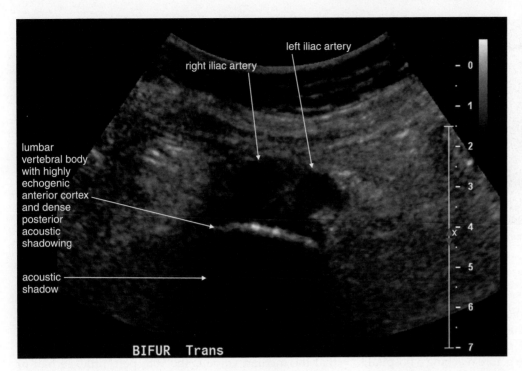

Figure 11-5. Normal ilioaortic bifurcation: Ultrasound. Transverse (short axis) view. Around the level of the umbilicus, the aorta bifurcates to form the iliac arteries. Do not confuse these with the aorta and vena cava—a normal iliac artery diameter may occur with an aneurysm of the more proximal aorta. Be sure to examine the aorta from xiphoid process to the iliac bifurcation.

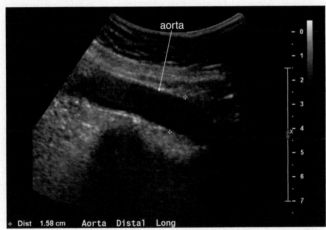

Figure 11-6. Normal abdominal aorta: Ultrasound. Sagittal (long axis) view. Should the aorta be measured in long axis cross section? This is a standard measurement made by ultrasonographers, but be wary as an emergency ultrasonographer: this is a source of a potential pitfall. If the ultrasound probe slides to the patient's right, the inferior vena cava (IVC), rather than the aorta, may be seen and measured. Though they do not look identical, the IVC might be mistaken for the aorta by a novice sonographer. Moreover, a long-axis view may not provide the maximal aortic diameter if the probe is positioned not in the midsagittal plane but, rather, slightly to the right or left of the midline diameter of the aorta. The diameter measured would then be a chord with a smaller length than the true diameter, underestimating the size of the aorta. See Figure 11-11 for an illustration.

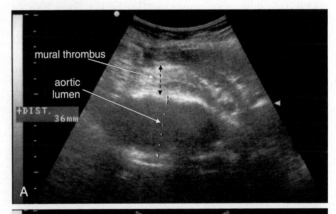

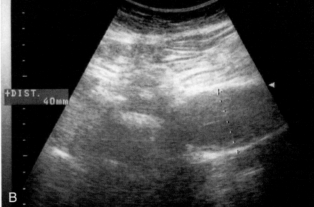

Figure 11-7. Large unruptured aortic aneurysm: Ultrasound. In a patient suspected of ruptured abdominal aortic aneurysm, detection of an aortic aneurysm on ultrasound has a high correlation with rupture. **A,** In this transverse (short-axis) image, the lumen of the aorta measures 36 mm, but the actual diameter is larger. Mural thrombus is visible, with a total aortic diameter of more than 50 mm. **B,** A long-axis image, the patent lumen measures 40 mm, but care must be taken to look for mural thrombus.

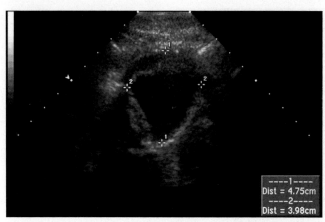

Figure 11-8. Unruptured abdominal aortic aneurysm: Ultrasound. A transverse view of the distal abdominal aorta. Again, adherent mural thrombus is present. This must be recognized to prevent undermeasurement of the aortic diameter.

of AAA rupture, but the majority of patients who have AAA ruptures with immediate hemodynamic instability never reach an emergency physician's care. Of those with AAA ruptures, 50% die before reaching a hospital,[5] and the overall mortality is greater than 50%.[6] In those patients surviving until hospital arrival, the clinical presentation is often more subtle. Fewer than half of those patients reaching the emergency department have the classic features of abdominal and back pain with hypotension.[7] In one study of patients dying from AAA rupture, only 20% of patients presented with abdominal and back pain with hypotension.[5] Hypotension with back or abdominal pain occurred in 60%.

Although a pulsatile abdominal mass is classically present, in several studies, the presence of a palpable pulsatile mass is unreliable. The sensitivity of abdominal palpation has been estimated from 15 studies of asymptomatic patients screened with ultrasound. For smaller AAAs, between 4.0 and 4.9 cm, the sensitivity of palpation is only around 50%, although these aneurysms have a low rate of rupture. The sensitivity of physical exam reaches 76% with an aortic diameter of 5 cm and greater, meaning that as many as one in four large AAAs in a size range at risk of acute rupture might be missed by palpation. The negative likelihood ratio for palpation in AAAs greater than 4.0 cm is only 0.51 with a 95% confidence interval (CI) of 0.38 to 0.67, making the absence of AAA by examination too unreliable for clinical use. The sensitivity of palpation is also compromised by increasing abdominal girth.[8] The sensitivity of physical examination in the setting of acute rupture is not well studied. Marston et al.[9] reported a pulsatile mass to be present in only about 60% of 152 patients with a ruptured AAA. In those patients who were initially misdiagnosed, only 26% had a pulsatile mass. It is possible that examination is even less sensitive once the AAA has ruptured. As a consequence, physical examination must never be used to rule out AAA rupture.

Historically, AAA rupture has been misdiagnosed initially in 30% to 60% of cases[9-11] or diagnosed after substantial delay. Many patients present with surprising apparent hemodynamic stability and lack of anemia.[10] Gaughan et al.[11] found that initial hemodynamic stability was associated with delay in diagnosis, perhaps reflecting the supposition among physicians that AAA rupture would ubiquitously result in shock. Common alternative diagnoses in cases of actual ruptured AAAs include renal colic, urinary tract infection, spinal disease, diverticulitis, and gastrointestinal hemorrhage.[9-12] Although these misdiagnoses may be less common today in an age of ubiquitous CT, the frequency of misdiagnosis in the past highlights the insensitivity of history and physical examination for the diagnosis. In one study of patients dying from AAA rupture within 2 hours of presentation, the median presenting systolic blood pressure was 110 mm Hg, the median presenting heart rate was 71 bpm, and the median presenting hemoglobin was 9.0 g/dL—all values that might be mistakenly interpreted as relatively reassuring.[5] Remember that the median value is the 50th percentile, so half of patients had laboratory or vital sign values less ominous than those listed above. That these values occurred in patients who ultimately died within 2 hours of emergency department arrival emphasizes that seemingly reassuring vital signs and laboratory values offer little prognostic reassurance. This also stresses the urgency of rapid imaging, as diagnosis using CT with oral contrast can result in delays as great as 140 minutes.[13] Although the time before diagnosis or death in some cases of AAA rupture can be greater than 24 hours, 12.5% of patients die within 2 hours of emergency department presentation without intervention.[5] In any individual patient, the moment of hemodynamic collapse cannot be predicted, and all urgency should be taken in making the diagnosis. Patients who are hemodynamically unstable at the time of surgery have a higher 30-day mortality rate than those who are not, emphasizing the need to identify patients with AAA rupture before physiologic collapse.[11]

Imaging for Suspected Ruptured Abdominal Aortic Aneurysm

Because of the potential for rapid and sudden hemodynamic collapse, imaging for suspected AAA must be performed as rapidly as possible. *Simultaneous with all diagnostic imaging should be patient resuscitation and surgical consultation.* As we discuss in detail later, ultrasound is a sensitive modality for the presence of AAA, although it is insensitive for detecting aneurysm rupture.[14] CT without any contrast, or with IV contrast if time allows, is usually definitive. X-rays play little role except in evaluating for other immediate surgical causes of abdominal pain such as free peritoneal air and should be avoided when possible to prevent dangerous delay.

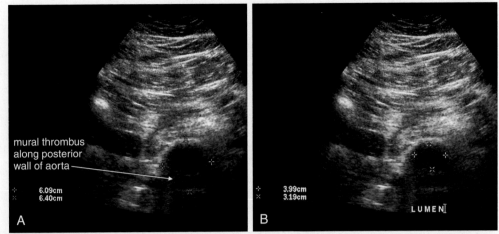

Figure 11-9. Abdominal aortic aneurysm (AAA): Ultrasound. Ultrasound is sensitive for detection of AAA when the aorta can be visualized. An aneurysm is defined by a diameter 1.5 times the upper limit of normal. Because the normal aorta is 2 cm or less, any diameter exceeding 3 cm defines an aneurysm. As described in the earlier figure on ultrasound of the normal aorta, it is essential to examine the aorta in short-axis cross section from the xiphoid process to the iliac bifurcation, because an aneurysm may be present anywhere along this course and could be missed by measurements only at the subxiphoid and umbilical levels. This figure demonstrates another potential pitfall for the inexperienced emergency sonographer. Many aortic aneurysms have a mural thrombus that may eccentrically or concentrically surround the residual lumen. If the lumen alone is measured, it may appear to be of normal caliber, or smaller than the 5-cm size at which aneurysmal rupture becomes more likely. The complete diameter of the aorta, including both the residual lumen and the mural thrombus, must be measured to determine the true size of the aorta. In this transverse view of the distal aorta, the aorta is 6 cm in diameter. A mural thrombus is present along the posterior wall of the aorta. The lumen measures between 3 and 4 cm. Although measurement of the lumen alone would allow recognition of aortic aneurysm, it would underestimate the size of the aorta. Look carefully for mural thrombus. **A,** Short-axis view. The full diameter, including the thrombus, is measured. **B,** Short-axis view. Only the lumen is measured, underestimating the aneurysm size.

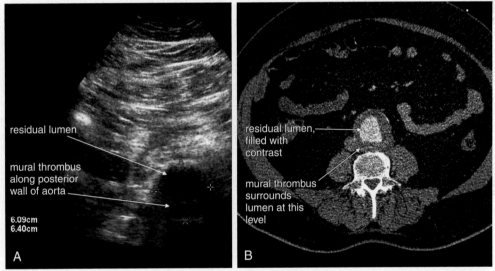

Figure 11-10. Abdominal aortic aneurysm: Ultrasound and CT with IV contrast, demonstrating mural thrombus. This figure compares the ultrasound from Figure 11-9 **(A)** with the intravenous contrast–enhanced CT scan **(B)** performed in the same patient, which clearly demonstrates the eccentric mural thrombus. We explore CT findings in more detail in the next several figures.

Ultrasound for Abdominal Aortic Aneurysm. Ultrasound is considered highly sensitive for the detection of AAA. Multiple studies have investigated ultrasound in the hands of emergency physicians. In the context of acute abdominal pain, the presence of AAA on emergency physician–performed ultrasound has a very high positive predictive value, allowing rapid triage to operative care without further imaging.[14-15] Ultrasound measurements of aortic diameter performed by emergency physicians correlate closely with measurements made using CT or MRI, differing by only around 4 mm.[16-17] Knaut et al.[17] reported that aortic measurements by emergency physicians closely estimated those from CT, differing by less than 1.5 cm at the superior mesenteric artery (SMA) and 1 cm at the aortic bifurcation in 95% of cases. Emergency physicians can perform the examination rapidly, in fewer than 5 minutes in most cases.[17] The examination is simple to learn as well, with physicians becoming proficient after brief training.[18] In one study of an abbreviated ultrasound examination performed in patients with suspected ruptured AAA, the sensitivity of ultrasound for detection of AAA is reported as 97%, with few indeterminate results in the hands of radiologists.[14] Tayal et al.[15] found that ultrasound performed by emergency physicians was 100% sensitive (95% CI = 89.5%-100%) with 98% specificity (95% CI = 92.8%-99.8%).

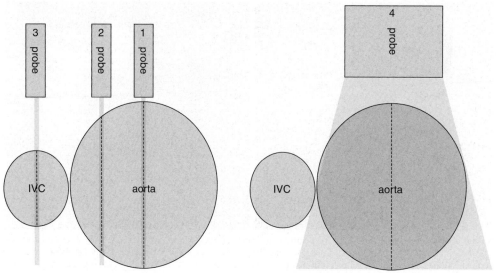

Figure 11-11. Abdominal aortic aneurysm: Ultrasound. This diagram illustrates a pitfall of attempting to measure the aorta using a long-axis view. (1) If the ultrasound probe is positioned in the midline of the aorta in a sagittal plane, a true diameter will be measured, accurately indicating the maximum size of the aneurysm. (2) A probe moved to the patient's right will measure a chord through the aorta, reflecting less than the maximum aortic diameter. (3) If the probe slides even farther to the right, the inferior vena cava (IVC) may be measured, giving a falsely reassuring value because the IVC is essentially always less than 3 cm in size. (4) Turning the probe 90 degrees to measure the aorta in short-axis cross section avoids this pitfall—though multiple cross sections from xiphoid process to the iliac bifurcation should be measured, because the aortic diameter may change drastically along its course.

In their study, 10 of 27 patients were taken to the operating room without further imaging following emergency physician ultrasound diagnosis of AAA.[15] Costantino et al.[16] similarly found that emergency medicine resident–performed ultrasound was 94% sensitive (95% CI = 86%-100%) and 100% specific (95% CI = 98%-100%).

The normal appearance of the aorta is simple to recognize on ultrasound (see Figures 11-4 to 11-6). The aorta occupies a uniform location anterior to the vertebral column, which serves as a reliable landmark. On transverse imaging, the aorta usually lies slightly left of the midline of the vertebral column. The inferior vena cava usually lies just to the patient's right of the aorta. The anterior bony cortex of the vertebral body appears as a bright or highly echogenic curve, deep to the aorta. Deep to this curve, dense black acoustic shadowing occurs, making the remainder of the vertebral body invisible. Anticipation of this appearance of the vertebral body prevents mistaking the vertebral body for a large aortic aneurysm. The abdominal aorta should not exceed 2-3 cm. Aortic aneurysm is defined by a diameter exceeding 3 cm, although rupture is unlikely below 5 cm in women and 6 cm in men.[2]

Several pitfalls in the ultrasound evaluation of AAA should be considered. First, the reported sensitivity for AAA rupture is a stunning 4%, according to a single study published in *Radiology* in 1988.[14] In this study, an abbreviated ultrasound examination was performed during the ongoing resuscitation of the patient, and only the peri-aortic region was examined for blood. Blood collecting in other abdominal areas such as Morison's pouch might have been missed by the abbreviated exam. The retroperitoneum, where aortic hematoma might collect following a contained aortic rupture, is generally not well-evaluated

with ultrasound. The sensitivity for AAA rupture today with modern ultrasound machines is unknown but must be assumed to be poor until proven otherwise. The second pitfall is undermeasurement of the aortic diameter because of the presence of circumferential mural thrombus (see Figures 11-7 to 11-10). Thrombus is common within aortic aneurysms and reduces the fluid-filled lumen visible on ultrasound. Although thrombus is usually visible on ultrasound, if it is not recognized, the fluid-filled channel may be measured without inclusion of the thrombus, underestimating the aneurysm size. A third pitfall is failure to image the abdominal aorta along its entire length from the xiphoid process to the umbilicus. Aortic aneurysms may occur anywhere along this length, although infrarenal aneurysms are most common. An additional pitfall is measuring the aorta in a longitudinal direction but failing to sample along the maximal diameter (see Figure 11-11). If a section of the aorta parallel to the long axis but not along the midpoint is measured instead, undermeasurement of the diameter may occur. Despite these concerns, in one study, longitudinal measurements correlated better with CT than did transverse measurements.[19] Finally, failure to recognize a nondiagnostic ultrasound resulting from overlying bowel gas can result in a missed aneurysm.

Contrast-Enhanced Ultrasound. Several new studies suggest a possible solution to the poor sensitivity of ultrasound for the diagnosis of ruptured AAA. Contrast agents originally developed for echocardiography provide a means of visualizing both the aortic lumen and extravasation of blood. A variety of agents approved by the U.S. Food and Drug Administration are available. They shared a common feature of containing highly reflective microscopic bubbles that are extremely echogenic on ultrasound. Studies in the context of acute abdominal trauma and acute

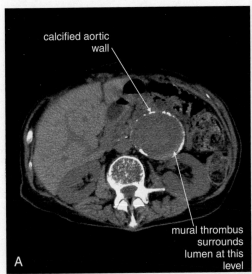
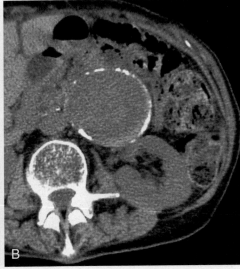

calcified aortic
wall

mural thrombus
surrounds
lumen at this
level

A   B

Figure 11-12. Unruptured abdominal aortic aneurysm (AAA): Noncontrast computed tomography (CT). A, noncontrast CT viewed on soft-tissue windows, demonstrating a very large AAA. **B,** Close-up from **A.** Characteristic features include a calcified rim and adherent mural thrombus, which is faintly visible on this noncontrast CT as a crescent-shaped rim along the aortic wall. Intravenous (IV) contrast better delineates this in the next figure. This patient does not have an aortic rupture, although it is difficult to be certain of this viewing this noncontrast CT. Retroperitoneal fat (nearly black) bounds the aorta posteriorly and on the patient's left, but the right and anterior margins of the aorta abut soft-tissue density, so a small amount of extraluminal bleeding could be missed on this scan. CT with IV contrast can evaluate for active bleeding, marked by contrast extravasation. In some cases, aortic rupture can be clearly identified on noncontrast CT. Examples of this are shown in Figures 11-15B and 11-16.

AAA rupture suggest improved sensitivity for extravasation of blood.[20-21] Contrast agents can be injected at the bedside with a single hand bolus, followed by immediate performance of ultrasound. Catalano et al.[22] reported the technique in the assessment of eight patients with ruptured AAA and visualized retroperitoneal hematoma and extravascular contrast leak in seven of the eight. The sensitivity has not been confirmed in larger series. Contrast-enhanced ultrasound has also been used to monitor aortic aneurysms for endoleak (discussed later in this chapter) following endovascular repair. In this setting, it has excellent sensitivity (100%) and specificity (93%) compared with multislice CT angiography. It outperforms color duplex ultrasound, which has a sensitivity of only 33.3% and specificity of 92.8%.[23] Ultrasound contrast agents can be used in patients with renal insufficiency, severe iodinated contrast allergy, or hemodynamic instability preventing use of CT scan.

Computed Tomography for Ruptured Abdominal Aortic Aneurysm.

CT scan without IV contrast can diagnose the presence of AAA and AAA rupture with high sensitivity and specificity (Figures 11-12 to 11-16).[24-25] An AAA is defined by an aortic diameter 3 cm or greater, but ruptures are rare in aneurysms of this size. The aorta is readily identified as a circular structure in cross section, anterior to the spine. On unenhanced CT, high-density retroperitoneal hematoma can be seen in the perinephric retroperitoneal space, sometimes displacing the kidney anteriorly.[26] Without IV contrast, blood shares the same density as the kidney and psoas muscle and can obscure the lower density fat plane that normally separates these two structures from one another and from the aorta. In addition, a high-attenuation crescent within

the aortic wall or within mural thrombus predicts rupture.[27-29] Without IV contrast, the crescent is considered to be "high attenuation" if its Hounsfield density exceeds that of unenhanced blood in the aortic lumen.[28] If time allows, CT scan with IV contrast provides more anatomic definition to allow open surgical or endovascular intervention (Figures 11-17 and 11-18; see also Figures 11-13 and 11-14). IV contrast also identifies ongoing hemorrhage at the time of CT. Oral contrast should never be used when AAA rupture is suspected, because it introduces an unacceptably long delay before imaging.[13]

Alternative Imaging Modalities for Abdominal Aortic Aneurysm Rupture.

Magnetic resonance imaging (MRI) and magnetic resonance angiography (MRA) can be used to diagnose AAA with excellent sensitivity and specificity, but the delay before imaging is unacceptably long in most institutions using this modality.[30] Noncontrast CT should always be preferred over MRI, because it is highly sensitive and specific for AAA and AAA rupture. Catheter-based formal angiography can be used to diagnose AAA with or without rupture, although in most institutions this has been replaced by ultrasound or CT imaging for diagnostic purposes, as angiography is both time-consuming and invasive. Plain radiographs play virtually no role in the diagnosis of AAA and should be avoided whenever possible, because they may introduce unacceptable diagnostic delay. Rarely, the calcified outline of an aortic aneurysm may be seen on x-ray, but the sensitivity is unknown and plain x-ray should not be used for this diagnosis (Figure 11-19). An exception to this rule is in the unstable patient in whom a competing diagnosis such as perforation of a hollow viscus is being considered. In this case, an

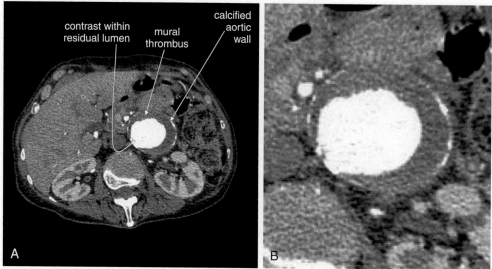

Figure 11-13. Unruptured abdominal aortic aneurysm: Computed tomography (CT) image enhanced by intravenous (IV) contrast. A, An IV contrast–enhanced CT scan performed immediately after the noncontrast CT in the same patient as Figure 11-12. **B,** Close-up from **A**. Both A and B are viewed on soft-tissue windows. With the administration of IV contrast, the true lumen can be clearly differentiated from the adherent mural thrombus, which is nearly circumferential in this patient. Calcifications in the aortic wall are visible. The contrast remains bounded within the rounded aortic contour, ruling out active bleeding from rupture (which would demonstrate contrast extravasation outside of the aortic contour). Oral contrast is not needed for evaluation of the abdominal aorta.

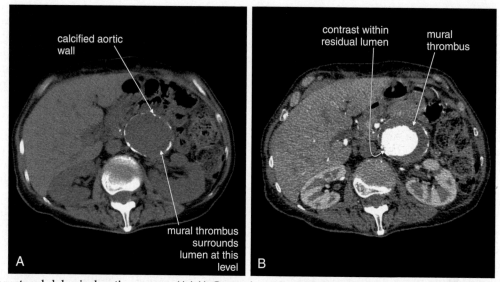

Figure 11-14. Unruptured abdominal aortic aneurysm (AAA): Comparison of noncontrast and intravenous (IV) contrast–enhanced computed tomography (CT). Noncontrast **(A)** and IV contrast–enhanced **(B)** CT scans were performed in the same patient on the same day. These slices are through the same level and demonstrate the additional value of IV contrast in delineating the lumen and adherent mural thrombus, which is faintly visible on the noncontrast scan. This patient does not have active rupture, so contrast is not seen leaving the aorta. **A,** The presence of an AAA can be confirmed or ruled out without IV contrast. IV contrast assists in the detection of active hemorrhage.

upright portable chest x-ray to assess for pneumoperitoneum can be rapidly performed (see Figure 11-1).

Angiography. Angiography is the historical gold standard for the diagnosis of AAA, aortic dissection, and mesenteric ischemia. Today, the wide availability of CT angiography has relegated catheter-based angiography to a purely therapeutic role following a diagnostic CT in most centers (discussed in more detail in Chapter 16). Angiography can be used for the treatment of even ruptured AAAs using endovascular stents.[31] Because the stent must be sized carefully to prevent occlusion of branch vessels

and to ensure that a leak does not occur at the margins of the stent, CT with IV contrast and multiplanar reconstructions is usually required (see Figures 11-17 and 11-18). Aortic dissection can also be diagnosed with angiography. Under angiographic guidance, stenting of dissections or fenestration of the intimal flap to restore blood flow to an occluded true lumen is sometimes used as a therapy. Angiography can be used to diagnose and treat mesenteric ischemia (see Figure 11-35 later in the chapter). Tissue plasminogen activator or similar thrombolytic agents can be infused through a catheter. Vascular stents can also be placed to restore blood flow. The urgency to restore bowel

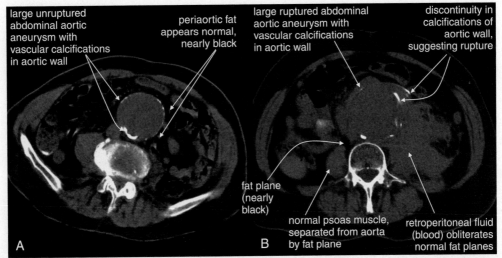

Figure 11-15. Unruptured and ruptured aortic aneurysms: CT without IV or oral contrast. A, An unruptured but large abdominal aortic aneurysm (AAA), identified by CT without IV contrast. CT without any contrast allows accurate identification of an aortic aneurysm. By definition, an aneurysm has a diameter of 3 cm or greater, though rupture is relatively rare under 4-5 cm. Increasing size is accompanied by increased rupture risk. Typical features include wall calcifications. The surrounding fat should appear nearly black on CT soft-tissue windows. Without IV contrast, blood within the aorta is dark gray on CT soft-tissue windows. **B,** A large ruptured AAA, identified on CT without IV contrast. Free peritoneal rupture has occurred, and blood is visible throughout the patient's left abdomen. Blood without contrast appears gray on CT. In this case, the extravasating blood appears slightly hyperdense (brighter) relative to blood in the aorta, despite the absence of injected contrast. This is a well-described phenomenon in the radiology literature. Rupture of an aneurysm can be detected without any contrast. Blood in the retroperitoneum obscures normal fat planes, such as that separating the aorta and psoas muscle. A retroperitoneal hematoma may also displace the kidneys.

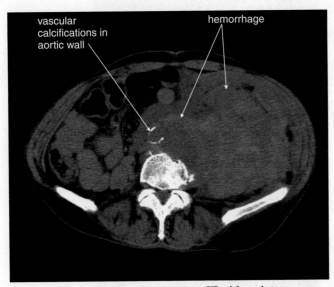

Figure 11-16. Ruptured aortic aneurysm: CT without intravenous or oral contrast. Free peritoneal rupture has occurred, and blood is visible throughout the patient's left abdomen.

perfusion cannot be overemphasized. Surgical consultation should be performed even if interventional radiology is the intended initial therapeutic approach. Death from delay in reperfusion can occur; increased time to surgery is strongly associated with poor outcome.[32]

Imaging of Patients With Prior Endovascular Abdominal Aortic Aneurysm Repairs: Endoleaks

Following endovascular repair of AAAs, an *endoleak* may occur (Figures 11-20 and 11-21).[33] An endoleak is defined as the continued flow of blood into the aneurysm sac. Endoleaks are graded as one of four types. *Type 1 endoleaks* occur immediately, at the time of placement of an endovascular graft, usually because of mis-sizing of the graft, such that the proximal or distal ends of the graft are not sealed against the aorta. This requires placement of a larger graft, because type 1 endoleak leaves the aneurysm sac subject to systemic vascular pressures with continued risk of acute rupture. *Type 2 endoleaks* result from retrograde flow of blood through collateral vessels into the aneurysm sac (see Figure 11-21). Common examples include filling of the aneurysm sac from lumbar perforating arteries. Type 2 endoleaks are often observed without treatment, because they do not subject the aneurysm sac to full systemic vascular pressures and are at relatively low risk of rupture. Type 2 endoleaks that do not resolve spontaneously can be treated with angiographic embolization. *Type 3 endoleaks* occur when a tear in the fabric of the graft occurs or if separation occurs between grafts consisting of multiple modules. This type of leak is relatively rare but leaves the aneurysm sac subject to systemic vascular pressures, requiring replacement of the graft because of continued risk of aneurysm rupture. *Type 4 endoleaks* occur from leaks through pores of the graft material and usually do not require repair.[33]

Definitive diagnosis of an endoleak can be made with IV contrast–enhanced CT (see Figures 11-20 and 11-21). Without IV contrast, the presence of an endoleak will go unrecognized on CT, because leaking blood will have a similar Hounsfield density to thrombus outside of the stent but contained within the aneurysm sac. With the addition of IV contrast, blood flow within the aneurysm sac outside of the stent is evident. Because retrograde filling of the aneurysm sac is often slow (e.g., with type 2 endoleaks described earlier), some endoleaks can be difficult to detect on arterial-phase CT with IV

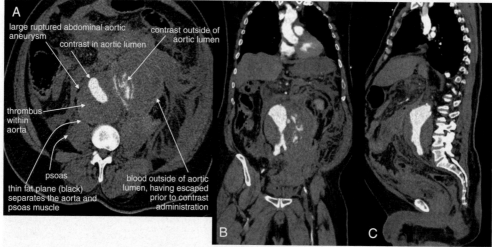

Figure 11-17. **Abdominal aortic aneurysm (AAA) rupture: CT with IV contrast. A,** Axial image. **B,** Coronal image. **C,** Sagittal image. All images are viewed on CT soft-tissue windows. Administration of IV contrast allows recognition of active contrast extravasation—ongoing hemorrhage at the moment of CT. However, IV contrast is not generally needed for recognition of AAA rupture. In this patient, blood is seen throughout the abdomen and retroperitoneum. Blood that escaped from the aorta before the administration of IV contrast appears dark gray. Abdominal and retroperitoneal fat appears nearly black on CT soft-tissue windows. Injected contrast appears bright white. Adherent thrombus within the aorta appears dark gray, whereas white contrast material defines the patent lumen. Contrast outside of the aorta indicates active hemorrhage. Compare the patient's right psoas muscle with the left. On the left, blood obscures the normal fat plane surrounding the psoas. The diagnosis of AAA rupture could have been made in this patient without any contrast. Multiplanar reconstructions with IV contrast are useful if the patient is sufficiently stable, because these allow sizing of endovascular grafts.

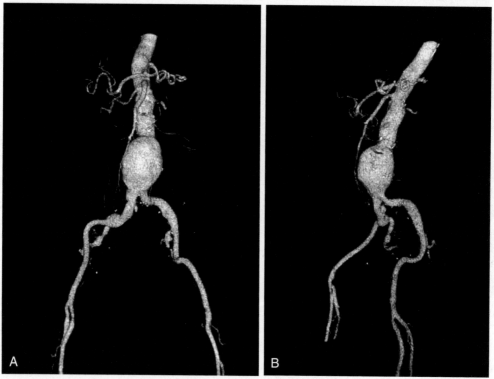

Figure 11-18. **Abdominal aortic aneurysm (AAA): Three-dimensional CT reconstructions.** Three-dimensional reconstructions can be generated and rotated in space to visualize the aorta for preoperative planning. Measurements from these three-dimensional models and from two-dimensional axial, coronal, and sagittal plane reconstructions are used to size endovascular grafts. Three-dimensional modeling requires fine CT slice acquisition, around 1.25 mm per slice, for high-quality rendering. Multiple software packages allow three-dimensional modeling from standard CT datasets. Here, a sacular AAA is viewed from the front **(A)** and side **(B).**

contrast. Additional delayed images (acquired approximately 5 minutes after initial contrast injection) may be required.[34-35] Some authors have argued against the need for delayed phase images, because most endoleaks detected with this technique resolve spontaneously without intervention.[36] Contrast-enhanced ultrasound can be used to assess for endoleak in patients with contraindications to IV contrast for CT. Contrast-enhanced ultrasound performs favorably compared with CT.[23,37] MRI can also be used to assess for endoleaks, because graft materials are MRI compatible. Contraindications to gadolinium contrast are discussed elsewhere in this chapter.

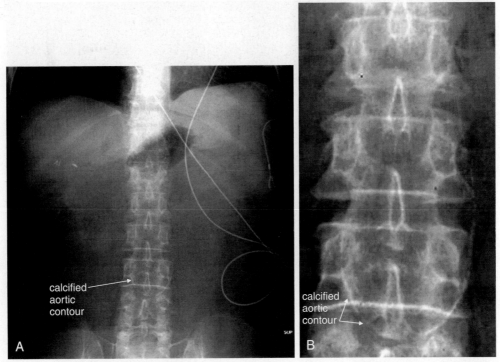

Figure 11-19. Abdominal aortic aneurysm (AAA): Plain radiograph. X-rays should not be used to diagnose the presence of AAA, because the sensitivity is unknown and the ability to detect rupture is likely poor. Occasionally, x-ray obtained for other suspected diagnoses may reveal a calcified aortic contour. **A,** Supine abdominal x-ray. **B,** Close-up from **A.**

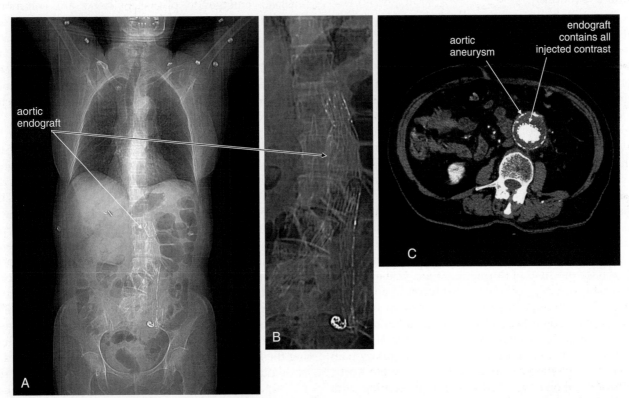

Figure 11-20. CT evaluation of patients with prior endovascular aortic aneurysm repair. A, B, CT scout images showing the radiodense graft. **C,** CT with intravenous (IV) contrast, showing contrast contained within the graft. CT is useful for assessment of patients with prior endovascular aortic aneurysm repair. Although the graft material is visible without IV contrast, detection of a leak of blood within the aneurysm sac but outside of the graft material (an endoleak) requires IV contrast. Here, contrast appears contained within the graft material.

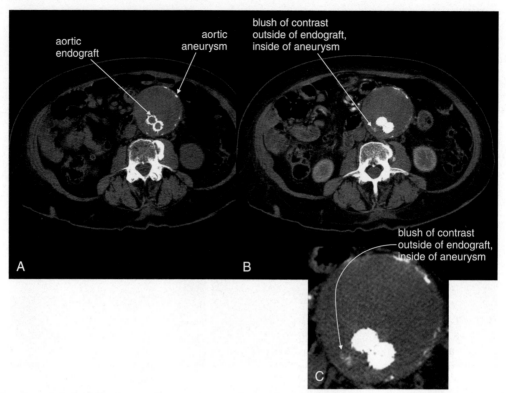

Figure 11-21. **Type 2 endoleak following aortic aneurysm endovascular repair: CT without and with intravenous (IV) contrast.**
A, A noncontrast CT shows the endograft within the aortic aneurysm but cannot detect an endoleak (leak of blood within the aneurysm sac, outside of the graft). **B, C,** IV contrast–enhanced CT shows contrast outside of the graft but within the aneurysm sac—confirming an endoleak. Some slow leaks are not seen on arterial phase imaging but are visible on delayed images.

Aortic Dissection

Dissection of the thoracic aorta presenting primarily with abdominal pain is rare, occurring in only 4.6% of cases in a large international registry.[38] However, mortality is increased in these patients, resulting from a delay in diagnosis because of atypical presentation.[38] Although type B aortic dissections (those affecting only the descending aorta) account for 37.5% of aortic dissections, only 1.3% of all aortic dissections affect solely the abdominal aorta.[39] Risk factors for aortic dissection include collagen vascular diseases such as Marfan's and Ehlers-Danlos syndrome, but these account for a minority of cases (2.9% of type B dissections) in the International Registry of Acute Aortic Dissection (IRAD), and a history hypertension is likely the greatest risk factor, occurring in 80%.[40] Pregnancy and the postpartum state are also risk factors, likely as a consequence of increased collagenase production during this time. Use of stimulant drugs such as cocaine can also result in aortic dissection.[41-42] Although the classic description of aortic dissection includes sudden tearing pain radiating to the back, the clinical presentation can be quite variable. Sudden pain is common (80% to 90%), as is migratory pain (25%).[38-40] In the International Registry of Acute Aortic Dissection, among type B dissections presenting with primarily abdominal pain, tearing pain was described in 25%, sharp pain in 44%, pressure-like pain in 33%, and burning pain in 6%.[38] The latter descriptors might

mislead emergency physicians who are commonly taught to seek "tearing" pain as a clue to aortic dissection. The age distribution for aortic dissection is skewed toward older patients, with a mean age of 65 years and with 42% of type B dissections occurring in patients 70 years or older. Patients with a personal or family history of connective tissue diseases must be suspected of dissection at a younger age.

Unlike aortic aneurysm rupture, which frequently leads to hemodynamic instability, aortic dissection can present without any substantial derangement of hemodynamics. Although hypertension is a risk factor for the development of aortic dissection, patients may present with normotension (28%), hypertension (69%), or hypotension (3%).[40] Initially, aortic dissection is a disease process involving only the intimal layer of the aorta. A tear in the intima develops, and blood typically undermines this layer, creating a flap that extends distally in the direction of blood flow. Proximal extension may also occur. Extension into branch vessels is the greatest threat, because it can disrupt perfusion to vital organs including the kidneys, mesentery, and bowel (21% in cases of abdominal aortic dissection); spinal perforating arteries (2.7%); and extremities (25% to 30%).[39-40] Proximal dissection can result in disruption of the aortic valve with acute valvular insufficiency. Dissection into the pericardium can occur, resulting in pericardial tamponade.

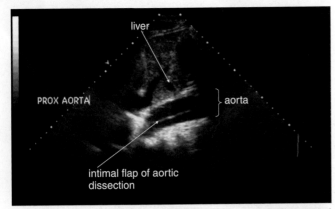

Figure 11-22. **Abdominal aortic dissection: Ultrasound.** This sagittal or long-axis ultrasound demonstrates the intimal flap of an aortic dissection in the proximal abdominal aorta.

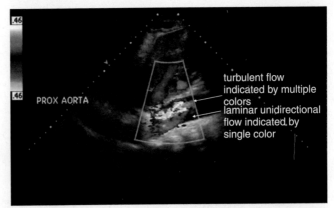

Figure 11-23. **Abdominal aortic dissection: Ultrasound with Doppler flow.** Same patient as Figure 11-22. Ultrasound demonstrates the intimal flap of an aortic dissection in the proximal abdominal aorta. Color Doppler shows differential blood flow in the true and false lumens. (*See Color Plate 1 for color Doppler image of this figure.*)

In none of these former cases does blood loss external to the aorta occur, accounting for the frequent relative hemodynamic stability of patients with aortic dissection.[38-40] This also accounts for the low sensitivity of chest x-ray for the diagnosis of thoracic aortic dissection and naturally for abdominal aortic dissection. In traumatic thoracic aortic injury, violation of all layers of the aorta may occur, leading to extravasation of blood and formation of a mediastinal hematoma, which can in turn lead to widening of the mediastinal silhouette on chest x-ray. In contrast, nontraumatic dissection may occur in an aorta of normal caliber and may be restricted to an intimal injury without formation of a mediastinal hematoma. This can result in a normal mediastinal silhouette on x-ray, occurring in as many as 20%, according to a large international registry.[40] Luker et al.[43] reported that only 25% of chest x-rays were prospectively interpreted as suggesting aortic pathology in cases of acute thoracic dissection.

Classic examination features such as pulse deficits are relatively rare in type B dissections, occurring in only about 20% to 30% of patients with type B thoracic or isolated abdominal aortic dissections.[39-40] The classic finding of a differential blood pressure between upper extremities is of unknown sensitivity and specificity. In a study of asymptomatic emergency department patients with a prior history of hypertension, 18% of patients had differences in the blood pressures obtained in the upper extremities exceeding 10 mm Hg.[44] This suggests that the finding is nonspecific, so its use as a screening tool would result in unnecessary diagnostic imaging in many patients. The sensitivity is also likely to be very low. If the intimal flap does not involve an extremity branch of the aorta, neither pulse deficits nor differential blood pressure might result. Reliance on this physical examination finding to prompt definitive imaging would result in failure to diagnose aortic dissection in many patients. Common features that should prompt evaluation for aortic dissection include sudden onset and migratory pain, which has been found to be a frequent, though not ubiquitous, feature. Abdominal pain in concert with back or chest pain is worrisome.

The presence of unilateral neurologic features also can suggest stroke from dissection involving the carotid arteries. Vertebral artery dissection can result in posterior circulation symptoms. Ischemic peripheral neuropathy occurs in a small minority of patients (2.2%).[40] Occlusion of spinal perforating arteries can result in neurologic deficits, including bilateral limb paralysis or sensory loss. Sometimes these symptoms can be transient, and they may be mistaken for patient malingering, sciatica, or spinal cord compression. Dissection of the mesenteric arteries can result in simultaneous mesenteric ischemia in as many as 5% of cases, and renal failure can result from dissection of the renal arteries in up to 13% (see Figures 11-25 and 11-26).[40] Limb ischemia (7%) may also result from abdominal aortic dissection involving the iliac arteries.[40]

Screening for aortic dissection using D-dimer measurement has been advocated by some authors, who have reported sensitivity of 93% to 100%.[45-52] A meta-analysis suggested a sensitivity of 94% (95% CI = 91%-98%).[53] However, other authors have reported sensitivities of 88% to 92%, with false-negative results reported in patients with thrombosed false aortic lumens. Moreover, the small size of most published studies results in wide 95% confidence limits. The lower confidence limits of sensitivity reported are as low as 67% to 85% in some studies; for this reason, some authors continue to raise concerns that D-dimer testing is too unreliable for clinical use, given the high mortality of aortic dissection.[54-55]

Imaging for Aortic Dissection

Because the clinical presentation of AAA rupture and abdominal aortic dissection can overlap substantially, diagnostic imaging for aortic dissection should begin with bedside ultrasound to assess for AAA. Ultrasound can sometimes visualize the intimal flap of dissection (Figures 11-22 and 11-23). However, the sensitivity is relatively low, around 70% with use of B scan and color Doppler techniques. Contrast-enhanced ultrasound has been reported to be 97% sensitive compared with CT, although the technique is not widely used.[56] CT without IV contrast cannot rule out aortic dissection, because the intimal flap typically shares the same density with blood in the true and false lumens (Figure 11-24). Rare case reports document aortic dissection on noncontrast CT, based on displacement of calcified atheromatous plaques or high attenuation clot within the false lumen, but the sensitivity of these findings is unknown and should not be relied upon.[57] Administration of a rapid bolus of IV contrast should be considered critical to the

diagnosis. Thus if a noncontrast CT is first performed to evaluate for AAA and is negative, CT with IV contrast must be performed if possible. With IV contrast, the intimal flap is highlighted as an unenhanced line separating the true and false lumens of the aorta (see Figure 11-24). A normal aorta is circular in cross section, filling uniformly with bright contrast. When an intimal flap is present, the circular cross section appears divided into two lumens. These may be unequal in size. Both lumens may enhance with contrast, or one or both lumens may be thrombosed and fail to enhance (Figure 11-25).

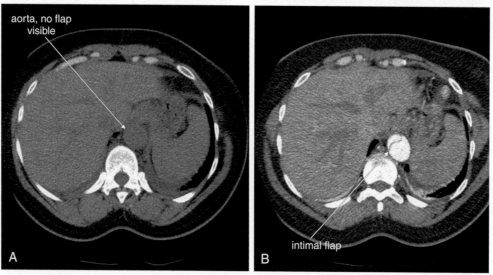

Figure 11-24. Aortic dissection involving the abdominal aorta: CT without and with intravenous (IV) contrast. Soft-tissue windows. **A,** On CT without IV contrast, the intimal flap of dissection is not visible. **B,** When IV contrast is administered, the intimal flap separating the true and false lumens of the aorta becomes visible. No oral contrast is needed to make this diagnosis.

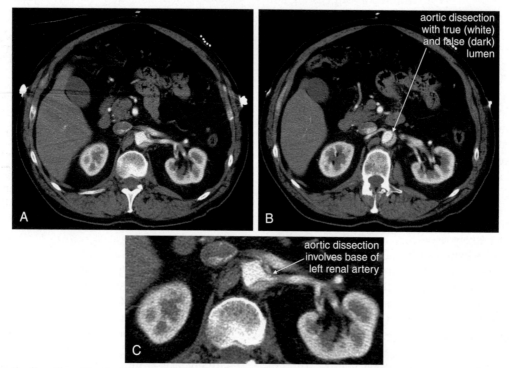

Figure 11-25. Aortic dissection: Stanford type B with involvement of the left renal artery. CT with IV contrast, soft-tissue windows. **A, B,** Sequential images at the level of the renal artery. **C,** Close-up from **A.** This patient has a dissection of the abdominal aorta. An intimal flap and false lumen appear to involve the origin of the left renal artery, although the kidney does enhance with contrast.

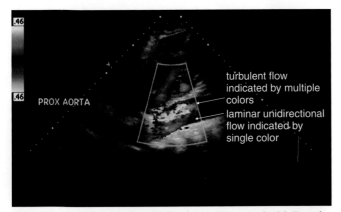

PROX AORTA

turbulent flow indicated by multiple colors

laminar unidirectional flow indicated by single color

Color Plate 1. Abdominal aortic dissection: Ultrasound with Doppler flow. Ultrasound demonstrates the intimal flap of an aortic dissection in the proximal abdominal aorta. Color Doppler shows differential blood flow in the true and false lumens.

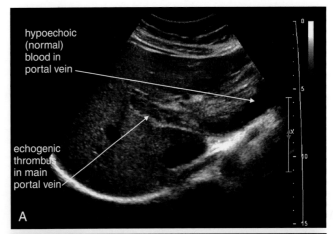

hypoechoic (normal) blood in portal vein

echogenic thrombus in main portal vein

A

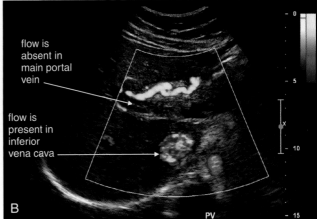

flow is absent in main portal vein

flow is present in inferior vena cava

B   PV

Color Plate 2. Portal vein thrombosis: Ultrasound. This 22-year-old female, 2 months postpartum, presented with 1 week of right upper quadrant pain. Ultrasound was performed to evaluate for suspected cholecystitis or symptomatic cholelithiasis. Instead, portal vein thrombosis was discovered. The postpartum state is a risk factor for this condition. Hypercoagulable states and inflammatory or neoplastic abdominal conditions, including pancreatitis and abdominal malignancies, also can result in portal vein thrombosis. **A,** Ultrasound grayscale image showing thrombus in the main portal vein. **B,** Doppler ultrasound showing no flow within the portal vein.

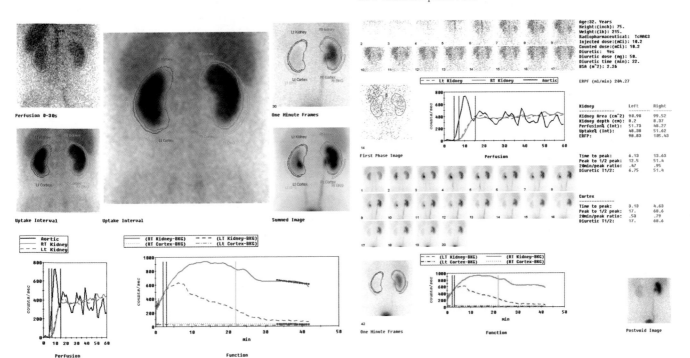

Color Plate 3. Lasix renal scan. Quantitative information about renal perfusion can be obtained from this study. In this patient, both kidneys were found to be well perfused despite poor excretion from right kidney, consistent with obstruction.

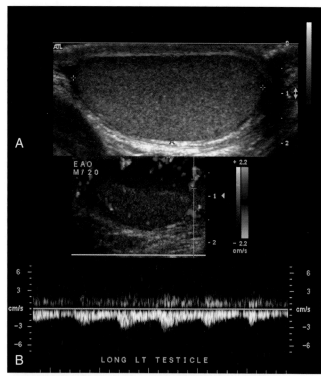

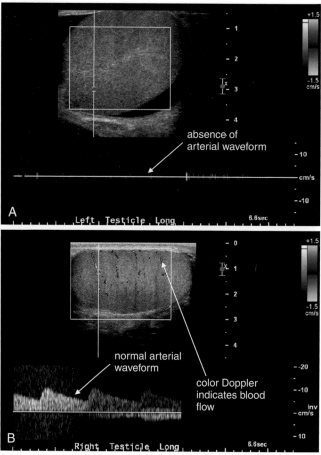

Color Plate 4. **Normal testicular ultrasound.** This 20-year-old male complained of a palpable nodule on the right testicle. These images of the left testicle are normal. **A,** The normal echo texture of the testicle is seen. No significant fluid surrounds the testicle. **B,** Arterial flow is normal, with a pulsatile waveform.

Color Plate 5. **Testicular torsion ultrasound. A** and **B,** Ultrasound has become the standard modality to assess for testicular torsion. In this 20-year-old male with left testicular pain, the left testicle has no blood flow, whereas the right testicle has normal arterial and venous blood flow by color Doppler assessment and a normal arterial waveform. The patient was taken to the operating suite, where left testicular torsion was confirmed. After rapid detorsion and orchiopexy, the left testicle reperfused and was viable.

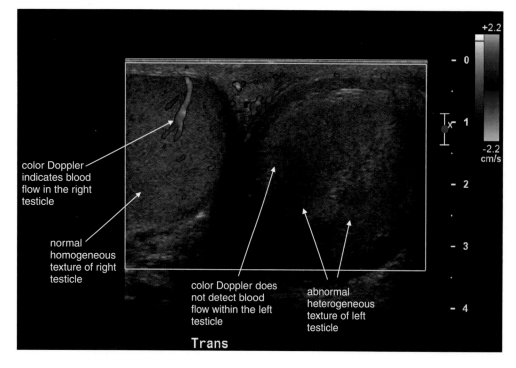

Color Plate 6. **Testicular infarct.** This patient had been treated for epididymitis without improvement. Ultrasound then revealed apparent testicular torsion, confirmed operatively. The patient underwent orchiectomy, and surgical pathology was consistent with hemorrhagic infarction. This case highlights the importance of imaging for testicular pain. Epididymitis, orchitis, and testicular torsion may have similar presentations. The ultrasound findings of note are an absence of blood flow in the left testicle by color Doppler, and a heterogeneous echotexture of the left testicle compared with the right, which is consistent with infarction.

Color Plate 7. Epididymitis. **A** through **C,** In addition to evaluating the more concerning diagnosis of testicular torsion, ultrasound can identify epididymitis and orchitis. In epididymitis, blood flow to the affected epididymis is increased. **A,** A hydrocele is visible (black) adjacent to the left testicle. **B** and **C,** The left epididymis shows increased blood flow compared with the normal right epididymis, based on color Doppler, consistent with epididymitis. In addition, the left epididymis is enlarged compared with the normal right epididymis. Blood flow to the testicles was normal.

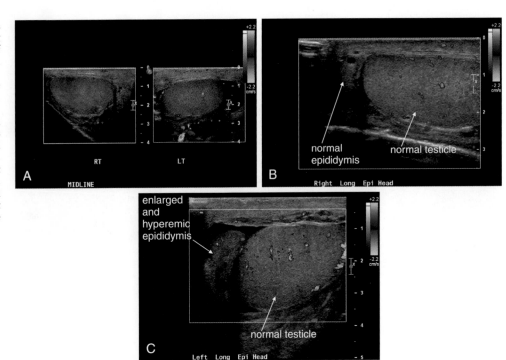

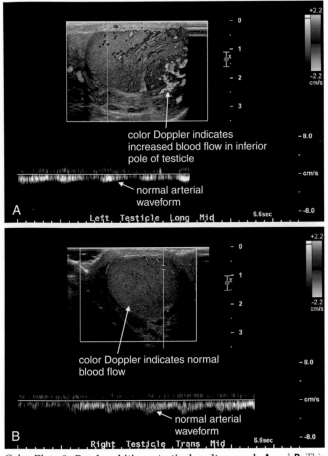

Color Plate 8. Focal orchitis on testicular ultrasound. A and **B,** This 45-year-old male was treated with antibiotics for epididymitis but had recurrent pain after completing treatment. Ultrasound was performed to rule out testicular torsion. Instead, the ultrasound suggested focal orchitis. Prominent flow is seen in the inferior portion of the left testicle, consistent with focal orchitis in that location. The right testicle shows normal blood flow.

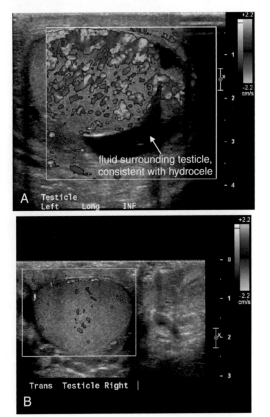

Color Plate 9. Orchitis, color Doppler ultrasound. A and **B,** This patient with left testicular pain shows markedly increased blood flow on color Doppler throughout the left testicle compared with the right, consistent with orchitis of the left testicle. A hydrocele is also seen surrounding the left testicle (black collection).

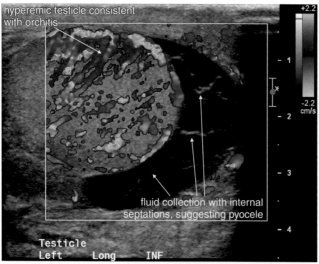

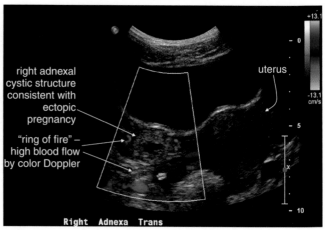

Color Plate 10. **Orchitis with pyocele: Testicular ultrasound.** The left testicle is markedly hyperemic on color Doppler ultrasound compared with the right testicle (not shown), consistent with orchitis. There is complex fluid collection with internal septations and internal echoes that is predominantly located inferior to the testicle and is concerning for a pyocele. Simple hydroceles are homogeneously black without internal echoes. Fluid collections with internal structure are more likely to represent infection or blood products, whereas simple fluid is more likely serous.

Color Plate 12. **Ectopic pregnancy confirmed in operating room: Transabdominal ultrasound.** This transverse transabdominal view shows the classic adnexal "ring of fire" sign—an adnexal cystic structure with high blood flow demonstrated by color Doppler.

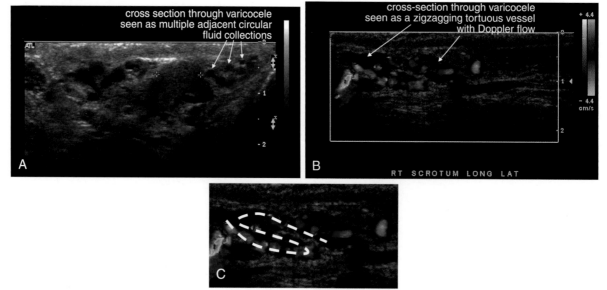

Color Plate 11. **Varicocele.** This 35-year-old male underwent ultrasound for evaluation of azoospermia. An incidental finding on this ultrasound was bilateral varicoceles. These tortuous veins may present as scrotal masses. **A** through **C,** Ultrasound confirms varicocele by demonstrating tortuous fluid-filled vessels with color Doppler flow consistent with venous blood flow. **A,** In the left scrotum, the vein passes in and out of the plane of the ultrasound image, giving the appearance of multiple adjacent circular cross sections. **B** and **C,** In the images from the right scrotum using color Doppler, a zigzagging vessel with flow is visible.

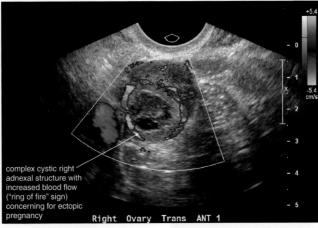

Color Plate 13. Possible ectopic pregnancy. A right ovarian complex cystic structure is seen, with increased blood flow consistent with the "ring of fire" sign—a sign described as concerning for ectopic pregnancy.

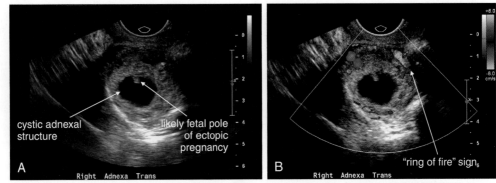

Color Plate 14. Ectopic pregnancy. A and **B,** These images of the right adnexa show an ovoid echogenic structure measuring approximately 4.6 × 4.0 × 3.3 cm with a central cystic region and an eccentric hyperechoic focus concerning for an ectopic pregnancy. Color Doppler shows increased blood flow around the structure, consistent with the "ring of fire" sign. At laparotomy, right adnexal ectopic pregnancy was confirmed.

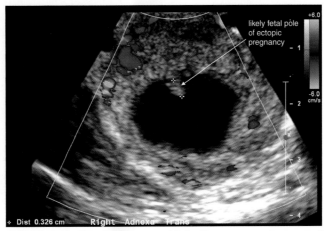

Color Plate 15. Ectopic pregnancy. No fetal heart rate was documented within the echogenic focus using motion mode. The echogenic focus measures approximately 3.3 mm.

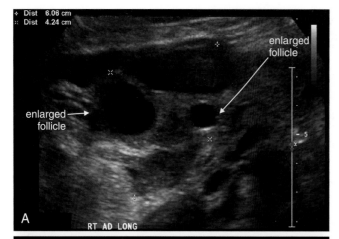

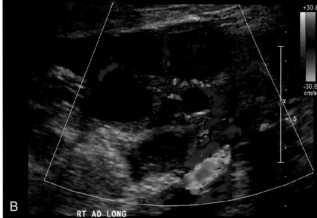

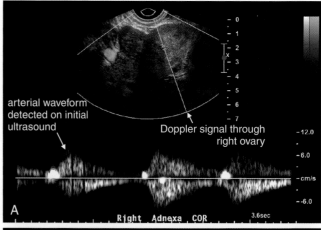

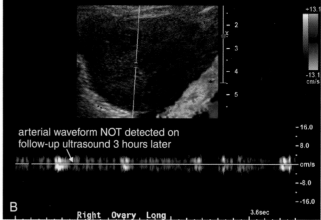

Color Plate 16. Hyperstimulated ovary. This 34-year-old female presented with abdominal pain and vomiting. The patient was 8 weeks pregnant after undergoing gonadotropin ovarian hyperstimulation therapy. **A** and **B,** The right ovary is enlarged, measuring at least 7.7 × 4.6 cm with hypoechoic structures consistent with follicles. Both arterial and venous blood flow were documented in the ovary. This is consistent with ovarian hyperstimulation. The left ovary had a similar appearance.

Color Plate 17. Ovarian torsion: Ultrasound. A and **B,** This patient was initially found to have normal arterial and venous flow in the right ovary, but the emergency physician remained concerned for ovarian torsion given the abrupt onset of severe lateralizing pelvic pain. Repeat ultrasound showed only dampened venous flow. The patient was confirmed to have ovarian torsion at laparotomy, with the ovary twisted four complete turns on its vascular pedicle. This case demonstrates an essential point for the emergency physician. Ultrasound has been reported to have a sensitivity for ovarian torsion of only approximately 60%. When torsion is strongly suspected, a normal ultrasound should not be interpreted as ruling out torsion.

In addition to initial arterial phase images, delayed images are usually obtained to assess the perfusion of organs such as the kidneys. Failure of the kidneys to enhance on delayed images indicates hypoperfusion related to the dissection and may require emergency surgery or intravascular techniques to fenestrate the dissection flap and restore blood flow (Figure 11-26).

MRI or MRA is also highly sensitive and specific for abdominal aortic disease, including aortic dissection.[58-59] In patients with contraindications to iodinated contrast for CT, such as renal insufficiency or iodinated contrast allergy, MRI or MRA is a reasonable alternative if its performance can be timely. Typical MRI or MRA for aortic dissection requires approximately 25 minutes to complete, compared with fewer than 6 minutes for CT.[60] This does not take into account the limited availability of MRI outside of normal business hours in many centers, with additional time often required for technicians to arrive. Three-dimensional MRA with injected gadolinium contrast is usually used to demonstrate the intimal flap.[58-59] In patients with renal insufficiency at risk for gadolinium-associated complications (discussed at the end of this chapter), MRI without IV gadolinium can be performed to assess for aortic dissection. New sequences that require no contrast material perform favorably compared with gadolinium-enhanced MRA.[58-61] These protocols include steady-state, two-dimensional, gradient–recall echo[60]; two-dimensional turbo spin echo; and two-dimensional, balanced, steady-state free precession.[61]

Mesenteric Ischemia

Mesenteric ischemia is not a single disease but a family of related disorders. These include acute and chronic occlusions of mesenteric arteries and acute, subacute, or even chronic occlusions of portal and mesenteric veins. Bowel ischemia can also be a consequence of small-bowel obstruction and intestinal volvulus. Vascular thrombosis most often afflicts patients at advanced age; however, rarely, conditions such as vasculitis, hypercoagulable states, or atrial fibrillation may underlie acute thrombosis in young patients.[32] We review here the mechanism and the presentation for each of these disease states, recognizing that these diseases are rare enough that large studies with good methodology are generally lacking.

Acute Mesenteric Artery Occlusion

Acute mesenteric artery occlusion and ischemia can occur from in situ thrombosis or embolic events. Atrial fibrillation is likely the most common cause, accounting for 95% of cases in one prospective study.[62] Dissection of mesenteric vessels can complicate aortic dissection or rarely may occur in isolation. The superior mesenteric artery (SMA) is the most commonly affected vessel in the setting of atrial fibrillation (see Figures 11-31 to 11-35).[63] Occlusion of the SMA may be more common than previously believed. In a population-based study using autopsy results, the incidence was 8.6 per 100,000 person years, with a cause-specific mortality of 6 in 1000 deaths. Suspicion of intestinal ischemia before death was noted in only 33%, possibly reflecting a variable presentation not fitting the classically described signs and symptoms.[64]

Classically, acute mesenteric ischemia from arterial occlusion is characterized by sudden and severe abdominal pain without significant abdominal tenderness. This is often described as "pain out of proportion to exam." This may be a misleading myth that could result in misdiagnosis or delayed diagnosis in many patients. In a retrospective review from Wake Forest University,[65] 63% of cases had a delay of greater than 24 hours from symptom onset until treatment, reflecting the difficulty of the diagnosis. Of 77 cases presenting with acute mesenteric ischemia, 64% were described in their initial emergency

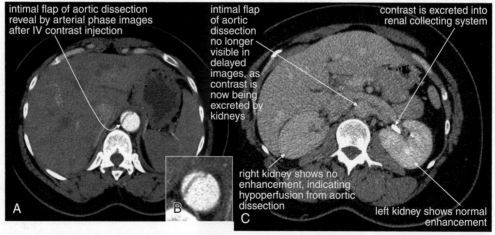

Figure 11-26. Aortic dissection with end-organ ischemia: Delayed phase, intravenous-contrasted CT images. Aortic dissection involving the abdominal aorta can result in ischemia of end organs, including bowel and kidneys. **A,** Arterial phase images obtained immediately following contrast administration can reveal the dissection flap, including major branch vessel involvement. In this case, the initial scan was terminated inadvertently above the level of the renal arteries. **B,** Close-up from **A** showing intimal flap in detail. **C,** Delayed images can show evidence of hypoperfusion. In this case, the right kidney does not show normal enhancement, indicating hypoperfusion. The left kidney enhances and shows contrast in the renal collecting system, indicating normal perfusion.

department record as having peritonitis–suggesting that exam findings were severe, not mild. In a second study of 43 patients with mesenteric ischemia, 48% had diffuse tenderness, and 52% had peritonitis by exam.[66] One explanation is that these are late findings and patients often present after a delay of many hours from onset of ischemia. In any case, mesenteric ischemia should never be ruled out because the physical examination demonstrates too much tenderness.

Lab abnormalities associated with mesenteric ischemia include substantial leukocytosis, elevated anion gap, elevated lactate level, and hyperphosphatemia, but small studies on the topic limit the value of these findings in ruling out a potentially lethal process. Ritz et al.[32] found that marked leukocytosis and elevated serum lactate occurred in 93% of patients with acute mesenteric ischemia and were prognostic of mortality. Lange and Jackel[67] found serum lactate to be elevated in 100% of 20 patients with mesenteric ischemia, although the specificity was only 42%. Merle et al.[68] found a serum lactate level of greater than 5 mmol/L to be associated with death within 72 hours. High inorganic phosphate levels have long been reported to be associated with mesenteric ischemia, based primarily on animal studies.[69-72] Phosphate is believed to originate from sloughing intestinal mucosa. The sensitivity has not been studied in well-designed human trials but is inadequate for screening in case series. May and Berenson[73] reported elevations in only 25% of cases of intestinal ischemia. Gorey and O'Sullivan[74] reported hyperphosphatemia in only 15% of 65 patients with extensive intestinal ischemia, leukocytosis in 65%, and metabolic acidosis in 67%.

Pitfalls in laboratory screening can occur. Although marked leukocytosis can suggest acute mesenteric ischemia, this is likely a late finding that may occur after frank bowel necrosis has occurred, in which case patient prognosis is poor. Thus patients with normal white blood cell counts should not be dismissed as not having mesenteric ischemia. Patients with significant leukocytosis may be mistakenly suspected of infectious or inflammatory conditions of the abdomen, such as diverticulitis, abdominal abscess, or appendicitis. Although these patients undoubtedly would undergo additional observation or diagnostic imaging, the absolute time criticality of the diagnosis of ischemia might be missed. For example, observation of several hours in the case of SMA thrombosis can result in complete loss of the small bowel, with high morbidity and mortality.

When considering the screening sensitivity of laboratory tests, it is extremely important to remember the methodologic limitations of most studies on the subject, which are usually small, retrospective reviews. In addition, mesenteric ischemia is a spectrum of disease including partial and incomplete vascular occlusions.

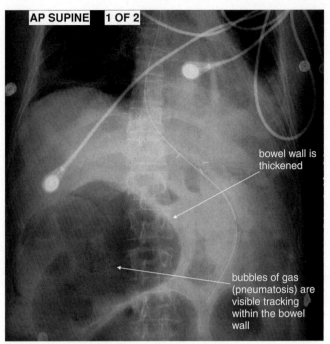

Figure 11-27. Bowel infarction (ischemic colitis with pneumatosis): X-ray. This image depicts classic findings of mesenteric ischemia, including gross distension of bowel, bowel wall thickening, and frank pneumatosis. Pneumatosis is a late finding, representing the penetration of gas-forming organisms into necrotic bowel wall. How can gas be recognized to be within the bowel wall? The gas is organized in a curved line—indicating that the gas is trapped within the bowel wall, not scattered at random as would be expected if gas were distributed in stool within the bowel. See magnified view, Figure 11-28.

The elapsed time from the moment of vascular occlusion until emergency department presentation, as well as the degree of bowel hypoperfusion, may affect the sensitivity of laboratory testing and diagnostic imaging.

Imaging for Mesenteric Ischemia

In any patient with suspected acute mesenteric ischemia, immediate surgical consultation and definitive imaging must be performed. Plain radiographs play a limited role in the diagnosis. In retrospective reviews of patients ultimately diagnosed with mesenteric ischemia, plain films are both insensitive and nonspecific.[75-76] In one study of 187 patients, 35% had normal plain films and 42% showed signs of small-bowel obstruction.[32] Common plain film abnormalities in acute mesenteric ischemia include an appearance of intestinal ileus, which should come as little surprise given that intestinal motility would be expected to cease in the absence of intestinal blood flow (Figures 11-27 and 11-28; see Figure 11-3). Findings in one small study included air–fluid levels (84%), dilated bowel loops (48%), thickened and unchanging loops (20%), gastric distension and gasless abdomen (12%), and small-bowel pseudo-obstruction (8%).[76] Findings of ileus may give false reassurance that no critical abnormality is present in the abdomen. The finding of intestinal pneumatosis is likely a relatively rare and late finding, occurring after the onset of intestinal necrosis (see Figures 11-3, 11-27,

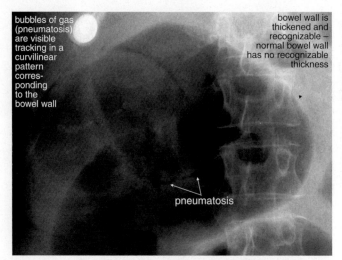

bubbles of gas (pneumatosis) are visible tracking in a curvilinear pattern corresponding to the bowel wall

bowel wall is thickened and recognizable – normal bowel wall has no recognizable thickness

pneumatosis

Figure 11-28. Bowel infarction (ischemic colitis with pneumatosis): X-ray. Close-up from Figure 11-27. This image depicts classic findings of mesenteric ischemia, including gross distension of bowel, bowel wall thickening, and frank pneumatosis.

and 11-28). In one study, only 4% of patients with mesenteric ischemia had pneumatosis on x-ray.[77] Although pneumatosis should prompt immediate surgical consultation, reliance on this finding likely results in diagnosis at such a late time that exceedingly high morbidity and mortality result.[78] Ironically, in addition to being insensitive for mesenteric ischemia, pneumatosis is not specific for the diagnosis, occurring sometimes from a variety of less emergent causes (see Figures 11-43 and 11-46).[78] As with other syndromes of acute abdominal pain, an upright portable chest x-ray is reasonable to detect pneumoperitoneum resulting from intestinal perforation (see Figure 11-1). A negative chest x-ray must be followed by immediate definitive imaging. Abdominal plain films should not be routinely obtained but should be considered in patients too unstable to undergo CT.

Computed Tomography for Mesenteric Ischemia. Definitive imaging for mesenteric ischemia is CT with IV contrast (Figures 11-29 to 11-34; see also Figures 11-36 to 11-43, 11-45, 11-46, and 11-48). Oral contrast is not necessary for the diagnosis and should be avoided because of substantial delay, more than 2 hours in some institutions, that can result.[13] Because of the overlapping presentation of AAA rupture, aortic dissection, and mesenteric ischemia, an immediate CT scan with no contrast agents can be performed to assess for AAA. If this test is negative, immediate CT with IV contrast should be performed unless the patient has significant contraindications to iodinated contrast. As with aortic dissection, the extreme morbidity and mortality of mesenteric ischemia means that the risks and benefits of IV contrast must be carefully weighed. Because this is a time-critical diagnosis with a mortality as high as 60% to 70%,[65-66] some patients with moderate or severe renal insufficiency or contrast allergies should receive immediate IV contrast after a discussion and informed consent from the patient

or patient family. Contrast allergies and renal insufficiency are discussed in more detail later.

If the patient has an absolute contraindication to administration of iodinated contrast, noncontrast CT can be performed to assess for mesenteric ischemia. There are no large trials of this approach. Several letters to the editors of radiology journals have commented on the ability to diagnose mesenteric ischemia based on the presence of mural pneumatosis, thickening of the bowel wall, free air, and fat stranding surrounding regions of the small bowel corresponding to vascular territories (see Figures 11-37 and 11-45).[79-81] It is likely that these findings occur relatively late in the presentation, so although their presence may be helpful, their absence does not rule out the possibility of acute mesenteric ischemia. A red flag for mesenteric ischemia is a normal noncontrast abdominal CT in the presence of significant abdominal pain or concerning laboratory findings, such as profound leukocytosis, anion gap, or elevated lactate (Figure 11-36).

When ordering CT for evaluation of mesenteric ischemia, it is important to communicate the diagnostic concern to the radiologist and CT technician so that the CT can be performed appropriately. Modern protocols specifically tailored for evaluation of mesenteric ischemia have been developed.[63,82-84] These use thin-section imaging through the region of the celiac, superior and inferior mesenteric, and middle colic arteries, as well as a rapid contrast bolus to ensure proper opacification of these vessels. Some protocols use arterial phase imaging to evaluate for acute arterial occlusion, followed by delayed images obtained approximately 60 seconds later to evaluate contrast filling of the mesenteric veins and portal venous system.[82] Kirkpatrick et al.[82] reported high sensitivity (96%) and specificity (94%) in a small study of 62 patients. Zandrino et al.[85] reported sensitivity of 92% and specificity of 100% using a similar protocol. However, because of the rarity of mesenteric arterial occlusion and resulting small studies, wide confidence intervals exist around these point estimates. In addition, no studies to date have evaluated the interobserver variability in recognizing these findings. In the setting of intestinal ischemia associated with small-bowel obstruction, the prospective sensitivity of CT for detecting ischemic changes is relatively low in clinical practice (15%),[86] in contrast to high sensitivity of CT in a pure research setting, which has been reported as high as 96%.[87] This may reflect the increased vigilance of radiologists when assessing specifically for ischemic changes in a research study.

What Are the CT Findings of Mesenteric Ischemia?

The CT findings of acute mesenteric ischemia include arterial vascular occlusion with an intravascular filling defect similar to that observed with pulmonary

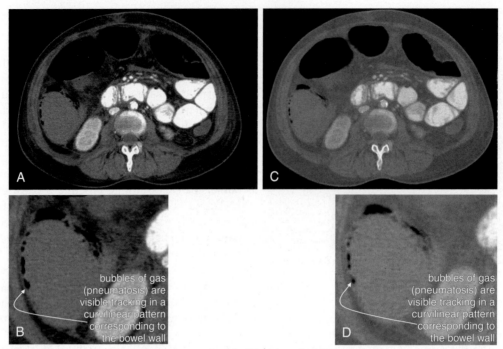

Figure 11-29. Bowel infarction (ischemic colitis with pneumatosis): CT with oral and IV contrast. Same patient as in Figures 11-27 and 11-28. **A,** A slice viewed on typical CT soft-tissue windows. **B,** Close-up from **A. C,** The same slice viewed on an intermediate window setting designed to highlight air. **D,** Close-up from **C.** Air is visible within the bowel wall, indicating a bowel segment with frank necrosis whose wall has been infiltrated with gas-forming organisms. This is a dire imaging finding that should prompt immediate surgical consultation. The mortality exceeds 70% for mesenteric ischemia. Why choose different CT window settings? Standard soft-tissue windows render fat dark—nearly black. This is useful because it allows the identification of subtle fat stranding, which lightens the color of fat. But air can be less noticeable on this setting, because air (black) and fat (nearly black) have little contrast with each other. The window settings in **C** and **D** make fat a lighter gray, helping to differentiate it from gas.

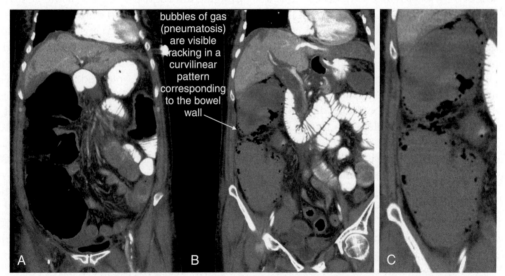

Figure 11-30. Bowel infarction (ischemic colitis with pneumatosis): CT with intravenous and oral contrast (soft-tissue windows). Same patient as Figures 11-27 through 11-29. This 61-year-old female presented with sepsis, lactic acidosis, and frank pneumatosis on x-ray caused by ischemic colitis. Unstable, on pressor medications, she underwent exploratory laparotomy, extensive lysis of adhesions, subtotal colectomy with end ileostomy, small-bowel resection with primary anastomosis, and splenectomy. Miraculously, she survived, given the severity of her illness on presentation. The operative findings suggested that her ischemia may have been caused by extensive adhesions rather than a single vascular obstruction. Coronal reconstructions show massive dilatation of the large bowel, as well as frank pneumatosis. **A,** An anterior slice shows the bowel to be dilated and air filled (remember, the patient was supine during CT, so an anterior coronal plane represents the superior portion of the abdomen). **B,** A more posterior coronal plane shows a dilated, fluid-filled ascending colon with gas infiltrating its wall—pneumatosis. **C,** Close-up from **B.**

embolism (see Figures 11-31 to 11-34 and 11-36). The normal celiac, superior mesenteric, and inferior mesenteric arteries fill uniformly with injected contrast. At their origins from the aorta, these are relatively large vessels with predictable locations. Failure of these vessels to fill, or partial filling, is generally readily recognized, and CT images correlate closely with formal angiography (see Figure 11-35). More distal branches are smaller and more difficult to assess. Secondary findings like bowel wall thickening, regional fat stranding, free air, and mural pneumatosis can be seen in advanced cases. Hypoperfused bowel may also fail to enhance with IV

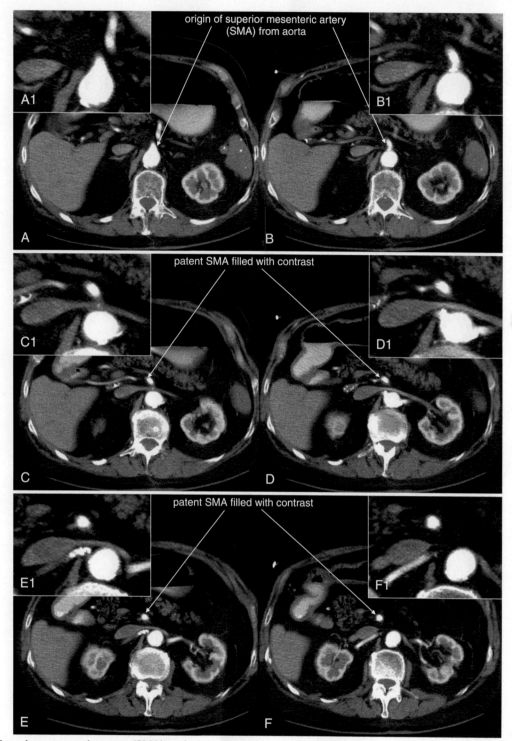

Figure 11-31. Superior mesenteric artery (SMA) occlusion: CT with intravenous (IV) contrast. This 77-year-old male presented in atrial fibrillation with abdominal pain and bright red blood from his colostomy, beginning abruptly after dinner. He had recently been discontinued from warfarin therapy because of falls. Mesenteric ischemia from an embolic occlusion was suspected, given the abrupt onset, atrial fibrillation, gastrointestinal bleeding, and an elevated lactate level (twice the upper limit of normal). CT with IV and oral contrast was performed. The SMA was noted to be completely obstructed with thrombus approximately 6 cm distal to its origin. No secondary bowel findings of ischemia were noted, likely because of the rapidity with which CT was performed after the onset of symptoms. This series of axial views follows the SMA from its origin (**A,** cephalad slice) to the point of thrombus obstruction (**N,** caudad slice). Because the SMA tracks anteriorly and diagonally from cephalad to caudad, it is visible in short-axis cross section in most of the slices. Note the sudden change from a widely patent, contrast-filled SMA to a completely unopacified vessel. The finding is the same one that would be noted with an occlusive pulmonary embolism.

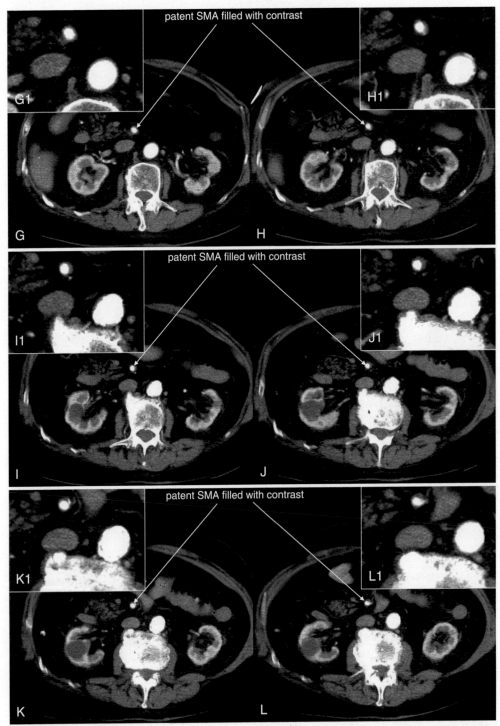

Figure 11-31, cont'd.

contrast. The portal venous system should be inspected for gas, which can also indicate mesenteric ischemia (Figures 11-38 to 11-40).[88]

Primary findings of a filling defect in mesenteric arteries are highly specific (see Figures 11-31 to 11-34 and 11-36). Unfortunately, some secondary CT findings of mesenteric ischemia are nonspecific and can sometimes be confused with those of inflammatory bowel disease such as Crohn's disease or ulcerative colitis. In addition, infectious causes such as infectious enteritis can cause bowel wall thickening and fat stranding, similar in appearance to ischemic changes (Figures 11-41 to 11-43; see also Figure 11-46). However, it is essential that the clinician consider ischemia and avoid delay in surgical consultation if the presentation remotely suggests an ischemic cause. If mesenteric ischemia is mistaken for a less dire condition such as inflammatory bowel disease, the outcome can be disastrous (see Figure 11-36).

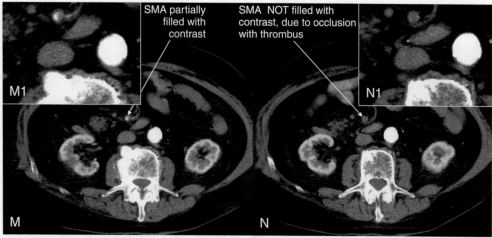

Figure 11-31, cont'd.

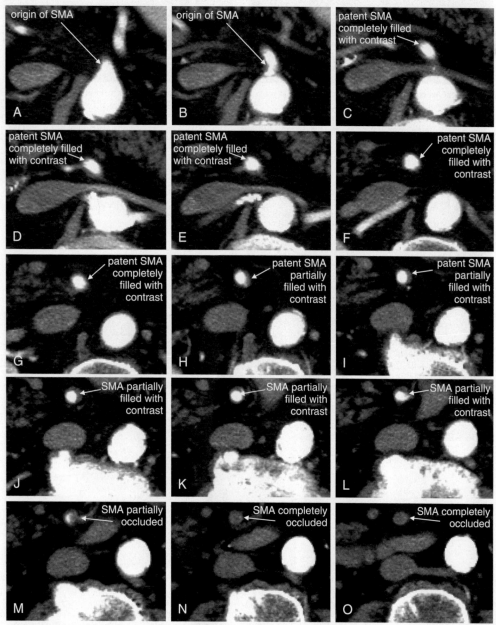

Figure 11-32. **Superior mesenteric artery (SMA) occlusion: CT with IV contrast.** Same patient as Figure 11-31. This series of axial views (cropped to the region of interest) tracks the SMA from its origin **(A)** to the point of thrombosis **(O)**.

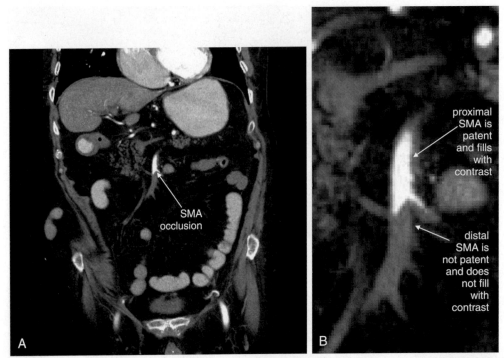

Figure 11-33. Superior mesenteric artery (SMA) occlusion: CT with IV contrast. Same patient as in Figures 11-31 and 11-32. This coronal CT captures the SMA at a point where it travels almost perfectly parallel to the coronal plane **(A).** The patent proximal portion is visible, and the abrupt thrombosed section is also seen. Compare with the angiogram in Figure 11-34. **B,** Close-up. Was contrast needed for this diagnosis? Oral contrast played no role here. This patient had a normal CT with the exception of the SMA thrombus, with no secondary bowel findings. IV contrast was essential to the diagnosis, because the SMA thrombosis would not have been visible without a well-timed, high-quality bolus through a large-bore IV catheter.

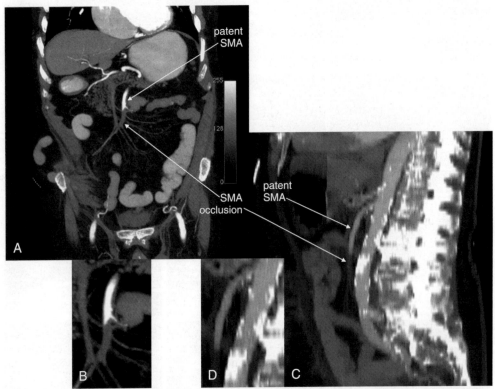

Figure 11-34. Superior mesenteric artery (SMA) occlusion: Computed tomography (CT) with intravenous contrast. Same patient as in Figures 11-31 through 11-33. Maximal intensity projection (MIP) images show the thrombosed SMA section in more detail. MIP images are created after the CT scan is performed using the original CT dataset. They "thicken" the image slab, allowing tortuous anatomic structures that cross through multiple routine CT slices to be seen in a single image. Your radiologist can create these upon request to improve diagnostic capabilities. Your local institution may already be performing this postprocessing "behind the scenes." **A,** Coronal reconstruction and enlargement. **B,** Close-up from **A. C,** Sagittal reconstruction and enlargement. **D,** Close-up from **C.**

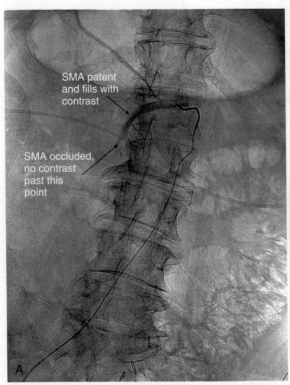
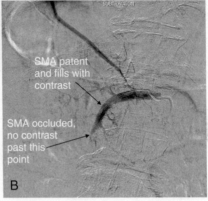

Figure 11-35. Superior mesenteric artery (SMA) occlusion: Angiogram. Same patient as in Figures 11-31 through 11-34. A catheter has been inserted into the aorta through a femoral artery. The catheter tip has been positioned at the origin of the SMA, and contrast has been injected. The proximal SMA fills, but contrast does not fill the vessel beyond approximately 6 cm—indicating complete thrombotic occlusion. Compare with Figure 11-34, a coronal maximal intensity projection image created from computed tomography reconstruction. **A,** Digital angiography. **B,** The same image using a digital subtraction technique, which digitally removes static portions of the image to allow better inspection of the dynamic contrast injection.

How Sensitive Is Ultrasound for the Diagnosis of Mesenteric Ischemia? What Are the Ultrasound Findings?

Doppler ultrasound can be used to assess thrombosis or stenosis of the celiac artery and SMA. The proximal portions of these vessels at their origins from the aorta are readily seen on ultrasound. The examination can be technically difficult but is a reasonable initial approach in patients with contraindications to CT with IV contrast. In one prospective study of 100 patients, Moneta et al.[89] reported that mesenteric duplex ultrasound was able to visualize 93% of superior mesenteric arteries and 83% of celiac arteries. Using a threshold of 70% or greater stenosis, duplex ultrasound was 92% sensitive and 96% specific for SMA stenosis and 87% sensitive and 80% specific for celiac stenosis. Danse et al.[90] reported that Doppler ultrasound confirmed mesenteric ischemia in 8 of 21 patients (38%) and suggested ischemia in an additional 11 of 21 patients (52%)—although this study did not include blinding to other clinical data. More recently, Hata et al.[19] assessed the performance of contrast-enhanced ultrasound for the diagnosis of bowel ischemia. In this study, patients with evidence of small-bowel dilatation were imaged using an injected ultrasound contrast agent. Rather than imaging blood vessels, the investigators assessed bowel wall for normal, diminished, or absent enhancement. The pooled sensitivity of diminished or absent enhancement was 85% (95% CI = 62%-97%), with a specificity of 100% (95% CI = 91%-100%). Contrast-enhanced ultrasound may gain a role in the assessment of unstable patients or those with contraindications to CT contrast agents.

How Sensitive Is Magnetic Resonance Imaging or Angiography for Mesenteric Ischemia?

MRI or MRA has excellent sensitivity and specificity for arterial mesenteric ischemia and for portal venous thrombosis.[30,58,63,84] Gadolinium contrast is generally given.[63,84] CT should be the first-line test because of higher spatial resolution and speed. Indications for MRI include nondiagnostic CT or contraindications for iodinated contrast, particularly severe allergy. Because mesenteric ischemia is extremely time dependent, no time should be wasted performing steroid prep for patients with iodinated contrast allergy (most protocols require 6 hours or more of delay); therefore, emergency MRI is sometimes required. Gadolinium is contraindicated in patients with renal insufficiency, as described later. In this circumstance, MRA can be performed without gadolinium contrast using special sequences as described earlier for aortic dissection—although the sensitivity of these sequences has not been extensively evaluated in mesenteric ischemia.

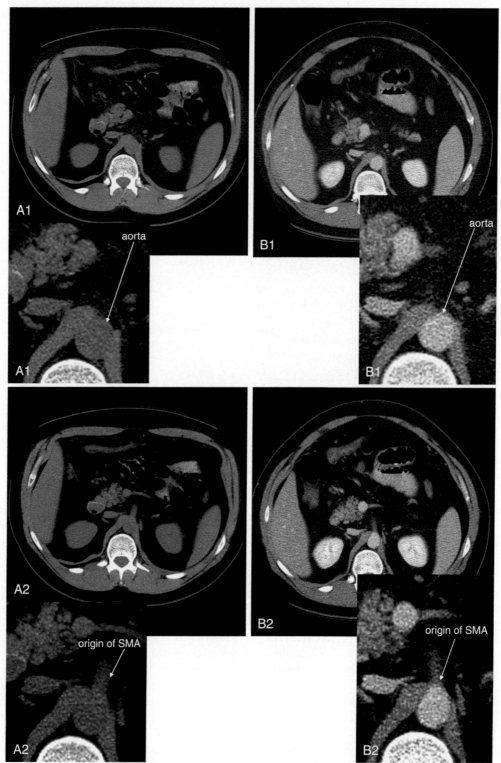

Figure 11-36. Mesenteric ischemia resulting from superior mesenteric artery (SMA) thrombosis: CT without and with contrast. This 37-year-old male with no prior medical or surgical history presented with abdominal pain with nausea, vomiting, and diarrhea. He underwent noncontrast CT that was interpreted as normal—despite a white blood cell count of 24.5 x 10^9, an anion gap of 19 mEq/L, and a lactate level of 3.5 mmol/L. The emergency physicians then suspected mesenteric ischemia. CT with contrast was performed, revealing complete thrombosis of the SMA near its origin from the aorta. The two CT scans are displayed side by side to allow comparison of the images. A key point is the need for injected contrast to allow recognition of filling defects within vascular structures. When reviewing the images, compare the noncontrast CT **(A)** to the CT with intravenous (IV) contrast **(B).** Slices are numbered from cephaladmost (1) to caudadmost (12). Each slice is shown with an enlarged view centered on the vascular structures of interest. Track the SMA from its origin off the aorta. Without IV contrast, patency of the SMA cannot be assessed, because liquid blood and thrombus have nearly identical density and appear dark gray. With the addition of IV contrast, the patent lumen appears bright white, whereas the filling defect resulting from a thrombus appears dark gray. Oral contrast is not needed for the diagnosis. In this patient, oral contrast was given but did not progress beyond the stomach—likely because of ileus in the face of bowel ischemia. Oral contrast results in unnecessary delay that can worsen the severe morbidity and mortality of mesenteric ischemia. Operatively, this patient was found to have SMA thrombosis with gangrene of the small intestine and right and transverse colon. He underwent resection of more than 200 cm of small bowel and was left dependent on total parenteral nutrition.

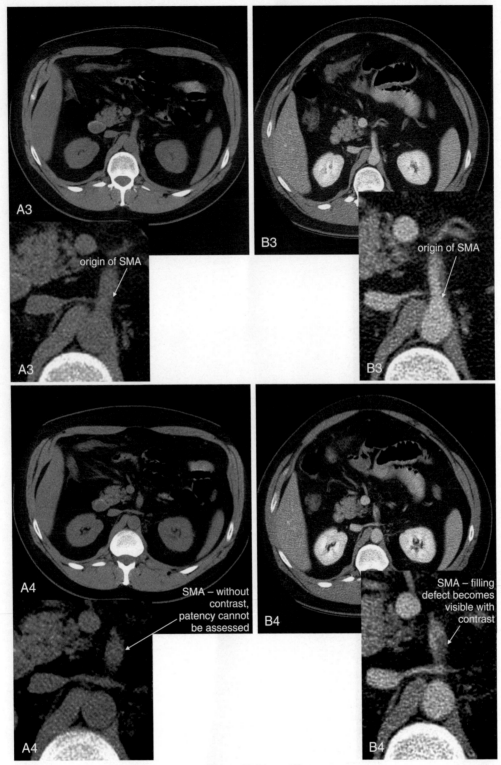

Figure 11-36, cont'd.

Variations in Mesenteric Ischemia

Ischemic Colitis. Ischemic colitis accounts for more than half of cases of intestinal ischemia, occurring in about 0.3% of acute hospital admissions. It particularly affects elderly patients with volume depletion and other medical illnesses. Ischemic colitis can also mimic infectious colitis such as *Clostridium difficile* colitis. Common features of ischemic colitis include hematochezia, abdominal pain, and diarrhea. Remarkably, many patients recover with IV fluid resuscitation and antibiotics. Nonetheless, morbidity is high, and mortality can occur in elderly patients with this condition. Emergent

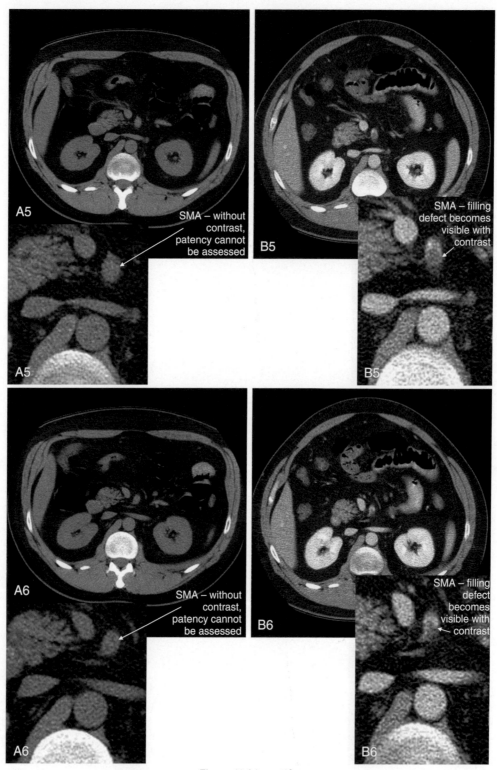

Figure 11-36, cont'd.

colectomy is sometimes required.[91] Moreover, the presentation can be indistinguishable from SMA occlusion, so the same urgency of diagnostic evaluation is essential. Ischemic colitis has similar noncontrast CT findings, with thickening of the large-bowel wall, surrounding regional fat stranding, pneumatosis, and sometimes pneumoperitoneum (Figures 11-45 and 11-46; see also Figures 11-29, 11-30, and 11-37 to 11-43). CT with IV contrast should be used when possible, because this may reveal a filling defect in vessels supplying the affected large bowel.[92] The findings are not specific and can mimic infectious colitis or inflammatory bowel disease.

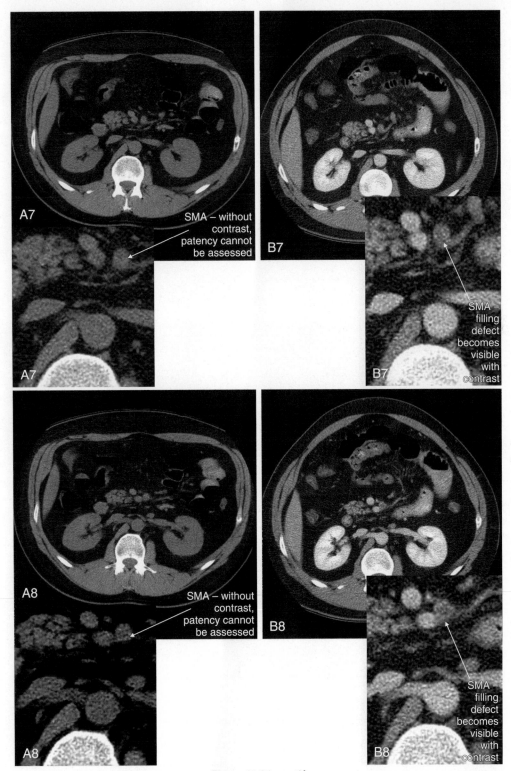

Figure 11-36, cont'd.

Chronic Mesenteric Ischemia. Chronic mesenteric ischemia has sometimes been called intestinal angina. Classically, the presentation is subacute or even chronic abdominal pain with a duration of weeks or even months. Patients develop weight loss and fear of eating, because they anticipate pain following a meal. Postprandial pain results from demand ischemia after a meal

challenge. Pathologically, this is caused by stenosis of a mesenteric vessel, resulting in diminished blood flow. This is not unlike stable angina developing in a patient with coronary artery disease. The presentation can overlap substantially with other disease processes, including intra-abdominal malignancies with weight loss and chronic pain, chronic pancreatitis, and ulcer disease. The

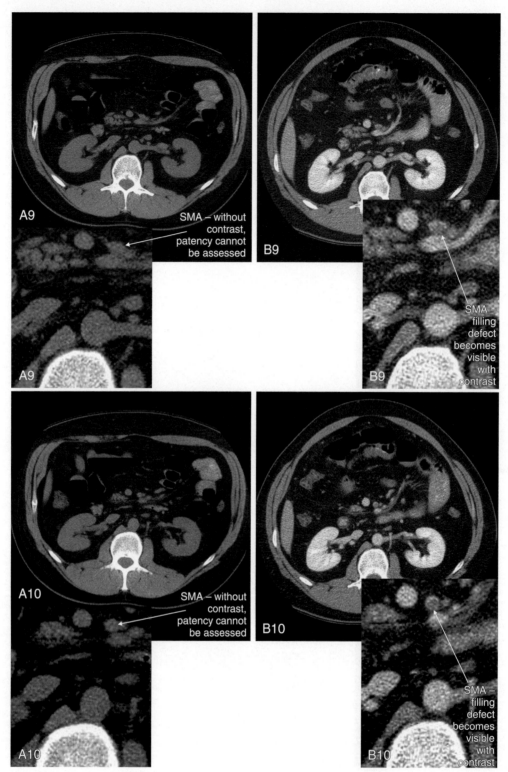

Figure 11-36, cont'd.

imaging workup is similar to acute mesenteric ischemia, with CT with IV contrast being the best test. CT is useful, because it can depict most other serious causes of abdominal pain, including malignancy, free air, appendicitis, diverticulitis, pancreatitis, and small-bowel obstruction. Ulcer disease is not well diagnosed by CT unless frank perforation has occurred, so a normal CT should not be considered to have eliminated the possibility. Because acute-on-chronic mesenteric ischemia can occur, a prodrome of several months of abdominal pain should not relieve the urgency to perform definitive imaging.

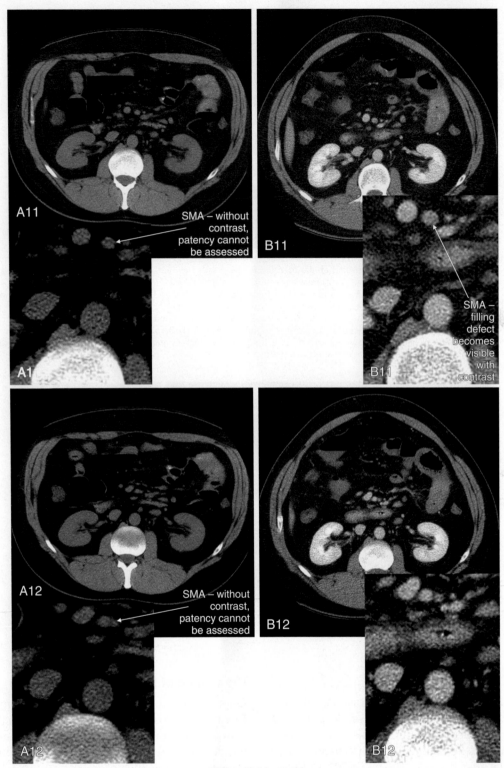

Figure 11-36, cont'd.

PORTAL VEIN THROMBOSIS

The presentation of portal vein thrombosis is variable, likely because of the variety of underlying pathology that can result in the condition. Many patients develop portal vein thrombosis in the setting of other acute or chronic abdominal conditions, including malignancies or acute inflammatory and infectious conditions within the abdomen such as pancreatitis. Symptoms may reflect the underlying disease process more than the acute or chronic thrombosis of the portal vein. Primary portal vein thrombosis can occur, with abdominal pain being

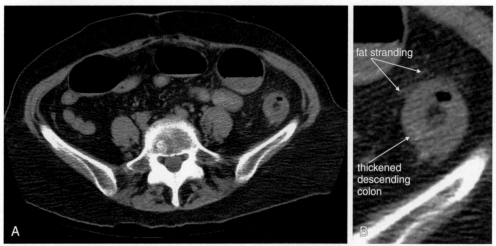

Figure 11-37. Ischemic colitis: CT without IV contrast. CT soft-tissue windows. This 86-year-old female presented with abdominal pain, vomiting, altered mental status, and hypotension. The patient had an elevated lactate level of 5.7 mmol/L, although this could represent sepsis, rather than mesenteric ischemia. **A,** The patient did not receive IV contrast because of renal insufficiency (creatinine 2 mg/dL), so vascular structures are not well seen. Although the patient received oral contrast, none reached the distal bowel before CT scan. **B,** Close-up. The descending colon shows circumferential wall thickening with a doughnut-like configuration, suggesting colitis, though the cause is not certain (ischemic or infectious). Some surrounding fat stranding is seen. Other images showed portal venous gas (Figure 11-38). The radiologist interpreted the CT scan as suggestive of ischemic colitis. Because of a concurrent non–ST-elevation myocardial infarction (NSTEMI), the patient was treated solely with fluid resuscitation and antibiotics. She survived the illness. Was the CT diagnosis correct? Was the portal venous gas real, or was it misrecognized air in biliary ducts? These questions remain unanswered. Perhaps this was a case of infectious colitis.

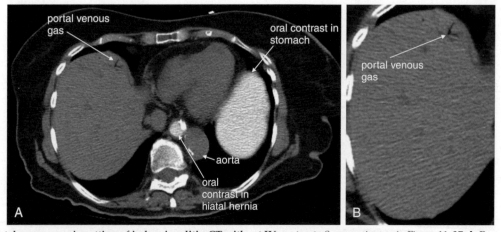

Figure 11-38. Portal venous gas in setting of ischemic colitis: CT without IV contrast. Same patient as in Figure 11-37. **A,** Portal venous gas does not require any contrast for identification. This patient had an elevated creatinine and received no IV contrast. She did receive oral contrast, but this did not contribute to the diagnosis. **B,** Close-up.

the predominant symptom. Hypercoagulable states can precipitate acute portal vein thrombosis. Portal vein thrombosis can be considered a type of deep venous thrombosis—"really deep vein thrombosis." The peripartum state is also a risk factor, with risk persisting for as long as 2 months after delivery. The morbidity and mortality of portal vein thrombosis is high, partly reflecting the underlying causes. Many patients with this condition are older, with chronic comorbidities contributing to the morbidity and mortality of portal vein thrombosis. Significant thrombosis of the portal venous system can result in mesenteric or bowel infarction, and death. The treatment is systemic anticoagulation. Late complications include upper gastrointestinal bleeding caused by portal hypertension.[93-95]

Ultrasound of Portal Vein Thrombosis

Doppler ultrasound can reveal portal vein thrombosis. In cases of gross thrombosis of the portal vein, ultrasound without use of Doppler imaging can reveal a filling defect (Figure 11-47). The normal patent portal vein appears anechoic (black) on ultrasound. Clot within the portal vein can appear hypoechoic or anechoic acutely but usually becomes echogenic with time.[96] Doppler imaging shows absence of flow in the portal vein. In cases of partial obstruction, some flow may be seen.

Computed Tomography for Portal Vein Thrombosis

CT with IV contrast can be performed to diagnose portal vein thrombosis.[97] Oral contrast is unnecessary and should not be used due to time delay. Ideally, CT should

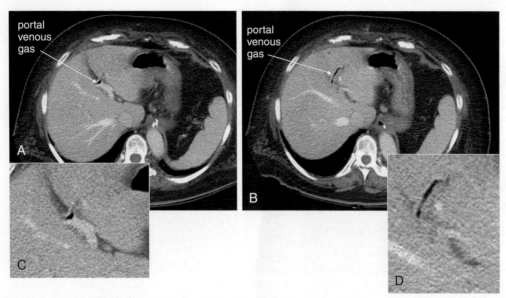

Figure 11-39. Portal venous gas and possible ischemic colitis. CT with IV contrast, soft-tissue windows. This 65-year-old female presented with nausea and epigastric pain. CT with intravenous contrast was performed and showed concerning findings, including thickening of the entire ascending colon, pneumatosis of the colon, and portal venous gas. Laparoscopy was performed because of concern for ischemic colitis—but after inspection of the entire bowel, no resection was performed. The patient was treated for likely infectious colitis. Stool cultures, *Clostridium difficile* testing, and fecal leukocyte testing were all negative. She recovered uneventfully. Look carefully at these images, which demonstrate portal venous gas. A collection of gas is seen at a branch point in the portal vein **(A)** and extending to the patient's left portal vein **(B). C,** Close-up from **A. D,** Close-up from **B.**

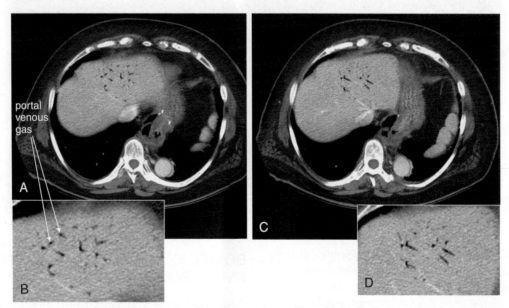

Figure 11-40. Portal venous gas and possible ischemic colitis. Same patient as Figure 11-39. Gas has spread through the portal system. Normally, this is an ominous sign, possibly indicating mesenteric ischemia. Remarkably, this patient had a nontherapeutic laparoscopy and recovered with fluids and antibiotic therapy. These images do not readily distinguish portal vein gas from gas in the biliary tree, which can have a similar appearance. However, Figure 11-39 showed gas more proximally in the portal vein, so these gas collections presumably are present in peripheral portal vein branches, not bile ducts **A** and **C,** two adjacent axial CT images through the cephalad portion of the liver, viewed on soft-tissue windows. IV contrast has been administered. **B,** Close-up from **A. D,** Close-up from **C.**

be performed with both arterial and portal venous phase images to rule out mesenteric arterial and venous thrombosis. This is accomplished by initiating CT scan early after contrast injection for arterial imaging. Additional CT images are then acquired after a delay of approximately 1 minute to allow filling of the portal venous system by the original injected contrast bolus. Portal venous thrombosis is marked by a failure of filling of the mesenteric and portal venous trees with IV contrast (Figure 11-48).[97-99] The imaging findings are similar

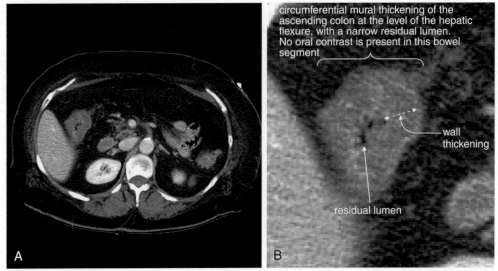

Figure 11-41. Thickening of right colon and ischemic colitis: CT with intravenous contrast only. Same patient as Figures 11-39 and 11-40. Did this patient have ischemic or infectious colitis? This is uncertain, but patients with her concerning constellation of CT findings should be pursued as possible mesenteric ischemia, because delay in treatment could be catastrophic. **A,** Axial CT viewed on soft-tissue windows. **B,** Close-up from **A**.

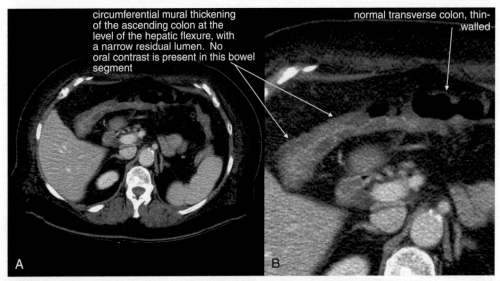

Figure 11-42. Thickening of right colon and ischemic colitis. Same patient as Figures 11-39 through 11-41. As the ascending colon transitions to the transverse colon beyond the hepatic flexure, it relatively rapidly resumes a normal wall thickness. **A,** Axial CT with IV contrast viewed on soft-tissue windows. **B,** Close-up from **A**.

to those found in pulmonary embolism. Some contrast may be seen distal to the filling defect if thrombosis is incomplete. Signs of bowel ischemia may also be present, including bowel wall thickening and regional mesenteric fat stranding. Other diagnostic imaging findings include air in the portal venous system. Depending on the underlying cause, other findings may include acute pancreatitis, regional lymph nodes, or intra abdominal mass lesions.

Magnetic Resonance of Portal Vein Thrombosis

MRI or MRA of the portal vein is highly sensitive and specific for portal vein thrombosis. As for other abdominal angiographic applications of magnetic resonance, gadolinium is usually given, although noncontrast methods are available.[100-102]

BOWEL ISCHEMIA COMPLICATING SMALL-BOWEL OBSTRUCTION

Bowel ischemia can complicate small-bowel obstruction. Frager et al.[103] found that intestinal ischemia complicated 48% of cases of high-grade obstruction from adhesions or hernias undergoing surgery—although selection bias undoubtedly inflates this number above what would be observed in patients with lower grades of obstruction being managed medically. Several mechanisms may account for ischemia in the setting of bowel obstruction. Volvulus of a segment of intestine may occur, or tight adhesive bands may reduce blood flow within the wall of the intestine. The possibility of bowel ischemia is one of the key reasons for CT, regardless of the x-ray appearance, when small-bowel

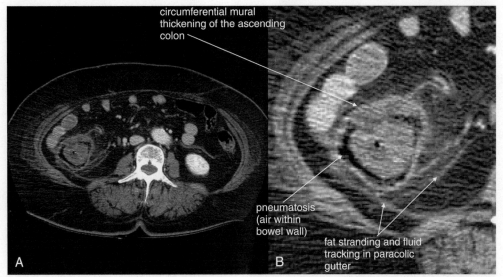

Figure 11-43. **Thickening of right colon and ischemic colitis.** Same patient as Figures 11-39 through 11-42. **A,** Axial CT with IV and oral contrast. **B,** Close-up from **A**. Bowel wall thickening is accompanied by an even more concerning finding—pneumatosis (air within the bowel wall). Normally, this finding is associated with bowel wall necrosis, usually in the face of ischemia. Remarkably, this patient recovered without bowel resection or revascularization, but pneumatosis should be treated as a possible surgical indication because of the extreme mortality of untreated mesenteric ischemia. Bowel wall thickening and inflammatory stranding may be seen in infectious, inflammatory, or ischemic colitis. *Yersina, Campylobacter,* and *Salmonella* have been described as causing pneumatosis. Remember that air appears black on all CT window settings. Fat also appears nearly black on soft-tissue window settings. When in doubt, inspect the same slice using lung or bone window settings, as fat appears gray on these window settings. In this case, a standard soft-tissue window setting has been adjusted slightly to make fat brighter in appearance, thereby making black gas more evident.

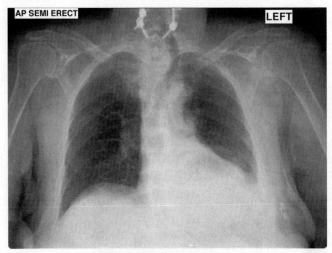

Figure 11-44. **Mesenteric ischemia with free air: Nondiagnostic chest x-ray.** This 81-year-old female presented with diffuse abdominal pain and vomiting. Her electrocardiogram showed new atrial fibrillation, and her lactate level was elevated. A chest x-ray was performed and showed no pneumoperitoneum. Compare this x-ray with the CT in Figure 11-45.

obstruction is suspected. For this indication, CT with IV contrast should be performed. Oral contrast is not necessary for the diagnosis of small-bowel obstruction or ischemia. Oral contrast may result in an unacceptable delay before imaging. Small-bowel obstruction is described in more detail in Chapter 9. Because a large vessel vascular occlusion is often not present, a filling defect should not be expected. A twisted vascular pedicle may be seen in some cases, with "whirling of the mesentery." CT findings of small-bowel ischemia

in the setting of small-bowel obstruction include thickening of bowel wall, stranding in surrounding fat, and decreased enhancement of a segment of the bowel following administration of IV contrast. Normally, the wall of well-perfused bowel enhances with IV contrast. When the blood supply is compromised, the bowel wall fails to enhance.[104]

In the pure research setting, CT has high sensitivity for the detection of ischemia complicating bowel obstruction. Mallo et al.[105] performed a meta analysis suggesting a sensitivity for ischemia of 83% (range = 63% to 100%) and a specificity of 92% (range = 61% to 100%). However, these studies may inflate the actual sensitivity, because the interpreting radiologists are specifically attuned to the possibility of ischemia. In studies investigating the sensitivity of CT in the hands of clinical radiologists interpreting CT in the course of usual patient care, the sensitivity is far lower, only around 15%.[86]

What Is Contrast Nephropathy? Which Patients Are at Risk?

Contrast nephropathy is defined as a 25% increase in baseline serum creatinine or an absolute rise of 0.5 mg/dL following administration of parenteral iodinated contrast.[106-107] It complicates 15% of contrast procedures, accounts for 10% of in-hospital renal failure, and affects more than 150,000 patients annually in the United States. Although a minority of these patients progress to permanent renal failure or require dialysis, contrast nephropathy is responsible for significant morbidity.[106]

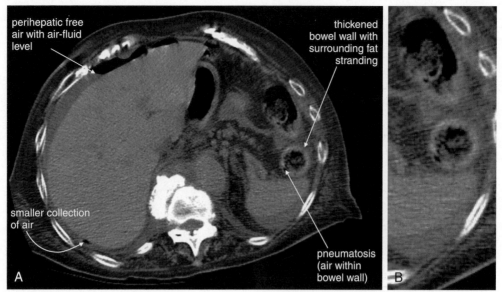

Figure 11-45. Ischemic colitis: CT without IV contrast. A, Axial CT, viewed on soft-tissue windows. **B,** Close-up from **A**. Same patient as Figure 11-44. The patient's presentation suggested mesenteric ischemia. Because of the patient's renal insufficiency, no IV contrast was given. Oral contrast was administered but did not progress beyond the small bowel before CT. This CT scan shows pneumoperitoneum, with a large amount of free air visible within a perihepatic fluid collection. Compare this with the chest x-ray in Figure 11-44, which showed no sign of pneumoperitoneum. Chest x-ray is relatively insensitive for pneumoperitoneum, whereas CT is exquisitely sensitive for this without any contrast agents. Also note the thickened descending colon with surrounding fat stranding. Pneumatosis is also visible in the wall of the descending colon, though no oral contrast has reached the colon. Laparotomy showed perforated ischemic colitis. The patient died of multiorgan failure and sepsis 4 days later.

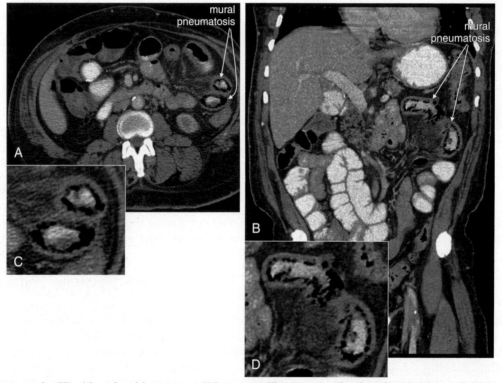

Figure 11-46. Pneumatosis: CT with oral and intravenous (IV) contrast. This 56-year-old male with end-stage renal disease on hemodialysis, diabetes, and peripheral vascular disease presented with abdominal pain. He reported similar episodes managed with antibiotics. His CT demonstrates pneumatosis intestinalis, concerning for ischemic bowel. Given his previous history, this patient was managed nonoperatively and improved with IV antibiotics (ciprofloxacin and metronidazole). CT findings of pneumatosis, though not specific for ischemic bowel, should prompt surgical consultation and consideration of surgical exploration. All panels are displayed with CT soft-tissue windows. Mesenteric ischemia has a mortality rate greater than 70%. **A,** Axial view. **B,** Coronal view. **C,** Close-up from **A. D,** Close-up from **B.**

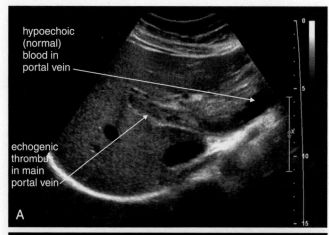

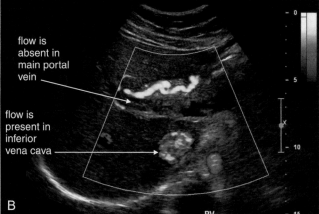

Figure 11-47. **Portal vein thrombosis: Ultrasound.** This 22-year-old female, 2 months postpartum, presented with 1 week of right upper quadrant pain. Ultrasound was performed to evaluate for suspected cholecystitis or symptomatic cholelithiasis. Instead, portal vein thrombosis was discovered. The postpartum state is a risk factor for this condition. Hypercoagulable states and inflammatory or neoplastic abdominal conditions, including pancreatitis and abdominal malignancies, also can result in portal vein thrombosis. **A,** Ultrasound grayscale image showing thrombus in the main portal vein. **B,** Doppler ultrasound showing no flow within the portal vein. *(See Color Plate 2 for color Doppler image of this figure.)*

Contrast nephropathy risk becomes significant at creatinine clearance rates below 60 mL per minute. Measured serum creatinine is a poor surrogate for creatinine clearance, because it is just one variable in the formula for creatinine clearance (Box 11-1), which is also affected by patient mass, age, gender, and race. In a study of 765 emergency department patients, of whom nearly 1 in 8 had a creatinine clearance rate of less than 60 mL per minute, a serum creatinine limit of 1.8 mg/dL missed 55% of at-risk patients.[108] Even using a highly conservative limit of 1.0 mg/dL would have failed to identify 9% of at-risk patients—highlighting the importance of using creatinine clearance rather than measured serum creatinine.

How Can Contrast Nephropathy Be Prevented?

Multiple means of reducing the risk of contrast nephropathy have been investigated. Early work suggested a benefit to hydration with sodium bicarbonate,[109] but a larger randomized, controlled trial showed no advantage over hydration with normal saline.[110] N-acetyl cysteine has been shown in some trials to reduce the incidence of contrast nephropathy, but studies have not demonstrated improvements in patient-oriented outcomes such as need for dialysis.[111] Most studies on N-acetyl cysteine focus on oral administration 24 hours before contrast administration and thus have no role in emergency department patients with suspected acute abdominal vascular catastrophes requiring immediate imaging. Only one study has investigated the use of IV N-acetyl cysteine 30 minutes before contrast administration and showed a small benefit.[112]

Low-osmolality and nonionic contrast agents have lower associated risks of contrast nephropathy than higher-osmolality and ionic contrast agents.[113] Hydration with sodium chloride has been shown to reduce the risk of contrast nephropathy and should be used whenever possible, unless contraindicated by comorbidities such as heart failure or anuria.[113-115] Reducing the volume of contrast administered is also beneficial.[106]

REACTIONS TO IODINATED CONTRAST

A history of reaction to iodinated contrast is a relative contraindication to its administration. Reactions to iodinated contrast agents are likely not true allergies but are treated clinically like allergic reactions. Allergies to seafood are generally related to protein allergens, not iodine allergy; however, severe allergy to any allergen increases the risk of a contrast reaction. Consequently, iodinated contrast should be used with caution in patients with any history of severe allergic reaction. When abdominal vascular catastrophe is suspected, contrast allergies present a particular dilemma. Vascular catastrophes including AAA rupture, aortic dissection, and mesenteric ischemia are time dependent and life threatening, making delay for prophylactic treatment of allergy hazardous. The best strategy in this scenario is likely immediate noncontrast CT. As discussed in this chapter and in Chapter 9, noncontrast CT has been shown to be sensitive and specific for a range of key abdominal disorders, including AAA and AAA rupture, pneumoperitoneum, small-bowel obstruction, renal colic, appendicitis, diverticulitis, and pancreatitis. If noncontrast CT provides a definitive diagnosis, the patient can be spared the risk of injected iodinated contrast. If noncontrast CT is nondiagnostic, a tailored risk–benefit decision must be made for the individual patient, weighing the suspicion of acute vascular catastrophe against the severity of prior allergic or contrast reactions. Other diagnostic options, including laparotomy without definitive imaging, delayed CT to allow time for prophylactic steroid treatment, MRA, and Doppler or contrast-enhanced ultrasound, must be considered. However, given the

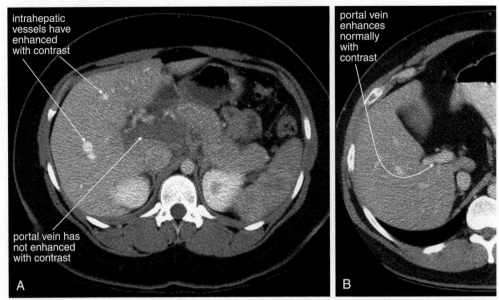

Figure 11-48. Portal vein thrombosis: CT with intravenous (IV) contrast. A, Same patient as Figure 11-47, with thrombosis of the portal vein. Notice how other vessels, including the aorta and intrahepatic vessels, have enhanced with IV contrast. The portal vein remains dark in appearance, because it has not enhanced with contrast because of lack of blood flow. Compare with ultrasound in the prior figure. For the CT diagnosis of portal vein thrombosis, IV contrast must be used, and delayed images must be obtained approximately 1 minute after contrast injection. Images acquired earlier could show lack of enhancement of the portal vein—even when the vein is patent—if contrast has not yet reached the portal vein, falsely simulating thrombosis. **B,** CT image from another patient showing normal enhancement of the portal vein, ruling out thrombosis. An advantage of ultrasound over CT for this diagnosis is that ultrasound does not require contrast administration and does not involve radiation exposure. However, CT may show secondary complications of portal vein thrombosis such as bowel wall ischemic changes.

Box 11-1: Cockcroft-Gault Formula for Estimating Creatinine Clearance

A serum creatinine clearance (glomerular filtration) rate of less than 60 mL per minute predicts an increased risk of contrast nephropathy following administration of IV contrast. Other formulas exist. Online creatinine clearance calculators are available.

$$\text{Creatinine clearance} = (140 - \text{age in years}) \times (\text{ideal body weight in kg}) / (\text{serum creatinine in mg}/\text{dL} \times 72)$$

- **Males: Ideal body weight = 50 kg + 2.3 kg for each inch over 5 feet**
- **Females: Ideal body weight = 45.5 kg + 2.3 kg for each inch over 5 feet**
- **Multiply creatinine clearance by 0.85 for females**

Box 11-2: Emergency Prophylaxis Regimens to Attenuate or Prevent Reaction to Iodinated Contrast Media[116]

Methylprednisolone 40 mg IV or hydrocortisone 200 mg IV or dexamethasone 7.5 mg IV or betamethasone 6 mg IV every 4 hours until contrast study is required, plus antihistamine.*[120-121]

---

*Diphenhydramine 50 mg intravenously 1 hour before contrast injection.

Lasser EC, Berry CC, Mishkin MM, et al. Pretreatment with corticosteroids to prevent adverse reactions to nonionic contrast media. *AJR Am J Roentgenol* 162:523-526, 1994.

---

mortality and morbidity risk of vascular catastrophes, in some cases the decision to proceed with IV contrast administration must be made, with informed consent from the patient.

Several prophylactic steroid protocols have been endorsed by the American College of Radiology (ACR) in its *Manual on Contrast Media* (Box 11-2).[116] Despite premedication, contrast reactions may occur. The evidence for benefit from premedication is relatively weak, based on small trials. The ACR recommends 6-hour pretreatment, with no study showing benefit from immediate steroid administration fewer than 3 hours before IV iodinated contrast.[113] Unfortunately, such a delay is unacceptable if an abdominal vascular catastrophe is strongly suspected.

MAGNETIC RESONANCE IMAGING AND GADOLINIUM-ASSOCIATED FATAL NEPHROGENIC SYSTEMIC FIBROSIS

Gadolinium contrast used in MRI is strongly contraindicated in patients with renal insufficiency, because it has been recently associated with the development of fatal nephrogenic systemic fibrosis (NSF), discussed extensively in Chapter 15.[117] The risks of NSF must be weighed against the risks of iodinated contrast for CT and a potentially fatal abdominal vascular catastrophe. Overall, the risk of NSF is very low after standard doses of gadolinium, occurring in none of more than 74,000 patients in one study.[118] Higher doses of gadolinium were associated with an overall risk of 0.17%, with all cases occurring in patients with glomerular filtration rates less than 30 mL per minute. In chronic dialysis patients, the risk was 0.4%. Patients with acute renal failure not receiving dialysis were at high risk, between 8% and 19%—and thus represent a group where gadolinium should be avoided whenever possible.[118] Dialysis patients and patients with acute renal failure should undergo dialysis immediately following MRI if possible to eliminate gadolinium.[119] This is in distinction to the scenario with iodinated contrast for CT, in which dialysis patients are not at risk of renal injury from contrast, as complete kidney failure is already present. Dialysis is not urgently needed following iodinated contrast administration.

SUMMARY

Abdominal vascular catastrophes must be considered early in the evaluation of patients with abdominal and back pain. Hemodynamic stability does not rule out a life-threatening vascular process, and imaging should be performed as quickly as possible before hemodynamic compromise. X-rays play little role and generally be should be avoided, with the occasional exception of upright chest x-ray to assess for free air. Ultrasound is a rapid and useful bedside screening modality for the presence of AAA. CT is the most rapid and definitive emergency department test for AAA rupture, aortic dissection, and mesenteric ischemia; oral contrast is not needed, though IV contrast is important to the diagnosis of aortic dissection, mesenteric ischemia, and active aortic aneurysm bleeding. Rarely, other modalities, including MRA, may be useful in stable patients with contraindications to CT.

CHAPTER 12 Imaging the Genitourinary Tract

Joshua Broder, MD, FACEP

Emergency conditions of the genitourinary tract include the life threatening, such as ruptured ectopic pregnancy and renal avulsion, and threats to organ function, such as testicular and ovarian torsion. The diversity of potential clinical scenarios and differential diagnoses means that our discussion is best presented in the context of the chief complaint or specific pathologic entities, rather than in a single algorithm to evaluate the entire genitourinary tract. We begin with nontraumatic urinary tract conditions. Next, we address conditions of the male and female reproductive organs, including conditions in the pregnant patient. Finally, we discuss imaging of genitourinary trauma.

CLINICAL PRESENTATIONS AND DIFFERENTIAL DIAGNOSIS

A variety of chief complaints may suggest genitourinary pathology. In some cases, no imaging is required. In other cases (such as back pain with suspected aortic aneurysm or renal colic), the nongenitourinary differential diagnosis is most important and drives imaging decisions. In still others, a targeted genitourinary differential requires emergency imaging. Table 12-1 outlines chief complaints, selected differential diagnoses, and appropriate imaging modalities.

IMAGING NONTRAUMATIC GENITOURINARY COMPLAINTS

Abdominal or Flank Pain With or Without Hematuria

Abdominal and flank pain with or without hematuria can suggest renal colic or pyelonephritis, although an array of other conditions can present with similar symptoms. Conditions such as abdominal aortic aneurysm (AAA), renal cell carcinoma, renal infarction, and perinephric abscess can cause flank and abdominal pain with hematuria. A variety of imaging options are available for evaluation of these signs and symptoms. The choice of imaging study should reflect the differential diagnosis under consideration, the clinical certainty of the diagnosis, radiation exposure concerns, contrast nephrotoxicity or allergy, time, and cost. In some cases, particularly in patients with recurrent urolithiasis, the diagnosis is virtually certain and no imaging may be required. Moreover,

in patients with recent prior imaging, other diagnostic concerns such as AAA can often be ruled out based on measurements made from existing images. Later, we discuss the imaging options with strengths and weaknesses of each. Noncontrast computed tomography (CT), CT with intravenous (IV) contrast, CT with IV and oral contrast, IV urography (IVU), x-ray, renal ultrasound, and rare tests such as Lasix renal scan all have roles in the evaluation of potential renal colic.

To select the best imaging test, the emergency physician should generate a differential diagnosis that is comprehensive yet tailored to the patient. If the differential diagnosis seriously includes entities other than renal colic, CT is likely the best test. If vascular abnormalities are considered, CT with IV contrast is useful, assuming the patient is stable and has an acceptable creatinine (because of concerns about nephrotoxicity of IV contrast). When the differential diagnosis is particularly broad, including renal, reproductive, vascular, bowel, and other abdominal pathology, CT with IV and oral contrast provides the most information. The decision to perform immediate noncontrast CT, CT with IV contrast, or oral and IV–contrasted CT should be based on the most dangerous pathology suspected. In young patients, in whom vascular disasters such as AAA are rare, radiation concerns may outweigh the impetus for rapid imaging. In these patients, the delay for oral contrast may be acceptable to avoid repeated radiation exposure if noncontrast CT were negative. In older patients with concern for vascular catastrophes, immediate CT without any contrast may be wise, with enhanced CT performed later if more information is needed. The danger of repeated radiation exposure in patients over the age of 50 pales in comparison with the risk for delayed diagnosis of AAA rupture. Vascular catastrophes are discussed in more detail in Chapter 11. If urolithiasis is the only suspected diagnosis, IVU can be performed. In pregnant patients, renal ultrasound can be used to assess for obstruction complicating urolithiasis, avoiding radiation exposure. This strategy may also be useful in patients of either gender with recurrent episodes of renal colic to avoid high cumulative radiation exposures from CT. Figure 12-1 shows an algorithm for CT imaging in acute flank and abdominal pain. Table 12-2 lists the information provided by the various imaging modalities, along with cost, time, and radiation information. We begin with a

TABLE 12-1. Chief Complaints, Differential Diagnosis, and Imaging Modalities for Genitourinary Pathology

Chief Complaint	Differential Diagnosis	Imaging Modalities
Nontraumatic Urinary Complaints		
Flank pain with or without abdominal pain	• Abdominal aortic aneurysm • Renal colic • Renal infarction • Pyelonephritis • Perinephric abscess	• Noncontrast CT (first line) • CT with IV contrast • Intravenous pyelogram • Ultrasound • X-ray • Lasix renal scan (rarely)
Painless hematuria	• Mass lesion of the genitourinary tract, such as renal cell or transitional cell carcinoma • Nephritis • Urinary infection • Renal infarction • Unlikely urolithiasis in absence of pain	• Depending on differential diagnosis, no emergency imaging • CT with and without IV contrast for neoplasm or infarct • Ultrasound
Dysuria	• Urinary tract infection, including cystitis and pyelonephritis	• No emergency imaging in most cases
Urinary retention	• Obstructive process at or distal to the bladder • Neurologic causes	• No emergency imaging in most cases • Spinal MRI for suspected neurologic causes
Abdominal pain	• Broad differential, including nongenitourinary causes • Ovarian torsion and ectopic pregnancy • Tuboovarian abscess	• Pursue most life-threatening abdominal and genitourinary diagnoses first • Perform transvaginal ultrasound early if ectopic pregnancy or ovarian torsion is suspected • CT and/or abdominal-pelvic ultrasound
Fever	• Infection • Drug reaction • Neoplasm • Inflammatory condition	• Rarely requires genitourinary imaging, unless additional symptoms such as pelvic, flank, or abdominal pain • Transvaginal ultrasound for suspected tuboovarian abscess
Perineal pain	• Fournier's gangrene • Perirectal abscess	• Surgical consultation, antibiotics, and fluid resuscitation take precedence over imaging for Fournier's gangrene • CT without contrast to show air and fluid collections • IV contrast for enhancement • Rectal contrast for delineation of perirectal abscess • Rarely, ultrasound and MRI
Male Genitourinary		
Testicular or scrotal pain	• Testicular torsion • Epididymitis • Orchitis • Abscess or Fournier's gangrene • Hernia • Hydrocele • Varicocele • Malignancy	• Scrotal ultrasound or nuclear scintigraphy for testicular torsion • Ultrasound or CT to evaluate hernia, abscess, or Fournier's gangrene
Testicular or scrotal mass	• Malignancy • Abscess • Hernia • Hydrocele • Varicocele	• Scrotal ultrasound • Possibly CT, if ultrasound suggests mass or abscess

TABLE 12-1. Chief Complaints, Differential Diagnosis, and Imaging Modalities for Genitourinary Pathology—cont'd

Chief Complaint	Differential Diagnosis	Imaging Modalities
Urethral discharge	• Urethritis	• No emergency imaging in most cases
Prostatic pain or suspected prostatic hypertrophy	• Prostatitis • Benign prostatic hypertrophy • Perirectal abscess • Prostatic abscess • Fournier's gangrene	• No emergency imaging in most cases for prostate • CT if perirectal or other abscess considered
Female Genitourinary		
Pregnant Patient		
Vaginal bleeding	• Ectopic pregnancy • Abortion (threatened, missed, complete, incomplete, inevitable) • Placenta previa • Placental abruption • Fibroids • Uterine or cervical malignancy • Ovarian cyst	• Abdominal or transvaginal ultrasound to evaluate for ectopic pregnancy in first-trimester presentations • Placental abruption cannot be ruled out by ultrasound
Abdominal or pelvic pain	• Ectopic pregnancy • Heterotopic pregnancy • Abortion (threatened, missed, complete, incomplete, or inevitable) • Endometritis • Benign causes such as round ligament pain • Other causes of abdominal pain unrelated to pregnancy	• Abdominal or transvaginal ultrasound to evaluate for ectopic pregnancy • Other imaging with caution, avoiding radiation exposure if possible • Abdominal ultrasound or MRI for diagnoses such as appendicitis
Fluid leak or vaginal discharge	• Normal pregnancy-related discharge • Infection or cervicitis • Amniotic fluid leak	• Ultrasound to assess fetal viability • Ultrasound to assess for oligohydramnios, which can result from membrane rupture
Recently Pregnant Patient		
Abdominal pain, vaginal bleeding or discharge, or fever	• Retained products of conception with endometritis • Uterine perforation • Peritonitis • Abscess • Other postsurgical complications • Septic pelvic thrombophlebitis • Other abdominal pathology unrelated to pregnancy	• Ultrasound for retained products or free pelvic fluid • CT for abscess or extrauterine pathology • MRI for septic pelvic thrombophlebitis
Nonpregnant Patient		
Vaginal bleeding	• Confirm pregnancy status—ectopic pregnancy • Normal menses • Fibroids • Uterine or cervical malignancy • Ovarian cyst • Ovarian malignancy • Dysfunctional uterine bleeding • Pelvic infection	• No emergency imaging in most nonpregnant patients • Follow-up endometrial biopsy and possible imaging in postmenopausal patient because of threat of malignancy • Routine follow-up for possible cervical malignancy (Pap smear)

TABLE 12-1. Chief Complaints, Differential Diagnosis, and Imaging Modalities for Genitourinary Pathology—cont'd

Chief Complaint	Differential Diagnosis	Imaging Modalities
Abdominal or pelvic pain	• Confirm pregnancy status—ectopic pregnancy • Other conditions not related to pregnancy, such as appendicitis • Fibroids • Uterine, ovarian, or cervical malignancy • Ovarian cyst • Dermoid or teratoma • Ovarian malignancy • Ovarian torsion • Pelvic inflammatory disease • Tuboovarian abscess • Endometriosis	• Ultrasound to assess for ectopic pregnancy • Transvaginal ultrasound to assess for ovarian torsion or tuboovarian abscess • Other imaging depending on differential diagnosis
Vaginal discharge	• Cervicitis • Pelvic inflammatory disease • Vaginal foreign body • Tuboovarian abscess (usually painful)	• Generally, no emergency imaging, unless additional symptoms such as adnexal pain • Transvaginal ultrasound to assess for tuboovarian abscess if pain is present
Trauma		
Blunt abdominal or torso trauma	• Nongenitourinary solid organ trauma such as spleen or liver injury • Important renal injury • Bowel, bladder, and diaphragm injuries	• Abdominal and pelvic CT with IV contrast • Delayed CT images for renal perfusion • CT or conventional cystogram
Traumatic hematuria (gross)*	• Renal injury • Ureteral injury • Bladder injury • Urethral injury	• Abdominal and pelvic CT with IV contrast for suspected renal or ureteral injury—delayed images should be obtained • CT or conventional cystogram for suspected bladder injury • Retrograde urethrogram for suspected urethral injury
Traumatic vaginal bleeding	• Penetrating vaginal laceration, possibly associated with pelvic fracture • Uterine trauma	• Vaginal examination to look for laceration • Pelvic radiography or CT to assess for underlying fracture
Direct genitourinary trauma	• Direct blunt trauma to the penis, scrotum, vaginal introitus, or urethral meatus • For blood at urethral meatus, consider urethral disruption, bladder rupture, renal or urethral injuries • Testicular vascular injury or hematoma	• Other injuries in a polytrauma patient take precedence • Bladder and urethral injuries, often with more life-threatening pelvic injuries • Significant renal injuries, usually in the context of significant abdominal injury, including spleen and liver injury • Imaging for these injuries takes precedence • Abdominal CT with IV contrast for renal injuries • Retrograde urethrogram for urethral injuries • Retrograde cystourethrogram—x-ray or CT—for bladder injuries • Ultrasound for testicular vascular injury

TABLE 12-1. Chief Complaints, Differential Diagnosis, and Imaging Modalities for Genitourinary Pathology—cont'd

Chief Complaint	Differential Diagnosis	Imaging Modalities
Abdominal or pelvic trauma in the pregnant patient	• Placental abruption • Uterine rupture • Other abdominal or pelvic injuries as in the nonpregnant patient	• Ultrasound is insensitive for placental abruption and cannot rule out the diagnosis; fetal heart monitoring is essential • Ultrasound for uterine rupture • Observation for stable patients with low clinical probability of abdominal or pelvic injury; abdominal CT should be avoided if possible • Abdominal CT if suspicion of injury is moderate or high, because the radiation dose does not measurably increase the rate of fetal malformations; mother's health is paramount
Penetrating abdominal or torso trauma	• Nongenitourinary solid or hollow organ trauma such as spleen, liver, or bowel injury • Important renal injury	• Abdominal and pelvic CT with IV, oral, and rectal contrast ("triple contrast")

*Microscopic hematuria generally does not require imaging in adults but does require it in pediatric patients.

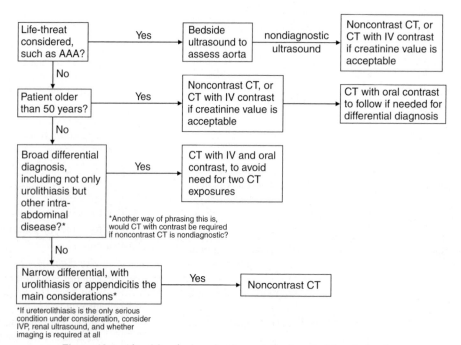

Figure 12-1. Algorithm for imaging in acute flank and abdominal pain.

discussion of CT scan, followed by descriptions of other imaging modalities.

Imaging Options for Suspected Renal Colic

Computed Tomography Scan. CT scan (Figures 12-2 to 12-15) is sensitive for many types of spontaneous disease of the kidneys, ureters, and bladder, including renal tumors and urolithiasis. It is less helpful in delineating disease such as transitional cell carcinoma within the ureters or bladder. For suspected renal colic, no IV or oral contrast is needed. A calcified stone within the kidney, ureters, or bladder usually is evident as a high-density (white) lesion on abdominal windows (see Figures 12-2 to 12-6). These lesions are easily seen without contrast because few other white structures should be present in the vicinity of the kidneys, ureters, or bladder. Calcified phleboliths in the pelvis may occasionally be confused with intraureteral stones.

TABLE 12-2. Common Diagnostic Imaging Modalities for Renal Colic

Modality	Information Provided	Radiation Dose	Contrast	Approximate Cost	Time
CT	• Renal stones, including size and position of stones and evidence of obstruction • Alternative diagnoses, such as AAA, appendicitis, and free air	4-10 mSv	No	$750-$1000	Less than 5 minutes to perform, 30 minutes for interpretation[94]
CT with IV contrast	• Same as noncontrast CT • Delineation of renal mass lesions • Additional information about vascular dissections and mesenteric ischemia	4-10 mSv[94-95]	Yes	$750-$1000	Less than 5 minutes, after delay to measure creatinine
CT with IV and oral contrast	• Same as CT with IV contrast • Potentially improved diagnosis of bowel abnormalities	4-10 mSv	Yes	$750-$1000	Less than 5 minutes, after delay of approximately 2 hours to ingest oral contrast
IVU	• Structural and functional information about obstruction • Rarely, identification of other pathology, such as AAA	1.5 mSv[95]	Yes	$350	Approximately 75 minutes[94]
X-ray	• Possible identification of stone, but not useful for hydronephrosis or most other pathology	0.5-1 mSv	No	$250	Less than 5 minutes
Ultrasound	• Identification of hydronephrosis or hydroureter • Possible identification of stone • Used to assess for AAA or biliary disease	No	No	$150	Approximately 15-30 minutes—bedside ultrasound is quicker

Noncontrast CT has become a test of choice because it can be performed immediately and provides several key pieces of information:

• Acute abdominal pathology outside of the urinary tract, such as ruptured AAA, appendicitis, bowel obstruction, and free air. Studies suggest that between 4% and 10% of CT scans performed for evaluation of suspected renal colic demonstrate alternative or additional diagnoses.[1]
• Presence of stones within the entire urinary tract, from kidneys to urethra.
• Size and location of urinary stones, information that is useful in predicting chance of spontaneous stone passage or need for urologic intervention.
• Presence of hydronephrosis or hydroureter resulting from an obstructing stone (see Figures 12-7 to 12-9).
• Additional stone burden within the kidney, which may predict future symptomatic urolithiasis. Stones currently in the kidney are rarely thought to cause symptoms, except in the case of staghorn calculi (see Figures 12-5 and 12-6).

Compared with IV urography, CT is also advantageous because it does not require contrast administration, which can cause nephrotoxicity in patients with already obstructed urinary systems. In addition, IVU does not routinely reveal nonurinary pathology. Studies comparing emergency department length of stay show an advantage to CT over IVU, the traditional standard.[2]

Is Intravenous or Oral Contrast Needed for Detection of Stones? Does Contrast Interfere With the Diagnosis of Urinary Stones?

For detection of intrarenal and intraureteral stones, no contrast of any form is needed. Administration of oral and IV contrast can interfere with diagnosis of urologic stone disease; for this reason, noncontrast CT is often performed immediately before an IV-contrasted study. This also allows comparison of the noncontrast and contrasted CT for identification of lesions that enhance with IV contrast. The addition of contrast makes identification of stones more difficult by providing an array of white (contrast-filled) structures among which a white urolith must be sought. The kidneys enhance intensely after administration of IV contrast, so stones within the kidneys may be difficult or impossible

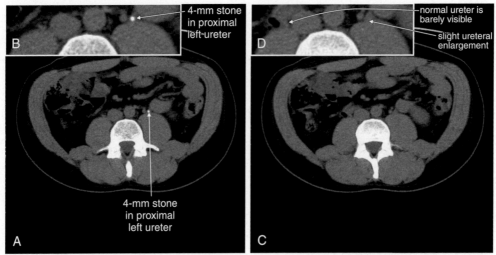

Figure 12-2. Urinary stones: Noncontrast CT on soft-tissue windows. Noncontrast CT has become the standard imaging modality for diagnosis of urinary tract stones and related complications. The study is useful because it can identify the size and location of stones, as well as complications such as hydronephrosis, hydroureter, or rupture of the renal collecting system as a consequence of obstruction. The size and location of stones have some prognostic power and can aid in planning of procedures to remove stones or relieve obstruction. Perhaps most importantly, noncontrast CT may reveal important alternative diagnoses such as aortic pathology and appendicitis. Noncontrast CT has the advantage of being available for rapid diagnosis, because it requires no preprocedural measurement of renal function and no preparation time for ingestion of oral contrast. In some institutions, the examination is performed with the patient in the prone position to allow bowel and other peritoneal organs to fall away from retroperitoneal urinary tract structures. In other institutions, the patient is scanned in a supine position. Thin slices (3 mm) are often obtained to allow detection of small stones. Because the abdomen does not usually contain calcified structures, calcified stones are readily visible against the background of soft tissues and fat, which are nearly black or dark gray on CT soft-tissue windows. Stones are bright white, as is calcified bone. Occasionally, other calcified structures may be found in the abdomen, including vascular calcifications in the aorta and its branches or pelvic vein calcifications called phleboliths. The latter can be difficult to distinguish from urinary stones. Some urinary stones are not visible on CT because they are not calcified. The classic example is indinavir stones—this relatively insoluble protease inhibitor used to treat human immunodeficiency virus infection can precipitate from solution, forming radiolucent stones. However, the sequela of obstruction, such as hydroureter or hydronephrosis, remains visible. Noncontrast CT can be viewed on soft-tissue or bone window settings to detect stones. Soft-tissue windows are appropriate for evaluating complications such as hydroureter and hydronephrosis, as well as perinephric stranding. In this 37-year-old man with left flank pain, a 4-mm stone is seen in the proximal left ureter **(A).** The ureter proximal to this is slightly dilated, consistent with hydronephrosis **(C,** one slice cephalad to **A). B,** Close-up from **A. D,** Close-up from **C.**

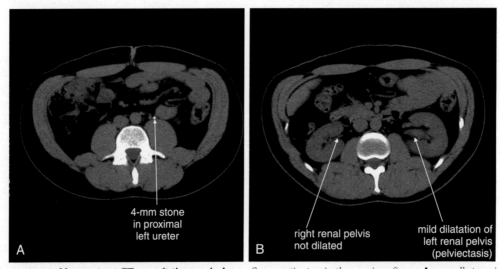

Figure 12-3. Urinary stones: Noncontrast CT on soft-tissue windows. Same patient as in the previous figure. **A,** a small stone is present in the left mid ureter. **B,** a slice cephalad to **A,** The left kidney is shows mild pelviectasis (enlargement of the renal pelvis) but no frank hydronephrosis.

to discern. Soon after IV contrast is administered, contrast is filtered and excreted by the kidneys and begins to fill the ureters, again potentially disguising stones within the ureters (see Figures 12-8 and 12-9). In cases of suspected high-grade obstruction, additional delayed images of the kidneys and ureters can be performed following IV contrast administration to assess for normal filling of the ureters, or pathologic nonfilling. This information is similar to that obtained from a standard intravenous pyelography (IVP) using conventional radiography. Oral contrast agents are not needed to detect urologic stone disease. Some CT protocols place the patient in a prone position, rather than the supine position commonly used for abdominal CT.

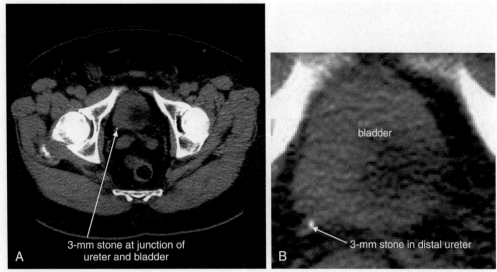

Figure 12-4. Urinary stone (small stone at ureterovesical junction): Noncontrast CT on soft-tissue windows. This patient presented with flank pain radiating to the right lower abdomen. **A,** A 3-mm stone is present at the right ureterovesical junction. **B,** Close-up. Stones of this size and location pass spontaneously in nearly all cases.

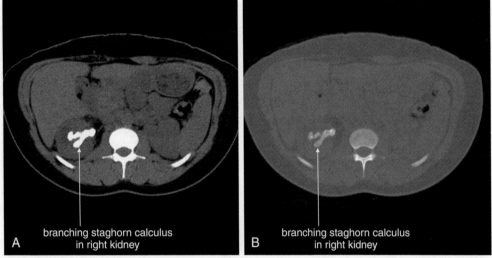

Figure 12-5. Urinary stones (staghorn calculus) noncontrast CT. Staghorn calculi are extensive branching urinary stones that may completely fill the intrarenal collecting system. Although small stones within the kidneys are not generally thought to cause pain, staghorn calculi are usually formed in the presence of chronic colonization or infection with the gram-negative rod *Proteus* and may cause pain. Occasionally, surgery is performed to remove these large stones. In this patient, a noncontrast computed tomography revealed a right staghorn calculus. Urine cultures grew *Proteus*. **A,** Soft-tissue window setting. **B,** Same slice viewed on a bone window.

This position leaves bowel and other intraabdominal organs in a dependent position, whereas ureters and kidneys are held tightly in their retroperitoneal position. Calcifications in the ureters may be more easily discriminated from nonurinary calcifications by this technique.

When Should Noncontrast CT Be Performed? When Should Noncontrast CT Be Followed by Contrasted CT?

This is a clinical decision, and it should be driven by the differential diagnosis. Several factors warrant consideration. First, is a life-threatening diagnosis, such as ruptured AAA or aortic dissection, under serious consideration? If so, immediate CT should be considered, perhaps without any contrast agents, depending on the stability of the patient (bedside ultrasound and surgery consultation may be appropriate in an unstable patient). AAA can be diagnosed without any contrast agents, whereas aortic dissection requires IV contrast for diagnosis. Second, is the patient old enough that the radiation exposure from multiple CT scans is *not* an important consideration? In patients older than 50 years, the radiation exposure from CT is unlikely to cause a clinically important cancer, and rapid diagnosis of an immediate life threat such as AAA easily trumps radiation risk. In younger patients, especially those in whom an imminent life threat is not suspected, it may be more reasonable to perform a single CT scan

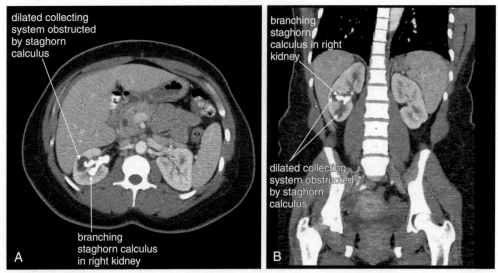

Figure 12-6. Urinary stones (staghorn calculus): Intravenous-contrasted CT soft-tissue windows. Same patient as in the previous figure. The patient received IV contrast. Now, the right kidney enhances, revealing a hypodense region of intrarenal collecting system that is obstructed by a branch of the staghorn. **A,** Axial image, **B,** Coronal image.

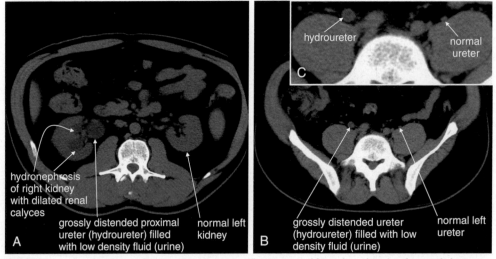

Figure 12-7. Hydronephrosis and hydroureter without urinary stones. This 32-year-old man has a history of ureteral obstruction resulting from past ureteral stones. He now presents with flank pain and hydronephrosis, but no stones were seen on noncontrast CT. A "dual renal scan"—noncontrast CT (this figure), followed by CT with intravenous (IV) contrast (see Figure 12-8)—was performed. This provides functional information, much like standard IV pyelography. **A** through **C,** In this noncontrast CT, the right kidney appears to have marked hydronephrosis whereas the left kidney is normal. High in the pelvis, the right ureter is readily recognized and has hydroureter, whereas the left ureter is barely visible in its normal position hugging the psoas muscle. When trying to locate the ureter using a digital picture archiving and communication system, start at the kidney and follow the ureter slice by slice to the bladder. Attempting to locate a normal ureter in midcourse is often difficult because of the small size of the normal ureter.

with IV and oral contrast to maximize the possibility of detecting nongenitourinary pathology. This strategy may be more beneficial to the patient in the long run than scanning without contrast and then scanning with contrast if no pathology is detected. At the same time, studies suggest that CT without contrast has good sensitivity for many conditions traditionally examined with contrast, including appendicitis. These studies are discussed in more detail in Chapter 9, Imaging of Nontraumatic Abdominal Conditions. Depending on the specific differential diagnosis being considered, noncontrast CT may be the only imaging needed—for example, contrasted CT may not be required if the appendix is well visualized on noncontrast CT. An additional factor to be considered is the patient's renal function and allergies—IV-contrasted CT should be avoided in patients with renal insufficiency or dye allergies, and noncontrast CT may be adequate to evaluate fully the differential diagnosis under consideration. Noncontrast CT generally is not performed after contrasted CT because orally administered agents may remain present for a day or more and IV contrast agents are visible for minutes to hours (in the case of urinary obstruction) within the renal collecting system, ureters, and bladder as they are excreted.

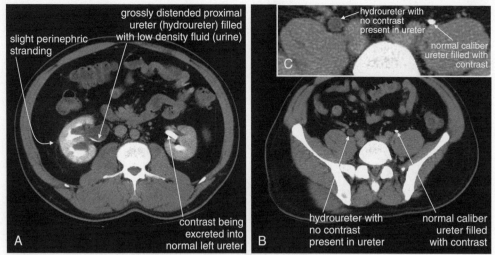

Figure 12-8. **Hydronephrosis and hydroureter without urinary stones: Intravenous-contrasted CT.** Same patient as in the previous figure. Now, the patient has received IV contrast. **A** through **C,** The right kidney is enhancing, but no contrast has been excreted into the ureter, which remains distended with low-density urine. The left kidney is enhancing, and contrast has been excreted from the kidney into the ureter and is present along its entire course, visible as a bright white dot in transverse cross section or as a linear bright structure in coronal section (see Figure 12-4).

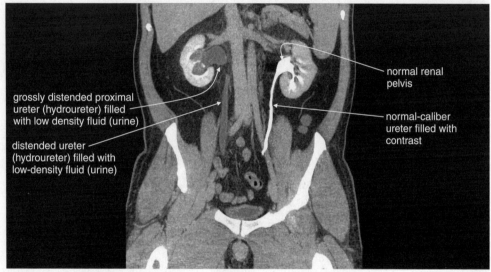

Figure 12-9. **Hydronephrosis and hydroureter without urinary stones: Intravenous-contrasted computed tomography.** Same patient as in the previous figures. A coronal image shows the kidneys and ureters. The right kidney has obvious hydronephrosis and hydroureter with no contrast in the ureter. The left kidney is excreting contrast normally, and the ureter is filled with contrast. Note the difference in caliber of the right and left ureters. The distal ureters and bladder are not seen because they lie in a more anterior plane. No stones were seen in the right ureter, and no extrinsic compression was witnessed. A stricture of the ureterovesical junction on the right was suspected, likely because of prior stones.

Besides the Presence of Stones, What Genitourinary Abnormalities Can Noncontrast CT Identify? What Genitourinary Abnormalities Can Be Seen With the Addition of IV Contrast?

Noncontrast CT can reveal the presence of ureteral obstruction.[3] **Hydronephrosis** is recognized by the presence of a dilated renal collecting system. The unobstructed contralateral side serves as a useful comparison (see Figures 12-7 to 12-9). Variation in size of the proximal ureter can occur because of the presence of a normal variant extrarenal pelvis, which can simulate significant proximal hydroureter. **Hydroureter** (see Figures 12-7 to 12-9) proximal to an obstructing stone can be detected on

noncontrast CT. The upper limit of normal diameter for an unobstructed ureter is 3 mm.[4] **Stranding** of perirenal fat (see Figures 12-8 and 12-11) can be seen without any contrast agents and can occur in the setting of obstruction or infection. Stranding is caused by lymphatic capillary leak, resulting in infiltration of fluid into the perirenal fat. This increases the density of the perirenal fat relative to normal fat. Increased density on CT results in a whiter appearance, compared with the usual dark gray appearance of fat. This finding may also occur in pyelonephritis, so the urinalysis should be examined for infection. Importantly, stranding alone does not indicate infection, unless other clinical

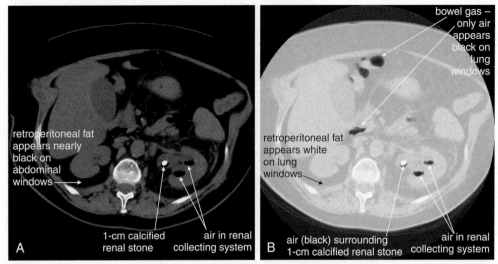

Figure 12-10. **Emphysematous pyelonephritis noncontrast CT. A, B,** Emphysematous pyelonephritis is a urologic emergency in which infection with gas-forming organisms affects the kidney. This patient has a large stone in the left renal pelvis. Notably, air is filling the renal collecting system. On typical soft-tissue windows, the black appearance of air may be difficult to distinguish from dark retroperitoneal and peritoneal fat. Lung windows make every tissue type except air white, leaving black air in stark relief.

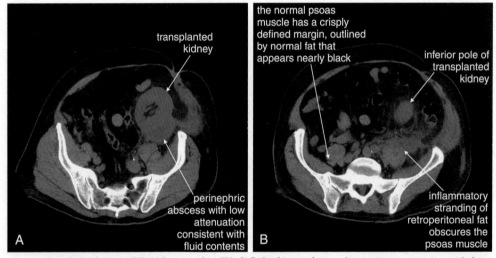

Figure 12-11. **Renal or perinephric abscess: CT with no oral or IV. A, B,** In this renal transplant patient presenting with fever and pain overlying his transplanted kidney, a noncontrast CT was performed because of concerns about potential contrast nephropathy. CT revealed perinephric abscess—although the patient's transplant had been performed more than 3 years prior. This collection was subsequently drained under CT guidance, and cultures of the fluid grew *Staphylococcus aureus*. In this case, CT findings suggesting perinephric abscess include regional fat stranding near the inferior pole of the kidney, extending to the left psoas muscle—which may also be involved in the abscess. The normally well-defined margins of the psoas are obscured by this fat stranding. Note that inflammatory fat stranding is visible without administration of any contrast. If IV contrast had been administered, rim-enhancement of the abscess would be expected.

indicators of infection (such as a positive urinalysis) are present. Emphysematous pyelonephritis (see Figure 12-10) can be observed on noncontrast CT because air appears black and does not require contrast for visualization. Perinephric abscess (see Figure 12-11) can be seen as a low-density (dark gray) fluid collection adjacent to the kidney, often with stranding. Addition of IV contrast enhances an abscess. Urine collections (urinomas) surrounding a kidney because of a leaking renal pelvis or ureter have a similar appearance to abscess on noncontrast CT but may lack stranding and do not enhance with IV contrast. Isolated simple renal cysts (see Figure 12-12) are visible on noncontrast CT. These structures have a low Hounsfield unit density near zero

because they contain fluid similar in density to water. The surrounding renal parenchyma is slightly denser and thus slightly brighter without contrast. When IV contrast is administered, renal cysts become more conspicuous because the surrounding normal kidney enhances dramatically but cysts do not. Solitary simple cysts are not usually diagnostically important because they are not typically a cause of acute pain. Polycystic kidneys may be the cause of acute or chronic pain and are readily seen on noncontrast CT. Unilateral, horseshoe, or pelvic kidneys are recognized on noncontrast CT, though these are not associated with acute abdominal or flank pain. Solid renal tumors such as renal cell carcinoma (see Figures 12-13 and 12-14) can

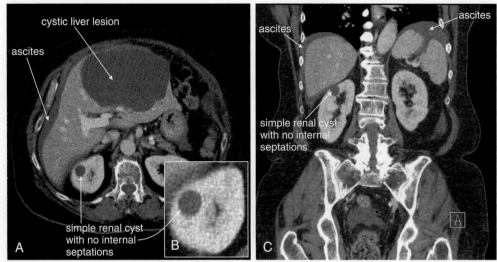

Figure 12-12. Simple renal cyst: CT with IV contrast on soft-tissue windows. A through **C,** Simple renal cysts have a rounded appearance without internal septations. They do not enhance with IV contrast because they are not vascular infectious or inflammatory lesions. This patient has a simple cyst in the right kidney, as well as an enormous cystic liver lesion and ascites. These share the same fluid density and thus have the same grayscale appearance on abdominal soft-tissue windows. On the Hounsfield scale used to measure density on CT, water is assigned a value of 0 Hounsfield units (HU), air is assigned a value of 0 HU, and the densest materials such as bone have values as high as +1000 HU. The density of the fluid in the simple renal cyst is around 30 Hounsfield units, similar to that of water.

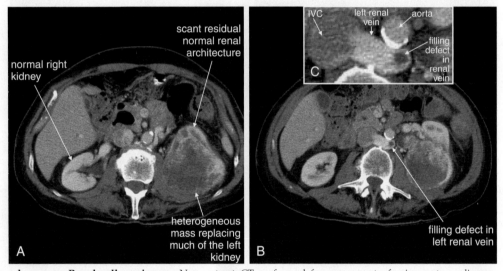

Figure 12-13. Renal masses: Renal cell carcinoma. Noncontrast CT performed for assessment of urinary stone disease sometimes reveals underlying renal malignancies. When a malignancy is suspected, intravenous contrast should be administered to further characterize the lesion. Flank pain and painless hematuria are both sometimes presenting symptoms of renal cell carcinomas (hypernephromas). **A** through **C,** In this patient, an aggressive renal cell carcinoma has nearly replaced the left kidney. A small amount of relatively normal renal architecture can be seen anteriorly, whereas the bulk of the tumor is heterogeneously enhancing, likely because of a degree of necrosis. Incidentally, the patient has a retroaortic left renal vein (the normal course being anterior to the aorta). This vein deserves attention because renal cell carcinomas are known to invade the renal vein, enter the inferior vena cava (IVC), and embolize to the lungs. In this patient, a filling defect is seen in the left renal vein, likely representing tumor invasion. The IVC is just beginning to fill with contrast and has a heterogeneous appearance due to mixing of contrast and normal blood, so it cannot be assessed for tumor invasion. Delayed images could be obtained to identify filling defects in the IVC once the contrast appearance of the IVC has become more uniform.

be difficult to identify on noncontrast CT when small. They may be exophytic and can invade adjacent structures (see Figure 7-56). Addition of IV contrast helps in detection of small lesions by allowing enhancement. Renal infarction is not easily identified on noncontrast CT but is readily apparent with IV contrast, as the infarcted region fails to enhance while normal renal parenchyma vividly enhances (see Figure 12-15).

Retroperitoneal hemorrhage (Figure 12-16), whether spontaneous or resulting from trauma, can be seen on noncontrast CT. Addition of IV contrast is important in these cases as it can reveal active bleeding.

IV contrast results in intense enhancement of the normal kidney because of the enormous blood flow to this organ. An abnormal kidney may fail to enhance compared with

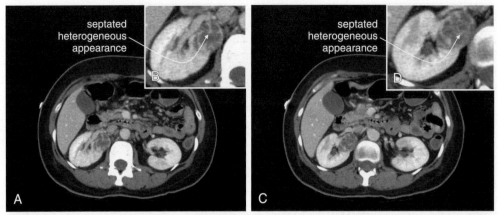

Figure 12-14. Renal masses: Smaller renal cell carcinoma identified on CT with IV contrast. A through **D,** A renal cell carcinoma is seen arising from the right kidney. Typical features of this malignancy include a septated or heterogeneous appearance with the administration of intravenous contrast. In comparison, benign simple renal cysts are homogeneous and have a single cyst cavity. Small renal cell carcinomas can be missed on CT without IV contrast, so IV contrast should be administered when malignancy is suspected, such as in adults with painless hematuria.

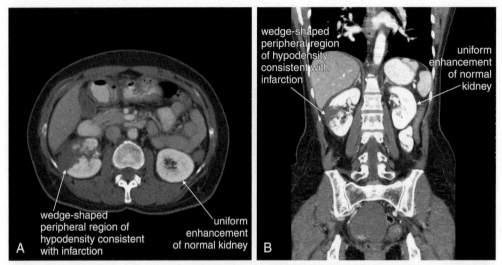

Figure 12-15. Renal infarcts: Contrast-enhanced CT on soft-tissue windows. A, B, CT with intravenous (IV) contrast gives important information on renal perfusion. This patient presented with flank pain and hematuria and was noted to be in new-onset atrial fibrillation. Renal infarction was suspected, and both oral and IV contrast were given because of a broad differential, including possible mesenteric ischemia. The renal findings could have been delineated using IV contrast alone. The left kidney enhances uniformly. The right kidney has a peripheral wedge-shaped area of hypodensity and nonenhancement, consistent with renal infarction. This appearance is similar to what might be seen with a traumatic renal contusion, but here no history of trauma exists. Severe focal pyelonephritis has been reported to have a similar appearance, but here the history of atrial fibrillation makes infarction the leading diagnosis. In the coronal image **(B),** the window level has been adjusted slightly, accounting for the brighter appearance of bone and solid organs.

the normal kidney. Examples include aortic dissection (see Figure 7-83) or renal artery dissection. In addition, hypoperfused renal segments may not enhance normally. Examples include renal infarcts in the context of atrial fibrillation (see Figure 12-15). Hypoperfusion of renal segments also is seen in some cases of pyelonephritis, although no clinical significance is known and contrasted CT is not recommended for this diagnosis.[5] As mentioned earlier, renal abscesses with rim enhancement may also be demonstrated on CT with IV contrast, though noncontrast CT or ultrasound may show a fluid collection around the kidney (see Figure 12-11). Perirenal fluid collections may also indicate urinomas because of a leaking urinary tract—these do not demonstrate rim enhancement with the addition

of IV contrast and can be seen on noncontrast CT. Renal masses such as renal cell carcinoma (hypernephroma; see Figures 12-13 and 12-14) are also detected as enhancing masses on contrasted CT (these lesions may be detected, though not as perfectly delineated, on noncontrast CT). Exophytic bladder lesions such as transitional cell carcinomas may become visible as IV contrast excreted by the kidneys fills the bladder. The tumor mass may be visible as a void or filling defect in the contrast-filled bladder. Clot may have a similar effect and appearance. Dense contrast settles in the dependent portion of the bladder. As a consequence, if the bladder is not completely filled with contrast, lesions in the nondependent portion of the bladder may not be visible.

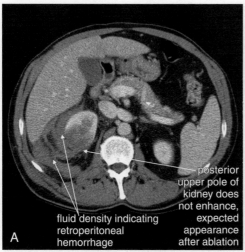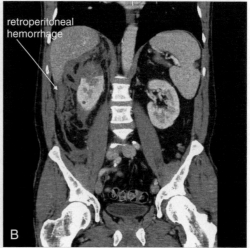

fluid density indicating retroperitoneal hemorrhage

posterior upper pole of kidney does not enhance, expected appearance after ablation

A

retroperitoneal hemorrhage

B

Figure 12-16. Retroperitoneal hemorrhage. CT with IV contrast gives important information on retroperitoneal hemorrhage. Blood that has escaped before the CT scan appears dark gray and can be seen on noncontrast CT. Addition of IV contrast allows recognition of active bleeding and demonstrates normal and abnormal renal perfusion. Oral contrast is not needed. This 50-year-old man on warfarin and enoxaparin for a Saint Jude aortic valve presented with flank pain after undergoing a CT-guided percutaneous ablation of a renal mass. The CT shows no enhancement in the upper pole of the right kidney, as expected following the ablation. Fluid density (blood) is seen in the retroperitoneum surrounding the right kidney. No blush of contrast is seen within this collection, indicating that no active bleeding is present. **A,** Axial view. **B,** Coronal view.

How Sensitive Is Noncontrast CT for Renal Stones?

CT is highly sensitive for most calcified ureteral stones. Its sensitivity and specificity approach 100%, with better positive and negative likelihood ratios than IVU.[6-7] In some cases, no stone is seen because the patient passed the stone just before CT scan.[3] Stones formed from indinavir, a poorly soluble protease inhibitor used in the treatment of human immunodeficiency virus infection, are not visible on CT because they are isodense with urine. However, findings of obstruction from these stones, such as hydroureter and hydronephrosis, are still readily recognized on CT. These stones can be seen by modalities such as ultrasound, and on IVU they create an obstruction picture identical to that seen with other stones.

What Is the Prognostic Value of CT for Renal Stones? What Size of Stone Will Pass? How Quickly can Stones Develop? What If the Patient Had a Scan Without Stones 1 Week Ago?

Stone size as measured on CT scan is predictive of the rate of spontaneous passage or need for surgical or procedural intervention. Only 2.2% of patients with stones smaller than 6 mm require a procedure, whereas 80% of patients with stones of at least 6 mm require a procedure. The rapidity with which stones can develop is not well studied, but in general, the absence of stones on recent CT imaging likely indicates that a large obstructing stone is unlikely.

Ultrasound. Ultrasound is a valuable tool for the assessment of obstruction of the ureters. Ultrasound has the advantage of being noninvasive, with no radiation exposure and no need for IV contrast. It is relatively inexpensive compared with CT[8] and can be repeated over time without harm to the patient. Ultrasound is portable, and it can be used to assess for important alternative causes of symptoms, from aortic aneurysm to appendicitis to complications of pregnancy. It is the standard test for suspected renal colic in the pregnant patient because it does not expose the fetus to ionizing radiation. Renal ultrasound assesses for hydronephrosis and hydroureter (Figures 12-17 and 12-18). It is limited to some extent by body habitus and operator experience, and it does not always allow visualization of the cause of the obstruction, whether that is an intraureteral stone or extrinsic compression of the ureter by a mass or retroperitoneal fibrosis. On ultrasound, calcified renal stones are hyperechoic (bright white) (see Figure 12-17), reflecting the ultrasound beam and preventing its transmission deep to the stone. As a consequence, they also create an acoustic shadow deep to the stone. Ultrasound can be used to detect other renal disease including atrophic kidneys, renal cysts including polycystic kidney disease, and renal masses. With the addition of Doppler ultrasound, flow in the renal arteries and renal artery stenosis can be diagnosed.

Studies comparing ultrasound and CT for the diagnosis of ureterolithiasis show comparable sensitivity and specificity (91% and 95%, respectively, for CT and 93% and 95%, respectively, for ultrasound).[8-9] Some studies have shown lower sensitivity of ultrasound (61%) compared with CT (96%).[9] Overall, ultrasound is a reasonable alternative to CT when the differential diagnosis is limited to ureteral stones and radiation reduction is a priority, as in pregnancy or young patients with multiple episodes of renal colic.

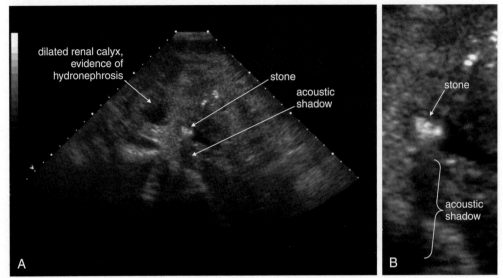

Figure 12-17. Ultrasound of renal stone. Ultrasound can be used to assess for renal stones and complications such as hydronephrosis. Stones can be difficult to detect, whereas hydronephrosis is usually readily observed. Because stones are dense, they reflect sound and prevent its through transmission. As a result, stones are echogenic (bright) on ultrasound, and cast an acoustic shadow (black). **A,** Short-axis view of kidney. **B,** Close-up.

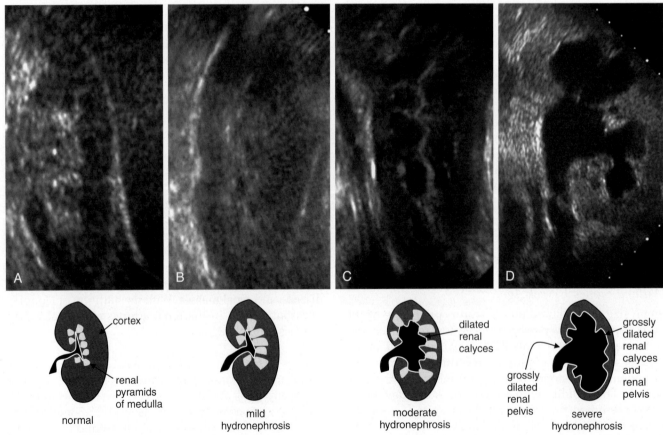

Figure 12-18. Hydronephrosis: Ultrasound. Ultrasound can detect hydronephrosis readily, whereas renal stones are not as easily observed. The normal kidney has a hypoechoic (dark gray) outer cortex, whereas the renal pyramids of the inner medulla are hyperechoic (bright). The renal calyces of a normal kidney are barely visible because urine drains from them readily in the absence of obstruction. As obstruction develops, the calyces fill with urine, which is hypoechoic (black). Normal kidney **(A)** and mild **(B),** moderate **(C),** and severe **(D)** grades of hydronephrosis. Kidneys are shown in the long-axis view.

Plain Film X-ray. Plain film x-ray plays a limited role in evaluation of nontraumatic urologic emergencies. In the setting of suspected renal colic, a single plain film of the abdomen was commonly performed before the era of CT. This x-ray is often called a KUB (for kidneys, ureters, bladder)—ironically, because none of these structures is usually visible, though they may be included in the field of view. X-ray is likely insensitive for detection of renal stones: 18.6% in one study compared with a gold standard of unenhanced CT. The specificity is high, around 95%.[10] This method may have some limited value when other imaging techniques are unavailable. It can demonstrate likely ureteroliths, although it may fail to detect noncalcified stones. In addition, extraurinary calcifications such as phleboliths may be misidentified as urinary stones (Figures 12-19 and 12-20*A*). Although the size of the stones may be measured, plain film does not allow assessment for obstruction. In addition, sensitivity for a broader differential diagnosis, including aortic aneurysm, appendicitis, and bowel obstruction, is quite limited. Perhaps the greatest benefit of a single plain film in this setting is that the radiation exposure to the patient is low—though the information gleaned from the study is so limited that no imaging is nearly as useful. Sometimes a single x-ray to evaluate for radiodense stones is combined with ultrasound to evaluate for hydronephrosis and hydroureter. When a stone has been visualized on a prior x-ray, x-ray can be used to monitor its progression. X-ray is also used to assess the position of medical devices such as ureteral stents.

Intravenous Urography. IVU (also called IVP) is a series of plain film images taken over time (see Figure 12-20). In addition to providing information about the structure of the urinary system, including the presence of stones or obstruction, this is a "functional study," because it provides a view of renal excretion of injected contrast. First, a plain film image of the abdomen and pelvis is obtained, before the administration of contrast. This image can be examined for radiopaque stones and medical devices such as ureteral stents, as described earlier. Occasionally, an alternative diagnosis such as appendicitis or AAA may be recognized, although this modality should never be relied on to exclude these diagnoses because it is insensitive. Next, around 50 mL of iodinated contrast is injected intravenously, and the plain film (KUB) is repeated after a delay of 5 minutes. Additional images are repeated at approximately 15-minute intervals until both kidneys have been observed to fill and then empty of contrast, allowing excretion of the contrast material to be observed over time. Depending on the speed of excretion, the examination usually takes less than 1 hour, though several hours may be required in cases of severe obstruction. A normal IVU demonstrates rapid and symmetrical enhancement of both kidneys, followed by complete filling of the ureters and

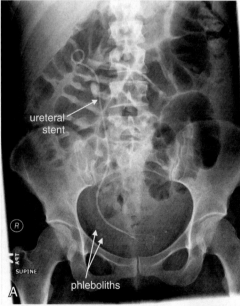

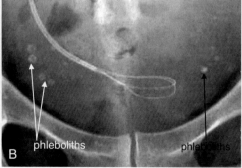

Figure 12-19. X-ray of renal stones. X-rays of the abdomen have been used historically to diagnose and monitor urinary stones. Unfortunately, x-rays are neither sensitive nor specific. Some renal stones are relatively radiolucent and not visible on x-ray. In addition, other calcifications in the abdomen and pelvis may be indistinguishable from ureteral stones. X-ray does not show complications of urinary stones, such as ureteral obstruction and hydronephrosis. In this patient, the right ureter has been stented to relieve obstruction. Calcifications are visible in the pelvis, but these are likely phleboliths (venous calcifications) rather than ureteral stones. Notice how they lie lateral to the position of the stent in the ureter. Some also have a radiolucent (dark) center, which is a common but not pathognomonic feature of phleboliths. **A,** X-ray, often called a KUB (for kidneys, ureters, and bladder) because these structures lie within the field of view. Ironically, none of these structures is well seen with plain x-ray. **B,** Close-up.

bladder. Several abnormalities may be observed. First, congenital anomalies may be observed, including duplications of the collecting system, and unilateral, horseshoe, or abnormally positioned (e.g., pelvic) kidneys. In the setting of ureteral obstruction from any cause, the kidney on the affected side may show delayed enhancement and delayed emptying, called a "delayed nephrogram" (see Figure 12-20E). This is because of diminished

renal filtration and excretion of contrast in the setting of obstruction. In addition, the affected ureter may fail to fill with contrast beyond the point of a complete obstruction, or the contrast may appear less intense beyond the point of a partial obstruction. IVU provides anatomic and functional information about the location and degree of obstruction, which may be important for planning urologic intervention.

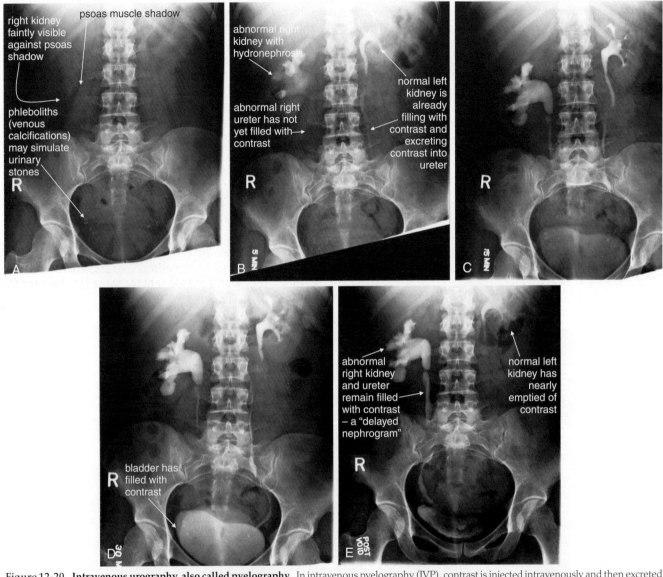

Figure 12-20. Intravenous urography, also called pyelography. In intravenous pyelography (IVP), contrast is injected intravenously and then excreted by the kidneys, providing a cast image of the renal calyces, pelvis, ureters, and bladder. This provides structural information because hydronephrosis, hydroureter, and points of ureteral stricture or obstruction are revealed. This also provides functional information because a nonfunctioning kidney does not excrete contrast. Together, delayed appearance of contrast in a renal collecting system and slow excretion from the collecting system is called a delayed nephrogram and is a sign of partial obstruction. An IVP consists of a preinjection plain x-ray of the abdomen and pelvis, followed by a series of x-rays of the same region conducted at intervals of 5, 15, and 30 minutes, as well as a final image after voiding of urine or contrast from the bladder. Additional delayed images may be obtained. Sometimes exophytic lesions in the bladder (neoplasms) are seen as filling defects. **A** through **E,** In this IVP series, the patient has a normal left kidney, with a collecting system that briskly fills with contrast and then empties. Structurally, this collecting system also appears normal, with no dilated calyces and a thin normal ureter. In contrast, the right renal calyces are slow to fill (because of high pressure in the collecting system from distal obstruction). The right kidney not only fills more slowly than the left but also is slower to empty, remaining markedly visible even on postvoid images. The right renal calyces and pelvis are extremely dilated consistent with hydronephrosis, and the proximal right ureter is dilated, consistent with hydroureter. There is relatively little contrast in the distal right ureter at the level of L3-L4, consistent with an obstruction proximal to this level. The patient had a ureteral stone at this level previously and likely has a stricture at this location. Phleboliths are also visible in the pelvis and may be mistaken for urinary stones.

Is Intravenous Urography Preferable to CT for Evaluation of Renal Colic or Ureteral Obstruction?

IVU and CT provide similar but not identical information. CT is superior in delineating a range of emergency alternative diagnoses, explaining its rapid incorporation into the imaging algorithm for suspected renal colic in the United States. CT also has the advantage of not requiring the administration of any contrast material, with the obvious benefit of not posing a threat of contrast nephropathy or dye allergy. In addition, CT can be performed immediately and diagnostic results are available within minutes, in comparison to IVU, which takes around 1 hour in most cases and longer in cases of severe obstruction. A number of studies have compared the time, expense, and radiation exposure of CT and IVU. CT generally results in slightly shorter emergency department length of stay, similar costs (depending on whether institutional or patient costs are compared), and somewhat higher radiation exposure, though new protocols have reduced radiation exposures.

Lasix Nuclear Medicine Scan: An Alternative Test for Ureteral Obstruction.

A patient with recurrent renal calculi may develop an appearance of chronic obstruction with a dilated renal pelvis and ureter by ultrasound, CT scan, or IVP. A Lasix nuclear medicine scan (Figures 12-21 and 12-22) can discriminate obstruction from a flaccidly dilated but currently unobstructed collecting system. Though rarely used in the emergency department, this test may be requested by a urologic consultant. In this test, a radiopharmaceutical, technetium-99m mercaptoacetyltriglycine, is administered intravenously. Dynamic blood flow phase images of the kidneys are obtained during bolus injection of the radiotracer. Sequential 2-minute acquisitions posteriorly over the abdomen are obtained through 30 to 60 minutes, allowing generation of graphs of radioactivity over time for the renal cortex and entire kidney. Lasix (50 mg IV) is administered after around 20 minutes. In a normal scan, rapid uniform excretion occurs after administration of Lasix. This is consistent with a flaccid but unobstructed collecting system. Lack of excretion

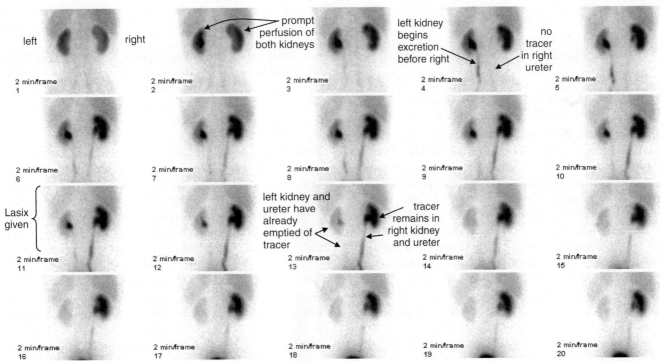

Figure 12-21. Lasix renal scan. Same patient as in the CT scan in Figures 12-7 to 12-9. A Lasix renal scan is a nuclear medicine study that provides quantitative information about renal perfusion and excretion. Though rarely used in the emergency department, this study may occasionally be requested by consulting urologists when uncertainty exists about the functional effect of a chronically dilated urinary system. Note that the right–left convention for this study is reversed from that used for CT. The frames are numbered sequentially and occur at 2-minute intervals. In this scan, 10.2 mCi of a radiopharmaceutical, technetium-99m mercaptoacetyltriglycine, are administered intravenously. Dynamic blood flow phase images of the kidneys are obtained during bolus injection of the radiotracer. Sequential 2-minute acquisitions posteriorly over the abdomen are obtained through 42 minutes. In addition to anatomic images, radioactivity can be graphed over time for the renal cortex and whole kidney, providing quantitative measurements of renal parenchymal perfusion. Lasix (50 mg intravenously) is administered at 22 minutes. In this patient, the dynamic blood flow images above demonstrate relatively prompt and symmetrical perfusion to the bilateral kidneys. On the initial renogram images, the right kidney appears slightly larger than the left kidney, and there is central photopenia in the right kidney that suggests hydronephrosis. On subsequent renogram images over 42 minutes, the left kidney demonstrates relatively prompt uptake, excretion, and clearance of radiotracer with no evidence of obstruction. The right kidney demonstrates mildly delayed uptake and excretion of radiotracer into a prominent collecting system, from which there is only minimal clearance of tracer activity until the administration of Lasix. After Lasix administration, there is somewhat better, though incomplete, clearance of tracer activity over the duration of the study, with residual tracer activity seen in the right collecting system and the right ureter to level of the urinary bladder on the postvoid image. These findings suggest partial obstruction of the right ureter.

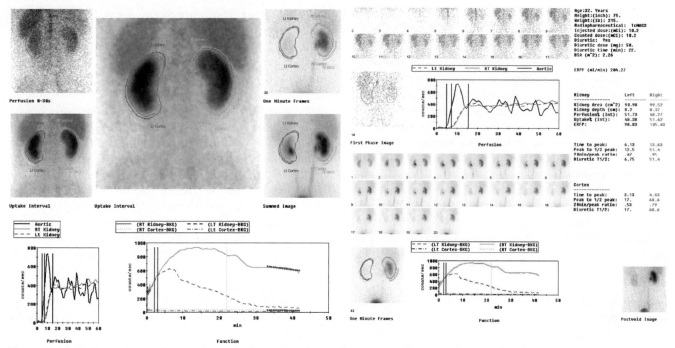

Figure 12-22. Lasix renal scan. Same patient as in the previous figure. Quantitative information about renal perfusion can be obtained from this study. In this patient, both kidneys were found to be well perfused despite poor excretion from right kidney, consistent with obstruction. *(See Color Plate 3 for color image of this figure.)*

of the tracer following Lasix administration suggests obstruction.

Is Any Imaging Needed for Suspected Renal Colic?

When a broad differential diagnosis is being considered, nongenitourinary diagnoses may drive the imaging strategy. Important diagnoses such as suspected AAA rupture or appendicitis may require CT or other imaging for diagnosis. In effect, though CT may confirm urolithiasis, the most important function of CT may be to exclude other diagnoses. When renal colic is the only serious diagnosis under consideration, the emergency physician should carefully consider whether any imaging is required. CT carries a moderately high radiation exposure, and patients with renal colic often have recurrent symptoms, resulting in multiple CT exposures over time. When complications such as infection or renal insufficiency are not present, deferring CT imaging may be reasonable. In first-time episodes of suspected renal colic, clinical judgment is incorrect in as many as 20% of cases, even when suspicion of stone is 90% or greater. Imaging of first episodes is likely warranted.[11] Alternative or additional diagnoses are reported in approximately 10% of patients undergoing CT for suspected renal colic, although not all of these diagnoses require specific emergency treatment.[1] In patients with recurrent symptoms, another reasonable strategy may be ultrasound to evaluate for hydronephrosis or hydroureter. Ultrasound may show a stone, though with lower sensitivity than CT. In patients older than 50 years, the risk of repeat CT radiation exposures may be relatively unimportant, and the risk of alternative causes of symptoms rises. CT may be a prudent strategy in this age group.

Painless Hematuria

Painless hematuria generally is not associated with urolithiasis because the latter condition is usually painful. Painless hematuria can indicate urinary infection, renal infarction, systemic illness such as glomerulonephritis or thrombocytopenia, or masses of the genitourinary tract, including renal cell carcinoma (see Figures 12-13 and 12-14) and transitional cell carcinoma of the ureters or bladder. Painless hematuria is an important complaint for this reason, but emergency imaging is only required in selected cases, depending on the specific differential diagnosis being entertained. For example, in the patient with atrial fibrillation, renal infarction (see Figure 12-15) should be considered. Imaging can alter patient management because confirmation of renal infarction can suggest a cardiac embolic source. When important but less urgent pathology such as renal mass is suspected, imaging can be deferred to an outpatient setting. Patients with poor follow-up may benefit from definitive imaging in the emergency department to allow appropriate referral. When the decision is made to perform imaging, CT without IV contrast followed by CT with IV contrast is most useful because it identifies enhancing renal masses such as renal cell carcinoma. CT with IV contrast can also demonstrate areas of abnormal renal parenchymal enhancement consistent with infarction. Noncontrast CT alone may fail to fully delineate these lesions. Oral contrast is not needed for these indications. CT scan does not evaluate intraluminal pathology of the bladder or ureters well, so additional follow-up for cystoscopy is indicated if transitional cell carcinoma is suspected. Exophytic bladder lesions such as transitional cell carcinomas may become visible as IV contrast excreted by the kidneys fills the bladder. Delayed CT images are often acquired to allow detection of such pathology. The tumor mass may be visible as a void or filling defect in the contrast-filled bladder. Clotted blood within the bladder may have a similar effect and appearance and may sometimes confuse the diagnosis. Renally excreted contrast within the ureters on CT or IVP may occasionally show a filling defect suggesting a ureteral mass.

Dysuria

Isolated dysuria can suggest urinary tract infection, infectious urethritis, or sterile urethritis such as Reiter's syndrome. This symptom generally does not require emergency imaging.

Urinary Retention

Obstruction of the bladder outlet and inability to urinate is a common emergency department complaint, particularly in men. Usual causes are benign prostatic hypertrophy and hematuria with clot formation leading to urethral obstruction. Ureteral obstruction rarely causes urine retention because bilateral ureteral obstruction would be required. Retroperitoneal causes such as retroperitoneal fibrosis or tumors may occasionally obstruct both ureters. Urinary retention from a neurologic cause should be considered, but in the absence of other neurologic signs or symptoms, back pain, or other red flags for spinal pathology, mechanical bladder outlet or urethral obstruction is the most common cause. Prostatic malignancies and bladder masses may also lead to obstruction, but emergency imaging is not generally required when symptoms are relieved by placement of a urinary catheter. Urologic follow-up is necessary. If a neurologic cause is suspected, spine magnetic resonance imaging (MRI) is usually required. Ultrasound of the bladder can be performed at bedside and reveals a full bladder in cases of urethral obstruction or neurogenic bladder. Renal ultrasound commonly reveals bilateral hydronephrosis but is not necessary if the obstruction is relieved by urinary catheter placement.

Nontraumatic Abdominal Pain

Nontraumatic abdominal pain can result from a host of serious and benign conditions. The chapters on abdominal imaging explore this in detail. Some causes of abdominal pain include genitourinary abnormalities, as described later in the sections on male and female genitourinary complaints. Flank pain with or without abdominal pain was discussed earlier.

Fever

Isolated fever without other genitourinary signs or symptoms rarely requires genitourinary imaging. Fever associated with abdominal, flank, or pelvic pain requires imaging as indicated for the evaluation of the associated pain. Serious genitourinary infections such as tuboovarian abscess, perinephric abscess (see Figure 12-11), or Fournier's gangrene (Figures 12-23 and 12-24), described in the next section, may have associated fever but are usually accompanied by localizing pain and examination findings that direct imaging. One exception is the obtunded septic patient with fever. Complicated urinary infections such as perinephric abscess and infected obstructing ureteral stone should be considered and may require imaging.

Perineal Pain

Perineal pain can result from a variety of conditions, including some serious and life-threatening causes. Local abscess formation may be difficult to detect by physical examination and can require emergency imaging. Most fearsome is Fournier's gangrene (see Figures 12-23 and 12-24), a polymicrobial infection resulting in soft-tissue necrosis and sepsis. When Fournier's gangrene is suspected clinically, empiric antibiotics, surgical consultation, and fluid resuscitation take precedence over imaging. CT without IV contrast can delineate the extent of infection and can show soft-tissue air and fluid collections. Addition of IV contrast can demonstrate enhancement typical of abscesses. When perirectal abscess is suspected, rectal contrast may assist in differentiating the bowel lumen from adjacent soft-tissue infectious fluid collections. MRI and ultrasound can also demonstrate local soft-tissue fluid and air collections but are rarely indicated in the emergency department. They can be used in the pregnant patient to avoid radiation exposure.

GENITOURINARY IMAGING IN THE MALE PATIENT

Several important genitourinary chief complaints may require imaging in male patients. The imaging approach varies with age and suspected differential diagnosis.

Testicular or Scrotal Pain

Testicular and scrotal pain can suggest testicular torsion, epididymitis, orchitis, local abscess, Fournier's gangrene, hernia, hydrocele, varicocele, and malignancy. Among these, testicular torsion, Fournier's gangrene, and incarcerated hernia are surgical emergencies. When these diagnoses are clinically suspected, immediate surgical or urologic consultation should be obtained, before or concurrent with imaging studies.

Testicular torsion is best evaluated with either ultrasound (Figure 12-25, normal ultrasound) (Figures 12-26

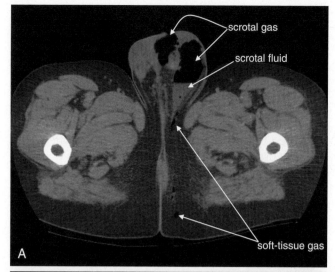

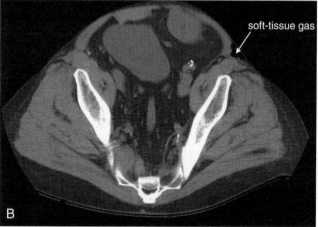

Figure 12-23. Fournier's gangrene. This 41-year-old man with a history of renal transplantation presented with diffuse scrotal pain and crepitus. He had first noted a "boil" in his perineal region several days prior. CT of the pelvis was performed without intravenous or oral contrast. **A,** A slice at the level of the scrotum shows an gas–fluid level in the left scrotum, as well as gas in the midline of the scrotum. Gas tracks posteriorly from this into gluteal subcutaneous fat. **B,** A slice from much higher in the pelvis and lower abdomen reveals that the patient does not have an isolated scrotal abscess. Here, gas remains visible in the subcutaneous space anterior to the left iliac wing. These findings are consistent with Fournier's gangrene. Coronal and sagittal images from the same patient illustrate the cephalad–caudad extent of the infection in the next figure. The patient was taken emergently to the operating room, and necrotic tissue was debrided from the scrotum, abdominal wall, and gluteal region. Two important points are illustrated by this case. First, arguably the clinical findings should have been acted upon without requiring any imaging. Fournier's gangrene requires emergent operative debridement. However, in this case, the CT findings prompted involvement of both urologists and general surgeons, whereas an isolated scrotal abscess may have been handled by a urologist alone. Second, CT without any contrast agents is exquisitely sensitive for the presence of soft-tissue gas. When necrotizing soft-tissue infections are suspected, noncontrast CT offers rapid assessment. Surgical consultation should not be delayed for imaging.

and 12-27, testicular torsion) or nuclear scintigraphy. Physical examination is relatively unreliable, with significant overlap in findings such as cremasteric reflex abnormalities between patients with torsion and epididymitis.[12] Ultrasound is moderately sensitive and highly specific for persistent torsion (nearly 100% sensitive and specific in some studies,[13-14] though others report

sensitivity of only 60% to 80% and specificity of only 80% to 90%[15-19]). Intermittent torsion may be one explanation for negative ultrasound results. Delayed presentations of torsion beyond 8 hours have been reported to lead to false-negative ultrasound interpretations.[20] Decreased blood flow demonstrated by Doppler ultrasound suggests or confirms torsion, whereas normal blood flow is reassuring. Complete loss of blood flow may not occur. Venous flow is often compromised first, followed by arterial flow. Emergency physician–performed ultrasound shows high agreement with studies performed by sonographers and interpreted by radiologists—reported as 95% sensitive and 94% specific in one study, though wide confidence intervals in this study may mean lower true sensitivity and specificity.[21] Nuclear scintigraphy detects abnormal testicular perfusion and has a sensitivity and specificity similar to that of ultrasound in studies directly comparing the two modalities, around 80% sensitive and 90% specific.[16,22] As stated earlier, consult a urologist as soon as torsion is suspected, before imaging. *Because false-negative imaging results are possible, when torsion is strongly suspected clinically, surgery may be appropriate despite normal ultrasound or scintigraphy.*

Epididymitis and orchitis (Figures 12-28 to 12-30) can be diagnosed by ultrasound. The usual indication for imaging is to rule out the diagnosis of testicular torsion. Increased Doppler blood flow signal in the epididymis or testicle suggests epididymitis or orchitis, respectively. The sensitivity and specificity are not well delineated, so other clinical factors should be incorporated into treatment decisions, rather than relying exclusively on imaging findings. Nuclear scintigraphy can also suggest increased blood flow consistent with epididymitis or orchitis.

Ultrasound of the scrotum can demonstrate loculated fluid collections consistent with abscess (Figures 12-31 to 12-33), although other fluids such as blood can have a similar appearance. Air in the scrotum from necrotizing infection causes dispersion of the ultrasound beam, disrupting the ultrasound image. Although this prevents a high-quality image, it can be diagnostic because air should never be found in the normal scrotum. As outlined earlier, Fournier's gangrene and local abscesses of the scrotum can be identified by CT without IV contrast. Air, fluid, and inflammatory soft-tissue stranding are evident without contrast. IV contrast improves diagnostic sensitivity and specificity by demonstrating rim enhancement of abscesses. Rectal contrast can delineate abscesses adjacent to the distal bowel, which may otherwise be difficult to distinguish from fluid-filled bowel.

Hydrocele (Figure 12-34), or fluid within the scrotum and outside of the testicle, is readily diagnosed by ultrasound. Because hydrocele can accompany a variety of other conditions, including infection, testicular torsion, and

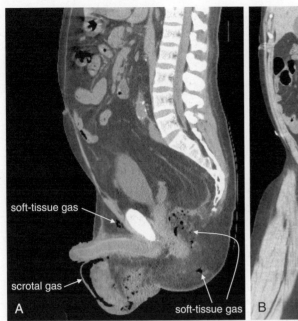
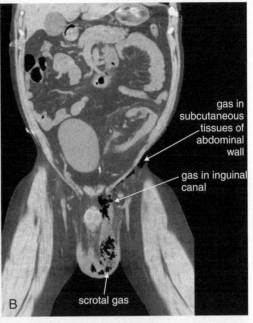

Figure 12-24. Fournier's gangrene. Same patient as in the previous figure. **A,** Sagittal view. **B,** Coronal view. These views demonstrate the cephalad–caudad and anterior–posterior extent of the infection. **A,** Gas is visible in the scrotum, as well as in soft tissues of the buttocks. **B,** Gas, and presumably infection, has tracked up the left inguinal canal from the scrotum and follows the muscles of the lower abdomen.

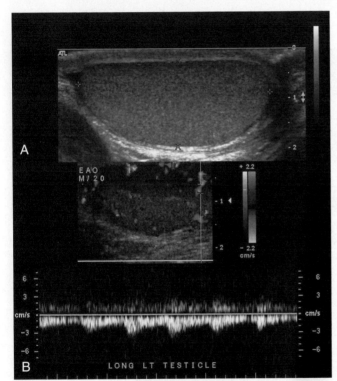

Figure 12-25. Normal testicular ultrasound. This 20-year-old male complained of a palpable nodule on the right testicle. These images of the left testicle are normal. **A,** The normal echo texture of the testicle is seen. No significant fluid surrounds the testicle. **B,** Arterial flow is normal, with a pulsatile waveform. *(See Color Plate 4 for color Doppler image of this figure.)*

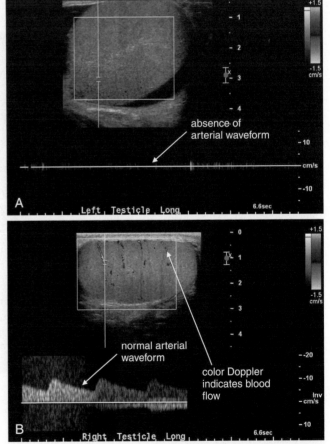

Figure 12-26. Testicular torsion ultrasound. A, B, Ultrasound has become the standard modality to assess for testicular torsion. In this 20-year-old male with left testicular pain, the left testicle has no blood flow, whereas the right testicle has normal arterial and venous blood flow by color Doppler assessment and a normal arterial waveform. The patient was taken to the operating suite, where left testicular torsion was confirmed. After rapid detorsion and orchiopexy, the left testicle reperfused and was viable. *(See Color Plate 5 for color Doppler image of this figure.)*

Figure 12-27. Testicular infarct. This patient had been treated for epididymitis without improvement. Ultrasound then revealed apparent testicular torsion, confirmed operatively. The patient underwent orchiectomy, and surgical pathology was consistent with hemorrhagic infarction. This case highlights the importance of imaging for testicular pain. Epididymitis, orchitis, and testicular torsion may have similar presentations. The ultrasound findings of note are an absence of blood flow in the left testicle by color Doppler, and a heterogeneous echotexture of the left testicle compared with the right, which is consistent with infarction. *(See Color Plate 6 for color Doppler image of this figure.)*

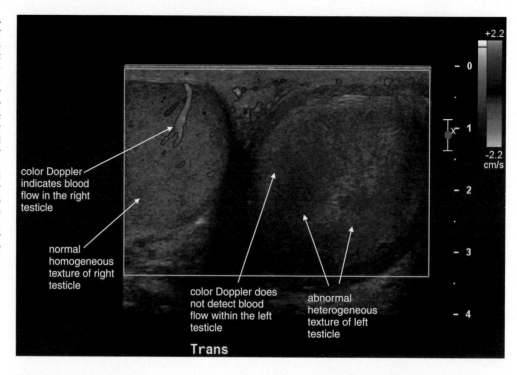

Figure 12-28. Epididymitis. A through **C,** In addition to evaluating the more concerning diagnosis of testicular torsion, ultrasound can identify epididymitis and orchitis. In epididymitis, blood flow to the affected epididymis is increased. **A,** A hydrocele is visible (black) adjacent to the left testicle. **B** and **C,** The left epididymis shows increased blood flow compared with the normal right epididymis, based on color Doppler, consistent with epididymitis. In addition, the left epididymis is enlarged compared with the normal right epididymis. Blood flow to the testicles was normal. *(See Color Plate 7 for color Doppler image of this figure.)*

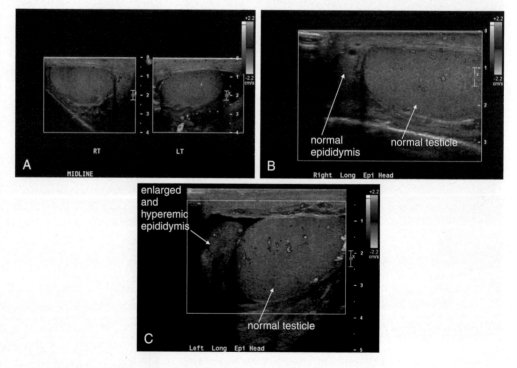

malignancy, its presence should not be used to exclude other diagnoses. Hydrocele can be simple fluid elaborated from an adjacent inflammatory process or communicating with abdominal ascites. Loculated or heterogeneous hydrocele can suggest infection or organizing hematoma, so the differential diagnosis should be considered carefully. Isolated hydrocele with otherwise normal imaging findings, including normal testicular blood flow, may not require additional emergency imaging, with the caveat that hydrocele can accompany both harmless and concerning conditions such as testicular torsion. Spermatocele (Figure 12-35) has a similar ultrasound appearance. CT without IV or oral contrast can also demonstrate hydrocele, although it generally should not be ordered for this indication because ultrasound conveys the same information without radiation exposure.

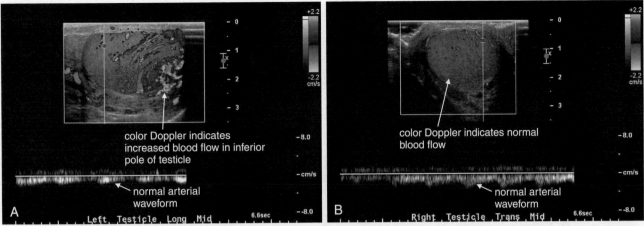

Figure 12-29. Focal orchitis on testicular ultrasound. A and **B,** This 45-year-old male was treated with antibiotics for epididymitis but had recurrent pain after completing treatment. Ultrasound was performed to rule out testicular torsion. Instead, the ultrasound suggested focal orchitis. Prominent flow is seen in the inferior portion of the left testicle, consistent with focal orchitis in that location. The right testicle shows normal blood flow. *(See Color Plate 8 for color Doppler image of this figure.)*

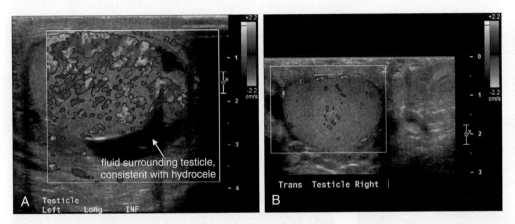

Figure 12-30. Orchitis, color Doppler ultrasound. A and **B,** This patient with left testicular pain shows markedly increased blood flow on color Doppler throughout the left testicle compared with the right, consistent with orchitis of the left testicle. A hydrocele is also seen surrounding the left testicle (black collection). *(See Color Plate 9 for color Doppler image of this figure.)*

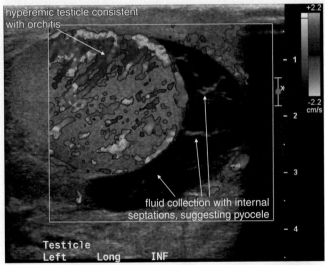

Figure 12-31. Orchitis with pyocele: Testicular ultrasound. The left testicle is markedly hyperemic on color Doppler ultrasound compared with the right testicle (not shown), consistent with orchitis. There is complex fluid collection with internal septations and internal echoes that is predominantly located inferior to the testicle and is concerning for a pyocele. Simple hydroceles are homogeneously black without internal echoes. Fluid collections with internal structure are more likely to represent infection or blood products, whereas simple fluid is more likely serous. *(See Color Plate 10 for color Doppler image of this figure.)*

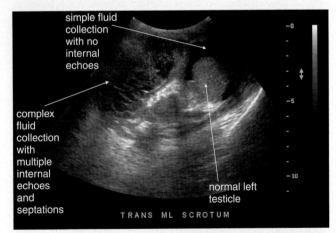

Figure 12-32. Scrotal hematocele after hernia repair. This patient developed increased right scrotal swelling after a hernia repair. Ultrasound was performed to evaluate the cause. This image shows the midline scrotum. The right scrotum is filled with a complex collection with multiple septa—no testicle is seen because the patient is known to have an undescended testicle on that side. The left scrotum shows a normal testicle surrounded by simple fluid collection, consistent with hydrocele. These findings are examined in more detail in the next figure. No bowel loops are seen to suggest a recurrent hernia.

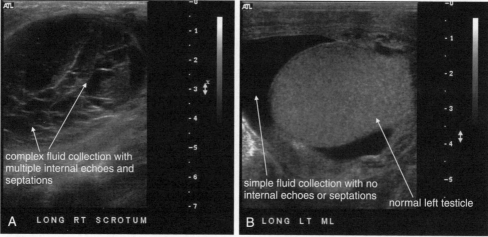

Figure 12-33. **Scrotal hematocele after hernia repair.** This patient developed increased right scrotal swelling after a hernia repair. Ultrasound was performed to evaluate the cause. **A,** The right scrotum with complex fluid collection with multiple internal septa. This is concerning for hematocele or pyocele—the two cannot be distinguished on ultrasound. **B,** The left scrotum with a normal testicle and simple fluid collection consistent with hydrocele. Note the absence of any internal septa or echoes within the fluid collection.

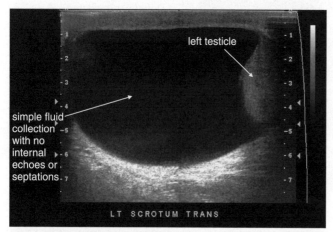

Figure 12-34. **Hydrocele.** This patient has a large left hydrocele. The fluid collection has no internal echoes or septations and likely represents serous fluid. Complex fluid collection with internal echoes and septations would be more concerning for infection or blood products.

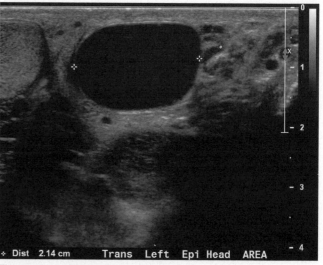

Figure 12-35. **Spermatocele.** This 41-year-old man noted a painless mass in his left scrotum. On examination, a firm nodular nontender mass was noted adjacent to but distinct from the left testicle. Ultrasound showed a cystic fluid–filled structure in the region of the left epididymis. Although this isolated image resembles a hydrocele, the structure is well circumscribed and does not surround the left testicle. The important feature here is the cystic quality, which makes this a likely benign lesion. A solid structure would be more suspicious for malignancy.

Varicocele (Figure 12-36) is a benign venous abnormality characterized by a palpable mass on examination, often described as a "bag of worms." Some patients may present with associated pain, usually not severe. Ultrasound readily confirms the diagnosis, demonstrating a series of low-flow channels using Doppler. Ultrasound is usually ordered to evaluate for other, more dangerous conditions, such as testicular torsion. CT can demonstrate this finding but is not generally indicated for its evaluation.

Malignancy can result in testicular or scrotal pain. Ultrasound can demonstrate solid testicular masses, which can include not only germ cell tumors but also metastatic and hematogenous malignancies such as lymphoma. Hydrocele may accompany these. CT may also demonstrate these abnormalities but is not the first-line imaging test because ultrasound provides accurate information without radiation. CT can be used to assess for metastatic involvement once an abnormality is confirmed with ultrasound.

Incarcerated hernia can be diagnosed using ultrasound and CT (see the chapter on imaging of nontraumatic abdominal conditions). Incarceration is largely a clinical diagnosis, based on pain, signs of bowel obstruction such as vomiting and absence of flatus, and inability to reduce the hernia on examination. However, both ultrasound and CT can confirm the presence of bowel within the scrotum. CT without IV contrast can demonstrate herniated bowel. Addition of IV contrast can illustrate bowel wall abnormalities such as abnormal enhancement suggesting

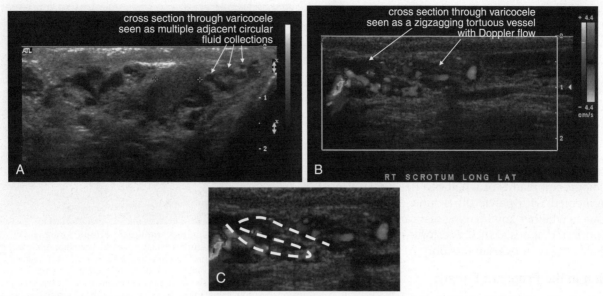

Figure 12-36. Varicocele. This 35-year-old man underwent ultrasound for evaluation of azoospermia. An incidental finding on this ultrasound was bilateral varicoceles. These tortuous veins may present as scrotal masses. **A** through **C,** Ultrasound confirms varicocele by demonstrating tortuous fluid-filled vessels with color Doppler flow consistent with venous blood flow. **A,** In the left scrotum, the vein passes in and out of the plane of the ultrasound image, giving the appearance of multiple adjacent circular cross sections. **B** and **C,** In the images from the right scrotum using color Doppler, a zigzagging vessel with flow is visible. *(See Color Plate 11 for color Doppler image of this figure.)*

ischemia. Oral contrast is rarely needed and not necessarily helpful because it may not reach the segment of herniated bowel. Ultrasound can demonstrate fluid- and air-filled bowel loops within the scrotum. Peristalsis may be visible, a reassuring finding suggesting preservation of bowel perfusion and viability. Air in the herniated bowel may scatter the ultrasound beam, disrupting the image. However, the presence of air in the scrotum is abnormal and can be recognized as suggestive of hernia.

Testicular or Scrotal Mass

Painless scrotal masses may include malignancy, hydrocele, varicocele, and nonincarcerated hernia. Infection (such as orchitis or abscess), testicular torsion, and incarcerated hernia usually result in a painful mass. The evaluation is with ultrasound as described earlier for evaluation of scrotal pain. Painless scrotal masses generally are not emergencies, although definitive diagnosis to exclude malignancy should be timely.

Urethral Discharge

As described earlier for dysuria, urethral discharge in men is a finding of urethritis, including infection with *Neisseria gonorrhea* and *Chlamydia trachomatis*. Inflammatory conditions such as Reiter's syndrome can also result in urethral discharge. Imaging is not generally required for this complaint.

Prostatic Pain or Urinary Retention From Suspected Prostatic Hypertrophy

Urinary retention from bladder outlet obstruction in male patients usually requires no emergency imaging. Bedside transabdominal ultrasound can demonstrate a distended bladder and an enlarged prostate. The prostate is visible on noncontrast CT, and abnormalities of the prostate are sometimes noted—although CT generally need not be performed in the emergency department for evaluation of suspected prostatic hypertrophy, prostate cancer, or bladder outlet obstruction from an enlarged prostate. If perineal pain is present, serious causes should be carefully considered, including perirectal abscess or Fournier's gangrene. CT with IV contrast and possible rectal contrast can be performed if these conditions are suspected. In patients who have undergone recent transrectal prostate biopsy, abscess may occur, best detected by CT with IV contrast, which can display abscess rim enhancement. Prostate calcifications may be noted on CT but do not distinguish benign from malignant disease.[23] Lytic lesions in the pelvis and spine may be indications of metastatic prostate cancer, although they are nonspecific and may be associated with other metastatic cancers, multiple myeloma, or other disease states.

GENITOURINARY IMAGING IN THE FEMALE PATIENT

Genitourinary complaints in the female patient mandate careful attention because they may indicate threats to life and fertility. The differential diagnosis and imaging approach hinge on pregnancy status and trimester of pregnancy, which form the framework for our discussion. Many presenting signs and symptoms of obstetric and gynecologic conditions, including abdominal pain, fever, and vomiting, overlap with abdominal and urinary conditions. In the patient with vaginal bleeding or discharge, and even in the known pregnant patient, a broad differential diagnosis must be entertained because pregnancy may be incidental to the patient's symptoms. Conditions such as appendicitis are common in pregnancy. In this section, we focus on the imaging diagnosis of several important obstetric and gynecologic emergencies, counting on your differential diagnostic skills to consider other conditions. We frame these as common chief complaints. In many cases, the question is whether a single imaging approach, such as abdominal CT or ultrasound, is adequate to evaluate both abdominal and gynecologic complaints or whether a negative CT must be augmented with pelvic ultrasound. In other cases, the issue is whether any imaging test can fully rule out an important diagnosis, such as ectopic pregnancy, placental abruption, or ovarian torsion.

Imaging in the Pregnant Patient

Urine pregnancy testing is the routine standard for determining pregnancy status. It is considered 99% sensitive for detection of intrauterine pregnancy. Rarely (less than 1% of cases), urine pregnancy tests may be false negative or ectopic pregnancy may occur with human chorionic gonadotropin (hCG) values below the detection limit of the urine test. Bearing this in mind, when a high suspicion of pregnancy exists (e.g., in the patient with a missed period, abdominal pain, vaginal bleeding, and hypotension), serum hCG testing is advisable.[24] Confirmation of pregnancy mandates imaging for several of the complaints that follow.

Perhaps the most common and important reason for abdominal and pelvic imaging in the pregnant patient is evaluation for potential ectopic pregnancy. Ultrasound has become the key diagnostic modality because of its safety in pregnancy. Ultrasound uses no ionizing radiation and can be repeated as often as is clinically indicated to monitor the patient's condition, response to treatment, and developmental phase of pregnancy.

Vaginal Bleeding in the Pregnant Patient

First-trimester vaginal bleeding or abdominal pain demands immediate imaging to evaluate for possible ectopic pregnancy, which occurs in about 1 in 100 pregnancies.[25] Once ectopic pregnancy is excluded, the differential diagnosis for vaginal bleeding can be explored in more detail.

Hemodynamically Unstable First-Trimester Pregnant Patient. Transabdominal ultrasound is the starting point for imaging to exclude ectopic pregnancy in a hemodynamically unstable patient. *In an unstable female patient with hypotension, tachycardia, altered mental status, or other findings of shock, ectopic pregnancy should be assumed and emergency obstetrical consultation should occur before or simultaneously with ultrasound. Fluid resuscitation, preoperative evaluation such as type and screen, and*

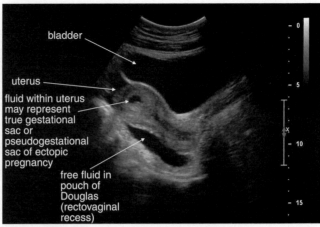

Figure 12-37. Suspected ruptured ectopic pregnancy: Transabdominal ultrasound. This 25-year-old pregnant patient presents with abdominal pain. According to the patient, she had visited Planned Parenthood the previous day and was told she might have an ectopic or molar pregnancy based on ultrasound at that time. Her human chorionic gonadotropin value is now 28,372 mIU/mL. The ultrasound shows a large amount of free fluid in the midline lower abdomen. In the midsagittal view, the bladder and uterus are seen with a large amount of free fluid in the pouch of Douglas (rectovaginal recess). Fluid within the uterus may represent a pseudogestational sac associated with an ectopic pregnancy or a true gestational sac—but in the absence of visible yolk sac or fetal pole, ruptured ectopic pregnancy must be assumed based on the other ultrasound findings and clinical presentation. An ectopic pregnancy need not be visualized to make the presumptive diagnosis. In the operating room, the patient was found to have a ruptured ovarian cyst with a large quantity of hemoperitoneum, although ectopic pregnancy was not confirmed.

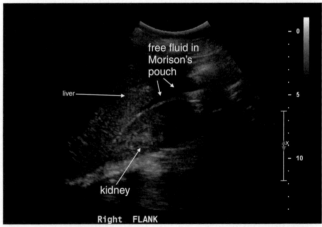

Figure 12-38. Suspected ruptured ectopic pregnancy: Transabdominal ultrasound. Same patient as in the previous figure. This right upper quadrant view shows fluid in Morison's pouch, indicating a large amount of hemoperitoneum. Given the clinical presentation of pregnancy, acute abdominal pain, and no visualized intrauterine pregnancy, ruptured ectopic pregnancy must be assumed.

transfusion should be considered before imaging confirms ectopic pregnancy. Bedside transabdominal ultrasound in the emergency department can be used to search for free abdominal or pelvic fluid, which is concerning for ruptured ectopic pregnancy and hemoperitoneum in this setting (Figures 12-37 to 12-42). As little as 100 mL of pelvic free fluid and as little as 200 to 600 mL in the hepatorenal space can be seen with transabdominal

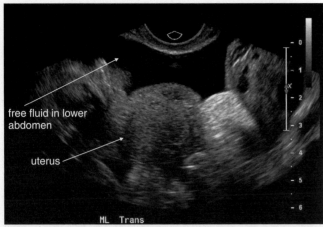

Figure 12-39. Suspected ruptured ectopic pregnancy: Transabdominal ultrasound. Same patient as in the previous figures. The ultrasound shows a large amount of free fluid in the midline lower abdomen. Given the absence of a visualized intrauterine pregnancy, ruptured ectopic pregnancy must be assumed.

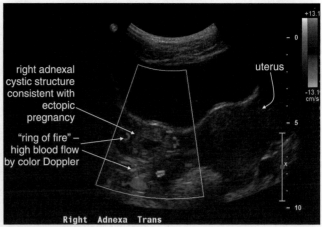

Figure 12-41. Ectopic pregnancy confirmed in operating room: Transabdominal ultrasound. Same patient as in the previous figure. This transverse transabdominal view shows the classic adnexal "ring of fire" sign—an adnexal cystic structure with high blood flow demonstrated by color Doppler. (*See Color Plate 12 for color Doppler image of this figure.*)

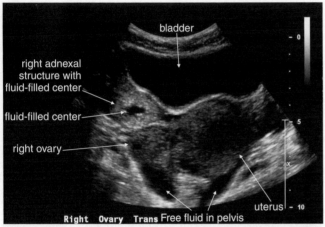

Figure 12-40. Ectopic pregnancy confirmed in operating room: Transabdominal ultrasound. This 23-year-old female presented with vaginal bleeding and a human chorionic gonadotropin value of 4680 mIU/mL. This transverse transabdominal view shows the uterus and right ovary—and an additional right adnexal structure with a fluid-filled cavity, concerning for ectopic pregnancy. Free fluid is also visible in the pelvis, suggesting possible ruptured ectopic pregnancy. No intrauterine gestational sac or fetal pole is seen on this or any other views.

ultrasound.[26] In patients with suspected ectopic pregnancy, free fluid detected in Morison's pouch by emergency-physician-performed bedside ultrasound predicts the need for operative intervention. Ultrasound may show gross evidence of an adnexal mass (see Figures 12-40 and 12-41), which may show high blood flow using Doppler (the so-called ring of fire of ectopic pregnancy). The uterus should be assessed for the presence of an intrauterine pregnancy (as described later), which markedly decreases the likelihood of a concurrent ectopic pregnancy.

Ultrasound Diagnosis of Ectopic Pregnancy. Two categories of ultrasound findings are used to diagnose ectopic pregnancy. The first category is failure to identify a normal intrauterine pregnancy. The second category is direct visualization of the ectopic pregnancy or related findings. We discuss both of these categories in detail later.

Ultrasound Findings of Normal Intrauterine Pregnancy. By about 8 weeks of pregnancy, an intrauterine pregnancy is usually readily recognized by transabdominal ultrasound as an early fetal pole with a visible heart beat. Earlier in pregnancy, an intrauterine pregnancy requires transvaginal ultrasound for detection and appears first as a gestational sac (4 to 5 weeks) (Figure 12-43), then as a gestational sac containing a yolk sac (5 weeks) (Figure 12-44), and then as a gestational sac with a fetal pole (6 weeks) (Figure 12-45). The combination of a gestational sac and yolk sac is considered sufficient to diagnose intrauterine pregnancy. On ultrasound, the gestational sac is a simple ovoid hypoechoic intrauterine structure. The yolk sac appears as a small hyperechoic ring with hypoechoic contents, contained within the larger gestational sac. *Without the yolk sac, a single ring gestational sac is not sufficient to diagnose normal intrauterine pregnancy and to exclude ectopic pregnancy, unless a double-decidual sign is seen* (see Figure 12-43). Although a single intrauterine ring may indicate the normal gestational sac of a very early pregnancy, it may also indicate the pseudogestational sac sometimes seen with ectopic pregnancy. A true gestational sac should have two decidual layers (the double-decidual sign) while a pseudogestational sac has only one decidual layer.[27] Identification of later pregnancy features such as the fetal pole, fetal cardiac activity, or fetal movement is not considered necessary to prove intrauterine pregnancy and exclude ectopic pregnancy.[28]

Human Chorionic Gonadotropin Values and Ultrasound: The "Discriminatory Zone." In the stable pregnant patient, transabdominal ultrasound

Figure 12-42. **Ectopic pregnancy confirmed in operating room: Transvaginal ultrasound. A, B,** This 23-year-old woman presented with vaginal bleeding and a human chorionic gonadotropin value of 4680 mIU/mL. An adnexal cystic structure was visualized, including a likely fetal pole. This is highly suggestive of ectopic pregnancy.

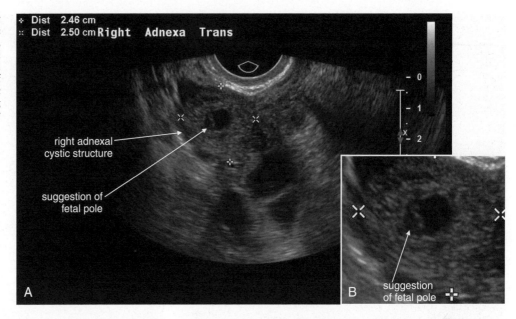

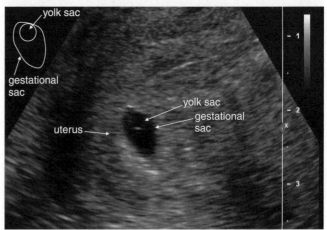

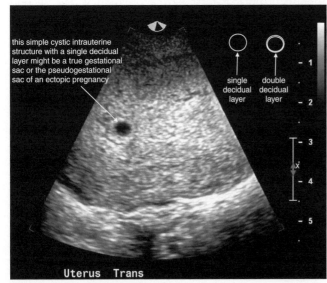

Figure 12-43. **Early gestational sac versus pseudogestational sac.** This young woman presented with vaginal bleeding in early pregnancy. Her human chorionic gonadotropin value was 3600 mIU/mL. An anechoic ovoid (simple cystic) structure is seen within the uterus. Is this an intrauterine pregnancy? We cannot be certain from this image. Because concurrent intrauterine and ectopic pregnancies are a rare event except in patients undergoing fertility therapy, the presence of an intrauterine pregnancy is used as a surrogate to exclude ectopic pregnancy. However, a simple cystic structure can be the gestational sac of a normal pregnancy or the pseudogestational sac of an ectopic pregnancy. A true gestational sac can sometimes be recognized by the presence of a two-layer deciduum (the double-decidual sign). Unless this double layer sac is seen, ectopic pregnancy remains possible. The sac in this image has only one visible layer. A definitive indication of intrauterine pregnancy is a gestational sac with a yolk sac (Figure 12-44).

Figure 12-44. **Normal intrauterine pregnancy—gestational sac with yolk sac: Transvaginal ultrasound.** This 24-year-old woman presented with right adnexal pain and vaginal spotting. Transvaginal ultrasound identified an intrauterine gestational sac containing a yolk sac. The combination of these findings confirms intrauterine pregnancy. Because heterotopic pregnancy is rare, occurring in approximately 1 in 10,000 patients, confirmation of intrauterine pregnancy effectively excludes ectopic pregnancy in all but the highest-risk patients. The presence of a gestational sac alone does not confirm intrauterine pregnancy and does not exclude ectopic pregnancy. The reason for this is simple: an intrauterine pseudogestational sac occurs with some ectopic pregnancies.

should be performed to assess for an intrauterine pregnancy, as described earlier. If an intrauterine pregnancy is confirmed by transabdominal ultrasound, additional imaging is usually not required, depending on the clinical scenario. When transabdominal ultrasound fails to demonstrate an intrauterine pregnancy, measurement of quantitative serum hCG is used in conjunction with transvaginal ultrasound to interpret imaging results, as described here.[29] Serum hCG rises rapidly during early pregnancy. Above a quantitative hCG value of 6000 mIU/mL, transabdominal ultrasound should show a normal intrauterine pregnancy, so failure to identify an intrauterine pregnancy with transabdominal ultrasound suggests abnormal pregnancy, including possible ectopic pregnancy or missed abortion.[30] At an hCG value between 1500 and 2000 mIU/mL, a normal intrauterine pregnancy should be visible with transvaginal ultrasound.[31] Failure to identify an intrauterine pregnancy

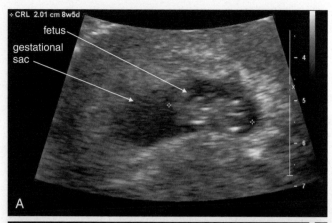

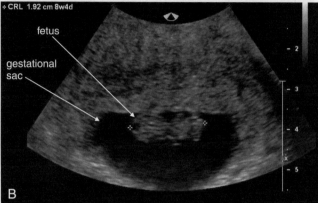

Figure 12-45. **Normal intrauterine pregnancy comparing trans-abdominal and transvaginal ultrasound appearance. A,** A transabdominal ultrasound performed in a young woman with abdominal pain. An intrauterine pregnancy is readily seen with both a gestational sac and a fetus. Crown–rump length measurement is consistent with 8 weeks, 5 days of gestation. **B,** A transvaginal ultrasound performed the same day shows higher resolution. Crown–rump length measurements closely match those made with transabdominal ultrasound in this case. In earlier pregnancy, transvaginal ultrasound can reveal a gestational sac, yolk sac, or even fetal pole when none is seen transabdominally.

TABLE 12-3. Ultrasound Findings and Ectopic Pregnancy

Ultrasound Finding	Implications for Ectopic Pregnancy
Intrauterine Findings	
Gestational sac	Does not exclude ectopic pregnancy unless double-decidual sign is definitely seen
Gestational sac with yolk sac	Excludes ectopic pregnancy (by confirming intrauterine pregnancy)
Gestational sac with fetal pole	Excludes ectopic pregnancy (by confirming intrauterine pregnancy)
Extrauterine Findings With Empty Uterus	
Fetal pole with heartbeat	Confirms ectopic pregnancy (100% specific)
Extrauterine gestational sac and yolk sac or fetal pole	Confirms ectopic pregnancy (100% specific)
Any adnexal mass other than a simple cyst	Highly suspicious for ectopic pregnancy (99% specific, 84% sensitive)
Pelvic free fluid	Suspicious for ectopic pregnancy
hCG > 6000 mIU/mL, no IUP on TAUS	Suspicious for ectopic pregnancy
hCG > 2000 mIU/mL, no IUP on TVUS	Suspicious for ectopic pregnancy

IUP, Intrauterine pregnancy; *TAUS,* transabdominal ultrasound; *TVUS,* transvaginal ultrasound.
Adapted from Brown DL, Doubilet PM. Transvaginal sonography for diagnosing ectopic pregnancy: Positivity criteria and performance characteristics. *J Ultrasound Med* 13:259-66,1994.

using transvaginal ultrasound strongly suggests ectopic pregnancy when hCG values exceed 2000 mIU/mL, although multiple gestations may lead to hCG values above 2000 mIU/mL with no visible intrauterine pregnancy.[32] An empty uterus with an hCG greater than 2000 mIU/mL is associated with a fivefold-higher relative risk for ectopic pregnancy.[33] The hCG values of 2000 and 6000 mIU/mL have been titled the "discriminatory zone," indicating the levels at which failure to visualize an intrauterine pregnancy with ultrasound becomes highly suspicious for ectopic pregnancy.[30] Normal intrauterine pregnancy is unlikely if no gestational sac is seen by transvaginal ultrasound in a patient with an hCG greater than 3000 mIU/mL.[34] Unfortunately, this has also led to misunderstanding of the utility of hCG and ultrasound in diagnosis of ectopic pregnancy. One misconception is that ultrasound need not be performed at hCG values less than 1500 to 2000 mIU/mL because a normal pregnancy would not be expected to be seen. Several studies have demonstrated that intrauterine pregnancy may be recognized by transvaginal ultrasound

with hCG values less than 1000 mIU/mL.[32,35-36] In addition, as many as 60% of ectopic pregnancies have hCG values lower than 1500 mIU/mL,[37] and ruptured ectopic pregnancies can be seen at values below 100 mIU/mL. As many as one third of ectopic pregnancies presenting with hCG values below 1000 mIU/mL will have a diagnostic initial transvaginal ultrasound.[38] *Consequently, ultrasound is indicated to evaluate for ectopic pregnancy regardless of hCG value. Failure to demonstrate an intrauterine pregnancy with transvaginal ultrasound suggests ectopic pregnancy when hCG exceeds 2000 mIU/mL.*

Ultrasound Findings of Ectopic Pregnancy. When ultrasound does not demonstrate an intrauterine gestational sac and yolk sac, proving intrauterine pregnancy, a diligent search must be conducted for other features of ectopic pregnancy, summarized in Table 12-3. A range of abnormal findings of ectopic pregnancy are shown in Figures 12-42 and 12-46 to 12-53 (see also Figures 12-37

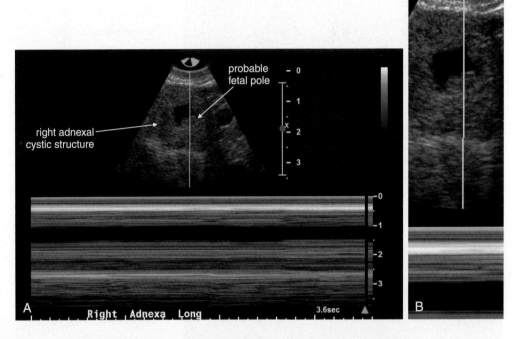

Figure 12-46. Ectopic pregnancy confirmed in operating room: Transvaginal ultrasound. A, B, Same patient as in the previous figure. Motion (M) mode ultrasound was used to assess for fetal cardiac activity. The familiar two-dimensional grayscale images of ultrasound use brightness (B) mode. In M mode, a line is placed through the two-dimensional B mode image *(top)*. A graph of motion along that line over time is generated along the bottom of the screen. If the line crosses through a beating fetal heart, a sinusoidal line will appear, and peak-to-peak or trough-to-trough measurements can be used to calculate fetal heart rate. In this case, no fetal cardiac activity was found.

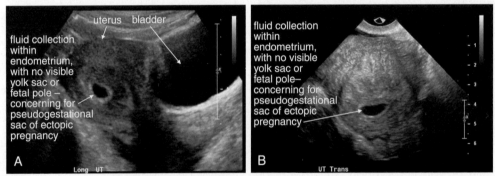

Figure 12-47. Possible ectopic pregnancy (found in the operating room to have a failed intrauterine pregnancy and two right ovarian cysts). This woman presented with lower abdominal pain and a menstrual period 4 to 5 weeks earlier. Her human chorionic gonadotropin value was 16,368 mIU/mL. An ultrasound in clinic was interpreted as suspicious for ectopic pregnancy. In these images of the uterus (**A,** long axis, and, **B,** transverse) a fluid collection is seen within the endometrium, with no visible yolk sac or fetal pole. This is concerning for a pseudogestational sac associated with ectopic pregnancy, given the hCG value greater than 16,000 mIU/mL. A normal intrauterine pregnancy (with a yolk sac or fetal pole) should be seen at an hCG value of around 6000 mIU/mL by transabdominal ultrasound and at an hCG value of around 2000 mIU/mL by transvaginal ultrasound. At laparotomy, the patient was found to have two right ovarian cysts. The absence of an intrauterine pregnancy in this case was felt to be because of failed intrauterine pregnancy, not ectopic pregnancy, although this is a retrospective determination. The described findings should be interpreted as concerning for ectopic pregnancy.

to 12-41). Diagnostic findings include direct visualization of an extrauterine fetal pole with a heart beat or an extrauterine gestational sac with a yolk sac or fetal pole. These findings have low sensitivity, around 20% to 60%, but nearly 100% specificity for ectopic pregnancy. Any adnexal mass other than a simple cyst is highly suspicious for ectopic pregnancy in the absence of an intrauterine pregnancy, with a sensitivity of 84% and specificity of nearly 99%.[39] When none of these findings is present, pelvic free fluid is suspicious for ectopic pregnancy. Isolated free fluid in the rectovaginal cul-de-sac suggests ectopic pregnancy; a moderate

amount of anechoic fluid has a positive predictive value of 22%, whereas a large amount of anechoic fluid or any echogenic fluid has a positive predictive value of 73%.[40] Moderate free fluid is defined as fluid tracking one third to two thirds up the posterior wall of the uterus without free-flowing fluid in the pelvis or abdomen. Large free fluid exceeds this amount, whereas small free fluid is less than this amount.

Even when no abnormal findings are noted, the absence of an intrauterine pregnancy on transabdominal ultrasound with an hCG above 2000 mIU/mL is concerning

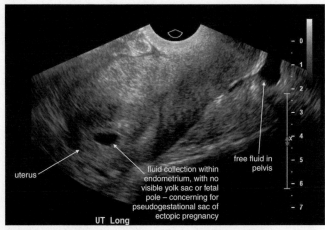

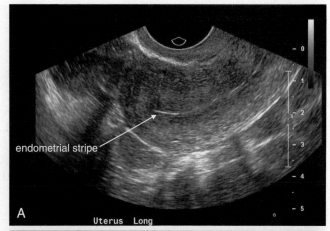

Figure 12-48. Possible ectopic pregnancy. Same patient as in the previous figure. Free fluid is seen in the pelvis, which could represent blood from a ruptured ectopic pregnancy.

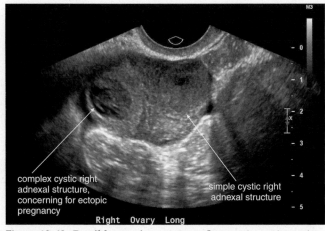

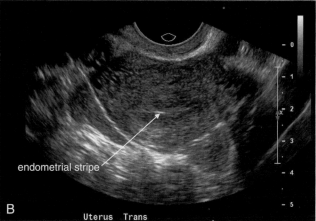

Figure 12-49. Possible ectopic pregnancy. Same patient as in previous figures. Two cystic structures are seen in the right adnexa. Given the absence of an intrauterine pregnancy, these are concerning for ectopic pregnancy.

Figure 12-51. Ectopic pregnancy. This 23-year-old female with abdominal pain had a human chorionic gonadotropin value of 27,000 mIU/mL. **A** and **B,** These images of the uterus show no intrauterine gestational sac, yolk sac, or fetal pole—very concerning absences given the hCG value. A definite intrauterine pregnancy with a gestational sac and yolk sac should be seen at an hCG value of 6000 mIU/mL by transabdominal ultrasound and at 2000 mIU/mL by transvaginal ultrasound.

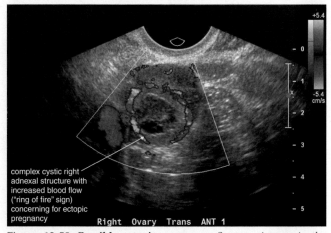

Figure 12-50. Possible ectopic pregnancy. Same patient as in the previous figures. A right ovarian complex cystic structure is seen, with increased blood flow consistent with the "ring of fire" sign—a sign described as concerning for ectopic pregnancy. (*See Color Plate 13 for color Doppler image of this figure.*)

for ectopic pregnancy. The differential diagnosis includes failed pregnancy such as blighted ovum, complete abortion not recognized by the patient, multiple gestation (with the total hCG being elevated but each gestation being too small to be seen), and ectopic pregnancy. The patient should be carefully followed for possible ectopic pregnancy, with repeat imaging and exams scheduled. In some cases, empiric therapy (methotrexate or laparoscopy) for possible ectopic pregnancy is initiated.

Heterotopic Pregnancy. In general, confirmation of intrauterine pregnancy is considered synonymous with exclusion of ectopic pregnancy, with one notable exception. Heterotopic pregnancy, the simultaneous occurrence of an intrauterine and an ectopic pregnancy, was once thought to be an extremely rare event, complicating 1 in 30,000 pregnancies. More recently, it is thought to occur in 1 in 2600 pregnancies in the United States. The risk is greatly increased by ovarian stimulation therapy, occurring in as many as 3% of these pregnancies.

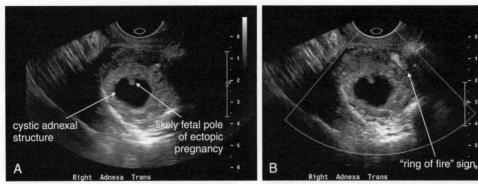

Figure 12-52. Ectopic pregnancy. Same patient as in the previous figure. **A** and **B,** These images of the right adnexa show an ovoid echogenic structure measuring approximately 4.6 × 4.0 × 3.3 cm with a central cystic region and an eccentric hyperechoic focus concerning for an ectopic pregnancy. Color Doppler shows increased blood flow around the structure, consistent with the "ring of fire" sign. At laparotomy, right adnexal ectopic pregnancy was confirmed. *(See Color Plate 14 for color Doppler image of this figure.)*

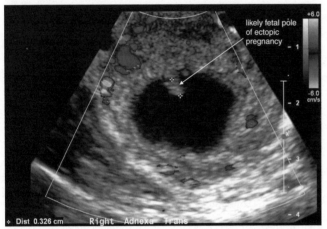

Figure 12-53. Ectopic pregnancy. Same patient as in previous figures. No fetal heart rate was documented within the echogenic focus using motion mode. The echogenic focus measures approximately 3.3 mm. *(See Color Plate 15 for color Doppler image of this figure.)*

High-risk patients for heterotopic pregnancy require more stringent imaging in an attempt to identify an ectopic pregnancy even when intrauterine pregnancy is confirmed.[41] Heterotopic pregnancy with concurrent gallstones is demonstrated in Figures 12-54 to 12-58, illustrating how caution must be taken to avoid ascribing symptoms in a pregnant patient to simultaneous abdominal disease or normal pregnancy.

Computed Tomography and Ectopic Pregnancy. CT is not the study of choice for ectopic pregnancy because of radiation exposure in the pregnant female. Occasionally, false-negative pregnancy testing or failure to obtain a pregnancy test before abdominal CT may lead to detection of ectopic pregnancy on CT scan. Findings may include an adnexal cystic structure, free pelvic and abdominal fluid consistent with hemoperitoneum, and active extravasation of IV contrast indicating active bleeding in the case of ruptured ectopic pregnancy (Figure 12-59).

Ultrasound and Spontaneous Abortion (Miscarriage). With first-trimester vaginal bleeding, once

ectopic pregnancy has been excluded, ultrasound and examination findings are correlated to diagnose the patient with some form of spontaneous abortion (miscarriage). We briefly review some basic definitions here. A spontaneous miscarriage can be divided into five types, summarized in Table 12-4. First, a **threatened abortion** describes a pregnancy that may spontaneously terminate but has the potential to continue to a live birth. By definition, a live intrauterine pregnancy must be present, and the cervical os must be closed. Depending on the gestational age ultrasound can be used to measure and document fetal heart rate (Figure 12-60) in this case. An **inevitable abortion** describes a live intrauterine pregnancy with an open cervical os, which uniformly results in miscarriage when this occurs in the first trimester. Again, ultrasound can document fetal heart rate. A **missed abortion** indicates an intrauterine fetal demise (nonviable intrauterine pregnancy, with no fetal cardiac activity) with a closed cervical os. **Incomplete abortion** (Figure 12-61) indicates an intrauterine demise with an open cervical os and some products of conception remaining in the uterus—a miscarriage in progress. As the name suggests, **complete abortion** indicates that the uterus is now empty and the cervical os is closed or preparing to close. Combined with physical examination to assess the cervical os, ultrasound can distinguish these entities, with a few important caveats. A complete abortion may be impossible to distinguish from an ectopic pregnancy because both may have an elevated hCG and an empty uterus. At very low hCG values (below 2000 mIU/mL), an intrauterine pregnancy may be so small that it is not seen on ultrasound, so spontaneous miscarriage and ectopic pregnancy cannot be reliably differentiated in some cases. These patients must be carefully followed with repeat examinations and ultrasound.

When an intrauterine pregnancy is confirmed in the first and second trimester, other common sonographic findings include subchorionic hemorrhage, which is associated with negative pregnancy outcomes.[42-43]

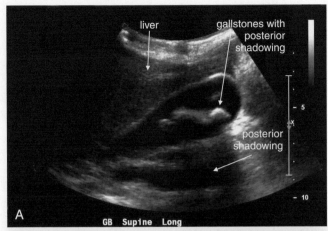

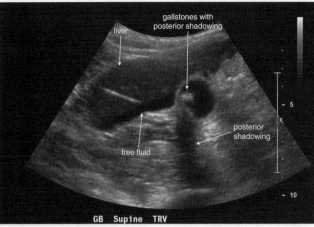

Figure 12-55. **Heterotopic pregnancy with gallstones.** Same patient as in the previous figure. A clue that more may be occurring in this patient than symptomatic cholelithiasis is the presence of free fluid in the right upper quadrant.

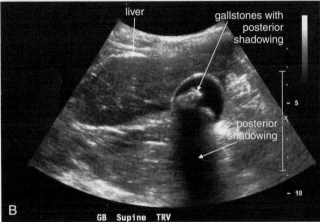

Figure 12-54. **Heterotopic pregnancy with gallstones.** This 34-year-old woman presented with acute diffuse abdominal pain and vomiting, beginning 3 hours after eating dinner. She was 8 weeks pregnant after undergoing gonadotropin ovarian hyperstimulation therapy. Her white blood cell count was 24,000 with 90% neutrophils. **A** and **B,** Bedside ultrasound shows gallstones. Additional ultrasound images were obtained confirming intrauterine pregnancy (see Figure 12-56)—and a right adnexal structure concerning for ectopic pregnancy. Heterotopic pregnancy, the simultaneous occurrence of an intrauterine and an ectopic pregnancy, was once thought to be an extremely rare event, complicating 1 in 30,000 pregnancies. It now is thought to occur in 1 in 2600 pregnancies in the United States. The risk is greatly increased by ovarian stimulation therapy, occurring in as many as 3% of pregnancies. Normally, the presence of an intrauterine pregnancy nearly "rules out" ectopic pregnancy. However, in a high-risk patient, heterotopic pregnancy must be considered, and the adnexa should be carefully inspected for evidence of ectopic pregnancy. Gallstones are a common incidental finding and may not be the cause of acute abdominal pain. Care must always be taken to consider other causes of acute abdominal pain when gallstones are found. The patient underwent a right salpingectomy and continued her intrauterine pregnancy to deliver a healthy infant 7 months later.

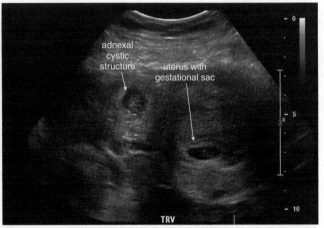

Figure 12-56. **Heterotopic pregnancy with gallstones.** Same patient as in previous figures. This transverse view of the uterus shows an intrauterine pregnancy, as well as a cystic right adnexal structure, concerning for ectopic pregnancy.

Imaging of Vaginal Bleeding in Second and Third Trimesters of Pregnancy.

Ectopic pregnancy is an event of the first trimester, so vaginal bleeding in the second and third trimesters suggests potential pregnancy failure. Throughout pregnancy, vaginal bleeding may threaten not only the fetus but also the mother. Ultrasound is used to assess for fetal viability and for conditions that may lead to maternal morbidity and mortality: placenta previa and placental abruption. Other causes of vaginal bleeding outside of pregnancy may also rarely be the cause of bleeding in pregnancy, including fibroids and uterine or cervical malignancy. Domestic violence is common during pregnancy, so inflicted trauma including vaginal injury should be considered.

Placenta previa indicates positioning of the placenta over the cervical os. A placenta in this location, may lead to pathologic bleeding. Vasa previa refers to a placenta vessel running directly over the cervical os. Both conditions can be diagnosed by ultrasound. Because the position of the placenta moves away from the cervical os during the late third trimester, some placentas previa detected during the second trimester resolve during the third trimester. Imaging with ultrasound serves an important role. First, identification of placenta previa should lead to planned surgical rather than vaginal delivery because vaginal delivery is not possible without severe hemorrhage. Second, placenta previa and particularly vasa previa are contraindications to digital vaginal examination

Figure 12-57. Heterotopic pregnancy with gallstones. Same patient as in previous figures. **A,** This sagittal view of the uterus shows gestational sac and fetal pole consistent with an intrauterine gestation of 6 weeks, 2 days. **B,** Close-up.

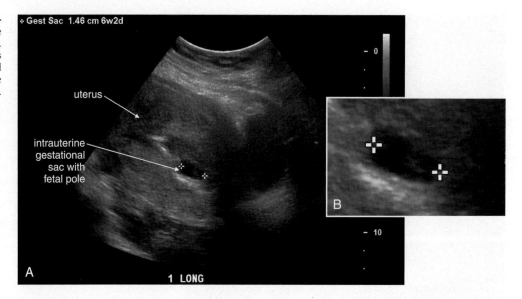

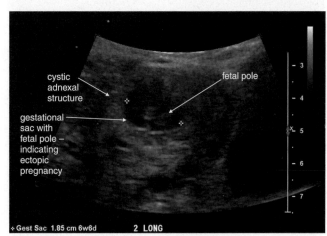

Figure 12-58. Heterotopic pregnancy with gallstones. Same patient as in previous figures. This adnexal cystic structure contains a gestational sac with a fetal pole, consistent with an ectopic pregnancy when the fetus is approximately 6 weeks in size. Fetal cardiac activity was detected in this ectopic pregnancy.

because manipulation of the cervix can result in hemorrhage from exposed vessels. The ultrasound findings are straightforward: a placenta and vessels overlying the cervix.

How Sensitive Is Ultrasound for Placental Abruption?

Placental abruption complicates 1% of pregnancies and can occur in the absence of significant abdominal trauma.[44] Abruption after minor trauma such as falls from standing or even apparently spontaneous abruption may occur. Beyond 25 weeks of gestation, when the fetus is potentially viable, any suspicion for abruption warrants immediate investigation. The chief complaint may be vaginal bleeding, abdominal pain, or diminished fetal movement. *Ultrasound is insensitive*

for the diagnosis of placental abruption (reported as low as 15% to 25% sensitivity) and cannot be used to rule out the diagnosis.[45-46] A variety of sonographic appearances may occur depending on the time from symptom onset, from hyperechoic to isoechoic to hypoechoic—thus a hematoma from abruption may be indistinguishable from the adjacent placenta.[47-49] *Abruption may be an ongoing dynamic process, and a single normal ultrasound should not be reassuring. However, an abnormal ultrasound showing abruption, fetal bradycardia or tachycardia, or decreased fetal movement is extremely concerning.* Diagnostic imaging thus can increase but not decrease concern for abruption. The specificity of ultrasound for abruption has been reported to be as high as 96%.[45] Continuous fetal monitoring for 6 hours or more is typically advised because the most sensitive signs of placental abruption may be uterine irritability and contractions and fetal tachycardia or bradycardia.

Fetal viability can be assessed with ultrasound. Fetal movements can be directly visualized, and fetal heart rate can be recorded. The typical two-dimensional ultrasound images are generated using brightness (B) mode. Motion (M) mode can be selected to allow measurement of fetal heart rate. Most modern ultrasound machines allow a split-screen mode with both B and M modes shown. On the B mode image, a line is positioned through the fetal heart. The M mode image then displays a waveform corresponding to both the frequency and the amplitude of motion along that line. Calipers positioned at two consecutive peaks or troughs allow automatic calculation of heart rate (see Figure 12-60). The American College of Obstetricians and Gynecologists defines a normal fetal heart rate as 110 to 160 bpm. Fetal bradycardia or tachycardia outside of these limits is concerning.

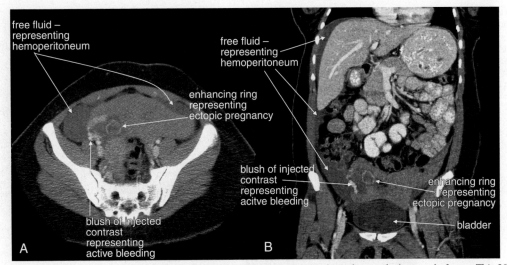

Figure 12-59. Ruptured ectopic pregnancy: CT with intravenous and oral contrast viewed on soft-tissue windows. This 20-year-old woman underwent abdominal CT for suspected appendicitis, given a history of right lower abdominal pain. A urine pregnancy test was not obtained before CT scan. **A** and **B,** Free fluid representing hemoperitoneum is seen in the pelvis and extending to a perihepatic subdiaphragmatic location (compare this dark fluid density with the urine-filled bladder). A ringlike enhancing structure is seen in the right pelvis. A bright blush of contrast is seen that is not contained within vessels or bowel—this represents active bleeding from a ruptured ectopic pregnancy. It is bright because of active extravasation of contrast, whereas blood that accumulated before contrast injection is dark. At laparotomy, 2 L of hemoperitoneum were evacuated and active bleeding from the right Fallopian tube was noted. A 4-cm structure that looked like a gestational sac with a possible tiny embryo within it was also found free in the abdomen.

TABLE 12-4. Ultrasound and Physical Exam in Evaluation of First-Trimester Pregnancy Status

Diagnosis	Intrauterine Pregnancy by Ultrasound?	Fetal Heart Beat by Ultrasound?	Cervical Os Closed?
Ectopic pregnancy	No	Yes or no	NA
Threatened abortion	Yes	Yes	Yes
Inevitable abortion	Yes	Yes	No
Missed abortion	Yes	No	Yes
Incomplete abortion	Yes*	No	No
Complete abortion	No	No	Yes or no†

NA, not applicable.
*At least some products of conception remain.
†Open initially but may then close.

Abdominal Pain in the Pregnant Patient

Abdominal pain in the pregnant patient requires a broad differential diagnosis, as with the nonpregnant patient. Complications of pregnancy, including ectopic pregnancy and spontaneous abortion, must be considered, with ultrasound used for assessment as described earlier. Endometritis should be considered, with imaging playing a limited role in its diagnosis, other than for assessment for intrauterine fetal demise, a risk factor for endometritis.

Once pregnancy-related considerations have been evaluated, conditions such as appendicitis and cholecystitis must be considered. Ultrasound can be used to assess for biliary disease with high sensitivity and specificity, as described in the chapter on abdominal imaging. Ultrasound and MRI can also be used to evaluate for appendicitis, as described in detail in the same chapter.

In general, ionizing radiation should be avoided when possible in the pregnant patient. However, many misconceptions about radiation and pregnancy exist. Regardless of the trimester, low levels of ionizing radiation likely contribute imperceptibly to the background rate of birth defects. While a truly safe threshold below which no effect occurs may not exist, the small contribution of medical radiation at low levels may pale in comparison to baseline levels of defects. Surveys of family physicians and obstetricians indicate that both groups overestimate the teratogenic effect of radiation from diagnostic imaging, with both groups believing in a significant risk from a single abdominal x-ray or CT scan. In reality, neither a single x-ray nor a single abdominal or pelvic CT scan is thought to convey sufficient radiation to increase teratogenic effects appreciably.[50] This is discussed in more detail at the end of this chapter.

This is not to say that radiation should be used with impunity in pregnancy. Radiation risks are based largely on theoretical models, and the precise effects are not well delineated in humans. Moreover, other more subtle but important effects may occur, including effects on cognition and rates of childhood malignancies. Finally, although only a single diagnostic imaging test may be planned during a patient's current medical evaluation, unforeseen events may lead to additional tests during the patient's pregnancy, so limiting ionizing radiation

Figure 12-60. Measurement of fetal heart rate: Motion (M) mode ultrasound. The familiar two-dimensional grayscale images of ultrasound are called brightness (B) mode. M mode images represent motion along a line and thus can be used to characterize moving structures such as the fetal heart. In the B mode image *(top)*, a line is placed by the user through the position of the fetal heart. M mode is then selected, and the bottom image is generated over a period of several seconds. Fetal heart motion creates the sine wave seen in the M mode image *(bottom)*. The user then places two markers at adjacent peaks or troughs in the waveform, and software calculates the fetal heart rate.

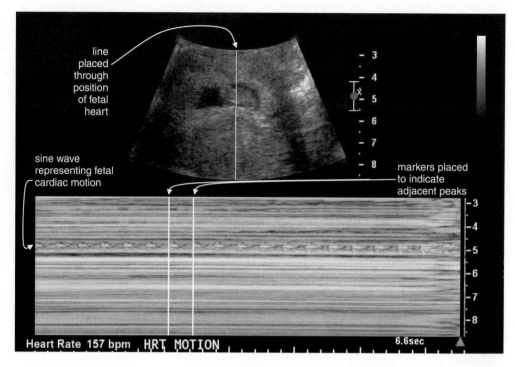

is prudent. A good guideline is that whenever possible, diagnostic strategies that do not use ionizing radiation should be employed. These can include ultrasound, MRI, and observation with serial physical examinations. Rarely, laparoscopy may be a better choice than diagnostic imaging. If the mother's health appears to be at significant risk, ionizing radiation should be used as needed.

Vaginal Discharge or Fluid Leak in the Pregnant Patient

In the first trimester, vaginal discharge or fluid leak may be normal or may be associated with vaginal or cervical infection. By the second and third trimesters, amniotic fluid leak must also be considered because this can lead to infection with fetal demise and maternal sepsis. Physical examination plays the largest role in this evaluation, but ultrasound can be used as an adjunct. Fetal viability assessment with ultrasound can be performed as described earlier. In addition, the quantity of amniotic fluid can be assessed with ultrasound. Formal measurements can be obtained and compared with standard definitions for polyhydramnios (>2000 mL, or single fluid pocket ≥8 cm in depth) and oligohydramnios (<500 mL, or no single fluid pocket ≥2 to 3 cm in depth) at 32 to 36 weeks of gestation. Bedside ultrasound by emergency physicians can provide a rough estimate of amniotic fluid levels. Low levels can be associated with intrauterine growth retardation. Oligohydramnios (Figure 12-62) may be a result of fetal anomalies including urinary obstruction or renal agenesis or, more emergently, of poor fetal perfusion or rupture of amniotic membranes with amniotic fluid leak. Polyhydramnios may result from multiple gestations, fetal gastrointestinal obstruction such as esophageal atresia, or fetal hydrops.[51]

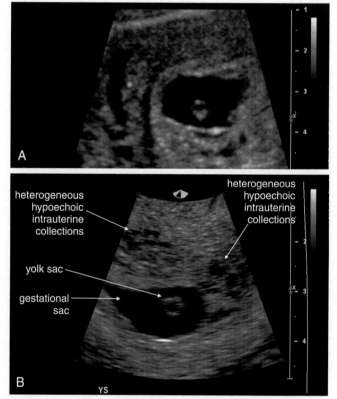

Figure 12-61. Intrauterine fetal demise: Pelvic ultrasound. This 22-year-old woman presented with heavy vaginal bleeding and a human chorionic gonadotropin value of 13,660 mIU/mL, with a last menstrual period 2 months prior. **A** and **B,** An intrauterine gestational sac and yolk sac were noted, with no definite fetal pole found. Hypoechoic regions found within the uterus surrounding the gestational sac could indicate hemorrhage associated with a failed intrauterine pregnancy. Another consideration would be partial mole—though the patient ultimately miscarried and pathology did not show a molar pregnancy.

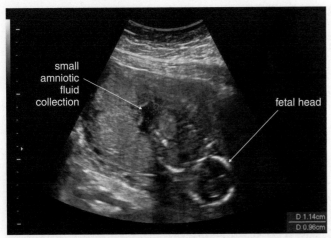

Figure 12-62. Oligohydramnios. Oligohydramnios can threaten pregnancy and should be recognized if present. This fetus has almost no amniotic fluid surrounding it—oligohydramnios. This can occur in the context of fetal renal disease or because of rupture of membranes, which is an obstetrical emergency requiring admission.

Recently Pregnant Patient

Abdominal pain, vaginal bleeding, or vaginal discharge in the recently pregnancy female should prompt consideration of retained products of conception and endometritis. Ultrasound can be used to assess for this condition. Fluid and solid debris within the uterus can support this diagnosis.

In the patient who has undergone pregnancy-related surgical procedures, peritonitis and abscess should be considered. Dilatation and curettage can rarely result in uterine perforation and peritonitis. Caesarean section can be complicated by abscess, bowel perforation, or injuries to the bladder and ureters. The litany of other causes of abdominal pain should also be considered. Ultrasound can be used to assess for free pelvic fluid. CT scan may be a better choice because of the wide differential diagnosis. CT can identify abnormalities of bowel, bladder, and ureters, as well as abscesses. If time allows, oral and IV contrast should be used because of the broad differential diagnosis. IV contrast alone can be used to allow enhancement of inflammatory or infectious processes.

Septic pelvic thrombophlebitis can complicate third-trimester pregnancy. It frequently presents following delivery, with fever, pelvic pain, and vaginal discharge. The diagnosis can be difficult with CT and ultrasound. MRI with gadolinium contrast can be used to confirm the diagnosis.

Diagnostic Imaging of Genitourinary Complaints in the Nonpregnant Female

Many of the same principles of imaging described earlier apply to the nonpregnant female. Always reconfirm pregnancy status because failure to recognize pregnancy can lead to missed ectopic pregnancy, as well as use of ionizing radiation in pregnancy.

Vaginal Bleeding in the Nonpregnant Female

Once pregnancy has been excluded, vaginal bleeding can be a sign of normal menses, dysfunctional uterine bleeding, ovarian cysts including polycystic ovarian syndrome, uterine leiomyomas (fibroids), uterine or cervical malignancy, or pelvic infection. In many cases, diagnostic imaging is not needed. Painless bleeding generally does not require emergency imaging in the premenopausal patient. In the postmenopausal patient, vaginal bleeding is always abnormal and may indicate malignancy. The workup usually includes endometrial biopsy. Imaging may be performed but is not generally required on an emergency basis.

Ultrasound and CT can both be used for assessment of pelvic pathology. Ultrasound is a reasonable first choice in many cases because it avoids radiation exposure and does not require administration of IV contrast, with its potential for allergy and nephrotoxicity. Ultrasound is the preferred diagnostic modality for some conditions because it provides dynamic information about blood flow. CT of the pelvis can be diagnostically ambiguous without contrast agents because many pelvic soft tissues have similar density. In thin patients, this problem can actually be worsened by the paucity of fat, which normally separates soft tissues and has a lower density, allowing fat to act as a form of intrinsic contrast.

The ovaries are generally readily imaged by transvaginal ultrasound. Ovarian follicles and cysts (Figures 12-63 to 12-66) are discussed later in the section on abdominal pain. Ovarian mass lesions and malignant ascites may be seen.

Uterine leiomyomas (fibroids) and malignant lesions are usually seen well on ultrasound. Fibroids may be exophytic or intramural, or it may project into the uterine cavity. Fibroids are usually well circumscribed, whereas malignant lesions may invade or adhere to surrounding structures. CT with IV contrast is useful in investigating extent of disease when malignancy is suspected. Metastatic lesions of the liver and malignant ascites may be seen. IV contrast leads to enhancement of metastatic lesions. Ultrasound may also demonstrate ascites, raising the possibility of malignancy.

Abdominal or Pelvic Pain in the Nonpregnant Female

In the nonpregnant patient with abdominal pain, an extensive differential diagnosis exists. Imaging of abdominal pain is described in detail in the dedicated chapter on abdominal imaging. Here, we discuss specific gynecologic pathology, although in reality an individual patient often requires consideration of a diverse range of pathology. The female patient with right lower-quadrant pain is a classic example, where appendicitis, large- and small-bowel pathology, ovarian pathology, and urinary pathology may all require evaluation.

Figure 12-63. Normal follicles in ovary. This 37-year-old female presented with negative pregnancy test and right lower abdominal pain. **A, B,** Her left ovary shows normal peripheral follicles. Characteristics include the absence of internal septations and small size (roughly 0.5 cm each).

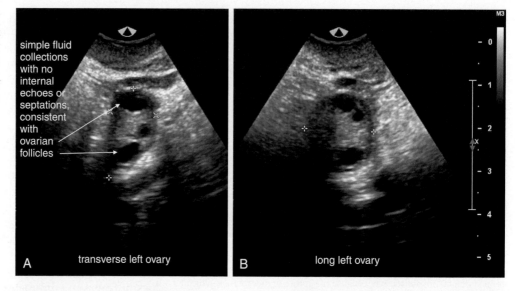

Figure 12-64. Ovarian cystic disease. Same patient as in the previous figure. **A, B,** Her ultrasound images are consistent with a hemorrhagic ovarian cyst. Characteristic features include internal septations and echoes. These suggest blood products within the ovary that have coagulated. Simple cysts typically have no internal echoes or septa. No calcifications are seen—these would produce shadowing deep to the ovary.

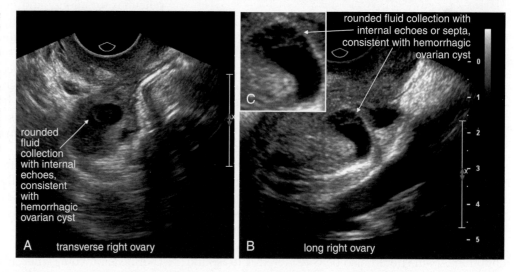

Figure 12-65. Ovarian cystic disease: Computed tomography (CT) with intravenous contrast on soft-tissue windows. Same patient as in the previous figures. She has a history of hysterectomy and bilateral salpingectomy. **A, B,** A peripherally enhancing cystic lesion is seen in the right pelvis, likely a corpus luteum. There is also a small amount of hyperdense fluid in the right and mid lower pelvis, likely hemoperitoneum. Ultrasound of the patient showed a hemorrhagic ovarian cyst. Other images from the patient's CT showed a normal appendix.

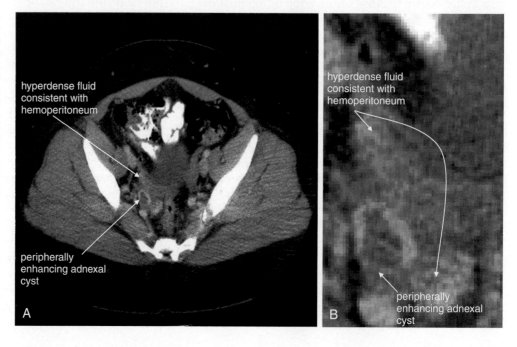

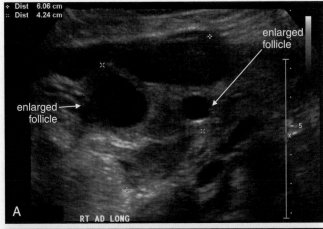

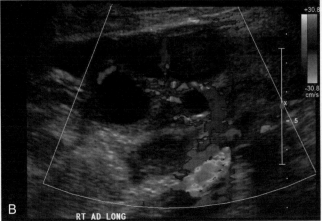

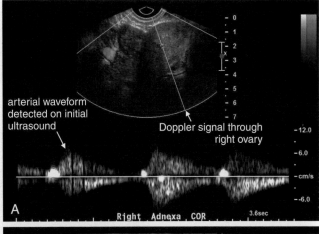

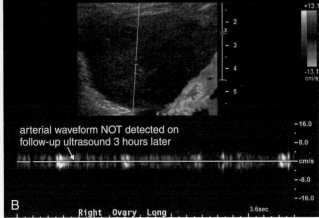

Figure 12-66. Hyperstimulated ovary. This 34-year-old female presented with abdominal pain and vomiting. The patient was 8 weeks pregnant after undergoing gonadotropin ovarian hyperstimulation therapy. **A** and **B,** The right ovary is enlarged, measuring at least 7.7 × 4.6 cm with hypoechoic structures consistent with follicles. Both arterial and venous blood flow were documented in the ovary. This is consistent with ovarian hyperstimulation. The left ovary had a similar appearance. (*See Color plate 16 for color Doppler image of this figure.*)

Figure 12-67. Ovarian torsion: Ultrasound. A and **B,** This patient was initially found to have normal arterial and venous flow in the right ovary, but the emergency physician remained concerned for ovarian torsion given the abrupt onset of severe lateralizing pelvic pain. Repeat ultrasound showed only dampened venous flow. The patient was confirmed to have ovarian torsion at laparotomy, with the ovary twisted four complete turns on its vascular pedicle. This case demonstrates an essential point for the emergency physician. Ultrasound has been reported to have a sensitivity for ovarian torsion of only approximately 60%. When torsion is strongly suspected, a normal ultrasound should not be interpreted as ruling out torsion. (*See Color Plate 17 for color Doppler image of this figure.*)

Again, after assessing clinical stability the next step in diagnostic planning is to reassess pregnancy status to avoid missing ectopic pregnancy. Once pregnancy has been excluded, two important forms of pelvic pathology deserve investigation: ovarian torsion and tuboovarian abscess. Other forms of gynecologic pathology may require imaging for diagnosis but are generally less emergent, including ovarian cysts, endometriosis, uterine fibroids, and pelvic malignancies.

Ovarian Torsion. Ovarian torsion (Figures 12-67 and 12-68) should be strongly considered in any patient with acute onset of lower abdominal pain, particularly when it is severe and accompanied by other signs and symptoms, such as diaphoresis or vomiting. Ultrasound is the preferred diagnostic test, but as we discuss later, *the presence of blood flow detected by ultrasound does not rule out ovarian torsion.* Like testicular torsion, ovarian torsion is time dependent, and delay in diagnosis and treatment can result in ovarian necrosis and loss. When ovarian torsion is strongly considered, gynecologic consultation

should occur before or concurrent with diagnostic imaging.

Transvaginal ultrasound assesses for arterial and venous blood flow, as well as nonspecific ovarian abnormalities such as cystic and solid ovarian lesions. Complete absence of arterial and venous blood flow by Doppler ultrasound is highly specific for the diagnosis of ovarian torsion. Conversely because normal ovaries without asymmetry or enlargement relatively rarely undergo torsion, a normal ovary (lacking cysts or masses) with normal arterial and venous blood flow nearly rules out ovarian torsion. Unfortunately, intermediate ultrasound results can be nondiagnostic and may fail to diagnosis ovarian torsion. Early in the course of torsion, low-pressure venous blood flow may be lost or diminished by twisting of the vascular pedicle, whereas higher-pressure arterial blood flow may be preserved. Later, arterial blood flow may diminish or be lost. In addition, the

Figure 12-68. **Ovarian torsion confirmed in the operating room: CT with IV contrast on soft-tissue windows. A,** There is a heterogeneous structure within the right lower quadrant that measures 6.0 × 5.0 cm, which is concerning for an enlarged right ovary. Ovarian torsion or mass are two important considerations given this appearance. An abnormally enlarged ovary is at increased risk for torsion. In addition, ovarian torsion of an initially normal ovary results in engorgement of the ovary and an enlarged appearance on imaging. **B,** Close-up.

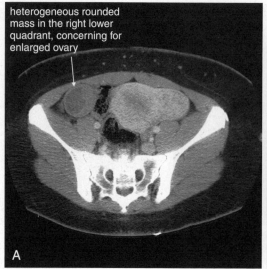

heterogeneous rounded mass in the right lower quadrant, concerning for enlarged ovary

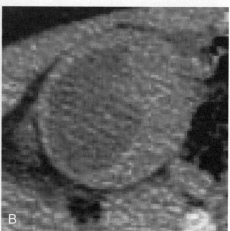

hypoperfused ovary may swell and appear enlarged on ultrasound. Preexisting ovarian cysts or masses may also be seen.

Ultrasound with Doppler evaluation of venous and arterial blood flow is the standard imaging modality for evaluation of suspected ovarian torsion (see Figure 12-67). However, multiple small studies suggest that the sensitivity of ultrasound is only moderate and that either arterial or venous flow may be present in a torsed ovary. Dane et al.[52] reported blood flow was present in 6 of 21 cases (28%). Shadinger et al.[53] reviewed 39 cases of pathologically proven ovarian torsion and found that 13 (33%) had venous flow and 21 (54%) had arterial flow. Pena et al.[54] reported normal Doppler findings in 6 of 10 patients with proven ovarian torsion. Pena[54] also noted delays in diagnosis when flow was present, likely reflecting undue confidence by physicians in use of ultrasound to rule out ovarian torsion. Although no large studies have examined ultrasound for the diagnosis of ovarian torsion, it appears that the sensitivity of abnormal blood flow by ultrasound is probably between 50% and 70%, quite inadequate to rule out the diagnosis.

Are Other Ultrasound Findings Useful in Evaluation for Ovarian Torsion?

Ovarian enlargement is reportedly a sensitive, though nonspecific, finding in ovarian torsion.[53] Kiechl-Kohlendorfer et al.[55] reported fluid–debris levels in 11 of 13 (85%) ovarian torsion cases, though the specificity of this finding is uncertain.

When ovarian torsion is strongly suspected, gynecologic consultation should be pursued despite negative ultrasound findings. Although diagnostic strategies such as repeat ultrasound or CT scan can be employed, diagnostic

delay can result in ovarian loss. In some cases, laparoscopy to visually inspect the ovary is preferable.

CT in ovarian torsion

The sensitivity and specificity of CT scan for ovarian torsion (see Figure 12-68) are not well studied. CT scan can demonstrate abnormal patterns of enhancement with IV contrast, as well as cystic and solid masses of the ovary. Case reports of ovarian torsion detected on unenhanced and enhanced CT describe an enlarged ovary, often displaced from the normal position, hyperdense compared with the normal ovary, and containing hypodense cystic regions. In a torsed cystic ovary, the cyst wall may exceed 10 mm in thickness. If IV contrast is given, the ovary may fail to enhance.[56] The uterus may be deviated toward the torsed ovary. Free fluid may also be seen.[57-61] Rarely, gas within the vessels of a torsed ovarian tumor may be seen.[62]

Tuboovarian Abscess. Tuboovarian abscess is an important cause of pelvic pain and can be evaluated with ultrasound or CT (Figures 12-69 and 12-70). Transvaginal ultrasound is more sensitive than is transabdominal ultrasound for this indication.[63] Ultrasound findings include an enlarged ovary and fallopian tube, often with multiple loculated, fluid-filled regions. Echogenic debris with a fluid–fluid level may be visible within the structures. High blood flow may be seen using Doppler ultrasound. These findings are not specific for tuboovarian abscess.[64] Because ultrasound cannot distinguish among blood, pus, and serous fluids, ultrasound does not prove the diagnosis of tuboovarian abscess. Sterile hydrosalpinx, hemosalpinx, and complex ovarian cysts could have similar appearances. A torsed ovary could have a similar ultrasound appearance, although confirmation of normal blood flow decreases the likelihood of this diagnosis. Overall, ultrasound findings can support the diagnosis of tuboovarian abscess, with clinical

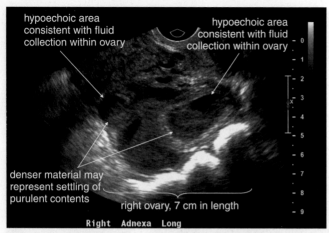

Figure 12-69. Tuboovarian abscess: Ultrasound. This 30-year-old woman presented with exquisite right lower abdominal pain. She later tested positive for *Trichomonas* and *Neisseria gonorrhea*. Ultrasound shows a 7 × 6.5 × 5.6 cm right ovarian mass with multiple heterogeneous hypoechoic areas, suggesting internal fluid collections of varying density. Both arterial and venous flow were normal. These findings are suggestive of tuboovarian abscess.

correlation required. Positive ultrasound findings in the context of some combination of adnexal pain and tenderness, fever, leukocytosis, and culture confirmation of pelvic infection confirm the diagnosis. A normal ultrasound is a reassuring sign that tuboovarian abscess is unlikely.

CT scan demonstrates similar findings of loculated ovarian and fallopian tube fluid collections.[65-67] In addition, hydroureter, increased presacral fat density (fat stranding), and increased presacral ligament density may be seen, though these are not specific for tuboovarian abscess.[65,67-68] These can be recognized without any form of contrast. IV contrast leads to rim enhancement of a tuboovarian abscess, helping to confirm the diagnosis, whereas fluid collections without infection or inflammation would not be expected to enhance. Oral contrast is not necessary, although it is frequently given to assist in the differential diagnosis of lower-quadrant abdominal pain, which can include appendicitis, diverticulitis, or inflammatory bowel disease. The role of oral contrast in abdominal CT is discussed in more detail in the chapter on imaging of nontraumatic abdominal complaints.

More than one diagnostic strategy for suspected tuboovarian abscess may be appropriate, depending on the differential diagnosis, the age of the patient, and the most important consideration for the specific patient, such as speed of diagnosis, accuracy, cost, or limitation of radiation exposure. For example, in an older patient where radiation exposure is of limited importance and conditions such as appendicitis, diverticulitis, or vascular pathology might cause lower abdominal pain, CT may be the most appropriate initial test. In a younger, sexually active patient, where radiation exposure is a significant concern, it may be appropriate to begin the

diagnostic workup using ultrasound, proceeding to CT scan if ultrasound is nondiagnostic. No formal decision rules exist for imaging patients for suspected tuboovarian abscess. One study suggests that an erythrocyte sedimentation rate greater than 50 mm per hour may predict tuboovarian abscess, but large and rigorous studies of this condition are lacking.[69]

Pelvic inflammatory disease (PID) may be difficult to distinguish clinically from tuboovarian abscess or ovarian torsion. Imaging is typically directed at ruling out these alternative diagnoses. Ultrasound or CT may show free fluid in the pelvis. CT may show inflammatory changes of fat surrounding pelvic structures, without focal or loculated fluid collections. Imaging may also be normal in the setting of PID, so treatment should be based on the overall clinical presentation. *Normal imaging does not rule out PID because the sensitivity of ultrasound and CT are not known.*

Ovarian cysts and masses such as dermoids (teratomas) (Figures 12-71 to 12-73) or ovarian cancer can cause abdominal or pelvic pain. Imaging in the emergency department is again aimed at detecting conditions such as tuboovarian abscess, ovarian torsion, or nongynecologic conditions such as appendicitis requiring emergency surgery, percutaneous drainage, or antibiotics. The choice of initial imaging study (ultrasound, CT, and rarely, MRI) depends on the most urgent potential surgical concern, with ovarian cyst being a diagnosis of exclusion in most cases. Rarely, ovarian cyst rupture can lead to significant hemoperitoneum, which can be detected by ultrasound or CT. Both modalities may demonstrate important mass lesions requiring follow-up. Dermoid tumors (see Figures 12-71 to 12-73) classically contain multiple tissue types derived from ectoderm, including skin, fat, hair, and even calcifications resembling teeth. These are visible on ultrasound as often-complex solid lesions. Calcifications or teeth are dense and cast acoustic shadows on ultrasound. On CT scan, low-density fat within dermoids is readily seen without any form of contrast; calcifications also are visible without contrast. Dermoids require follow-up and typically are electively removed because of a small risk for malignant transformation (1% to 2%). They may bleed internally, causing pain, and torsion of a dermoid may occur.[70] Simple ovarian cysts are usually recognized on ultrasound or CT as simple fluid collections without loculations. On ultrasound, these appear hypoechoic. On CT, they are low-attenuation fluid density, with Hounsfield units around or slightly greater than zero (water density). Polycystic ovaries can be seen on ultrasound or CT scan. Ovarian malignancy can be detected by ultrasound and CT, but differentiation from benign lesions is difficult except in advanced cases in which local invasion or metastasis has occurred. Solid ovarian masses seen by ultrasound

Figure 12-70. Tuboovarian abscess: CT with oral and IV contrast. Same patient as in the previous figure. CT with oral and IV contrast demonstrates a 7.4 × 6.4 cm right adnexal mass with multiple septations and fluid-filled cavities, concerning for tuboovarian abscess. The rim enhances with IV contrast, which is typical of infectious abscess. The abscess was treated with CT-guided percutaneous drainage and IV antibiotics. **A,** Axial image. **B,** Coronal reconstruction.

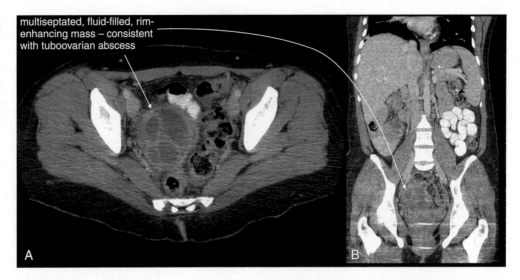

multiseptated, fluid-filled, rim-enhancing mass – consistent with tuboovarian abscess

Figure 12-71. Dermoid with calcifications: Noncontrast CT on soft-tissue windows. This 46-year-old woman presented with right lower-quadrant pain and a negative pregnancy test. A CT scan was performed to evaluate for possible renal colic. **A, B,** Within the pelvis, a lobulated mixed attenuation mass (predominately fat attenuation, with soft-tissue components and punctate calcific foci) measures at least 8.1 × 5.2 cm. This is consistent with a dermoid cyst (teratoma). There is a small to moderate amount of free fluid within the pelvis.

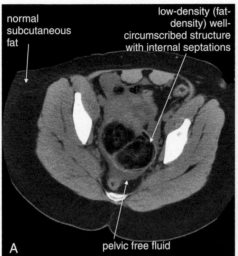

normal subcutaneous fat

low-density (fat-density) well-circumscribed structure with internal septations

pelvic free fluid

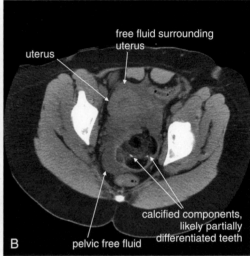

free fluid surrounding uterus

uterus

calcified components, likely partially differentiated teeth

pelvic free fluid

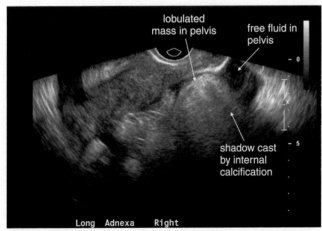

lobulated mass in pelvis

free fluid in pelvis

shadow cast by internal calcification

Long Adnexa Right

Figure 12-72. Dermoid. Same patient as in the previous figure. In the expected location of the right adnexa, a large heterogeneous hyperechoic bi-lobed structure measures at least 8.3 × 4.3 × 6.7 cm. This demonstrates posterior shadowing because of internal structures (calcifications), seen best on CT scan in the previous figure. Free fluid is seen surrounding the structure, as on the prior CT.

or CT require follow-up because malignancy is always a possibility.

Fibroids (Figures 12-74 and 12-75) and uterine malignancy may cause pelvic pain. Imaging is key to diagnosing these conditions, but in most cases emergency imaging is directed at ruling out ovarian torsion or tubo-ovarian abscess. Ultrasound and CT can demonstrate fibroids or uterine malignancy. Imaging does not reliably distinguish a fibroid from an early malignancy—for this reason, patients should always be advised to follow up, and the possibility of malignancy must be considered. Doppler ultrasound is somewhat more specific for malignancy than is conventional ultrasound, but it cannot rule out malignancy.[71-73] MRI can provide additional differentiation but is not completely specific.[74] Advanced malignancy may demonstrate invasion or entrapment of adjacent structures, as well as ascites or metastasis. In contrast, fibroids remain confined to the uterus and do not invade locally or remotely.

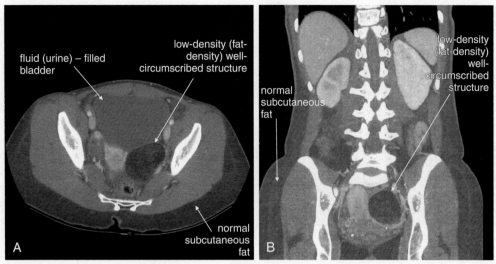

Figure 12-73. Dermoid: CT with IV contrast, soft-tissue windows. This 25-year-old woman presented with right lower abdominal pain and underwent CT, which showed a normal appendix. **A, B,** Incidentally, a 5.9 × 4.1 cm fat-containing lesion was identified in the left adnexa, most compatible with a dermoid. Dermoid cysts are neoplasms, usually benign but with rare potential for malignant transformation. Because they are derived from tissues with the ability to differentiate into multiple ectoplasm tissues, they frequently contain fat, skin, hair, or even teethlike structures. Typical features in this patient include a well-circumscribed appearance and low density. Because the structure is largely composed of fat, it is less dense than the adjacent bladder, which is filled with urine. Compare with normal subcutaneous fat. The window level has been adjusted from a typical soft tissue setting to make fat appear brighter.

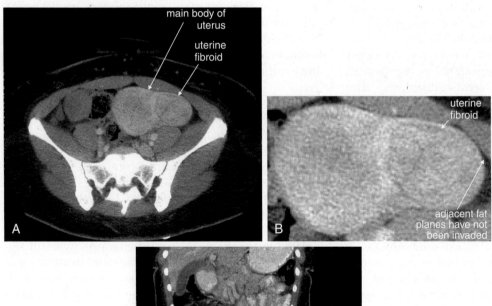

Figure 12-74. Fibroid uterus: CT with IV contrast on soft-tissue windows. A through **C,** Although ultrasound is the primary modality used for evaluation of uterine fibroids (leiomyomas), these benign neoplasms are often detected on CT scan performed for evaluation of abdominal pain. Typical features are a well-circumscribed appearance and enhancement with contrast. Because uterine malignancies can also occur, a careful search of the abdomen for lymphadenopathy is required. Malignant uterine tumors may invade adjacent structures, whereas a fibroid is contained within the uterine serosa. Uterine tumors, both benign and malignant, can show central necrosis, which has a nonenhancing, dark appearance. **A,** axial image. **B,** close-up from **A. C,** coronal image.

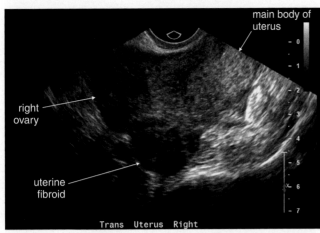

Figure 12-75. Fibroid uterus: Endovaginal ultrasound. Ultrasound is the primary modality used for evaluation of uterine fibroids (leiomyomas). Typical features include a well-circumscribed appearance. Fibroids may be hypoechoic or hyperechoic relative to the uterus. They may be exophytic or intramural, or they may project into the uterine cavity. Malignant uterine tumors may invade adjacent structures, whereas a fibroid is contained within the uterine serosa. Uterine tumors, both benign and malignant, can show central necrosis, which usually appears hypoechoic with ultrasound. In this 38-year-old woman, the fibroid is exophytic. The right ovary lies adjacent and is difficult to distinguish in this case.

Fibroids can be exophytic but remain bounded by the uterine serosa.

Endometriosis is not easily detected by imaging. Findings are nonspecific and can include pelvic free fluid, which has a broad differential diagnosis, including normal physiologic free fluid, blood, ascites, and infection. Ectopic endometrial tissue itself may be seen by either ultrasound or CT, but the appearance is nonspecific, with a broad radiographic differential diagnosis.[75] The diagnosis is usually confirmed laparoscopically. Imaging in the emergency department is usually aimed at evaluating for other acute surgical disease, rather than detecting or excluding endometriosis.

Vaginal Discharge in the Nonpregnant Patient

In the nonpregnant patient, vaginal discharge can be a finding of vaginal or pelvic infection or, rarely, malignancy. In the absence of adnexal pain or tenderness, focal infection such as PID or tuboovarian abscess is unlikely. Retained vaginal foreign bodies are possible but are usually detected by physical examination, not imaging. Imaging is usually not required for isolated vaginal discharge in the nonpregnant female.

IMAGING OF GENITOURINARY TRAUMA

Following blunt trauma, injuries to the kidneys, ureters, bladder, urethra, scrotum, and uterus and vagina are possible. The imaging evaluation depends on the presentation. Common presentations are blunt or penetrating abdominal trauma with or without flank pain, traumatic hematuria, traumatic vaginal bleeding, direct perineum or scrotal injury, and abdominal or pelvic trauma in pregnancy.

Blunt Abdominal or Pelvic Trauma With Suspected Genitourinary Injury

Blunt torso trauma can result in injury to the kidneys, ureters, and bladder, best diagnosed with CT (described in more detail later). In the patient with blunt trauma, genitourinary injuries are rarely immediately life threatening, so patient stabilization and diagnosis of more imminently dangerous injuries should take priority. Significant traumatic injuries to the kidneys usually do not occur from low-energy trauma—even from direct blows, as may occur in an assault. Instead, major renal lacerations are usually found in the setting of high-energy trauma, such as falls from great height or deceleration injuries in motor vehicle collisions. Renal injuries are often noted incidentally, accompanying major injuries to the liver, spleen, pelvis, and spine. Many renal injuries require no specific treatment, exceptions being those involving the renal pedicle because these may threaten renal blood supply, result in major hemorrhage, or disrupt the ureter. The decision to image a patient to identify a traumatic renal injury should be made largely on the basis of other suspected injuries. Traumatic ureteral injuries occur in the same setting of major trauma. CT with IV contrast can identify these injuries, with additional delayed images obtained to allow time for renal excretion of injected contrast. Contrast leak from the ureters confirms injury. Bladder injuries are discussed later but usually occur in the setting of pelvic fracture. In patients receiving anticoagulation, retroperitoneal hematomas may occur with relatively minor trauma and are diagnosed by CT.

Traumatic Hematuria and Other Indications for Genitourinary Imaging

Gross traumatic hematuria may indicate injury to the kidneys, ureters, bladder, or urethra. The likely source of bleeding can be deduced from a combination of history, physical examination, and simple imaging studies. Additional imaging is then performed to evaluate selected portions of the urinary system, as described later.

Isolated traumatic microscopic hematuria (without significant abdominal, flank, or pelvic pain) in adults generally does not require specific imaging evaluation. If the patient does not require torso imaging for considerations such as spleen, liver, or bowel injury, microscopic hematuria alone should not drive renal imaging for trauma in adults because the injuries identified are generally low-grade renal contusions that do not require therapy. An example would be a stable patient struck in the flank by a baseball and noted to have microscopic hematuria on urinalysis. The patient would require imaging only if concerns existed for significant injuries to other organs, such as the spleen. In children, microscopic hematuria is considered an independent indication for imaging evaluation, as discussed later.

Miller and McAninch[76] found only three significant renal injuries in 1588 adult blunt trauma patients with microscopic hematuria and no hemodynamic shock; consequently, they recommend against imaging for renal injury. The authors recommend imaging only for gross hematuria, shock, or other suspected abdominal injury. The case in pediatric patients is less clear. Abou-Jaoude et al. found that a threshold of more than 20 red blood cells per high-power field would have missed 28% of patients with a spectrum of renal anomalies, including minor and major trauma and congenital anomalies. However, this threshold would have missed only 2 of 8 patients with major injuries, out of 100 patients evaluated. Despite the investigators' warnings, microscopic hematuria with less than 20 red blood cells per high-powered field had a negative predictive value of 98% for significant renal injury.[77] Morey et al.[78] found a low incidence of significant renal injuries in children (2%) with fewer than 50 red blood cells per high-power field.

Which Patients Require Imaging for Bladder and Urethral Injury?

Traditionally, microscopic hematuria greater than 50 red blood cells per high-power field was considered an indication for genitourinary imaging for renal, ureteral, bladder, and urethral injury.[79] More recent studies in adults suggest that gross hematuria, not microscopic hematuria, is the indication for renal,[76] bladder, and urethral imaging. In children, microscopic hematuria (>20 red blood cells per high-power field) is still cited as an indication for genitourinary imaging for trauma. Although pelvic fractures are associated with bladder injuries, when gross hematuria is absent, pelvic fractures alone do not appear to predict bladder and urethral injuries.

Morey et al.[80] investigated risk factors for bladder injury to establish guidelines for imaging. The authors point out that imaging studies for suspected genitourinary injury add time to the patient workup, which could adversely affect patients requiring rapid operative repair of other injuries. The authors performed a retrospective chart review spanning a 4-year period using the trauma registries from four level-I trauma centers. They identified 53 patients (37 male and 16 female) with bladder rupture from blunt trauma. All presented with gross hematuria. Blood at the urethral meatus was identified in 6 patients (11%), all with coexisting urethral injuries. In addition, 45 patients (85%) had pelvic fractures. The authors suggest revision of older guidelines that called for cystography in all patients with either gross or microscopic hematuria. They propose mandatory cystography in all patients with gross hematuria with pelvic fracture. They argue that gross hematuria without pelvic fracture and microscopic hematuria with or without pelvic fracture are only relative indications, requiring imaging only in the presence of other findings, such as suprapubic pain and tenderness, inability to void, perineal hematoma, blood at the urethral meatus, free fluid on CT, or altered mental status.

Fuhrman et al.[81] also found gross hematuria to be the only indication for lower genitourinary imaging because they found no bladder injuries in 120 patients without gross hematuria, whether or not pelvic fractures were present. Bladder injuries were found only in the 31 patients with gross hematuria, one quarter of whom had pelvic fractures. The authors argue against cystography in the absence of gross hematuria, even when pelvic fractures are present.[81] Pao et al.[82] found that the absence of pelvic free fluid on routine trauma CT (without CT cystography) made bladder rupture unlikely, though its presence was not specific for bladder injury.

CT Scan Evaluation of Suspected Renal and Ureteral Injury

Renal and ureteral injuries are possible whenever major blunt abdominal or torso trauma has occurred. In the setting of gross hematuria, a renal and ureteral injury is the likely source in the absence of a pelvic fracture, which is usually required for bladder or urethral injury to occur. CT for evaluation of renal and ureteral trauma is performed with IV contrast, just as for other blunt traumatic abdominal injuries (Figure 12-76). Extravasation of contrast during the initial CT indicates active bleeding from a renal parenchymal or an arterial or venous injury. Extravasated contrast appears as an amorphous bright white blush, often surrounded by a darker collection representing retroperitoneal blood that has already escaped from the kidney before administration of contrast (see Figure 12-16). This dark fluid collection may be subcapsular, extrarenal, or contained within the renal parenchyma as a contusion or renal laceration. A kidney that does not enhance with injected contrast during this initial phase is poorly perfused and may represent a complete renal pedicle avulsion requiring emergency repair or nephrectomy (see Figure 7-84 for example of poor renal perfusion resulting from aortic dissection).

Hypoattenuated (dark) perinephric fluid may also represent urine that has leaked from an injury to the renal pelvis or ureter. To evaluate this, additional CT images are obtained following a short delay, allowing time for injected contrast to be filtered and excreted by the kidneys. These CT nephrograms and ureterograms provide important information by demonstrating renal perfusion and by allowing contrast to fill the ureters. Contrast extravasation from the ureter into the retroperitoneum indicates ureteral injury (Figures 12-77 and 12-78), which is then investigated with retrograde urography using a cystoscope (Figure 12-79). In this procedure, a cystoscope

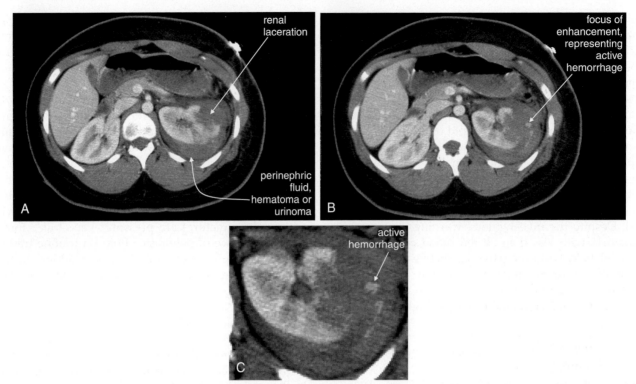

Figure 12-76. Renal laceration: CT with IV contrast on soft-tissue windows. A, B, CT through the level of the kidneys. **C,** Close-up from **B.** Renal injuries often occur in the context of other significant torso trauma. In this CT scan with IV contrast, the majority of the left kidney is seen to enhance normally with contrast, excluding a significant vascular injury to the pedicle. The lateral left kidney has a deep laceration with surrounding perinephric hypoattenuated fluid. This represents blood that had already accumulated before the moment of CT scan acquisition—although urine from a renal pelvis or ureteral injury would have a similar appearance. Small foci of enhancement are seen beyond the apparent margin of the kidney within the perinephric hematoma. These represent small areas of continuing hemorrhage at the moment of CT scan. Delayed images were performed to assess for possible urine leak, but none was noted. Urine leaks are discussed in the next figure.

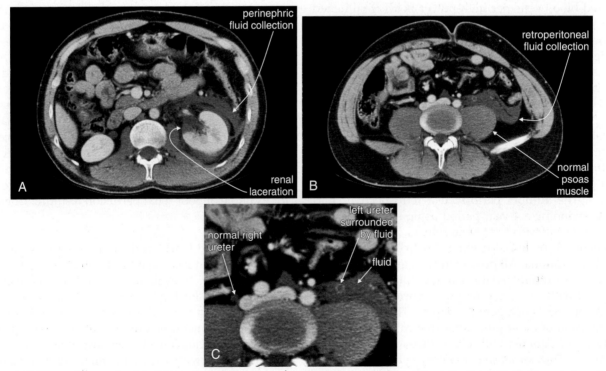

Figure 12-77. Ureteral or renal pelvis injury. A, CT through the level of the kidneys. **B,** CT just above the iliac crest. **C,** Close-up from **B.** This 30-year-old man was ejected from a vehicle. Initial CT images with IV contrast show a left perinephric fluid collection and evidence of renal contusion. Is the perinephric fluid blood, urine, or both? These initial images (obtained when the injected contrast was within arteries) do not show extravasation of contrast, suggesting that active bleeding was not occurring. Delayed CT images (obtained several minutes later, when contrast was being excreted by the kidneys) were obtained to evaluate for urine leak (next figure).

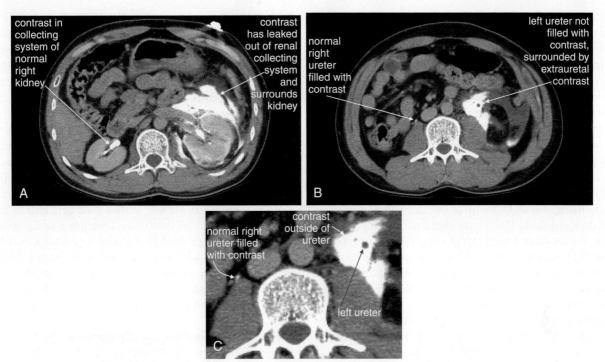

Figure 12-78. Ureteral or renal pelvis injury. A, CT through the level of the kidneys. **B,** CT just above the iliac crest. **C,** Close-up from **B.** Same patient as in the previous figure. These delayed CT images (obtained several minutes later, when intravenously injected contrast is being excreted by the kidneys) now show contrast collecting around the kidney and in the retroperitoneal space anterior to the psoas. The right ureter is filling normally with or contrast. The left ureter is not filled with contrast and is seen as a filling void (dark), surrounded by retroperitoneal contrast (bright white). A leaking renal pelvis or ureter is the likely culprit. Retrograde urography was performed by the urology service, demonstrating leaking contrast from the renal pelvis (next figure).

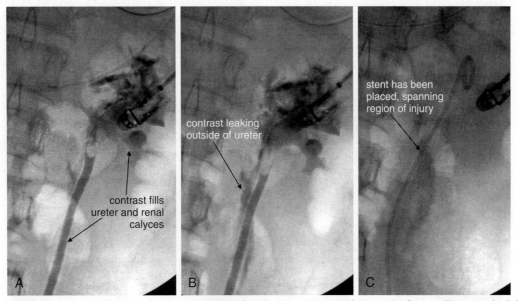

Figure 12-79. Ureteral or renal pelvis injury: Retrograde urography. Same patient as in the previous figures. CT images had demonstrated an apparent urine leak. **A,** Retrograde urography (injection of contrast material into the ureter from the ureteral orifice in the bladder using a cystoscope) shows filling of the ureter and renal pelvis. **B,** A moment later, contrast is seen accumulating outside of the renal pelvis and ureter, indicating a urine leak. **C,** A stent has been placed to treat the apparent injury to the proximal ureter and renal pelvis.

is inserted into the bladder, the affected ureter is cannulated, and contrast is injected through the ureter to the kidney to identify the location of a discontinuity or leak. Ureteral injuries may be treated by placement of a stent or with surgery.

Suspected Bladder Injury

Hematuria may also indicate bladder injury, which usually occurs in the setting of pelvic fracture. Standard CT with IV contrast yields several clues to this diagnosis. First, pelvic fractures are detected with great sensitivity using bone windows from standard abdominal-pelvic CT or reconstructions using specialized bone algorithms. Second, a pelvic hematoma often accompanies pelvic fracture. This hematoma may exert mass effect on the bladder, compressing and deforming the bladder from its usual symmetrical shape and midline position. Extravasation of urine from the bladder into the peritoneum (intraperitoneal rupture) or outside of the peritoneum (extraperitoneal rupture) may be suggested by the presence of low-density fluid in the pelvis or abdomen, but it may be difficult or impossible using the standard CT images to be certain that this fluid is urine. Measurement of the density of the fluid in Hounsfield units (HU) may demonstrate the fluid to be less dense than blood. Urine should be water density, or 0 Hounsfield units. Blood varies in density but is typically between 30 and 50 HU. Preexisting ascitic fluid can be indistinguishable from urine on CT, with a density near 0 HU. Additional CT images can confirm bladder rupture. This study, a **CT cystogram** (Figures 12-80 and 12-81), takes the place of the conventional cystogram used in the past to detect bladder injury. CT cystogram is best explained by comparison with a conventional cystogram.

Conventional Cystogram. In a conventional (plain film) cystogram (Figures 12-82 and 12-83), an x-ray of the pelvis is performed before the administration of contrast material. This x-ray can demonstrate the presence of pelvic fractures (see Figure 12-84). Next, a Foley or urinary catheter is placed, and contrast material is instilled into the bladder, usually under gravity pressure only. An x-ray of the pelvis is repeated, and an uninjured bladder appears symmetrically distended, with no contrast material present beyond its sharply demarcated but smooth borders. An injured bladder may have several abnormalities noted. First, a pelvic hematoma adjacent to the bladder may deform the bladder and displace it from the midline. Second, in the instance of bladder rupture, contrast instilled through the Foley catheter may be seen extending outside the confines of the bladder. The conventional cystogram is then completed by evacuating the contrast material from the bladder through the Foley catheter and repeating a plain x-ray of the pelvis. This step allows recognition of subtle contrast extravasation deep or posterior to the bladder. Extravasation in this location can be masked on the x-ray performed with the bladder distended with contrast because the full bladder may be directly in front of the contrast leak. A normal x-ray at this point should show no or little residual contrast. Linear or irregular streaks of residual contrast may indicate rupture.

Computed Tomography Cystogram. In a CT cystogram (see Figures 12-80 and 12-81), the bladder is filled with contrast through a Foley catheter under gravity pressure, just as with a conventional cystogram.[80] In addition, previously administered IV contrast begins to fill the bladder as it is filtered and excreted by the kidneys. As with conventional cystogram, extravasation of contrast from the bladder can then be detected on CT images taken of the bladder and pelvis. Unlike conventional cystogram, additional images of the empty bladder are not needed because CT can detect contrast leak deep to the bladder. Contrast outlining bowel or other intraperitoneal structures indicates intraperitoneal

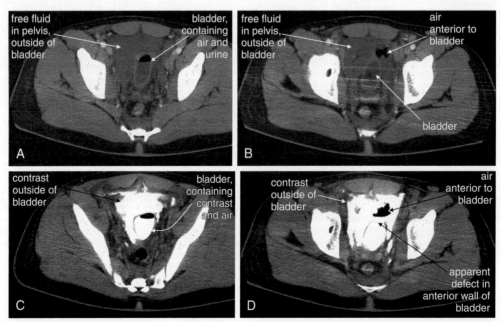

Figure 12-80. Bladder rupture: Extraperitoneal. This 18-year-old man was an unrestrained driver in a car that struck a tree. He had multiple pelvic fractures. **A** through **D,** His intravenous-contrasted abdominal and pelvic CT scan **(A, B)** showed free fluid and air in the extraperitoneal pelvic space, suggesting extraperitoneal bladder rupture. However, blood or other fluid in this space could have a similar appearance, particularly given the presence of pelvic fractures that could have associated bleeding. CT cystogram was performed after contrast was instilled into the bladder through a urinary catheter. This confirmed extravasation of contrast from the bladder through an anterior bladder wall defect.

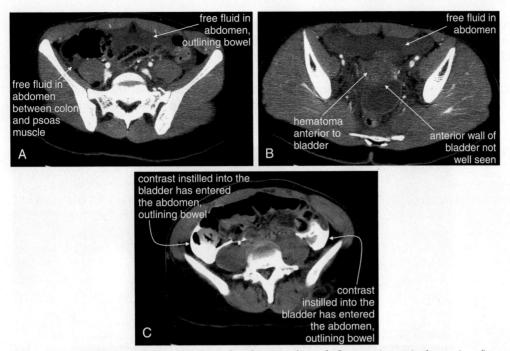

Figure 12-81. Bladder rupture: Intraperitoneal and extraperitoneal. Same patient as in the previous figure. Her intravenous-contrasted CT scan showed pelvic fractures, as well as free fluid in the abdomen and pelvis **(A, B)**. Although theoretically this fluid could be from multiple sources, no solid organ injuries were seen. The anterior bladder appeared possibly ruptured. **C,** CT cystogram was performed, confirming that contrast instilled into the bladder through a urinary catheter entered the peritoneal cavity and outlined bowel loops—an intraperitoneal bladder rupture. Some extraperitoneal extravasation was also seen. This patient also had a vaginal laceration. Consider vaginal-penetrating injuries when complex pelvic fractures or bladder injuries are present. The patient underwent operative repair of her bladder and vaginal injuries.

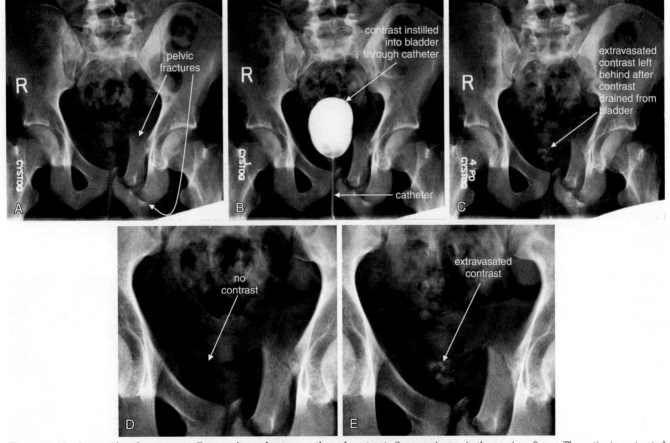

Figure 12-82. Conventional cystogram: Extraperitoneal extravasation of contrast. Same patient as in the previous figure. The patient was treated nonoperatively with Foley catheter drainage for an extraperitoneal bladder rupture. This conventional cystogram was obtained 2 weeks after the original injury and computed tomography scan. **A,** First, an x-ray of the pelvis is obtained. **B,** Contrast is instilled into the bladder through a catheter. **C,** Contrast is drained from the bladder, and an x-ray is again obtained—this shows abnormal irregular collections of contrast, indicating persistent bladder leak. **D,** Close-up from **A. E,** Close-up from **C,** emphasizing the extravasated contrast.

bladder rupture. CT cystography has been found to be highly accurate when the bladder is distended with at least 300 mL of dilute contrast (usually 50 mL of Hypaque or similar contrast, mixed with 450 mL of saline) and can replace traditional cystography in patients undergoing CT.[81-82]

Suspected Urethral Injury

Following blunt trauma, several clinical factors may predict urethral injury, and retrograde urethrogram before bladder catheterization is indicated when urethral injury is suspected. Blood at the urethral meatus or high-riding prostate on rectal examination are clinical

Figure 12-83. **Conventional cystogram: No extravasation of contrast.** Same patient as in the previous figures. This conventional cystogram was obtained 4 weeks after the original injury and computed tomography scan. **A,** First, an x-ray of the pelvis is obtained. **B,** Contrast is instilled into the bladder through a catheter. **C,** Contrast is drained from the bladder, and an x-ray is again obtained. A small amount of contrast appears to be retained within the bladder. Notice the regular rounded appearance, unlike in the previous figure, where extravasated contrast had an irregular appearance. This indicated complete healing of the bladder rupture. **D,** Close-up from **C.** If doubt remained, the bladder could be gently irrigated to wash out retained contrast, and x-ray could be repeated.

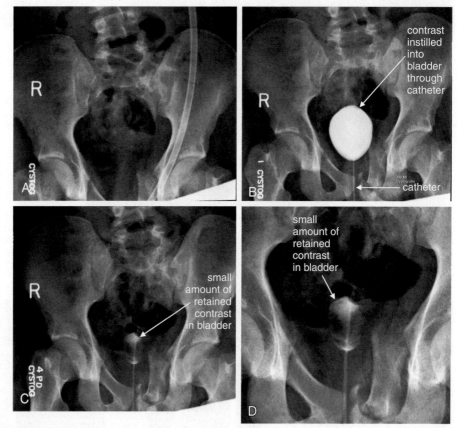

Figure 12-84. **Bladder rupture: Intraperitoneal and extraperitoneal.** This 19-year-old woman was an unrestrained back seat passenger in a motor vehicle collision. **A,** Her pelvis x-ray shows displaced fractures of the right and left superior and inferior pubic rami fractures, as well as left pubic symphysis. **B,** Careful inspection reveals a left sacral fracture. Associated genitourinary injuries are discussed in the figure that follows.

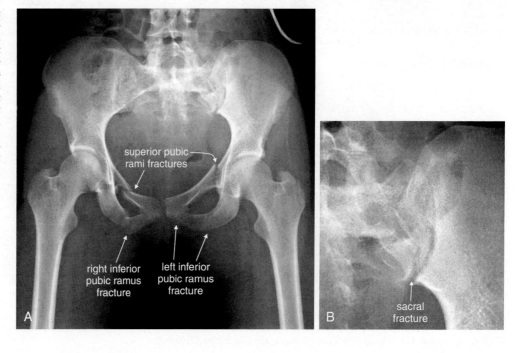

predictors of this injury. Urethral injuries are rare in the absence of pelvic fracture, although straddle injuries can damage the urethra without fracture. Fractures through the inferior and superior pubic rami may suggest urethral injury, particularly when the symphysis pubis is disrupted.[76] Remember that similar findings and mechanisms of injury may result in perforation of the vagina, so speculum pelvic examination may also be important when pelvic fractures are suspected or detected on imaging.

Retrograde Urethrogram. Urethrogram (Figures 12-85 and 12-86) is performed by placement of the tip of a Foley catheter into the entrance of the urethra, followed by instillation of 50 mL of contrast under low pressure (usually gentle hand injection or gravity).[86] A plain x-ray of the region is then performed. An uninjured urethra should show a smooth linear contour and filling of the bladder. An injured urethra may have an irregular contour, end abruptly without filling of the bladder, or show extravasation of contrast into surrounding tissues. In the case of a normal study, the Foley catheter can be advanced as usual. In the case of an abnormal study, suprapubic catheterization may be performed.

Traumatic Vaginal Bleeding

Traumatic vaginal bleeding can indicate injury to the uterus or vagina. In the pregnant patient, vaginal bleeding can indicate uterine rupture, **placental abruption,**

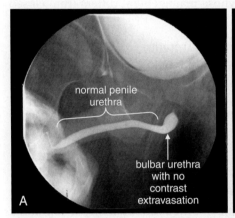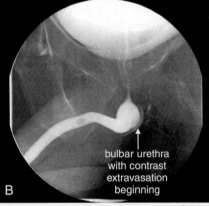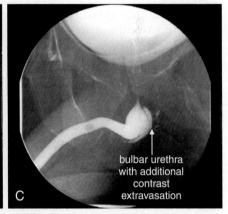

Figure 12-85. Urethral tear of the bulbar urethra: Retrograde urethrogram with contrast material. When blood is detected at the urethral meatus after blunt torso trauma, injury to the urethra, bladder, ureters, or kidneys may be the source. If a urethral injury is present, insertion of a urinary catheter may create a false passage or complete a partial urethral tear. A retrograde urethrogram can be performed to evaluate for urethral injury before catheter placement. This study is performed by sterilely cannulating the urethral meatus with a small-caliber urinary catheter and slowly instilling 15 to 20 mL of Renografin or similar contrast into the urethra while a series of fluoroscopic images are acquired over several minutes. In this patient, the bladder is already filled with contrast because the patient had undergone computed tomography scan with intravenous contrast. This injected contrast material was filtered by the kidneys and filled the bladder normally, excluding kidney, ureteral, and bladder injury. The penile urethra appears normal in caliber, with no tears present. The bulbar urethra shows slight ballooning, a nonspecific finding. Over approximately 5 minutes (from **A** to **C**), contrast is seen extravasating from the bulbar urethra. A small amount of contrast is seen in the membranous and prostatic urethra, with no evidence of extravasation above the urogenital diaphragm.

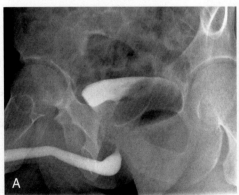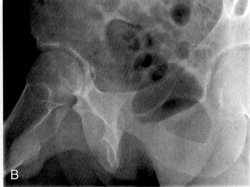

Figure 12-86. Normal retrograde urethrogram. This retrograde urethrogram was performed in the patient from the previous figure, 2 weeks after the initial injury. The image is an oblique lateral projection of the pelvis. It now shows normal contours of the penile and bulbar urethra with no extravasation. **A,** The urethra is filled with contrast and has a normal contour. Some contrast is seen filling the bladder. **B,** Contrast has been allowed to drain out of the bladder and urethra after dwelling there for several minutes. No residual contrast is seen after this, consistent with the absence of any residual tear. If a tear were present, contrast would be expected to have leaked into adjacent tissues and be visible on the delayed images.

and fetal distress—*so pregnancy status should be immediately assessed in all female patients.* In the pregnant patient fetal monitoring should be initiated as soon as possible.

Uterine injuries are rare except in pregnant patients because the uterus is usually small and protected within the bony pelvis, deep to the bladder. As pregnancy advances, the uterus rises out of the pelvis and is more subject to blunt and penetrating injury. Uterine injury and placental abruption are real possibilities in second- and third-trimester patients with abdominal and pelvic trauma. Concurrent with maternal stabilization, immediate abdominal ultrasound can be performed to assess fetal heart rate. Fetal bradycardia and tachycardia are ominous signs that may accompany maternal blood loss and shock or may indicate placental abruption. Abruption itself is not detected with high sensitivity by ultrasound as described earlier, so false reassurance should not be taken from a normal ultrasound. Continuous fetal monitoring should be initiated as soon as possible, regardless of normal ultrasound findings. Abnormal ultrasound should prompt consideration of immediate surgical delivery, as well as further assessment of the mother for sources of hemorrhage and shock.

Initial evaluation for uterine rupture should be conducted with ultrasound and external fetal monitoring, with the focus being on fetal viability and assessing the mother for other potentially life-threatening injuries. CT is quite sensitive for findings of uterine trauma or even uterine rupture and can be performed if other trauma considerations warrant abdominal or pelvis CT in the pregnant patent. However, uterus rupture is almost always associated with placental abruption and fetal distress, and CT diagnosis of uterine rupture likely would occur with too large a delay to allow emergency delivery of a live infant. Again, early ultrasound and fetal monitoring are imperative. Radiation and fetal safety considerations for CT in pregnant patients are discussed later. Descriptions of CT findings in critically injured pregnant patients include avascular (nonenhancing) regions of the placenta indicating placental abruption and infarction. Findings of uterine rupture include free abdominal fluid and extrauterine fetal parts. Normal changes in pregnancy, including heterogeneous placental enhancement, hydronephrosis from uterine compression of ureters, and enlarged ovarian veins, may be mistaken for pathological abnormalities.[87]

X-ray is of little utility in evaluating uterine rupture, although it may detect important findings such as pelvic fracture that may coexist with uterine injury. In some cases, x-ray may show the fetal skeleton in an abnormal location, indicating uterine rupture—but x-ray should not be relied upon for this diagnosis for a multitude of

reasons, including radiation exposure, poor sensitivity, and diagnostic delay that would likely result in fetal demise.

What Are the Best Tests for Cervical–Vaginal Trauma? What Other Imaging Findings Should Raise Concern for These Injuries?

Cervical and vaginal trauma is not easily detected by diagnostic imaging modalities. Instead, these injuries should be suspected when bony injuries to the pelvis are present. When pelvic fractures are detected by x-ray or CT scan, vaginal perforation should be considered and speculum pelvic examination should be performed. This is particularly the case for anterior pelvic fractures such as injuries to the superior or inferior pubic rami. Pelvic examination may prove these to be open fractures whose management differs from closed pelvic injuries.

Direct Genitourinary Trauma

Direct blunt trauma to the scrotum can result in testicular injury, including vascular injury and scrotal hematoma. Ultrasound can assess for these injuries, much as in the setting of testicular torsion. CT may demonstrate scrotal soft-tissue swelling and fluid, as well as testicular dislocation.[88]

Abdominal-Pelvic Trauma in the Pregnant Patient: Balancing Radiation Risk With Risk for Injury

The pregnant patient with abdominal or pelvic trauma requires dual evaluation of the mother and the fetus. In the first trimester, uterine and fetal injuries are rare; moreover, the fetus is not yet viable, so maternal evaluation should proceed much as in the nonpregnant female. In the late second and the third trimesters, the enlarged uterus rises out of the pelvis and is more subject to injury. In addition, beyond 25 weeks of gestation, the fetus may be viable; therefore, if fetal distress occurs, emergency delivery may be indicated. Consequently, assessment and stabilization of the fetus should occur concurrently with stabilization of the mother. Maternal safety takes precedence over that of the fetus, so imaging studies should be performed as needed for maternal evaluation, with appropriate clinical risk stratification.

No single x-ray or CT is thought to exceed the threshold to increase birth defects measurably—regardless of trimester (Tables 12-5[96] and 12-6[97]). However, trauma patients often undergo multiple imaging tests with significant cumulative radiation exposure. Therefore, whenever reasonable, ultrasound or clinical examination and observation should be substituted for ionizing radiation imaging studies. In unstable patients, fetal radiation concerns are overridden by maternal safety concerns. In stable patients, minimizing radiation exposure to the fetus should be a relative priority. Ionizing radiation exposure

TABLE 12-5. Effects of Radiation Exposure on Prenatal Development

Gestational Stage	Time After Conception	Fetal Dose	Potential Effect
Preimplantation	0-14 days	50-100 mSv	• Prenatal death
Major organogenesis	1-8 weeks	200-250 mSv	• Growth retardation
	2-15 weeks	200-250 mSv	• Small head size • Exposure before 8 weeks does not cause an intellectual deficit, despite small head size • Most sensitive period for induction of childhood cancer
Rapid neuron development and migration	6-15 weeks	>100 mSv	• Small head size, seizures, decline in intelligence quotient (25 points per 1000 mSv)
After organogenesis and rapid neuron development	15 weeks to term	>100 mSv	• Increased frequency of childhood cancer
	15 weeks to term	>500 mSv	• Severe mental retardation

Adapted from Bentur Y, Horlatsch N, Koren G. Exposure to ionizing radiation during pregnancy: Perception of teratogenic risk and outcome. *Teratology* 43:109-12,1991; Ratnapalan S, Bentur Y, Koren G. "Doctor, will that x-ray harm my unborn child?" *CMAJ* 179:1293-6, 2008.

TABLE 12-6. Estimated Radiation Doses From Common Diagnostic Imaging Procedures

Imaging Test and Body Region	Fetal Dose
Radiographs	
Upper extremity	0.01 mSv
Lower extremity	0.01 mSv
Upper gastrointestinal series (barium)	0.48-3.60 mSv
Cholecystography	**0.05-0.60 mSv**
Chest (two views)	<0.1 mSv
Lumbar spine	3.46-6.20 mSv
Pelvis	0.40-2.38 mSv
Hip and femur series	0.51-3.70 mSv
Retrograde Pyelogram	8.00 mSv
Abdomen (kidneys, ureter, and bladder)	2.00-2.45 mSv
Urography (IVP)	3.58-13.98 mSv
Barium enema	7.00-39.86 mSv
CT Scan	
Head	<0.5 mSv
Chest	1.0-4.5 mSv
Lumbar spine	35.0 mSv
Abdomen (10 slices)	2.4-26.0 mSv
Pelvis	7.3 mSv
Abdomen and pelvis	6.4 mSv
Ventilation–Perfusion Scan	0.6-10.0 mSv
Potentially Teratogenic Dose	**50 mSv**

Adapted from Ratnapalan S, Bentur Y, Koren G. "Doctor, will that x-ray harm my unborn child?" *CMAJ* 179:1293-6, 2008.

can be limited by using clinical parameters to determine the need for imaging. As discussed in the chapter on imaging the bony pelvis, clinical decision rules exist that can identify patients who do not require imaging of the bony pelvis. The pelvis x-ray can be avoided in patients without altered level of consciousness, complaint of pelvic pain, pelvic tenderness on examination, distracting injury, or clinical intoxication.[89] In the stable patient with no significant abdominal pain or tenderness, observation with serial physical exams can be performed to avoid abdominal or pelvic irradiation with CT. Serial ultrasound of the abdomen can assess for free fluid or development of hemoperitoneum. Monitoring of vital signs for tachycardia and serial measurement of hematocrit can be used to observe for blood loss, rather than using immediate CT. This strategy of maternal observation is particularly reasonable because patients in the late second and the third trimesters require admission for extended fetal monitoring due to the risk of placental abruption, whether or not other maternal injuries are suspected.

Penetrating Trauma

Penetrating genitourinary trauma has a more straightforward imaging approach than blunt trauma. In many cases, laparotomy may be needed to assess for other abdominal and pelvic injuries. In these cases, additional imaging studies to assess for genitourinary injury occur later, outside of the emergency department.

High-energy penetrating abdominal or pelvic trauma, such as gunshot wounds, traditionally requires laparotomy for assessment. Injuries to retroperitoneal and pelvic vascular structures and bowel are major concerns. Although most often the approach is surgical exploration, limited experience with "triple contrast" CT (IV, oral, and rectal contrast) has been described and is discussed in more detail in the chapter on torso trauma.[90-92] As in blunt trauma, CT can demonstrate renal hemorrhage, extravasation of contrast from the renal collecting system or ureters, and bladder perforation, as well as associated abdominal injuries. In hemodynamically stable patients, CT imaging may be a reasonable approach if operative care is being deferred for reasons such as operating room availability. In most cases, simple x-rays of the chest, abdomen, and pelvis are performed in the trauma bay, although these provide little information about genitourinary injuries. Later, specific studies such as CT, cystogram, and IVP or retrograde urography can be performed to assess the kidneys, ureters, and bladder. In unstable patients requiring immediate laparotomy, IV urography can be performed in the operating room to assess for renal injuries. overall, the imaging plan for patients with penetrating trauma should be a team decision involving the emergency physician and surgical consultants.

Lower-energy-penetrating trauma, such as stab wounds to the flank, is increasingly investigated with triple-contrast CT.[91] Initial studies suggest high sensitivity for injuries, but extreme caution should be used following a negative CT scan. Although CT may accurately identify genitourinary injuries requiring therapy, such as significant renal or ureteral injury, concurrent bowel injuries such as penetration of the retroperitoneal colon may be missed, with significant associated morbidity. Patients may develop sepsis from missed bowel injuries. Imaging in this setting is discussed in more detail in the chapter on abdominal trauma.

RADIATION EXPOSURES FROM DIAGNOSTIC IMAGING IN PREGNANCY

Diagnostic imaging in the pregnant patient raises particular concerns related to radiation and fetal safety. Approximate fetal radiation doses associated with harmful clinical effects are shown in Table 12-5. The fetal radiation doses from individual diagnostic imaging exams are shown in Table 12-6. *Note that no single common examination exceeds the threshold known to cause teratogenic effects, although the cumulative dose of multiple imaging studies should be considered.* High levels of radiation exposure may lead to fetal demise. Lower levels of radiation exposure may lead to fetal malformation. Although very low levels of radiation exposure, such as those encountered in most emergency diagnostic imaging, are not thought to pose any specific fetal risk, some researchers have raised concerns that fetal irradiation may lead to increases in childhood leukemia or other subtle abnormalities, such as developmental delay or cognitive defects. Certainly radiation exposures in pregnancy contribute to maternal anxiety. However, as emergency physicians, we must balance the risk for immediate danger to fetus and mother from an ongoing and undiagnosed emergency medical condition against small and delayed risks posed by medical radiation. How accurately do physicians and patients characterize these risks? Physicians likely overestimate and underestimate risk.

In 2004, Lee et al.[93] conducted a survey of radiologists, emergency physicians, and patients regarding radiation exposure and cancer risk. At that time, only about 50% of radiologists, 10% of emergency physicians, and 3% of patients recognized that radiation exposure from CT scan might pose any future risk for cancer development. In a survey of family physicians and obstetricians, Ratnapalan et al.[96] asked each subject group to estimate the risk for fetal malformation resulting from a single exposure during pregnancy to abdominal x-ray or abdominal CT scan (neither of which is thought to pose a radiation exposure high enough to result in fetal harm after a single exposure, regardless of gestational age). As a follow-up question, the researchers asked each subject group to indicate their practice of advising a patient about elective termination of pregnancy following such exposure, based on fetal risk from radiation. 44% of family physicians and 11% of obstetricians believed that the fetal malformation risk from x-ray exceeded 5%. In addition, 61% of family physicians and 34% of obstetricians believed a single abdominal CT exceeded a 5% fetal malformation risk. Finally, 6% of family physicians and 5% of obstetricians recommended elective abortion following a single abdominal CT scan—a recommendation unjustified by current risk estimates.[50]

It is often said that maternal health must take precedence over any concerns for fetal risk from medical diagnostic radiation exposures. Although this is certainly true, this statement is sometimes used as carte blanche to perform whatever diagnostic imaging tests might be used in a nonpregnant female. Instead, consider the following approach. First, determine what life-threatening conditions are strongly considered in the mother. Truly life-threatening considerations probably warrant the same diagnostic imaging approach that would be used in a nonpregnant patient. Second, determine what other important diagnoses must be evaluated but could be diagnosed in a more measured fashion because they do not pose an immediate risk. Examples could include such diagnoses as appendicitis or even intraabdominal solid organ injury in a stable patient, which is often managed nonoperatively. Many diagnoses that might initially seem to fit into the first category actually fall into the second on further consideration. For these diagnoses, consider alternative diagnostic imaging tests that do not involve ionizing radiation. Ultrasound or MRI for appendicitis diagnosis may be appropriate; these are discussed in more detail in the chapter on abdominal imaging. Strategies for the pregnant trauma patient are discussed earlier. Finally, a third category of diagnostic considerations should be entertained. These diagnoses likely pose no significant threat to the mother at any time but are often worked up in the nonpregnant patient for purposes of closure or for exclusion of other, more dangerous diagnoses. Examples might include renal colic or simple ovarian cysts. In the pregnant patient, exclusion of dangerous causes of symptoms may be sufficient, and careful explanation to the patient of those diagnoses that are not being evaluated may take the place of diagnostic imaging. Perhaps we can learn a lesson from pregnant patients, resulting in less indiscriminate use of diagnostic imaging in nonpregnant patients for these relatively nonemergent diagnoses.

SUMMARY

Genitourinary complaints can include life- and organ-threatening conditions. A variety of imaging modalities are available for diagnosis. For patients with significant trauma, and in the nontrauma patient with a broad differential diagnosis including abdominal pathology, CT is the most valuable modality for most complaints. Ultrasound is the key modality for assessment of complications in the pregnant patient. Ultrasound is also useful in the diagnosis of testicular and ovarian torsion but is not 100% sensitive—thus a negative imaging result does not rule out these conditions when clinical suspicion is high. No imaging modality is sensitive for placental abruption, so fetal monitoring is essential. In the pregnant patient, reasonable steps should be considered to reduce radiation exposures through clinical observation and use of modalities such as ultrasound that do not use ionizing radiation. When the mother's life is at risk, imaging should be performed as for the nonpregnant patient. No single imaging test exceeds the threshold known to induce fetal malformation.

CHAPTER 13 Imaging of the Pelvis and Hip

Joshua Broder, MD, FACEP

Imaging of the pelvis can be required following minor or major trauma and for nontraumatic painful conditions. In this chapter, we review a systematic approach to interpretation of the standard pelvis x-ray, correlating abnormalities with computed tomography (CT) findings. We also discuss high-risk pelvic bony injuries associated with soft-tissue and vascular injuries—which are examined in detail in related chapters on genitourinary imaging (Chapter 12), abdominal trauma (Chapter 10), and interventional radiology (Chapter 16). Because fractures of the proximal femur are often clinically indistinguishable from fractures of the pelvis, we illustrate these injuries here, with more discussion in the chapters on extremity injuries (Chapter 14) and musculoskeletal magnetic resonance imaging (MRI, Chapter 15). Along the way, we consider a number of critical clinical questions:

1. How common are pelvic injuries?
2. What injuries are associated with pelvic trauma?
3. How dangerous are pelvic injuries?
4. What are the techniques for pelvic x-ray and CT?
5. How should x-ray and CT of the pelvis be interpreted?
6. Who needs pelvic x-ray following trauma?
7. When pelvic x-ray is normal, who needs CT?
8. If CT is planned for evaluation of other abdominal and pelvic soft-tissue injuries, is x-ray needed? If so, in which patients?
9. Why is MRI recommended for some injuries and CT for others?
10. If CT is used in the setting of major trauma, why is MRI called upon for minor mechanisms of injury?
11. What associated injuries must be suspected and evaluated when pelvic fractures are detected?
12. What special imaging tests should be considered for pelvic fractures?
13. What is the role of interventional radiology and angiographic embolization?

How Common Are Pelvic Injuries? What Injuries Are Associated With Pelvic Trauma?

An 8-year retrospective review of the trauma registry at the Los Angeles County and University of Southern California trauma center found that 9.3% of 16,630 adult admissions sustained some type of pelvic fracture. In patients with pelvic fractures, 16.5% had associated abdominal injuries, including liver (6.1%), bladder and urethra (5.8%), spleen (5.2%), diaphragm (2.1%), and small bowel (2%). In severe pelvic fractures (defined by an Abbreviated Injury Scale score ≥4), intrabdominal injuries rose in frequency to 30.7% of patients, and the bladder and urethra were most commonly injured, in 14.6% of patients.[1] Aortic rupture was seven times more common in patients with pelvic fracture than in those without, although still rare (1.4%, compared with 0.2%).

How Dangerous Are Pelvic Injuries?

Mortality in patients with pelvic fractures is high—13.5% in adults in one large study. However, only about 0.8% of deaths are directly attributed to pelvic injuries. These are high-energy injuries that frequently coexist with severe injuries to the head, chest, abdomen, spine, and extremities. When pelvic injuries are noted on imaging studies, careful attention should be given to determining the presence of other injuries.[1] The low mortality directly attributed to pelvic injuries should not suggest that these injuries themselves are unimportant. This low mortality is achieved when patients are treated at major trauma centers and receive aggressive therapy for pelvic injuries, including blood transfusion, orthopedic fixation, and angiographic embolization of pelvic vascular injuries. In one study, 38.5% of pelvic fracture patients received blood transfusion, with a mean transfusion of nearly 1 L.[1] In severe pelvic fracture patients, 60.6% received transfusion, with a mean of more than 3.5 L. When severe pelvic injury was the only significant injury, more than 50% received transfusion, with a mean of 2.7 L. Overall, 16.6% of pelvic fracture patients required more than 2 L of blood in transfusion. Angiography (discussed in detail in Chapter 16) was performed in 4.7% of patients with pelvic injuries, and therapeutic embolization was performed in 2.3%, or half of those undergoing angiography.

PELVIC X-RAY AND COMPUTED TOMOGRAPHY TECHNIQUES

The routine initial view of the pelvis is the anterior–posterior (AP) x-ray (Figure 13-1). This image is obtained with the patient supine and the x-ray beam oriented 90 degrees to the patient's long axis, passing through the patient from anterior to posterior. Additional plain films can be obtained when injuries are seen on the AP image or if occult injuries are suspected with a normal AP view. These include oblique (Judet) views for characterization of acetabular fractures (Figure 13-2), and inlet and outlet views for characterization of pelvic ring fractures (Figure 13-3). Inlet views are obtained with the patient supine and the x-ray tube positioned at the

patient's head, angled 45 degrees toward the patient's feet. This allows assessment of pelvic brim integrity, AP displacement of the hemipelvis, internal or external rotation of the hemipelvis, and anterior displacement of the sacrum. Outlet views are also obtained with the patient supine, with the x-ray tube at the patient's feet and angled 45 degrees toward the head. This provides an excellent view of the sacrum, which is perpendicular to the x-ray beam in this position. The sacral neural foramina are seen well in this view, and vertical displacement of the hemipelvis may be evident. These additional views may be unnecessary if CT of the pelvis is planned, particularly if multiplanar two-dimensional images or three-dimensional models can be constructed, which depends on local software. Most modern picture archiving and communication system (PACS) software allows multiplanar two-dimensional reconstructions from multidetector CT image data, and three-dimensional capability is becoming routine. Three-dimensional reconstruction (Figure 13-4) depends on high-quality original image data but is otherwise a postprocessing function and does not require a different CT protocol during the image acquisition phase.

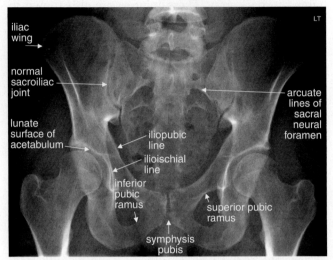

Figure 13-1. The normal anterior–posterior pelvis. This normal pelvis x-ray is from a 24-year-old with no history of direct trauma. Normal findings are labeled. Patients commonly have subtle asymmetry from right to left. Overlying bowel gas frequently hides portions of the bony pelvis, and you will have to make careful judgments about abnormal lucency indicating fracture versus overlying gas.

Fracture detection with CT does not require the administration of IV or oral contrast. However, in most cases, IV contrast is given because the pelvic CT is obtained with the abdominal CT for detection of visceral injury. IV contrast allows recognition of active bleeding from

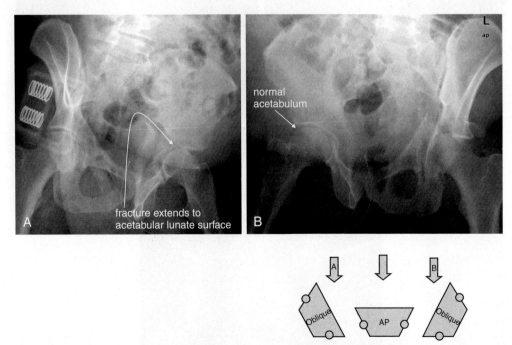

Figure 13-2. Oblique (Judet) views of the pelvis for evaluation of the acetabulum. Oblique (Judet) views of the pelvis are useful for evaluation of the acetabula for fractures. The patient is rolled onto the left and right side at a 45-degree angle, which isolates the hemipelvis and acetabulum, removing posterior pelvic structures from the x-ray path. This provides an en-face view of the dependent iliac wing and places the acetabular lunate surface in relief, preventing overlap by other lines that may simulate or obscure fractures. In this patient, an obvious left acetabular fracture is present, but more subtle fractures may be revealed by this technique. A, An oblique view with left hip in dependent position (called LPO for left posterior oblique) allows evaluation of the left acetabulum. B, An oblique view with right hip in dependent position (called RPO for right posterior oblique) allows evaluation of the right acetabulum. The schematic shows the position of the pelvis relative to the x-ray tube (block arrow).

pelvic vascular structures. Oral contrast is often not administered in the setting of trauma because it has little impact on diagnosis of bowel injuries (see the chapter on imaging of abdominal trauma, Chapter 10). A single CT scan of the pelvis can provide information about both soft-tissue and bony injuries. Urinary tract injuries require special CT techniques for diagnosis, as mentioned later and explored in more detail in the chapter on genitourinary imaging (Chapter 12). When more detail of fractures is needed, fine-cut, dedicated "bony pelvis" CT can be performed without contrast, although not all injuries mandate this. In the past, dedicated bony pelvis CT was often obtained to characterize pelvic fractures in greater detail when fractures were seen on body CT performed for evaluation of visceral injury. Today, thin-slice multidetector body CT images offer good resolution of fractures, and bony pelvis CT may not be routinely required. CT images can be reconstructed in three dimensions for further characterization of fractures and dislocations (see Figure 13-4).

INTERPRETATION OF THE PELVIC X-RAY

The bony pelvis is a ring structure in which isolated fractures are rare. When reviewing a pelvic x-ray, detection of a single break in the ring mandates search for a second injury. Certain injury patterns are common, and detection of one component of a pattern logically guides your evaluation for the remaining components of the injury. In the figures that follow, a number of frequently encountered fracture patterns are described and illustrated. Figure 13-1 shows a normal pelvis x-ray with labels. Figures 13-5 to 13-19 show common patterns of injury schematically, with displaced fragments highlighted in dark gray. These injuries are also shown in actual x-rays and CTs in the figures that follow. In many cases, multiple injury types are present, so review the schematics first to understand the simplified key features of isolated injuries. Table 13-1 lists the injury patterns and associated figures in this chapter.

We begin with the normal AP pelvis x-ray (labeled, see Figure 13-1). Each structure examined on x-ray should also be reviewed when interpreting CT scan. Stepwise inspection of the AP pelvic x-ray should include evaluation of the following (see Figure 13-5):

1. Inspect the pubic symphysis for widening, overlap, or vertical dislocation, which may be seen with the injury patterns described later. The normal pubic symphysis is usually about 4 to 5 mm in width and does not exceed 1 cm. Figures 13-6 and 13-7 illustrate some common patterns of abnormality of the symphysis pubis.

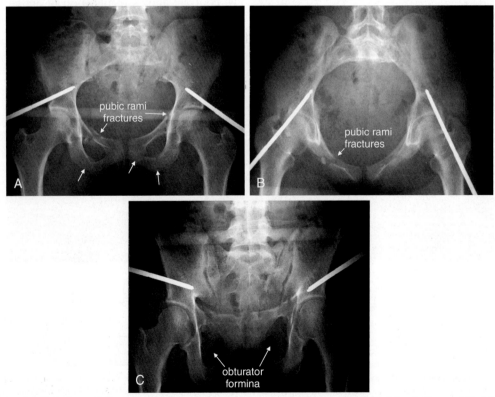

Figure 13-3. Inlet and outlet views of the pelvis for evaluation of pelvic ring fractures. This patient has fractures of the bilateral superior and inferior rami and a vertical sacral fracture seen on computed tomography (arrows in panel **A**). An external fixator has been placed. **A,** Standard anterior–posterior (AP) view for comparison. **B,** The inlet view reveals the pelvic ring in detail, allowing assessment of pelvic brim integrity, AP displacement of the hemipelvis, internal or external rotation of the hemipelvis, AP displacement of the sacrum, and AP displacement of pubic rami fractures. **C,** The outlet view provides a good view of the sacrum, which is perpendicular to the x-ray beam in this position. The sacral neural foramina are seen well in this view, and vertical displacement of the hemipelvis may be evident when present. The obturator foramina are also seen well in this view.

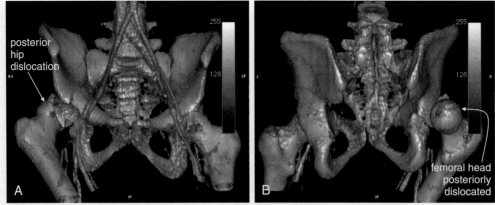

Figure 13-4. Three-dimensional computed tomography (CT) reconstruction of the pelvis. CT images can be reconstructed in three dimensions using postprocessing software. These CT images were created using axial images from a standard CT scan with intravenous contrast performed for the evaluation of trauma. The patient has a right posterior hip dislocation **(A),** more evident a posterior view of the pelvis **(B)**, where the femoral head is exposed rather than hidden within the acetabulum. The acetabulum is also fractured posteriorly. While this model is of high quality, a stair-step pattern is visible in the pelvis because of the relatively thick two-dimensional slices used to reconstruct the three-dimensional model. Higher-quality models can be rendered when thinner slices are acquired during CT. Models can be rotated in three dimensions, and structures can be digitally removed. The aorta, inferior vena cava, and iliac arteries and veins have intentionally been left visible to emphasize the potential for vascular injuries when bony pelvic injuries occur.

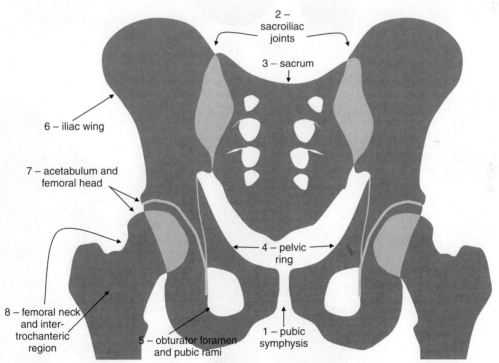

Figure 13-5. The normal pelvis. This schematic shows a normal pelvis. When reviewing a pelvis x-ray, take the following steps.

1. Inspect the pubic symphysis for widening, overlap, or vertical dislocation, which may be seen the injury patterns described below. The normal pubic symphysis is usually about 4 to 5 mm in width and does not exceed 1 cm.

2. Inspect the sacroiliac joints for widening, excessive overlap, or vertical off-set. The normal sacrum and iliac wing share a thin zone of overlap defining the sacroiliac joint. Widening of this joint space is abnormal and suggests joint injury and diastasis. The joints should be bilaterally symmetrical. The normal sacroiliac joint is 2 to 4 mm in width.

3. Examine the sacrum for fractures, which may intersect the normal neural foramina. If the sacroiliac joints are intact but the right and left pelvis are malaligned vertically, suspect a vertically oriented sacral fracture.

4. Follow the ring formed by the inferior portion of the sacrum and the medial portion of the ilium and ischium, sweeping down the pubic bone to the pubic symphysis and back up the opposite side to your starting point. This should form a smooth continuous ring without cortical irregularities.

5. Inspect the smaller ring formed between the inferior and superior pubic rami, called the obturator foramen. This should be a smooth continuous circle. The opposite side usually provides an excellent comparison view, unless bilateral injuries are present. Inspect the superior and inferior pubic rami for discontinuities.

6. Inspect the iliac wings for fractures. Overlying bowel gas may create rounded lucencies overlying the iliac bones, whereas linear lucencies are more suggestive of fracture. Follow lucencies to determine whether they intersect the outer border of the iliac bones, which should be smooth continuous curves without cortical stepoffs.

7. Inspect the acetabula bilaterally, noting whether the femoral heads are located appropriately or dislocated. The curved concave surface of the acetabulum, called the lunate surface, should be a smooth continuous curve, matching the curve of the femoral head. Clues to acetabular fractures include disruption of the iliopubic line, ilioischial line, and lunate surface. The joint spaces separating the femoral head and lunate surface of the acetabulum should be bilaterally symmetrical.

8. Inspect the femur, including the femoral head, neck, and intertrochanteric region, as these are common sites of fracture, particularly in elderly patients.

Figure 13-6. Open-book pelvis. This schematic of an open-book pelvis shows separation of the pubic symphysis and right sacroiliac joint. Diastasis of the pubic symphysis, combined with either diastasis of one or both sacroiliac joints or fractures of the pelvis ring, allows the pelvis to "open" anteriorly, with a hinge joint posteriorly. The darkened region indicates the portion of the pelvis that has become traumatically displaced.

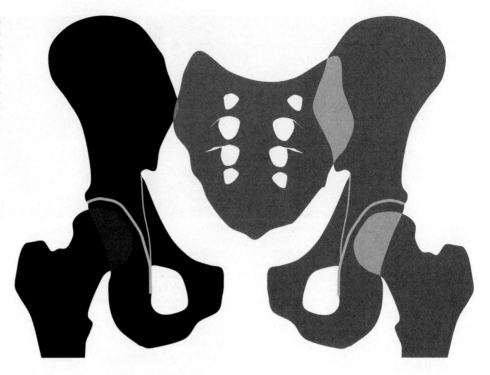

Figure 13-7. Vertical shear injury. Vertical shear can separate the pubic symphysis and sacroiliac joints in a cephalad–caudad direction. Alternatively, fractures may occur vertically, allowing vertical offset of the pelvis. In this schematic, the right sacroiliac joint and pubic symphysis are diastatic. The darkened region indicates the portion of the pelvis that has become traumatically displaced.

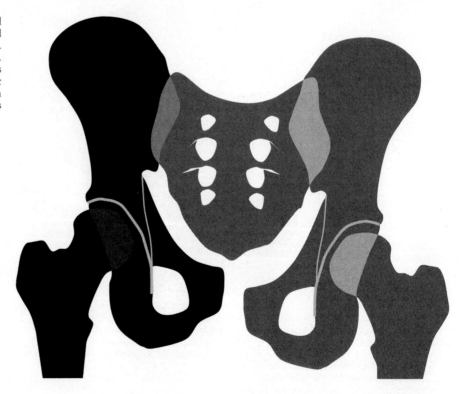

2. Inspect the sacroiliac joints for widening, excessive overlap, or vertical offset. The normal sacrum and iliac wing share a thin zone of overlap defining the sacroiliac joint on the AP view. Widening of this joint space is abnormal and suggests joint injury and diastasis. The joints should be bilaterally symmetrical. The normal sacroiliac joint is 2 to 4 mm in width. Figures 13-6 to 13-9 show abnormal sacroiliac joints.

3. Examine the sacrum for fractures, which may intersect the normal neural foramina. If the sacroiliac joints are intact but the right and left pelvis are malaligned vertically, suspect a vertically oriented sacral fracture. Transverse sacral fractures may sometimes occur in isolation and may not disrupt the integrity of the pelvic ring. Figures 13-10 and 13-11 depict sacral fractures.

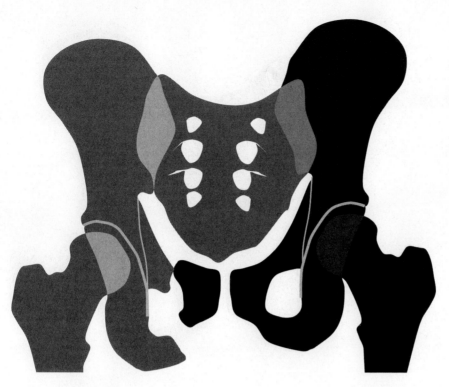

Figure 13-8. **Pubic ramus fractures with vertical shear: Bucket-handle pattern.** When pubic rami fractures and sacroiliac joint diastasis are contralateral, a bucket-handle pattern is present. In this schematic, the right pubic rami are fractured, and the left sacroiliac joint is diastatic. Because the pubic symphysis is intact, the left pelvis carried the small right pubic fragment with it in its cephalad migration. The darkened region indicates the portion of the pelvis that has become traumatically displaced.

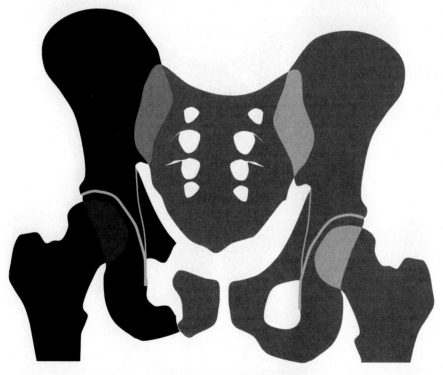

Figure 13-9. **Pubic ramus fractures with vertical shear: Malgaigne pattern.** When pubic rami fractures and sacroiliac joint diastasis (or sacral fracture) are ipsilateral, a vertical shear injury called a Malgaigne fracture is present. A common mechanism is landing from height on an outstretched leg. In this schematic, the right sacroiliac joint is diastatic and the right pubic rami are fractured. Because the pubic symphysis is intact, the small right pubic bone fragment remains attached to the left pelvis, whereas the entire right pelvis moves cephalad. The darkened region indicates the portion of the pelvis that has become traumatically displaced.

4. Follow the ring formed by the inferior portion of the sacrum and the medial portion of the ilium and ischium, sweeping down the pubic bone to the pubic symphysis and back up the opposite side to your starting point. This should form a smooth, continuous ring without cortical irregularities. Figures 13-6 to 13-13 show abnormalities in this contour associated with different fracture patterns.

5. Inspect the smaller ring formed between the inferior and the superior pubic rami, called the obturator foramen. This should be a smooth, continuous circle. The opposite side usually provides an excellent comparison view, unless bilateral injuries are present. Inspect the superior and inferior pubic rami for discontinuities. Figures 13-8, 13-9, 13-12, and 13-13 show fractures involving the pubic rami and obturator foramen.

Figure 13-10. Sacral fractures. Sacral fractures may occur in isolation or with other fractures. Vertical sacral fractures can occur with vertical pelvic shear, and commonly other fractures or diastasis of the pubic symphysis are seen. Transverse fracture of the sacrum may be seen in isolation and may not compromise the integrity of the pelvic ring. In this schematic, a vertical sacral fracture is depicted with vertical offset of the pubic symphysis. The darkened region indicates the portion of the pelvis that has become traumatically displaced.

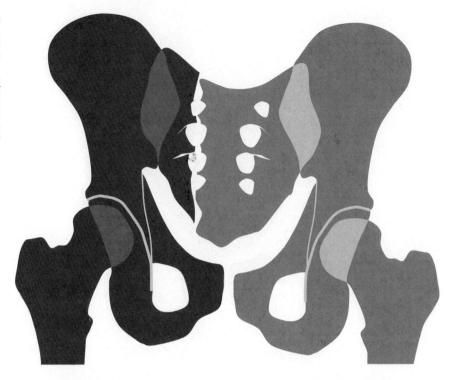

Figure 13-11. Transverse sacral fracture. Transverse sacral and coccygeal fractures may occur with little clinical consequence because they do not affect the structural integrity of the pelvic ring. Transverse sacral fractures may intersect sacral nerve foramen, with potential for nerve injury. In this schematic, a transverse sacral fracture is depicted intersecting sacral foramen.

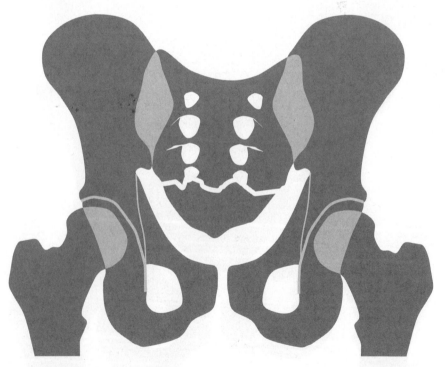

6. Inspect the iliac wings for fractures. Overlying bowel gas may create rounded lucencies overlying the iliac bones, whereas linear lucencies are more suggestive of fracture. Follow lucencies to determine whether they intersect the outer border of the iliac bones, which should be smooth, continuous curves without cortical step-offs. Figure 13-14 depicts an isolated iliac wing fracture.
7. Inspect the acetabula bilaterally, noting whether the femoral heads are located appropriately or dislocated.

The curved concave surface of the acetabulum, called the lunate surface, should be a smooth, continuous curve, matching the curve of the femoral head. Clues to acetabular fractures include disruption of the iliopubic line, ilioischial line, and lunate surface (Figure 13-15). The joint spaces separating the femoral head and lunate surface of the acetabulum should be bilaterally symmetrical. Figures 13-16 and 13-17 depict posterior and anterior dislocations of the femoral head (hip).

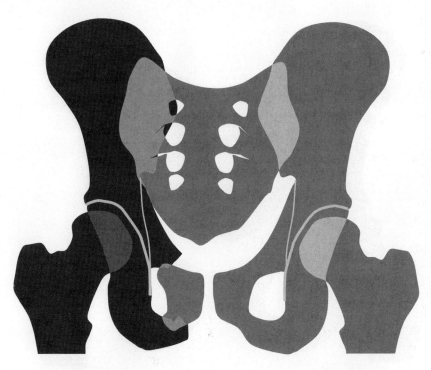

Figure 13-12. **Lateral compression of the pelvis.** Lateral compression of the pelvis can disrupt the pelvic ring anteriorly and posteriorly. Commonly, one sacroiliac joint folds inward, although sacral or iliac wing fractures may occur. Anteriorly, pubic rami fractures are common, as well as disruptions of the sacroiliac joint. In this schematic, the right sacroiliac joint has folded inward and the right superior and inferior pubic rami have fractured. The darkened region indicates the portion of the pelvis that has become traumatically displaced.

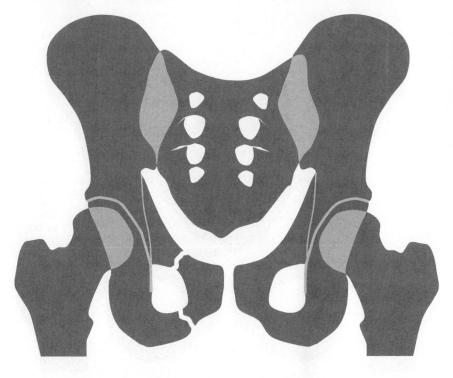

Figure 13-13. **Pubic ramus fractures.** Pubic ramus fractures, as in this schematic, either occur singly or involve the superior and inferior pubic rami. Usually, a single fracture occurs only if minimally displaced. An offset of a single fracture usually creates tension in the pelvic ring that is relieved through a second fracture or diastasis of a joint.

8. Inspect the femur, including the femoral head, neck, and intertrochanteric region because these are common sites of fracture, particularly in elderly patients. Figures 13-18 and 13-19 illustrate some common patterns of proximal femur fracture.

PATTERNS OF PELVIC INJURY

Fractures of the pelvis can range from innocuous, requiring no treatment, to immediately life threatening. Their appearance on x-ray can be subtle or overt,

and the emergency physician must be able to recognize key injuries immediately to take appropriate stabilization measures, plan interventions such as angiographic embolization, consider additional imaging, and arrange safe disposition. We examine a number of common fracture patterns, recognizing that often a mixture of injury patterns may be present in the same patient.

Two major systems of classification of pelvic fractures are the Young-Burgess classification and the Tile classification systems (Tables 13-2 and 13-3). The Young-Burgess

Figure 13-14. Iliac wing fracture. Inspect the iliac wings for fractures. Overlying bowel gas may create rounded lucencies overlying the iliac bones, whereas linear lucencies are more suggestive of fracture. Follow lucencies to determine whether they intersect the outer border of the iliac bones, which should be smooth continuous curves without cortical step-offs.

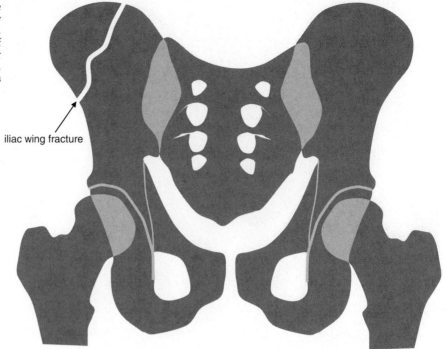

Figure 13-15. Acetabular fractures. Acetabular fractures can be subtle on x-ray and are best diagnosed by computed tomography. Clues to the diagnosis are disruptions of the iliopubic line, which forms the medial border of the anterior column of the acetabulum; disruption of the ilioischial line, which forms the medial border of the posterior column of the acetabulum; and disruptions of the articular surface of the acetabulum, called the lunate surface. In this schematic, defects in each of these lines are shown by short arrows on the patient's right, whereas the patient's left side is normal. In an actual x-ray, fracture fragments may or may not be visible.

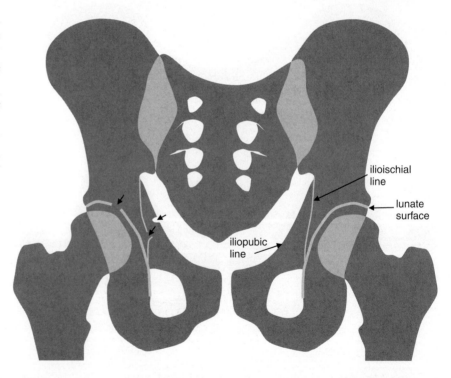

classification[2] describes injuries in terms of mechanism and type of injury, direction of hemipelvis displacement, and stability. The Tile classification[3] divides fractures into three main categories, each with multiple subtypes, including stable fractures with an intact posterior arch (type A), unstable anterior and lateral compression fractures with incomplete disruption of the posterior arch (type B), and vertical shear injuries with complete disruption of the posterior arch (type C). While these are useful for orthopedists in surgical planning, emergency physicians can understand injuries and communicate them clearly to specialty colleagues with simple descriptions, based on recognition of several common injury patterns.

Two primary categories of injury should be considered from an emergency medicine perspective: fractures that disrupt the major pelvic ring and those that do not. Fractures that compress or open the pelvis ring can disrupt blood vessels passing through the pelvis. In addition,

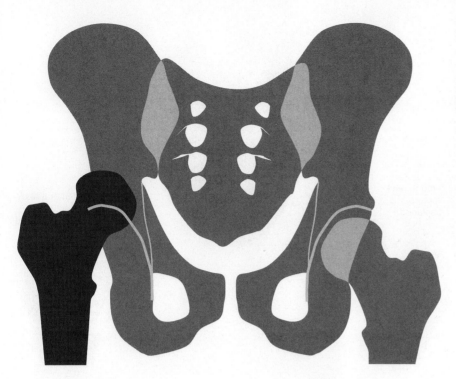

Figure 13-16. Posterior hip dislocation. Hip dislocation most frequently occurs in a posterior direction, with a common scenario being anterior-posterior force directly against a flexed and adducted hip in a seated patient in a vehicle collision. If the hip is abducted at the moment of impact, anterior dislocation sometimes occurs. Once dislocated posteriorly, as in this schematic, the femur is usually pulled cephalad by hip flexors. The darkened region indicates the traumatically dislocated hip.

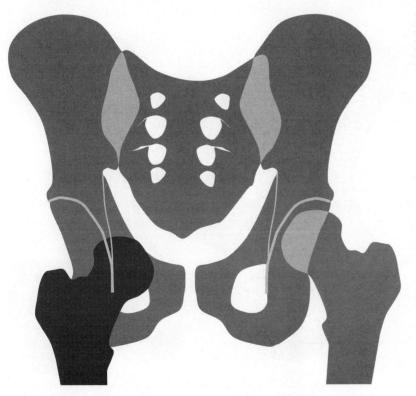

Figure 13-17. Anterior hip dislocation. Anterior hip dislocation, shown in this schematic, is less common than posterior dislocation but may position the femoral head medially relative to the acetabulum. The darkened region indicates the traumatically dislocated hip.

because they change the geometry of the pelvis from a stable cone with a fixed volume to an expandable structure with the ability to increase in size, substantial bleeding can occur in the pelvis from these fracture types. Identification of a fracture in this group should prompt pelvic stabilization, preparation for potentially massive transfusion, and consideration of angiographic embolization. Fractures that do not affect the pelvic ring in this

way can be important for other reasons, but rarely are they as immediately life-threatening. For example, fractures near the pubic symphysis involving the inferior or superior pubic rami may be associated with bladder and urethral injuries, as well as vaginal lacerations in female patients. Acetabular fractures, while associated with disability from posttraumatic arthritis, do not pose an immediate life-threat to the patient.

Figure 13-18. Femoral neck (hip) fracture. Fractures of the femoral neck can be overt or subtle. Often, these occur in older patients with osteopenia, making cortical and trabecular abnormalities more difficult to see. In this schematic, an obvious fracture is diagrammed on the right, whereas a more subtle fracture is depicted on the left. Sometimes all that is seen is a faint band of increased density in nondisplaced fractures. Magnetic resonance imaging, computed tomography, or bone scan can clarify equivocal fractures.

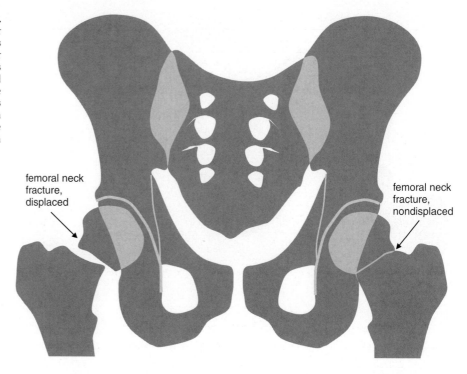

femoral neck fracture, displaced

femoral neck fracture, nondisplaced

Figure 13-19. Intertrochanteric femoral (hip) fracture. Intertrochanteric hip fractures are a common form of fracture in patients over the age of 65 years, with relatively minor mechanisms of injury, such as falls from standing, predominating. As the name suggests, they typically run between the greater and the lesser trochanters. They may be comminuted and displaced. Sometimes, these fractures are more subtle and require magnetic resonance imaging, computed tomography, or bone scan for confirmation. In this schematic, an overt intertrochanteric fracture is depicted on the patient's right, with a more subtle abnormality on the left.

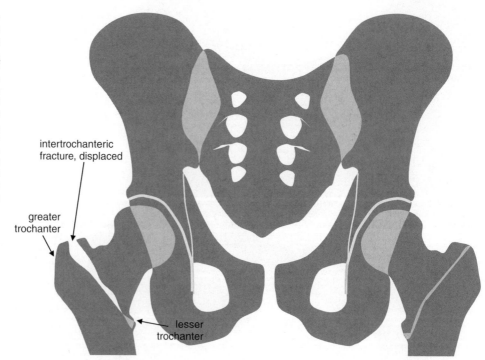

intertrochanteric fracture, displaced

greater trochanter

lesser trochanter

Forces That Disrupt the Major Pelvic Ring

Fractures that affect the stability of the pelvic ring can be subcategorized in several additional ways—for example, by mechanism of injury. In theory, fractures that compress the pelvic ring laterally may be less likely to stretch and tear vascular structures, compared with structures that involve AP compression, opening the pelvis at the pubic symphysis and sacroiliac joints.

Vertical shear injuries to the pelvis may disrupt vascular structures and result in damage to nerve roots at the level of the sacrum. Important pelvic ring disruptions involve fractures or diastasis of joints at two or more sites of the anterior and posterior pelvic arcs. Separation of the pubic symphysis and diastasis of the sacroiliac joints can cause pelvic ring disruption in the absence of a fracture. Two or more fractures can also result in pelvic

TABLE 13-1. Guide to Figures in This Chapter

Content	Figure Number
Approach to pelvic image interpretation	
• Normal pelvis, AP view	13-1, 13-5
• Oblique (Judet) views	13-2
• Inlet and outlet views	13-3
• Three-dimensional CT reconstruction	13-4
• Schematic figures of common injury patterns	13-5 to 13-19
Pelvic ring pathology	
• AP compression injury, including open-book pelvis	13-6, 13-20 to 13-30
• Vertical shear injury	13-7 to 13-10, 13-36 to 13-41
• Lateral pelvic compression injury	13-12, 13-31 to 13-35
• Sprung pelvis	13-38
• Pubic ramus fractures	13-8, 13-9, 13-12, 13-13, 13-31, 13-33, 13-39, 13-40, 13-44, 13-51, 13-55 to 13-57
• Sacral fracture	13-10, 13-11, 13-40, 13-41, 13-52 to 13-54
• Iliac wing fracture	13-14, 13-28, 13-31, 13-32, 13-43
• Penetrating pelvic injury	13-42
• Soft-tissue injuries and pelvic hematoma	13-30
Injuries of the hip	
• Acetabular fracture	13-15, 13-28, 13-29, 13-43 to 13-46, 13-48 to 13-50, 13-62, 13-64, 13-65
• Hip dislocation, posterior	13-4, 13-16, 13-62 to 13-65
• Hip dislocation, anterior	13-17, 13-34, 13-66, 13-67
• Hip dislocation, prosthetic	13-68
• Femoral neck fracture	13-18, 13-69, 13-70
• Intertrochanteric femoral neck fracture	13-19, 13-71
• Femoral head fracture	13-72, 13-73
• Femoral subcapital fracture	13-74
Low-mechanism pelvic injuries	
• Anterior superior iliac spine avulsion	13-58
• Anterior inferior iliac spine avulsion	13-59
• Ischial tuberosity avulsion	13-60, 13-61
Nontraumatic hip pathology	
• Avascular necrosis	13-75, 13-76
• Slipped capital femoral epiphysis	13-77 to 13-79

ring disruption. A combination of one fracture and one diastatic joint may also occur. Because the bony pelvis is a ring, a single disruption usually does not occur; rather, a disruption in one location results in fracture or diastasis at a second point in the ring. When one disruption in the pelvis ring is seen, a second should be suspected and sought. Sometimes the second disruption is at the pubic symphysis or sacroiliac joint and may be unapparent on x-ray because these joints can open and close with repositioning of the patient once the joint has been destabilized.

Anterior-posterior compression injuries

AP compression of the pelvic ring typically separates the pubic symphysis anteriorly while opening the sacroiliac joint posteriorly (Figures 13-20 to 13-30; see also Figure 13-6). This fracture pattern is often called an open-book pelvic fracture and can be a life-threatening injury. It results from substantial force and can shear pelvic veins and arteries. Significant bleeding into the pelvis often occurs with this injury. Because this injury increases the volume of the potential space within the pelvis, tamponade of bleeding does not occur, and the patient's entire

TABLE 13-2. Young-Burgess Classification of Pelvic Fractures

Classification (Based on Injury Mechanism, Hemipelvis Displacement, and Stability)		Characteristics	Stability
AP compression with external rotation of hemipelvis	Type I	Pubic diastasis <2.5 cm	Stable
	Type II	Pubic diastasis >2.5 cm and anterior sacroiliac joint disruption	Rotationally unstable, vertically stable
	Type III	Type II plus posterior sacroiliac joint disruption	Rotationally and vertically unstable
Lateral compression with internal rotation of hemipelvis	Type I	Ipsilateral sacral buckle fractures or ipsilateral horizontal pubic rami fractures (or disruption of symphysis pubis with overlapping pubic bones)	Stable
	Type II	Type I plus ipsilateral iliac wing fracture or posterior sacroiliac joint disruption	Rotationally unstable, vertically stable
Vertical shear with cranial–caudal displacement of hemipelvis		Vertical pubic rami fractures and sacroiliac joint disruption with or without adjacent fractures	Rotationally and vertically unstable

blood volume can be accommodated within the pelvis. When this injury is recognized on x-ray or on CT scan, the pelvis should be closed using some type of external compression device. Urethral injuries are also associated with this type of pelvic injury. Evaluation of urethral injury is discussed in detail in the chapter on the genitourinary system (Chapter 12).

Lateral compression injuries
Lateral compression of the pelvis may result in a posterior injury in which the sacroiliac joint on the affected side folds inward or the iliac wing or sacrum fractures (Figures 13-31 to 13-35; see also schematic Figure 13-12). Often, the posterior injury is matched anteriorly by fractures of the superior and inferior pubic rami or pubic symphysis (see Figures 13-31 and 13-33). Again, injury to the urethra may occur, and *vaginal penetrating injuries may be sustained in female patients—consider these injuries when pubic rami fractures are present. A vaginal exam should be performed to evaluate for laceration.* Bladder injuries are also possible with this fracture pattern. Serious pelvic bleeding is somewhat less common with this injury pattern because pelvic blood vessels are folded rather than stretched and sheared. The volume of the pelvis may be decreased, contributing to tamponade effect that may limit bleeding. Nonetheless, this is an extremely high-energy injury, frequently associated with other injuries to the head, chest, abdomen, spine, and extremities. Vascular injury should be considered as a possible complication.

Vertical shear injuries
Vertical shear injuries are also a common injury pattern (Figures 13-36 to 13-41; see also schematic Figures 13-7 to 13-10). These may occur with falls from great height or deceleration injuries with a single outstretched leg, which distributes force asymmetrically to the pelvis. The pelvic ring is disrupted at a posterior and an anterior location, commonly one sacroiliac joint posteriorly and the pubic symphysis anteriorly. Alternatively, the sacrum or the pubic rami may fracture vertically. Spinal and lower extremity injuries are common with pelvic vertical shear injuries.

While blunt mechanisms are the most frequent cause of serious pelvic trauma, penetrating trauma can also result in severe pelvic injury; Figure 13-42 shows an open pediatric pelvic injury resulting from a riding lawn mower.

Fractures That Do Not Disrupt the Major Pelvic Ring

Fractures that may not affect the stability of the pelvic ring include sacral transverse fractures (Figures 13-52 to 13-54; see schematic Figure 13-11), some lateral iliac wing fractures (see schematic Figure 13-14), some acetabular fractures (see schematic Figure 13-15), isolated inferior and superior pubic ramus fractures (Figures 13-55 to 13-57; see also schematic Figure 13-13), and avulsion fractures.

Acetabular fractures
Acetabular fractures can occur in isolation or in combination with other pelvic fractures (Figures 13-43 to 13-51; see also schematic Figure 13-15). Fractures of the acetabulum can be difficult to recognize on plain x-ray but are readily evident with CT. Clues to the diagnosis are disruptions of the iliopubic line, which forms the medial border of the anterior column of the acetabulum; disruption of the ilioischial line, which forms the medial border of the posterior column of the acetabulum; and disruptions of the articular surface of the acetabulum, called the lunate surface.

TABLE 13-3. Tile Classification of Pelvic Fractures

Classification			Characteristics	Hemipelvis Displacement	Stability
Type A—posterior arch intact	A1—pelvic ring fracture (avulsion)	A1.1	Anterior iliac spine avulsion	None	Stable
		A1.2	Iliac crest avulsion		
		A1.3	Ischial tuberosity avulsion		
	A2—pelvic ring fracture (direct blow)	A2.1	Iliac wing fracture		
		A2.2	Unilateral pubic ramus fracture		
		A2.3	Bilateral pubic rami fracture		
	A3—transverse sacral fracture	A3.1	Sacrococcygeal dislocation		
		A3.2	Nondisplaced sacral fracture		
		A3.3	Displaced sacral fracture		
Type B—incomplete posterior arch disruption	B1—AP compression	B1.1	Pubic diastasis and anterior sacroiliac joint disruption	External rotation	Rotationally unstable, vertically stable
		B1.2	Pubic diastasis and sacral fracture		
	B2—lateral compression	B2.1	Anterior sacral buckle fracture	Internal rotation	
		B2.2	Partial sacroiliac joint fracture or subluxation		
		B2.3	Incomplete posterior iliac fracture		
	B3.1—AP compression	B3.1	Bilateral pubic diastasis and bilateral posterior sacroiliac joint disruption	External rotation	
	B3.2—AP and lateral compression	B3.2	Ipsilateral B2 injury and contralateral B1 injury	Ipsilateral internal rotation and contralateral external rotation	
	B3.3—bilateral lateral compression	B3.3	Bilateral B2 injury	Bilateral internal rotation	
Type C—complete posterior arch disruption	C1—vertical shear	C1.1	Displaced iliac fracture	Vertical	Rotationally and vertically unstable
		C1.2	Sacroiliac joint dislocation or fracture and dislocation		
		C1.3	Displaced sacral fracture		
	C2—vertical shear and AP or lateral compression	C2	Ipsilateral C1 injury and contralateral B1 or B2 injury	Ipsilateral vertical (cranial) and contralateral internal or external rotation	
	C3—bilateral vertical shear	C3	Bilateral C1 injury	Bilateral vertical (cranial)	

Avulsion fractures

Avulsion fractures of the pelvis, common in pediatric and adolescent patients, occur at points of muscle attachment. Avulsion fractures can transpire with surprisingly modest mechanisms of injury, such as stretching, lifting, and sporting events with forceful contraction of a muscle without direct trauma. Consequently, they are not usually associated with other serious injuries but are important sources of continued pain and dysfunction if not recognized and treated. Examples include avulsion of the anterior superior iliac spine by contraction of the sartorius muscle (Figure 13-58), avulsion of the anterior inferior iliac spine by contraction of the rectus femoris (Figure 13-59), and avulsion of the ischial tuberosity by contraction of the hamstring muscles (Figures 13-60 and 13-61). Some pelvic injuries, such as fractures of the coccyx, require no imaging because their management is not influenced by radiographic findings.

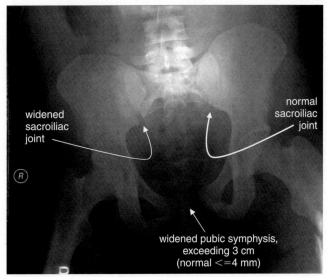

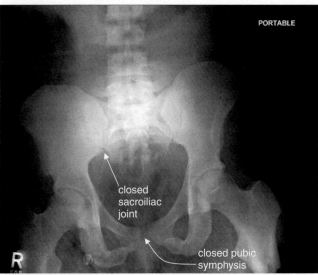

Figure 13-20. Open-book pelvis. This patient has substantial widening of the pubic symphysis without an evident fracture. Given the usual stability of the pelvic ring, there must be at least one additional point of motion to allow the pelvic ring to open to this degree. The most likely locations in the absence of fracture are one or both sacroiliac joints. Look carefully at the right sacroiliac joint, which appears wide compared with the left. Compare with Figure 13-21, showing the patient's pelvis minutes later—after application of an external binder—and with the computed tomography that follows in Figure 13-22. How much force is required to open the pelvis? This patient also suffered an aortic tear and diaphragm rupture. He was a Jehovah's Witness, refused blood transfusion, and expired.

Figure 13-21. Open-book pelvis. Same patient as in Figure 13-20 and 13-22. An external pelvic binder has been applied, and the right sacroiliac joint has flexed closed, in turn closing the pubic symphysis. Compare with Figure 13-20. This x-ray looks essentially normal—beware of unstable pelvis diastasis that can be missed on x-ray if external pelvic stabilization has been performed.

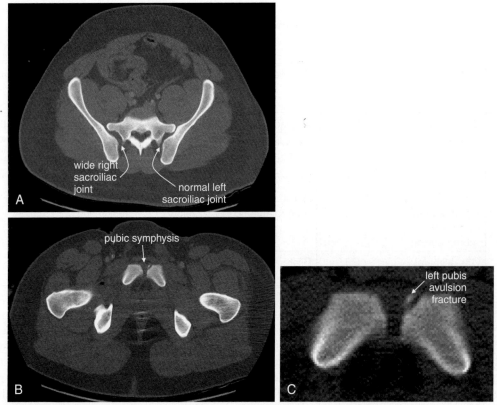

Figure 13-22. Open-book pelvis. Same patient as in Figures 13-20 and 13-21. What are the CT findings of an open-book pelvis injury? Remarkably, in this patient with an apparent open-book pelvis on initial x-ray, the external binder has closed the pelvis almost completely. The patient's pelvis injury is primary ligamentous, affecting the pubic symphysis and right sacroiliac joint, with no significant fractures. **A,** The right sacroiliac joint continues to look slightly widened. **B,** The pubic symphysis is normal in appearance, with the exception of a tiny avulsion fracture from the left pubis. **C,** Close-up from **B**.

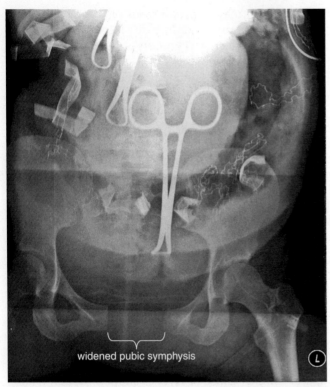

widened pubic symphysis

L

Figure 13-23. **Pelvic ring disruption.** This 20-year-old female was near term in her pregnancy when she was pinned in a motor vehicle collision. In the emergency department, her pelvis was found to be unstable and ultrasound showed fetal bradycardia. An emergency Cesarean section was performed in the trauma bay. Once the fetus was delivered, this x-ray was performed, showing a dramatically open pubic symphysis.

Hip Dislocations

Hip dislocations of native (nonprosthetic) hips usually occur only following extremely high-energy mechanisms of injury because this weight-bearing joint is one of the most stable mobile joints in the body. Acetabular fractures are common with hip dislocation. Commonly, the hip dislocates posteriorly when a seated motor vehicle passenger sustains AP force to the flexed and adducted hip (Figures 13-62 to 13-65; see also Figures 13-4 and 13-16). This injury is associated with posterior acetabular fractures. The femoral head usually appears cephalad to the acetabulum and may be laterally displaced. Anterior hip dislocations are less common but can occur if the hip is flexed and abducted at the time of an AP force (Figures 13-66 and 13-67; see Figure 13-17). The femoral head appears medially and is often inferiorly displaced relative to the acetabulum. Dislocations of prosthetic hips can occur with trivial force, such as flexion of the hip beyond 90 degrees. The acetabular component of the prosthetic hip usually remains in appropriate position while the femoral component dislocates. Posterior dislocation is most common, and the prosthetic femoral head appears cephalad and medial to the acetabulum (Figure 13-68).

Hip Fractures

Fractures of the proximal femur, often called hip fractures, commonly occur with low-energy mechanisms such as falls from a standing position in osteoporotic

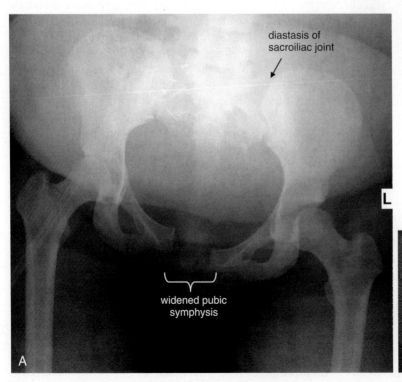

diastasis of sacroiliac joint

widened pubic symphysis

A

L

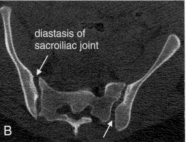

diastasis of sacroiliac joint

B

Figure 13-24. **Open-book pelvis. A,** Another x-ray from the same patient as in Figure 13-23 shows persistent dramatic diastasis of the pubic symphysis despite an external stabilizer. The sacroiliac joints are diastatic (compare with CT in **B**). Remarkably, no other fractures were present. The patient had surgical fixation performed (Figure 13-25).

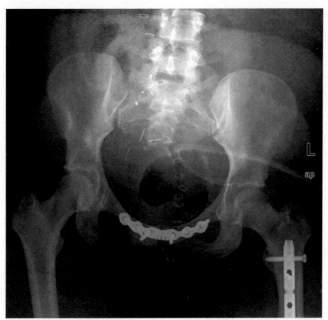

Figure 13-25. Open-book pelvis after fixation. Same patient as in Figures 13-23 and 13-24 after stabilization of the pubic symphysis.

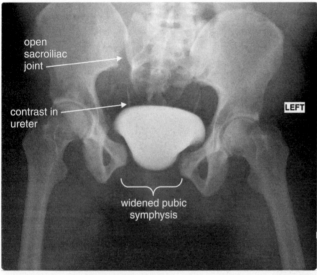

Figure 13-26. Pelvic ring disruption. This patient has an open pubic symphysis and complete disruption of the right sacroiliac joint. The left sacroiliac joint also appears wide. Contrast material is seen in the bladder and both ureters from computed tomography performed at an outside hospital before transfer to the trauma center. Pelvic stabilization with an external binder could have been helpful in this patient to contain the pelvic volume and limit bleeding.

patients age 65 years and older. Consequently, they are not highly associated with other serious pelvic soft-tissue injuries, such as vascular injuries, although dangerous injuries including cervical spine fractures and traumatic intracranial injury can occur. Common sites of fracture are the femoral neck and intertrochanteric region (Figures 13-69 to 13-71; see also Figures 13-18 and 13-19). Fractures through the femoral head (Figures 13-72 and 13-73) and at the juncture between the femoral head and the femoral neck (subcapital fractures, as in

Figure 13-74) may also occur. All of these injuries can be subtle on x-ray when nondisplaced because osteoporotic bone makes recognition of the cortical and trabecular defects more difficult. A detailed discussion of the evidence for MRI and CT in the evaluation of these injuries is included in the chapter on musculoskeletal MRI (Chapter 15).

Nontraumatic hip abnormalities

Nontraumatic abnormalities of the hip are an important cause of hip pain or limping in pediatric patients. Avascular necrosis (AVN) of the femoral head (Figures 13-75 and 13-76) may present with hip pain or limp. AVN may occur from previous trauma with disruption of the blood supply to the hip, from chronic steroid use, from sickle cell anemia with microvascular infarction, or as an idiopathic form, Legg-Calvé-Perthes disease. The latter occurs at a rate of 1 in 1200 children under the age of 15 years in the United States, most commonly in patients ages 3 to 12 years. It is a cause of limp in toddlers, and a frequent pitfall is x-ray of the distal leg without consideration of the hip. X-ray findings of AVN of any cause include a moth-eaten, irregular, and flattened femoral head and narrowed joint space. Another cause of AVN is slipped capital femoral epiphysis (SCFE) (Figures 13-77 to 13-79), a rare condition seen in around 1 in 10,000 U.S. children. Obesity and male gender are risk factors, with males developing the condition at 2.4 times the female rate. The common age range at diagnosis is 10 to 16 years. Bilateral involvement is common, occurring in up to 20% initially and 40% with passage of time, so both hips should be imaged when the diagnosis is suspected. SCFE may present with hip pain or with referred pain to the knee. Frog-legged x-ray views can assist in detection. Internal fixation is usually performed in an attempt to prevent further displacement and AVN. The x-ray findings of SCFE include a widened physis (growth plate) and a femoral epiphysis medially displaced relative to the femoral neck. A line drawn along the lateral aspect of the femoral neck should intersect the normal femoral capital epiphysis but will not intersect a SCFE, because the epiphysis is displaced medially. This appearance is sometimes described as resembling an ice cream cone with the scoop of ice cream (femoral epiphysis) slipping off of the cone (femoral neck). This injury is a Salter-Harris I fracture. The Salter-Harris classification system is described in detail in the chapter on the extremities (Chapter 14).

Other nontraumatic hip abnormalities include osteoarthritis, rheumatoid arthritis, and septic arthritis; gout; and toxic synovitis. Ultrasound is the preferred diagnostic imaging modality when joint infection is suspected because it can confirm joint effusion and guide joint aspiration, which is diagnostic. Less common imaging studies of the hip include nuclear medicine studies and MRI. These are discussed in more detail in the chapter on musculoskeletal MRI (Chapter 15).

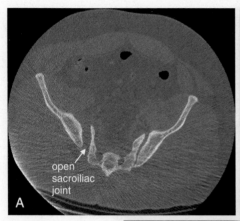

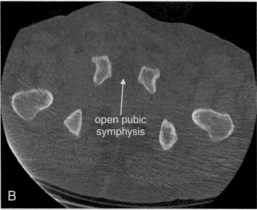

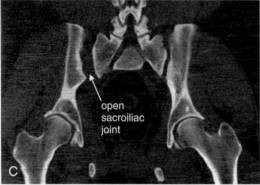

Figure 13-27. Open-book pelvis. CT images, bone windows. This patient has complete separation of the right sacroiliac joint and marked diastasis of the pubic symphysis. Remarkably, no other pelvic fractures are present. A large hematoma is present anterior to the pubic symphysis. Was this pelvis stable on examination? Naturally, it should not have been, but 10 cm of soft tissue separates the skin surface from the iliac crest. The examination may have been difficult to interpret. **A, B,** Axial views. **C,** Coronal view.

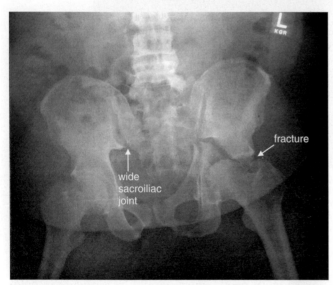

Figure 13-28. **Pelvic ring disruption with sacroiliac joint diastasis and iliac wing fracture.** Both sacroiliac joints are widened, the right more so than the left. The left iliac bone has fractured transversely with extension into the left acetabulum. This likely resulted from significant anterior–posterior compression of the pelvis. Compare with the CT in Figure 13-29.

INTERPRETATION OF PELVIC COMPUTED TOMOGRAPHY

Pelvic CT for evaluation of bony injuries should be evaluated using a bone window setting. The evaluation of soft-tissue injuries to pelvic organs requires the use of soft-tissue windows and is discussed in more detail in the chapters on genitourinary imaging (Chapter 12) and abdominal trauma (Chapter 10). Axial images are routinely available and should be evaluated first. The pelvis has a complex structure, and the rings seen on plain x-ray are not fully oriented in the axial plane. It may take some time for you to feel comfortable recognizing injuries by tracking an obliquely oriented portion of the pelvic ring through several adjacent CT slices. Nonetheless, axial images are excellent for detecting the range of pelvic injuries described earlier on x-ray. Review of sagittal and coronal planar images can clarify some injury patterns. The key to diagnosis of fractures on CT is identification of a cortical discontinuity, which may be the only evidence of a nondisplaced fracture. Displaced fractures are readily apparent on CT. The pubic symphysis and sacroiliac joints can be measured using digital PACS tools. In the figures throughout this chapter, plain x-ray and multiplanar CT images depicting the same pelvic injuries are shown, allowing you to develop your skills in recognition of important fractures and dislocations. CT images should be reviewed for the same abnormalities as described earlier for x-ray. The figures in this chapter contain detailed guidance on CT interpretation, not repeated here. Pelvic fractures are often associated with important vascular injuries, seen best on soft-tissue windows. These are described in detail in the chapter on interventional radiologic procedures in emergency medicine (Chapter 16). Bladder and urethral injuries may accompany pelvic fractures. These are seen best on

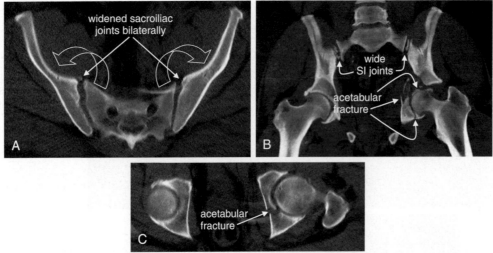

Figure 13-29. Widened sacroiliac joints and iliac wing fracture involving left acetabulum. CT, bone windows. Again, take a moment to appreciate the sacroiliac joint widening on CT, and look again at the x-ray from the same patient in Figure 13-28. The iliac wing fracture is impressive, but sacroiliac joint diastasis is also a significant contributor to the instability of this pelvis, which has open-book characteristics, although the pubic symphysis appears narrow. **A,** Axial CT reconstruction showing bilateral sacroiliac joint diastasis. Imagine the two iliac wings as the covers of a book being opened. Anterior–posterior compression of the pelvis can have this effect. **B,** Coronal CT reconstruction. The wide sacroiliac joints are still visible. This image suggests a competing or additional mechanism of injury: lateral compression applied to the left pelvis. The femoral head has been driven like a hammer into the acetabulum, fracturing the medial wall and pushing it medially into the pelvis. **C** shows this in axial section.

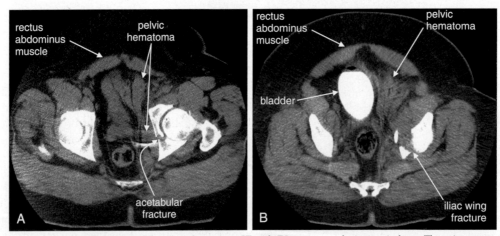

Figure 13-30. Soft-tissue injuries associated with pelvic fractures. CT with IV contrast, soft-tissue windows. These images are in fact taken from the same scan as in Figure 13-29, but displayed using a different window setting. CT offers the ability to assess both bony and soft-tissue injuries. **A,** Soft-tissue injuries of the bladder and pelvic blood vessels are discussed in more detail in the genitourinary and abdominal trauma sections. However, recognize that it is the hemorrhage associated with major pelvic fractures that can make them an immediate life threat. The large pelvic sidewall hematoma is associated with the iliac fracture shown in Figure 13-29. On soft-tissue windows, this hematoma is the same intermediate gray as the rectus abdominus muscles. **B,** The hematoma displaces the bladder (filled with contrast).

soft-tissue CT windows and are described in more detail in the chapter on genitourinary imaging (Chapter 12).

How Reliable Is a Physical Examination for Detecting Pelvic Injury?

When does a blunt trauma patient require imaging of the pelvis? Can some patients avoid pelvic imaging altogether? Advanced Trauma Life Support guidelines have historically called for pelvis x-ray in all blunt trauma patients,[4] but selective imaging based on patient history and examination could improve the yield, saving time and money and reducing radiation exposure. Clinical predictors of pelvic injury would be particularly helpful in pregnant women, in whom pelvic irradiation is especially undesirable. Numerous studies suggest that in awake, alert patients, a normal examination of the pelvis combined with a normal neurologic examination eliminates the need for pelvic x-ray. We review several of these studies here.

In 2004, Sauerland et al.[5] conducted a meta-analysis of the reliability of the clinical examination in detection of pelvic fractures in blunt trauma patients. The authors identified 12 studies with 5454 patients and found a pooled sensitivity of 90%, with a 95% confidence interval (CI) of 85% to 93%, and a specificity of 90% (95% CI = 84%-94%). They found that clinically relevant injuries were extremely rare in patients with a normal Glasgow Coma Score (GCS) and a normal examination of the pelvis and concluded that in stable and alert trauma patients, pelvic x-ray is unnecessary when examination is normal. Many individual studies included in this meta-analysis are examined later because the details of their methods are important to us in deciding their applicability to our patients.

In 2008, Duane et al.[6] prospectively compared clinical examination and x-ray against a gold standard of CT scan for the diagnosis of pelvic fracture. They evaluated 1388 patients undergoing pelvic x-ray and CT scan for hip pain, internal rotation of the leg, or tenderness over the sacrum, hip, or diffuse pelvis. The authors reported the sensitivity of x-ray as 79% (133 of 168 fractures). All injuries detected by x-ray were also detected by physical examination, and examination was 96.4% sensitive compared with CT (detecting 162 of 168 patients with fractures). The authors recommended that x-ray be eliminated as a routine screening tool in patients with GCS greater than 13. This study follows an earlier publication by the same group in 2002,[6a] which prospectively evaluated

520 patients for whom a detailed physical examination questionnaire had been completed. In that study, 45 patients were found to have fractures by x-ray, and the gold standard in patients not undergoing x-ray was absence of clinical symptoms until hospital discharge. The investigators considered the presence of any of the questionnaire history or examination findings a "positive" history and physical. The sensitivity of a positive history and physical was 100%, and the specificity was 37.2%. The absence of any pelvic complaints or examination findings had a negative predictive value of 100% for pelvic fracture, and would have safely eliminated the need for pelvis x-ray in two-thirds of patients.

Gross and Niedens[7] prospectively validated a clinical decision rule for imaging the pelvis following blunt trauma. Fractures were classified as significant or insignificant, following the previously published Tile classification,[3] which focuses on pelvic stability. All blunt trauma patients undergoing pelvic x-ray were enrolled and rated upon five criteria, similar to those of the

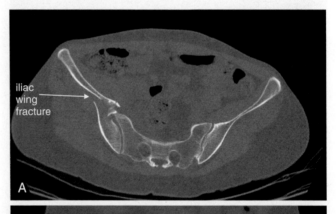

A

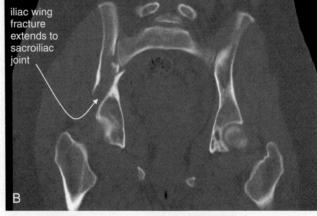

B

Figure 13-32. Iliac wing and pubic rami fractures. Same patient as in Figure 13-31. This CT viewed with bone windows shows a fairly dramatic right iliac wing fracture. The sacroiliac joint itself appears intact on the axial view **(A)**, but in the coronal reconstruction **(B)** the fracture appears to extend to the right sacroiliac joint. How could this be so plain on CT yet so subtle on x-ray? Although the fracture is complete, the fragments are not fully distracted from one another, and on a frontal projection they overlap and are nearly invisible. Additional x-ray views such as inlet and outlet views could throw these into relief, but in the trauma patient, CT is the preferred modality because it can simultaneously evaluate internal soft-tissue injuries.

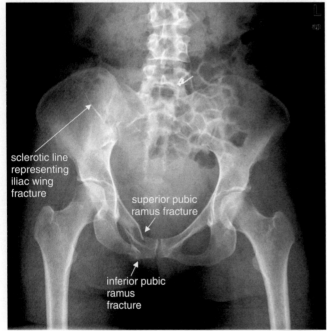

Figure 13-31. Iliac wing fracture with superior and inferior pubic rami fractures. This young female was involved in a motor vehicle collision. As is frequently the case, an injury to one portion of the pelvis is accompanied by a second injury in this patient. Deformation in one part of the pelvic ring builds tension elsewhere, which is relieved by fracture or joint diastasis. Two separate types of injuries are visible here, one obvious and the second more subtle. First, the right superior and inferior pubic rami are fractured and deformed. Compare with the normal left side. Second, a fine sclerotic line crosses the right iliac wing—a fracture line. An isolated fracture of a single iliac wing is called a Duverney fracture. These fractures do not disrupt the pelvic ring, though hemorrhage may occur from injury to vessels hugging the iliac bone, particularly the internal iliac arteries. Compare with the CT in Figure 13-32.

National Emergency X-radiography Utilization Study (NEXUS) cervical spine criteria (discussed in Chapter 3): altered level of consciousness, complaint of pelvic pain, pelvic tenderness on examination, distracting injury, or clinical intoxication. The Gross and Niedens study enrolled 973 patients, of whom 62 (6.4%) had pelvic

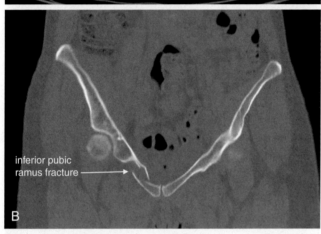

Figure 13-33. Pubic ramus fractures. Same patient as in Figure 13-31 and 13-32. These CT images show the pubic ramus fractures in more detail. **A,** Axial view. **B,** Coronal reconstruction. This injury alone would not significantly affect the stability of the pelvic ring.

fractures. The sensitivity of the five criteria was 96.8% for any pelvic fracture (95% CI = 92.4%-100%). If only clinically significant fractures were included, the sensitivity was 100% (95% CI = 95.2%-100%). Application of the five criteria would have eliminated 44% of x-rays. A larger prospective sample is required for external validation and to narrow confidence intervals.[7]

An earlier study by Gonzalez et al.[8] reached similar conclusions. In this prospective study including 2176 patients (14 years or older) with a GCS of 14 or 15, patients were evaluated for pelvic pain, neurologic complaints or deficits, and pelvic examination abnormalities, including abrasions or contusions over bony prominences; ecchymosis about the pubis, perineum, or scrotum; or blood at the urethral meatus. In addition, pelvic examination included medial and posterior compression of the iliac wings, compression of the pubic symphysis, inspection for limb length discrepancies, hip flexion, internal and external hip rotation, and rectal examination for gross blood. The gold standard for diagnosis was pelvic fracture based on final readings of all radiologic studies by board-certified attending radiologists. Physical examination detected 90 of 97 pelvic fractures (sensitivity = 93%, 95% CI = 85%-97%). X-ray detected 84 of 97 pelvic fractures (sensitivity = 87%, 95% CI = 78%-92%). Application of the clinical criteria would have reduced x-ray utilization by 88%. In the subgroup of 185 patients with a GCS of 14, clinical examination missed two of nine pelvic fractures (22%). Among the 1991 patients with a GCS of 15, only 5 of 88 patients with fracture were missed by examination (sensitivity 94%). The authors noted that none of the 7 injuries missed by physical examination required surgical intervention, and only 2 were treated with non-weight-bearing status. This study also included 463 patients with ethanol levels greater than 100 mg/dL.

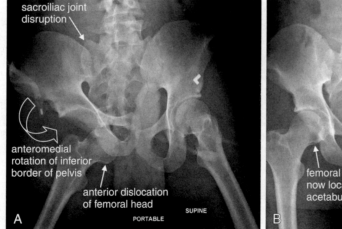
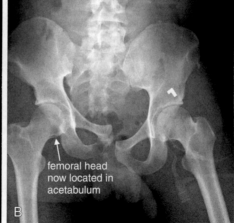

Figure 13-34. Pelvic ring disruption with sacroiliac and symphysis pubis disruption, as well as anterior hip dislocation. This patient has complete separation of the right sacroiliac joint, as well as disruption of the symphysis pubis. **A,** The right hip is dislocated anteriorly. The right hemipelvis has rotated in an anterior, as well as a medial, direction. **B,** The right hip has been reduced, and the anterior rotation of the hemipelvis is somewhat reduced. Compare with the CT in Figure 13-35.

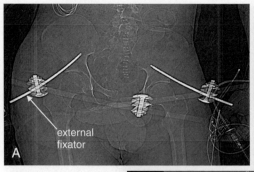

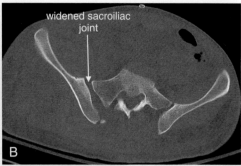

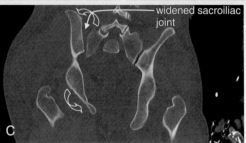

Figure 13-35. **Unstable pelvis with complete diastasis of right sacroiliac and symphysis pubis joints. A,** The CT scout image shows an external fixator has been placed, with fixators placed into the ischium. **B,** An axial image shows widening of the right sacroiliac joint. **C,** A coronal image shows a wide right sacroiliac joint with medial angulation of the lower right hemipelvis. The right pelvis has rotated counterclockwise on the fulcrum of the lower right sacroiliac joint *(open curved arrows).* **B** and **C,** Bone windows.

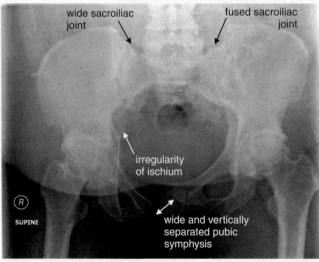

Figure 13-36. **Vertical shear injury.** This patient presented with chronic pain after a pelvic fracture 20 years earlier. Her x-ray shows a markedly abnormal pelvis, with a horizontally widened and vertically distracted pubic symphysis. The left sacroiliac joint is obscured, and the left iliac wing appears to be riding somewhat high in relationship to the sacrum. Her original injury was probably a vertical shear injury along the left sacroiliac joint, which fused long ago in this abnormal position. The right sacroiliac joint appears widened. The right ischium and pubic bone are irregular along their medial border, likely indicating an old fracture. Compare with the CT in Figure 13-37.

Clinical examination identified 19 of 20 patients with pelvic fractures (95% sensitivity). The undiagnosed injury was an acetabular fracture. The authors concluded that routine pelvic x-ray in awake and alert blunt trauma patients is unnecessary and not cost-effective, and that ethanol intoxication does not substantially alter the sensitivity of examination.

These results are concordant with numerous earlier studies. Yugueros et al.[9] published a retrospective study of 608 Colombian blunt trauma patients. They asserted that physical examination detected 57 of 59 patients (96.6%) with pelvic fractures and that the 2 patients with missed injuries were stable and required no treatment. They advocated that x-ray is not required in hemodynamically stable adult patients with normal pelvis examination, no spinal injury, and a GCS greater than 10.

Koury et al.[10] reported a prospective study of 125 alert and oriented blunt trauma patients and concluded that a normal physical examination of the pelvis eliminated the need for x-ray, with no injuries detected on x-ray in this group.

Salvino et al.[11] reported on 810 prospectively evaluated blunt trauma patients with a GCS of 13 or greater. They found that only 3 of 743 patients (0.4%) with neither pain nor abnormal pelvis physical examination findings had fractures. Among 39 patients with fractures, pelvis pain by history or abnormal pelvis examination findings were 92% sensitive for fracture.

Civil et al.[12] prospectively evaluated 265 blunt trauma patients for pelvic fracture. Patients were classified as unconscious; impaired; awake, alert and symptomatic; or awake, alert, oriented, and asymptomatic for pelvic fracture. No fractures were identified in 110 patients in the category of awake, alert, oriented, and asymptomatic.

Gillott et al.[13] argued for routine pelvic x-ray during the early resuscitation of blunt trauma patients, noting a 16.7% incidence of pelvic injury among 669 patients and a higher requirement for blood transfusion, higher injury severity scores, and a higher incidence of chest and abdominal injuries in patients with pelvic injury on

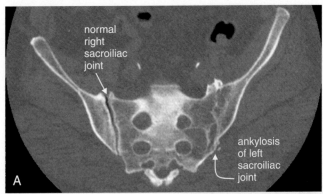

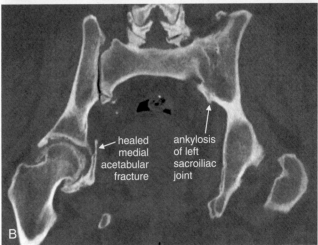

Figure 13-37. Old sacroiliac joint injury. CT, bone windows. Same patient as in Figure 13-36. **A,** An axial image shows a normal right sacroiliac joint but an abnormal left sacroiliac joint with ankylosis. **B,** The coronal view also shows this sacroiliac joint abnormality. The right acetabulum does have an old healed fracture, as suggested on the x-ray in Figure 13-36.

x-ray. However, the authors did not investigate the predictive value of history and physical examination.

In summary, medical literature supports the use of clinical assessment to determine the need for pelvic x-ray in adult blunt trauma patients. X-ray appears unnecessary in patients with normal mental status and normal pelvis physical examination findings.

How Common Are Pelvis Injuries in Children? How Serious Are These Injuries in Pediatric Patients? Could a Clinical Decision Rule Reduce Unnecessary Imaging in This Group?

Pelvis fractures are rarer in children than in adults, occurring in only 2.4% to 7.5% of serious trauma,[14-15] with lower associated mortality in children.[14] Naturally, when an injury or disease process is rare, many normal x-rays would need to be obtained to identify a single injury. As a consequence, the published negative predictive value of the pediatric physical examination is reported to be high, but the more important clinical

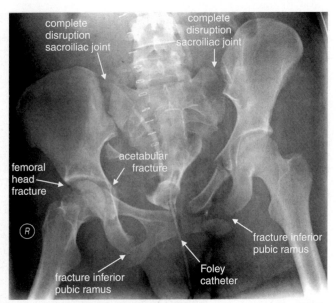

Figure 13-38. Pelvic ring disruption. This patient has remarkable disarticulation of the pelvic ring—sometimes called a "sprung pelvis." The bilateral sacroiliac joints have separated completely, leaving the sacrum and lumbar spine free of the iliac wings. The bilateral inferior pubic rami have displaced fractures. The right femoral head is fractured, associated with a fracture of the medial wall and anterior column of the right acetabulum. The left acetabulum also has a fracture through its anterior column at the junction with the superior pubic ramus. Is any portion of the pelvis intact? The pubic symphysis is not diastatic because tension in the pelvic ring was dissipated through other fractures and disruption of the sacroiliac joints. This x-ray was taken after other emergency interventions. The patient has a Foley catheter in place, and some contrast is seen in the bladder and right ureter. Skin staples are also visible. Packing material is visible overlying the lower pelvis.

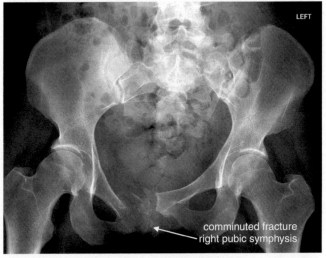

Figure 13-39. Pubic symphysis fracture with pelvic ring disruption. This 30-year-old female experienced a vertical shear and lateral compression injury in a horse-riding accident. She has a comminuted fracture of the right medial pubic bone. Be wary of fractures in this region. This was an open fracture, with lacerations extending into the patient's vagina. Fractures near the pubic symphysis should raise consideration of vaginal and urethral injuries. The orientation of the right pelvis does not match that of the left; the right pubic bone points obliquely down, compared with the nearly horizontal position of the left pubic bone. Another pelvic injury must exist that has not yet been identified. Is it diastasis of one or both sacroiliac joints? Bowel gas obscures these regions and the sacrum. Computed tomography (Figure 13-40) reveals the answer.

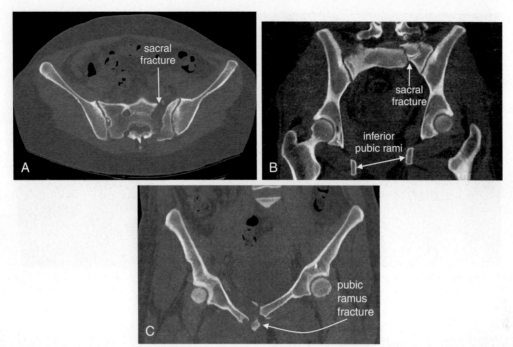

Figure 13-40. Sacral fracture with pubic rami fractures. Same patient as in Figure 13-39. CT viewed on bone windows reveals the explanation for the odd orientation of the right pelvis relative to the left on the previous x-ray. A complete vertical fracture through the left sacrum is present. The sacroiliac joints are intact. **A,** Axial view. This fracture is seen running nearly in a perfect anterior–posterior direction, separating the left ilium and a piece of the sacrum from the bulk of the sacrum and right pelvis. **B,** Coronal reconstruction. The left pelvis and attached sacral fragment are seen to be displaced vertically compared with the right pelvis—accounting for the x-ray appearance. Note the relative positions of the right and left femoral heads and inferior pubic rami. The entire left pelvis and femur have moved cephalad relative to the right. The left femoral neck is not visible; this is not a fracture but simply the result of the plane of this slice not intersecting the femoral neck. **C,** Coronal view. The pubic rami fractures are again seen. This is a bucket-handle type injury pattern, with vertical shear through contralateral injury sites.

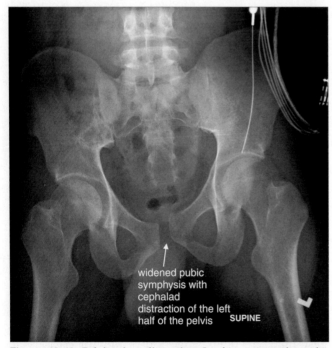

Figure 13-41. Pelvic ring disruption. In this patient, the pubic symphysis is widened, and the left pubic symphysis is positioned cephalad relative to the right. No other fractures or disruptions are seen on this x-ray, although you will recognize by now that an isolated disruption of the pelvic ring is extremely unlikely. If no other fractures are present, a discontinuity through the sacroiliac joint is likely. Not surprisingly, CT showed a similar left sacral fracture to the one explored in Figure 13-40.

question is the sensitivity of the examination. Numerous studies have assessed the value of clinical indications for pelvic x-ray in pediatric patients, although the strength of evidence is poorer than in adults because of the small numbers of patients enrolled, the wide age range of patients, and frequently retrospective methods.

Ramirez et al.[16] published a retrospective chart review using case-control design of 33 pediatric patients with pelvic fractures and 63 patients without fracture, all with GCS of 14 or 15. Blunt trauma patients 14 years and younger were included. The authors found that pelvic contusion or abrasion, hip or pelvic pain, abdominal pain and distention, back pain, hip held in rotation, and femur deformity or pain independently predicted pelvic fracture. They noted that the absence of all these findings has a negative predictive value of 87% and concluded that clinical findings could be useful in assessing the need for pelvic x-ray in awake and alert pediatric blunt trauma patients. The sensitivity of a simple four-part rule incorporating the absence of hip or pelvic pain, pelvic abrasions or contusions, abdominal pain or distention, and thigh pain or deformity was 73%, with a specificity of 92%. They estimated a reduction in x-ray use by 73% using this rule. Their study is quite limited by its retrospective methods because it

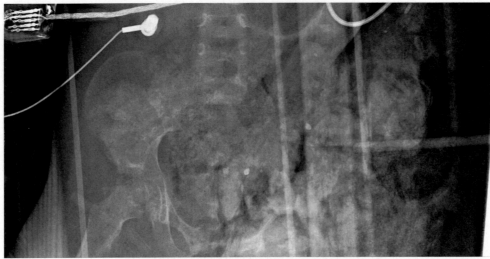

Figure 13-42. Pelvic ring disruption from penetrating lawn mower accident. This 3-year-old was run over by a riding lawn mower and has transsection of the pelvic. The left pelvis is absent. Dressing materials obscure much of the detail of the pelvis.

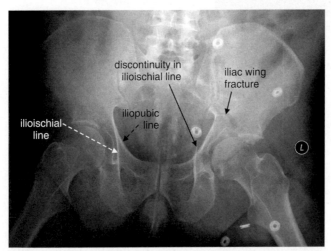

Figure 13-43. Acetabular fractures. Two lines help to define the normal acetabulum. The anterior column of the acetabulum is defined by the iliopubic line, a curve from the medial ilium to the pubic symphysis. The posterior column of the acetabulum is bounded by the ilioischial line, a nearly vertical line from the medial ilium to the ischial tuberosity. These two lines are labeled on the patient's right, where they are normal. On the patient's left, the ilioischial line is disrupted, indicating a fracture of the posterior column of the acetabulum. In addition, a transverse fracture of the left ilium is visible and runs toward the left sacroiliac joint. The left superior and inferior pubic rami are fractured. Compare with the computed tomography images in Figures 13-44 and 13-45.

is uncertain whether the absence of documentation of these physical examination findings truly represents their absence in a given patient.

Junkins et al.[17] reported a prospective study of 140 pediatric blunt trauma patients. An abnormal pelvic examination identified 11 of 16 patients with pelvic fractures (69% sensitivity). The specificity and negative predictive value were 95% and 91%, respectively. However, a lack of standardization of the pelvic examination

and broad age ranges make this study difficult to apply clinically. Moreover, the reported sensitivity is inadequate to exclude fracture; the reported negative predictive value is more a reflection of the rarity of pelvic fractures in the group (11%) than of the strength of the diagnostic test.

In a separate retrospective study of 174 patients between the ages of 3 months and 18 years (median age = 8 years), Junkins et al.[18] classified the pelvic examination as normal or abnormal. Using this binary classification, the sensitivity of examination was 92% (95% CI = 89%-95%), with a specificity of 79% (95% CI = 74%-84%). The positive predictive value was 84%, with a negative predictive value of 89%. The authors noted that examination appeared unreliable in patients with a GCS of less than 15 and those with distracting injury. However, retrospective methods such as those in the study may be unreliable. For example, it is possible that physical examination abnormalities were not written in the chart, although they may have been noted at the time of examination. In addition, it is unclear whether the reviewers abstracting the charts were blinded to the study question, an important practice to reduce bias in this type of study.[19]

Rees et al.[20] performed a retrospective chart review of 444 pediatric blunt trauma patients in Auckland, New Zealand. The 347 performed x-rays identified only one pelvic fracture, which appeared clinically obvious from documentation in the medical record. The authors suggest that screening pelvic x-rays are unnecessary in patients without findings of injury. Pelvic fractures were extremely rare in this group, concordant with other studies of pediatric blunt trauma. However, this study does not provide rigorous proof that physical examination is sensitive for detection of pelvic injury. A larger

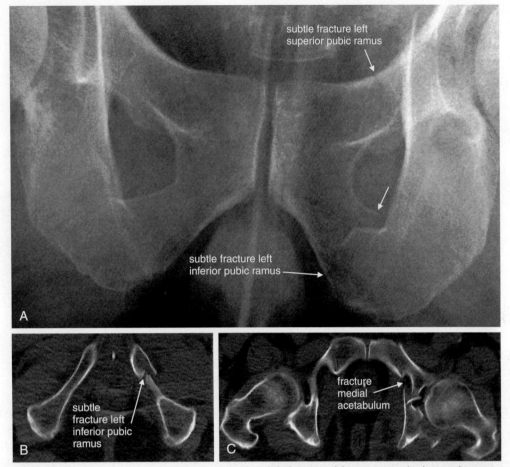

Figure 13-44. **Acetabular fractures.** Same patient as in Figure 13-43. **A,** Subtle fractures of the superior and inferior pubic rami appear to be present on the original x-ray, magnified. Are these real? Look at the axial computed tomography slices, seen on bone windows **(B, C).**

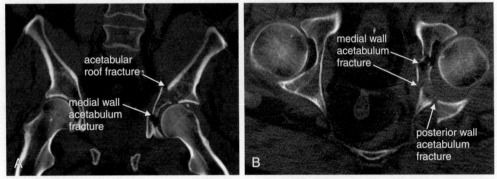

Figure 13-45. **Acetabular fracture.** Same patient as in Figures 13-43 and 13-44. These CT images explore the left acetabular fracture in more detail. The fracture fragments have been pushed medially by the impact of the femoral head into the acetabular cup. **A,** Coronal view, bone windows. **B,** Axial view, bone windows. The lunate surface (the articular surface of the acetabulum) has been disrupted by the fractures. The acetabular cup has increased in size because of radial spread of fragments in **B.** Acetabular fractures are frequently associated with femoral head dislocations.

number of injured patients are required for this purpose. Two research methods could enrich the number of injured patients. First, a case-control study could be conducted, ensuring that a target number of injured patients is included. However, this would require retrospective methodology, which would fall prey to the same limits of chart review mentioned earlier, including uncertainty about the meaning of undocumented physical examination findings. Second, a large prospective

multicenter trial could be conducted to assess physical examination sensitivity. This is unlikely to occur given the cost of such a study.

Soundappan et al.[21] retrospectively reviewed charts of 274 blunt trauma patients under the age of 16 years and argued for selective rather than routine use of pelvic x-ray. However, the limitations of the retrospective methods and the small number of patients with pelvic

Figure 13-46. Pelvic ring disruption with acetabular fracture. Multiple patterns of injury may combine in a given patient. **A,** This patient has both a widened pubic symphysis and a widened right sacroiliac joint. In addition, the right acetabulum is slightly irregular. A fracture also extends into the left acetabulum from the curve of the pelvis (**B,** Close-up). Compare with the CT in Figure 13-47.

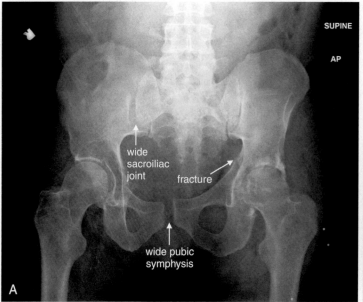

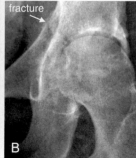

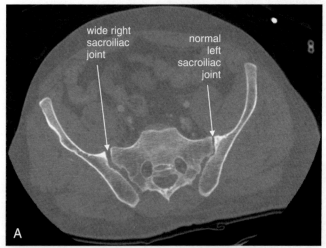

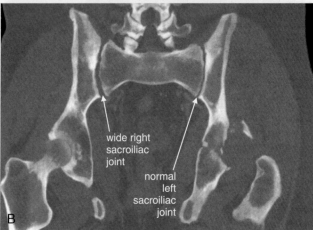

Figure 13-47. Widened sacroiliac joint. CT, bone windows. Same patient as in Figure 13-46. Sacroiliac joint injuries are extremely important to recognize. They allow opening of the pelvic "book," with the potential for serious hemorrhage as pelvic vessels are stretched. Look carefully at the CT images and refer back to the x-ray in Figure 13-46. **A,** Axial image showing a widened sacroiliac joint. **B,** Coronal reconstruction indicating the same finding.

injuries reduce the validity of this study in assessing physical examination.

Quick and Eastwood[22] reviewed the pediatric pelvic trauma literature and recommended against pelvic screening x-ray in hemodynamically stable pediatric patients with GCS greater than 10, no spinal cord injury, a normal pelvic examination, and no hematuria. Overall, it appears likely that clinical exam can reliably exclude pelvic fractures in older adolescents using criteria similar to those demonstrated for adults. However, younger children are less well-studied and routine pelvis x-ray may be warranted at this time.

Have Airbags and Seatbelts Changed the Rate of Pelvic Fracture? Is a Patient Less Likely to Have a Pelvic Injury If Airbags and Seatbelts Are in Use?

Data from 1988 to 2003 suggest that airbags and seatbelts in use at that time were not protective against pelvic fractures. However, newer side-impact airbags were not evaluated in these studies.[23-25]

When Pelvic X-ray Is Normal, Who Needs CT? In Other Words, How Sensitive Is X-ray for Fracture?

As described earlier, x-ray is likely not indicated in alert and awake patients with no pelvic pain and no abnormal physical examination findings. If x-rays are obtained in this group and are normal, no further imaging is generally required for evaluation of the bony pelvis. Other clinical concerns for abdominal injuries may warrant abdominal and pelvic CT; these are reviewed in detail in the chapter on imaging of abdominal trauma (Chapter 10).

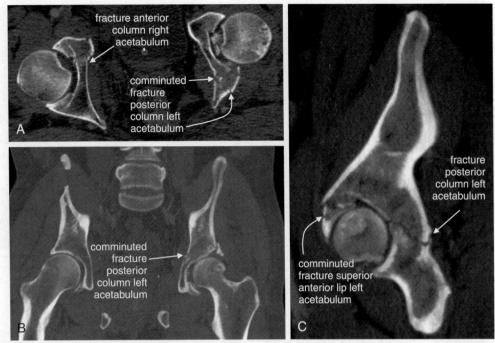

Figure 13-48. Acetabular fracture. CT, bone windows. Same patient as Figures 13-46 and 13-47. Spend a moment gaining a better understanding of acetabular fractures on x-ray by studying the CT images. **A,** Axial image showing bilateral acetabular fractures. The left is more obvious than the right. **B,** Coronal reconstruction showing the same injury. You begin to sense the three-dimensional destruction of the left acetabular cup. **C,** Sagittal reconstruction illustrating the same abnormality.

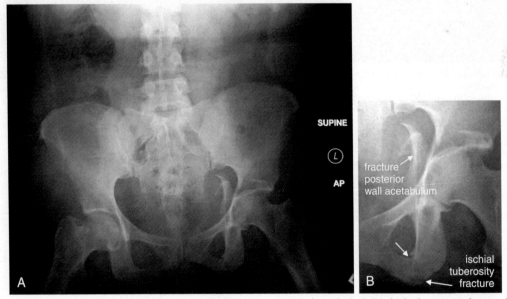

Figure 13-49. Pelvic ring disruption with acetabular fracture. A fracture extends through the left ischial tuberosity. A fracture fragment from the posterior wall of the left acetabulum has been displaced medially into the pelvis. Compare with the CT in Figure 13-50. **A,** AP pelvis x-ray. **B,** Close-up from **A.**

In the Patient With Pelvic Pain or Abnormal Pelvis Physical Examination Findings after Blunt Trauma, Does a Negative X-ray Rule Out Fracture?

Numerous studies have shown x-ray to be relatively insensitive for pelvis fractures, compared with a gold standard of CT scan. Gonzalez et al.[8] found x-ray to be only 87% sensitive for fracture, including both positive and "equivocal" x-rays. When only x-rays prospectively read as positive for fracture are considered "true positives," the sensitivity was only 79%. As described earlier, Duane et al.[6] also reported the sensitivity of x-ray to be only 79%, compared with CT.

Vo et al.[27] found that x-ray detected only 81% of fractures detected by CT scan and 87% of patients with

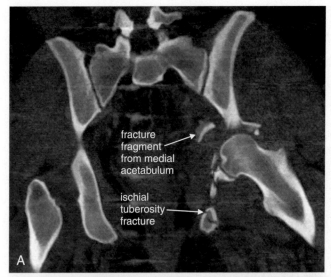

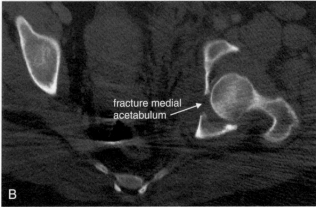

Figure 13-50. **Acetabular and inferior pubic ramus fractures.** CT, bone windows. Same patient as Figure 13-49. **A,** A coronal reconstruction shows both the ischial tuberosity fracture and a comminuted fracture of the medial wall of the left acetabulum. **B,** An axial view shows the same acetabulum fracture.

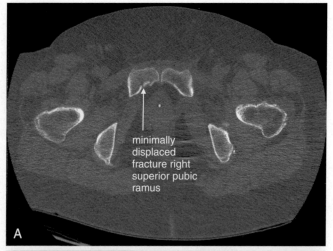

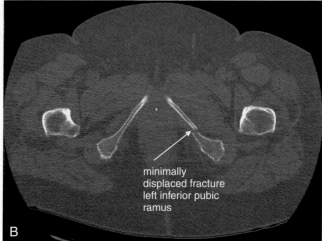

Figure 13-51. **Right superior and left inferior pubic rami fractures.** Axial CT images, bone windows. **A, B,** CT shows a right superior pubic ramus fracture and a left inferior pubic ramus fracture. Remember to look for a second pelvic fracture when one is detected. However, in this case, either of these fractures might have occurred in isolation. When fractures are quite minimally displaced, they may not introduce enough tension into the pelvic ring to result in a second fracture. Certainly, the right superior ramus fracture is minimally displaced. Typically, fractures such as this are not associated with significant additional injuries.

injuries detected by CT. This retrospective study, like many studies of diagnostic imaging, had no independent gold standard. CT was assumed to be correct when injuries are detected. Moreover, it is not certain that all pelvic injuries missed on x-ray but detected on CT scan had any clinical significance. Nonetheless, it does suggest that x-ray misses a substantial number of bony pelvic injuries.

These studies suggest that when a specific concern for pelvic fracture exists, based on patient complaints or physical examination findings, x-ray is insufficient to rule out fracture. Additional pelvic imaging should be performed. In the major trauma patient, CT is the routine test of choice because of its ability to detect other abdominal and pelvic soft-tissue and vascular injuries. The proper follow-up test for suspected pelvis or hip fracture following lower-energy injuries, such as falls from standing, is in debate. We consider some evidence for MRI in comparison to CT and nuclear medicine studies in the chapter on musculoskeletal MRI (Chapter 15).

If CT Scan Is Planned for Evaluation of Other Abdominal and Pelvic Soft-Tissue Injuries, Is Pelvis X-ray Needed? If so, in Which Patients?

CT of the abdomen and pelvis provides detailed information about the bony pelvis. It would appear redundant to obtain pelvic x-ray in a stable patient if CT of the abdomen and pelvis is planned for evaluation of other injuries. Multiple studies have investigated the utility of pelvic x-ray in this scenario and conclude that it is unnecessary.

Kessel et al.[26] performed a retrospective trauma registry review of all stable blunt trauma patients at two trauma centers from 2001 through 2004. Compared with a gold standard of CT, x-ray was only 64.4% sensitive and

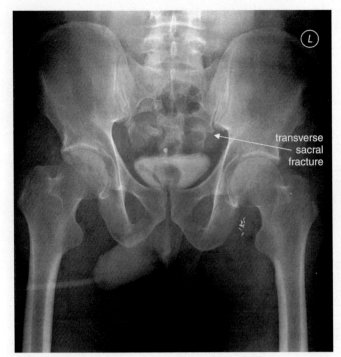

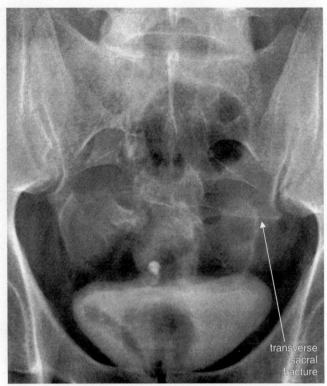

Figure 13-52. Transverse sacral fracture. Sacral fractures may or may not disrupt the pelvis ring. Vertically oriented fractures through the body of the sacrum can disrupt the ring, as can disruptions of the sacroiliac joints. This patient has an isolated transverse fracture of the sacrum, approximately at the level of the inferior margin of the left sacroiliac joint. This runs through the neural foramen of the sacrum so that the arcuate lines of the foramen do not form a complete circle. Because the fracture only separates the caudad portion of the sacrum from the cephalad portion, the sacrum continues to form a complete bridge between the iliac wings, and the pelvis remains stable. A close-up view is seen in Figure 13-53.

Figure 13-53. Transverse sacral fracture. Close-up from the same patient as in Figure 13-52. This patient has an isolated transverse fracture of the sacrum, approximately at the level of the inferior margin of the left sacroiliac joint. This runs through the neural foramen of the sacrum, so that the arcuate lines of the foramen do not form a complete circle. Because the fracture only separates the caudad portion of the sacrum from the cephalad portion, the sacrum continues to form a complete bridge between the iliac wings, and the pelvis remains stable. Compare with the CT in Figure 13-54.

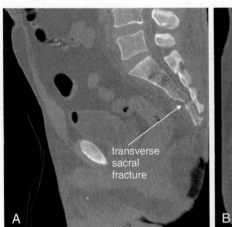

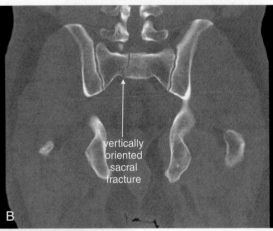

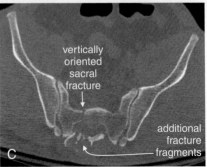

Figure 13-54. Comminuted sacral fracture. Same patient as in Figures 13-52 and 13-53. CT, bone windows. Fracture patterns in real patients can be far more complex than textbook examples. This 40-year-old male fell 25 feet from a roof onto an air-conditioning unit, sustaining a comminuted sacral fracture. The x-ray in the earlier figures suggested an isolated transverse fracture, but CT shows otherwise. The fracture runs in multiple planes and cannot be fully appreciated on a single CT series. **A,** A midsagittal view suggests a transverse fracture through the distal sacrum. **B,** A coronal view shows a vertically oriented fracture line through the proximal sacrum. **C,** Axial view. A comminuted sacral fracture is visible.

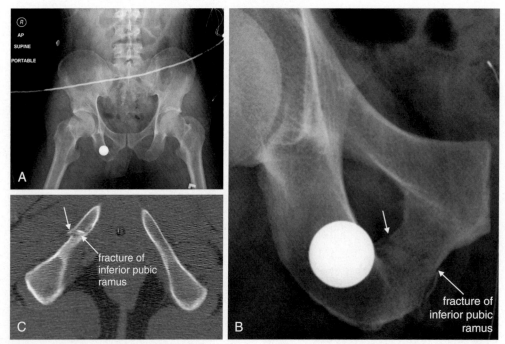

Figure 13-55. **Isolated inferior pubic ramus fracture.** We have argued that an isolated fracture of the pelvic ring is rare. This patient has an apparently isolated fracture of the inferior right pubic ramus (AP x-ray **A,** and **B**). Is there a second occult injury? No, this fracture is so minimally displaced that it does not introduce tension elsewhere in the pelvic ring. Compare with the axial CT image in **C.** No other injuries were found on CT.

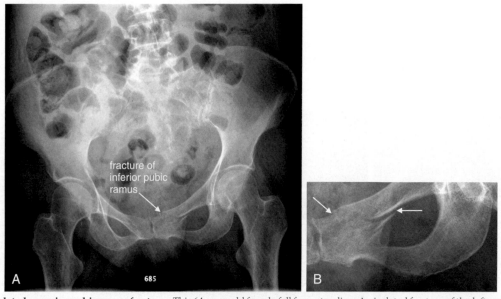

Figure 13-56. **Isolated superior pubic ramus fracture.** This 64-year-old female fell from standing. An isolated fracture of the left superior pubic ramus is seen. Again, careful inspection for a second fracture should occur. Radiology recommended CT, but magnetic resonance imaging was performed—showing the same left pubic ramus fracture and a left sacral alar fracture. This pattern is commonly called a pelvic insufficiency fracture. It is attributed to weakened bone giving way under stress induced by a second injury. In this case, presumably the fall caused the sacral fracture, introducing stress into the pelvic ring that resulted in the anterior arch fracture. **A,** AP pelvis. **B,** Close-up from **A.**

90% specific. The authors suggested eliminating routine pelvic x-ray when CT is planned in a stable patient.

Vo et al.[27] conducted a retrospective study of 509 patients undergoing both CT scan and x-ray. CT identified 163 pelvic injuries in 60 patients, whereas x-ray identified only 132 injuries in 52 patients. No patient with a negative CT scan had an injury detected on x-ray. In contrast, 8 patients with negative x-rays had injuries detected on CT scan. Compared with CT scan, the sensitivity of x-ray was only 81% on a per-fracture basis and 87% on a per-patient basis. The authors concluded that x-ray should be eliminated in stable blunt trauma patients who will undergo CT.

Stewart et al.[28] retrospectively reviewed 397 patients undergoing both pelvic x-ray and abdominopelvic CT.

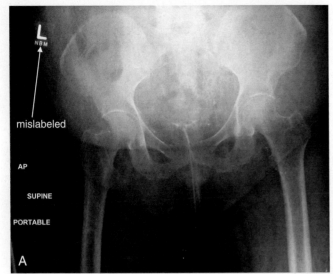

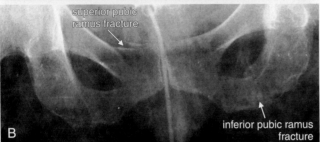

Figure 13-57. Pubic ramus fracture and labeling error. A, AP pelvis x-ray. **B,** Close-up from **A**. This x-ray demonstrates several teaching points. First, the x-ray is mislabeled—an "L" is visible in the upper right corner. Technically, we cannot determine this from this x-ray, but this is a firm reminder to confirm your orientation before performing an invasive procedure. Second, this patient is quite osteopenic, making fractures more difficult to identify. Remember to look for two or more areas of discontinuity if one is found. Inspect the close-up, and you will see a fracture of the right superior pubic ramus, as well as one of the left inferior pubic ramus. Compare this with the CT in Figure 13-58, which confirms our suspicion about the labeling error.

Compared with a gold standard of CT, the portable pelvic x-ray detected only 58 of 109 fractures (sensitivity = 53%) and did not identify 9 of 43 injured patients (sensitivity = 79%). X-ray was particularly insensitive for detection of sacroiliac fractures. Investigators reported four "false-positive" x-rays, blaming reporting errors and film artifact for these. As with other studies we have discussed, the lack of an independent diagnostic standard limits the study results; however, from a practical standpoint, CT is the current clinical gold standard in major trauma patients. It appears unlikely that pelvis x-ray provides clinically useful information in stable trauma patients undergoing abdomen and pelvis CT.

Guillamondegui et al.[29] performed a retrospective review of all blunt trauma patients undergoing immediate abdominal and pelvic CT scan. The sensitivity and specificity of portable pelvis x-ray were 68% and 98%, respectively, compared with the gold standard of CT scan. The authors concluded that portable pelvis x-ray should not be performed in hemodynamically stable patients who will undergo immediate CT scan of the abdomen and pelvis. They recommended x-ray in unstable patients and those who cannot or will not undergo CT scan because of other clinical interventions.

Using a pediatric trauma registry, Guillamondegui et al.[15] performed a retrospective review of 130 pediatric patients younger than 18 years with pelvic fractures over an 8-year period. In this series, x-ray detected only 81 of 151 fractures noted on CT (54% sensitivity). The authors recommended against pelvic x-ray in pediatric patients for whom CT scan is planned. They continued

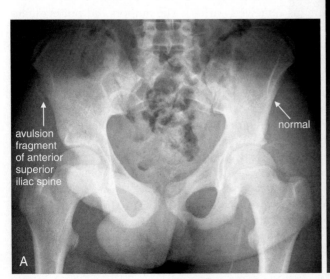

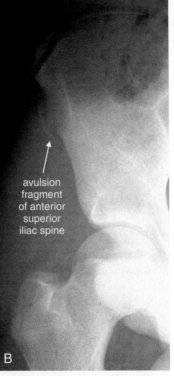

Figure 13-58. Avulsion fracture of anterior superior iliac spine by sartorius muscle. This 15-year-old boy had acute right hip pain accompanied by a "popping" sound while running the first 100 m of a 400-m track race. He was unable to continue running and was brought to the emergency department for evaluation. **A,** The right anterior superior iliac spine is avulsed—compare with the normal left side. The fracture fragment appears as an ossified crescent. This is the insertion site of the origin of the sartorius muscle and may be avulsed by forceful contraction of the sartorius, which flexes the hip and knee. **B,** Close-up. Do not confuse this avulsion fracture with the lucent growth plates along the iliac crest, which are normal in this adolescent. Use symmetry to assist you here.

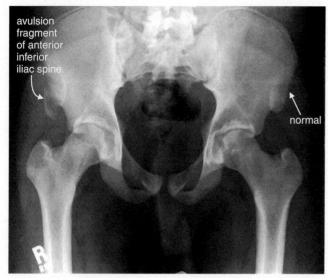

Figure 13-59. **Avulsion of the anterior inferior iliac crest apophysis by the rectus femoris muscle.** This 16-year-old male presented with right hip pain after lifting a heavier person 2 days earlier. Since the incident, the patient has had trouble flexing his leg at the hip. He complains of pain in the right lateral and anterior hip. The x-ray shows an avulsion fracture fragment from the anterior inferior iliac spine. The donor site is clearly visible. This is the attachment point for the rectus femoris muscle. With forceful contraction of this muscle, the apophysis can be pulled off. Compare with the normal left. No clinical action was taken, though the patient's cause of pain was now clear.

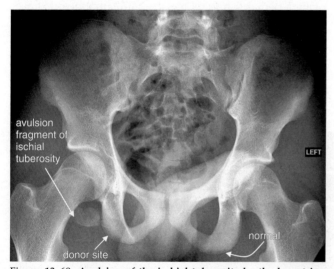

Figure 13-60. **Avulsion of the ischial tuberosity by the hamstring muscles.** This 15-year-old male complained of pain in his right buttock and numbness in his right groin after doing an accidental "complete split." He had slipped while walking at school, and his right hip flexed and left hip extended. During the split, he states that he heard something "pop." His x-ray shows an avulsion fragment from the ischial tuberosity at the point of attachment of the hamstring muscles. Compare with the opposite normal side. The patient underwent operative repair of this injury to restore the function of the hamstring muscles (Figure 13-61).

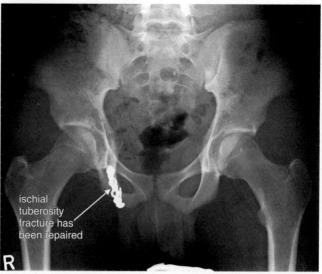

Figure 13-61. **Avulsion of the ischial tuberosity by the hamstring muscles.** Same patient as in Figure 13-60. His x-ray in the previous figure showed an avulsion fragment from the ischial tuberosity at the point of attachment of the hamstring muscles (semitendinosus, semimembranosus, and biceps femoris). Because this muscle group is functionally important for hip flexion and knee extension, the bony fragment was repositioned and fixed in place with the muscle origins still intact.

Are Clinical Factors Useful in Identifying a Subset of Patients With Unstable Fractures? Should These Patients Undergo X-ray for Early Diagnosis, Even If Computed Tomography Will Be Performed?

Even if CT of the abdomen and pelvis will be performed, it is possible that x-ray in the trauma bay could provide immediate information with clinical utility. A prospective study of 979 emergency department trauma patients examined a binary rating of the pelvic examination as stable or unstable. Unstable pelvis on physical examination was 99% specific for fracture, indicating that when a physician finds the pelvis to be unstable on examination, a pelvic injury is almost certain to be present. However, the sensitivity of pelvic instability for fracture was only 44%.[30] The authors concluded that pelvic radiography should be routine, a practice not supported by other trauma literature (as reviewed earlier). The authors did not evaluate the sensitivity of a more detailed history and examination, including factors such as pelvic tenderness, pelvic pain, or examination findings such as ecchymosis or abrasion. Some patients in this study were clinically difficult to assess because of severe injuries and endotracheal intubation. The authors did note a higher rate of blood transfusion requirements in patients with pelvic instability on examination, suggesting that when this finding is present, an early aggressive plan for blood products and potential pelvic embolization should be considered.

A second retrospective study of 1502 consecutive patients found that unstable pelvic ring on physical examination was poorly sensitive (26%, 95% CI = 15%-43%) but highly specific (99.9%, 95% CI = 99%-100%)

to advocate for x-ray in unstable patients or those in whom CT will not be performed.

Overall, in the hemodynamically stable blunt trauma patient, it is probably reasonable to forgo pelvic x-ray when pelvic CT is planned, saving both time and money.

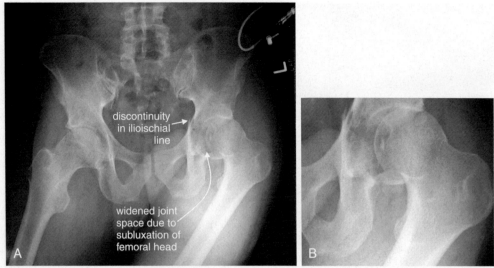

Figure 13-62. **Posterior hip dislocation with acetabular fracture. A,** This patient has a comminuted left-sided acetabular fracture with discontinuity of the ilioischial line and a lucency extending into the acetabulum. The ilioischial line marks the posterior column of the acetabulum, so we should predict a posterior column fracture on CT. There is apparent subluxation or dislocation of the left femoral head—likely a posterior dislocation, explaining the posterior acetabular fracture. Disbelieve this finding? Note the unusual position of the femur. Compare with the CT in Figure 13-63. **B,** Close-up.

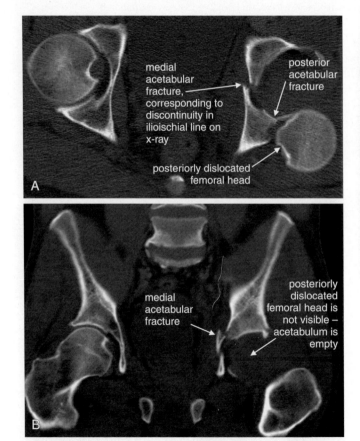

Figure 13-63. **Posterior hip dislocation with acetabular fracture, CT bone windows.** Same patient as in Figure 13-62. **A,** Axial view. The left femoral head is positioned completely posterior to the cup of the acetabulum, which is fractured medially and posteriorly. Because the femoral head was displaced in a posterior direction but remains aligned in a cephalad–caudad direction, the x-ray in Figure 13-62 is deceptive. Remember that two orthogonal views are needed to rule out dislocation on x-ray. **B,** Coronal view. The left femoral head is not visible because it lies behind the coronal plane of this image.

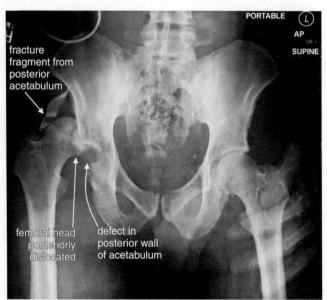

Figure 13-64. **Hip dislocation with posterior acetabular fracture.** Dislocations of the hip are often accompanied by fracture of the acetabulum. In this case, the femoral head has dislocated posteriorly, fracturing the posterior wall of the acetabulum. The fracture fragment is visible cephalad to the femoral head Compare with the CT in Figure 13-65.

for mechanically unstable pelvic fractures. Pelvic deformity was 55% sensitive (95% CI = 38%-70%) and 97% specific (95% CI = 96%-98%) for mechanically unstable pelvic fractures. Although the authors focused on the poor sensitivity of physical examination, the high specificity implies that when these examination abnormalities are present, an unstable fracture is virtually certain. In awake and alert trauma patients with a GCS of more than 13, pelvic pain or tenderness was highly

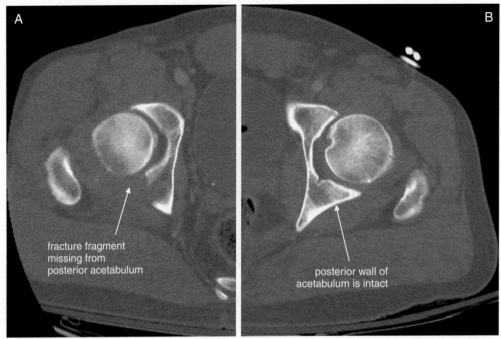

Figure 13-65. **Posterior acetabular fracture.** Same patient as in Figure 13-64. The hip dislocation has been reduced before CT scan. **A,** A large fracture fragment is missing from the posterior wall of the right acetabulum. Because the patient was not aligned well in the CT scanner, the two acetabula did not appear in the same CT slice, but the same level through the left acetabulum has been selected and displayed for this illustration **B.**

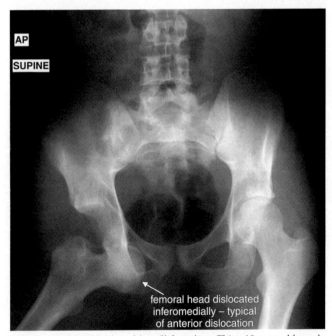

Figure 13-66. **Anterior hip dislocation.** This 18-year-old male was involved in a motor vehicle collision. The femoral head is dislocated medially and inferiorly—typical of anterior dislocation. This pattern is less common than posterior dislocation, which may happen when a patient seated in a vehicle with the hip flexed and adducted impacts the knee on a dashboard, forcing the femur posteriorly. The mechanism of anterior dislocation is believed to be force along an abducted and flexed hip. Remarkably, this patient had no pelvic fractures on CT (Figure 13-67).

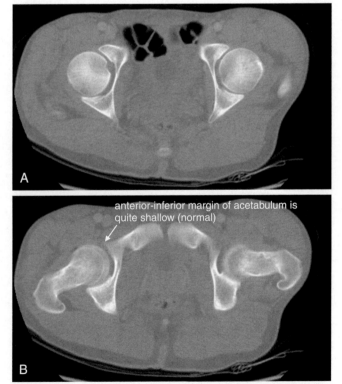

Figure 13-67. **Anterior hip dislocation: Postreduction CT, bone windows.** Same patient as in Figure 13-66. These images, acquired following reduction, show no fractures of the acetabulum. **A,** Axial slice at the cephalad–caudad midpoint of the acetabulum. **B,** Slice at the level of the pubic symphysis, corresponding to the inferior margin of the acetabulum. Notice how shallow the anterior inferior rim of the acetabulum is, allowing dislocation without fracture if forces are applied in the correct vector.

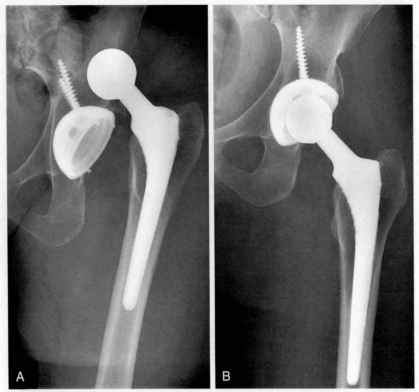

Figure 13-68. Hip dislocation: Prosthetic. Dislocation of a prosthetic hip may occur with relatively little force. Simple hyperflexion of the hip is often sufficient. The femoral head is then drawn cephalad and posterior by contraction of the hip muscles. **A,** The femoral component of the prosthesis is dislocated, while the acetabular cup remains in normal position. **B,** the femoral component has been reduced.

sensitive (100%, 95% CI = 85%-100%) for unstable pelvic fracture.[31]

Overall, evidence supports the presence of an unstable or deformed pelvis on examination as a specific though insensitive sign of an unstable pelvic fracture. It may be reasonable to perform portable pelvic x-ray in the trauma room of patients with pelvic instability on examination to identify gross fractures and allow earlier pelvic stabilization. The insensitivity of the physical examination for mechanically unstable pelvic fracture may make bedside portable pelvic x-ray a good choice in patients with unstable vital signs. Alternatively, if CT scan can be rapidly performed, patients with an unstable pelvis on examination or unstable vital signs could be treated empirically with external pelvic binding and fluid resuscitation. If CT will not be performed because of hemodynamic instability, pelvic x-ray should be performed.

How Much Does Pelvic X-ray Cost? How Long Does a Pelvic X-ray Take To Obtain?

In 2008, an AP pelvis x-ray cost $245, with an additional $22 fee for radiologist interpretation.[6] Duane et al.[6] calculated substantial savings by elimination of routine pelvic x-ray. X-ray of the pelvis is rapid to obtain because only a single view is performed. However,

given the number of tasks that must be accomplished in the trauma patient, every effort should be made to eliminate unnecessary steps with little clinical benefit. When CT is planned as part of the evaluation, x-ray appears of little value in stable patients, and even the minimal time required for pelvic x-ray may be wasteful. In less stable patients, pelvic x-ray can provide rapid and valuable information by identifying or excluding the pelvis as a probable source of hemorrhagic shock as described in more detail in Chapter 10.

When Pelvic Fractures Are Detected, Should Bladder and Urethral Injuries Be Evaluated?

Pelvic fractures are associated with bladder and urethral injuries, which occur in about 6% of all pelvic fractures and almost 15% of severe pelvic fractures in adults.[1] Do all pelvic fractures mandate additional radiographic evaluation for these injuries, or are some fractures riskier than others with regard to genitourinary injuries? The indications for imaging and the specific features of the diagnostic tests used for evaluation of these injuries are reviewed in detail in the chapter on genitourinary imaging (Chapter 12). However, because pelvic fractures are one potential predictor of bladder and urethral injury, we discuss the implications of pelvic fractures and the appropriate genitourinary imaging tests here. Briefly,

Figure 13-69. **Fractures of the proximal femur: Neck, transcervical.** Compare the normal right side **(A)** to the subtle fracture of the left femoral neck, which is complete but nondisplaced **(B).** Bearing weight on this injury would likely lead to a displaced fracture. Minute cortical defects are visible, and the zone of fracture appears slightly denser because of impaction **(C,** close-up from **B).**

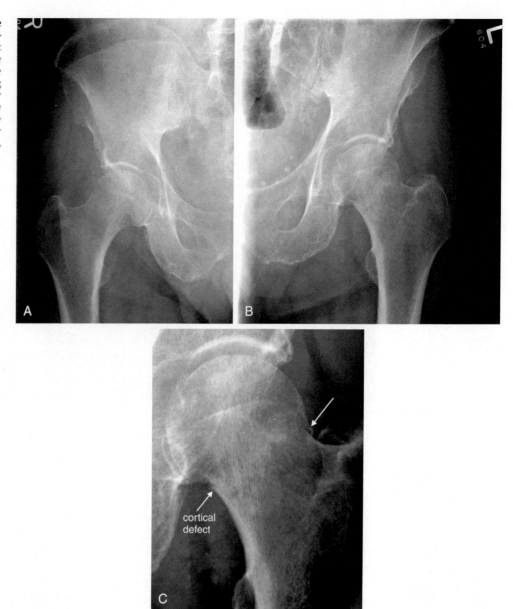

Figure 13-70. **Femoral neck fracture.** This 84-year-old female had an unwitnessed fall. **A,** Normal right hip, osteoporotic. **B,** Left hip, another relatively subtle femoral neck fracture. Note the smudging of the trabeculae of the femoral neck. In addition, the distal fragment has shifted medially, creating an overhanging ledge of the femoral head not seen on the opposite normal side. Some femoral neck fractures are more obvious.

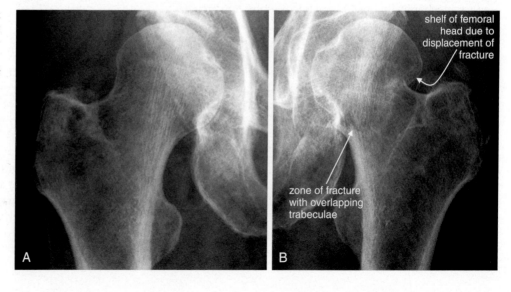

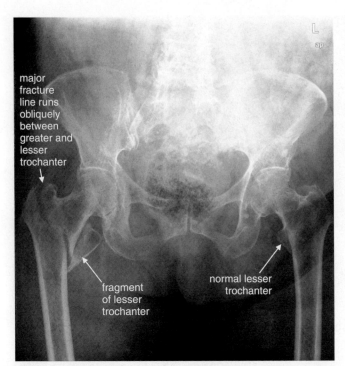

Figure 13-71. Intertrochanteric femur fracture: Three parts (proximal, distal, and one trochanter). Intertrochanteric femur fractures are common, with the mechanism often being a fall from standing in an elderly patient. The major fracture line usually runs obliquely between the greater and the lesser trochanters. These fractures may have two, three, or four parts classically, although badly comminuted combinations are also possible. Two-part fractures consist of the proximal and distal fragments. Three-part fractures also include a fragment of one trochanter. Four-part fractures include fragments of both trochanters. This 86-year-old female had an unwitnessed fall. She has a typical three-part fracture, with a fragment of the lesser trochanter visible. Note her generalized severe osteopenia.

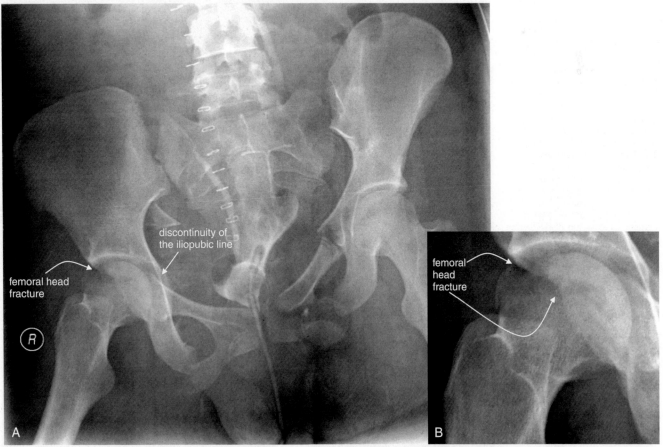

Figure 13-72. Fractures of the proximal femur: Femoral head fracture. A, AP pelvis x-ray. **B,** Close-up from **A.** Fractures of the femoral head are usually associated with hip dislocation or acetabular fracture. We have already seen this radically comminuted pelvis, a reminder of the forces that often are associated with these injuries. Note the discontinuity of the iliopubic line on the right, indicating fracture of the anterior column of the acetabulum. Compare with the CT in Figure 13-73.

Figure 13-73. Femoral head fracture. CT, bone windows. Same patient as in Figure 13-72. **A,** Coronal reconstruction showing fracture of femoral head. Note the scalloped defect in the femoral head. **B,** Axial view showing fractures. Two fractures are visible. **C,** Close-up from **B**. **D,** Close-up from **A**.

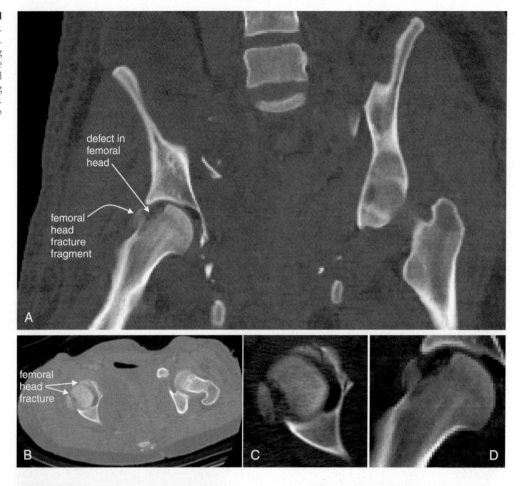

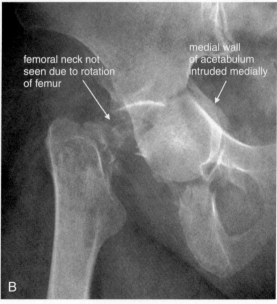

Figure 13-74. Subcapital femoral fracture. A subcapital femoral fracture separates the femoral head from the femoral neck. This patient had an unwitnessed fall and sustained an impacted fracture of the right acetabulum. The femoral head remains in the acetabulum, the medial wall of which appears intruded into the pelvis. The femoral neck is not clearly seen because the femur has rotated, placing the femoral neck perpendicular to the plane of the x-ray. **A,** AP x-ray. **B,** Close-up from **A**.

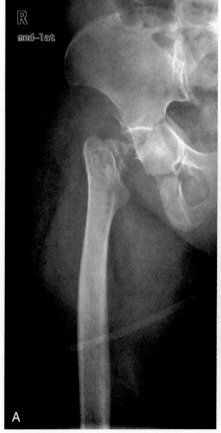

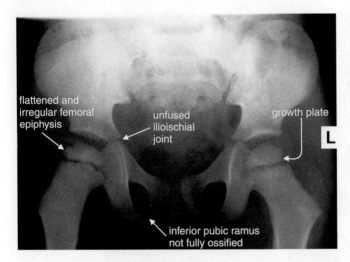

Figure 13-75. Avascular necrosis (AVN), Legg-Calvé-Perthes disease: Pediatric. This 4-year-old male had persistent limping on his left lower extremity for 2 months. The patient had been seen by his primary care physician and an urgent care for the same problem. The father suggested the child might have fallen from a bicycle. This x-ray shows the classic signs of AVN of the bilateral proximal femoral epiphyses, or Legg-Calvé-Perthes disease. The epiphyses appear irregular and flattened with some sclerosis. The history is typical as well, with diagnostic delay. Notice that the findings are bilateral, slightly worse on the right than left, though clinically the patient was thought to be favoring the left leg. Incidentally, the patient has normal skeletal immaturity. The ilium and ischium have not fully fused, the femoral growth plates remain open, and the inferior pubic rami have not fully ossified. These should not be mistaken for fractures.

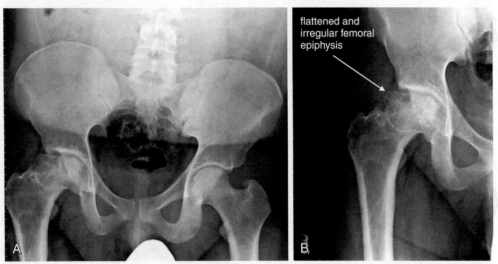

Figure 13-76. Avascular necrosis (Legg-Calvé-Perthes): Pediatric, advanced. A, B, This 17-year-old male shows advanced findings of Legg-Calvé-Perthes disease. The femoral head is collapsed and flattened with subchondral lucencies. Notice how the acetabulum has also remodeled.

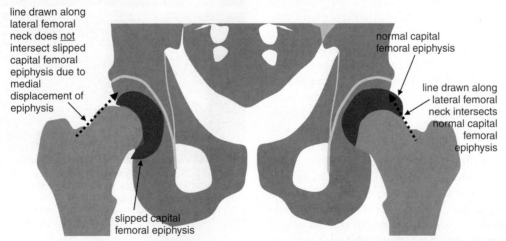

Figure 13-77. Slipped capital femoral epiphysis (SCFE). SCFE is a rare condition of adolescents and preteens. Obesity and male sex are risk factors. The x-ray findings include a widened physis (growth plate) and a femoral epiphysis medially displaced relative to the femoral neck. A line drawn along the lateral aspect of the femoral neck, as in this schematic, should intersect the normal femoral capital epiphysis but will not intersect a SCFE because the epiphysis is displaced medially. This appearance is sometimes described as resembling an ice cream cone with the scoop of ice cream (femoral epiphysis) slipping off of the cone (femoral neck). Frog-legged x-ray views can assist in detection. Because bilateral involvement occurs in 20% at initial presentation, both hips should be x-rayed. Internal fixation is usually performed in an attempt to prevent further displacement and avascular necrosis. This is a Salter-Harris I injury. The Salter-Harris classification is described in detail in Chapter 14.

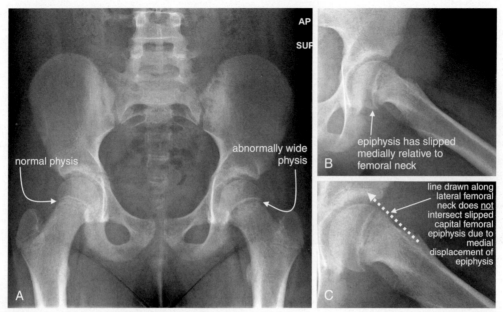

Figure 13-78. **Slipped capital femoral epiphysis (SCFE).** This 10-year-old female presented with 6 weeks of nontraumatic left hip pain, starting insidiously around the thigh. She limps occasionally and is unable to participate in sports. **A,** The anterior–posterior pelvis shows widening of the physis, concerning for SCFE (a Salter-Harris I fracture). **B,** A frog-leg view reveals subtle posteromedial displacement of the epiphysis, consistent with SCFE. **C,** A close-up frog-leg view shows that a line drawn along the lateral aspect of the femoral neck does not intersect the physis as it normally would.

retrograde urethrogram is used to assess for urethral injury, whereas conventional or CT cystogram assesses for bladder rupture. Some authors believe that anterior pelvic injuries including pubic rami fractures and pubic symphysis diastasis mandate imaging of the urethra and bladder.

Basta et al.[32] evaluated the subtypes of pelvic fracture most associated with genitourinary injury. Using a retrospective nested case-control method, the investigators reviewed x-rays and CT scans and recorded location, displacement, and estimated direction of force in 119 male patients with pelvic fractures. They detected 25 patients with urethral injuries, all with anterior pelvic fractures or diastasis of the symphysis pubis. No urethral injuries were found in isolated acetabular fractures. The authors performed logistic regression and found an increased risk for urethral injury in patients with displaced fractures of the inferomedial pubic bone (odds ratio = 6.4, 95% CI = 1.6-24.9) and symphysis pubis diastasis (odds ratio = 11.8, 95% CI = 4.0-34.5). The authors noted a 10% increase in risk for urethral injury with each millimeter of diastasis or displacement in these two pelvic injury patterns.[32] Limits of this study include the small sample of injured patients (because of the overall rarity of this injury) and exclusion of female patients. The urethra is shorter in females and less prone to injury, and it is uncertain whether the risk for urethral injury would follow the same trends in female patients. Urethral injuries occur in as many as 25% of males with pelvic injury but only 4.6% of female patients with pelvic injury. This study is concordant with previous

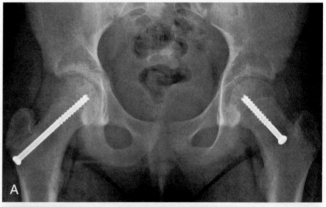

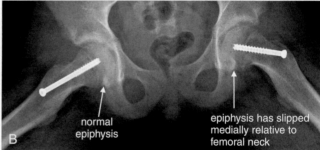

Figure 13-79. **Slipped capital femoral epiphysis.** Same patient as in Figure 13-78, 1 month later, after internal fixation of both capital femoral epiphyses. **A,** Anterior–posterior view. **B,** Frog-legged view. Note the subtle medial displacement of the left femoral capital epiphysis, compared with the normal right, which was pinned prophylactically.

studies suggesting that urethral injuries are restricted to patients with fractures of the anterior pelvic arch. However, the study is too small to establish with certainty whether some anterior pelvic injuries do not require follow-up evaluation for urethral injury. Other studies are reviewed in Chapter 12.

In the Presence of Pelvic Fractures, When Should Additional Imaging Be Performed To Detect Pelvic Vascular Injury? What Is the Role of Angiographic Embolization?

In cases of stable pelvic fractures from low energy mechanisms, such as as pubic rami fractures following a fall from a standing position, no further imaging may be required. These injuries are almost never associated with pelvic vascular or abdominal injuries. In contrast, severe pelvic fractures from high energy blunt trauma often are complicated by vascular injuries and significant pelvic bleeding. Treatment is generally nonsurgical, using angiographic embolization to achieve hemostasis. CT with IV contrast should be performed, providing detailed information about both fractures and vascular injuries. In most cases, active extravasation of parenteral contrast on CT scan is considered an indication for embolization. See the chapter on interventional radiologic techniques in emergency medicine (Chapter 16) for a detailed discussion of angiographic treatment of pelvic vascular injuries.

Why Is Magnetic Resonance Imaging Recommended for Some Pelvic Injuries and CT for Others? Is This an Evidence-Based Practice?

As described earlier, x-ray is known to be relatively insensitive for the detection of pelvic fractures. Fractures of the hip (proximal femur) may also be missed with x-ray. CT is routinely used to exclude pelvic fractures in major trauma patients, without recourse to MRI. In contrast, MRI is often used rather than CT in the evaluation of osteoporotic patients with hip pain and negative x-rays after relatively minor trauma, such as falls from standing. The evidence basis for this practice is critically examined in the chapter on musculoskeletal MRI (Chapter 15).

SUMMARY

Pelvic fractures are a common source of serious morbidity and less commonly mortality in trauma patients. X-ray provides an initial screening examination for the symptomatic patient, with CT providing a highly sensitive assessment of fractures and associated vascular injuries. A normal pelvis physical examination in a neurologically intact and asymptomatic trauma patient likely is sufficient to rule out pelvic fractures.

CHAPTER 14 Imaging the Extremities

Joshua Broder, MD, FACEP

Evaluation of extremity injuries and nontraumatic abnormalities is one of the most common indications for diagnostic imaging in the emergency department. This chapter considers the modalities available for evaluation of a range of extremity conditions, including fractures, dislocations, arterial and venous vascular anomalies, infections, and foreign bodies. We review standard fracture terminology and discuss the interpretation of common imaging tests by the emergency physician. We also discuss selected indications for diagnostic imaging using validated clinical decision rules. We review the Salter-Harris classification of pediatric fractures. We highlight high-risk extremity injuries that may be difficult to diagnose by physical examination and are sometimes missed despite diagnostic imaging. We also describe and illustrate with detailed figures the most common and serious extremity conditions.

Chapter 15 highlights the use of magnetic resonance imaging (MRI) and computed tomography (CT) in evaluation of wrist and hip injuries. Hip dislocations, fractures, and pediatric pathology including slipped capital femoral epiphysis and Legg-Calvé-Perthes disease are discussed in Chapter 13.

IMAGING MODALITIES

X-ray

By far the most common imaging modality for the extremities is x-ray. X-ray is useful in evaluation of fractures, dislocations, bony tumors, soft-tissue air, and radiopaque foreign bodies. Although x-ray can give some indication of the presence of joint effusions and soft-tissue pathology, its sensitivity is quite limited for these indications.

Computed Tomography

CT scan has seen growing applications in recent years for evaluation of complex periarticular fractures, such as fractures of the tibial plateau, and for evaluation of areas with a confluence of overlapping bones that make evaluation with plain x-ray difficult. Examples include bony injuries to the ankle and wrist. The three-dimensional capability of CT scan is particularly useful in demonstrating the relationship of fracture fragments and dislocations. Modern CT scan has submillimeter resolution, allowing detection of even subtle nondisplaced fractures in many cases. Technical features of CT

relevant to fracture detection are discussed in detail in Chapter 15.

CT angiography (CTA) has also become a first-line imaging modality for evaluation of extremity arterial injuries and arterial insufficiency caused by atherosclerotic disease. CT venography has become an option for evaluation of **deep venous thrombosis (DVT),** as described in Chapter 7. CT is highly sensitive for detection of soft-tissue gas and foreign bodies that differ in density from surrounding tissues.

Magnetic Resonance Imaging

The excellent soft-tissue contrast of MRI makes it a first-line imaging modality for evaluation of ligamentous, tendon, cartilage, and muscle injury. However, these injuries rarely require specific emergent treatment, and in most cases MRI can be deferred to the outpatient setting. MRI is also exquisitely sensitive for detection of soft-tissue foreign bodies and serves an important role when a foreign body is suspected but not detected with x-ray. Ironically, although MRI is quite insensitive for detection of cortical bone because of the absence of resonating protons, MRI has become a preferred test in evaluation of subtle fractures of the hip and scaphoid bone, because it can detect marrow edema associated with these injuries. The evidence for use of MRI in this setting is discussed in detail in Chapter 15. Magnetic resonance angiography (MRA) also offers an alternative to CTA for evaluation of extremity vascular conditions. In general, MRA is reserved for patients with contraindications to CT with iodinated contrast. MRI is also sensitive for infections and tumors of bone and soft tissue —although it lacks specificity to distinguish the etiology of some conditions such as joint effusions. MRI does not expose patients to ionizing radiation.

Ultrasound

Ultrasound is the first-line test for detection of DVT, and it can be used to assess for vascular injuries such as pseudoaneurysm occurring after arterial catheterization. Ultrasound also clearly delineates soft-tissue fluid collections and can be used to differentiate cellulitis from abscess. Ultrasound is useful in the evaluation of intraarticular fluid collections and plays an important role in evaluation of pediatric conditions such as septic hip. Joint aspiration and drainage of abscesses can be performed under real-time ultrasound guidance. Ultrasound can detect soft-tissue foreign bodies, including materials that are too low in density to be detected by x-ray. Recent research demonstrates the accuracy of ultrasound for evaluation of fractures and soft-tissue injuries including injuries to muscles, tendons, and ligaments. Ultrasound has advantages that include portability and a lack of exposure to ionizing radiation.

Catheter Angiography

Catheter angiography was once the primary test used in assessment of arterial injuries and arterial insufficiency. Today, some of these diagnostic applications have been supplanted by the use of CTA and MRA. However, catheter angiography under fluoroscopic guidance remains a useful diagnostic tool in some instances and offers therapeutic interventions that cannot be performed with CTA or MRA. Disadvantages of catheter angiography include the requirement for arterial catheterization, the use of contrast agents with potential for nephrotoxicity and allergic reaction, and the requirement for an interventional radiologist, whose services may not be available in all institutions at all hours.

Fluoroscopy

Fluoroscopy is used in some institutions to provide real-time visualization of fractures and joints during reduction and immobilization. The advantage of live visualization during a procedure is offset by a relatively high radiation exposure to both the patient and the health care provider.

Nuclear Medicine

Nuclear medicine imaging tests (scintigraphy) are relatively rarely used today in the emergency department for extremity imaging. These tests can detect metabolically active regions of bone and soft tissue (as seen in some malignancies, infections, and healing fractures). In a nuclear medicine **bone scan,** a radioisotope (technetium-99m–methylene diphosphonate) is administered and taken up by osteoblasts in areas of bone construction. Areas characterized by net bone destruction such as the lytic lesions of multiple myeloma may not be seen with this technique.[1a] A gamma camera detects emitted radiation, creating a low-resolution, two-dimensional image. Increased activity in bone indicates osteoblast activity, although it does not specifically differentiate malignancy, infection, and fractures. Smaller lesions (<1 cm) can be detected using **single photon emission CT.**

Some lesions not seen with bone scan (because of an absence of osteoblast activity) require **[18F]-2-fluoro-2-deoxy-D-glucose–positron emission tomography (FDG-PET),** which detects metabolic activity based on metabolism of a radioactive glucose analogue (FDG). Glucose is present in high concentrations in metabolically active tissues. Decay of the radioisotope results in emission of a positron, the antiparticle of an electron. The positron travels a short distance before interacting with an electron, resulting in annihilation of both particles and emission of gamma photons, which are then detected and used to localize their source. Three- and four-dimensional images (three-dimensional images with changes depicted over a fourth dimension, time) can be constructed from this data.

Following radioisotope injection, three phases of uptake are described. Phase 1 immediately following injection demonstrates blood flow, phase 2 during the first 30 minutes after injection depicts the blood pool, and phase 3 two to three hours following injection indicates bone uptake. Tumor detection with bone scan usually is performed by imaging 2 to 3 hours after radioisotope injection. For detection of osteomyelitis, a three-phase bone scan is performed, with imaging performed during the first 20 to 30 minutes after radioisotope injection (phases 1 and 2) and again at 2 to 3 hours after injection (phase 3).

Variations of these techniques can be used for other applications. In a leukocyte scintigraphy scan, a sample of the patient's white blood cells is extracted, labeled with a radioisotope (e.g., indium-111), and reinjected. These white blood cells then travel to sites of inflammation or infection. Decay of the radioisotope is detected with a gamma camera, allowing localization of processes such as osteomyelitis.[1] In a gallium scan, radioactive gallium-67 is injected intravenously, and images are acquired with a gamma camera 18 to 72 hours later (rendering the technique of no value in the emergency department). Gallium scanning is preferred to leukocyte scanning in some sequestered infections, such as intervertebral disc space infection. In addition, the technique is sometimes used to localize the source of infection in patients with fever of unknown origin, because whole-body surveys can be performed with a wide field-of-view gamma camera.[2] New techniques for whole body MRI may compete with some applications of nuclear medicine.[2a]

Nuclear medicine techniques are compared later in this chapter in the section on diagnosis of osteomyelitis.

CLINICAL DECISION RULES

Several well-validated clinical decision rules are available for imaging extremities. As described in Chapter 3, a clinical decision rule is a bedside instrument that allows the health care provider to determine the need for further diagnostic testing based on readily available data from the history and physical examination. The Ottawa foot and ankle rules and the Pittsburgh and Ottawa knee rules provide reliable guidance for radiography. Compared with clinical judgment, these rules have the potential to reduce imaging utilization while detecting nearly all important fractures. Application of these rules can save time and money and can reduce radiation exposure. Unfortunately, studies suggest that health care providers rarely use these valuable clinical aids.

Ottawa Foot and Ankle Rules

The Ottawa foot and ankle rules were originally derived and validated in an adult population with the intent of reducing unnecessary radiography to distinguish ankle sprains from fractures of the ankle and midfoot. The rules consist of four criteria, with ankle and foot x-rays required only if pain in the malleolar zone or midfoot is accompanied by one of the four findings (Box 14-1). Figure 14-1 graphically demonstrates these rules. The rules have been extensively studied in children and adults, in multiple countries (including the United Kingdom, United States, Canada, France, Greece, Germany, Netherlands, Spain, New Zealand, Singapore, and Hong Kong), and in the hands of a variety of practitioners, including attending physicians, house officers, nurse-practitioners, and nurses. A systematic review published in the *British Medical Journal* in 2003 analyzed 27 studies of these rules that included 15,581 patients.[151] Only 47 patients (0.3%) had a false-negative result. Results were similar in adults and children. Table 14-1 demonstrates the performance of the rule in important subgroups, including adults, children, and patients presenting within or after 48 hours of injury. Application of the rules would reduce radiography by 30% to 40%. Assuming a typical prevalence of fracture of 15%, the probability of a fracture after application of the rules is less than 2%. Although the Ottawa foot and ankle rule is one of the best-validated clinical rules in all of medicine, many emergency physicians do not use the rule appropriately, adding to their assessment factors such as swelling that have been shown to have no predictive value. In addition, only 30% of physicians correctly remember the rule, and many do not review the rule at the time of application or use memory aids.[3]

Ottawa Knee Rule

Stiell et al.[4] found that 74% of adult patients presenting with knee injuries underwent x-ray but only 5% had fractures. From the x-rays of the knee and patella ordered, 92% were negative for fracture. The same group of investigators subsequently derived and then validated

---

Box 14-1: Ottawa Ankle and Foot Rules

Ankle x-ray series is required if the patient complains of pain in the malleolar zone or midfoot and has any of the following findings:

- **Tenderness at the posterior edge or tip of the lateral or medial malleolus, distal 6 cm**
- **Navicular tenderness**
- **Tenderness at the base of the fifth metatarsal**
- **Inability to bear weight both immediately and in the emergency department**

Adapted from Bachmann LM, Kolb E, Koller MT, et al: Accuracy of Ottawa ankle rules to exclude fractures of the ankle and midfoot: Systematic review. *BMJ* 326:417, 2003.

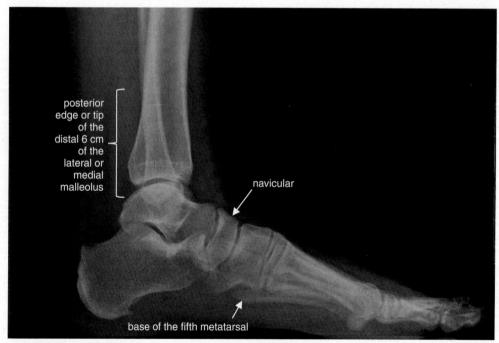

Figure 14-1. Ottawa ankle and foot rule. Ankle x-rays are needed only if the patient has pain in the malleolar zone and any of the following is true:
- The patient is unable to bear weight immediately and is in the emergency department
- The patient has bone tenderness at the posterior edge or tip of the distal 6 cm of the lateral or medial malleolus

Foot x-rays are needed only if the patient has pain in the midfoot zone and any of the following is true:
- The patient is unable to bear weight both immediately and in the emergency department
- The patient has tenderness at the navicular bone or base of the fifth metatarsal

a clinical decision rule, now known as the Ottawa knee rule (Box 14-2). In a derivation set of 1047 adults, the rule was 100% sensitive (with a 95% confidence interval [CI] of 95%-100%) and 54% specific (95% CI = 51%-57%). Application of the rule would have reduced radiography from 68.6% to 49.4%, a 28% relative reduction.[5] In a prospective validation study of 1096 adults, sensitivity was 100% (95% CI = 94%-100%) and the estimated relative reduction in radiography use was 28%. There was virtually no probability of fracture if the rule was "negative" (95% CI = 0%-0.4%). The rule also had excellent interobserver agreement, with a kappa of 0.77 (values greater than 0.5 are generally accepted to represent a high degree of agreement).[6] A subsequent prospective study in 1522 adults showed 100% sensitivity (95% CI = 96%-100%), reductions in radiography as great as 49%, and no estimated probability of fracture with a negative rule (95% CI = 0%-0.5%).[7] A systematic review found six studies, with 4249 adult patients, with high sensitivity (Table 14-2).[8]

Limitations of the Ottawa Knee Rule: Insensitivity in Children?

One study in children suggests inadequate sensitivity of the Ottawa knee rule. In a prospective study of 234 children 18 years and younger, the rule identified 12 of 13 patients with fractures (sensitivity = 92%, 95% CI = 64%-99%), missing a nondisplaced proximal tibia fracture in an 8-year-old male.[9] Other studies find the rule to be highly sensitive.[9a] Subsequent meta-analyses suggest sensitivity of 99% in children over the age of

5 years.[9b] Other authors have suggested that children be assessed using the Pittsburgh knee rule, described later. This rule in its original form mandates imaging of children younger than 12 years, although studies in patients as young as 6 years show high sensitivity.

Pittsburgh Knee Rule

Seaberg and Jackson[10] retrospectively derived a clinical decision rule for knee radiography in 201 consecutive patients with knee injuries. They then prospectively validated the rule (Box 14-3) in 133 consecutive patients with knee injuries. Sensitivity was 100%, specificity was 79%, and x-ray utilization using the rule would be reduced by 78%. The same investigators prospectively compared the Ottawa and Pittsburgh rules in a sample of 934 patients, ages 6 to 96 years.[9c] The Pittsburgh rule was 99% sensitive (95% CI = 94%-100%) and 60% specific (95% CI = 56%-64%). The Ottawa rule was 97% sensitive (95% CI = 90%-99%) and 27% specific (95% CI = 23%-30%).

Identifying Fractures: What Do Fractures Look Like on X-ray?

Complete and displaced fractures in adults are usually overt—readily recognized by lay people, as well as nonradiologist physicians. Let's take a moment to articulate what we are seeing when we recognize an overt fracture, because some of the same characteristics may be present in subtler fractures. In an overt fracture,

---

TABLE 14-1. Diagnostic Accuracy of the Ottawa Foot and Ankle Rules

Category (n = studies)	Sensitivity (95% CI)	Median Specificity (interquartile range)	Negative Likelihood Ratio (95% CI)	Fracture Probability With Negative Rule, Assuming 15% Prevalence of Fracture (95% CI)
All studies (n = 39)	97.6% (96.4%-98.9%)	31.5% (23.8%-44.4%)	0.10 (0.06-0.16)	1.73% (1.05%-2.75%)
Type of Assessment				
Ankle (n = 15)	98.0% (96.3%-99.3%)	39.8% (27.9%-47.7%)	0.08 (0.03-0.18)	1.39% (0.53%-3.08%)
Foot (n = 10)	99.0% (97.3%-100%)	37.8% (24.7%-70.1%)	0.08 (0.03-0.20)	1.39% (0.53%-3.41%)
Combined (n = 14)	96.4% (93.8%-98.6%)	26.3% (19.4%-34.3%)	0.17 (0.10-0.30)	2.91% (1.73%-5.03%)
Population				
Children (n = 7)	99.3% (98.3%-100%)	26.7% (23.8%-35.6%)	0.07 (0.03-0.18)	1.22% (0.53%-3.08%)
Adults (n = 32)	97.3% (95.7%-98.6%)	36.6% (22.3%-46.1%)	0.11 (0.06-0.18)	1.90% (1.05%-3.08%)
Time to Referral (in hours)				
< or =48 (n = 5)	99.6% (98.2%-100%)	27.9% (24.7%-31.5%)	0.06 (0.02-0.19)	1.05% (0.35%-3.24%)
>48 (n = 34)	97.3% (95.9%-98.5%)	36.6% (19.9%-46.8%)	0.11 (0.07-0.18)	1.90% (1.22%-3.08%)

Pooled sensitivity, specificity, negative likelihood ratio, and probability of fracture using the Ottawa ankle and foot rules. Note that although 27 published studies were analyzed, these provide 39 separate comparisons when foot and ankle are separately considered.
Adapted from Bachmann LM, Kolb E, Koller MT, et al: Accuracy of Ottawa ankle rules to exclude fractures of the ankle and mid-foot: Systematic review. *BMJ* 326:417, 2003.

Box 14-2: Ottawa Knee Rule for Adults

Radiography of the knee is indicated if any of the criteria are met. Sensitivity is 100%.
- **Age greater than or equal to 55 years**
- **Isolated tenderness of the patella**
- **Tenderness at the fibular head**
- **Inability to flex knee to 90 degrees**
- **Inability to bear weight both immediately and in the emergency department (four steps)**

Adapted from Stiell IG, Wells GA, Hoag RH, et al: Implementation of the Ottawa knee rule for the use of radiography in acute knee injuries. *JAMA* 278:2075-2079.

TABLE 14-2. Performance of the Ottawa Knee Rule

	Performance	95% CI
Sensitivity	98.5%	93.2%-100%
Specificity	48.6%	43.4%-51.0%
Negative likelihood ratio	0.05	0.02-0.23

From a systematic review of 4249 adult patients.
Adapted from Bachmann LM, Haberzeth S, Steurer J, ter Riet G: The accuracy of the Ottawa knee rule to rule out knee fractures: A systematic review. *Ann Intern Med* 140:121-124, 2004.

Box 14-3: Pittsburgh Knee Rule

Knee radiography is required if
- **Blunt trauma or a fall is the mechanism of injury and either of the following is true:**
  - **Age <12 years or >50 years**
  - **Inability to walk four weight-bearing steps in the emergency department**

Adapted from Seaberg DC, Jackson R: Clinical decision rule for knee radiographs. *Am J Emerg Med* 12:541-543, 1994; Seaberg DC, Yealy DM, Lukens T, et al: Multicenter comparison of two clinical decision rules for the use of radiography in acute, high-risk knee injuries. *Ann Emerg Med* 1998;32:8-13, 1998.

the cortex of bone is disrupted and the trabecular bone is fragmented. The cortex of bone, usually a smooth continuous line on plain x-ray, is discontinuous. A line indicating the fracture connects the defect on one cortex with the cortex on the opposite side. If the fracture fragments are displaced, space divides one fragment from the other (Figure 14-2).

Unfortunately, from the perspective of diagnostic simplicity, this scenario does not always occur. Let's examine some scenarios in which fractures can be more occult.

Decreased bone density can mask cortical and trabecular abnormalities. In the case of young children, the growth plate or physis is an area of lucency, making

fractures through this zone difficult to recognize—as discussed in the later section on Salter-Harris fractures. In the youngest children, entire regions of bone are not calcified, so fractures of these regions are invisible. Minimally calcified bones are flexible and may bend rather than undergo frank fracture, much like a young tree branch. In this case, one cortex undergoes compression and the opposite side experiences stretch or extension stress. The result can be a **greenstick fracture,** a common fracture type in children. In this fracture type, a cortical defect is seen in the side of the bone undergoing extension, whereas no fracture is typically seen in the side undergoing compression (Figures 14-3 and 14-4; see also Figure 14-2). Alternatively, the cortex undergoing compression may demonstrate another common fracture pattern, the **buckle** or **torus fracture** (Figures 14-5 and 14-6; see also Figure 14-2). These injuries typically occur with a compression injury, such as a fall on an outstretched hand (often abbreviated FOOSH) and thus are often seen in the distal forearm. The relatively soft cortex can crumple under compression rather than undergoing complete fracture, resulting in a small bump or irregularity in both cortices of a long bone. The fracture zone is sometimes visible as a lucency through the bone (see Figure 14-6). In some cases, if the compression is unequally distributed to one cortex, the typical "buckle" cortical irregularity is visible only in one cortex.

At the opposite extreme of age, significant osteoporosis or osteopenia can develop and complicate detection of fracture. Osteopenic bones in the elderly lack the pliable characteristics of young bones, with their flexible cartilaginous scaffolding. Instead, osteopenia contributes to brittle bones that easily fracture rather than bending. However, the paucity of calcium makes the cortex and trabecula relatively radiolucent on x-ray. Against this backdrop, the additional lucency of a cortical fracture, or injuries to trabecular bone, may be difficult to recognize. A common clinical scenario in the osteopenic patient is suspected hip fracture without clear x-ray findings. Chapter 15 discusses imaging options for this scenario in detail. Osteopenia and osteoporosis can develop in patients with chronic steroid use or who cannot bear their own weight (e.g., in nonambulatory patients with neuromuscular disease) at an earlier age.

At any age, nondisplaced fractures can be difficult to recognize on x-ray. If the fracture zone is impacted, it may appear somewhat denser than normal bone on x-ray, though a definite cortical abnormality may not be seen. Extension in the fracture zone may make this area more lucent, without a definite visible cortical abnormality. In the case of nondisplaced fractures, other secondary signs of injury may be present and can indicate the presence of fracture. A classic example is the **pathologic fat pad sign** of fractures about the elbow

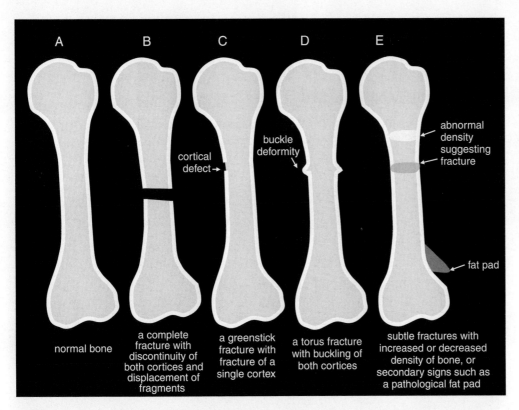

Figure 14-2. Identifying a fracture. Some fractures are readily recognizable, whereas others are subtle or apparent only based on secondary signs of injury, rather than specific bony findings. **A,** Normal bone. **B,** Bone with an obvious complete fracture. **C,** Greenstick fracture, with disruption of only one cortex. **D,** Torus (buckle fracture). **E,** Subtle fractures, sometimes seen only as areas of increased or decreased density. A sail sign resulting from displacement of a fat pad by hematoma may be the only sign of an otherwise-invisible fracture.

Labels in figure: A — normal bone; B — cortical defect → a complete fracture with discontinuity of both cortices and displacement of fragments; C — buckle deformity → a greenstick fracture with fracture of a single cortex; D — a torus fracture with buckling of both cortices; E — abnormal density suggesting fracture, fat pad → subtle fractures with increased or decreased density of bone, or secondary signs such as a pathological fat pad

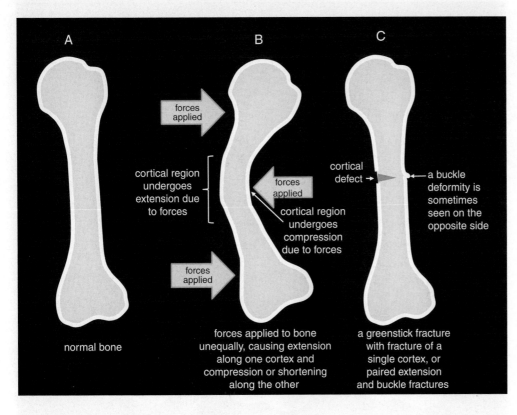

Figure 14-3. Greenstick mechanism. Immature and partially calcified bone is soft and pliable, like a green stick from a young tree. The bone can tolerate significant bending before fracture occurs. During bending, one cortex elongates and may fracture. The other cortex shortens and may not fracture or may buckle. **A,** Normal bone at rest. **B,** Forces are applied unequally to the bone. **C,** Pliable bone returns to its static position, but the cortex that experienced extension has fractured, like a green stick.

Labels in figure: A — normal bone; B — forces applied, cortical region undergoes extension due to forces, cortical region undergoes compression due to forces, forces applied to bone unequally, causing extension along one cortex and compression or shortening along the other; C — cortical defect →, a buckle deformity is sometimes seen on the opposite side, a greenstick fracture with fracture of a single cortex, or paired extension and buckle fractures

(Figure 14-7; see also Figure 14-2; this sign is also discussed later in this chapter). A fat pad is normally hidden from view on the lateral x-ray, because it is recessed in a groove of the distal humerus. When fracture occurs, a hematoma may infiltrate the groove, displacing the fat pad, which then becomes visible as a lucency called the "sail" sign on the lateral x-ray. A visible fat pad implies the presence of a hematoma, which in turn suggests a fracture. A serous joint effusion has the same radiographic appearance. Fat pads and other secondary signs of injury, such as soft-tissue swelling, are not specific for fracture. An exception is lipohemarthrosis. In the case

Figure 14-4. **Greenstick radius fracture and complete transverse ulnar fracture.** This 11-year-old male fell on his left arm while tackling another football player. The ulna demonstrates a complete transverse fracture, whereas the radius appears to have a greenstick fracture pattern, with one cortex bending rather than showing a complete fracture. This fracture shows both dorsal and ulnar angulation. **A,** Anterior–posterior view. **B,** Lateral view. **C,** Close-up from **A.**

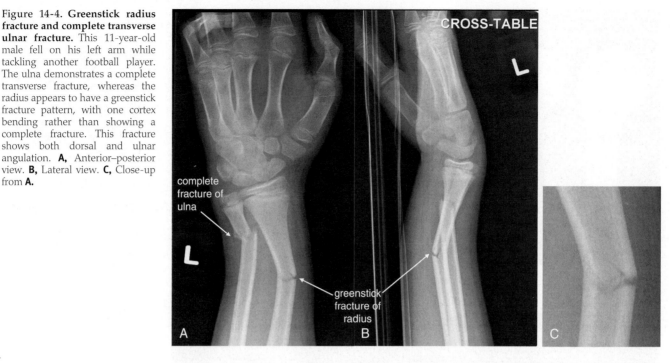

Figure 14-5. **Buckle fracture mechanism.** Immature and partially calcified bone is soft and pliable. Under compression forces, the cortices may buckle rather than shattering like more heavily calcified bone. Buckle fractures can be visible along one or both cortices. The distal radius is a common location for this fracture pattern, following a fall on an outstretched hand. These fractures are typically stable as a result of impaction of the two fragments and incomplete fracturing of the cortices. **A,** Normal bone at rest. **B,** Forces are applied, compressing the pliable bone. **C,** Pliable cortices buckle under compressive forces. Buckle fractures can also occur with unequal application of forces to immature bone, as seen in Figure 14-3.

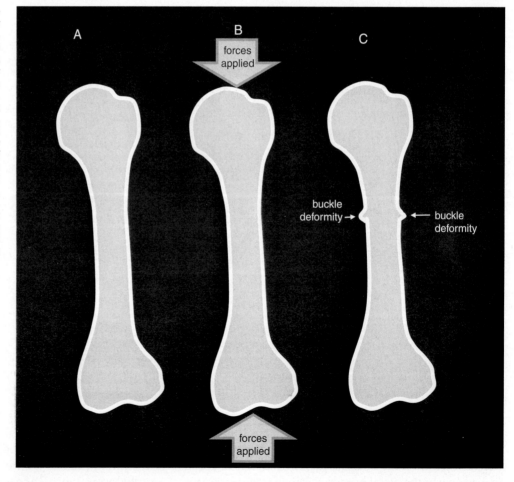

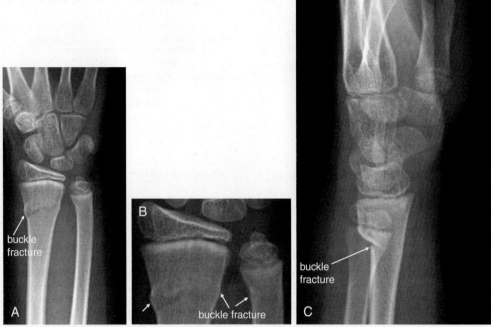

Figure 14-6. Buckle (torus) fracture of distal radius and ulna. This 12-year-old male fell while ice-skating, landing on his outstretched left arm. Anterior–posterior **(A, B)** and lateral **(C)** views show buckle fractures of the distal radius and ulna. Buckle fractures are pediatric fractures resulting from the soft, partially mineralized cortex of immature bone. Rather than breaking completely under stress, the cortex bends or buckles, with a characteristic rounded shape.

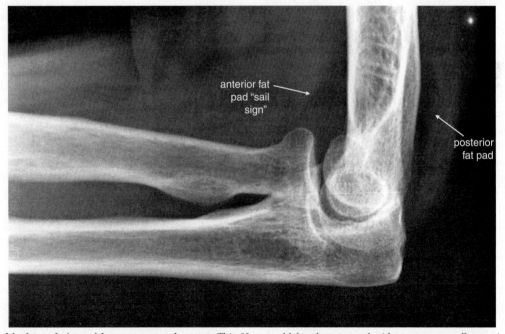

Figure 14-7. Double fat pad sign with no apparent fracture. This 83-year-old female presented with spontaneous elbow pain without trauma. Large anterior and posterior fat pads are visible, consistent with a joint effusion displacing fat pads from their usual hidden positions. In the setting of trauma, visible fat pads suggest hemarthrosis, often associated with occult fractures about the elbow. In the absence of trauma, this finding can indicate a serous effusion or even septic joint in the correct clinical context.

of distal femur or proximal tibia fracture, fat and blood from the bone marrow space may enter the joint space of the knee, forming a fat–fluid level that is visible on x-ray. Although the absence of this finding does not rule out fracture, the presence of lipohemarthrosis on x-ray is highly specific for fracture.[11]

Some acute nondisplaced fractures are not visible on x-ray and display no secondary signs to betray their presence. When a fracture is highly suspected on clinical grounds but is invisible on x-ray, several options are available. The patient can undergo advanced imaging such as CT, MRI, or bone scan if immediate management demands a definitive diagnosis. In many cases, however, immobilization of the injured region based on the suspected injury is sufficient. Follow-up x-rays in 1 to 2 weeks may demonstrate evidence of healing fracture, such as **callus formation** or **sclerosis,** an increase in density in the fracture zone.

DESCRIBING FRACTURES IDENTIFIED ON X-RAY: STANDARD TERMINOLOGY

Fractures and dislocations identified on plain x-ray should be described using standard terminology to allow clear communication among the radiologist, emergency physician, and orthopedist or other consultant. Table 14-3 presents an algorithm for describing a fracture.

The **anatomic location** of a fracture should be described by naming the bone and identifying the location of the fracture within the proximal, middle, or distal third of a long bone (Figure 14-8). Extension to the **articular surface** of a bone should also be noted.

The **direction of fracture lines** should be described. A transverse fracture extends perpendicular to the long axis of the bone. An oblique fracture is in neither the long axis nor the short axis of the bone but rather extends in a diagonal plane. A spiral fracture extends in a helical pattern, generally along the long axis of a bone (see Figure 14-8).

A **nondisplaced fracture** is one in which the fracture fragments maintain their normal anatomic positions. The fracture surfaces are described as having 100% or full apposition. A **displaced fracture** is one in which the fracture fragments no longer are in their normal anatomic positions relative to one another. Their fractured surfaces may be in partial contact (also called apposition), or they may no longer have contact (Figure 14-9). *Displacement may not be evident from a single radiograph. For example, marked displacement perpendicular to the plane of the x-ray may be undetectable. Consequently, two orthogonal-view x-rays are necessary to rule out displacement of a fracture* (Figure 14-10). The distance of fracture displacement should be measured. The displacement of the distal fragment is usually described relative to the proximal fragment. Displacement can be described as AP, medial–lateral, or relative to the normal anatomic position of a limb. For example, a fragment may be described as displaced in a volar or dorsal direction, relative to the proximal fragment in the normal anatomic position. Another example of a description of a fracture fragment by anatomic relationship would be to state that a fragment is displaced in an ulnar direction, rather than describing this as medial displacement. This use of the standard anatomic position to describe fracture displacement can prevent confusion that results from less specific terms

TABLE 14-3. Standard Terminology to Characterize Fractures

Characteristic	Example
Anatomic location (including affected bone and location specified by the proximal, middle, or distal third of a long bone)	• Proximal humerus • Distal femur
Articular surface involvement	Distal humerus fracture with articular extension
Direction of fracture lines	• Transverse • Oblique
Distance and direction of displacement	• Nondisplaced • 10-mm proximal displacement of distal fragment
Impaction, distraction, or apposition (including bayonet apposition, in which two fracture fragments overlie one another like the blade and muzzle of a bayonet)	• The fracture fragments are impacted. • The fragments show 2 cm of distraction. • The fragments show close apposition.
Angulation or alignment	20 degrees of anterior angulation
Severity of comminution	• Two-part comminution • Three-part comminution • Severely comminuted
Presence or absence of an overlying skin laceration or wound	A soft-tissue defect overlies the fracture.
Presence of foreign bodies or air	Radiopaque foreign bodies are present. Lucencies suggesting air are present.

such as medial and lateral, whose meaning can vary depending on limb position.

Impaction or distraction of the distal fragment is described relative to the proximal fragment. If the distal fragment has not moved proximally or distally relative to the proximal fragment, neither impaction nor distraction is present. If the distal fragment has moved proximally relative to the proximal fragment with the two fracture zones in direct contact because of compression, **impaction** is present. A distal fragment that has been proximally and medially or laterally dislocated is sometimes called an **overriding fragment.** If the distal fragment has moved distally relative to the proximal fragment so that a gap is present between the fracture fragments, **distraction** is present (Figure 14-11).

Angulation of the distal fragment is described relative to the proximal fragment. In a long bone divided into two fracture fragments, the distal fragment is not angulated if the long axis of the distal fragment remains parallel to

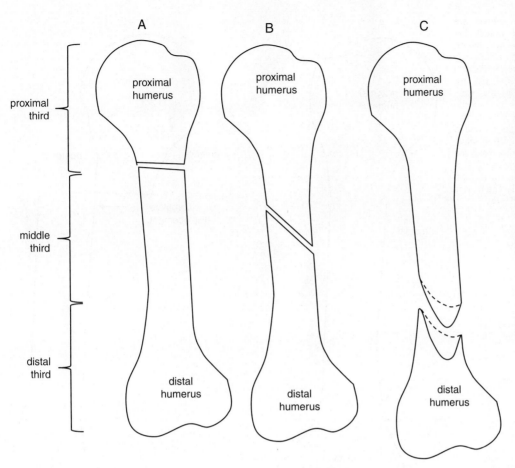

Figure 14-8. **Fracture location and direction of fracture lines.** Fractures are described by naming the affected bone and identifying the position of the fracture by the proximal, middle, or distal third of a long bone. In the case of flat or irregular bones such as the scapula, a fracture may instead be described by its involvement of named structures, such as the scapular spine or glenoid fossa. The direction of a fracture relative to the long axis of the bone should be described using terms such as transverse, oblique, or spiral. If a fracture extends to an articular surface, this should be noted. **A,** Transverse fracture of the proximal third of the humerus. **B,** Oblique fracture of the middle third of the humerus. **C,** Spiral fracture of the distal third of the humerus. Spiral fractures result from torsion of the bone. The fracture does not lie in a single plane; rather, it creates a curved surface.

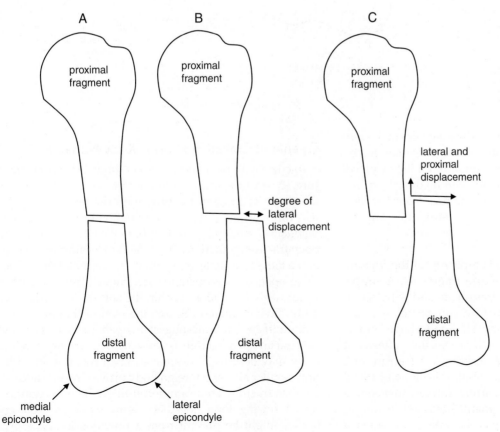

Figure 14-9. **Apposition or displacement.** The distance and direction of displacement of fracture fragments should be noted. **A,** The proximal and distal fragments maintain their normal relationship, and no displacement is present. **B,** The distal fragment has moved laterally relative to the proximal fragment. Displacement is present and can be measured. **C,** The distal fragment has moved both laterally and proximally relative to the proximal fragment.

Figure 14-10. **Two orthogonal views are needed to detect fracture and assess for dislocation.** A fracture line may be invisible on a single view, and displacement of a fracture may not be evident. Two orthogonal (perpendicular) views are required to minimize the risk for missing a fracture or dislocation in this way. **A,** In this stylized view of a humerus fracture, the fracture line is only faintly visible on the anterior–posterior (AP) view as a cortical discontinuity. No displacement is visible. **B,** In this lateral view, the distal fragment is seen to be fully displaced posterior relative to the proximal fragment. This gross displacement was not visible on the AP view, because the direction of displacement was perpendicular to the plane of the AP x-ray.

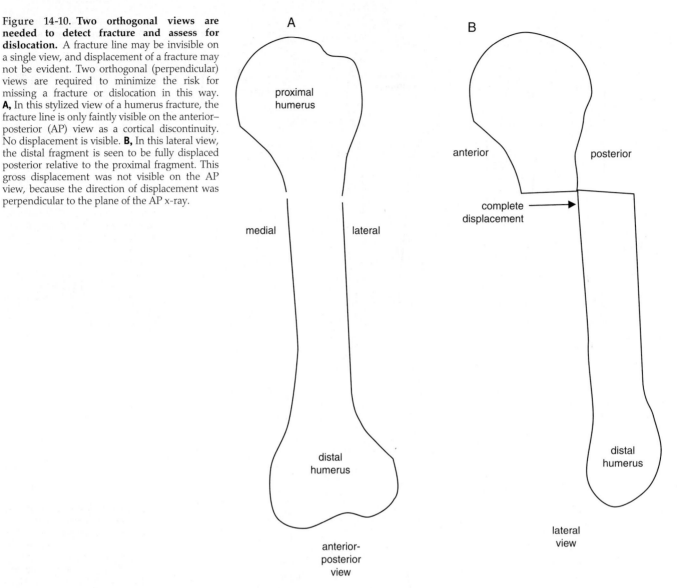

that of the proximal fragment. If the long axes of the two fragments are no longer parallel, the angle subtended by the two axes is the degree of angulation. Like displacement, the direction of angulation can be described in a number of ways, including AP, medial–lateral, volar–dorsal, or relative to other anatomic structures, such as adjacent bones (Figure 14-12).

Comminution describes the complexity of the fracture based on the number of fracture fragments. A simple fracture results in only two fragments and is not comminuted. A complicated fracture can result in many fracture fragments of varying size and shape and is comminuted (Figure 14-13). Other specific patterns of comminution are sometimes described. A fracture that divides a long bone into proximal, middle, and distal fragments is a **segmental fracture.** A fracture that results in a triangular fracture fragment, bounded by larger proximal and distal fragments, is sometimes called a **butterfly fracture.**

Open and Closed Fractures: X-ray Findings

A fracture with no associated lacerations is a **closed fracture.** A fracture that communicates with an overlying laceration is an **open fracture,** with risk for osteomyelitis. Although the physical examination often makes this distinction evident, radiographic clues can suggest an open fracture, sometimes with the skin laceration appearing relatively remote in location on examination. Clues to an open fracture include radiopaque foreign material visible on x-ray and air within the soft tissues visible on x-ray, having entered through the wound (Figure 14-14). Although an x-ray can suggest an open fracture, it cannot rule out an open fracture, because neither air nor a foreign body may be present despite an open fracture. In addition, neither air nor a foreign body proves the presence of an open fracture. For example, air might have been introduced during local anesthetic administration. Foreign bodies might be present from a previous injury. X-ray, examination, and patient history must be correlated.

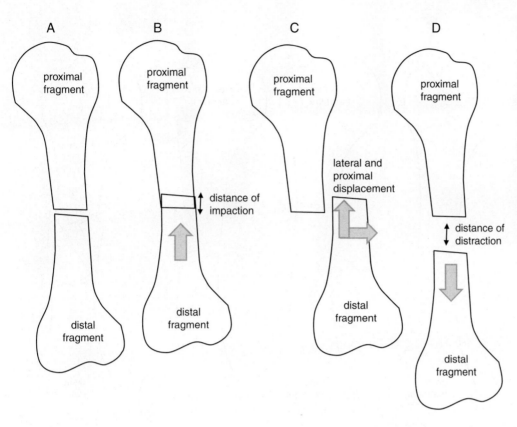

Figure 14-11. **Impaction or distraction. A,** The proximal and distal fragments maintain their normal relationship, and neither impaction nor distraction is present. **B,** The distal fragment has moved proximally relative to the proximal fragment. Impaction is present and can be measured. **C,** The distal fracture fragment has been displaced both proximally and laterally and is therefore not impacted. Instead, it is described as overriding. **D,** The distal fragment has moved distally relative to the proximal fragment. Distraction is present. The distance of distraction can be measured.

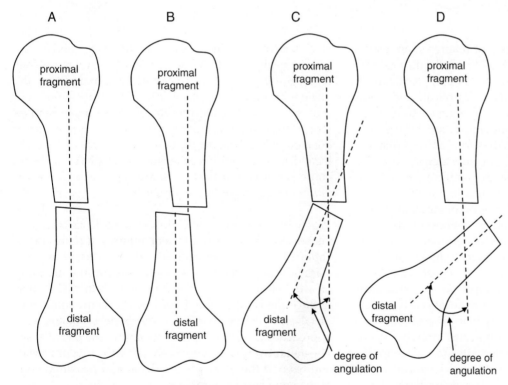

Figure 14-12. **Angulation.** The degree of angulation of the distal fracture fragment relative to the proximal fragment should be described. **A,** The long axes of bone fragments remain aligned, with no angulation. **B,** Despite displacement of the distal fragment, the long axes of the two fragments are parallel, so no angulation is present. **C,** The long axes of the two fragments are no longer aligned. The angle between the two axes can be measured. **D,** An even greater degree of angulation is present.

DESCRIBING JOINT DISLOCATIONS IDENTIFIED ON X-RAY: STANDARD TERMINOLOGY

Joint dislocations identified on x-ray can be described using terminology similar to that applied to fractures. A **joint dislocation** suggests complete loss of apposition of the articular surfaces of the bones comprising a joint. **Joint subluxation,** in which partial contact of the articulating surfaces of the bones comprising a joint is preserved, may also be seen. The involved joint should be identified and named. Dislocation is described based on the location of the distal bone, relative to the proximal bone of the joint. Dislocations can be described as

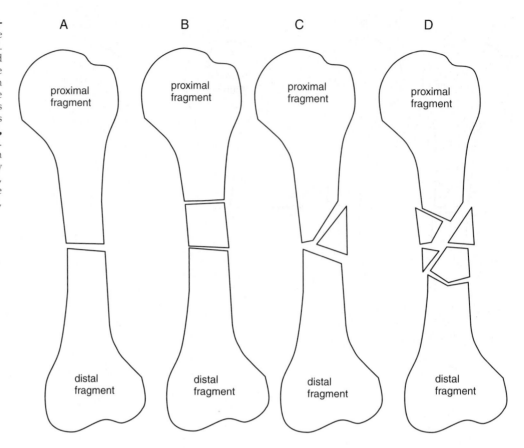

Figure 14-13. Number of fragments. The number of fracture fragments should be described. **A,** The fracture has resulted in only two fragments. **B,** The fracture is comminuted, with three fragments. When the three fragments are arranged in this way, the pattern is sometimes called a segmental fracture. **C,** Another comminuted fracture. This fragmentation pattern, with a triangular fragment bounded by the proximal and distal fragments, is called a butterfly fracture. **D,** The fracture is severely comminuted, with multiple fragments.

medial–lateral, AP, volar–dorsal, or relative to an associated anatomic structure, such as "radially dislocated." Associated fractures should be noted, particularly intraarticular fractures that may complicate reduction or require surgical fixation. Some fractures and dislocations are commonly seen in tandem and are discussed in later sections of this chapter; therefore when a dislocation is seen, a fracture should be considered, and vice versa. Dislocations can result in significant neurovascular injury, and normal anatomic alignment on x-ray does not rule out the presence of neurovascular injury. For example, an x-ray showing no dislocation does not exclude the possibility of a dislocation that has undergone spontaneous reduction. This is extremely important to recognize, because some dislocations pose substantial risk for vascular injury. For example, **knee dislocation** (not to be confused with patellar dislocation) is associated with **popliteal artery injury** that can result in limb ischemia, compartment syndrome, and limb loss if not recognized and treated (depicted later in this chapter). Spontaneous reduction of a dislocated knee can occur and may have no visible fractures or dislocations.

PEDIATRIC CONSIDERATIONS

Salter-Harris Classification

When evaluating pediatric patients, the emergency physician must consider the possibility of injury to the growth plate, also called the physis. The physis closes at a variable age in patients of differing gender and genetic background. Before physeal closure, the physis represents a point of relative weakness. In addition, the normal lucency of the physis can prevent recognition of fractures involving the growth plate. To make matters worse, these often-occult injuries can result in arrest of bone growth; consequently, they are a source of medical–legal risk. A key point for the emergency physician bears emphasis: *a normal radiograph does not rule out a physis injury in a symptomatic pediatric patient.*

The Salter-Harris classification is used to characterize visible and suspected physeal injuries (Figure 14-15; Table 14-4 gives a mnemonic). Before describing this classification system, let's briefly review the anatomy of a developmentally immature long bone. The shaft of the bone is called the diaphysis. At the proximal and distal ends of the diaphysis, the bone broadens as it approaches the growth plate, becoming the metaphysis. The metaphysis is capped by the growth plate or physis, and beyond the physis at the distal and proximal ends of the bone lies the epiphysis.

A **Salter-Harris type I fracture** is a fracture through the physis, involving neither the epiphysis nor the metaphysis. Salter-Harris I fractures can occur with or without displacement. Displaced Salter-Harris I fractures are generally readily evident because of the misalignment of the epiphysis and metaphysis. The fracture itself is often not seen, because it lies through the radiographically

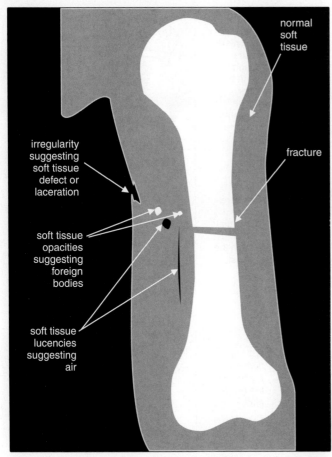

normal
soft
tissue

fracture

irregularity
suggesting
soft tissue
defect or
laceration

soft tissue
opacities
suggesting
foreign
bodies

soft tissue
lucencies
suggesting
air

Figure 14-14. **Clues to open fracture.** X-ray does not rule out open fracture, nor does it prove the presence of an open fracture. However, x-ray can yield clues to the presence of an open fracture. Air within soft tissues near a fracture suggests open fracture. Soft-tissue foreign bodies also suggest open fracture. However, an open fracture may demonstrate neither of these x-ray findings. If these findings are present, must an open fracture be present? Not necessarily. For example, air might have been introduced during local anesthetic administration. Foreign bodies might be present from a previous injury. Examination and x-ray findings should be correlated. This figure represents schematically some typical x-ray findings that may suggest open fracture. On x-ray, air outside the patient is generally black. Soft-tissue air appears nearly black as well. Soft-tissue air may track along tissue planes, giving a linear lucency appearance. A soft-tissue defect suggesting a laceration is present near the fracture. Radiopaque foreign bodies are visible, though these could represent tiny bone fragments rather than introduced foreign material.

lucent physis. Salter-Harris I fractures without displacement can be radiographically normal—with the only clinical clues to their presence being extremity pain, tenderness to palpation, and awareness on the part of the emergency physician that these injuries can be radiographically occult. *Thus a normal x-ray does not rule out a Salter-Harris I fracture in a symptomatic patient.* A classic example of a Salter-Harris I injury is **slipped capital femoral epiphysis (SCFE),** an injury demonstrated in Chapter 13.

Salter Harris type II fractures involve a fracture of the physis, extending to the metaphysis. These may occur with or without displacement. When no displacement along the physis occurs, the physeal injury itself may not be apparent but must be inferred by the visible

metaphyseal fracture intersecting the growth plate. Remember that these fractures involve the metaphysis—be careful in using the terms *proximal* and *distal* to describe the extension of the fracture, because the position of the physis relative to the metaphysis is not fixed. At the proximal end of the bone, the physis is proximal to the metaphysis, so the fracture extends distally from the physis into the metaphysis. At the distal end of the bone, the physis is distal to the metaphysis, so the fracture extends proximally from the physis into the metaphysis.

Salter-Harris type III fractures extend from the physis into the epiphysis. As with type II fractures, they can be displaced or nondisplaced. Nondisplaced Salter-Harris III fractures can appear to involve only the epiphysis, but the fracture line extends to the physis—and a fracture through the physis must be inferred. Growth plate involvement is usually evident in displaced Salter-Harris III fractures, because displacement in the plane of the physis is visible.

Salter-Harris type IV fractures extend from the metaphysis, through the growth plate, and into the epiphysis. These fractures can occur with or without displacement. In some cases, the fracture line crosses directly through the growth plate, clearly connecting the epiphyseal and metaphyseal fractures. In other cases, the metaphyseal fracture line enters the physis, extends laterally in the plane of the physis, and exits at a different location into the epiphysis In these cases, the emergency physician must recognize that a type IV fracture is present and that the growth plate is involved, rather than interpreting the image as two isolated fractures without physis injury.

A **Salter-Harris type V** injury is a crush or compression injury of the growth plate. As with type I injuries, this injury can be radiographically occult, with a normal appearance or an appearance of modest loss of height of the normal growth plate. Consequently, a type V fracture should be specifically considered in a symptomatic patient with a normal x-ray.

Later in this chapter, figures depicting Salter-Harris fractures are labeled with icons to assist you in recognizing the fracture pattern.

Further Imaging of Pediatric Fractures: Is Computed Tomography or Magnetic Resonance Imaging Useful in Detection of Radiographically Occult Salter-Harris Injuries?

Suspected or radiographically confirmed Salter-Harris injuries are often followed today with additional advanced imaging (CT or MRI) to further characterize injuries. Such imaging provides additional diagnostic information, but it does so at a high economic cost. In addition, in the case of CT, the additional imaging results

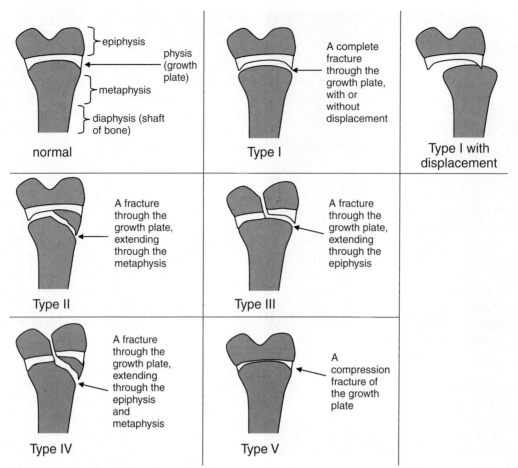

Figure 14-15. Salter-Harris fracture classification. The Salter-Harris classification is used to describe fractures involving the growth plate. Importantly, if the clinical scenario suggests fracture (with trauma and bony tenderness), a Salter-Harris I fracture may be present, even with normal x-rays. This classification scheme is used to describe injuries in pediatric patients in whom the growth plate is not yet closed. The scheme does not apply to adult patients. Refer to this figure when reviewing the x-rays that follow.

TABLE 14-4. A Mnemonic for the Salter Harris Classification: SALTER*

Mnemonic	Meaning	Salter Harris injury type	Prognosis
Straight Across	Involving only the growth plate	Salter Harris I	Good, little risk of growth arrest
Above	Involves the metaphysis as well as growth plate	Salter Harris II	Good
Lower bone	Involves the epiphysis as well as growth plate	Salter Harris III	Moderately good
Two bones	Involves the metaphysis and epiphysis as well as growth plate	Salter Harris IV	Moderately poor, treated surgically
End	Axial force to the "end" of the bone crushes the growth plate	Salter Harris V	Worst prognosis
Remember	Remember the mnemonic	—	—

Adapted from Tandberg D, Sherbring M: A mnemonic for the Salter-Harris classification. *Am J Emerg Med* 17:321, 1999.
*This mnemonic supposes that the Salter Harris injury has occurred at the distal end of the bone, giving meaning to the relationships "above" and "lower" below. For a Salter Harris injury of the proximal end of a bone, these relationships are reversed.

in substantial radiation exposure, an issue of increasing concern because of higher carcinogenic potential in children. The effective dose of a conventional ankle x-ray is approximately 0.01 to 0.05 mSv, whereas CT of the lower extremity results in an exposure as high as 2.7 mSv. Low-dose CT protocols have been developed to minimize radiation exposure while obtaining the additional information necessary for operative planning; one such protocol reduces the exposure to a dose range equivalent to that from plain film.[12]

A limitation of studies of MRI and CT in the setting of suspected injury is that no clear diagnostic reference standard is available; consequently, there is no simple method to determine whether MRI or CT findings represent true-positive, false-positive, true-negative, or false-negative results. This limitation is discussed in detail in Chapter 15.

Lemburg et al.[13] compared x-ray findings against a gold standard of CT to determine the sensitivity of x-ray and to estimate the additional diagnostic yield of CT for distal tibia growth plate injuries. X-ray underestimated the presence of metaphyseal fractures, articular surface dehiscence, and intraarticular fragments. It overestimated the presence of metaphyseal and epiphyseal fractures, and it was not specific for fractures of the growth plate and articular surface. As a result of overstimulation and underestimation of metaphyseal involvement, x-ray misclassified the Salter-Harris type in 30% of fractures. The importance of misclassifications of growth plate fractures based on x-ray to therapeutic planning is less clear, though therapeutic decisions often rest on the x-ray interpretation. Prospective studies comparing therapeutic plans and patient outcomes based on x-ray alone or the addition of CT have yet to be performed.

MRI provides a radiation-free means of assessing growth plate fractures and suspected fractures. An additional advantage of MRI is that it may diagnose ligamentous injuries that may clinically simulate fracture but do not require extended immobilization. In one study of 18 suspected Salter-Harris I fractures of the distal fibula, MRI revealed no Salter-Harris fractures but instead identified 14 ligamentous injuries, 11 bony contusions, and a fibular avulsion fracture that did not involve the growth plate.[14]

Pediatric Patterns of Ossification

Assessment of pediatric x-rays for fracture is complicated because bones in young children are not fully ossified and large segments of bones may be invisible on x-ray. Variations in the age at which ossification occurs have been described with both gender and ethnicity. The temporal patterns of ossification are described in detail in dedicated pediatric radiology texts and are beyond the scope of this text. However, the occurrence of incomplete ossification must be borne in mind when reviewing pediatric x-rays.

Pediatric Bony Tumors and Infections

Pediatric bony tumors, including both benign conditions such as bone cysts and malignant conditions such as sarcomas, must be suspected when fractures occur in the absence of significant trauma or when bony pain occurs in the absence of trauma. Although the multitude of radiographic features that assist in distinguishing these conditions is beyond the scope of this text, some general points of distinction can be made. Benign bony tumors are usually well circumscribed, whereas malignant bony tumors may have indistinct margins. A classic finding of malignant bony tumors is **periosteal reaction.** A triangular appearance of new periosteal bone called the **Codman triangle** may occur when tumor raises the periosteum away from cortical bone. Osteosarcoma, Ewing sarcoma, and subperiosteal abscesses may all create this appearance. Periosteal reaction can also be seen as a normal finding of bone healing, usually about 3 weeks into the healing process. Osteomyelitis can also lead to periosteal reaction, so the patient history must be considered. The possibility of a malignancy or bony infection should be entertained when reviewing pediatric orthopedic x-rays. Emergency physicians frequently review orthopedic x-rays and make clinical decisions without the immediate assistance or availability of a radiologist. Losses to follow-up can create medical and legal risk when a malignant or infectious lesion is not recognized in the emergency department. When uncertainty about the nature of a bone lesion exists, careful follow-up should be arranged.

Nonaccidental Trauma

Orthopedic injuries are common in **nonaccidental trauma** in children, with fractures being second only to skin lesions in frequency.[15] Humerus and femur fractures are the most common nonaccidental orthopedic injuries and are most frequent in children younger than 2 years.[16] When reviewing pediatric orthopedic x-rays, several clues should be sought that may support or confirm the diagnosis of nonaccidental trauma. Fractures that are inconsistent with the reported mechanism of injury should raise suspicion of nonaccidental trauma (Figure 14-16). The presence of multiple healing fractures, sometimes revealed only by the presence of callus at the location of an older and incompletely healed fracture, also is concerning. Long-bone fractures in nonambulatory infants are suspicious though not pathognomonic for abuse. **Corner fractures** are avulsion fractures (most commonly of the distal femur and proximal tibia), which result from violent shaking of a small infant (Figure 14-17). These injuries are considered pathognomonic for nonaccidental trauma, because they do not occur with other injury mechanisms such as falls or direct blows and are rarely seen with other inherited conditions.[15] Spiral fractures of extremities were once thought to be highly suspicious for nonaccidental trauma, but the link between this injury pattern and abuse has been questioned. A **toddler's fracture** is a spiral fracture of the tibia that can occur during a fall in the absence of nonaccidental trauma (Figure 14-18). Unfortunately, physicians may fail to consider a nonaccidental cause of trauma in young children, potentially leaving patients susceptible to continued injury or

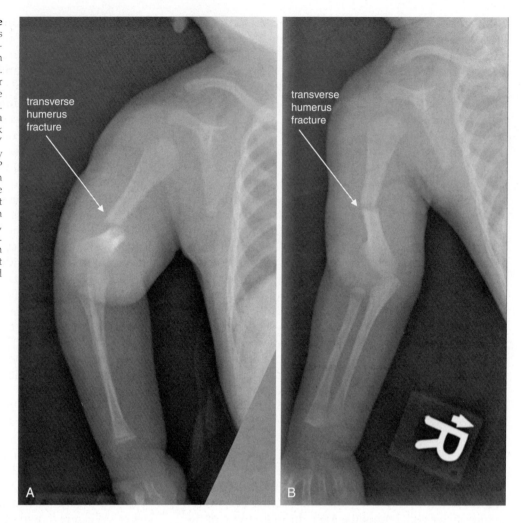

Figure 14-16. Humerus fracture from nonaccidental trauma. This full-term 7-week-old male presented with 1 day of crying when his right arm was manipulated. The mother stated that the father had accidentally rolled onto the child while asleep the prior night. The father had reported hearing a "popping sound" and then "shook the child to make sure he was OK." **A,** AP view of the upper extremity with the forearm pronated. **B,** AP view of the upper extremity with the forearm supinated. A complete transverse distal diaphyseal right humeral fracture is present, with anterior and medial displacement, as well as 2 mm of bony overlap. Delay in presentation after an injury and a history inconsistent with the observed injury are typical of nonaccidental trauma.

death. Racial disparities in reporting of potential abuse exist. In one study of children younger than 3 years admitted for skull or long-bone fracture, only 22.5% of white children versus 52.9% of minority children underwent evaluation for abuse.[17] Emergency physicians must consider nonaccidental trauma in every case of pediatric fracture.

Slipped Capital Femoral Epiphysis, Legg-Calvé-Perthes Disease, and Pediatric Pelvic Avulsion Fractures

Other common disorders of bone occur in skeletally immature children. SCFE is a displaced Salter-Harris I fracture of the physis of the proximal femur, occurring spontaneously in children, which can lead to avascular necrosis of the hip if not recognized and surgically treated. Legg-Calvé-Perthes disease is spontaneous avascular necrosis of the femoral head, which can lead to debilitating degenerative joint disease of the hip. A number of other avulsion fractures can occur at points of muscular attachment to the bony pelvis in young athletes, resulting from incomplete ossification. The preceding injuries are discussed and demonstrated in figures in Chapter 13.

PATHOLOGY ARCHIVE WITH FIGURES

Upper Extremity Imaging

In this section, we discuss upper extremity injuries and nontraumatic pathology, beginning with the proximal upper extremity and proceeding distally.

Scapulothoracic Dissociation

Scapulothoracic dissociation is a rare life- and limb-threatening injury because of the possibility of associated injuries to vessels such as the subclavian and axillary arteries. Neurologic injury accompanies this, with disruption of the brachial plexus or cervical nerve root avulsion. The flail extremity is consequently irreparably disabled, and amputation is commonly recommended.[18-20] The scapula may appear laterally displaced on chest x-ray, and the acromioclavicular (AC) joint is often disrupted. Clavicle fracture can accompany this injury, as can other upper extremity fractures. Based on a case series of eight patients, other findings such as apicolateral pleural cap and axillary or mediastinal hematoma may be seen.[21] The injury is so rare that large studies to delineate the common radiographic findings do not exist. When the injury is suspected, emergency

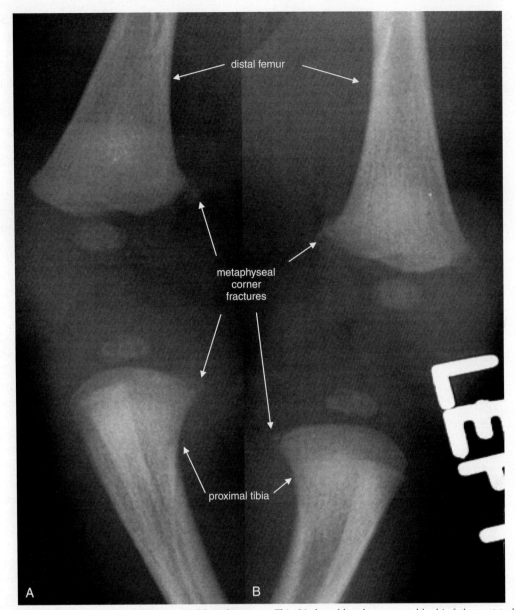

Figure 14-17. Metaphyseal corner fracture from nonaccidental trauma. This 21-day-old male was noted by his father not to be using his right arm normally after being dressed. No history of trauma was reported. A midshaft clavicle fracture was noted on x-ray (not shown). Although clavicle fractures can result from birth trauma during vaginal delivery, this injury is not compatible with birth trauma given the patient's age of 21 days and no evidence of healing on x-ray. A skeletal survey was performed. Close-ups from the patient's lower extremity x-rays are shown here. **A,** Right distal femur and proximal tibia. **B,** Left distal femur and proximal tibia. Multiple lower extremity metaphyseal corner fractures are present. These involve the bilateral distal femurs and proximal tibias. Corner fractures are highly suspicious for nonaccidental trauma. When multiple injuries are present without a history of trauma, nonaccidental trauma should be suspected. Formal skeletal survey radiographs should be performed, although this may be deferred until obvious acute injuries have been stabilized.

catheter angiography or CTA should be performed and preparation made for surgery.

Clavicle Fractures

Clavicle fracture (Figures 14-19 and 14-20) is commonly seen following motor vehicle collisions and bicycling injuries. Fractures are typically classified into three groups: fractures of the middle third (group I), the distal third (group II), and the medial third (group III), as shown in Table 14-5. Fractures of the middle third of the clavicle are most common. Fractures of the distal third of the clavicle account for 10% to 15% of injuries but are usually managed nonoperatively, unless significant displacement is present. Fractures of the medial third of the clavicle are rare and are associated with significant multisystem trauma, but the fractures themselves require little management and heal without sequelae following nonoperative management.[22]

Clavicle fractures are generally not radiographically or clinically occult. A standard frontal projection chest x-ray can reveal these fractures, and the asymptomatic side provides a normal image for comparison. Evaluation should include a search for other injuries, such as

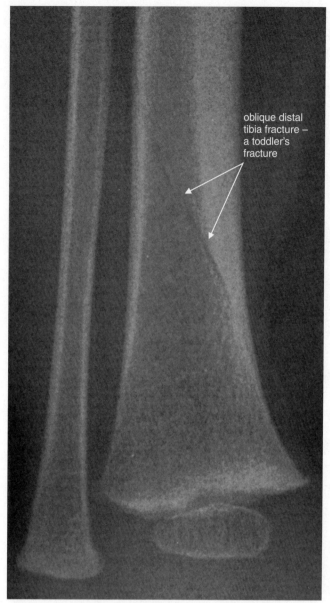

oblique distal tibia fracture – a toddler's fracture

Figure 14-18. Toddler's fracture. This 16-month-old male fell. The patient's mother attempted to catch him but lost her grip on his leg. He has been unable to bear weight without crying. Anterior–posterior view of the distal tibia and fibula. An oblique fracture is seen through the distal tibia, consistent with a toddler's fracture. This injury is usually not caused by nonaccidental trauma.

pneumothorax, scapula injury, and glenohumeral joint injuries. Dedicated clavicle x-rays can be obtained that provide an AP image with the x-ray beam angled 30 degrees cephalad. A serendipity view is a supine AP x-ray with the x-ray beam angled 40 degrees cephalad to evaluate the sternoclavicular joints. Indications for surgery in clavicle fractures are based more on clinical factors than on radiographic findings. Open fractures, gross fracture displacement with skin tenting, and fractures with significant medial displacement of the shoulder girdle are managed operatively. Less serious injuries in performance athletes may be surgically repaired to speed return to play.

Sternoclavicular Joint Dislocations. Sternoclavicular dislocations are discussed in Chapter 6.

Acromioclavicular Joint Dislocations. AC joint dislocations (also called separations) commonly occur with mechanisms similar to those for clavicle fractures. Although the name conventionally given to these injuries is *AC joint injury,* a second articulation is present in the same region and may be injured simultaneously. The acromion process of the scapula is attached medially to the distal clavicle by the AC ligament. The coracoid process of the scapula lies inferior to the clavicle and is attached to the clavicle by two coracoclavicular ligaments. AC joint separations can be classified by several grading systems (Table 14-6).

Standard shoulder radiographs, including nonstress (non-weight-bearing) AP, axillary, and lateral projections of the shoulder, can be used if AC or glenohumeral joint injury is suspected. The normal AC joint distance in the coronal plane is variable, usually 1-3 mm, and decreases with age (Figure 14-21). An AC joint distance of more than 7 mm in men and 6 mm in women is generally considered pathologic (Figure 14-22). The normal coracoclavicular distance is 11-13 mm; an increase of 50% suggests complete AC joint dislocation.[23] Stress views of the AC joint, consisting of an AP projection of the shoulder obtained with 10-15 pounds of weight attached to the arm, have been advocated to demonstrate ligamentous injury when subluxation is not evident on routine nonstress images. Normal AC joints show laxity of no more than 3 mm between the coracoid process and the clavicle with stress.[24] Stress images are not necessary if subluxation is readily evident on routine images. Because management is not significantly altered in most cases by the occurrence of subluxation on stress images, it is not clear that patients benefit from this additional imaging, which can cause pain in the setting of an acute injury. If stress images are obtained, the patient should not hold the weight, because this can decrease the amount of subluxation visible radiographically because of recruitment of muscles.[25] Bossart et al.[26] found that weighted or "stress" x-rays only identified Grade III injuries (see Table 14-6) in 4% of cases in which the injury was not evident on routine imaging and recommended that this imaging technique be abandoned.

MRI can differentiate between Rockwood type II and Rockwood type III injuries when these cannot be distinguished clinically or by x-ray findings.[23] However, studies suggest even type III injuries have good outcomes when managed nonoperatively, so specific diagnosis is likely unnecessary.[27]

Glenohumeral Joint (Shoulder) Dislocations
Glenohumeral joint dislocations are evaluated using three standard x-ray views: an AP x-ray of the shoulder, a lateral view called the **scapular "Y" view,** and an

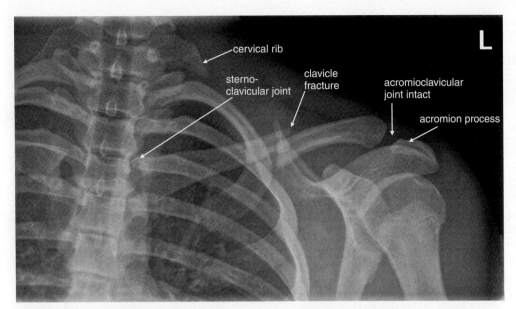

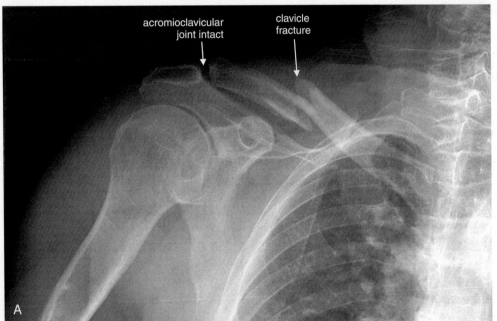

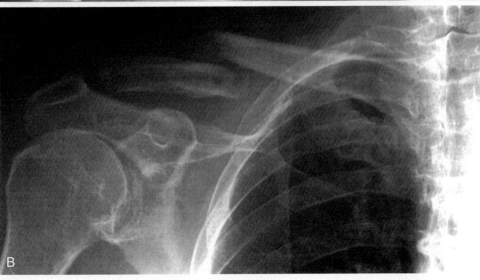

Figure 14-19. Clavicle fracture. This 15-year-old male wrestler presented with left clavicle pain after a second wrestler fell on his left shoulder. His x-ray shows a mildly displaced midclavicular fracture with inferior displacement of the lateral fragment. The acromioclavicular (AC) joint appears intact. The sternoclavicular joint also appears normally aligned. Remember to look for clavicle fractures, sternoclavicular joint, and AC joint alignment on chest x-rays after trauma. Incidentally, this patient has vestigial cervical ribs.

Figure 14-20. Clavicle fracture. This 77-year-old male presented after being hit by a car on his bike. **A,** The patient has a fracture of the distal third of the clavicle, with displacement of the fragments. Using typical nomenclature, the distal fragment would be described as inferiorly displaced relative to the proximal fragment. In this case, the radiologist described the proximal fragment as superiorly displaced relative to the distal fragment, which communicates the same information. **B,** Three months later, this fracture shows minimal callus formation and demonstrates continued displacement and nonunion.

TABLE 14-5. Clavicle Fractures

Group	FRACTURE LOCATION		Frequency (% of all clavicle fractures)	Outcomes
I	Middle third of the clavicle		80%-85%	The medial fragment is usually displaced cephalad by the sternocleidomastoid muscle.
II	Distal third of the clavicle	Type I—minimal displacement	10%-15%	Despite a high incidence of nonunion, most nonunions are asymptomatic and do not require surgery. Type II fractures may require surgery because of displacement.
		Type II—fracture medial to the coracoclavicular ligaments, leading to upward displacement of the medial fragment		
		Type III—articular surface fractures of the AC joint, which may be confused with AC joint separation		
III	Medial third of the clavicle		5%-10%	These fractures are associated with other serious traumatic injuries but have little significance themselves. Most heal with nonoperative management.

Adapted from Post M: Current concepts in the treatment of fractures of the clavicle. *Clin Orthop Relat Res* 245: 89-101, 1989.

TABLE 14-6. Classification of Acromioclavicular Dislocations or Separations

Injury Grade	Description	X-ray Findings
I	Sprain or incomplete tear of the AC ligament	Findings are normal, without subluxation even with application of stress.
II	Subluxation of the AC joint with disruption of the AC ligament, but the coracoclavicular ligaments remain intact	Routine x-rays of the shoulder are normal. Subluxation of the AC joint occurs in stress views. Separation of the clavicle from the acromion process is no more than half of the clavicle diameter. The distance from the clavicle to the coracoid process is preserved.
III	Complete disruption of the AC and coracoclavicular ligaments, with upward displacement of the distal clavicle	Routine x-rays show widening of the AC and coracoclavicular joints. Stress views are unnecessary.
Rockwood Type	**Description**	**Typical Treatment**
I	Sprain of the joint without a complete tear of either ligament	Nonoperative management
II	• Tear of AC ligaments with coracoclavicular ligaments intact • No visible marked elevation of the lateral end of the clavicle • May display >5-mm elevation of the AC joint without weights (consistent with severe type II injury)	Nonoperative management except most severe cases
III	• Both AC and coracoclavicular ligaments are torn • >5-mm elevation of the AC joint without weights	Controversial management; nonoperative management encouraged
IV	Distal clavicle impaled posteriorly into the trapezial fascia	Operative management
V	Disruption of all ligaments with the clavicle displaced superiorly toward the base of the neck	Operative management
VI	Inferior dislocation of the clavicle with the lateral end displaced down	Operative management

Adapted from Alyas F, Curtis M, Speed C, et al. MR imaging appearances of acromioclavicular joint dislocation. *Radiographics* 28:463-479, 2008; quiz 619.

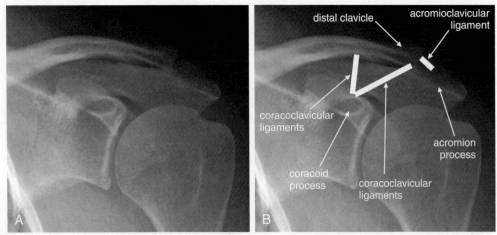

Figure 14-21. Normal acromioclavicular (AC) and coracoclavicular joints. A normal AC joint shows close apposition of the distal clavicle and the acromion process of the scapula. These are joined by the AC ligament, which is invisible on x-ray. A second joint is also present: the corococlavicular ligament joins the coracoid process of the scapula to the distal clavicle. Injuries to these ligaments can lead to separation of these joints, as shown in Figure 14-22. **A,** Normal AC joint. **B,** Same image with the position of the AC and coracoclavicular ligaments shown.

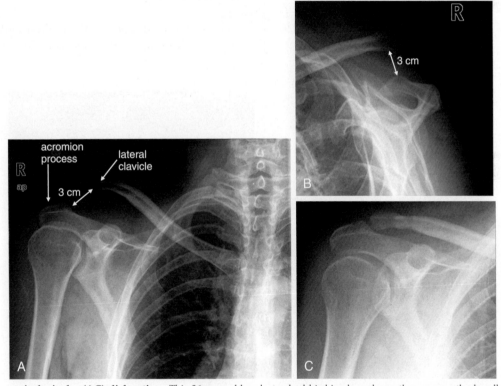

Figure 14-22. Acromioclavicular (AC) dislocation. This 36-year-old male crashed his bicycle and was thrown over the handlebars, sustaining a Rockwood type V AC separation. Nearly 3 cm of separation is present. This was surgically repaired 2 weeks later with a hamstring tendon graft. His postoperative x-ray shows a normal AC joint. **A,** Anterior–posterior (AP) view. **B,** Lateral view. **C,** Postoperative AP view.

axillary view. It is important to recognize that dislocation can be excluded only by examining two orthogonal views. The functions of each of these views are described in Table 14-7. The normal glenohumeral joint is shown in Figure 14-23.

The most common dislocations of the glenohumeral joint (more than 90%) are **anterior shoulder dislocations.**[28] In this injury pattern, the humeral head is typically displaced anteriorly, medially, and inferiorly relative to the glenoid fossa (Figures 14-24 and 14-25). On the AP view, the humeral head usually lies medial to the glenoid fossa, inferior to the coracoid process. It also may commonly be seen in a subglenoid position. On the AP view, the AP alignment of the humeral head with the glenoid fossa cannot be determined —so a normal appearing AP x-ray does not exclude pure anterior dislocation. On the scapular "Y" view, the humeral head is seen anterior to the center of the scapular "Y".

TABLE 14-7. Standard Radiographic Views of the Shoulder, With the Functions in Evaluation of the Glenohumeral Joint

X-ray View	Description or Function
AP	This view allows evaluation of medial–lateral and inferior–superior dislocation of the humeral head relative to the glenoid fossa. *It does not allow evaluation of AP displacement of the humeral head.* It does allow evaluation of humerus, scapula, and clavicle fractures.
Scapular "Y" or lateral shoulder	The glenoid fossa is located at the convergence of a "Y" formed by the body of the scapula inferiorly, the scapular spine and acromion process posteriorly, and the coracoid process anteriorly. A normally located humeral head overlies this intersection. *This view allows evaluation of AP displacement of the humeral head.*
Axillary	This view confirms apposition of the humeral head and glenoid fossa articular surface.

Posterior shoulder dislocations are rarer, constituting only a few percent of all glenohumeral dislocations.[28] The appearance on an AP x-ray is similar to that seen with an anterior dislocation, with the humeral head often lying inferior to the glenoid fossa. As with anterior dislocation, the AP x-ray cannot determine the AP location of the humeral head relative to the glenoid fossa, so a normal AP x-ray cannot exclude pure posterior dislocation. The scapular "Y" view confirms or excludes posterior dislocation of the humeral head (Figure 14-26). An axillary view can clarify uncertain findings on AP and "Y" views.

Rarer still are **inferior shoulder dislocations (luxatio erecta)** and **superior dislocations.** Inferior dislocations are usually clinically evident because of the position of the arm, with the humerus abducted, the elbow flexed, and the hand behind or atop the patient's head (Figure 14-27). The humeral head again appears inferior to the glenoid fossa on the AP view.

Glenohumeral dislocations are frequently associated with two fractures: the **Bankart lesion** and **Hill-Sachs**

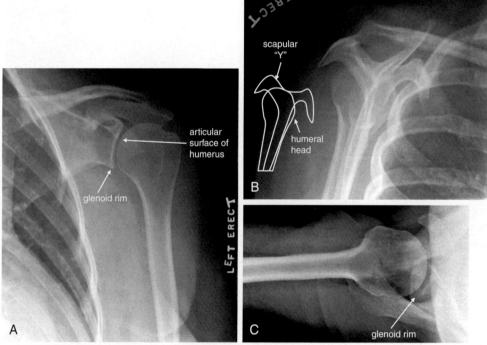

Figure 14-23. Normal shoulder. This 68-year-old female presented with shoulder pain without trauma. This x-ray shows the configuration of the normal glenohumeral joint. On the frontal projection **(A),** the curve of the humeral head is seated in the shallow curve of the glenoid fossa and overlaps slightly with the coracoid and acromion processes of the scapula. A scapular "Y" view **(B)** was obtained by aligning the x-ray beam laterally so that it is in the plane of the scapular body. This perspective places the glenoid fossa en face to the x-ray beam. The glenoid fossa lies at the center of the "Y" formed by the union of the scapular spine and acromion process posteriorly, the body of the scapula inferiorly, and the coracoid process anteriorly. A normally positioned humeral head should lie at the center of the glenoid fossa in this view. The coracoid process can be seen projecting anteriorly. In an axillary view **(C),** the x-ray beam is oriented up into the axilla and the humerus is slightly abducted. Again, the humeral head can be seen articulating with the surface of the glenoid fossa. In an anterior shoulder dislocation, the frontal projection usually shows medial and sometimes inferior displacement of the humeral head. The "Y" view shows the humeral head is anterior to the center of the "Y." In a posterior dislocation (see Figure 14-24), the frontal projection occasionally appears normal, but the "Y" view shows the head is posterior to the center of the "Y."

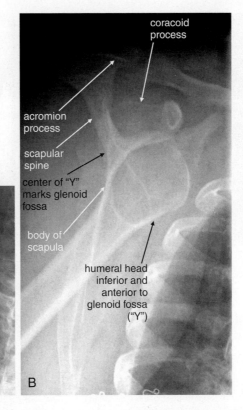

Figure 14-24. Anterior shoulder (glenohumeral joint) dislocation. This 50-year-old female fell from standing, landing on her right shoulder. **A,** Anterior–posterior view. The humeral head is medially and inferiorly displaced—typical of anterior dislocation. A *dashed line* has been added to show the normal position of the humeral head. **B,** Scapular "Y" view. The humeral head is anterior to the confluence of the "Y" of the scapular body inferiorly, scapular spine and acromion process posteriorly, and coracoid process anteriorly. This "Y" marks the location of the glenoid fossa. The humeral head should be centered there.

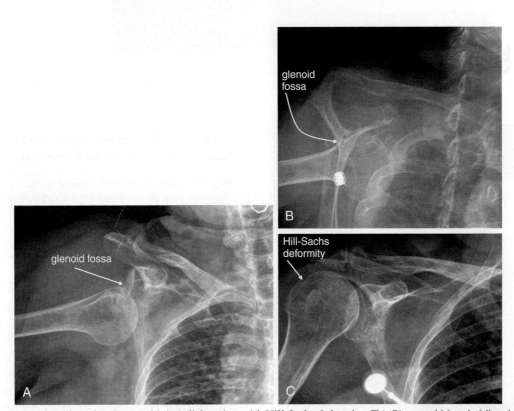

Figure 14-25. Anterior shoulder (glenohumeral joint) dislocation with Hill-Sachs deformity. This 71-year-old female fell on her right shoulder from a standing position. Again, notice the inferior position of the humeral head relative to the glenoid fossa on the anterior–posterior (AP) view **(A).** In a scapular "Y" view **(B),** the humeral head is anterior to the "Y" marking the glenoid fossa. On the postreduction AP view **(C),** a cortical irregularity of the posterolateral humeral head is seen—a Hill-Sachs lesion (named for Harold Arthur Hill and Maurice David Sachs, the radiologists who described this lesion and its mechanism of injury). This is a compression deformity of the humeral head that occurs as the soft humeral head impacts against the glenoid rim during anterior shoulder dislocation. The lesion is felt to be quite specific for anterior shoulder dislocation. However, the clinical relevance is less evident. Unless large and symptomatic (causing clicking or catching of the joint), most do not require treatment.

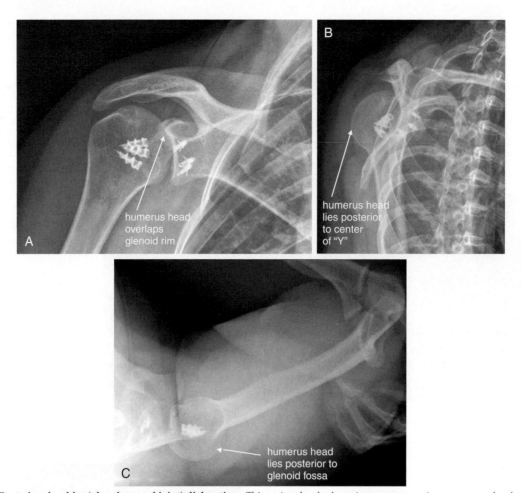

Figure 14-26. Posterior shoulder (glenohumeral joint) dislocation. This patient has had previous reconstructive surgery, and orthopedic hardware is visible. **A,** Anterior–posterior view. The humeral head looks nearly normal in position, but it overlaps the glenoid rim more than usual. **B,** Scapular "Y" view. The humeral head is slightly posterior to the center of the "Y," indicating posterior dislocation. **C,** Axillary view. The humeral head is again posteriorly subluxed.

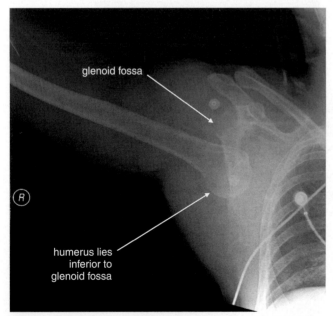

Figure 14-27. Inferior shoulder (glenohumeral joint) dislocation with luxatio erecta. This patient presented with a classic appearance of luxatio erecta (inferior glenohumeral joint dislocation) following a motorcycle collision. The arm is abducted, and the patient's hand was raised above his head.

Box 14-4: Fractures Associated With Glenohumeral Joint Dislocation

- **Bankart fracture (lesion)—fracture of inferior rim of glenoid fossa, associated with avulsion of the labrum**
- **Hill-Sachs deformity—depression fracture of posterolateral humeral head, associated with anterior humerus dislocation**

deformity (Box 14-4 and Figure 14-28; see also Figure 14-25). These fractures have little immediate clinical significance. However, the Bankart fracture is associated with tears of the anterior-inferior labrum of the shoulder (visible with MRI), and thus is associated with repeated dislocation.[29] MRI is considered more sensitive than x-ray[30] but has no role for this indication in the emergency department. Ultrasound is also sensitive (95.6%) and specific (92.8%). CT arthrogram (using intra-articular contrast injection) can also diagnose this condition but would rarely be needed in the ED.[31]

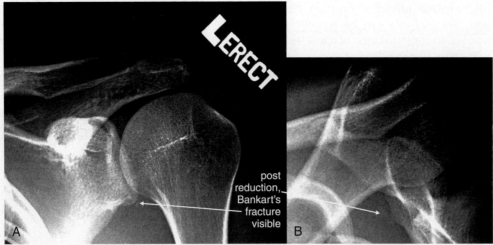

Figure 14-28. Bankart fracture. This patient presented with his arm held in abduction and elevation, clinically appearing to be a case of luxatio erecta associated with inferior glenohumeral dislocation. His x-rays showed a more typical anterior dislocation appearance. On this postreduction x-ray, a small fragment is seen consistent with a Bankart fracture. A Bankart fracture is an avulsion of the anteroinferior glenoid labrum that usually occurs with inferior–anterior dislocation. Although subtle in appearance, the lesion is thought to be significant because it indicates stretching of the anteroinferior glenohumeral ligament, which is not visible on x-ray. Disruption of the joint capsule associated with the Bankart lesion results in continued anterior instability and a predisposition to recurrent dislocation.

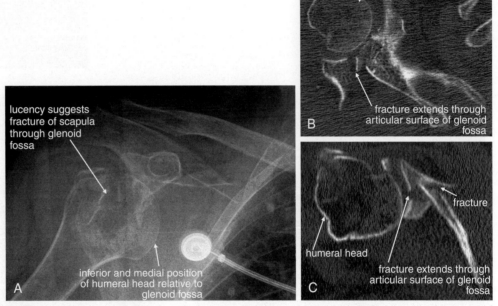

Figure 14-29. Scapular fracture with glenoid fossa involvement. Scapula fractures are often associated with high-energy mechanisms and multisystem trauma, but sometimes relatively minor trauma can result in such injuries. This 85-year-old female fell from a standing position and complained of shoulder pain. **A,** Her x-ray shows anterior dislocation of the humeral head. The glenoid fossa is partially obscured behind the humerus, but a lucent area centered on the humeral head suggests a scapula fracture. CT shows a comminuted intraarticular fracture of the scapula involving the glenoid fossa. **B,** Axial reconstruction. **C,** Coronal CT reconstruction. Fractures of the scapula can be difficult to evaluate with x-ray. CT scan with multiplanar reformations can provide detailed information about the scope of scapula injury. In particular, CT provides information about intraarticular injury to the glenoid fossa, which may require surgical intervention.

Scapular Fractures

Scapula fractures (Figures 14-29 through 14-31) are classically high-energy injuries, usually caused by mechanisms such as motor vehicle collision or falls from height. They can be associated with significant multisystem trauma, including mediastinal injury, so careful interpretation of images should be performed, with attention paid to the possibility of other injuries.

A standard AP or posterior–anterior chest x-ray can reveal scapular fracture. Overlying skin folds can simulate fracture, and the medial border of the scapula can be mistaken for the pleural line of a pneumothorax (or vice versa). A standard shoulder series (described earlier) should also be obtained to allow inspection of the scapular spine, body, and glenoid fossa. CT scan is more sensitive and should be obtained when scapular injury is strongly suspected or when fractures identified on x-ray require further delineation. The scapula can be reconstructed from CT datasets acquired for evaluation of chest trauma, so additional CT imaging is generally not required if the patient has undergone chest CT. If the patient does not require CT imaging for other indications, scapular CT can be performed without intravenous (IV) contrast. Thin-section CT (1-mm to 2.5-mm slice thickness) with multiplanar reformations is useful in characterizing fractures.[32-33] Haapamaki et al.[33] compared x-ray and CT

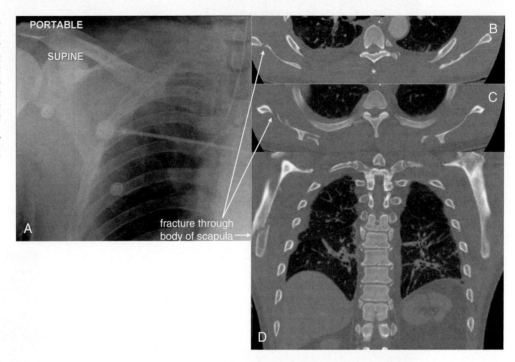

Figure 14-30. Scapular fracture. This 56-year-old male has a scapular fracture following major trauma. His chest x-ray did not reveal this injury. He underwent pan–CT for associated injuries. His chest CT provides clear anatomic detail of his scapular fracture. He died soon after from traumatic brain injury and herniation. **A,** Chest x-ray. **B, C,** Axial chest CT images, bone window. **D,** Coronal reconstruction.

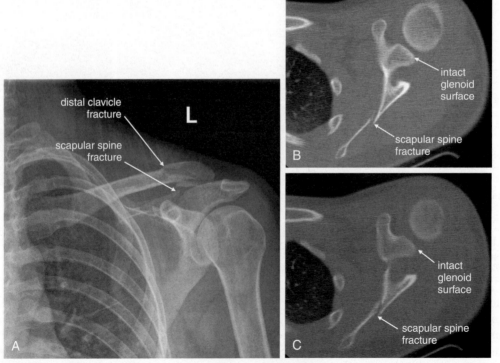

Figure 14-31. Scapula fracture. This 19-year-old female presented after hydroplaning her car on a wet road at 60 mph, spinning the vehicle into a tree. Her sole complaint was left shoulder pain with tenderness over her left scapula and distal clavicle. **A,** X-ray reveals fractures of the distal clavicle and scapular spine. Avoid the error of stopping your evaluation after identifying the first fracture. **B, C,** Axial CT images show the fracture extends through the scapular spine and body, sparing the glenoid fossa. This injury was treated nonoperatively. Although scapular fractures in the setting of high-speed mechanisms of injury, as in this case, are associated with other major injuries, this patient had none and did well on follow-up.

for the diagnosis of scapular fractures in 210 patients. Compared with CT, x-ray was insensitive in diagnosis of many fracture types (Table 14-8).

Humerus Fractures

Humerus fractures are most commonly evaluated with two orthogonal x-rays: an AP and a lateral view. Fractures of the head, neck, and shaft are generally not radiographically occult, with the exception of Hill-Sachs lesions, described earlier in the section on shoulder dislocation. As we discuss later, fractures of the distal humerus can be radiographically subtle, particularly in children. These injuries can have neurovascular repercussions and are often treated operatively, so careful attention to x-ray findings and the possibility of hidden injury is essential.

TABLE 14-8. Sensitivity of X-ray for Scapular Fracture, Compared With Diagnostic Standard of Computed Tomography

Fracture Type	X-ray Sensitivity (CT = assumed to be 100%)
Glenoid	88%
• Anterior inferior part of glenoid	95%
• Glenoid fossa	65%
Acromion	86%
Coracoid process	40%
Scapular neck	82%
Scapular wing	94%
Scapular spine	57%

Adapted from Haapamaki VV, Kiuru MJ, Koskinen SK: Multidetector CT in shoulder fractures. *Emerg Radiol* 11:89-94, 2004.

Proximal Humerus Fractures (Head and Neck). Fractures of the anatomic neck of the humerus are uncommon but can jeopardize the blood supply of the articular surface, leading to ischemic necrosis. Fractures of the surgical neck of the humerus (Figures 14-32 through 14-34), or proximal diaphyseal fractures, also threaten the blood supply of the articular surface. These injuries typically require surgical fixation if displaced or angulated, whereas less-displaced fractures are sometimes treated nonoperatively with a sling. Avulsion fractures of the greater and lesser humeral tuberosities may also be seen. Greater tuberosity fragments are often laterally and superiorly displaced, whereas lesser tuberosity fragments are usually pulled inferomedially by the attached muscles.

Humeral Shaft Fractures. The humeral shaft most commonly fractures in its middle third (Figure 14-35). Neurovascular injuries can result and should be assessed on physical examination when humeral diaphyseal fractures are identified on x-ray. Brachial artery and vein and radial, median, and ulnar nerve injuries should be suspected. Nerve and vascular injury can result from the initial injury or from attempts at reduction.

Fractures of the Elbow

Fractures of the elbow are technically fractures of the distal humerus, proximal radius, and proximal ulna. In children, supracondylar fractures are most common (55%), followed by radial neck fractures (14%) and lateral humeral condyle fractures (12%).[34] We begin our discussion with fractures of the distal humerus.

Supracondylar Humerus Fractures. Supracondylar humerus fractures (Figures 14-36 through 14-40 and 14-42) are rare in adults, accounting for only about 3%

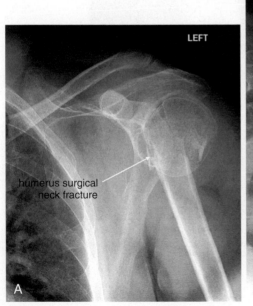

A

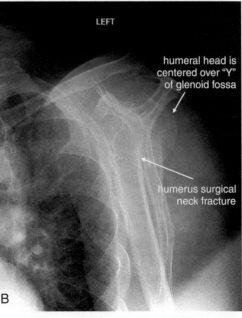

B

Figure 14-32. **Humerus fracture (surgical neck).** This 60-year-old male presented with right shoulder pain after slipping on a wet floor and landing directly on his left shoulder. **A,** His anterior–posterior x-ray shows the humeral head to be appropriately located in the glenoid fossa. However, the surgical neck of the humerus shows a complete fracture through both cortices. The distal fragment is overriding the proximal fragment and is dislocated slightly medially. **B,** The lateral (scapular "Y") view confirms these findings. The shaft of the humerus does not intersect the humeral head in the expected location. This injury was treated nonoperatively.

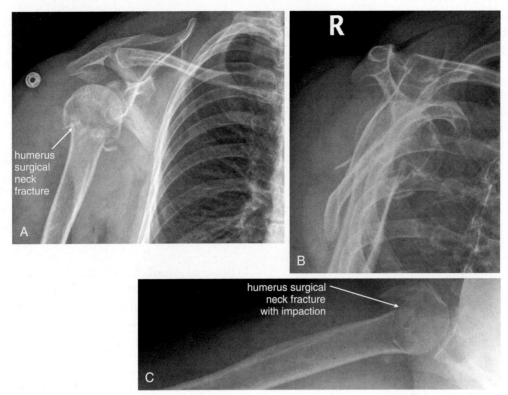

Figure 14-33. Humerus fracture (surgical neck). This 60-year-old female presented with right shoulder pain after falling onto her right arm while intoxicated. X-ray shows a humeral neck fracture with the distal fragment impacted. The humeral head is seated in the glenoid fossa normally. **A,** Anterior–posterior view. **B,** Scapular "Y" view. **C,** Axillary view.

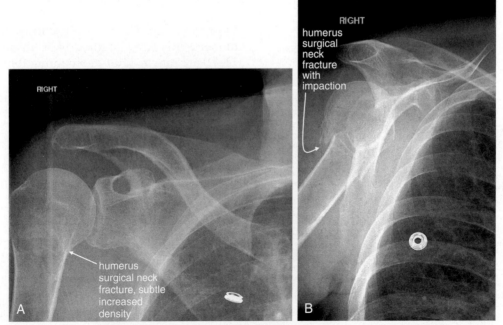

Figure 14-34. Humerus fracture (surgical neck). This 54-year-old female fell onto her right arm. Her x-rays show the importance of obtaining appropriate orthogonal views to avoid missing a fracture. **A,** Anterior–posterior view. A subtle band of sclerosis is seen but might be missed—this represents the fracture zone. **B,** Lateral (scapular "Y") view. A complete fracture of the humeral neck is visible, and there is impaction of the distal fragment. The overlap of the fragments accounts for the increased density seen in **A.**

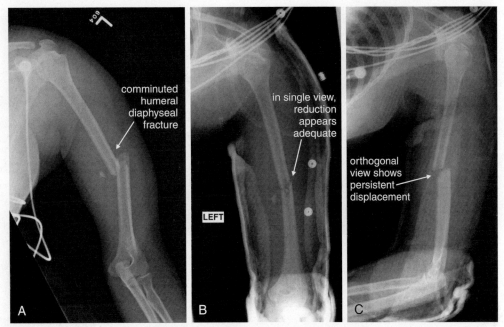

Figure 14-35. Humerus fracture (diaphyseal). This 17-year-old female was struck by a car while crossing a road. Her x-ray shows a comminuted midshaft humerus fracture with angulation of the distal fragment. **A,** Only a single x-ray was obtained before reduction, so additional displacement in the perpendicular plane cannot be assessed. **B,** After splinting, reduction appears adequate in a single view. **C,** An orthogonal view demonstrates persistent fracture displacement. Two perpendicular views are needed to assess alignment in fractures and dislocations. As a rule, midshaft long-bone fractures are easily recognized, because they do not involve the overlap of other bones and normal structures such as growth plates that can make proximal and distal fractures near joints more difficult to assess.

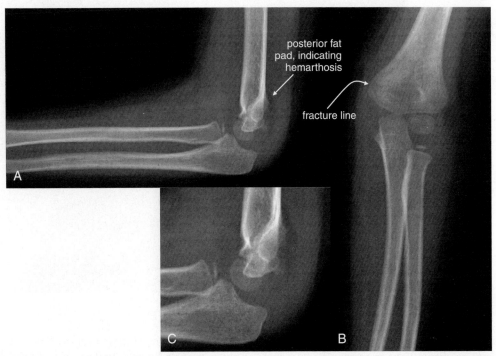

Figure 14-36. Distal humerus fracture (medial condylar fracture with pathologic fat pad sign). This 3-year-old female fell while jumping on a trampoline and landed on her left elbow. Her x-ray shows a nondisplaced medial condylar fracture with mild dorsal angulation of the distal fracture fragment. A large posterior fat pad is visible—a sign of hemarthrosis that should alert you to possible fracture even if no fracture is seen. Fat pads are normally hidden from sight in bony grooves on the lateral view. Blood tracking in these grooves can elevate the fat pad, making it visible. An anterior fat pad can be normal, but a posterior fat pad is a pathologic sign of joint effusion or hemarthosiosis (though not always associated with fracture). **A,** Lateral view. **B,** Anterior–posterior view. **C,** Close-up from **A.**

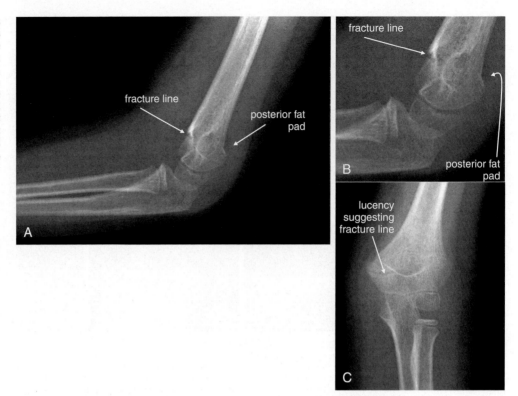

Figure 14-37. Distal humerus fracture (medial condyle). This 5-year-old female fell while playing and complained of pain and tenderness above her elbow. As in the last case (Figure 14-36), a cortical defect is seen in the humerus, involving the medial condyle. Note the posterior fat pad, a sign of hemarthrosis often associated with fracture. **A,** Lateral view. **B,** Close-up from **A. C,** Anterior-posterior view.

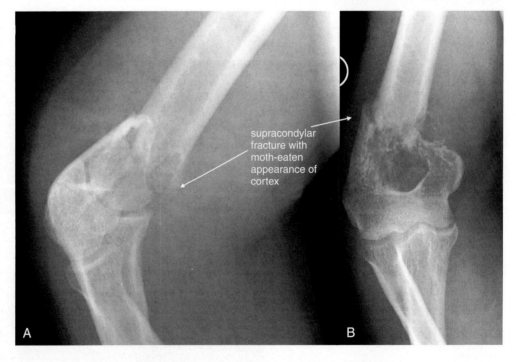

Figure 14-38. Distal humerus fracture (pathologic supracondylar fracture). This 46-year-old male complained of severe pain in his right arm after skeet shooting. He stated that the shotgun recoiled against his right arm and that he heard a "pop" emanating from his arm. His x-ray shows an obvious fracture proximal to the humeral condyles. The history is concerning for pathologic fracture, given a modest injury mechanism. Look carefully at the lateral view **(A).** The proximal fragment has a thinned and irregular cortex, suggesting that a lytic lesion may have been present before the fracture. **B,** Anterior–posterior view. The patient underwent further workup, revealing multiple myeloma. His CT scan is reviewed in Figure 14-39.

of adult fractures. In children, these fractures are more common and can be difficult to diagnose because of skeletal immaturity. Most supracondylar fractures are extension injuries, resulting from falls on outstretched arms. The distal fracture fragments are often posteriorly displaced. *Displaced supracondylar humerus fractures can result in brachial artery and median, radial, and anterior interosseous nerve injury, so this fracture pattern must be recognized and associated neurovascular injuries must be investigated. Volkmann ischemic contracture can result from postfracture edema and forearm compartment syndrome.* As the name implies, these injuries occur proximal to the humeral condyles and may be extraarticular. However, they often require internal fixation to prevent vascular compression and ischemia and to allow stabilization and early mobilization of the elbow.

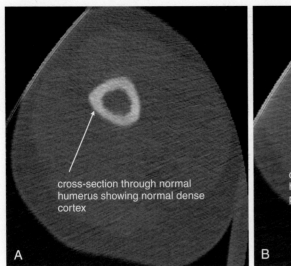

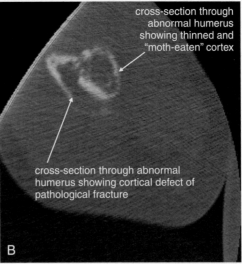

cross-section through
abnormal humerus
showing thinned and
"moth-eaten" cortex

cross-section through normal
humerus showing normal dense
cortex

cross-section through abnormal
humerus showing cortical defect of
pathological fracture

Figure 14-39. **Humerus fracture (pathologic fracture with multiple myeloma), CT.** Same patient as in Figure 14-38. **A,** Axial section through the normal humerus proximal to the fracture zone. **B,** Slice through the fracture zone. In addition to the obvious cortical defect, note the moth-eaten appearance of the bony cortex compared to **A.** The patient was diagnosed with multiple myeloma on further workup.

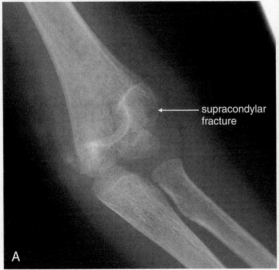

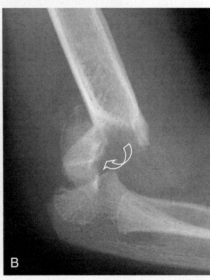

supracondylar
fracture

Figure 14-40. **Distal humerus fracture (supracondylar fracture).** This 4-year-old female fell from a couch onto her outstretched hand, sustaining a supracondylar humeral fracture. **A,** An anterior–posterior view shows a fairly subtle lucency through the distal humerus. Although you may recognize this as a fracture, the degree of displacement appears minimal. In contrast, the lateral view **(B)** shows dramatic posterior displacement and angulation of the distal fracture fragment, emphasizing the importance of obtaining perpendicular views when evaluating for fracture or dislocation. The *curved arrow* is meant to convey the rotation of the fracture fragment to reach its current position. The patient underwent closed reduction and percutaneous pinning, followed by long arm cast application.

Several classification schemes have been proposed to describe supracondylar fractures, specifically with preoperative planning in mind. For emergency physicians, recognizing subtle indicators of fracture and characterizing the radiographic abnormalities by usual descriptive terms (see Table 14-3) may suffice. AP and lateral x-rays of the elbow are usually obtained to evaluate these injuries. In complex fractures, CT can assist in delineating injuries.

Medial Epicondylar Humerus Fractures. Fractures of the medial epicondyle are common in children between the ages of 9 and 14. Most are extraarticular, because the medial epicondyle forms an apophysis of the humerus and is not part of the articular surface. The injury can be confused with medial condyle fracture, particularly in children with incomplete ossification. An isolated medial epicondyle fracture is not associated with a positive **fat pad sign,** because the medial epicondyle is largely outside of the joint capsule. In contrast, a medial condyle fracture is included within the joint capsule and can result in a pathologic fat pad sign. Displacement of the epicondyle greater than 5 mm is considered an indication for surgical fixation, and functional outcomes are good with this treatment.[35] Most fractures with lesser degrees of displacement are treated nonoperatively with casting, with good outcomes.[36] Ulnar nerve contusion can occur with this injury. Dislocation of the elbow commonly results in epicondylar fracture.[35,37]

Medial Humeral Condylar Fractures. Medial humeral condyle fractures (Figure 14-43) separate the medial metaphysis and epicondyle from the remainder of the humerus. The fracture is intraarticular, involving the trochlea (the grooved surface of the distal humerus that articulates with the ulna), and thus compromises the stability of the elbow. The injury is rare and can be difficult to distinguish from medial epicondyle fracture, caused by incomplete ossification in children, the common population for this injury. When x-rays are inconclusive, arthrography,[38] CT, or MRI can be diagnostic. A clue to the injury is the fat pad sign, resulting from displacement of normal fat by hematoma. A Milch type I fracture splits the trochlear groove, leaving the lateral ridge of the trochlea attached to the proximal portion of the humerus. This injury is somewhat more stable than the Milch type II fracture, which includes the entire trochlea in the distal fracture fragment and is unstable, requiring open reduction and internal fixation. These injuries are particularly serious in children because they are Salter-Harris IV injuries (by definition, involving the growth plate) and are intraarticular. Complications include growth arrest and arthritis.[39]

Lateral Humeral Condylar Fractures. Lateral humerus condylar fractures are common in young children between the ages of 5 and 10 years. They are often radiographically subtle or occult, because the distal humerus is primarily cartilage at this age. Because of this subtlety, lateral and oblique x-rays of both elbows are usually recommended to provide a normal comparison view. The typical course of the fracture line is from the lateral metaphysis proximal to the condyle, traveling distally and exiting through the articular surface in either the medial trochlear notch or the capitellotrochlear groove.[40]

Lateral condyle fractures can be characterized by the Milch or Jakob systems (Table 14-9).[41-42] When considering the importance of lateral condyle fractures, recognize that the lateral condyle includes the capitellum and the lateral portion of the trochlea. The capitellum articulates with the radius and is thus important to forearm supination and pronation but not to elbow stability. The trochlea articulates with the ulnar and must be intact for stability of the elbow joint. Thus lateral condyle fractures that extend to the lateral trochlea can render the elbow unstable.

When the diagnosis is uncertain from x-ray, CT or MRI can be performed to confirm or exclude lateral humeral condyle fracture. Complications of this injury include nonunion, malunion, valgus angulation, and avascular necrosis—all potentially affecting elbow function. Fractures with greater than 2 mm of displacement are treated surgically, with percutaneous pinning or open reduction and internal fixation.[40]

TABLE 14-9. Classifications of Lateral Humerus Condyle Fractures

Milch Type	Description
I (less common)	• Extends through the ossification center of the lateral condyle and exits at the radiocapitellar groove • Salter-Harris IV fracture • Relatively stable, because the lateral portion of the trochlea is intact
II (more common)	• Extends across the physis and exits through the apex of the trochlea • Salter-Harris II or IV fracture • Lateral trochlea is part of the fracture fragment, rendering the elbow unstable
Jakob Stage	**Description**
I	Nondisplaced, extraarticular
II	Intraarticular fracture, with moderate rotational displacement
III	Complete displacement and capitellar rotation with elbow instability

Adapted from Milch H: Fractures and Fracture Dislocations of the Humeral Condyles. *J Trauma* 4:592-607, 1964; Jakob R, Fowles JV, Rang M, Kassab MT: Observations concerning fractures of the lateral humeral condyle in children. *J Bone Joint Surg Br* 57: 430-436, 1975.

Intercondylar Humerus Fractures. Intercondylar humerus fractures can occur in adults following major trauma or with falls on an outstretched arm. These can be complex injuries requiring surgical fixation and even total elbow replacement. Numerous classification systems have been proposed, but none fully describe all possible fracture patterns. Involvement of the articular surface should be described, noting injuries to the lateral and medial condyles.

Assessment of Injuries Involving the Trochlea and Capitellum. In addition to the preceding considerations, the trochlea and capitellum should be assessed on the lateral and AP radiographs. Subtle abnormalities in alignment may be visible, revealing an otherwise occult fracture, particularly in children with incomplete ossification. On the lateral x-ray, the anterior humeral line should intersect the middle third of the capitellum. In case of fracture, posterior angulation of the distal fracture fragment can displace the capitellum posterior to the anterior humeral line. A second line, the radiocapitellar line, is drawn down the center of the long axis of the radius and should intersect the capitellum on both AP and lateral x-rays (Figure 14-41). Displacement of the radial head, or fractures or dislocations of the capitellum (including supracondylar humerus fractures), can disrupt this normal alignment (see Figure 14-42). Fractures of the trochlea and capitellum are intraarticular and may result in a pathologic fat pad (see Figures 14-7 and 14-42).

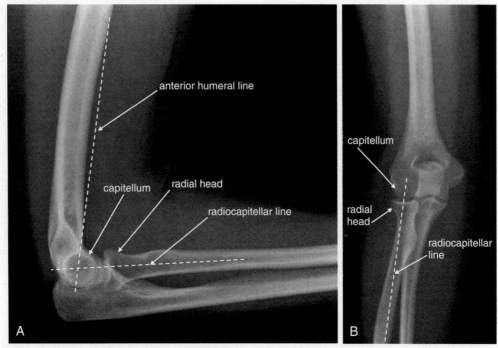

Figure 14-41. Normal alignment of radial head and capitellum. The radial head and capitellum (the rounded portion of the distal humerus with which the radius articulates) should be aligned when no fracture or dislocation is present. On the lateral view **(A)**, the anterior humeral line should intersect the middle third of the capitellum. Failure of this line to intersect the capitellum can occur when a supracondylar fracture is present, with posterior displacement of the distal humerus, including the capitellum. In this case, the capitellum may lie posterior to the anterior humeral line or be intersected in its anterior third. On both the lateral **(A)** and the anterior–posterior **(B)** view, a line drawn down the center of the long axis of the radius should intersect the capitellum, indicating normal radial head alignment with the capitellum. Failure of this alignment indicates radial head dislocation.

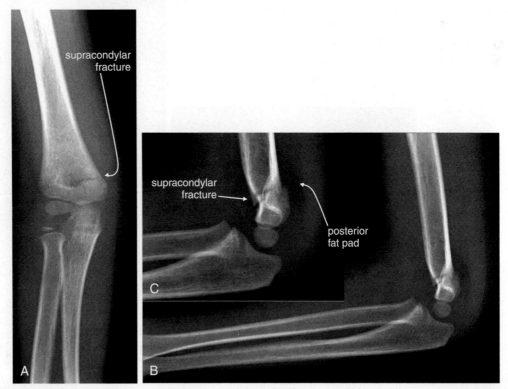

Figure 14-42. Distal humerus fracture (supracondylar fracture with fat pad). This 4-year-old female fell onto an outstretched right upper extremity from a playhouse. Her x-ray shows a supracondylar humerus fracture. Although the fracture itself is quite evident in this case, notice the posterior fat pad, a sign of hemarthrosis. This may be your only clue to more occult supracondylar fractures. **A,** Anterior–posterior view. **B,** Lateral view. **C,** Close-up from **B.** The patient underwent closed reduction with percutaneous pinning to limit the risk for later hyperextension deformity, which could occur if the fragment becomes dorsally displaced and angulated. This fracture also poses a threat of vascular injury. Finally, the anterior humeral line does not intersect the capitellum in the expected location. This is because of mild posterior displacement and angulation of the fracture fragment. Compare this with the normal appearance in Figure 14-41. Always assess the intersection of the anterior humeral line with the capitellum. If the normal intersection does not occur, suspect a dorsally displaced supracondylar fracture, even if the fracture line is not seen.

In adults, fractures about the elbow are also common following mechanisms such as falls on an outstretched arm. O'Dwyer et al.[43] performed MRI in 20 consecutive patients (ages 15-71 years) with fat pad signs but no visible fracture on elbow x-ray. Fractures were detected by MRI for 75% of the patients, with 87% being radial head, 6.7% lateral epicondyle, and 6.7% olecranon. The sensitivity of the fat pad sign for occult fracture was 70% with a specificity of 80%. However, the authors noted that no change in management occurred in these patients as a consequence of this additional imaging.

Elbow Dislocations

Elbow dislocations (Figures 14-43 through 14-45) most commonly result from a fall on an outstretched arm; consequently, the most common pattern is posterior dislocation of the forearm relative to the humerus. Dislocation of the ulna from the humerus is usually accompanied by radial head dislocation. The elbow is a stable joint that requires significant force to dislocate; consequently, elbow dislocations are commonly associated with fractures, including injuries to the distal humerus, radial head, articular processes of the ulna, distal forearm, and wrist.

Nursemaid's Elbow (Radial Head Subluxation)

Nursemaid's elbow is subluxation of the radial head, usually seen in children between the ages of 1 and 3 years. The common mechanism of injury is traction on the arm by an adult. The patient may present with failure to use the arm, rather than overt pain. In some cases, the injury reduces spontaneously, may reduce during manipulations for physical examination, or may become reduced during x-ray. X-rays are generally not needed for the diagnosis or to confirm reduction if the patient regains normal use of the arm after reduction. However, when concern exists about other fractures or dislocations, x-rays should be obtained, including x-rays of the humerus, elbow, and forearm, depending on the examination and history.

Forearm Fractures and Dislocations

The forearm is one of the most commonly injured body regions, with mechanisms including FOOSH and defensive injuries. Injuries in this location require careful evaluation,

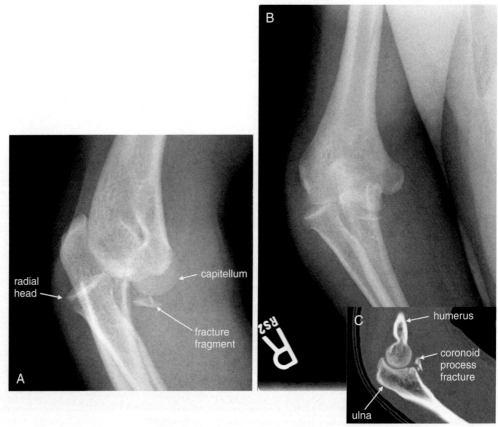

Figure 14-43. Elbow dislocation with medial condyle humerus fracture and ulnar coronoid process fracture. This 32-year-old male was standing on a chair when he fell on his outstretched right arm, sustaining a deformity at the elbow. He was unable to flex, extend, pronate, or supinate. **A,** A lateral x-ray shows posterior dislocation of the radial head with respect to the capitellum. The olecranon appears posteriorly displaced with respect to the trochlea, although this image is not a true lateral but a slightly oblique view, which makes this evaluation difficult. For comparison, look at the images of the normal elbow earlier in this chapter. A bone fragment is visible distal to the distal humerus. The source is not completely clear on x-ray, although the coronoid process is a likely suspect given the apparent elbow dislocation. **B,** Anterior-posterior view. Again, the articular surface of the radial head is not appropriately aligned with the capitellum. After joint reduction, computed tomography confirmed a coronoid process fracture **(C).**

because multiple injuries may be present from the distal humerus, to the elbow and proximal forearm, and continuing to the distal forearm and wrist. In this section, we discuss common injuries and pitfalls to be avoided.

Forearm Fractures

Radial Head Fractures and Dislocations.   Radial head fractures accompany about 20% of cases of elbow fracture or dislocation, and radial head dislocation can accompany

other injuries, as in the Monteggia pattern described later in this chapter. Alignment of the **radiocapitellar line** (described earlier) should be assessed, and the articular surface of the radius should be carefully inspected. Assessment of both AP and lateral views is essential to avoid missing radial head fracture or dislocation (Figures 14-46 and 14-47, see also Figures 14-59, 14-61, and 14-62).

Proximal Ulna Fractures.   Ulnar fractures commonly occur along the proximal third of the ulna, often in association with radial injuries, as in the Monteggia pattern described later in this chapter. The **coronoid process** of the ulna can be fractured during a forceful landing on an outstretched arm (Figures 14-48 and 14-49). Coronoid fractures are associated with elbow dislocation, because the distal humerus can shear the coronoid process if the ulna is dislocated posteriorly. Fractures of the olecranon can occur with FOOSH mechanisms or direct trauma.[44] The fracture is usually transverse (Figures 14-50 and 14-51).

Distal Radius Fractures.   Distal radius fractures occur following a FOOSH mechanism. Five common patterns are described in Table 14-10. In addition to describing the fracture by these patterns, several measurements can be useful in determining orthopedic treatment. The radial height should be measured, as demonstrated in Figure 14-52. Normal radial height is 10-13 mm in adults. Radial shortening of more than 2 mm can disrupt normal wrist mechanics, leading to altered loading and osteoarthritis. Radial inclination (normal = 21-25 degrees) and volar tilt (average = 11 degrees, range =

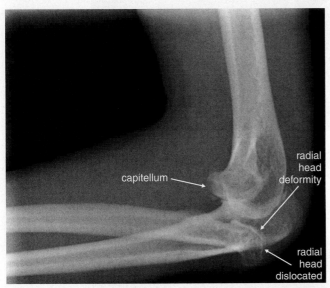

Figure 14-44. Elbow dislocation or fracture. This 33-year-old female fell onto her left arm and noted immediate pain in her elbow. This patient has degenerative changes of the radial head, which is posteriorly dislocated relative to the capitellum. This may reflect a prior radial head fracture and dislocation. Compare with the normal alignment demonstrated in Figure 14-41.

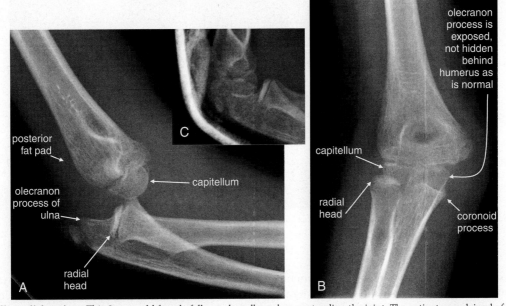

Figure 14-45. Elbow dislocation. This 8-year-old female fell onto her elbow, hyperextending the joint. The patient complained of pain and swelling of the elbow. **A,** Lateral x-ray. Posterior dislocation of the elbow is evident. The anterior and posterior fat pads are visible, indicating joint effusion or hemarthrosis, although no fractures are seen. The radial head is not aligned with the capitellum. The trochlea and olecranon are not aligned. **B,** AP view. The radial head does not articulate normally with the capitellum, and the coronoid process of the ulna is not seated against the trochlea of the humerus. **C,** Postreduction x-ray. The expected normal alignment is now seen.

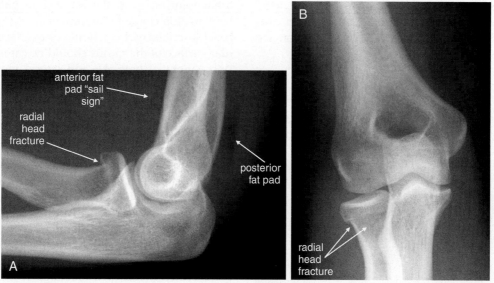

Figure 14-46. **Radial head fracture and double fat pad sign.** This 28-year-old female complained of left elbow pain after falling onto her outstretched forearm. Her flexion and extension were quite limited by pain, and she was unable to supinate or pronate. Her x-ray shows a subtle fracture of the radial head. The anterior and posterior fat pads indicate a hemarthrosis associated with this fracture. Look for abnormal fat pads—and an underlying fracture when they are present. **A,** Lateral x-ray. **B,** AP view.

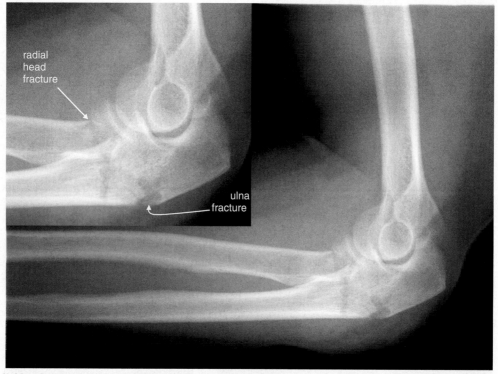

Figure 14-47. **Radial head and proximal ulnar fractures.** This 66-year-old female presented after falling directly on her left elbow. Her lateral x-ray shows fractures through the proximal radius and ulna.

2-20 degrees) should also be measured. Radial inclination less than 10 degrees and dorsal tilt greater than 20 degrees are associated with decreased wrist range of motion, reduced grip strength, and pain with forearm supination and pronation.[45] Common radial fractures are shown in Figures 14-53 through 14-58.

Nightstick Fractures. Nightstick fractures are isolated fractures of the ulnar diaphysis. The classic mechanism, from which the name derives, is a defensive injury sustained when the patient attempts to ward off a blow by presenting the ulnar aspect of the forearm in the path of a weapon such as a club or nightstick.

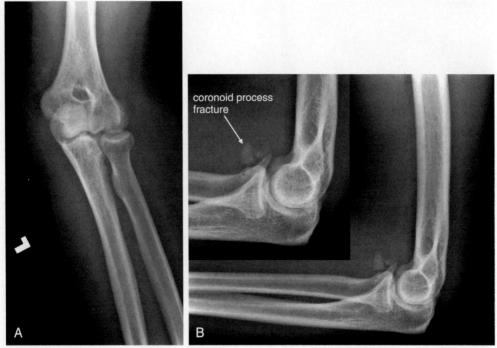

Figure 14-48. Ulnar fracture (coronoid process fracture). This 35-year-old female fell from standing, landing directly on her left elbow. **A,** Anterior–posterior view, showing a normal appearing elbow with normal alignment and no visible fracture. **B,** Lateral view (with close-up), revealing a fracture of the coronoid process of the ulna. This fracture may appear trivial but actually undermines the stability of the elbow joint, allowing posterior subluxation of the ulna relative to the humeral condyles. The patient underwent CT (Figure 14-49), which defined this fracture in more detail.

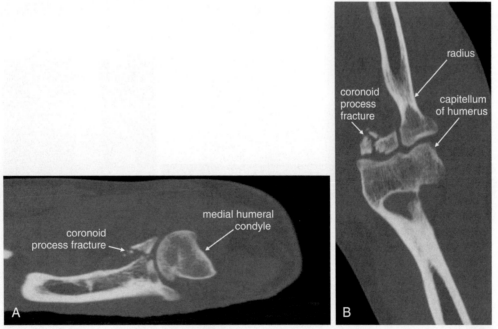

Figure 14-49. Ulnar fracture (coronoid process fracture). Same patient as in Figure 14-48. **A,** Sagittal view. This CT reconstruction shows a fracture through the base of the coronoid process of the proximal ulna. Without this lip to restrict posterior motion of the ulna relative to the humeral condyle, the ulna may sublux posteriorly. **B,** Coronal view. The radius articulates normally with the humerus.

Single-Bone Forearm Fractures With Associated Dislocation of the Unfractured Bone. The close anatomic relationship of bones in the forearm results in an association between single-bone fractures and dislocations of the unfractured bone. The Monteggia and Galeazzi injury patterns (Tables 14-11 and 14-12 and Figures 14-59 through 14-62) are classic examples of this fracture–dislocation injury. The dislocations are easily overlooked because of the obvious fracture, and the emergency physician must use a disciplined

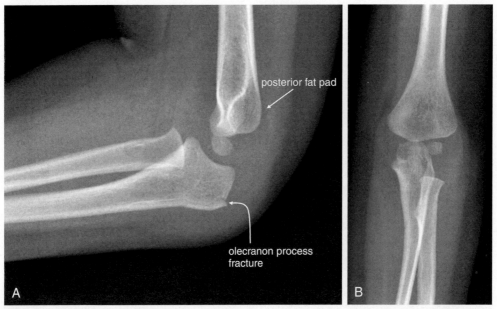

Figure 14-50. Olecranon process fracture with posterior fat pad sign. This 2-year-old female fell on her left elbow and was not using her left arm. Her lateral x-ray **(A)** showed a posterior fat pad and a subtle olecranon process fracture. This was not visible on the anterior–posterior view **(B)**.

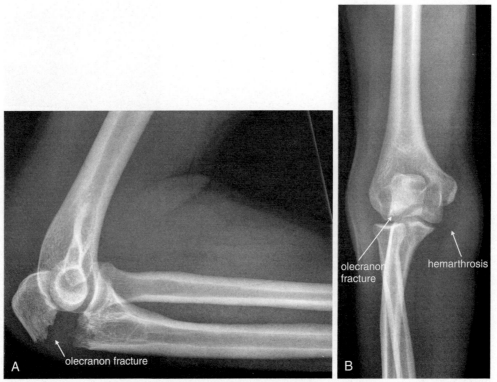

Figure 14-51. Olecranon fracture. This 17-year-old male complained of right elbow pain after falling off his bike. The x-ray shows a proximally displaced fracture of the ulnar olecranon process, with angulation of the proximal fragment. **A,** Lateral view. **B,** Anterior–posterior view, with a large hemarthrosis visible. The olecranon fracture is also visible, though far less obvious than on the lateral image. The radial head is normally aligned with the capitellum.

TABLE 14-10. Common Distal Radius Fractures Occurring With the FOOSH Mechanism

Name or Eponym	Description	Common X-ray Findings
Colles fracture	Distal radius fracture with dorsal displacement of the distal fracture fragment and wrist; occurs with a fall onto an extended wrist	• Transverse radius fracture • Dorsal displacement and angulation • Radial angulation of the wrist • Location 1 inch proximal to the radiocarpal joint • Radial shortening • Ulnar styloid fracture • Salter-Harris fractures (in children)
Smith (also called reverse Colles) fracture	Distal radius fracture with volar displacement of the distal fracture fragment and wrist; occurs with a fall onto a flexed wrist	• Transverse radius fracture • Volar displacement and angulation • Location 1 inch proximal to the radiocarpal joint • Radial shortening • Salter-Harris fractures (in children)
Barton fracture	Intraarticular distal radius fracture, with dislocation of the radiocarpal joint; shearing mechanism	• Intraarticular radius fracture • Dislocation of the radiocarpal joint in either the volar or the dorsal direction
Hutchinson (chauffeur) fracture	Oblique intraarticular distal radius fracture, including the radial styloid in the distal fracture fragment; shearing mechanism	• Variable size of the fracture fragment • Associated carpal ligament injuries, including scapholunate dissociation visible on x-ray
Die-punch radiolunate fossa fracture	Depressed fracture of the articular surface of the distal radius, resulting from impacting of the lunate; the name *die punch* comes from the similarity to the depression created by a die-punch tool in a surface when struck by a hammer	• Subtle irregularity and depression of the lunate fossa (articular surface) of the distal radius • Irregularity of one of the three carpal arcs

Adapted from Goldfarb CA, Yin Y, Gilula LA, et al: Wrist fractures: What the clinician wants to know. *Radiology* 219:11-28, 2001.

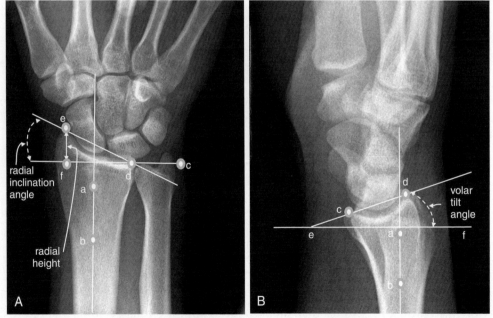

Figure 14-52. Measurement of radial height, radial inclination, and volar or doral tilt. Several measurements assist in description of distal radial injuries. First, draw three lines on the anterior–posterior x-ray **(A):**
- *Line ab,* Parallel to the radial axis.
- *Line cd,* Perpendicular to *line ab* and intersecting the ulnar edge of the lunate fossa of the radius (*point d*).
- *Line ed,* Connecting the distal radial styloid (*point e*) to the ulnar edge of the lunate fossa of the radius (*point d*).

  Radial height is then measured as the shortest distance from the distal tip of the radial styloid (*point e*) to *line cd*. This is *line ef* in the figure. A normal value is 10 to 13 mm in adults. The radial inclination angle is the angle formed between *line ed* and *line cd*. A normal value is 21 to 25 degrees. Next, draw three lines on the lateral x-ray **(B):**
- *Line ab,* Parallel to the radial axis.
- *Line cd,* Connecting the volar (*point c*) and dorsal (*point d*) rims of the distal radius.
- *Line ef,* Any line perpendicular to *line ab* and intersecting *line cd*.

  The angle created between *line cd* and *line ef* is the volar tilt angle, which averages 11 degrees and normally has a range of 2 to 20 degrees.

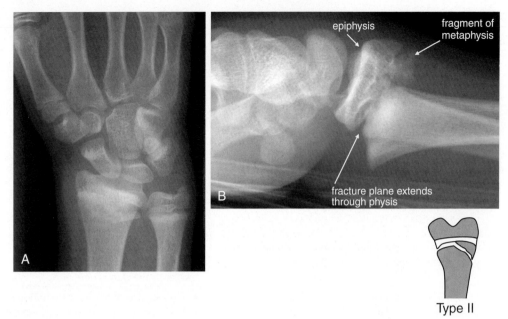

Figure 14-53. Distal radius (Colles) fracture. This 14-year-old male fell while skateboarding, landing on his outstretched right arm. **A,** Anterior–posterior view. A band of increased density suggests fracture. This view does not reveal any degree of displacement. Remember that a perpendicular view may be needed to determine displacement of a fracture. **B,** Lateral view. The patient has a distal radial fracture, with dorsal displacement of the fracture fragment. This is consistent with the Colles fracture pattern. This fracture extends through the physis (growth plate), as well as through the distal metaphysis, making this a Salter-Harris II fracture. This was treated with closed reduction and percutaneous pinning, following by short-arm casting.

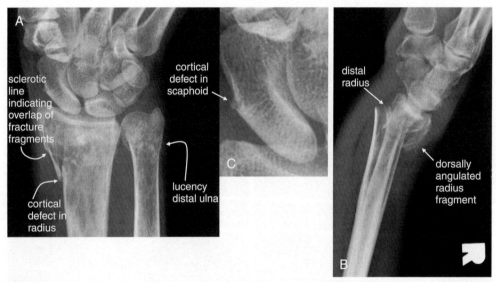

Figure 14-54. Distal radius (Colles) fracture. This 54-year-old female fell on her outstretched right upper extremity. **A,** Anterior–posterior (AP) view. A cortical defect is seen in the distal radius, and a lucent band extends across the distal ulna, consistent with transverse fractures of both bones. Again, the AP view does not provide evidence of the degree of angulation or displacement. **B,** Lateral view. Dorsal displacement of the radial fracture fragment is seen, consistent with Colles fracture. The AP view also shows a cortical irregularity of the scaphoid, possibly indicating scaphoid fracture as well. **C,** Close-up.

approach to review the entire x-ray, rather than stopping evaluation after detection of a single injury. A common medical error is to recognize the obvious fracture while failing to identify the associated joint dislocation.

The Galeazzi and Monteggia patterns share a common feature: one forearm bone is fractured, either proximally or distally, whereas the second forearm bone is dislocated. (see Tables 14-11 and 14-12). These injuries should

be specifically considered and sought on x-ray when a forearm injury has occurred. The **Galeazzi fracture–dislocation** is a fracture at the junction of the middle and distal third of the radius with distal dislocation of the ulna, or distal radial–ulnar joint (see Figures 14-59 and 14-60). Conversely, the **Monteggia fracture–dislocation** is a fracture of the proximal third of the ulna, associated with proximal dislocation of the radial head from its articulation with the capitellum (see Figures 14-61 and 14-62).

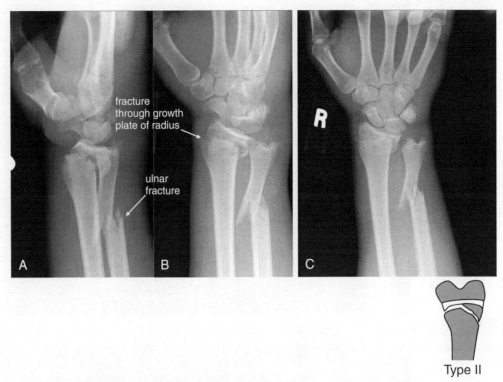

Type II

Figure 14-55. Distal radius and ulna fractures. This 15-year-old male crashed his motorbike and sustained multiple injuries. The distal ulna is fractured, displaced, and angulated. In addition, a fracture extends through the growth plate of the radius, with dorsal angulation of the distal fragment. This is a Salter-Harris II injury. **A,** Lateral view. **B, C,** Anterior–posterior views.

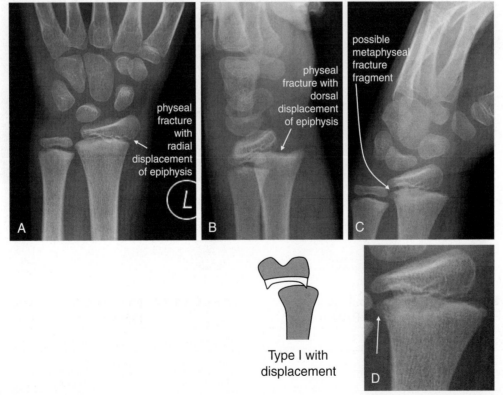

Type I with displacement

Figure 14-56. Distal radius (Colles) fracture. This 9-year-old male fell while roller skating, landing on his outstretched hand. His x-rays show a displaced fracture through the radial physis. The dorsal displacement of the distal radius fits a Colles fracture pattern. Let's also describe this using the Salter-Harris classification. **A,** Anterior–posterior view, showing radial displacement of the epiphysis. **B,** Lateral view, showing additional dorsal displacement of the epiphysis. **C,** Oblique view, showing a possible tiny metaphyseal fracture fragment. Without this additional finding, this would be a Salter-Harris I fracture. With this finding (see the close-up, **D**), it would be classified as a Salter-Harris II fracture. More importantly, the displacement requires reduction.

Figure 14-57. Distal radius (Colles) fracture. This 15-year-old male fell on his outstretched left wrist 6 days prior while playing basketball. He presented with continued wrist pain. His x-rays show a transverse physeal fracture of the radius with a large metaphyseal fragment—a Salter-Harris II fracture. Given the dorsal displacement of the distal fracture fragment, this also fits a Colles fracture pattern. **A,** Anterior–posterior view, showing radial displacement of the fracture fragment. **B,** Lateral view, showing dorsal displacement. Minimal dorsal angulation is also seen.

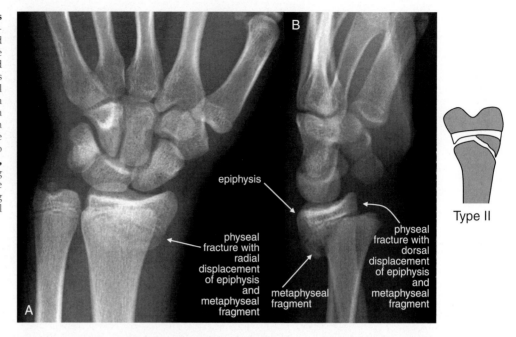

Figure 14-58. Distal radius (Smith's) fracture. This 12-year-old male fell from a scooter, landing prone on his outstretched right arm. He has a Salter-Harris II fracture of the distal right radius, with slight volar displacement of the distal fragment, consistent with a Smith's fracture. An ulnar styloid fracture is also visible. **A, B,** Anterior–posterior views. **C,** Lateral view, showing the volar displacement characteristic of Smith's fracture.

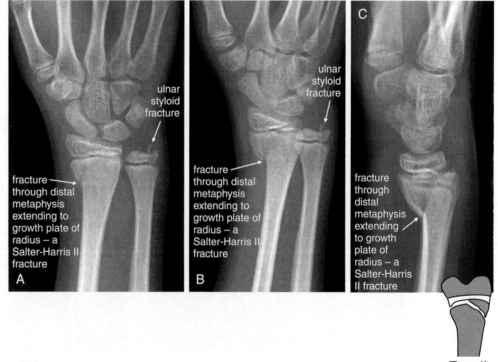

TABLE 14-11. Mnemonic for the Monteggia Fracture–Dislocation Pattern

Say the phrase…	To remember…
Michigan	Monteggia is an
University	Ulnar fracture with
Police	Proximal
Department	Dislocation of the radius (radial head)
Pitfall	*Recognizing the obvious fracture while missing the associated dislocation*

TABLE 14-12. Mnemonic for the Galeazzi Fracture–Dislocation Pattern

Say the phrase…	To remember…
Great	Galeazzi is a
Rays	Radius fracture with
Down	Distal
Deep	Dislocation of the ulna (radial–ulnar joint)
Pitfall	*Recognizing the obvious fracture while missing the associated dislocation*

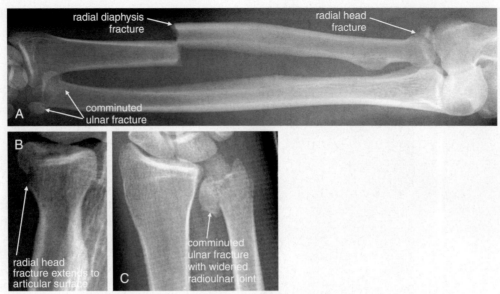

Figure 14-59. Galeazzi fracture (radius fracture with distal ulnar dislocation) variation. This 43-year-old male was playing baseball when he slid into a base, deforming his right arm. As with many of the other cases we have reviewed, several different injuries are present—review the x-ray systematically to avoid missing injuries. **A,** Anterior–posterior (AP) view of forearm. **B,** Close-up from AP elbow. **C,** Close-up from AP wrist. The most obvious injury here is a transverse fracture of the distal third of the radial diaphysis. This shows ulnar displacement of the distal fracture fragment. Remember that fractures in this location are associated with dislocation of the radioulnar joint, a Galeazzi pattern of injury. A normal distal radioulnar joint should measure 2 mm. The distal radioulnar joint does appear wide in this case, and a comminuted fracture of the distal ulna is present. Also inspect the elbow for abnormal fat pads, alignment, and fracture. In this case, the patient has an intraarticular fracture of the radial head. All of these injuries were repaired with open reduction and internal fixation.

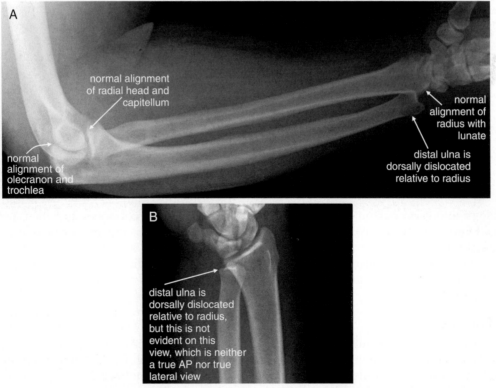

Figure 14-60. Distal radioulnar joint dislocation. This 36-year-old male was injured when a baling machine entrapped his right forearm. He sustained a crush injury to his distal forearm and wrist. His x-rays show no fractures, but look carefully at the anterior–posterior (AP) and lateral x-rays. **A,** The lateral x-ray shows an abnormal position of the distal ulna. Look back at the previous forearm cases and note that a true lateral x-ray should place the radius and ulna in overlapping positions at the wrist. Instead, this patient has evidence of dorsal dislocation of the distal ulna at the radioulnar joint. Is this simply an artifact of positioning for x-ray? No, the patient's forearm is supinated, the usual position for the lateral x-ray. The lunate bone of the wrist can be seen in its usual cup-shaped configuration, which is its appearance on a lateral x-ray in supination. The radial head articulates normally with the capitellum and the olecranon with the trochlea at the elbow. This is a case of true radioulnar dislocation. **B,** This view does not reveal this dislocation clearly because the dislocation is perpendicular to the x-ray plane. This image was intended to be a true AP view, but the patient was obliquely positioned at the time of image acquisition.

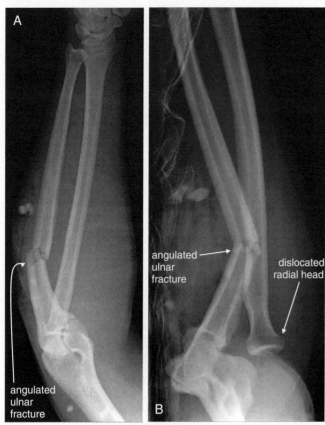

Figure 14-61. Monteggia fracture. This 29-year-old male rolled his car over and was found walking at the scene of the collision. The patient has a classic Monteggia pattern of injury, with proximal ulnar fracture and dislocation of the radial head. The x-rays are a little confusing because neither a true anterior–posterior (AP) nor a true lateral x-ray was obtained. **A,** Near-AP view. The ulna appears to articulate normally with the distal humerus. The radial head is not seen well. An angulated ulnar fracture is seen, involving the proximal third of the ulna. **B,** Near-lateral view. The angulated ulnar fracture again draws our attention, but note the dislocation of the radial head from its normal interface with the capitellum. Whenever a proximal ulnar fracture is identified, look carefully for radial head dislocation. Inspect two perpendicular views of the elbow to avoid missing this injury. If x-rays are inadequate, insist on repeat imaging.

A third example of a forearm fracture–dislocation pattern is the **Essex-Lopresti fracture,** a radial head fracture with dislocation of the distal radioulnar joint, resulting in disruption of the interosseous membrane.[46-47] A lateral x-ray of the wrist may show subtle dorsal subluxation of the ulna (see Figure 14-60).

Carpal Bone Fractures

FOOSH mechanisms commonly result in fractures and dislocations of carpal bones. Although any carpal bone can be fractured, the most common and potentially serious fractures are those of the scaphoid bone.[45] These injuries have a high rate of nonunion, resulting from the poor blood supply of the proximal scaphoid bone, which enters the proximal pole from the dorsal aspect near the waist of the scaphoid and may be disrupted by fractures through that region. This can result in avascular necrosis of the proximal pole, with persistent pain.

Scaphoid fractures can be difficult to identify on initial x-rays. Evaluation of radiographically occult scaphoid injuries with MRI, CT, and bone scan is discussed in detail in Chapter 15.

The normal wrist is shown in Figure 14-63.

Scaphoid Fractures

The scaphoid bone articulates between the distal radius proximally, the trapezium and trapezoid distally, and the capitate and lunate on its ulnar border. Clinically, scaphoid fractures manifest with wrist pain, tenderness to palpation of the anatomic snuffbox, and pain with axial loading of the thumb, which transmits force to the scaphoid. On x-ray, scaphoid fractures may be obvious, with complete disruption of both cortices and displacement of fragments on AP views of the wrist. In other cases, only subtle irregularity of the cortex is visible, or no radiographic abnormality may be apparent. An AP "scaphoid view" can be obtained, with the fist clenched and the wrist held in ulnar deviation. In this position, the scaphoid assumes an elongated position and displacement of scaphoid fracture fragments is exaggerated. When fracture is not apparent on x-ray but is suspected clinically, immobilization should be performed until repeat x-rays, repeat examination, MRI, CT, or bone scan excludes or confirms fracture, as discussed in Chapter 15.

Figures 14-64, 14-66, and 14-69 demonstrate scaphoid fractures.

Fractures of Other Carpal Bones

Recognition of carpal fractures can be difficult for the emergency physician, resulting from the complexity of overlapping bones in the wrist. Some simple strategies can assist in recognition. First, the emergency physician should become familiar with the normal appearance of the wrist in AP and lateral views, including the normal alignment of carpal bones and their articulations with the radius, ulna, and metacarpals (see Figure 14-63). Second, true AP and lateral x-rays of the wrist should be obtained in the patient with suspected injury. Both views should be reviewed to exclude or confirm injury. The perimeter of each carpal bone should be traced, with attention to any cortical irregularity. The spacing between carpal bones should be reviewed, and any excessively narrow or wide spaces should be noted, because these can indicate injury. Figure 14-67 demonstrates triquetrum fracture.

Carpal Dislocations and Malalignments

Carpal bone dislocations and malalignments are common injuries occurring with the familiar FOOSH mechanism. We review the three most common injury patterns (Table 14-13), although other variants may be seen. Because they share the FOOSH mechanism with

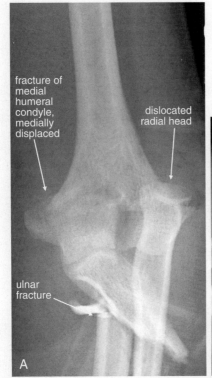

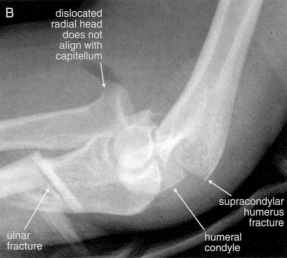

Figure 14-62. Monteggia fracture and transcondylar or supracondylar fracture of the humerus. This 24-year-old male collided his car with a tree, sustaining a left upper extremity injury. He has a complex fracture pattern, including both a supracondylar humerus fracture and a Monteggia pattern forearm fracture. A Monteggia fracture consists of a proximal ulnar fracture with dislocation of the radial head. **A,** Anterior–posterior view, showing radial head dislocation, ulnar fracture, and medial condyle humerus fracture. **B,** Lateral view, showing the same injuries but clarifying the humerus fracture. The trochlea of the humerus remains seated in the distal ulna, which is dislocated anteriorly relative to the distal humerus.

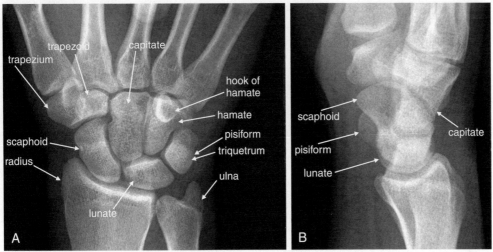

Figure 14-63. Normal wrist. Knowledge of the normal appearance of the wrist is necessary when evaluating for wrist injuries, which can be quite subtle. Evaluate the anterior–posterior (AP; **A**) and lateral **(B)** views in all cases. On the AP view, the triquetrum and pisiform overlap. The spaces between carpal bones should be uniform on the AP view. The distal radius, lunate, capitate, and third metacarpal should align in the AP and lateral views. The alignment of the carpal bones is discussed in detail in later figures demonstrating common injuries. Refer to this figure for a normal comparison.

common fractures of the wrist and forearm, these dislocations can coexist with fractures. A common diagnostic error is recognition of either a fracture or a dislocation but failure to recognize the second injury. Figures 14-64 through 14-66 demonstrate concomitant wrist (scaphoid and radius) fractures and perilunate dislocation.

Two keys to recognition of carpal bone dislocations are an understanding of the normal alignment of these bones and a familiarity with the common patterns of dislocation. The carpal bones are arrayed in two parallel curved rows of 4 bones each, visible on the AP radiograph. The carpal bones form 3 arcs. Carpal arc I is defined as a smooth curve tracing the proximal convexities of the

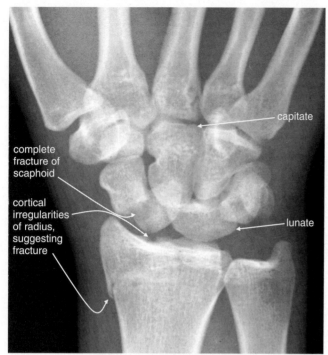

Figure 14-64. Scaphoid fracture (also distal intraarticular fracture of radius and perilunate dislocation). This 18-year-old male was struck by a truck while riding a dirt bike. His anterior–posterior wrist x-ray shows multiple abnormalities that should immediately catch your attention. First, the spacing of the bones of the wrist is not uniform; instead, some bones overlap in unexpected ways. To recognize this abnormality, you must understand that the spacing of carpal bones is normally quite regular. Second, the proximal carpal row appears to contain five bones rather than the normal four—because of a complete fracture of the scaphoid. Third, the normal alignment of wrist bones is disturbed, without the usual alignment of lunate with capitate. In addition, the scaphoid and lunate do not have their normal separation but overlap with each other. The distal radius also shows a cortical irregularity, suggesting an intraarticular fracture. The patient's lateral x-ray is reviewed in Figure 14-65. Computed tomography from the same patient is shown in Figure 14-66. Also compare with the normal wrist in Figure 14-63.

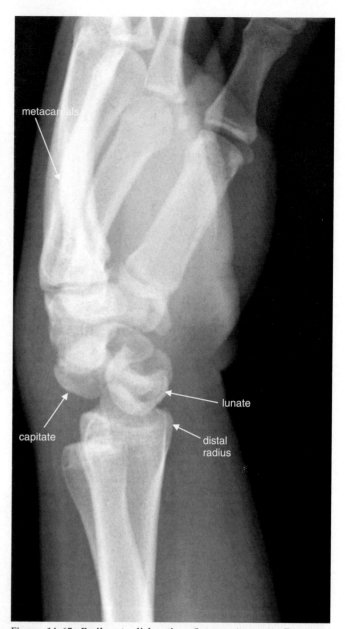

Figure 14-65. Perilunate dislocation. Same patient as in Figure 14-64. His lateral wrist x-ray shows a perilunate dislocation. The lateral view is typically the most informative for this injury pattern. What is a perilunate dislocation? In general, think of a perilunate dislocation as a dorsal dislocation of the entire wrist and hand distal to the lunate and radius, which maintain their usual alignment. Normally, the capitate sits in the cup of the lunate, with a straight line formed by the distal radius, lunate, capitate, and metacarpal bones. In the case of a perilunate dislocation, the capitate and metacarpals "hop" as a unit out of the lunate cup, moving dorsally. The lunate remains in its normal location. This is in contrast to a lunate dislocation, in which the lunate tips in a volar direction. The usual mechanism of injury for a perilunate dislocation is a fall on an outstretched hand, with force directed dorsally through the wrist. A CT scan from the same patient is shown in Figure 14-66. Also compare with the normal wrist in Figure 14-63. Figure 14-68 compares perilunate and lunate discolorations.

scaphoid, lunate, and triquetrum. Carpal arc II follows the distal concavity of these same three carpal bones. Carpal arc III is a smooth curve joining the proximal convexities of the capitate and hamate—overlapping carpal arc II. Disruption of the carpal arcs suggests fracture or dislocation. The spaces between the carpal bones are usually uniform on a true AP x-ray, measuring a few millimeters in adults. Dislocations of these bones may result in abnormal widening of the intercarpal spaces in one location and abnormal narrowing of spaces or overlap of bones in other locations. Unfortunately, if the wrist x-ray is obtained at a slight oblique angle rather than in a true AP projection, a false appearance of dislocation may result. Assessment of the plane of projection thus is an essential step in interpretation of wrist x-rays. The lateral x-ray must also be assessed, because some dislocations are most evident on this projection, as described later.

Three dislocation patterns of the wrist are most common: lunate dislocation, perilunate dislocation, and scapholunate dissociation (Figures 14-68 through 14-71). Table 14-13 compares these patterns.

Lunate dislocation occurs when the lunate bone rotates out of its normal anatomic position. The lunate is named for its crescent-moon appearance, with its concave

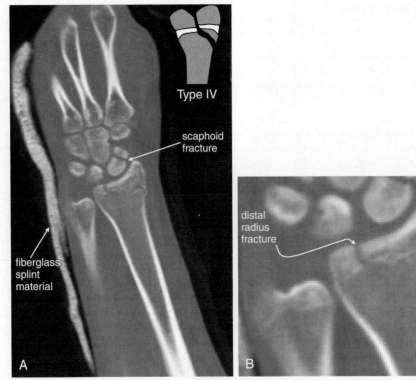

Figure 14-66. Scaphoid fracture (also distal intraarticular fracture of radius and perilunate dislocation), CT. Same patient as Figures 14-64 and 14-65. **A,** Coronal reconstruction of the wrist and distal forearm. **B,** Enlarged view of **A.** The arm is intentionally positioned obliquely in the CT scanner, because this increases the number of detector lines through the region of interest, increasing sensitivity. CT is felt to be quite sensitive for bony wrist injuries using 0.625-mm slice thickness. This CT confirms a distal radius fracture involving the growth plate and epiphysis. In addition, the fracture appears to cross the physis to involve the distal metaphysis, which would make this a Salter-Harris IV fracture if it were to occur in a skeletally immature patient. In this patient, the growth plate appears closed. This CT was performed after reduction of the scaphoid fracture and perilunate dislocation described in Figures 14-64 and 14-65.

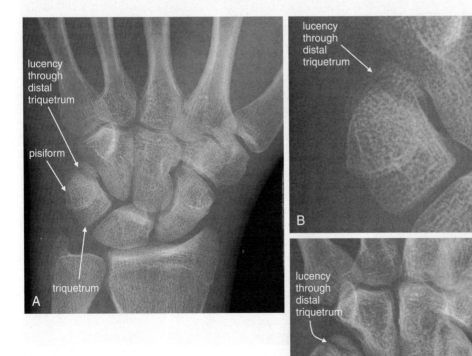

Figure 14-67. Triquetrum fracture. This 17-year-old male fell while playing soccer, trapping his left wrist under his body. An anterior–posterior view of the wrist **(A)** shows normal spacing between carpal bones. The scapholunate distance is normal, and no cortical defects are seen in the scaphoid. The triquetrum and pisiform overlap as usual, but a subtle lucency is seen through the distal triquetrum—a fracture **(B,** close-up from **A).** Is CT needed to confirm this subtle abnormality? No, a slightly oblique view **(C)** uses parallax to move the pisiform to a nonoverlapping position, revealing the fracture in more detail.

TABLE 14-13. Carpal Bone Dislocations

Carpal Dislocation	Description	Eponym	Best Seen on
Lunate dislocation	The lunate is dislocated, usually tipped in a volar direction. The remainder of the hand, wrist, and forearm are in normal alignment.	Tipped teacup sign, for the cuplike appearance of the lunate, tipped on its side	Lateral x-ray. On the AP view, the dislocation is not directly seen, but the normal spacing of carpal bones is disrupted.
Perilunate dislocation	The lunate remains upright and in normal anatomic alignment with the forearm proximal to it (the "teacup" is not tipped). The capitate has "hopped" out of the teacup shape of the lunate and is dislocated in a dorsal direction relative to the lunate. The remainder of the hand and wrist distal to the capitate moves with the capitate, remaining aligned with it.	As the name implies, dislocation around the lunate	Lateral x-ray. On the AP view, the dislocation is not directly seen, but the normal spacing of carpal bones is disrupted.
Scapholunate dissociation	During the FOOSH event, the scaphoid and the lunate are driven apart, tearing the scapholunate ligament. The space between these carpal bones is widened, relative to the spaces separating the other carpal bones from one another. These spaces are normally uniform.	Terry Thomas or David Letterman sign, for the gap-toothed appearance created by this injury on AP views of the wrist	AP x-ray.

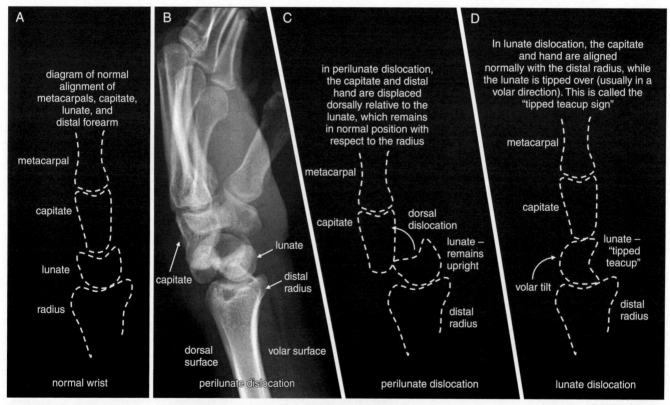

Figure 14-68. Perilunate versus lunate dislocation. This lateral view of the wrist demonstrates a perilunate dislocation. Perilunate dislocations are characterized by translation of the capitate and bones of the hand, usually in a dorsal direction relative to the radius. The lunate remains aligned with the distal radius, whereas the capitate no longer is aligned with the radius and does not sit within the cup of the lunate. In contrast, a lunate dislocation occurs when the lunate tips on its side (the tipped teacup sign), whereas the capitate remains aligned with the distal radius. **A,** Normal wrist, lateral projection. **B, C,** Perilunate dislocation. **D,** Lunate dislocation.

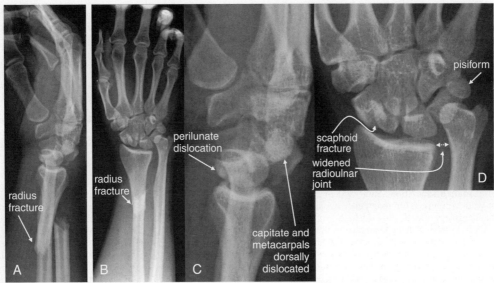

Figure 14-69. Perilunate dislocation, scaphoid fracture, and radial fracture with radioulnar dislocation (Galeazzi fracture). This 20-year-old male fell from a tree and sustained the injuries to his right arm. His blood alcohol level was 260 mg/dL. His x-rays show several important findings. First, a radial shaft fracture is present. The fracture is transverse, with volar and proximal dislocation of the distal radius relative to the proximal fragment (lateral view, **A** and **B**). Resist the temptation to stop your assessment after identifying this injury. Look at the close-up views of the wrist from the same radiographs. On the lateral image **(C)**, the lunate appears slightly tipped in a volar direction, which suggests lunate dislocation. However, the capitate and metacarpals are dorsally dislocated relative to the lunate while maintaining their relationship to one another. This is a perilunate dislocation. On the anterior–posterior view **(D)**, the radioulnar joint appears wide. In combination with the radial fracture, this is a Galeazzi pattern of injury. Continue your assessment of the wrist. Count the bones of the proximal carpal row, and you will note five instead of the usual four. Two bones are located to the radial side of the lunate—actually two fragments of the scaphoid, which is fractured at its midpoint.

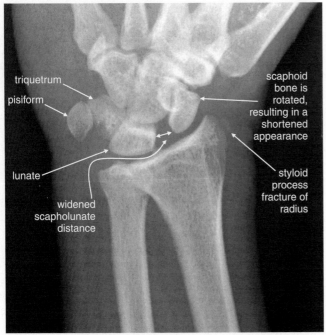

Figure 14-70. Scapholunate dislocation. This 37-year-old male caught his arm in a grinding machine, twisting the wrist as it was drawn into the machine. Fortunately, the machine was turned off before significant crush injury occurred. On the anterior–posterior (AP) view, a styloid process radius fracture is seen with a small avulsion fragment. However, look carefully at the AP x-ray. The scapholunate interval is wide. In addition, the scaphoid bone appears shorter than usual, in this case because of volar rotation of the bone. Also, this is not a true AP view but rather a slightly oblique view. As a result, the pisiform does not appear to overlie the triquetrum. Ideally, the x-ray should be repeated to evaluate the spacing of other carpal bones, which appear to overlap because of the oblique view. Compare with additional images in Figure 14-71.

surface usually facing distally and articulating with the convex surface of the proximal capitate bone. In lunate dislocation, the lunate typically rotates 90 degrees in a volar direction, with the concave surface facing the volar wrist. *On the lateral x-ray,* this gives the dislocated lunate the appearance of a "tipped teacup." The distal structures of the wrist remain in normal anatomic position.

Perilunate dislocation occurs when the capitate bone and the distal wrist and hand dislocate as a unit, usually in a dorsal direction. The capitate, which normally rests in the concavity of the distal lunate, "hops" out of the cup. The lunate retains its upright teacup appearance relative to the distal radius. *This injury is seen best on the lateral x-ray.* Figure 14-68 demonstrates a perilunate dislocation and compares it with a lunate dislocation.

Scapholunate dissociation occurs when a FOOSH drives apart the scaphoid and the lunate, which normally articulate with each other in the concavity of the distal radius. X-ray is relatively insensitive (57%, 95% CI = 41%-72%) but specific (98%, 95% CI = 91%-100%). Fluoroscopy can be used to assess instability at the scapholunate articulation and is more sensitive (85.7%, 95% CI = 71.5%-94.6%).[48] *This injury is best seen on the AP x-ray.* Figures 14-70 and 14-71 demonstrate a scapholunate dissociation.

A final reminder and admonition: wrist dislocations typically occur with a FOOSH mechanism. This mechanism

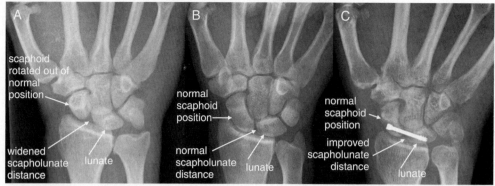

Figure 14-71. Scapholunate dissociation. Same patient as in Figure 17-40. This 37-year-old male was working with a grinding machine when his right hand and wrist were entrapped. On emergency department arrival, diffuse swelling and tenderness of the wrist were noted. This patient has evidence of scapholunate dissociation. Findings include a widened scapholunate distance, as well as rotation of the scaphoid out of its normal position. Familiarity with the normal radiographic appearance of the wrist allows recognition of this injury. A normal wrist should demonstrate narrow and uniform spaces between all carpal bones. In addition, the normal scaphoid has a ship-like profile on an anterior–posterior (AP) view (hence its other name, *navicular*). A widened scapholunate distance indicates disruption of the scapholunate ligament. This gap-toothed appearance has been called the Terry Thomas sign, named for the British comedian with this famous characteristic. Scapholunate dislocation is easily missed on plain x-ray, which has a reported sensitivity of around 50%. However, a widened scapholunate distance is more than 90% specific. Posttraumatic osteoarthritis is a common result of scapholunate dissociation, so early recognition and repair is important. This patient underwent open repair of a complete scapholunate ligament tear, as well as carpal tunnel release. Despite this and additional surgical repairs of associated cartilaginous injuries, he did not regain full wrist palmar flexion or dorsiflexion. He had permanent partial loss of median nerve sensation. **A,** Initial AP x-ray. **B,** Normal wrist from another patient for comparison. **C,** Same patient as in **A,** after surgical fixation.

is also common to scaphoid bone fractures, distal radius and ulna injuries, and other extremity trauma. Beware of the temptation to cease the search for injuries once a single abnormality, such as a wrist dislocation, is identified. A comprehensive evaluation of the radiograph for other injuries is necessary. Sometimes multiple patterns of dislocation and fracture are present.

Can a Clinical Decision Rule Reduce Radiography Following Pediatric Wrist Trauma?

Earlier in this chapter, we discussed clinical decision rules, including well-validated rules for imaging of knee, ankle, and foot injuries. Studies of indications for wrist radiography are more limited. Webster et al.[49] prospectively evaluated criteria for wrist radiography in 227 children. A rule incorporating radial tenderness, focal swelling, and abnormal supination or pronation of the forearm had sensitivity of 99.1% but specificity of only 24%, with a resulting radiography rate of 87% compared with standard practice in this study. This rule has not been externally validated, and more work is needed to identify clinical factors that exclude fracture and eliminate the need for imaging.

Metacarpal Fractures

Metacarpal fractures can occur with a variety of mechanisms, including offensive and defensive postures by the patient. Clinically important injuries include the boxer's fracture; extraarticular fractures of the base, shaft, and neck; and intraarticular fractures. Metacarpals are conventionally numbered one through five, beginning with the thumb and ending with the small finger.

Boxer's (Fighter's) Fractures

A **boxer's** or **fighter's fracture** (Figures 14-72 through 14-74) occurs with a clenched fist striking an immobile object, often a wall or another person. The fracture usually involves the neck of the fifth or sometimes fourth metacarpal. Open fractures in this location are common, and air and foreign bodies such as teeth may be seen on x-ray—resulting from punching an opponent's mouth. Infection of such open injuries is common and has gained a specific name, the "fight bite" or "clenched fist" injury. Boxer's fractures should be assessed for air and foreign bodies, degree of angulation, and rotational deformity (see Figure 14-74). Typically, the metacarpal head is angulated in a volar direction, as measured using the lateral radiograph. The normal angle of the metacarpal neck is 15 degrees. Angulation greater than 30 degrees interferes with fist closure or flexion at the metacarpophalangeal (MCP) joint, giving a "clawed" appearance and resulting in functional impairment of flexion caused by shortening of intrinsic muscles of the hand.[50] If closed reduction cannot decrease angulation below this threshold, percutaneous fixation may be required.

Rotational deformity along the long axis of the metacarpal results in an MCP joint that is rotated off-axis with respect to the other MCP joints. Consequently, when the affected joint is flexed, the affected finger crosses other fingers, interfering with normal grip. Any degree of malalignment on AP x-ray of the hand suggests an axial or rotational deformity. Intraarticular fractures of the metacarpal head require operative management.

A **Bennett fracture** is an oblique intraarticular fracture at the base of the first metacarpal (metacarpal of the thumb),

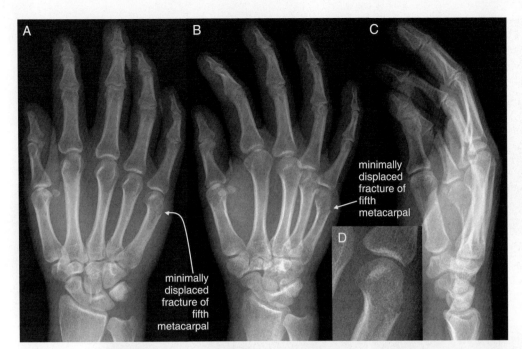

Figure 14-72. Boxer's fracture. This 23-year-old female sustained a hand injury in a motor vehicle collision. Her x-rays show a minimally displaced fracture of the distal fifth metacarpal, without intraarticular extension. The injury fits a boxer's fracture pattern, although her mechanism of injury is not typical. The anterior–posterior **(A)** and oblique **(B)** views demonstrate this injury clearly, though it is not clearly seen on the lateral view **(C).** Minimal angulation is present, and splinting without further reduction would have an acceptable outcome. Importantly, no rotational deformity is evident, because this would require reduction. **D,** Close-up from **A.**

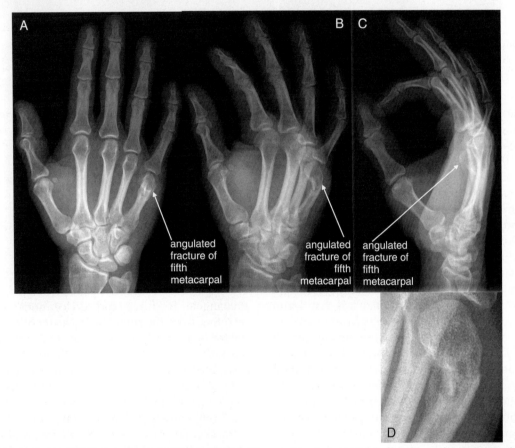

Figure 14-73. Boxer's fracture (fifth metacarpal neck fracture). This 39-year-old male complained of hand pain after dropping a brake rotor on his hand. His x-rays show a volar angulated fracture of the distal fifth metacarpal. The anterior–posterior (AP) view **(A)** may appear confusing—a cortical break is not definitely seen, although the fifth metacarpal head appears abnormally positioned. The fifth metacarpal seems short. On the oblique view **(B),** both the cortical defect and the degree of angulation are evident. The lateral view **(C)** shows the fifth metacarpal head to be tilted in a volar direction and projecting anterior to the other distal metacarpals. **D,** Close-up from **B.** Reduction of this injury is necessary because it exceeds 30 degrees of angulation on the lateral view. Normally, the angle between the neck and the head of the metacarpal is 15 degrees on the lateral view. Measurement of this angle is shown in Figure 14-74. No lateral angulation on the AP view should be accepted, nor should a rotational deformity, because these will lead to the patient's fifth finger crossing the others when flexed at the metacarpophalangeal joint. If the fracture is not reduced, range of motion at the metacarpophalangeal joint will be impaired. Did the patient report the true mechanism of injury? This is a boxer's fracture, with the most common mechanism being blunt trauma from punching a hard object with a clenched fist.

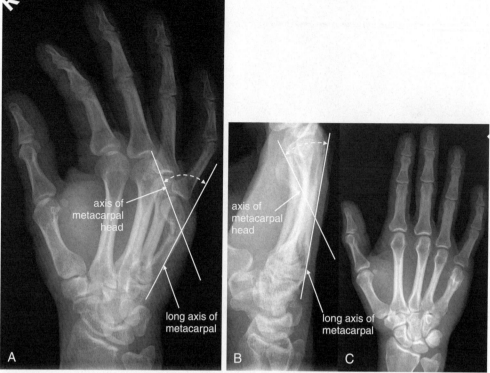

Figure 14-74. Boxer's fracture, measurement of angulation. Normal angulation of the distal metacarpal head relative to the long axis of the metacarpal is 15 degrees. Angulation greater than 30 degrees results in functional deficits of flexion at the metacarpophalangeal joint and should be reduced. **A,** Oblique view. **B,** Lateral view. **C,** AP view.

extending into the carpometacarpal joint. Subluxation or dislocation of the carpometacarpal joint may also be seen. The proximal fracture fragment is typically small but includes the insertion site of the anterior oblique ligament, which typically maintains the fragment in its normal anatomic position. The distal fracture fragment includes the majority of the metacarpal bone, including most of the proximal articular surface. This fragment is typically subluxed from its normal anatomic position by the actions of the abductor pollicis longus and adductor pollicis muscles. The trapeziometacarpal joint is unstable with this fracture and requires immobilization: thumb spica casting when subluxation of less than 1 mm is present, percutaneous pinning for subluxation of 1 to 3 mm, and open fixation for subluxation greater than 3 mm. Failure to diagnose and treat appropriately can lead to posttraumatic arthritis and pain, which are common sequelae even with treatment. Normal, painless thumb range of motion is critical to hand function, making deficits resulting from Bennett fractures particularly disabling.[51-52] Figure 14-75 demonstrates a Bennett fracture.

A **Rolando fracture** is a comminuted intraarticular fracture of the base of the first metacarpal. The fracture has three fragments, with a characteristic "T" or "Y" shape. The two proximal fracture fragments involve the articular surface with the trapezium. The distal fracture fragment is largest and consists of the remainder of the metacarpal. Rarer than Bennett fracture, this injury

has a worse prognosis. Operative fixation is required to restore the articular surface.[53] Figure 14-76 demonstrates a Rolando fracture.

Figures 14-77 and 14-78 demonstrate other metacarpal fractures.

Fractures at other locations along the course of metacarpals are possible but more rarely pose diagnostic or therapeutic dilemmas.

Phalangeal Fractures and Dislocations
Phalangeal fractures and dislocations are common, resulting from the constant exposure of hands to potential trauma. Simple dislocations of interphalangeal joints are radiographically obvious (Figure 14-79), although associated ligamentous injuries may be present and are not visible on plain radiographs. Follow-up radiographs can demonstrate the development of deformities resulting from untreated ligamentous injury (Figure 14-80). Intraarticular fractures may occur with or without dislocations (Figure 14-81; see also Figure 14-145 later in the chapter). Following reduction of a dorsal or lateral dislocation of the proximal interphalangeal (PIP) joint, the joint is usually splinted in 10 to 30 degrees of extension to prevent additional volar plate injury.

Boutonniere deformities are characterized by flexion at the PIP joint and hyperextension at the distal

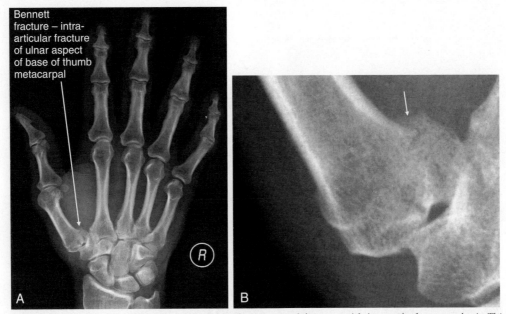

Figure 14-75. **Bennett fracture of the right thumb (proximal thumb metacarpal fracture with intraarticular extension).** This 45-year-old male was a restrained driver in a rollover motor vehicle collision. He complained of pain with movement of his right thumb. **A,** His anterior–posterior x-ray shows a fracture at the base of the right thumb metacarpal, with 2-mm displacement. This extends to the carpometacarpal joint on the ulnar side. The lateral x-ray did not reveal the fracture. **B,** Close-up. An intraarticular fracture in this location is called a Bennett fracture. The most common of thumb fractures, it involves a proximal metacarpal fragment that remains attached to the palmar beak ligament (also called deep anterior oblique ligament). This keeps the proximal metacarpal fragment in normal anatomic position, while the distal fragment is often dislocated by the action of its attached muscles. Repair is required to maintain stability and mobility of the thumb.

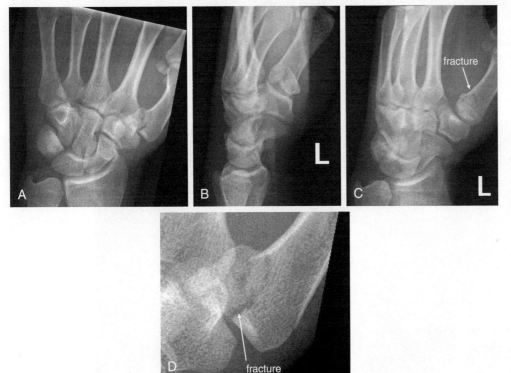

Figure 14-76. **Rolando or Bennett fracture?** This 23-year-old male was a pedestrian struck by a police car. X-rays of his left wrist show a comminuted fracture of the base of first metacarpal, which extends intraarticularly. From these images, it is difficult to distinguish this injury from a Bennett fracture, which is not comminuted. The radiologist characterized this as a Rolando fracture; the orthopedist called it a Bennett fracture. Because of the minimal degree of displacement, the patient was treated with thumb spica splinting with good results. **A,** Anterior–posterior view. **B,** Lateral view. **C,** Oblique view. **D,** Close-up from **A.**

interphalangeal (DIP) joint. These deformities may occur after volar dislocations of the PIP joint, closed injuries with axial loading ("jammed finger"), or forced flexion of the PIP with the PIP in extension. The mechanism resulting in boutonniere deformity is disruption of the central slip, a structure of the extensor hood of the finger. An intact central slip maintains the lateral bands of the extensor hood in a location dorsal to the axis of rotation of the PIP. Once the central slip is disrupted, the lateral bands migrate volar to the axis of rotation of

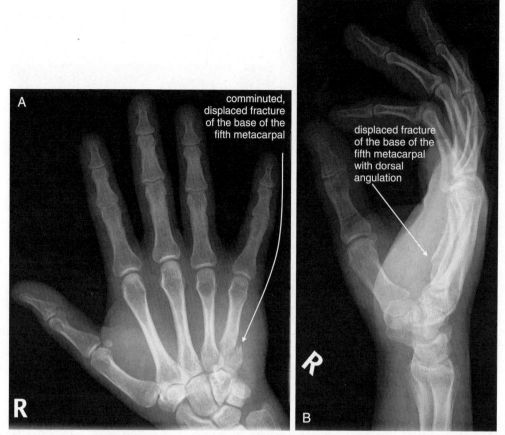

Figure 14-77. Displaced, comminuted fracture of base of fifth metacarpal. This 26-year-old male fell from a skateboard the previous evening and complained of pain and swelling in the ulnar aspect of his right hand. **A,** Anterior–posterior view, showing a comminuted, displaced fracture of the base of the fifth metacarpal. This does not appear to extend intraarticularly. **B,** Lateral view, also demonstrating some dorsal angulation of the fracture. This injury was treated with open reduction and internal fixation.

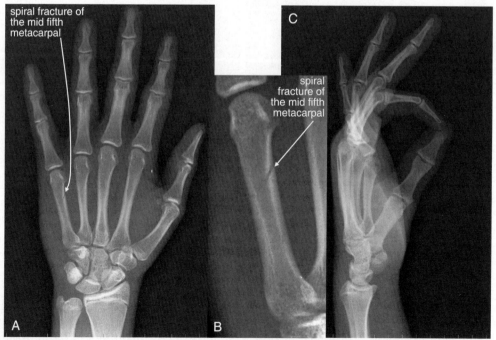

Figure 14-78. Nondisplaced spiral fracture of the middle third of the fifth metacarpal. This 16-year-old male blocked a blow from a piece of lumber using the ulnar aspect of his hand. He has a subtle spiral fracture of the fifth metacarpal without displacement, visible on the anterior–posterior view (**A; B,** close-up) but not on the lateral view (**C**).

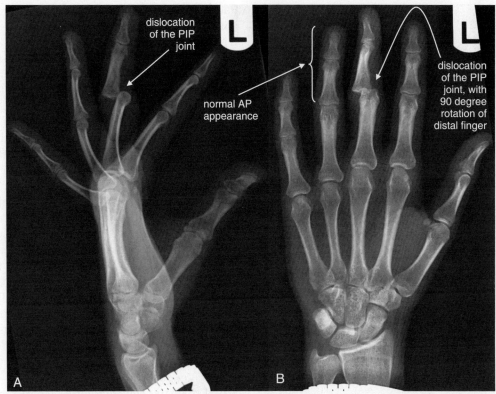

Figure 14-79. Dislocation proximal interphalangeal (PIP) joint. This 26-year-old female fell while dancing at a nightclub, injuring her left hand. There is a dislocation at the level of the third PIP joint. The middle phalanx is dislocated a complete shaft width dorsally and a half shaft width in the ulnar direction. In both **A** and **B,** the middle and distal phalanx of the involved finger have a different profile from the other digits—this is caused by rotation of the middle phalanx relative to the proximal phalanx by nearly 90 degrees. As a result, the distal finger appears to have a lateral configuration on the AP view and an AP configuration on the lateral view. The dislocation was reduced, but on follow-up 3 months later the patient was noted to have a marked boutonniere deformity of the left middle finger, consistent with central slip injury (Figure 14-80). Interphalangeal dislocations warrant orthopedic follow-up because of the possibility of ligamentous injuries not directly visible on x-ray. **A,** Lateral view. **B,** Anterior–posterior (AP) view.

the PIP, forcing it into flexion and causing extension of the DIP. Patients with volar dislocations of the PIP and even radiographically normal fingers with a "jamming" mechanism should be warned of the possibility of this deformity and advised to follow-up. Extension splinting of the PIP joint is usually performed.[54]

Mallet deformity occurs with stretch of the extensor tendon of the finger or its avulsion from the distal phalanx. Forced flexion of an extended DIP joint can result in this injury. The injury is usually delayed in presentation, but injuries to the DIP joint, including axial loading injuries, distal phalanx fractures, intraarticular fractures, and dislocation or volar subluxation of the distal phalanx should raise suspicion of this injury. Bony mallet injuries include avulsion of the proximal articular surface, whereas ligamentous mallet injuries have no visible fracture. Large avulsion articular fragments may be associated with the development of mallet deformity, according to a cadaver model.[55]

Transverse fractures of phalanges are common (Figure 14-82), as are **tuft fractures.** Tuft fractures (Figure 14-83) are fractures of the distal tip of the distal phalanx, usually because of a crush mechanism. These injuries may

be open or closed. Finger amputations are clinically obvious but are usually evaluated with x-ray for foreign body and to delineate fractures (Figure 14-84).

Soft-tissue gas is visible as a lucency on plain x-ray. Hand injuries and infections can result in penetration of gas into deep tissue planes, including tendon sheaths (Figure 14-85).

Lower Extremity Injuries and Pathology

Hip Injuries and Conditions of the Femoral Head
Hip fractures, hip dislocations, SCFE, and Legg-Calvé-Perthes disease (avascular necrosis of the femoral head) are discussed in detail in Chapter 13. MRI and CT of occult hip fracture are discussed in Chapter 15.

Femoral Shaft Fractures
Fractures of the femoral shaft are usually readily evident on x-ray (Figure 14-86). As with other fractures, the injury should be characterized by its location, angulation, distraction or overriding of fracture fragments, comminution, plane of fracture lines, involvement of articular surfaces, and evidence of open fracture or foreign body (see Table 14-3). The femur is a strong, weight-bearing bone that resists fracture except in cases

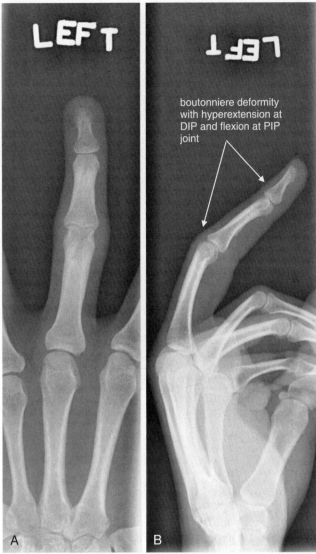

Figure 14-80. Dislocation proximal interphalangeal (PIP) joint with subtle boutonniere deformity. Same patient as Figure 14-79. In these 3-month follow-up x-rays, a boutonniere deformity of the left middle finger is visible, consistent with central slip injury. This injury is visible on the lateral **(B)** but not on anterior–posterior **(A)** view. DIP, Distal interphalangeal.

of significant force, severe osteoporosis, or underlying pathology. Some bony tumors affect the femoral diaphysis (shaft), including Ewing sarcoma and osteosarcoma. When fracture occurs without a history of significant force, be sure to examine the x-ray for lytic bone lesions, periosteal reaction, and soft-tissue densities suggesting benign or malignant neoplasm.

Femoral Condyle Fractures

In adults, **femoral condyle fractures** are also usually readily evident on x-ray (Figures 14-87 through 14-90). In addition to standard AP and lateral views, oblique x-rays may assist in detection of fractures. When uncertainty exists about the presence of a fracture, CT can be performed to provide additional delineation of injury.

Patella Fractures and Dislocations

Patella fractures (Figures 14-91 and 14-92) can occur with direct force to the patella or with avulsion of the quadriceps or patellar tendon insertion sites. A lateral knee radiograph can demonstrate fractures in the axial plane. Patellar fractures can be difficult to visualize on AP views of the knee, because the patella overlies the denser distal femur. A **sunrise view** of the patella is obtained with the knee in flexion and the x-ray beam tangential to the patella, throwing the patella into relief by eliminating overlap of the patella with the femur and tibia. This can demonstrate vertical fractures not seen on an AP or lateral view. A bipartite patella is a normal variant that can simulate fracture. In the case of bipartite patella, the two patellar portions are usually rounded and smooth, rather than showing the irregular borders typical of fracture. **Patella dislocation** (Figure 14-93) is a common injury that does not require radiographic confirmation, because it is usually clinically evident and readily reduced at the bedside with simple knee extension. If x-rays are obtained, the patella usually appears laterally displaced on AP views.

Tibial Plateau Fractures

Tibial plateau fracture (Figures 14-94 through 14-98) is a clinically important and sometimes relatively occult injury on plain radiographs. An important complication of tibial plateau fracture is compartment syndrome, occurring in up to 10% of cases.[56] In addition, because the tibial plateau is a weight-bearing surface, fractures in this location typically require operative reduction to ensure the best possible anatomic alignment of fracture fragments. Although most tibial plateau injuries are seen on x-ray, subtle depressions of the tibial plateau surface may be difficult to recognize on AP and lateral x-rays. Obliquely oriented vertical fractures may be invisible on these views, and oblique projections should be obtained when injuries are suspected but not seen on standard views. CT of the tibial plateau can provide exquisite detail to delineate the fracture in multiple planes or even three-dimensionally and to aid in operative planning.[57] In one study, CT modified the surgical plan in almost 60% of operative cases of tibial plateau fracture.[58] Fractures with depression of greater than 5 mm typically require elevation and grafting.

On the AP view, the **intercondylar eminence** (also called the **tibial spine**) is visible in the center of the tibial plateau. This structure serves as the attachment point for the anterior and posterior cruciate ligaments (on the anterior and posterior portions of the intercondylar eminence) and the medial and lateral menisci. Avulsion of this spine can occur with anterior and posterior cruciate ligament injuries (Figures 14-99 through 14-101). This relatively innocuous x-ray finding is clinically significant, because avulsion of the attachment point of these ligaments can render the knee unstable and often

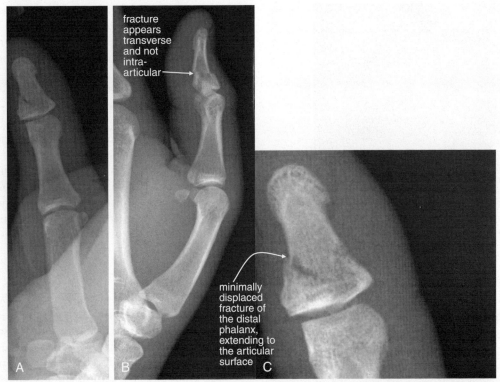

Figure 14-81. Intraarticular phalangeal fracture. This 18-year-old male complained of left thumb pain after falling off of his dirt bike and jamming his thumb into the ground. **A,** Anterior–posterior view. A minimally displaced fracture of the distal phalanx is seen, extending to the articular surface (see close-up, **C**). **B,** Lateral view. This fracture is not seen to involve the joint. Two perpendicular views are necessary to evaluate fracture displacement, angulation, dislocation, and potential articular involvement.

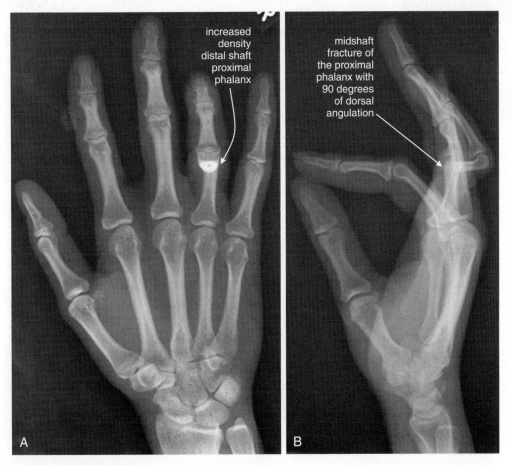

Figure 14-82. Transverse fracture of fourth proximal phalanx. This 28-year-old female was struck on her right ring finger with a hammer. **A,** Anterior–posterior x-ray, showing a high-density area of the distal shaft of the fourth proximal phalanx. Is this increased density a ring on the finger? No fracture or dislocation is seen in this view although the fourth proximal phalanx appears rather short. In stark contrast, the lateral view **(B)** reveals the area of increased density to be caused by a middiaphyseal fracture that is angulated dorsally by 90 degrees. This case illustrates the key importance of obtaining two orthogonal views when assessing for fracture or dislocation.

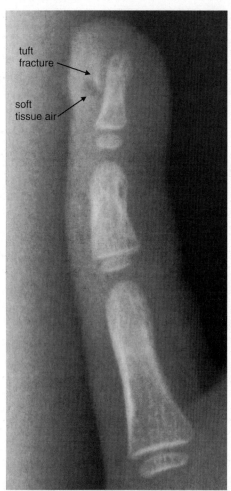

Figure 14-83. Tuft fracture. This 3-year-old female closed her left small finger in a door. Her x-ray shows a bone fragment along the distal phalanx, consistent with tuft fracture. Soft-tissue air is also seen, introduced through an associated laceration. The patient had an overlying laceration and nail bed injury that was repaired in the operating room. Should a nail bed injury associated with a tuft fracture be treated as an open fracture? Controversy exists, but antibiotics may be indicated. Osteomyelitis is a rare but published complication.

requires surgical fixation.[59] Other subtle radiographic abnormalities can suggest important injuries. **Lipohemarthrosis** (fat–fluid level) can occur when a fracture has allowed marrow fat to enter the joint space. This is seen in the suprapatellar recess on a horizontal-beam lateral knee radiograph. On the AP projection, increased trabecular density beneath the lateral tibial plateau is abnormal. The trabecular density is normally greater beneath the medial plateau surface, because this region bears a greater load. Nonalignment of the femoral condyles and tibia on the AP view can also suggest tibial plateau fracture. In difficult cases, x-rays of the contralateral knee can reveal asymmetry suggesting fracture. These images are also useful in restoring leg length and alignment. Traction radiographs and a tibial plateau radiograph (an AP projection angled 15 degrees caudally) can reveal the depth of tibial plateau depression.[60]

Ligamentous and Meniscus Injuries of the Knee

Ligamentous and meniscus injuries of the knee are common and may be completely occult on x-ray. Joint effusion may be visible but is not specific for ligamentous or meniscus injury. Avulsion of the tibial spine may be seen (see Figures 14-99 through 14-101). MRI is the current optimal imaging test for these injuries according to the American College of Radiology (ACR),[57] but imaging need not be performed to assess for these injuries in the emergency department. Management is not acutely affected by results of imaging tests in most cases. Immobilization of the knee and outpatient follow-up are generally adequate. Timing of repair of anterior cruciate ligament injury is controversial, with studies suggesting that outcomes are no better with early than with late surgery in adults.

Knee Dislocations

Traumatic dislocation of the knee usually occurs with significant blunt trauma such as motor vehicle collisions, falls from height, and pedestrians struck by vehicles, although the injury can rarely occur with sports mechanisms such as football injuries and even with simple falls.[61] This is a limb-threatening injury, associated with popliteal artery and nerve injuries, as well as disruption of all major ligaments of the knee. Spontaneous reduction of this unstable injury can occur, so x-rays demonstrating normal knee alignment do not rule out these important associated injuries. Vascular injury may occur in 20% of patients with posterior knee dislocation.[62] On x-ray, posterior dislocation of the tibia relative to the distal femur is most often seen, although anterior dislocation can occur (Figures 14-102 through 14-105).

Can Physical Examination Exclude Vascular Injury, or Is Arterial Imaging Required in All Cases of Knee Dislocation?

Physical examination cannot adequately exclude arterial injury requiring surgery, according to a metaanalysis of seven studies with 284 injuries. Abnormal pedal pulses had a sensitivity of 79% (95% CI = 64%-89%) with a specificity of 91% (95% CI = 78%-96%).[63] Scattered case series suggest higher sensitivity of physical examination for clinically significant injuries requiring surgery. Dennis et al.[62] found absent pulses to be 100% sensitive for popliteal injuries requiring surgical repair, though some subtler intimal injuries and stenoses occurred in the presence of diminished or normal pulses. Abou-Sayed and Berger[64] reported abnormal pedal pulses to be 100% sensitive for vascular injuries requiring intervention, but this small retrospective study of 52 patients does not prove the sensitivity of examination. At this time, imaging for arterial injury is prudent in patients with suspected or confirmed knee dislocation.

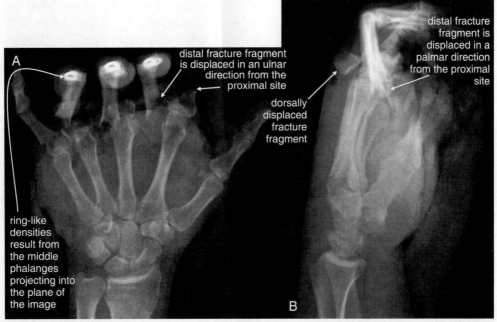

Figure 14-84. Phalangeal amputation. This 39-year-old male sustained a crush injury to the left hand between the rollers of an industrial machine. **A,** Anterior–posterior view. Complete fracture of the proximal phalanges of the second through fifth digits is seen. Significant ulnar displacement of the distal fragments is seen for the second through fourth fingers. The PIP joints are held in flexion, resulting in the ringlike densities seen in these digits, which are projecting into the plane of the image. **B,** Lateral view. Additional palmar displacement of the proximal phalanx fractures is seen.

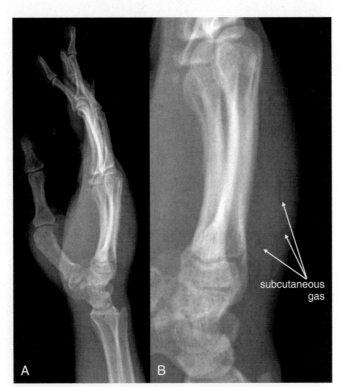

Figure 14-85. Subcutaneous emphysema, first metacarpal fracture. This 25-year-old female was assaulted with a barbecue fork and sustained a stab injury to the right palm. X-rays were taken on the date of the injury. **A,** Lateral x-ray, demonstrating lucencies representing air tracking in the dorsum of the hand. These were not visible on the anterior–posterior view (not shown). **B,** Close-up, with contrast and brightness adjusted. Because of the risk for extensor tendon tenosynovitis from inoculation of the tendon sheath, the patient underwent exploration and irrigation in the operating room.

What Imaging Modalities Can Be Used to Evaluate Lower Extremity Vascular Injuries, Particularly of the Popliteal Artery?

The ACR gives conventional angiography, MRA, and CTA equal appropriateness (7 on its 1-to-9 scale) for evaluation of popliteal artery injury.[57] No large studies exist directly comparing these modalities for popliteal artery injury. Because this injury can be time sensitive, with ischemia of the distal extremity a consideration, the most rapidly available test may be most appropriate. In most U.S. emergency departments, CTA is more widely available at all hours. MRA has the advantages of causing no radiation exposure and allowing simultaneous assessment of other structural damage to the knee, but it is relatively time-consuming and may interfere with other resuscitative actions for the patient. Conventional angiography is invasive but offers treatment options such as endovascular stenting in the case of isolated vascular flaps.[65-66]

Rieger et al.[67] retrospectively reviewed 87 cases of suspected traumatic extremity arterial injury and found the sensitivity of CTA to be 95% with 87% specificity, compared with a mixed diagnostic standard including surgery, angiography, clinical follow-up, and radiologic follow-up. Other small studies suggest high sensitivity and specificity of CTA.[67a-c]

In a review article, Fleiter and Mervis[68] concluded that CTA can replace conventional angiography in patients with both blunt and penetrating extremity injuries.

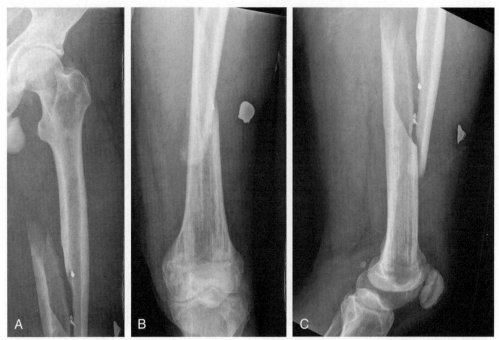

Figure 14-86. Midfemoral shaft fracture. This 44-year-old male presented after a gunshot wound to the left thigh. His x-rays show a comminuted oblique fracture through the middiaphysis. The distal fragment is angulated. Radiopaque material representing shrapnel is visible. The *small arrows* on the images are radiopaque wound markers placed in the emergency department, not labels placed by the author. This patient was taken to the operating room for repair, at which time tight anterior and posterior thigh compartments were noted. The patient underwent anterior and posterior thigh fasciotomies, as well as intramedullary nail fixation of his femur fracture. Compartment syndrome is not a radiographic diagnosis; nonetheless, long-bone fractures of the lower extremities should prompt consideration of this diagnosis. Remember that compartment syndrome can also occur in the absence of fracture. **A, B,** Anterior–posterior (AP) views. **C,** Lateral view.

Potter et al.[69] compared the results of MRA and conventional angiography in six patients with severe multiligament knee injuries and found 100% agreement, though only two arterial injuries were identified, leaving wide CIs. However, MRA compares favorably with CTA and conventional angiography for vessels of similar size in the head and neck, suggesting that it would be accurate in the setting of extremity trauma.

Tibial Stress Fractures

Tibial stress fractures can occur with repetitive exercise in runners and other athletes, particularly in young patients. The tibia accounts for nearly 50% of stress fractures in athletes. Initial x-rays are abnormal in only about 10% of cases[70] but should be performed to evaluate for competing diagnoses, including complete fracture, osteomyelitis, or malignancy.[71] Later in the course, the x-ray appearance of healing stress fractures includes localized periosteal reaction, endosteal thickening, and radiolucent cortical lines. Stress fractures in cancellous bone may be visible as a radiolucent fracture line, whereas in cortical bone, cortical thickening may be the only evidence of fracture.[71] Bone scan and MRI can be used for diagnosis in uncertain cases; the primary emergency indication for these studies is not to confirm stress fracture but to exclude more serious causes of pain such as bone infection or tumor, which can have similar x-ray appearances.[72]

Tibial and Fibular Shaft Fractures

The tibia is the most commonly fractured long bone, with an incidence of 2 per 1000 annually. Tibial and fibular shaft (diaphyseal) fractures are typically radiographically evident on plain x-ray (Figure 14-106). These fractures should be characterized using standard terms as described in Table 14-3, although more specific classification schemes are described in the orthopedic literature and used for prognosis and therapeutic planning. Often, fractures of both the tibial and the fibular shaft occur together. Tibial shaft fractures are high-energy injuries and can be associated with compartment syndrome in up to 7% of cases.[73] *The presence of tibial fracture does not guarantee compartment syndrome, nor does the absence of fracture exclude it.*

Open tibial fractures are surgical emergencies and should generally undergo debridement and irrigation within 6 hours.

Ankle Mortise Injury

The ankle mortise is the true ankle joint formed by the articulation of the distal fibula, distal tibia, and talus. The fibula forms the lateral border of the mortise, whereas the tibia forms the proximal and medial borders. Mechanisms leading to fractures of this structure include inversion injuries and impaction. Fractures can be described as unimalleolar, bimalleolar, or trimalleolar. Trimalleolar fractures include the lateral malleolus (distal fibula),

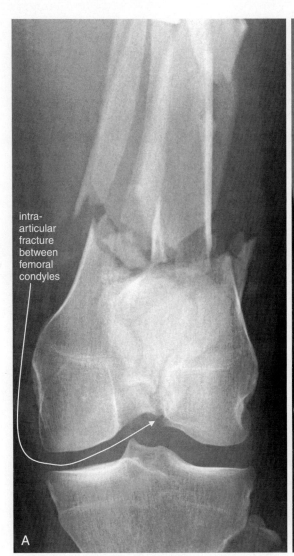

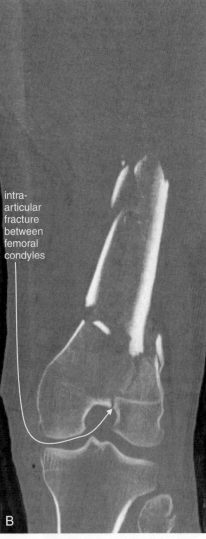

medial malleolus (medial distal tibia), and posterior malleolus (posterior distal tibia). More specific classification schemes are described in the orthopedic literature. A variety of eponyms are applied to describe various ankle mortise fracture patterns, including Maisonneuve fractures, pilon fractures, bimalleolar (Pott) fractures, trimalleolar (Cotton) fractures, triplane fractures, and snowboarder's fracture. In children, Salter-Harris fractures of the distal tibia, including Tillaux fractures, are common and often radiographically subtle.

Maisonneuve Fractures. Maisonneuve fractures involve the proximal third of the fibula and the distal tibia, usually the medial malleolus (Figure 14-107). In some cases, the deep deltoid ligament ruptures, sparing the medial malleolus from fracture. Tearing through the interosseous membrane and distal tibiofibular syndesmosis also occurs. This pattern of injury resembles the Galeazzi and Monteggia patterns seen in the forearm (discussed earlier in this chapter). As with those injury patterns, care must be taken not to overlook the second injury.

Tibial Plafond Fractures (Pilon Fractures). Fractures of the distal tibia are sometimes called **pilon fractures,** for hammer, referring to the compression nature of these injuries (Figure 14-108). Common mechanisms include vertical loading from falls from height, motor vehicle collision, and sporting mechanisms such as skiing. The talus is driven into the distal tibia, usually resulting in intraarticular injury, including comminuted fractures of the medial malleolus, anterior margin of the distal tibia, and transverse fractures of the posterior tibia. Of these injuries, 20% to 25% are open, and 75% are associated with fibula fractures. Other associated injuries include vertebral compression fractures, pelvic and acetabular injuries, vascular injuries, and compartment syndrome.[74]

A variety of classification schemes have been described and are used to plan surgical reconstruction and fixation. For the purposes of the emergency physician, describing these fractures using standard terminology is sufficient.

Figure 14-88. Distal femur fracture and proximal tibia fracture (tibial plateau). This 39-year-old male crashed his car into a tree while intoxicated and complained of left leg pain. **A,** Anterior–posterior view. **B,** Lateral view. The patient's fractures are not subtle, but some finer points are worth noting. First, the distal femur fracture not only is comminuted but also shows the distal fragment to be proximally dislocated, with the distal femoral shaft now overriding the femoral condyles. Both the distal femur and the proximal tibia are comminuted with intraarticular extension. Injuries such as these pose significant threat of arterial injury and compartment syndrome. Associated ligamentous injuries are likely but do not require emergency diagnosis. Compare with CT images in Figures 14-89 and 14-90.

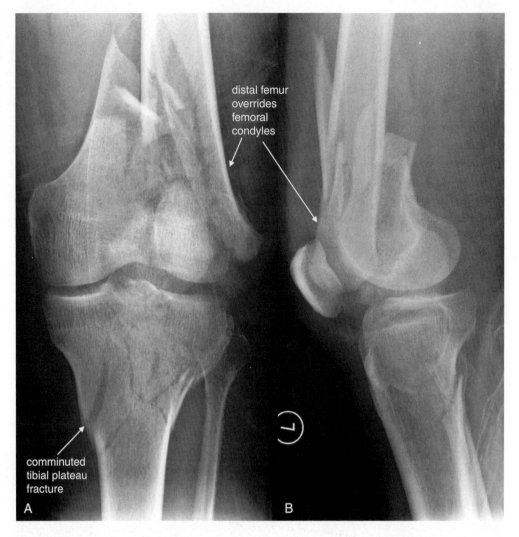

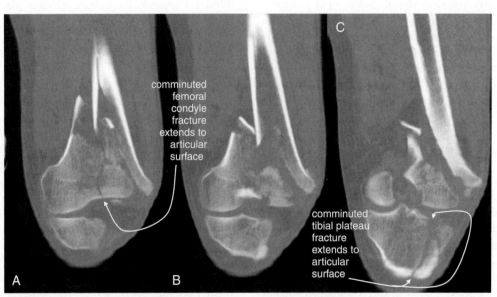

Figure 14-89. Distal femur fracture and proximal tibia fracture (tibial plateau), CT bone windows. Same patient as in Figure 14-88. **A** through **C,** This series of coronal reconstructions shows the degree of comminution and intraarticular extension of both the tibial plateau and the distal femoral fractures. Although not performed in this case, CT angiography can be performed concurrently if vascular injuries are suspected.

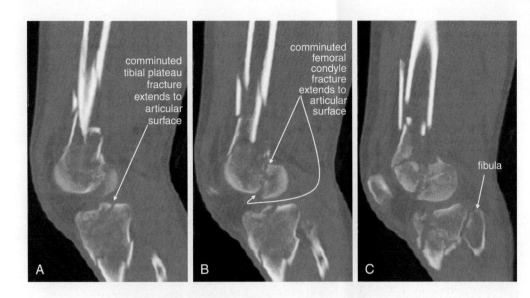

comminuted tibial plateau fracture extends to articular surface

comminuted femoral condyle fracture extends to articular surface

fibula

Figure 14-90. **Distal femur fracture and proximal tibia fracture (tibial plateau), CT bone windows.** Same patient as in Figures 14-88 and 14-89. **A** through **C,** This series of sagittal reconstructions shows the degree of comminution and intraarticular extension of both the tibial plateau and the distal femoral fractures.

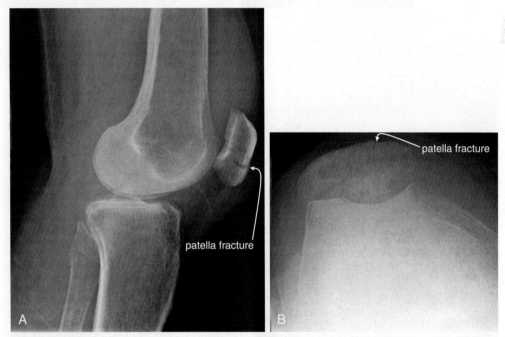

patella fracture

patella fracture

Figure 14-91. **Comminuted patellar fracture.** This 74-year-old female with a history of osteoarthritis fell directly on her right knee. Anterior–posterior (AP), lateral, and sunrise views of the knee were obtained for suspected patellar fracture. The AP view (not shown in this case) is often unhelpful for this injury, because the patella overlaps with the distal femur. **A,** The lateral view projects the patella clear of the femur and reveals a comminuted, mildly displaced transverse fracture. **B,** The sunrise view, obtained with the knee in flexion, also projects the patella clear of the femur and shows an oblique fracture. The patient was treated with a knee immobilizer, with weight bearing as tolerated.

CT scan is valuable in delineating these complex injuries and planning surgical repair. Conventional angiography or CTA should also be performed if associated vascular injury is suspected.

Other Ankle Mortise Fracture Patterns. **Bimalleolar (Pott) fractures** involve two of three malleoli: lateral (fibula), medial (tibia), and posterior (tibia). These unstable fractures require orthopedic fixation. **Trimalleolar (Cotton) fractures** involve all three malleoli and are unstable, requiring fixation (Figure 14-109).

A **Tillaux fracture** is Salter-Harris III injury of anterolateral tibial epiphysis caused by eversion and lateral ankle rotation, most common in adolescents, in whom the medial epiphyseal plate has closed, whereas the lateral physis remains open (Figure 14-110).[75] Other Salter-Harris injuries of the distal tibia and fibula are shown in Figures 14-111 through 14-113.

A **triplane fracture** combines distal tibial fractures in coronal, sagittal, and transverse planes. Distal fibula fractures commonly occur with these injuries. Like

Figure 14-92. Patella fracture. Like the patient in Figure 14-91, this patient fell directly on the knee, striking the patella. **A,** Anterior–posterior (AP) knee. **B,** Lateral knee. **C,** Close-up from **B**. **D,** Sunrise view. In this case, the orientation of the fracture is primarily horizontal or transverse to the long axis of the leg. Consequently, the fracture line is not seen on the sunrise view. It is visible in the lateral view. On the AP view, the density of the femur obscures the fracture of the patella.

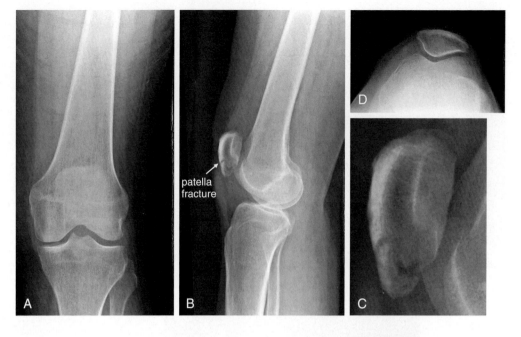

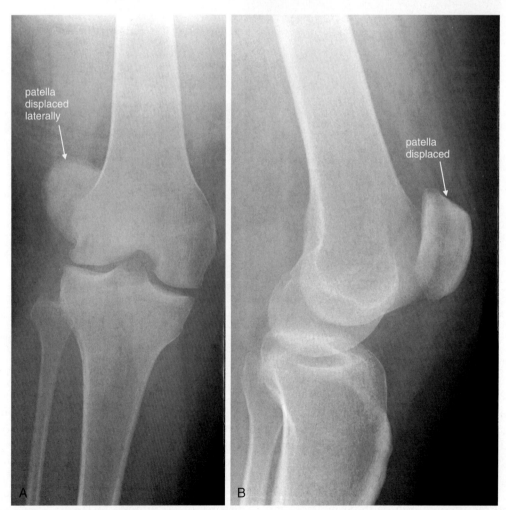

Figure 14-93. Patella dislocation. This 34-year-old female was playing Nintendo Wii baseball when she swung the controller, twisting and falling on her right knee. The patella is subluxed laterally, evident in the anterior–posterior view **(A).** In the lateral view **(B),** the patella overlaps with the distal femur in an abnormal manner, because it has subluxed off of the patellar surface, a groove on the anterior surface of the distal femur between the medial and the lateral femoral condyles. Patellar dislocation does not usually require x-ray for diagnosis, nor are postreduction x-rays usually required. If fracture of the patella or other injuries are suspected, x-rays may be useful. The patient's patella was reduced uneventfully. She also sustained a distal fibula fracture (not in field of view of these x-rays).

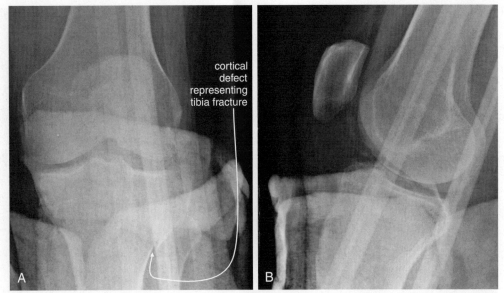

Figure 14-94. Tibial plateau fracture. This 42-year-old male was struck by a car while riding a moped. He presented with leg pain and a pretibial wound. **A,** Anterior–posterior view of left knee. **B,** Lateral left knee. Although stabilization of open extremity fractures is of key importance, remember to remove unnecessary external foreign material whenever possible. These x-rays are quite limited because of splint materials in the field. Nevertheless, a fracture of the proximal tibia can be seen extending from the lateral metaphysis toward the articular surface. Computed tomography was performed to evaluate this injury further (Figure 14-95).

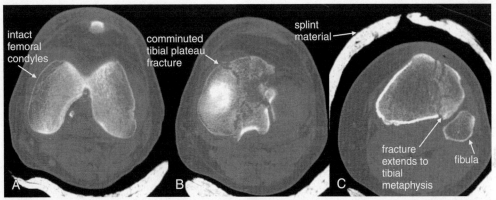

Figure 14-95. Tibial plateau fracture. Same patient as in Figure 14-94. CT provides detailed information about articular fractures. These images taken from the axial CT series show the distal femoral condyles to be intact **(A).** The tibial plateau is comminuted **(B),** and the fracture extends to the lateral tibial metaphysis **(C),** as seen on the x-ray in Figure 14-94. Another advantage of CT is that it can image bone through overlying splint material. Because of its cost and radiation exposure, CT should not be used if adequate clinical information can be gathered with x-ray, so unnecessary splint materials should be removed before plain x-ray when possible to allow the best diagnostic images to be obtained.

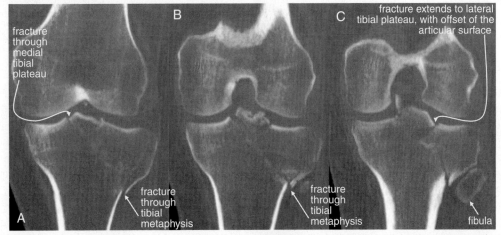

Figure 14-96. Tibial plateau fracture. Same patient as in Figures 14-94 and 14-95. **A** through **C,** Coronal CT reconstructions demonstrate this tibial plateau fracture in more detail. For assessment of fractures, the scan is performed using 0.625-mm axial imaging with multiplanar reconstructions. There is a comminuted fracture involving the tibial plateau. The fracture line can be seen extending from the medial tibial plateau obliquely to the lateral tibial metaphysis. A branch of the fracture extends to the lateral tibial plateau as well. The articular surface of the lateral tibial plateau is slightly offset.

Figure 14-97. **Tibial plateau fracture.** Same patient as in Figures 14-94 through 14-96. Here, sagittal computed tomography reconstructions reveal severe comminution of the posterior tibial plateau. In addition, a proximal fibula fracture is visible. **A** represents a lateral parasagittal plane. **B** and **C** progress medially.

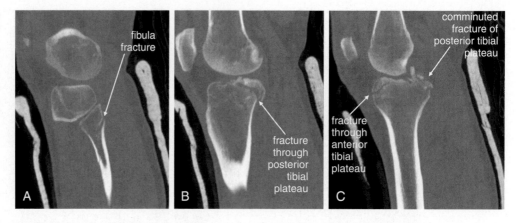

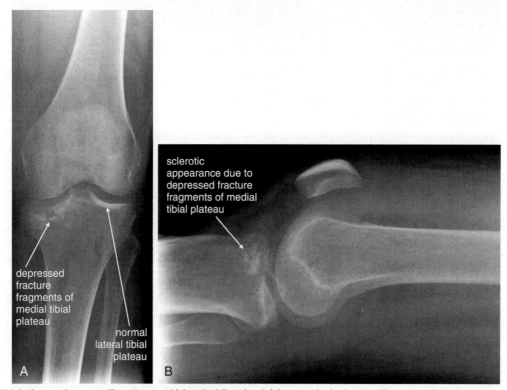

Figure 14-98. **Tibial plateau fracture.** This 48-year-old female fell on her left knee in the bathroom. This relatively low-energy mechanism resulted in a depressed medial tibial plateau fracture—probably a complication of osteoporosis related to end-stage renal disease. **A,** Anterior–posterior view. Compare the smooth articular surface of the lateral tibial plateau with the medial plateau, which is irregular, comminuted, and depressed. The cortex appears discontinuous. **B,** Lateral view. The fracture is less evident here, but the anterior tibia appears sclerotic and dense because of overlapping depressed fracture fragments. CT (not shown) was performed to evaluate the injury more completely and to allow operative planning. The patient was treated with open reduction and internal fixation.

the Tillaux fracture, this injury usually occurs in early adolescence, when the medial tibial physis has closed but the lateral physis remains open. The coronal fracture line is typically best seen on the lateral x-ray and involves the posterior tibial metaphysis and a portion of the epiphysis. The sagittal fracture is seen best on AP views and is a vertically oriented fracture through the epiphysis, usually at a midportion of the tibial plafond. It can occur at any portion of the anterior epiphysis and extends in variable directions. The axial fracture occurs through the physis and is often difficult to see on x-ray. CT is useful to characterize these fractures further.

Triplane fractures can occur as two-, three-, and four-part fractures. Two-part fractures are most common and are a Salter-Harris IV fracture of the distal tibia. Two fracture fragments are produced: (1) the lateral portion of the epiphysis attached to a posterior metaphyseal spike and (2) the distal tibia with the anteromedial epiphysis attached.

Three-part triplane fractures appear as Salter-Harris III fractures on AP view and as Salter-Harris II fractures on lateral view. Three fracture fragments are produced: (1) a rectangular fragment of the anterolateral epiphysis,

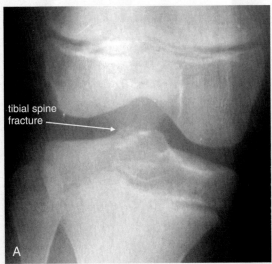

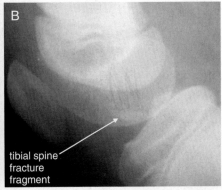

Figure 14-99. Tibial spine avulsion fracture. This 7-year-old female fell while riding a bicycle. She complained of right knee pain and swelling. **A,** Anterior–posterior knee. **B,** Lateral knee. X-rays of the right knee show a subtle intercondylar eminence (tibial spine) fracture. Don't believe it? Look carefully at her CT in Figure 14-100, and then return to these images. This injury may appear relatively innocuous, but it is a disabling injury requiring surgical repair. This is the tibial attachment point for the anterior cruciate ligament (ACL). Particularly in children, avulsion of the bony attachment, rather than ACL tear, may occur. Postoperative x-rays are shown in Figure 14-100. The patient underwent attempted arthroscopic repair, which was subsequently converted to an open repair.

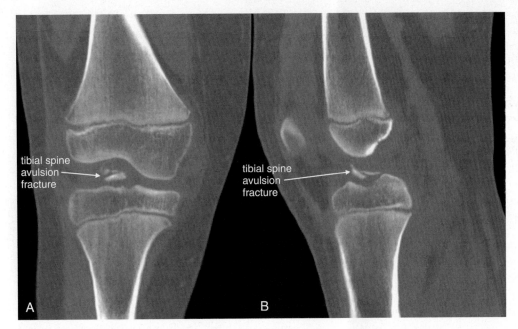

Figure 14-100. Tibial spine avulsion fracture. Same patient as in Figure 14-99. **A,** Coronal CT reconstruction. **B,** Sagittal reconstruction. The tibial spine is avulsed at the insertion point of the anterior cruciate ligament (ACL). Compare with the x-rays in Figure 14-99. Clinically, this injury simulates ACL tear. Magnetic resonance imaging was not performed in this patient before operative therapy, because a tear of the ACL is unlikely to occur when the attachment has avulsed. Moreover, because operative repair with direct visualization is required, additional imaging is unnecessary.

(2) the remainder of the epiphysis with an attached posterior spike of the distal tibial metaphysis, and (3) the tibial shaft with the anteromedial epiphysis.[76-77]

Four-part triplane fractures are similar to three-part fractures, with the addition of a fourth fragment from the medial malleolus.

Talus Fractures

Talus fractures (Figures 14-114 and 14-115) can occur in association with other ankle mortise or pilon injuries. In addition, a lateral talus process fracture called a **snowboarder's fracture** can occur with extreme dorsiflexion

of the ankle. X-rays are normal in 40% of cases.[78] CT is often needed for diagnosis of this occult injury and should be considered in snowboarders with lateral ankle pain and normal plain films.[79]

Tibiotalar and Subtalar Dislocations

Forceful plantar flexion and inversion or eversion stress can result in **tibiotalar dislocation** (often called ankle dislocation) or **subtalar dislocation** (Figures 14-116 and 14-117). Motor vehicle collisions or falls from height are common causes, though forceful lateral motion during sports occasionally can result in this injury, because the ankle joint bears a force equal to several times the body

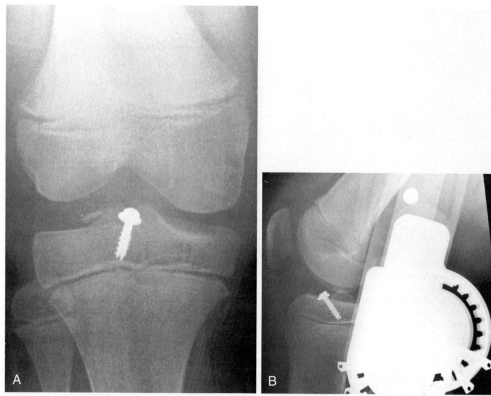

Figure 14-101. Tibial spine avulsion fracture. Same patient as in Figures 14-99 and 14-100. Here, the tibial spine fracture fragment has been fixed in position with a surgical screw. **A,** Anterior-posterior view. **B,** Lateral view.

weight during these activities. Fractures of the talus and of the tibial or fibular malleoli are commonly present, resulting from the high energy required to dislocate the tibiotalar joint. Posterior dislocation is most common. These injuries can be open, and vascular injury can result even from closed injuries. High-degree ligamentous injuries occur with this dislocation.[80]

Calcaneal Fractures

Calcaneal fractures (Figures 14-118 through 14-120) classically occur with falls from height, although motor vehicle collisions are another common cause. Associated injuries include lumbar and thoracic compression fractures. Compartment syndrome of the foot can complicate high-energy calcaneus fracture. Stress fractures of the calcaneus without associated injuries can result from long marches, such as by military personnel. Compression of the calcaneus results in loss of height, visible on lateral x-ray as a decrease in the **Bohler (sometimes spelled *Boehler* or *Böhler*) angle** (see Figures 14-118 and 14-119).[81] The Bohler angle is determined by drawing a line from the posterior superior aspect of the calcaneus through the highest point of the posterior subtalar articular surface (the apex of the calcaneus). A second line is drawn from the highest point of the anterior process of the calcaneus to the posterior margin of the subtalar surface of the calcaneus. The angle formed by the intersection of the two lines is the Bohler angle. A normal Bohler angle is 20-40 degrees, with values less than 20 degrees

strongly suggesting fracture. Isaacs et al.[82] studied 212 patients with calcaneus fracture and 212 normal controls. A Bohler angle less than or equal to 20 degrees was 99% sensitive and specific for calcaneus fracture, with a positive likelihood ratio of 110. However, larger Bohler angles, although 100% sensitive, were less specific for fracture: an angle below 25 degrees was only 82% specific, with a positive likelihood ratio of 5, and below 23 degrees was 89% specific, with a positive likelihood ratio of 9. Knight et al.[83] found the Bohler angle to have excellent interrater reliability for emergency physicians. However, emergency physicians in this study were highly accurate (97.9%) in diagnosing calcaneus fractures without the assistance of the Bohler angle. The accuracy of emergency physicians in this study may not reflect real-world practice, because the physicians were specifically asked to evaluate x-rays for the presence of calcaneal fracture.

In uncertain cases, CT is valuable in identifying and characterizing these fractures, which are often comminuted and intraarticular.[84]

Achilles Tendon and Ligamentous Injuries of the Ankle

As described earlier, clinical decision rules can guide ordering of x-rays of the foot and ankle, allowing x-rays to be avoided in many cases of sprain without fracture. Ligamentous injuries of the ankle are common, accounting for about 85% of ankle injuries. In most cases, diagnostic imaging is not indicated in the emergency

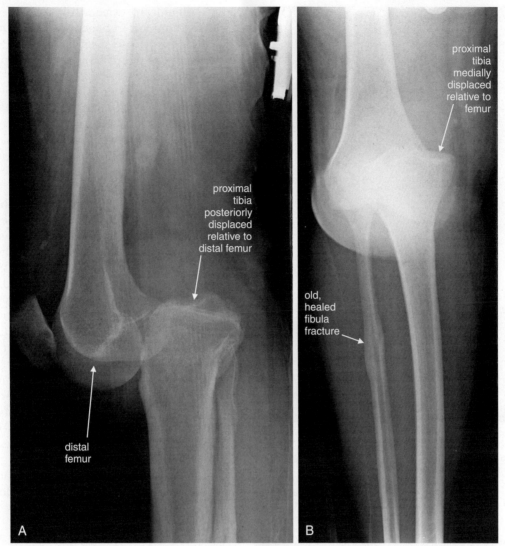

proximal
tibia
medially
displaced
relative to
femur

proximal
tibia
posteriorly
displaced
relative to
distal femur

old,
healed
fibula
fracture

distal
femur

A

B

Figure 14-102. Knee dislocation, posterior. This 29-year-old male fell down an embankment while intoxicated and was transported by emergency medical services to the emergency department, where he was noted to have no palpable pulses in his right foot. His knee appeared posteriorly dislocated on examination. He was unable to move his toes or ankle. Emergent knee reduction was performed in the emergency department, but the distal pulses remained absent even when sought by Doppler ultrasound. **A,** A lateral knee x-ray before reduction shows definite posterior dislocation of the tibia relative to the femur. **B,** An anterior–posterior view shows medial displacement of the tibia and fibula relative to the distal femur. Incidentally, the patient has an old, healed fibula fracture. This patient underwent angiography, shown in Figure 14-103.

department to confirm these injuries. MRI is considered by the ACR the diagnostic imaging standard for ligamentous injury.[85]

Tarsal Fractures
Tarsal fractures (Figure 14-121) can be difficult to diagnose by plain x-ray, resulting from the confluence of the outlines of the tarsal bones, talus, and calcaneus. The tarsal bones include the navicular (named for its sail shape on AP x-ray), cuboid (named for its cubelike shape), and three cuneiform bones: the medial, intermediate (sometimes called middle), and lateral. When fracture is suspected but is not seen on plain x-ray, CT scan can provide fine anatomic detail to delineate fractures. No large studies have compared the sensitivity of x-ray and MRI for tarsal fractures, but small studies suggest x-ray to be insensitive.

Preidler et al.[86] prospectively compared x-ray (including resting and stress views), CT, and MRI in 49 patients with acute hyperflexion injuries of the foot. The authors did not report sensitivity and specificity values, because a well-defined diagnostic standard was not available in all patients. However, x-ray revealed only 33 metatarsal and 20 tarsal fractures, whereas CT revealed 53 metatarsal and 41 tarsal fractures in the same patients. Magnetic resonance revealed 41 metatarsal fractures and 18 metatarsal "bone bruises," with 39 tarsal fractures and 9 tarsal bone bruises. The authors concluded that conventional x-ray is inadequate and that CT should be the primary imaging technique for patients with acute hyperflexion foot injuries. Presumably, other acute midfoot injuries might show similar patterns of greater diagnostic sensitivity of CT and MRI.

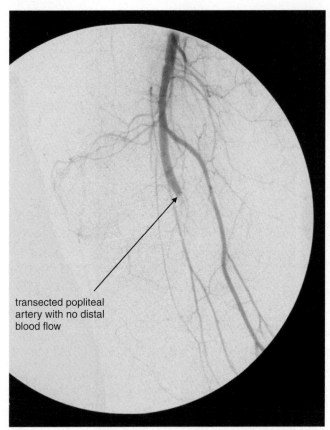

transected popliteal
artery with no distal
blood flow

Figure 14-103. Knee dislocation with popliteal arterial injury. Same patient as in Figure 14-102, with posterior knee dislocation. An arteriogram shows no flow beyond the popliteal artery at the level of the knee, consistent with severe arterial injury. Popliteal arterial injury is a limb-threatening injury associated with knee dislocation. When knee dislocation is known or suspected, popliteal artery injury must be strongly suspected and thoroughly evaluated. Spontaneous reduction of a dislocated knee can occur before emergency department arrival and should be suspected in cases of severe knee trauma. As described in the text, a meta-analysis suggests that physical examination is inadequate to exclude popliteal artery injury, although some small studies conclude otherwise. The gold-standard radiographic method for evaluation of popliteal arterial injury remains arteriogram. CT angiography appears to have sensitivity and specificity approaching that of conventional angiography. The sensitivity and specificity of ultrasound in this setting are not well characterized in the literature.

Peicha et al.[87] prospectively compared x-ray with stress views, CT, and MRI in 75 consecutive patients with acute hyperflexion foot trauma. X-ray revealed 48 metatarsal and 24 tarsal fractures, CT showed 86 metatarsal and 74 tarsal fractures, and MRI detected 85 metatarsal and 100 tarsal fractures. The authors concluded that x-ray is inadequate in diagnosis of acute hyperflexion foot injuries.

Tarsometatarsal Joint Fractures and Dislocations (Lisfranc Fracture)

Hyperflexion injuries to the foot can result not only in fractures but also in dislocations of the tarsometatarsal joint, called the **Lisfranc joint** (Figures 14-122 and 14-123). This injury is both notoriously difficult to diagnose radiographically and clinically important,

because significant osteoarthritis and poor long-term outcomes can occur in patients with this injury who do not undergo adequate surgical fixation. Poor outcomes are common even in patients who are properly treated, but misdiagnosis is a source of medical–legal liability for emergency physicians. Normally, the tarsometatarsal joint is well aligned, with little separation of the first and second metatarsals and closely apposed medial and middle cuneiform bones. The lateral aspect of the first metatarsal should align with the lateral aspect of the medial cuneiform bone. The medial border of the second metatarsal should align with the medial border of the middle cuneiform bone. Ligaments join the second and third metatarsals, the third and fourth metatarsals, and the fourth and fifth metatarsals at their bases. However, no ligament stabilizes the space between the first and the second metatarsals, making this a potentially unstable region. Instead, a ligament joins the medial cuneiform bone to the base of the second metatarsal—called the **Lisfranc ligament** (see Figure 14-122). This ligament is often disrupted in the Lisfranc injury. The Lisfranc injury is characterized on x-ray by splaying of the distance between the first and the second metatarsals and often of the space between the medial and the middle cuneiform bones. Fractures may also be seen. Traditionally, if resting x-rays do not show splaying of the joint space, stress (weight bearing) x-rays are obtained to exaggerate the joint distance if an unstable joint is present.

Several small studies have examined advanced imaging techniques in comparison with x-ray for detection of the Lisfranc joint injury.

Preidler et al.[88] retrospectively reviewed MRI findings in 11 patients with Lisfranc injuries, 5 with x-rays for comparison. X-ray showed tarsometatarsal joint widening in all 5 patients, and tarsal and metatarsal fractures were seen in 4 patients. MRI showed Lisfranc joint malalignment in all 11 patients and a disrupted Lisfranc ligament in 8. In the 3 patients with intact Lisfranc ligaments, an avulsion fracture was seen either in the second metatarsal base or in the medial cuneiform bone at the site of ligament insertion. MRI also showed metatarsal base and tarsal bone fractures in 10 patients. This small series proves little about the sensitivity of x-ray or MRI, but the authors suggested MRI should be used in patients with inconclusive x-ray findings.

Preidler et al.[86] then prospectively compared x-ray with stress views, CT, and MRI in 49 patients with hyperflexion foot injuries, as described earlier in the section on tarsal fractures. Resting and stress x-ray each revealed 8 cases of Lisfranc joint malalignment; stress views did not detect any cases not seen already with resting x-ray. CT scan revealed 16 Lisfranc joint malalignments. MRI showed Lisfranc joint malalignment in 16 patients, including 11 cases with Lisfranc ligament disruption.

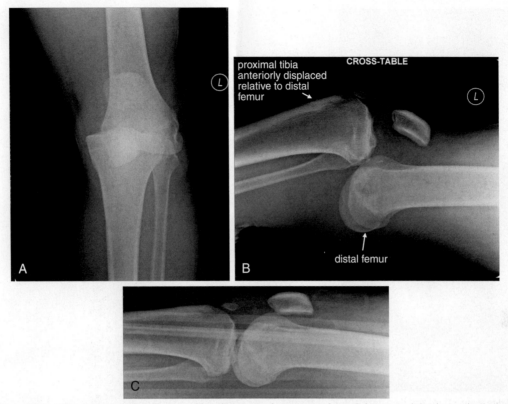

Figure 14-104. Knee dislocation, anterior. This 18-year-old male sustained an anterior knee dislocation while playing football. Compare with the posterior knee dislocation in Figure 14-102. **A,** Anterior–posterior view before reduction. **B,** Lateral view before reduction. **C,** Lateral view after reduction. Beware of the possibility of spontaneous reduction of this unstable injury, which may then look normal on x-ray. If a knee dislocation is suspected, evaluate for popliteal artery injury. See the CT angiogram image from this patient in Figure 14-105.

The authors concluded that x-ray is inadequate for detection of this injury. Assuming that CT and MRI were correct in all cases, x-ray was only 50% sensitive for detection of this important injury.

Peicha et al.[87] prospectively compared x-ray with stress views, CT, and MRI in 75 consecutive patients with acute hyperflexion foot injuries. Resting x-ray showed 17 cases of Lisfranc joint injury, and stress views showed no additional injuries. CT showed 31 cases of Lisfranc joint malalignment and 4 cases of bony avulsion of the Lisfranc ligament. MRI detected 31 cases of Lisfranc joint malalignment and 22 partial or complete tears of the Lisfranc ligament. Again, x-ray was inadequate to detect Lisfranc joint injury, with a sensitivity of only 55% compared with a standard of CT or MRI.

Crim[89] reviewed the literature and concluded that data on the diagnostic accuracy of MRI was lacking. This is because of the paucity of studies in which MRI findings are confirmed against an independent diagnostic standard, such as surgical findings.

Metatarsal Fractures
Metatarsal fractures (Figures 14-124 and 14-125) can occur from a variety of mechanisms, including hyperflexion foot injuries, as described earlier; direct foot blunt or penetrating trauma; or ankle inversion injuries. Fractures can occur at any point along the course of the metatarsal. However, certain patterns are most clinically important. Metatarsal base fractures may occur in conjunction with Lisfranc joint injuries, as described earlier. Metatarsal fractures are common and occur as much as 10 times more often than Lisfranc injuries.

Fractures of the first metatarsal typically require internal fixation (sometimes percutaneously), because the first metatarsal bears significant weight compared with the other metatarsals. Fractures of the second through fourth metatarsals also often require internal fixation because of their role in weight-bearing.[90] As described later, fractures of the fifth metatarsal may not require internal fixation.

The fifth metatarsal is prone to fractures at its base. A normal anatomic feature, the proximal apophysis or tuberosity, may be mistaken for fracture by novice interpreters. The apophysis is a bony projection on the lateral base of the fifth metatarsal; its growth plate is oriented parallel to the long axis of the metatarsal and may appear as a lucent (dark) or sclerotic (white) line on x-ray—simulating a fracture. In contrast, many true fractures in this location are transverse, though avulsion fractures of the apophysis can occur. Important fifth

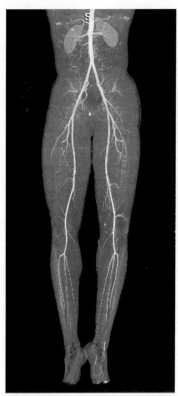

Figure 14-105. **Knee dislocation, anterior, normal CT.** Same patient as in Figure 14-104. Because of suspected popliteal artery injury, the patient underwent CT angiography (CTA). Studies suggest that CTA is similar in sensitivity and specificity to conventional angiography for lower extremity injuries. Magnetic resonance angiography is an alternative with similar diagnostic ability for vascular injuries. In CTA, an intravenously injected contrast bolus is followed from the aorta into the lower extremities. Images can be reconstructed in any plane, and three-dimensional computer models can be rapidly built and manipulated. In this case, no vascular injury was found.

metatarsal fractures with eponyms include the Jones, pseudo-Jones, and dancer's fractures.[91]

A **Jones fracture** (see Figure 14-125) is an acute transverse fracture of the fifth metatarsal at the junction between the proximal diaphysis and the adjacent metaphysis (1-2 cm distal to the proximal tip of the metatarsal). The mechanism is believed to be indirect, with inversion of the foot coincident with plantar flexion. Fracture may result from stress at the insertion point of the peroneus tertius. Poor blood supply to the region is believed to increase the risk for nonunion. This injury is radiographically similar to a proximal diaphyseal fifth metatarsal stress fracture, an overuse injury that is located immediately distal to the site of Jones fractures. Standard texts continue to distinguish these conditions and to differentiate their treatments. Jones fractures are typically treated with 6-8 weeks of non-weight-bearing immobilization, with operative treatment reserved for competitive athletes and failures of nonoperative therapy. In contrast, proximal diaphyseal stress fractures are reported to have healing times as long as 21 months in nonoperative cases, with

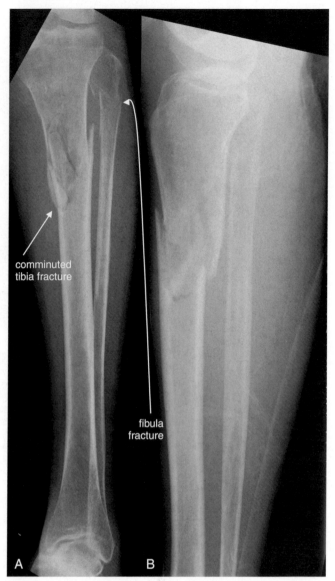

Figure 14-106. **Tibial and fibular shaft fractures.** This 54-year-old female with a history of chronic steroid use slipped on water in her home and sustained a left lower extremity injury. Her x-rays show a proximal tibial diaphysis fracture that is comminuted. The distal fragment is somewhat anteriorly displaced relative to the proximal fragment. In addition, the proximal fibula has a transverse fracture. **A,** Anterior–posterior view. **B,** Lateral view. Diaphyseal fractures of long bones in adult patients are usually not a diagnostic challenge on plain x-ray. Important points for this case are the association of tibial fractures with fibular fractures. Because of the strong syndesmosis (intraosseous membranous joint), these two bones act like a ring under stress, and force transmitted through one bone often generates tension resulting in fracture of the other. Moreover, tibial fractures are associated with lower extremity compartment syndrome. Patients should be carefully instructed on symptoms and signs of compartment syndrome, and monitoring with repeated examinations or actual compartment pressure measurements should be considered. This patient underwent closed reduction and intramedullary fixation of the tibial fracture. Her compartment pressures were monitored but did not become elevated.

nonunion rates as high as 25%; consequently, operative therapy is usually recommended.[92] Chuckpaiwong et al.[93] reviewed clinical outcomes in Jones fractures and proximal fifth metatarsal fractures and found no difference in therapy or outcomes in the two groups.

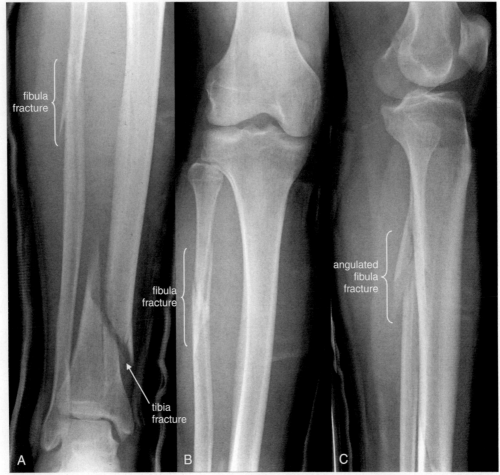

Figure 14-107. Maisonneuve fracture. This 29-year-old male was tackled playing rugby and complained of right lower extremity pain. His x-rays show an obvious fracture of the distal tibial metaphysis. His proximal fibular diaphysis fracture is subtler. On the anterior–posterior views **(A, B),** this appears minimally displaced and angulated, although the lateral view **(C)** tells a different tale. A fibular fracture fragment is displaced and angulated. The combination of a distal tibial fracture and a proximal fibula fracture fits the Maisonneuve fracture pattern. Often, this pattern involves the medial or posterior malleoli of the tibia, or the tibia itself may not be fractured but a significant ankle sprain with injuries of the deltoid ligament or anterior talofibular ligament may be present. When injuries to the distal tibia or ankle ligaments are present, inspect the proximal fibula carefully for fracture. The proximal fibula fracture does not require surgical fixation, but long leg casting is typical. This patient had an external fixator placed because of the severity of his tibial fracture.

Consequently, the authors suggest that efforts to distinguish the two conditions are unnecessary, because they do not appear to be associated with differences in treatment or prognosis.

Avulsion fractures of the base of the fifth metatarsal (see Figure 14-125) may occur from tension at the insertion point of the peroneus brevis, although a competing theory suggests the lateral band of the plantar aponeurosis may be responsible.[90] These injuries are sometimes called **pseudo-Jones fractures,** because of their location in the proximal fifth metatarsal, grossly similar to Jones fractures. However, unlike the Jones fracture, which is a transverse fracture of the proximal diaphysis, the pseudo-Jones fracture is an avulsion fracture of the base of the fifth metatarsal involving the lateral apophysis (also called tuberosity). This fracture site is proximal to the site of a Jones fracture and may appear incomplete, involving only the lateral cortex on x-ray. Most are extraarticular. In some series, pseudo-Jones fractures are

the most common fifth metatarsal base fracture, accounting for more than 90% of these fractures. Patients with pseudo-Jones fractures can weight bear as tolerated and heal in around 4 weeks, unlike patients with Jones fractures, who are treated with non-weight-bearing status.[92,94] A below-knee cast is unnecessary for fifth metatarsal avulsion fractures.[95]

A **dancer's fracture** is a spiral or oblique fracture of the distal shaft or neck of the fifth metatarsal, resulting from inversion of the foot from a demipointe ballet position (plantar-flexed ankle, with dorsiflexion of the metatarsophalangeal joints). The injury is common in ballet dancers, as the name implies. The fracture line usually begins proximally along the medial aspect of the fifth metatarsal and extends distally to the lateral surface. Mildly displaced fractures heal in 6 to 8 weeks with short-leg casting or a CAM walker boot. Fractures with displacement of 3 to 5 mm may require open reduction and internal fixation, although recent series

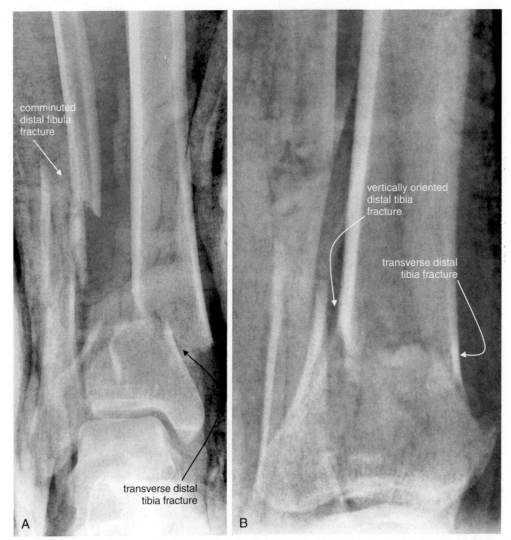

Figure 14-108. Tibial plafond fracture (pilon fracture). Tibial plafond or pilon fractures are compression injuries of the ankle and distal tibial metaphysis, often with intraarticular comminution. The medial malleolus (tibia), anterior tibia, and posterior tibial surfaces are usually fractured. The fibula is also fractured in about 75% of cases. These injuries occur from major trauma mechanisms and are associated with compartment syndrome, vertebral compression fractures, pelvic injuries, and vascular injuries. Pilon fractures are often open injuries. This 30-year-old male fell 30 feet from the roof of a house, landing on his feet. He had an open ankle injury on emergency department arrival, with protrusion of the medial malleolus. **A,** Anterior–posterior view. **B,** Lateral view. Fiberglass cast material partially obscures bony detail. However, a transverse comminuted, laterally displaced distal tibia fracture is present. A vertically oriented fracture of the posterior tibia is also present. The patient was treated with an external fixator.

document good clinical outcomes with nonoperative therapy.[96]

Toe Fractures
Fractures of the toes are common—not surprisingly, given their exposure to trauma. Fractures in adults are usually readily apparent on x-ray. In children, Salter-Harris I fractures can occur with stubbing of the toe and are often radiographically occult if nondisplaced (Figure 14-126). Moreover, these may be open fractures, with the laceration obscured under the nail. Clinical clues may include subungual hematoma, bleeding from the eponychium (cuticle), and a laceration proximal to the nail bed. Cases of osteomyelitis resulting from such presumably open Salter-Harris I fractures have been reported (see Figures 14-140 and 14-141).[97-98]

Consequently, antibiotics should be considered when a stubbing injury occurs in children, even if no radiographic abnormality is visible.

Muscle Injuries

Muscle injuries are not visible on x-ray, though in some cases they may be suspected based on patterns of bony injury. In general, these injuries do not require diagnostic imaging in the emergency department. When management requires specific diagnosis, MRI is the optimal imaging test because of its excellent soft-tissue contrast.

Neoplasms and Soft-Tissue Masses

Bony extremity tumors include primary bone malignancies such as osteosarcomas and Ewing sarcoma, as well as a variety of metastatic tumors, such as lung,

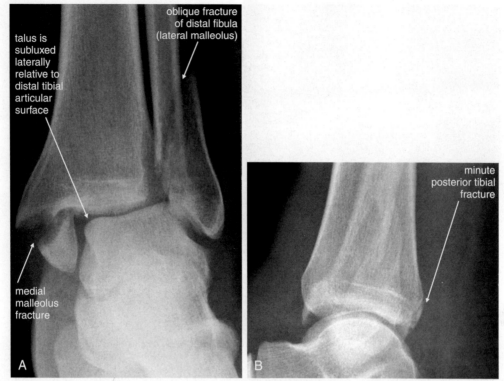

Figure 14-109. Ankle mortise injury (trimalleolar). This 48-year-old male fell from his bicycle while intoxicated and was unable to bear weight on his left ankle. His examination showed significant swelling of both malleoli. **A,** Anterior–posterior x-ray. The medial malleolus of the tibia is fractured and displaced. The lateral malleolus (composed of the distal fibula) is also obliquely fractured, with lateral displacement of the fracture fragment. The talus is laterally displaced with respect to the distal tibia. This is a highly unstable fracture, because the bony attachment sites of multiple ligaments of the ankle are avulsed. **B,** Lateral x-ray. The posterior distal tibia also appears to have a small fracture, making this a trimalleolar fracture. The patient underwent open reduction and internal fixation.

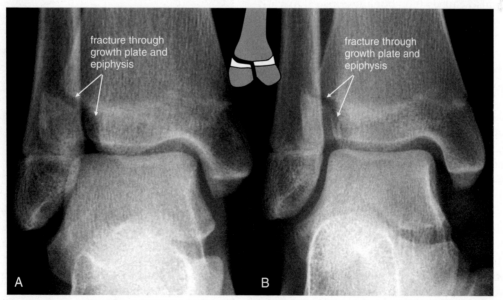

Figure 14-110. Tillaux fracture, a Salter-Harris III tibial fracture. This 12-year-old female was playing softball when she slid into home plate and injured her ankle. She has been unable to ambulate because of pain. Her x-rays show a Tillaux fracture, an eponym for an anterolateral tibial epiphyseal fracture, extending to the physis (growth plate). This is a Salter-Harris III injury. The mechanism is external foot rotation with avulsion fracture because of the strength of the anterior tibiofibular ligament. This is common in adolescents but rare in adults, in whom rupture of the ligament usually occurs, rather than fracture. This patient underwent open reduction and internal fixation of the right anterolateral tibial epiphysis. **A,** Anterior–posterior view. **B,** Oblique view.

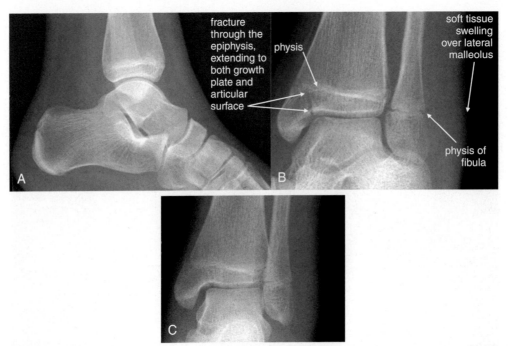

Figure 14-111. Nondisplaced Salter-Harris III fracture of the tibia, with nondisplaced Salter-Harris I fibula fracture. This 14-year-old basketball point guard inverted her ankle during a game and was unable to walk. **A,** Lateral view. **B,** Oblique view. **C,** Anterior–posterior view. A lucent fracture line runs through the medial malleolus of the tibial epiphysis and extends to the physis. This is nondisplaced but extends to the articular surface as well. Though fracture through the physis cannot be directly seen, extension of the fracture through the growth plate should be assumed, making this a Salter-Harris III fracture. Note the significant swelling overlying the lateral malleolus. Although no fracture is seen, a nondisplaced Salter-Harris I distal fibula fracture may be present, and empiric treatment should be instituted. Remember that ankle sprains in children should be assumed to represent Salter-Harris I fractures, which are fractures through the growth plate only. When nondisplaced, these are radiographically occult. The patient was placed in a bivalved, short-leg cast to allow for swelling.

breast, thyroid, testicular, kidney, and prostate. Multiple myeloma also causes lytic bone lesions often visible on x-ray. Figures 14-127 and 14-128 demonstrate bone abnormalities concerning for neoplasm. Pathologic fractures may also be seen at the site of a bone neoplasm, whether benign or malignant (see also Figure 14-38).

Soft-tissue masses do not routinely require emergency diagnostic imaging, although abscesses may masquerade as solid masses. Abscesses are usually readily identified by ultrasound when superficial; deeper collections may require CT for diagnosis. Solid soft-tissue masses can be extremely serious, including malignancies such as sarcomas. Although the workup can often be deferred to the outpatient setting, there may be patients whose follow-up cannot be assured and for whom a definitive diagnosis in the emergency department is preferred. MRI is the optimal imaging test for these patients. The ACR recommends x-rays in the initial evaluation of soft-tissue masses, while noting their limited utility and the possible need for advanced imaging such as MRI, regardless of x-ray results. X-rays may indicate an underlying bony lesion such as infection or bone neoplasm. X-ray findings of neoplasms can include lytic or sclerotic lesions, pathologic fractures, soft-tissue calcifications, and periosteal reaction.[99,99a] Detailed diagnostic imaging of extremity neoplasms is beyond the scope of this text.

SPECIAL TOPICS

Although orthopedic injuries including fractures and dislocations constitute some of the most common reasons for extremity imaging in emergency medicine, other conditions of the extremities can be dangerous to the patient and diagnostically challenging to the physician, creating medical–legal risk. In this section, we consider these conditions, discuss the limits of diagnostic imaging, and point out diagnostic pitfalls that may arise during evaluation.

Arterial Injuries and Other Arterial Pathology

We discussed in other sections of this chapter the evaluation of arterial vascular injuries in the context of knee dislocation. Vascular injury can result from a variety of other blunt and penetrating trauma mechanisms. In addition, the emergency physician may encounter nontraumatic cases of suspected vascular insufficiency, requiring confirmation with diagnostic imaging. Although x-ray may reveal extensive vascular calcifications related to peripheral arterial disease, it does not provide information about the patency of the vessel (Figure 14-129). Diagnostic modalities for assessing vascular structures include ultrasound, conventional angiography, CTA, and MRA.

Advantages of ultrasound include portability, lack of ionizing radiation exposure, and absence of the need for vascular contrast agents, with their attendant risks for

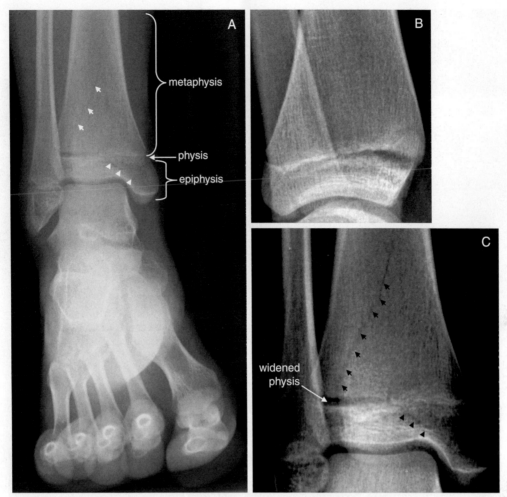

Figure 14-112. Nondisplaced Salter-Harris IV fracture of the tibia. This 12-year-old female tripped while running and twisted her right ankle. She had immediate pain and was unable to bear weight. Examination showed swelling and tenderness over both malleoli. **A,** Anterior–posterior view of the ankle. **B,** Lateral view of the ankle. **C,** Close-up from **A,** with contrast altered to emphasize fracture lines. The x-ray shows a Salter-Harris IV fracture, defined as a fracture crossing through the physis (growth plate) and involving both the metaphysis and the epiphysis. Salter-Harris IV fractures may interfere with normal growth, even with perfect reduction. Displaced fractures of this type require open reduction and internal fixation. In this case, an oblique fracture extends from the distal tibial metaphysis *(short arrows)*, through the growth plate, and into the epiphysis *(arrowheads).* Also notice the widened physis in the lateral tibia. Computed tomography of the same injury is shown in the Figure 14-113. The patient underwent posterior splinting followed by 6 weeks of cast treatment with good outcome. Because of the risk for poor outcomes even in optimally treated cases, clear discussion of the natural history of the injury with the patient, documentation of the discussion, and orthopedic consultation or referral are advised.

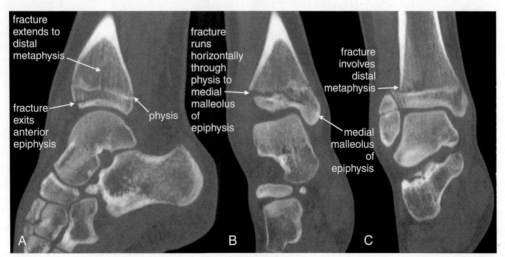

Figure 14-113. Nondisplaced Salter-Harris IV fracture of the tibia. Same patient as in Figure 14-112. Computed tomography reconstructions in sagittal **(A)** and coronal **(B, C)** planes reveal the extent of the fracture. **A,** The fracture line is seen running through the distal metaphysis, crossing the physis, and then exiting the anterior epiphysis without involving the articular surface. **B,** The fracture extends horizontally through the growth plate and into the medial malleolus of the epiphysis. **C,** In another coronal plane, the fracture is seen extending into the distal metaphysis. Injuries extending from the metaphysis, through the physis, and into the epiphysis are Salter-Harris IV fractures.

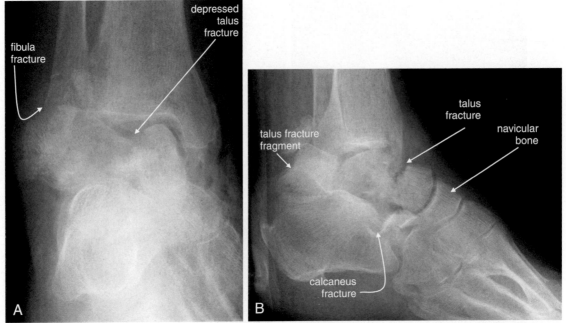

Figure 14-114. Talus and calcaneal fractures. This 80-year-old female was in a severe motor vehicle collision and presented with injuries to her distal right lower extremity. **A,** Anterior–posterior view. **B,** Lateral view. A depressed talus fracture is visible. In **B,** this fracture is seen to run through the midbody of the talus. **A** also demonstrates a distal fibula fracture, whereas in **B,** a calcaneal fracture is seen. The patient underwent CT to characterize these fractures further (Figure 14-115).

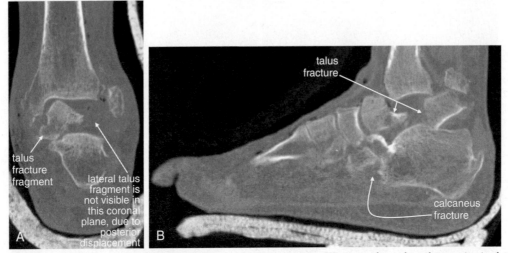

Figure 14-115. Talus and calcaneal fractures, CT. Same patient as in Figure 14-114. CT was performed to characterize in detail fractures seen on x-ray. **A,** Coronal reconstruction. The lateral half of the talus is missing from the image because it has been retropulsed, as seen in **B. B,** Sagittal reconstruction. The talus and calcaneus fractures are shown in detail. A large talar fragment is dislocated posteriorly. Axial, coronal, and sagittal CT reconstructions can make the three-dimensional detail of fractures evident. This CT also revealed a cuboid fracture not seen on the x-ray.

allergy, renal dysfunction, and other systemic toxicity (see Chapter 7 for a discussion of iodinated contrast and Chapter 15 for a discussion of gadolinium). In the extremities, ultrasound can assess flow and identify aneurysms and intimal flaps. Some structures can be difficult to visualize, depending on the patient's body habitus. In addition, ultrasound does not allow ready imaging of the complete course of vessels from their origins at the aorta, which may be important in cases such as vascular insufficiency from aortic dissection or atherosclerotic disease.

Conventional angiography (Figure 14-130), although the historical criterion standard, has the disadvantages of being an invasive procedure requiring a team of specialist interventional radiologists, high radiation exposure, and use of iodinated contrast. However, it allows imaging of the aorta and extremity branch vessels. In addition, some lesions such as intimal flaps or vascular stenoses can be treated with endovascular stenting. Some vascular thromboses can be treated with local administration of thrombolytic agents during angiography.

CTA has multiple advantages, including multiplanar and three-dimensional imaging of vessels from the aorta to the distal extremities (Figure 14-131; see also Figure 14-105). CTA of the extremities in the setting of injury

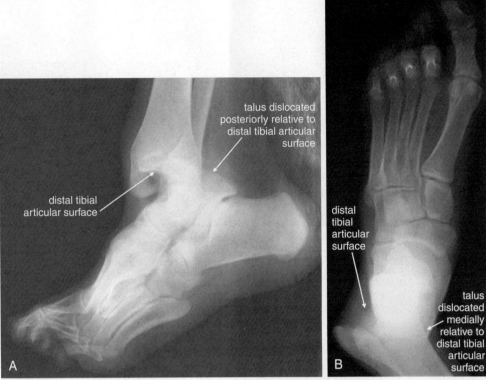

Figure 14-116. Tibiotalar dislocation. This 17-year-old male landed on his left ankle after dunking a basketball, sustaining a deformity. His tibiotalar joint is dislocated, with the talus dislocated posteriorly (visible on the lateral view, **A**) and medially (visible on the anterior–posterior view, **B**). No fractures are present in this case, although fractures are commonly associated with this injury because of the amount of force required to dislocate the ankle. This was an open injury, and the patient underwent exploration, irrigation, and debridement with primary closure.

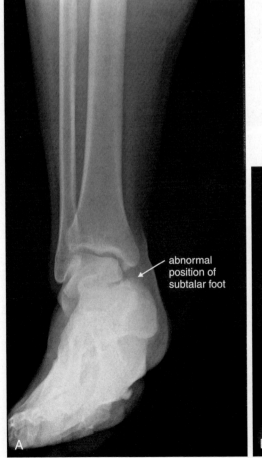

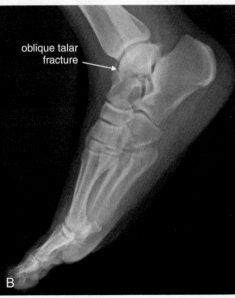

Figure 14-117. Subtalar dislocation with talar fracture. This 38-year-old male presented with an ankle deformity following a motorcycle collision. **A,** Anterior–posterior ankle, obtained on ED arrival. The talus is positioned normally in the ankle mortise. The alignment of the talus with the calcaneus is abnormal, with the calcaneus and remainder of the distal foot displaced medially. This is a subtalar dislocation and was reduced immediately because of concern for vascular compromise. **B,** Lateral foot, obtained after reduction. An oblique fracture through the talus is visible.

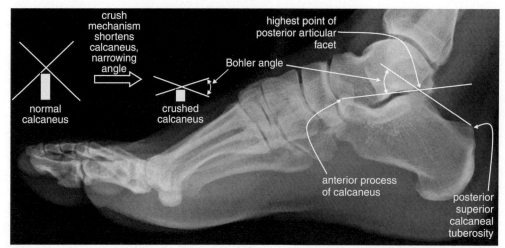

Figure 14-118. Normal calcaneus and the Bohler angle. Most calcaneal fractures are compression injuries from falls from height. The Bohler angle is a measurement used to identify subtle compression fractures. To measure the Bohler angle, first draw a line from the posterior superior calcaneal tuberosity to the highest point of the posterior articular facet. Next, draw a second line from the posterior articular facet to the anterior process. The intersection of these lines forms the Bohler angle, which is normally between 20 and 40 degrees. With compression fracture of the calcaneus Figure 14-119), the posterior articular facet is usually crushed into the body of the calcaneus and is not as tall as normal. As a result, the lines crossing at this point form a narrower angle. Values of the Bohler angle that are less than 20 degrees are considered abnormal. Sometimes the calcaneus is flattened so much that the Bohler angle is 0 degrees, though these injuries are usually not so subtle as to require measurement of the Bohler angle for recognition.

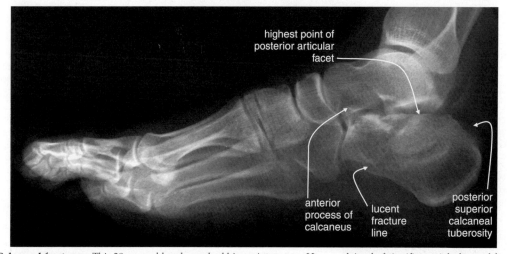

Figure 14-119. Calcaneal fractures. This 39-year-old male crashed his car into a tree. He complained of significant right leg and foot pain. His x-rays show a comminuted fracture of the calcaneus. For an obvious fracture such as this, measurement of the Bohler angle may be unnecessary, but it is helpful to consider this extreme case to understand the value of the measurement for subtler cases. Look at the normal calcaneus in the prior figure. The apex of the posterior articular facet normally forms a peak atop the calcaneus. In this case, the peak has been flattened. The two lines would each be horizontal and would form an angle of 0 degrees. This is a comminuted fracture, with a lucent fracture line running obliquely from the inferior margin of the anterior calcaneus to the superior margin of the posterior calcaneus. Computed tomography was also performed to define this fracture in more detail.

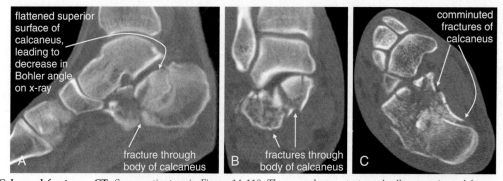

Figure 14-120. Calcaneal fractures, CT. Same patient as in Figure 14-119. The scan demonstrates a badly comminuted fracture of the calcaneus. **A,** Sagittal reconstruction. As in the lateral x-ray in Figure 14-119, the normal apex of the posterior articular facet can be seen to be depressed as a consequence of the fractures, giving the calcaneus a flattened upper contour. For this reason, the Bohler angle on the lateral x-ray was nearly 0 degrees. A coronal reconstruction **(B)** and an axial reconstruction **(C)** show the calcaneus to be severely fragmented.

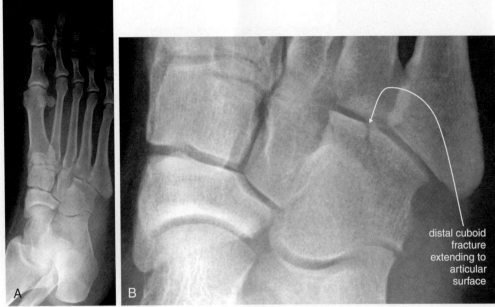

distal cuboid
fracture
extending to
articular
surface

Figure 14-121. Cuboid fracture. This 41-year-old fell, twisting her right foot. She was unable to walk because of pain in her lateral foot. **A,** An oblique view of the foot, shown for context. **B,** Close-up. A fracture of the distal cuboid is visible, extending to the articular surface with the metatarsals. This is nondisplaced. This fracture was not readily seen on the anterior–posterior and lateral views (not shown). The patient was treated with a CAM walker boot and without bearing weight for 4 to 6 weeks. This figure also demonstrates a normal Lisfranc joint. Abnormalities of the Lisfranc joint are discussed in Figures 14-122 and 14-123.

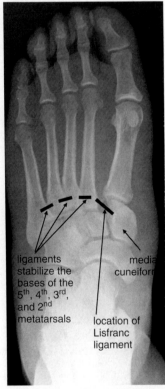

ligaments
stabilize the
bases of the
5th, 4th, 3rd,
and 2nd
metatarsals

media
cuneiform

location of
Lisfranc
ligament

Figure 14-122. Tarsometatarsal joint fracture dislocations (Lisfranc fracture). The tarsometatarsal joint is subject to fracture and dislocation with hyperplantar flexion of the foot. Ligaments join the fifth and fourth, the fourth and third, and the third and second but not the second and first metatarsal bases. Instead, a ligament joins the second metatarsal and medial cuneiform bones. This is called the Lisfranc ligament and can be disrupted, as in this image. Though the ligament itself is not visible on x-ray, disruption widens the space between the first and the second metatarsals and between the second metatarsal and the medial cuneiform. Compare with the normal Lisfranc joint in Figure 14-121, as well as the abnormal joint in Figure 14-123.

is comparable in sensitivity to conventional angiography (around 95%), with moderate specificity (87%).[67] Chapter 7 describes principles of CTA in the setting of pulmonary embolism and aortic dissection, which also apply to peripheral CTA. In CTA of the extremities, the contrast bolus is followed as it passes through the aorta to the vessels of the upper or lower extremities. Unlike conventional angiography, a single contrast bolus can be used to construct a detailed map of an entire vascular system. Other advantages of CTA include wide availability and the ability to assess other injuries, including thoracoabdominal and bony injuries with the same modality.

MRA is less readily available in many emergency departments, especially outside of normal business hours. However, it offers three-dimensional imaging capability, accuracy similar to CT and conventional angiography, an absence of radiation exposure, and outstanding soft-tissue evaluation for concurrent injuries to muscle and joint structures.

Deep Venous Thrombosis

Diagnostic imaging for DVT is discussed extensively in Chapter 7, in association with a discussion of pulmonary embolism diagnosis. Ultrasound remains the primary modality for assessment (Figure 14-132). Serial compression of the deep venous system is performed from the inguinal ligament to the popliteal fossa. Normal veins are readily compressible, whereas thrombosed veins may be deformed but do not compress with pressure applied with the ultrasound probe. In a metaanalysis of studies of ultrasound, the sensitivity of

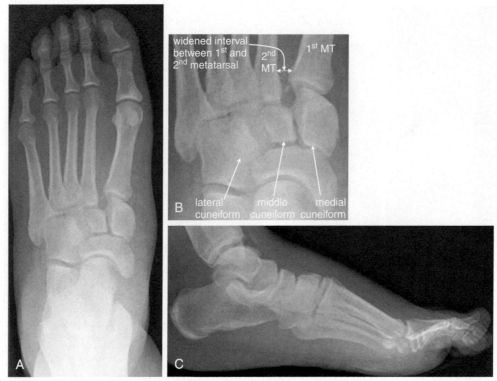

Figure 14-123. Tarsometatarsal joint fracture dislocations (Lisfranc fracture). This 29-year-old female presented with pain in the left midfoot after falling down two steps. She was unable to bear weight because of pain. **A,** Anterior–posterior view of the foot (**B,** close-up). Look carefully at the metatarsal–tarsal joints. The medial aspect of the second metatarsal (MT) does not align with the medial aspect of the *middle* cuneiform, and a small osseous fragment is seen. The distance between the first and the second MTs is wider than normal. This subtle injury is a Lisfranc joint fracture dislocation. The lateral film **(C)** does not reveal this injury. The patient underwent open reduction and internal fixation.

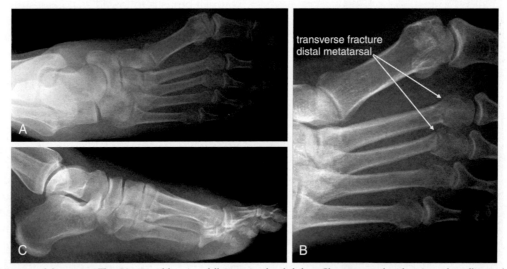

Figure 14-124. Metatarsal fractures. This 50-year-old patient fell, inverting her left foot. She presented with pain and swelling in her distal midfoot. **A,** Anterior–posterior view, showing transverse fractures of the distal second and third metatarsal diaphyses, with slight lateral angulation but without intraarticular extension. **B,** Close-up. **C,** Lateral view, which does not show these injuries. The patient was treated with a posterior short-leg splint and non-weight-bearing status.

compression ultrasound for proximal DVT was 93.8% (95% CI = 92.0%-95.3%) with specificity of 97.8% (95% CI = 97.0%-98.4%).[100] Addition of color Doppler techniques improves sensitivity slightly, to around 96% for proximal DVT, but reduces specificity to around 94%.[100] Repeated ultrasound 1 to 2 weeks after an initial negative study has been recommended in the past, but detects DVT in only about 1% of patients with initial negative studies. Withholding anticoagulation in patients with negative ultrasound appears safe, with only 0.6% of patients with normal ultrasound having interval development of thromboembolism at 3-month

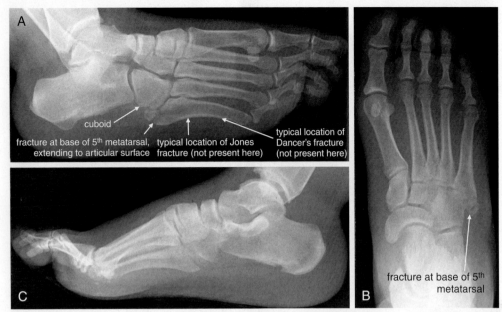

Figure 14-125. Fifth metatarsal fractures. This 29-year-old woman fell down two steps, inverting her right foot and ankle. She complained of pain with weight bearing and was unable to walk four steps in the emergency department. She had tenderness over the proximal fifth metacarpal. Because she failed the Ottawa ankle rule, x-rays were obtained. **A,** Oblique view. **B,** Anterior–posterior view. **C,** Lateral view. A proximal fracture of the fifth metatarsal is seen in **A** and **B** but not in **C**. This extends to the cuboid articulation **(A).** This fracture is an avulsion fracture of the apophysis, sometimes called a pseudo-Jones fracture. Proximal fifth metatarsal fractures are common ankle inversion injuries. Fractures at the metaphysis–diaphysis junction (Jones fractures) have a poorer prognosis for healing and traditionally have been treated with casting and non-weight-bearing status for 6-8 weeks. More distal fractures of the fifth metatarsal are common ballet-dancing injuries and are called dancer's fractures. This patient was treated with a CAM walker boot weight-bearing status.

follow-up.[101] CT venography has comparable sensitivity and specificity to ultrasound (Figure 14-133). CT allows assessment for pelvic thrombus that cannot be detected with ultrasound but also exposes the patient to substantial radiation and to iodinated contrast, neither of which occurs with ultrasound. Magnetic resonance venography is an alternative in patients with suspected pelvic thrombus and contraindications to radiation or iodinated contrast exposure. See Chapter 7 for additional details.

Sutter et al.[102] reported that important incidental findings were found in about 3% of patients undergoing lower extremity ultrasound for suspected DVT, including pseudoaneurysms, arterial occlusive disease, vascular graft complications, compartment syndrome, and tumor. The authors noted that low clinical probability of DVT, in conjunction with a negative D-dimer, is often used to avoid the use of ultrasound but question whether other important causes of lower extremity signs and symptoms might be missed with this approach.

Compartment Syndrome

Compartment syndrome, an increase in the pressure of a fascial compartment, leading to decreased perfusion and potential ischemic infarction of compartment contents, *is not a radiologic diagnosis. Compartment syndrome can occur in the absence of fractures,* although the most common injury resulting in compartment syndrome is

fracture of the tibial diaphysis, which should prompt consideration of compartment syndrome (Figures 14-134 and 14-135). Research has examined the role of MRI, ultrasound, nuclear scintigraphy, and infrared imaging, but these techniques are not well validated.[103]

Magnetic Resonance Imaging in Compartment Syndrome
Rominger et al.[104] performed a case-control study with 15 patients with compartment syndrome (10 "described as "manifest," and 5 described as "imminent") and 5 normal volunteers. In the 10 advanced cases of compartment syndrome, MRI demonstrated abnormalities of muscle architecture on T1-weighted images and increased signal on spin–echo T2-weighted sequences. Affected compartments showed increased enhancement with gadolinium. However, in 4 of the 5 patients with earlier manifestations of compartment syndrome, MRI was normal. The ability of MRI to identify early changes of compartment syndrome and to distinguish these changes from local muscle edema caused by trauma is not established, and MRI should not be used to exclude or confirm compartment syndrome at this time.

Ultrasound in Compartment Syndrome
Standard ultrasound is likely not useful in excluding or confirming compartment syndrome. In a study of healthy athletes, measurements with ultrasound were not reproducible.[105] Experimental techniques show promise but are not ready for clinical application.[103]

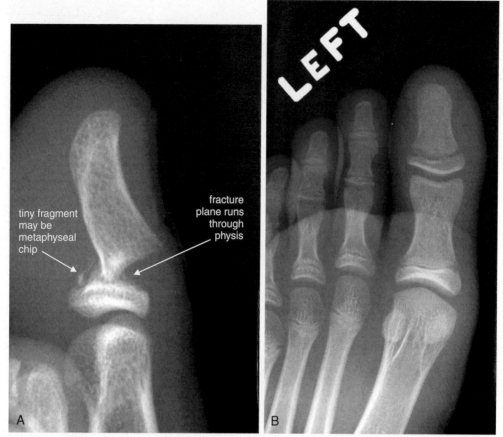

Figure 14-126. Salter-Harris II fracture of great toe. This 12-year-old male sustained a great toe injury when an adult stepped on his foot. The patient had a subungual hematoma on examination. **A,** Lateral x-rays show a displaced fracture through the physis, with plantar angulation of the distal fragment. A tiny bone chip is visible, possibly representing part of the metaphysis. Note how normal the anterior–posterior view **(B)** is. If the separation of the physis is the only injury, this would be characterized as a Salter-Harris I injury. Involvement of the metaphysis makes this a Salter-Harris II fracture. However, the bottom line for the emergency physician should be that this is a displaced fracture through a growth plate and potentially an open fracture given the subungual hematoma. Immediate orthopedic consultation is appropriate. This patient underwent operative repair with pinning of the fracture and repair of the nail bed.

Figure 14-127. Osteosarcoma. This 13-year-old male complained of 4-6 weeks of left shoulder pain, with no history of trauma. X-rays were obtained. **A,** Internal rotation, AP view. **B,** Close-up in external rotation. The proximal humerus shows both sclerotic (*dense white*) and lucent (*black*) areas with ill-defined margins. These extend from the physis to the metaphysis. Periosteal reaction is also present, with new bone formation occurring in the uplifted subperiosteal space—a finding called Codman's triangle. These findings are extremely concerning for osteosarcoma in this age group. This was confirmed on bone biopsy. Bony pain without trauma in children should prompt evaluation for malignancy or bone infection. Immediate follow-up is needed for abnormal findings such as in this patient. Sadly, this patient already had lung metastases and died despite aggressive treatment.

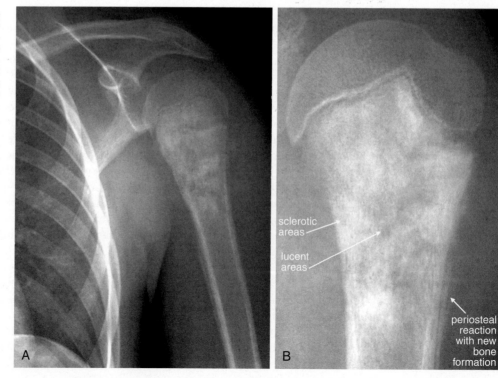

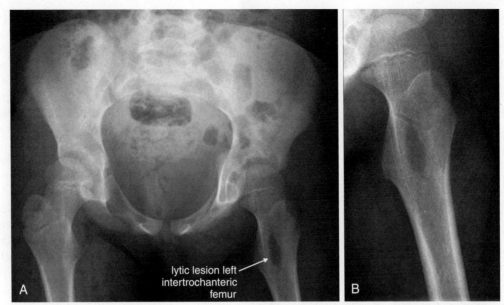

Figure 14-128. Lytic lesions. This 6-year-old female presented with left proximal femur pain for 5 days, with no history of trauma or fever. **A,** Anterior–posterior pelvis. **B,** Close-up. X-rays of the hip show a lytic lesion in the intertrochanteric left femur. No periosteal reaction is visible, which would be typical of some bony malignancies, such as osteosarcoma. Radiologists can generate a differential diagnosis for lesions such as this based on their appearance—this lesion was felt to be suspicious for Langerhans cell histiocytosis. However, infection or benign or malignant neoplasm is possible with lesions that have this appearance. Pathologic fracture through lytic bone lesions can occur spontaneously or with minor trauma. The emergency physician should recognize the general appearance of such lesions and understand the importance of timely follow-up. Spontaneous bony pain, particularly in children, can indicate neoplasm or infection. This patient underwent next-day magnetic resonance imaging showing a heterogeneous mass with cortical destruction and a soft-tissue component. Surgical excision was performed, and biopsy fortunately showed a benign fibroosseous lesion with multiple giant cells but no evidence of malignancy.

Nuclear Scintigraphy in Compartment Syndrome

In the setting of chronic exertional compartment syndrome, nuclear scintigraphy with 99- technetium-99m–methoxyisobutylisonitrile was 80% sensitive and 97% specific in 46 patients.[106] However, the sensitivity and specificity in acute compartment syndrome, in which traumatic injuries to limbs may cause additional imaging abnormalities, is unknown. The technique should not be used to exclude acute compartment syndrome until validated through further research.

Infrared and Near-Infrared Noninvasive Monitoring for Compartment Syndrome

Infrared imaging of lower extremities shows promise in detection of compartment syndrome. In a study of 164 trauma patients, 11 with compartment syndrome, anterior surface temperatures of affected extremities showed greater differences between proximal and distal measurements than did unaffected extremities.[107] However, the technique requires further validation. Near-infrared spectroscopy provides a continuous transcutaneous measure of tissue oxygenation and may offer a future method of early detection of compartment syndrome.[108]

Necrotizing Fasciitis and Other Soft-Tissue Infections

Imaging of necrotizing soft-tissue infections, including necrotizing fasciitis, has not been examined in large methodologically rigorous studies because of the relative rarity of the condition. X-ray, ultrasound, and MRI all have been described as having utility, but the sensitivity and specificity of the modalities is not known.

X-ray findings of necrotizing fasciitis include soft-tissue air tracking along muscle fascial boundaries (Figure 14-136).

Ultrasound can demonstrate adipose tissue, fascial, and muscle changes in necrotizing fasciitis. Parenti et al.[109] reported results in 32 patients with confirmed necrotizing fasciitis but found sensitivity of only 47% for muscle changes and 56% for fascial changes when ultrasound was performed by operators noted to be particularly skilled at soft-tissue examination. Because no normal group was examined in this study, the specificity could not be calculated.

Contrast-enhanced CT can demonstrate the extent of disease, although no contrast is needed to demonstrate soft-tissue air (Figure 14-137).[109] Wysoki et al.[110] reviewed CT scans in 20 patients with pathologically confirmed necrotizing fasciitis. Soft-tissue air tracking along fascial planes (sensitivity = 55%), asymmetrical fascial thickening and fat stranding (sensitivity = 80%), and associated deep abscesses (sensitivity = 35%) were seen. Again, the specificity cannot be calculated, because no disease-free patients were included in this study. Other case reports suggest utility of CT in diagnosis.[111-112]

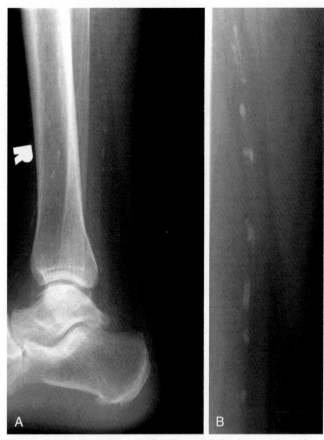

Figure 14-129. Vascular calcifications. Calcifications within blood vessels betray the presence of peripheral arterial disease in this patient. However, plain x-ray does not reveal essential information about the patency of the vascular lumen. Ultrasound, conventional angiography, CT angiography, and magnetic resonance angiography provide this information. **A,** Lateral ankle. **B,** Close-up.

Small studies have explored the role of MRI for the diagnosis of necrotizing fasciitis. Seok et al.[113] compared MRI findings in 11 patients with surgically confirmed necrotizing fasciitis and 8 patients with pathologically confirmed pyomyositis. MRI findings in necrotizing fasciitis included a peripheral, bandlike, hyperintense signal in muscles on fat-suppressed, T2-weighted images (73%) and peripheral, bandlike, contrast enhancement of muscles, neither of which were seen in pyomyositis patients. In addition, necrotizing fasciitis patients showed thin, smooth enhancement of deep fascia in 82% of cases, compared with 13% of pyomyositis patients. In all necrotizing fasciitis patients, the superficial and deep fascia and muscle showed hyperintense signals on T2-weighted images and contrast enhancement on fat-suppressed, contrast-enhanced, T1-weighted images. However, the small size of this study and the absence of a normal control group limit the findings.

Brothers et al.[114] reported results of MRI in nine patients with suspected necrotizing fasciitis of the lower extremity. Absence of gadolinium enhancement on T1-weighted images was seen in six patients with surgically proven fascial necrosis. MRI showed fascial inflammation (defined as low signal intensity on T1-weighted images and high signal intensity on T2-weighted images) in all nine patients, including three who ultimately did not have a clinical diagnosis of necrotizing fasciitis.

Schmid et al.[115] compared MRI findings with surgical findings, autopsy, and clinical outcomes in 17 patients with suspected necrotizing fasciitis. MRI detected all 11

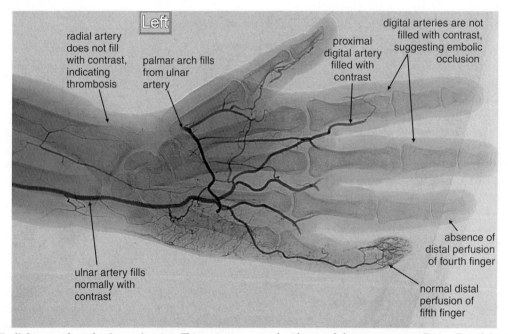

Figure 14-130. Radial artery thrombosis, angiogram. This patient presented with acute left arm pain, as well as pallor of the palm and fingers. The patient had no palpable radial pulse. An angiogram was performed to determine the site of vascular occlusion. The radial artery does not fill with contrast, indicating proximal occlusion. The digital arteries of the second through fourth fingers do not fill with contrast, suggesting embolic occlusion. The digital artery on the lateral aspect of the fifth finger fills with contrast. The palmar arch fills from the patient's ulnar artery.

surgically proven cases of necrotizing fasciitis, based on imaging findings of deep fascial involvement with fluid collections, thickening, and enhancement after contrast administration. MRI was false positive in one case of cellulitis. Other case reports suggest utility of MRI in identifying early necrotizing fasciitis.[116-117]

Because necrotizing fasciitis is a time-sensitive and life-threatening infection, operative therapy should never be delayed for imaging when the diagnosis is strongly suspected.[118] Studies of MRI are too limited at this time to determine whether MRI can exclude early necrotizing fasciitis. Presumably, imaging findings early in the course of disease might be subtler and less sensitive. MRI may not be perfectly specific and might prompt unnecessary operation in some patients.

Septic Arthritis

Septic arthritis is typically proven by culture of joint aspirates, in conjunction with clinical examination findings, synovial fluid Gram stain, and cell counts. The role of diagnostic imaging includes guidance of joint aspiration (e.g., using ultrasound in aspiration of the hip) and assessment of joints that are not successfully aspirated.

Can Ultrasound Rule Out Septic Arthritis of the Hip?

Zawin et al.[119] reviewed results in 96 children with suspected septic arthritis of the hip. Among 40 with normal ultrasound of the hip, none had septic arthritis (95% CI = 0%-9%). Ultrasound detected hip effusions in 56 children; 31 had attempted ultrasound-guided joint aspiration, 29 successfully. Of these patients, 15 had joint aspirates consistent with septic arthritis. The authors concluded that a normal ultrasound of the hip rules out septic arthritis. Ultrasound-guided joint aspiration was highly successful in this series.

Can Magnetic Resonance Imaging Distinguish Septic Arthritis From Other Causes of Inflammation?

Karchevsky et al.[120] reviewed 50 consecutive cases of MRI of septic arthritis and described the frequency of various findings (Table 14-14). Graif et al.[121] compared MRI findings in 19 patients with septic joint and 11 with uninfected inflamed joints. Although combinations of findings made the diagnosis of septic joint more likely, no single MRI abnormality could confirm or exclude joint infection, because the findings in both conditions were similar and none showed statistically significant differences between the two groups (Table 14-15).

Lee et al.[122] retrospectively compared imaging findings in 9 pediatric patients with septic arthritis and 14 with transient synovitis of the hip. The authors documented signal intensity changes in bone marrow of the femoral head and neck on fat-suppressed, T1- and T2-weighted image sequences in patients with septic joint but not in those with transient synovitis. Similarly, Kwack et al.[123] reviewed MRI findings in 9 patients with septic hip arthritis and 11 with transient

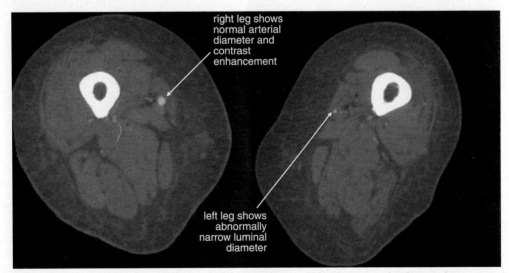

Figure 14-131. Peripheral arterial disease, CT angiography (CTA). This 60-year-old female presented with severe lower extremity pain, left greater than right. Although this had been going on intermittently for some months, the pain was now present at rest. She had developed bilateral purpura of her toes extending to her midfoot in the past few hours. The patient underwent CTA, which demonstrated a short segment of nearly complete occlusion of the left common femoral artery and proximal superficial femoral artery. The patient underwent surgical thrombectomy. CTA can provide detailed three-dimensional or multiplanar images of the lower extremities for assessment of arterial injury or peripheral vascular diseases including dissections, aneurysms, and occlusions. Advantages of CT include its speed and accessibility. It compares favorably with digital angiography in sensitivity and specificity, but it offers no therapeutic options, unlike formal angiography that offers the possibility of clot lysis, extraction, or stenting. CTA of the extremities requires approximately 150 mL of injected contrast material. Consider the full diagnostic and therapeutic plan for patients with renal disease before ordering this test. If the treatment plan will not be influenced by CTA, avoid unnecessary risk for contrast nephropathy.

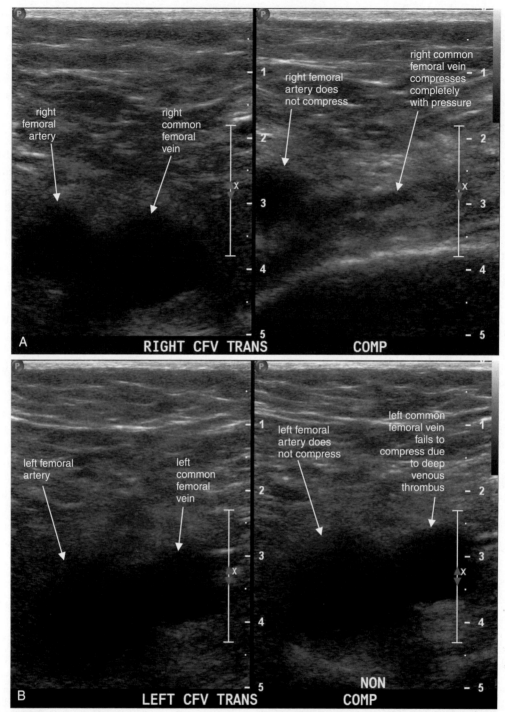

Figure 14-132. Deep venous thrombosis (DVT). This 61-year-old male presented with abdominal pain and a history of adenocarcinoma of the colon. He underwent abdominal CT, which incidentally suggested DVT of the left common femoral vein. Ultrasound of his lower extremities is shown. **A,** Normal ultrasound of the patient's right common femoral vein. The same location is shown without compression *(left)* and with application of compression *(right)*. The artery remains visible in both images, because the degree of compression is insufficient to compress the high-pressure artery. In contrast, the normal common femoral vein is easily compressed. **B,** Abnormal ultrasound of the patient's left leg. This documents left common femoral vein DVT. Again, the artery and vein are seen without compression *(left)*, and compression is applied yet the vein does not compress *(right)*. This is because of the presence of an acute deep venous thrombus. New thrombus is generally hypoechoic *(black)* like liquid blood. As thrombus ages, it may become hyperechoic *(white)* and recognizable even without compression. In this case, a DVT is diagnosed without use of Doppler ultrasound. Although it is common for emergency physicians to refer to "Dopplering the legs" to detect DVT, in reality serial compression ultrasound along the length of a vein is usually sufficient to evaluate for thrombus. Doppler technology can be useful in equivocal cases to document augmentation of venous flow with squeezing of the calf muscles. The patient's CT scan is shown in Figure 14-133 for comparison.

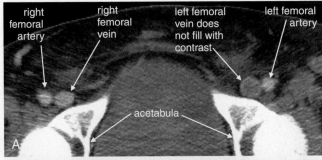

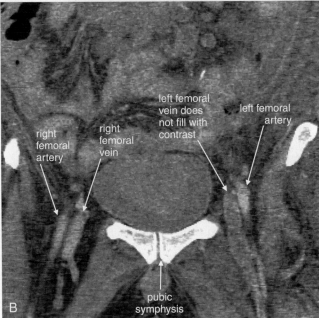

Figure 14-133. Deep venous thrombosis (DVT). This 61-year-old male presented with abdominal pain and a history of adenocarcinoma of the colon. He underwent abdominal CT, which incidentally suggested DVT of the left common femoral vein. Ultrasound of his lower extremities is shown in Figure 14-132. Although DVT was an unexpected finding in this patient, who was undergoing CT for abdominal pain, computed tomography venography (CTV) is sometimes used intentionally to diagnosis DVT. Proponents of CTV have encouraged its use in conjunction with pulmonary computed tomography angiography (CTA) for the diagnosis of pulmonary embolism. However, others have argued that CTV is unnecessary because it adds cost and radiation exposure to a patient's evaluation. Ultrasound remains the standard modality for diagnosis of DVT. In selected circumstances, CTV may be the best test available. For example, if a patient's legs are inaccessible to ultrasound because of cast material or overlying soft-tissue wounds, CTV can provide diagnostic information. External orthopedic fixators that interfere with ultrasound diagnosis of DVT may also prevent CTV from making the diagnosis because of metallic streak artifact. CTV does potentially provide information not available from ultrasound, including evaluation of the pelvic veins. Diagnostic CTV requires the same conditions as pulmonary CTA: a rapid injection of a large volume of iodinated contrast material. Patients with poor renal function or contrast allergies may be unable to undergo the procedure. DVT is diagnosed when a filling defect is visualized, resulting from an obstructing DVT preventing contrast from entering a segment of vessel. **A,** Axial section showing a filling defect in the left femoral vein. This slice has been cropped to show the region of interest. **B,** Coronal reconstruction. This image shows the extent of the thrombus.

synovitis. The authors found statistically significant differences in the frequency of some findings between the two groups. These two small studies suggest but do not prove that MRI can distinguish between the two conditions.

Osteomyelitis

Osteomyelitis can occur in the absence of any plain radiographic changes in its early phases. Later changes of osteomyelitis include osteolysis and soft-tissue swelling (Figures 14-138, 14-139, and 14-141). Soft-tissue air may also be seen. Unfortunately, by the time that these late findings develop, significant clinical deterioration and irreversible bone damage may be present. A prospective study of 110 consecutive patients with suspected diabetes-related osteomyelitis of the foot found the sensitivity of x-ray to be 63%, with specificity of 87%.[124]

Earlier detection of osteomyelitis can be performed with MRI or bone scan. Nawaz et al.[124] reported MRI to be 91% sensitive and 78% specific for diabetic osteomyelitis of the foot. In a study of 78 children, unenhanced MRI was equal to enhanced MRI in sensitivity and specificity for osteomyelitis, although use of gadolinium-enhancement increased reader confidence.[125] Johnson et al.[126] retrospectively reviewed 74 consecutive cases of MRI of the foot for suspected osteomyelitis and found that confluent decreased T1 marrow signal in a medullary distribution was 95% sensitive and 91% specific for osteomyelitis. Kan et al.[127] retrospectively reviewed MRI following surgical interventions in 34 pediatric cases and 96 controls and concluded that iatrogenic soft-tissue and bone edema resulting from recent surgical intervention did not affect the diagnostic accuracy of MRI.

In a study of 51 patients with suspected osteomyelitis, Morrison et al.[128] reported that fat-suppressed, contrast-enhanced MRI was more sensitive (88%) and specific (93%) for osteomyelitis than was nonenhanced magnetic resonance (sensitivity = 79%, specificity = 53%) or three-phase bone scan (sensitivity = 61%, specificity = 33%).

Earlier studies suggest that combining multiple nuclear scintigraphy tests (e.g., gallium and technetium-99m) can increase the accuracy for osteomyelitis in children. However, nuclear scintigraphy scans can be falsely positive in conditions such as fracture and juvenile rheumatoid arthritis.[129]

FDG-PET has been investigated in prospective comparison with MRI. Its sensitivity and specificity were 81% and 93%, respectively. In patients with contraindications to MRI, FDG-PET is an alternative. Its specificity is higher than that of MRI and can complement MRI when the diagnosis is uncertain.[124]

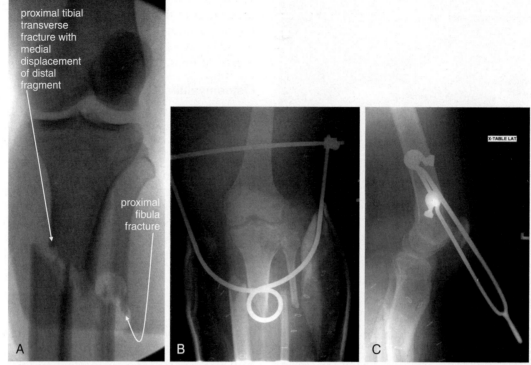

Figure 14-134. Compartment syndrome with tibial fracture. This 25-year-old pregnant female presented with life-threatening injuries, including an open book pelvic fracture. After an emergency Cesarean section in the trauma bay, she was taken to the operating room, where additional stabilization was performed. **A,** Fluoroscopy of her deformed left lower leg showed proximal tibial and fibular transverse fractures with significant medial displacement. Her calf compartments were noted to be taut. Compartment pressures were 55 mm Hg for the deep posterior compartment, 39 mm Hg for the superficial posterior compartment, 42 mm Hg for the anterior compartment, and 46 mm Hg for the lateral compartment. Emergency fasciotomy was performed. **B, C,** Postoperative x-rays show persistently displaced tibial and fibular fractures. The radiopaque device is a traction pin through the distal femur. Although compartment syndrome is not a radiographic diagnosis, remember that proximal tibial fractures are associated with the development of compartment syndrome.

Which Imaging Modality Is Best for Diagnosis of Chronic Osteomyelitis?

The many studies of imaging of osteomyelitis makes selection of the best imaging test difficult. From 3384 studies identified in Medline, Embase, and Current Contents databases, a systematic review and meta-analysis identified only 23 clinical studies meeting strong methodologic standards and addressing diagnostic imaging of chronic osteomyelitis, defined as osteomyelitis requiring more than one episode of treatment or lasting more than 6 weeks.[130] The results are summarized in Table 14-16. According to this metaanalysis, FDG-PET appears most sensitive and specific, but is not widely used in the emergency department setting. However, controversy remains about the best diagnostic modality, with some authors advocating MRI.[131]

Foreign Bodies

Dense foreign bodies, such as those composed of metal, stone, or glass, are usually visible on plain x-ray, because they are considerably denser than body soft tissues and similar to bone density (Figure 14-142). Multiple orthogonal views may be required to identify such foreign bodies, because they may not be visible if projected directly over bone of similar density. Less dense foreign bodies, such as those composed of wood, rubber, plastic, or other organic material (e.g., the defensive spines of marine organisms) pose a greater dilemma (Figure 14-143). These materials are often invisible on x-ray but can sometimes be detected using ultrasound and MRI. No large studies comparing these modalities exist.

In a case series of eight patients, rubber foreign bodies from puncture wounds through rubber-soled shoes were not detected by x-ray in 50% of cases, with serious wound complications including osteomyelitis arising in some patients.[132]

In a controlled study using simulated wounds in chicken thighs, x-ray using standard extremity exposures had no sensitivity for wood and was 10% sensitive for rubber foreign bodies, with 90% specificity in both cases. Soft-tissue exposure x-ray was 10% sensitive for detection of wood and rubber foreign bodies, with 90% specificity. In comparison, high-frequency ultrasound was 90% sensitive and 80% specific.[133] Imaging was interpreted by blinded radiologists in this study.

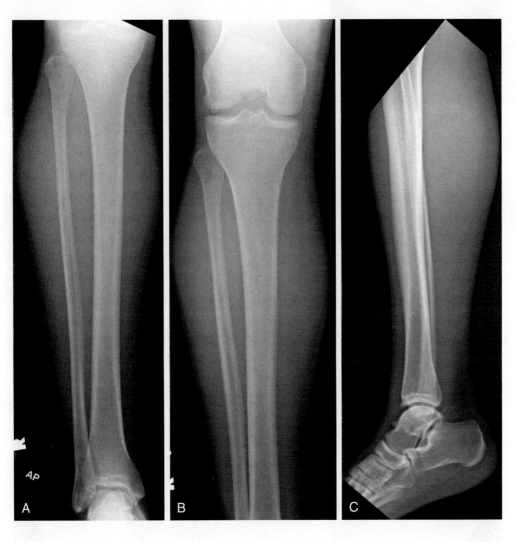

Figure 14-135. Compartment syndrome. This 22-year-old male presented with calf pain and swelling 2 days after his right calf was stepped on during a rugby match. He complained of numbness in the lateral aspect of his foot. In addition, his dorsalis pedis pulse was diminished to palpation and his right calf was extremely tense. **A, B,** Anterior–posterior views. **C,** Lateral view. X-rays were obtained, showing no fractures. The patient's posterior compartment pressures were elevated to 70 mm Hg, and he underwent four-compartment fasciotomy for compartment syndrome. This revealed necrosis of the medial third of the gastrocnemius, which was surgically debrided. Compartment syndrome can occur in the absence of fractures. Normal radiographs do not rule out the diagnosis.

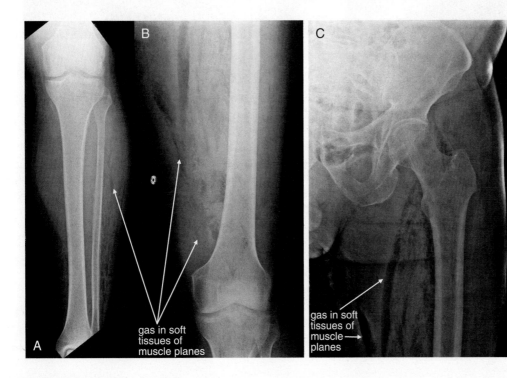

gas in soft tissues of muscle planes

gas in soft tissues of muscle planes

Figure 14-136. Necrotizing fasciitis. This 71-year-old male with aplastic anemia presented with fevers to 38.9°C, leg weakness, and extreme leg pain. Initially, the patient was felt to have neuropathic pain and weakness, possibly indicating spinal pathology such as epidural abscess. He rapidly developed crepitus of his legs. X-rays of the patient's legs were obtained, followed by noncontrast CT (Figure 14-137) **A,** Anterior–posterior (AP) tibia and fibula. **B,** AP femur. **C,** AP hip. Air is seen dissecting in muscle planes of the legs. On x-ray, air appears *black*. Given the wide distribution of air, a focal abscess is unlikely, and necrotizing fasciitis with gas-producing organisms should be suspected.

Figure 14-137. **Necrotizing fasciitis.** Same patient as in Figure 14-136, where x-rays of the patient's legs are shown. Noncontrast CT is shown here. **A,** Soft-tissue window. **B,** Lung window, same slice. If the diagnosis is highly suspected and x-rays are nondiagnostic, noncontrast CT is very sensitive for air. Air appears *black* on all CT window settings and is particularly evident on lung window, which makes all other tissues *white*. However, do not delay surgical consultation, antibiotic therapy, and surgical debridement to obtain diagnostic imaging once the diagnosis is suspected. This patient was taken to the operating room, and disarticulation of the hips was performed. He died of septic shock hours later. Blood cultures grew *Clostridium perfringens*—the feared gas gangrene organism of trench warfare in World War I.

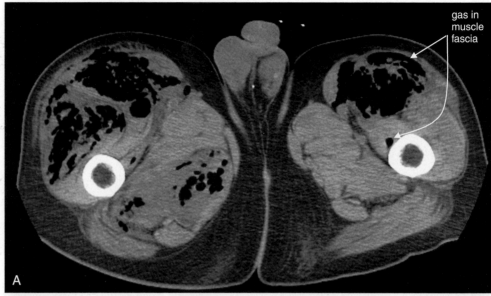

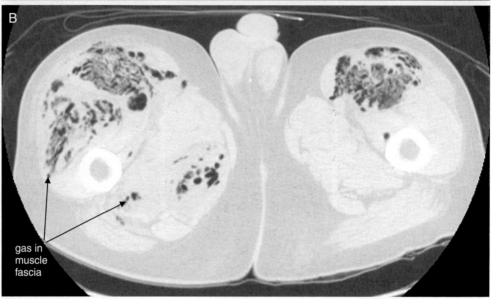

Case reports suggest value of ultrasound in detection of radiolucent soft-tissue foreign bodies, including small fragments not detected with CT.[134-138] In a prospective human study of 131 wounds in pediatric patients, sensitivity and specificity for foreign body detection were 67% and 97%, respectively, for bedside ultrasound performed by an attending pediatric emergency physician and 58% and 90%, respectively, for x-ray interpreted by a radiologist.[139] However, in a prospective cadaver study involving 900 ultrasound examinations, ultrasound performed by trained emergency physicians was only 52.6% sensitive and 47.2% specific for detection of a variety of small foreign bodies composed of wood, metal, plastic, or glass.[140] Why this low sensitivity and specificity? Several factors may account for the discrepancy between this study and studies in living humans. First, the gold standard in the preceding cadaver study

was extremely strong, because foreign bodies were placed in the cadavers by the investigators. In contrast, in the preceding pediatric human study, the gold standard is less robust, because the diagnostic standard was removal of a foreign body. It is possible that x-ray and ultrasound both missed some foreign bodies, which were then not detected and removed from the wound.[139] Thus the pediatric study may overestimate the sensitivity of x-ray and ultrasound. In addition, the cadaver study examined the sensitivity and specificity of ultrasound for detection of very small foreign bodies—2.5 mm^3 or less in total volume and 5 mm or less in longest dimension, with insertion depths of up to 3 cm.[140]

In case reports, MRI has been reported to demonstrate soft-tissue foreign bodies, though no large studies validate its sensitivity and specificity.[141-142] CT also has been reported to be useful in detection of radiolucent foreign bodies, though large studies are lacking.[134,143]

Do All Glass-Inflicted Wounds Require X-ray for Evaluation of Foreign Body?

A common principle in emergency medicine practice is to x-ray all wounds resulting from glass because of concern for an unrecognized retained foreign body. In a prospective study of 264 wounds, glass foreign bodies were found in 8.7%. In 2 (1.5%) of 134 superficial wounds (no deeper than subcutaneous fat), a foreign body was detected on x-ray but not on examination. In 10 (7.7%) of 130 deeper wounds, glass was detected with x-ray but not on examination. Consequently, in superficial wounds amenable to adequate exploration, x-ray may be unnecessary to evaluate for a glass foreign body.[144]

Gout

Gout is not typically a radiographic diagnosis, but x-rays are sometimes obtained to assess for competing diagnoses, including septic joint, osteomyelitis, and retained foreign body. In advanced cases (Figure 14-144), gout can create a characteristic appearance of periarticular and articular bony erosions, which must be recognized to avoid mistaken diagnosis of lytic lesions of osteomyelitis. Other x-ray findings associated with gout include soft-tissue opacities (less dense than bone but denser than surrounding soft tissue), representing tophi, and osteophyte formation at the margins of bony erosions and soft-tissue opacities. X-ray sensitivity for gout is reported to be 31%, with specificity of 93%, although small study sizes result in wide CIs. In addition, the diagnostic standard in some studies is poor, casting uncertainty on the reported diagnostic characteristics of x-ray. Ultrasound has a reported sensitivity of 96% but a lower specificity (73%). Ultrasound findings of gout include bright stippling and hyperechoic soft tissues, consistent with tophi.[145]

Rickets

Rickets, the demineralization of bone at growth plates in children most commonly because of vitamin D deficiency, can be an incidental radiographic diagnosis in the emergency department.[146] Risk factors include dark skin color and prolonged breast feeding, which predispose a child to vitamin D deficiency. X-ray findings can include decreased bone density, bowing of weight-bearing long bones, greenstick fractures from low bone density, metaphyseal lucencies, a coarsened trabecular pattern, and cortical tunneling from secondary hyperparathyroidism. The metaphyses of long bones may demonstrate splaying. Anterior rib ends may appear expanded.[147] The findings can be subtle; an emergency physician may recognize that an abnormality is present, but the specific diagnosis may require the interpretation of a pediatric radiologist. Emergency physicians should be attuned to the possibility of this diagnosis, which is

TABLE 14-14. Magnetic Resonance Imaging Findings of Septic Arthritis and Associated Osteomyelitis

Finding	Frequency
Synovial enhancement	98%
Perisynovial edema	84%
Joint effusions	70%
Fluid outpouching	53%
Fluid enhancement	30%
Synovial thickening	22%
Marrow bare area changes	86%
Marrow abnormal T2 signal	84%
Marrow abnormal gadolinium enhancement	81%
Marrow abnormal T1 signal	66%

Adapted from Karchevsky M, Schweitzer ME, Morrison WB, Parellada JA. MRI findings of septic arthritis and associated osteomyelitis in adults. *AJR Am J Roentgenol* 182:119-122, 2004.

TABLE 14-15. Magnetic Resonance Imaging Findings in Septic and Nonseptic Arthritis

Finding	Septic Arthritis Frequency	Nonseptic Arthritis Frequency
Effusion	79%	82%
Fluid outpouching	79%	73%
Fluid heterogeneity	21%	27%
Synovial thickening	68%	55%
Synovial periedema	63%	55%
Synovial enhancement	94%	88%
Cartilage loss	53%	30%
Bone erosions	79%	38%
Bone erosions enhancement	77%	43%
Bone marrow edema	74%	38%
Bone marrow enhancement	67%	50%
Soft-tissue edema	63%	78%
Soft-tissue enhancement	67%	71%
Periosteal edema	11%	10%

Adapted from Graif M, Schweitzer ME, Deely D, Matteucci T: The septic versus nonseptic inflamed joint: MRI characteristics. *Skeletal Radiol* 28:616-620, 1999.

still seen in developed countries including the United States, particularly in immigrant populations who may lack vitamin D supplementation.[148] Moreover, in pediatric fractures occurring with minimal force, the possibility of rickets and rare conditions such as **osteogenesis imperfecta** should be considered, along with nonaccidental trauma (described earlier).[146]

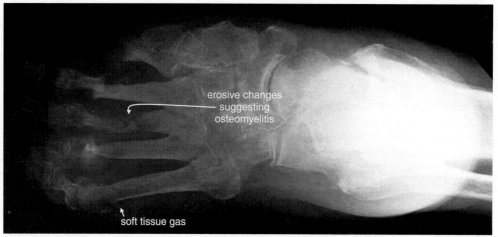

Figure 14-138. Charcot foot with osteomyelitis. This 81-year-old male with diabetes was noted to have a foul-smelling foot wound by his daughter. She noted maggots in the wound, prompting an emergency department visit. The patient had wounds on the distal third, fourth, and fifth toes. He denied having any foot pain. There are extensive erosive changes of the metatarsals with fractures through the second and third distal metatarsal diaphyses—findings concerning for osteomyelitis. Gas is present in the soft tissues around the lateral aspect of the distal fifth metatarsal diaphysis, which could indicate gas-forming organisms or air entering through a wound. A number of other findings are present. The fourth proximal interphalangeal joint is subluxed. There has been great toe and first metatarsal amputation. There is diffuse degenerative joint disease, osteopenia, and soft-tissue swelling.

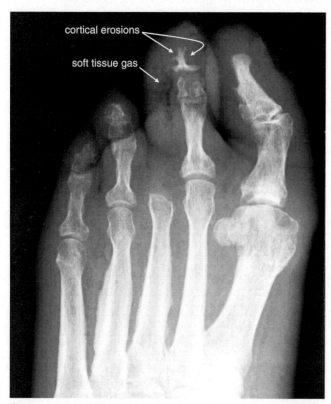

Figure 14-139. Diabetic foot infections. This 61-year-old female with diabetes presented with fever, foot pain, and a foul-smelling foot wound with erythema and purulent discharge. This anterior–posterior view shows cortical irregularities of the second toe's distal and middle phalanges, with adjacent soft-tissue swelling. A collection of rounded lucencies in the soft tissues are gas bubbles. The patient underwent amputation of her left second toe.

Lead

Chronic lead toxicity may result in a radiodensity in the distal metaphyseal plate in children. So-called lead lines in the long bones of children represent growth arrest lines. They are not pathognomonic of lead toxicity but may be seen with long-standing lead levels greater than 40 μg/dL.[149] X-ray should not be used to rule out lead toxicity because of poor sensitivity with acute ingestions. Instead, a whole-blood lead level is the criterion standard.[150]

SUMMARY

Extremity imaging is an essential part of emergency medicine practice. In some common clinical scenarios such as ankle injury, clinical decision rules can assist in imaging decisions and reduce the need for radiography. Although x-rays suffice for evaluation of many extremity injuries and nontraumatic pathology, in selected cases such as scaphoid fracture and injuries to the Lisfranc joint, the emergency physician must be aware of the poor sensitivity of x-ray and the potential necessity of advanced imaging such as MRI. Emergency physicians must recognize patterns of high-risk injuries and understand when imaging is required for associated conditions including vascular trauma. MRI, CT, ultrasound, angiography, and nuclear scintigraphy play specialty roles for evaluation of subtle but important conditions such as osteomyelitis. Some important extremity conditions such as compartment syndrome remain clinical diagnoses at this time, with little added diagnostic value of imaging.

TABLE 14-16. Summary of Diagnostic Sensitivity and Specificity of Diagnostic Imaging Modalities for Chronic Osteomyelitis

Modality	Studies	Sensitivity (95% CI)	Specificity (95% CI)
Radiography	2 (33 patients)*	60% (28%-86%) 78% (40%-96%)	67% (36%-89%) 100% (16%-100%)
MRI	5	84% (69%-92%)	60% (38%-78%)
CT	1 (8 patients)	67% (24%-94%)	50% (3%-97%)
Bone scintigraphy	7	82% (70%-89%)	25% (16%-36%)
Leukocyte scintigraphy, peripheral skeleton	13	84% (72%-91%)	80% (61%-91%)
Gallium scintigraphy	1 (22 patients)	80% (44%-96%)	42% (17%-71%)
Combined bone and leukocyte scintigraphy	6	78% (72%-83%)	84% (75%-90%)
Combined bone and gallium scintigraphy	3	Not reported; graph estimate = 55% with broad 95% CI	Not reported; graph estimate = 75% with broad 95% CI
FDG-PET	4	96% (88%-99%)	91% (81%-95%)

*Metaanalysis authors chose not to pool these two small studies, with 22 patients and 11 patients, respectively.
Adapted from Termaat MF, Raijmakers PG, Scholten HJ, et al: The accuracy of diagnostic imaging for the assessment of chronic osteomyelitis: A systematic review and meta-analysis. *J Bone Joint Surg Am* 87:2464-2671, 2005.

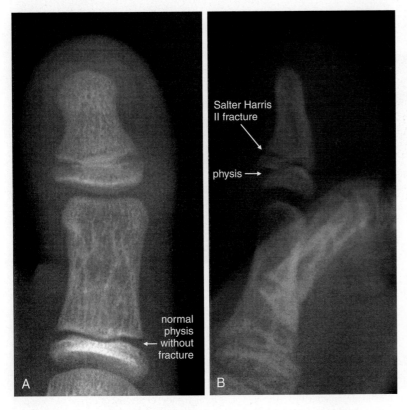

Figure 14-140. **Stubbed toe with Salter-Harris II fracture.** This 8-year-old male presented with left great toe pain after stubbing his toe. Examination showed an abrasion just proximal to the cuticle, which the patient reported was bleeding before emergency department arrival. **A,** Anterior–posterior (AP) view of the great toe. **B,** Lateral view. Lateral x-ray shows a fracture line extending through the metaphysis to the physis—a Salter-Harris II fracture. The AP view does not clearly reveal this injury. Two perpendicular views should be assessed when evaluating for fracture. Abrasions or lacerations overlying fractures constitute open fractures, with risk for osteomyelitis. See Figure 14-141.

Figure 14-141. Stubbed toe osteomyelitis. Same patient as in Figure 14-140. X-rays obtained 2 weeks after initial injury. **A,** Anterior–posterior view of the great toe. **B,** Lateral view. A lucency is visible in the metaphysis at the site of the prior Salter-Harris II fracture, suggesting osteomyelitis. Subtle soft-tissue injuries such as abrasions and subungual hematoma can indicate the presence of an open fracture. Given that Salter-Harris injuries can be radiographically occult, consider antibiotics when soft-tissue defects overlie physes in pediatric patients.

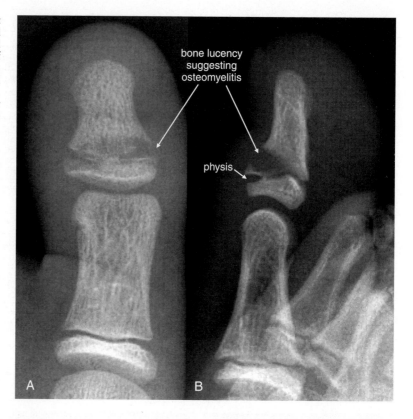

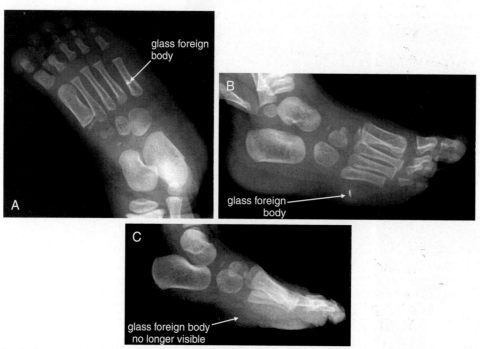

Figure 14-142. Foreign body x-ray, glass. This 20-month-old female presented with a suspected glass foreign body. One week prior, she had stepped on a broken drinking glass and had been favoring her left foot since that time. Her parents had noted pus draining from the wound on the day of presentation. **A,** Anterior–posterior view of the foot. **B,** Oblique view of the foot. **C,** Lateral x-ray obtained after foreign body removal. Ordinary glass foreign bodies are typically visible on x-ray. Glass need not be of an unusual type, such as leaded glass, to be seen on x-ray. Two orthogonal views should be obtained to localize the foreign body. **A,** The foreign body appears to overlie the fifth metatarsal. **B,** The foreign body is visible in the plantar soft tissues. Exploration of the wound in the left foot showed one glass fragment, which was removed. **C,** No foreign body is visible.

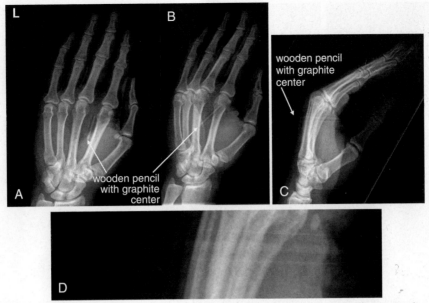

Figure 14-143. Foreign body x-ray, wood. This 49-year-old right-hand-dominant teacher fell on a pencil while wrestling with a student. The pencil pierced the left hand from a volar to dorsal direction. **A,** Anterior–posterior x-ray. **B,** Oblique x-ray. **C,** Lateral x-ray. **D,** Expanded view from **C.** A pencil fragment pierces the soft tissues between the second and the third metacarpals without underlying bone fracture. The pencil appears intact. The graphite rod in the center of the pencil is visible as an opacity because of its high density, whereas the wood is seen as a lucency against the soft tissues, resulting from its low density. Wood is often not visible on x-ray. The paint on the pencil is faintly visible as lines parallel to the graphite center.

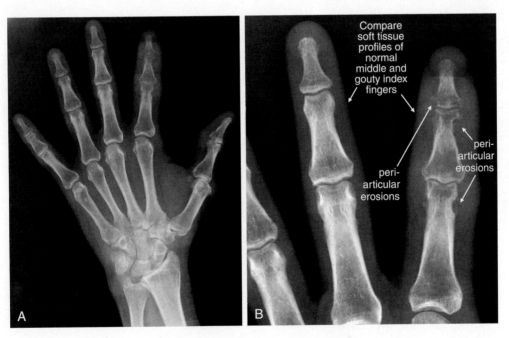

Figure 14-144. Gout. This 58-year-old male with a history of gout complained of left index finger swelling, erythema, and pain. His x-rays show well-defined periarticular erosions with overhanging edges at the index finger proximal interphalangeal (PIP) and distal interphalangeal (DIP) joints. Soft-tissue swelling is also seen at DIP and PIP joints of the index finger. These are characteristic findings of crystalline deposition disorders such as gout. **A,** Anterior–posterior view of the hand. **B,** Close-up.

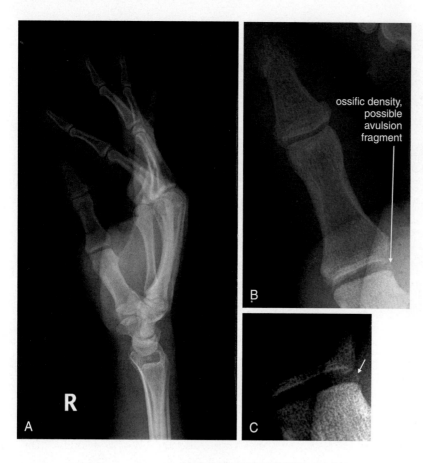

ossific density,
possible
avulsion
fragment

Figure 14-145. Gamekeeper's thumb. A 36-year-old male, with pain at the metacarpophalangeal (MCP) joint of the thumb after a bicycling accident. **A,** Lateral view of the hand. **B, C,** Close-ups. Gamekeeper's thumb refers to avulsion of the ulnar collateral ligament (UCL) from the base of the thumb, usually occurring from forced thumb abduction. An avulsion fracture of proximal thumb at the MCP joint may accompany this injury. The avulsion fragment may be seen at the ulnar aspect of the proximal portion of the proximal phalanx of the thumb. When no fracture is seen, stress views of the thumb are sometimes used to assess the integrity of the UCL. Normal neutral position x-rays do not rule out this ligamentous injury. In this patient, a tiny ossific density is seen at the ulnar thumb base, possibly representing a tiny avulsion fragment.

ONLINE CHAPTER 15 Emergency Department Applications of Musculoskeletal Magnetic Resonance Imaging: An Evidence-Based Assessment

Joshua Broder, MD, FACEP

For the complete chapter text, go to expertconsult.com. To access your account, look for your activation instructions on the inside front cover of this book.

Magnetic resonance imaging (MRI) is a relatively rarely used modality in the emergency department, most often applied to acute neurologic conditions such as stroke and spinal cord injury.[1] MRI offers outstanding soft-tissue contrast and can be used to evaluate acute musculoskeletal complaints when other imaging modalities do not provide the diagnosis. Most musculoskeletal MRI can be deferred to the outpatient setting, but certain high-risk musculoskeletal complaints may warrant emergent imaging. In this chapter, we review basic principles and technical features of MRI relevant to its emergency department use, exploring its potential benefits and limitations. We discuss the cost and time required for MRI, which are significant barriers to its emergency department use. We examine the scientific evidence for the diagnostic accuracy of MRI, comparing the performance of MRI to other imaging modalities, including computed tomography (CT) and nuclear medicine. We review the role of MRI in the diagnosis of occult hip and scaphoid fractures and spinal epidural abscess, which remain clinically challenging. Because of the expense and limited availability of MRI, we review alternative imaging strategies when MRI cannot be readily performed. Finally, we discuss the role of gadolinium contrast agents and the risks associated with their use, and we consider contraindications to MRI.

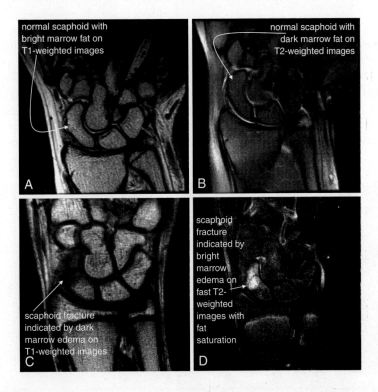

ONLINE CHAPTER 16
"Therapeutic Imaging:" Image-Guided Therapies in Emergency Medicine

Joshua Broder, MD, FACEP

For the complete chapter text, go to expertconsult.com. To access your account, look for your activation instructions on the inside front cover of this book.

Medical imaging serves first to diagnose disease or injury, but imaging techniques are increasingly used to guide temporizing or definitive therapy for a range of conditions. Depending on the practice setting, medical treatments guided by imaging techniques may be performed by interventional radiologists, cardiologists, and surgeons. In many cases, emergency physicians perform image-guided procedures, using ultrasound to guide procedures as diverse as peripheral and central venous catheter placement, abdominal paracentesis, thoracentesis, lumbar puncture, and joint aspiration. Fluoroscopic guidance of fracture reduction is a standard practice for orthopedists and many emergency physicians.

In this chapter, we discuss some selected applications of image-guided procedures, as well as the evidence supporting their use. At their best, image-guided procedures are definitive treatment, with strong evidence suggesting equivalent or superior clinical outcomes compared with other medical and surgical approaches. In other cases, the evidence disappoints the medical community, showing no benefit to a therapy with great initial expectations. Many applications of image-guided therapies have surprisingly little evidence to support them, despite having been widely accepted by the medical community. Other applications are rarely used today but offer "heroic" options in moribund patients with few treatment options for their life-threatening conditions. The emergency physician must be familiar with the available interventions, their indications and contraindications, and the class of supporting evidence.

We begin with a brief overview of imaging modalities used to guide procedures, with their advantages and disadvantages. We then discuss some important methodologic issues to consider when reviewing the evidence for any treatment, including image-guided therapies. Although most of us may never design or conduct research, we all must be capable of understanding research and recognizing when research is so seriously flawed that we can no longer trust the conclusions drawn by investigators. We provide some basic background so that we can draw appropriately limited conclusions from flawed research when possible. Finally, with this background, we grapple with some important image-guided procedures, comparing those with excellent evidence to those with more modest support.

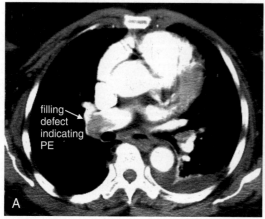

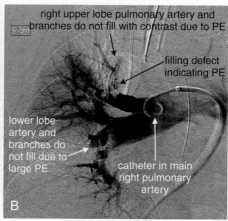

Index

Page numbers followed by *f* indicate figures; *t*, tables; *b*, boxes.

Broad Estimates of Cancer Risk Resulting From Diagnostic Imaging

Example Diagnostic Imaging Exams	Approximate Effective Doses	Equivalent Natural Background Radiation	Approximate Additional Lifetime Cancer Risk per Exam[*]
Ultrasound MRI	0 mSv	None	None
Chest x-ray Extremity x-rays Dental x-rays	0.01 mSv	A few days	Negligible
Cervical spine x-ray	0.1 mSv	A few weeks	Minimal risk (1 in 1,000,000 to 1 in 100,000)
Pelvis x-ray Abdominal x-ray CT head	1 mSv	A few months to 1 year	Very low risk (1 in 100,000 to 1 in 10,000)
IV urogram CT chest CT abdomen CT pelvis Ventilation-perfusion scan	10 mSv	A few years	Low risk (1 in 10,000 to 1 in 1000)

Modified from *Radiation and your patient: A guide for medical practitioners*. International Commission on Radiological Protection.

[*]This risk is superimposed on the baseline population risk of cancer, which is approximately 1 in 3, and thus represents a small incremental risk to the individual patient. However, when large populations are subjected to this risk, a substantial number of additional cancers may result in the population.

Estimated Lifetime Risk of Radiation-Induced Cancer from Computed Tomography Based on Age at Exposure, Gender, and Median Radiation Dose[*]

Anatomic Region	Median Effective Dose	Age 20 Years, Female	Age 20 Years, Male	Age 40 Years, Female	Age 40 Years, Male	Age 60 Years, Female	Age 60 Years, Male
Head	2 mSv	1 in 4360 (0.02%)	1 in 7350 (0.01%)	1 in 8100 (0.01%)	1 in 11,080 (0.01%)	1 in 12,250 (0.01%)	1 in 14,680 (0.01%)
Neck	4 mSv	1 in 2390 (0.04%)	1 in 4020 (0.02%)	1 in 4430 (0.02%)	1 in 6058 (0.02%)	1 in 6700 (0.01%)	1 in 8030 (0.01%)
Chest (CT pulmonary angiogram protocol)	10 mSv	1 in 330 (0.30%)	1 in 880 (0.11%)	1 in 620 (0.16%)	1 in 1333 (0.08%)	1 in 930 (0.11%)	1 in 1770 (0.06%)
Abdomen/pelvis with contrast	16 mSv	1 in 470 (0.21%)	1 in 620 (0.16%)	1 in 870 (0.11%)	1 in 942 (0.11%)	1 in 1320 (0.08%)	1 in 1250 (0.08%)

Modified from Smith-Bindman R, Lipson J, Marcus R, et al: Radiation dose associated with common computed tomography examinations and the associated lifetime attributable risk of cancer, *Arch Intern Med* 169(22):2078–2086, 2009.

[*]This risk is superimposed on the baseline population risk of cancer, which is approximately 1 in 3, and thus represents a small incremental risk to the individual patient. However, when large populations are subjected to this risk, a substantial number of additional cancers is believed to result in the population.

Estimated Mean Lifetime Cancer Risk (%) from Computed Tomography by Body Region, Patient Age at Exposure, and Gender*

Age At Exposure (years)	Head	Head Angiography	Cervical Spine	Chest	Chest Angiography	Coronary Artery Angiography	Thoracic Spine*	Lumbar Spine†	Abdomen/ Pelvis
Females									
3	0.08	NA	0.70	0.40	NA	NA	0.70	0.20	0.20
15	0.04	0.30	0.50	0.30	0.60	0.10	0.40	0.10	0.20
30	0.02	0.04	0.05	0.10	0.20	0.06	0.10	0.07	0.10
50	0.01	0.02	0.02	0.07	0.10	0.05	0.09	0.06	0.08
70	0.01	0.01	0.01	0.03	0.05	0.03	0.03	0.02	0.03
Males									
3	0.09	NA	0.10	0.10	NA	NA	0.20	0.20	0.20
15	0.05	0.10	0.10	0.09	0.20	0.10	0.08	0.10	0.20
30	0.03	0.05	0.03	0.05	0.08	0.06	0.05	0.07	0.10
50	0.02	0.03	0.02	0.04	0.08	0.05	0.04	0.06	0.09
70	0.01	0.02	0.01	0.03	0.05	0.03	0.03	0.04	0.05

Modified from Berrington de Gonzalez A, Mahesh M, Kim KP, et al: Projected cancer risks from computed tomographic scans performed in the United States in 2007. *Arch Intern Med* 169(22):2071-2077, 2009.

*This risk is superimposed on the baseline population risk of cancer, which is approximately 1 in 3, and thus represents a small incremental risk to the individual patient. However, when large populations are subjected to this risk, a substantial number of additional cancers is believed to result in the population.

†If reconstructions of the spine are performed using data acquired from chest and abdominal imaging, no additional radiation exposure occurs. Values here assume separate dedicated spinal imaging.

Effect of *in utero* Radiation Exposure on Prenatal Development

Gestational Stage	Time After Conception	Fetal Dose (millisieverts)	Potential Effect
Pre-implantation	0-14 days	50-100	Prenatal death
Organogenesis	1-8 weeks	200-250	Growth retardation
Organogenesis	2-15 weeks	200-250	• Small head size • Exposure before 8 wk does not cause an intellectual deficit despite small head size • Most sensitive period for induction of childhood cancer
Rapid neuron development and migration	6-15 weeks	> 100	Small head size, seizures, decline in intelligence
After organogenesis and rapid neuron development	15 weeks to term	>100	Increased frequency of childhood cancer
After organogenesis and rapid neuron development	15 weeks to term	>500	Severe mental retardation (16-25 wk)

Note that the fetal doses at which deleterious effects are believed to occur exceed those seen with any single common diagnostic imaging procedure (next table), although the cumulative dose from multiple imaging tests during pregnancy should be considered.[1]

[1]Ratnapalan S, Bentur Y, Koren G "Doctor, will that x-ray harm my unborn child?" *CMAJ*. 179(12):1293-1296, 2008.